Assisted Ventilation
of the NEONATE

AN EVIDENCE-BASED APPROACH TO
NEWBORN RESPIRATORY CARE

Assisted Ventilation of the NEONATE

AN EVIDENCE-BASED APPROACH TO NEWBORN RESPIRATORY CARE

SIXTH EDITION

JAY P. GOLDSMITH, MD, FAAP
Clinical Professor
Department of Pediatrics
Tulane University School of Medicine
New Orleans, Louisiana

EDWARD H. KAROTKIN, MD, FAAP
Professor of Pediatrics
Neonatal/Perinatal Medicine
Eastern Virginia Medical School
Norfolk, Virginia

MARTIN KESZLER, MD, FAAP
Professor of Pediatrics
Warren Alpert Medical School
Brown University
Director of Respiratory Services
Department of Pediatrics
Women and Infants Hospital
Providence, Rhode Island

GAUTHAM K. SURESH, MD, DM, MS, FAAP
Section Head and Service Chief of Neonatology
Baylor College of Medicine
Texas Children's Hospital
Houston, Texas

ELSEVIER

ELSEVIER

1600 John F. Kennedy Blvd.
Ste 1800
Philadelphia, PA 19103-2899

ASSISTED VENTILATION OF THE NEONATE: AN EVIDENCE-BASED
APPROACH TO NEWBORN RESPIRATORY CARE, SIXTH EDITION

ISBN: 978-0-323-39006-4

Notices

Knowledge and best practice in this field are constantly changing. As new research and experience broaden our understanding, changes in research methods, professional practices, or medical treatment may become necessary.

Practitioners and researchers must always rely on their own experience and knowledge in evaluating and using any information, methods, compounds, or experiments described herein. In using such information or methods they should be mindful of their own safety and the safety of others, including parties for whom they have a professional responsibility.

With respect to any drug or pharmaceutical products identified, readers are advised to check the most current information provided (i) on procedures featured or (ii) by the manufacturer of each product to be administered, to verify the recommended dose or formula, the method and duration of administration, and contraindications. It is the responsibility of practitioners, relying on their own experience and knowledge of their patients, to make diagnoses, to determine dosages and the best treatment for each individual patient, and to take all appropriate safety precautions.

To the fullest extent of the law, neither the Publisher nor the authors, contributors, or editors, assume any liability for any injury and/or damage to persons or property as a matter of products liability, negligence or otherwise, or from any use or operation of any methods, products, instructions, or ideas contained in the material herein.

Previous editions copyrighted 2011, 2003, 1996, 1988, and 1981.

Library of Congress Cataloging-in-Publication Data

Names: Goldsmith, Jay P., editor. | Karotkin, Edward H., editor. | Keszler, Martin, editor. | Suresh, Gautham, editor.
Title: Assisted ventilation of the neonate : an evidence-based approach to newborn respiratory care / [edited by] Jay P. Goldsmith, MD, FAAP, Clinical Professor, Department of Pediatrics, Tulane University School of Medicine, New Orleans, Louisiana, Edward H. Karotkin, MD, FAAP, Professor of Pediatrics, Neonatal/Perinatal Medicine, Eastern Virginia Medical School, Norfolk, Virginia, Martin Keszler, MD, FAAP, Professor of Pediatrics, Warren Alpert Medical School, Brown University, Director of Respiratory Services, Department of Pediatrics, Women and Infants Hospital, Providence, Rhode Island, Gautham K. Suresh, MD, DM, MS, FAAP, Section Head and Service Chief of Neonatology, Baylor College of Medicine, Texas Children's Hospital, Houston, Texas.
Description: Sixth edition. | Philadelphia, PA : Elsevier, [2017]
Identifiers: LCCN 2016029284 | ISBN 9780323390064 (hardback : alk. paper)
Subjects: LCSH: Respiratory therapy for newborn infants. | Artificial respiration.
Classification: LCC RJ312 .A87 2017 | DDC 618.92/2004636--dc23 LC record available at
https://lccn.loc.gov/2016029284

Executive Content Strategist: Kate Dimock
Publishing Services Manager: Hemamalini Rajendrababu
Senior Project Manager: Beula Christopher
Designer: Renee Duenow
Marketing Manager: Kristin McNally

Printed in Canada

Last digit is the print number: 9 8 7 6 5 4 3 2 1

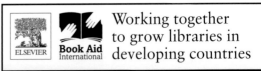

This book is dedicated to my wife, Terri, who has supported
me through six editions of this text and my many nights away
from home while caring for sick neonates.

JPG

I would like to dedicate this sixth edition of *Assisted Ventilation
of the Neonate* to the numerous bedside NICU nurses, neonatal nurse
practitioners, and respiratory therapists, and all of the other ancillary
health care providers I have had the honor of working with over
the past nearly 40 years at the Children's Hospital of
The King's Daughters. Without your commitment to providing
the best of care to our patients I could not have done my job.

EHK

I dedicate this book to my wife, Mary Lenore Keszler, MD,
who has been my lifelong companion, inspiration, and best friend.
Without her incredible patience and unwavering support, none of this
work would have been possible. The book is also dedicated to the many tiny
patients and their families who taught me many valuable lessons, and to the
students, residents, and Fellows whose probing questions inspired me to seek
a deeper understanding of the problems that face us every day.

MK

I dedicate this book to my teachers and mentors over the years,
who taught me and guided me. I also thank my wife, Viju Padmanabhan,
and my daughters, Diksha and Ila, for their support and patience
with me over the years.

GKS

CONTRIBUTORS

Kabir Abubakar, MD
Professor of Clinical Pediatrics
Neonatology/Pediatrics
Medstar Georgetown University Hospital
Washington, DC

Namasivayam Ambalavanan, MBBS, MD
Professor, Pediatrics
University of Alabama at Birmingham
Birmingham, AL

Robert M. Arensman, BS, MD
Head, Division of Pediatric Surgery
Department of Surgery
University of Illinois at Chicago
Chicago, IL

Eduardo Bancalari, MD
Professor of Pediatrics, Obstetrics, and Gynecology,
Director, Division of Neonatology,
Chief, Newborn Service
Department of Pediatrics, Division of Neonatology
University of Miami School of Medicine
Miami, FL

Keith J. Barrington, MB, ChB
Neonatologist and Clinical Researcher
Sainte Justine University Health Center,
Professor of Paediatrics
University of Montréal
Montréal, Canada

Jonathan F. Bean, MD
Chief Resident
Department of General Surgery
University of Illinois Hospital and Health Sciences Center
Chicago, IL

Edward F. Bell, MD
Professor of Pediatrics
Department of Pediatrics
University of Iowa
Iowa City, IA

David M. Biko, MD
Assistant Professor
The Children's Hospital of Philadelphia,
Pediatric Radiologist
Pennsylvania Hospital
The University of Pennsylvania Health System
Philadelphia, PA

Laura D. Brown, MD
Associate Professor
Pediatrics
University of Colorado School of Medicine
Aurora, CO

Jessica Brunkhorst, MD
Assistant Professor of Pediatrics
Children's Mercy Hospital
University of Missouri - Kansas City
Kansas City, Missouri

Waldemar A. Carlo, MD
Edwin M. Dixon Professor of Pediatrics
University of Alabama at Birmingham,
Director, Division of Neonatology
University of Alabama at Birmingham
Birmingham, AL

Robert L. Chatburn, MHHS, RRT-NPS, FAARC
Clinical Research Manager
Respiratory Institute, Cleveland Clinic,
Director, Simulation Fellowship
Education Institute, Cleveland Clinic,
Adjunct Professor of Medicine
Lerner College of Medicine of Case Western Reserve
    University
Cleveland, OH

Nelson Claure, MSc, PhD
Research Associate Professor of Pediatrics,
Director, Neonatal Pulmonary Research Laboratory
Department of Pediatrics, Division of Neonatology
University of Miami School of Medicine
Miami, FL

Clarice Clemmens, MD
Assistant Professor of Pediatric Otolaryngology
Medical University of South Carolina
Charleston, SC

Christopher E. Colby, MD
Associate Professor of Pediatrics
Mayo Clinic
Rochester, MN

Sherry E. Courtney, MD, MS
Professor of Pediatrics
Department of Pediatrics
University of Arkansas for Medical Sciences
Little Rock, AR

Peter G. Davis, MBBS, MD, FRACP
Professor/Director of Neonatal Medicine
The University of Melbourne and The Royal Women's
    Hospital
Melbourne, Victoria, Australia

Eugene M. Dempsey, MBBCH BAO, FRCPI, MD, MSc
Clinical Professor
Paediatrics and Child Health
University College Cork,
Department of Neonatology
Cork University Maternity Hospital
Wilton, Cork, Ireland

Robert Diblasi, RRT-NPS, FAARC
Seattle Children's Research Institute - Respiratory Care
Center for Developmental Therapeutics
Seattle, WA

Jennifer Duchon, MDCM, MPH
Clinical Fellow
Pediatric Infectious Disease
Columbia-Presbyterian Medical Center
New York, NY

Jonathan M. Fanaroff, MD, JD
Associate Professor of Pediatrics
Case Western Reserve University School of Medicine,
Co-Director, Neonatal Intensive Care Unit,
Director, Rainbow Center for Pediatric Ethics
Rainbow Babies and Children's Hospital
Cleveland, OH

William W. Fox, MD
Attending Neonatologist
Division of Neonatology
Medical Director
Infant Breathing Disorder Center
Children's Hospital of Philadelphia,
Professor of Pediatrics
University of Pennsylvania Perelman School of Medicine
Philadelphia, PA

Debbie Fraser, MN, RNC-NIC
Associate Professor
Faculty of Health Disciplines
Athabasca University
Athabasca, Alberta, Canada,
Advanced Practice Nurse
NICU
St Boniface Hospital
Winnipeg, Manitoba, Canada

John T. Gallagher, MPH, RRT-NPS, FAARC
Critical Care Coordinator
Pediatric Respiratory Care
University Hospitals, Rainbow Babies and Children's Hospital
Cleveland, OH

Jay P. Goldsmith, MD, FAAP
Clinical Professor
Pediatrics
Tulane University
New Orleans, LA

Malinda N. Harris, MD
Assistant Professor of Pediatrics
Mayo Clinic
Rochester, MN

William W. Hay, Jr., MD
Professor
Pediatrics
University of Colorado School of Medicine
Aurora, CO

Robert M. Insoft, MD
Chief Medical Officer and Attending Neonatologist
Women and Infants Hospital
Alpert Medical School of Brown University
Providence, RI

Erik A. Jensen, MD
Instructor of Pediatrics
The University of Pennsylvania,
Attending Neonatologist
The Children's Hospital of Philadelphia
Philadelphia, PA

Jegen Kandasamy, MBBS, MD
Assistant Professor
Pediatrics
University of Alabama at Birmingham
Birmingham, AL

Edward H. Karotkin, MD, FAAP
Professor of Pediatrics
Neonatal/Perinatal Medicine
The Eastern Virginia Medical School
Norfolk, VA

Martin Keszler, MD, FAAP
Professor of Pediatrics
Alpert Medical School of Brown University,
Director of Respiratory Services, Pediatrics
Women and Infants Hospital
Providence, RI

John P. Kinsella, MD
Professor of Pediatrics
Department of Pediatrics
Section of Neonatology
University of Colorado School of Medicine and Children's
    Hospital Colorado
Aurora, CO

Haresh Kirpalani, BM, MRCP, FRCP, MSc
Professor
The University of Pennsylvania,
Attending Neonatologist and Director
Newborn and Infant Chronic Lung Disease Program
The Children's Hospital of Philadelphia
Philadelphia, PA;
Emeritus Professor
Clinical Epidemiology
McMaster University
Hamilton, Ontario, Canada

Derek Kowal, RRT
Supervisor NICU, Respiratory Services
Foothills Medical Centre
Alberta Health Services
Calgary, Alberta, Canada

Satyan Lakshminrusimha, MBBS, MD
Professor of Pediatrics
Director, Center for Developmental Biology of the Lung
University at Buffalo,
Chief of Neonatology
Women and Children's Hospital of Buffalo
Buffalo, NY

John D. Lantos, MD
Director of Bioethics
Children's Mercy Hospital Professor
Pediatrics University of Missouri - Kansas City
Kansas City, MO

Krithika Lingappan, MD, MS, FAAP
Assistant Professor
Section of Neonatology
Department of Pediatrics
Texas Children's Hospital
Baylor College of Medicine
Houston, TX

Akhil Maheshwari, MD
Professor of Pediatrics and Molecular Medicine
Pamela and Leslie Muma Endowed Chair in Neonatology,
Chief, Division of Neonatology,
Assistant Dean, Graduate Medical Education Pediatrics
University of South Florida
Tampa, FL

Mark C. Mammel, MD
Professor of Pediatrics
Department of Pediatrics
University of Minnesota
Minneapolis, MN

George T. Mandy, MD
Associate Professor of Pediatrics
Baylor College of Medicine
Houston, TX

Richard J. Martin, MBBS
Professor
Pediatrics, Reproductive Biology, and Physiology and
    Biophysics
Case Western Reserve University School of Medicine,
Drusinsky/Fanaroff Professor
Pediatrics
Rainbow Babies and Children's Hospital
Cleveland, OH

Kathryn L. Maschhoff, MD, PhD
Assistant Professor of Clinical Pediatrics
The University of Pennsylvania,
Attending Neonatologist
The Children's Hospital of Philadelphia
Philadelphia, PA

Bobby Mathew, MD
Associate Program Director
Assistant Professor of Pediatrics
University at Buffalo
Women and Children's Hospital of Buffalo
Buffalo, NY

Patrick Joseph McNamara, MD, MRCPCH, MSc
Associate Professor
Pediatrics and Physiology
University of Toronto,
Staff Neonatologist
Pediatrics
Hospital for Sick Children
Toronto, Ontario, Canada

D. Andrew Mong, MD
Assistant Professor
The University of Pennsylvania,
Pediatric Radiologist
The Children's Hospital of Philadelphia
Philadelphia, PA

Colin J. Morley, DCH, MD, FRCPCH
Professor
Neonatal Research
Royal Women's Hospital
Melbourne, Cambridge, Great Britain

Leif D. Nelin, MD
Dean W. Jeffers Chair in Neonatology
Nationwide Children's Hospital,
Professor and Chief,
Division of Neonatology
The Ohio State University and Nationwide Children's Hospital
Columbus, OH

Donald Morley Null Jr., MD
Professor of Pediatrics
Department of Pediatrics
University of California Davis
Sacramento, CA

Louise S. Owen, MBChB, MRCPCH, FRACP, MD
Neonatologist
Newborn Research
Royal Women's Hospital,
Honorary Fellow
Murdoch Childrens Research Institute
Melbourne, Victoria, Australia

Allison H. Payne, MD, MSCR
Assistant Professor
Pediatrics
Division of Neonatology
UH Rainbow Babies and Children's Hospital
Case Western Reserve University
Cleveland, OH

Jeffrey M. Perlman, MBChB
Professor of Pediatrics
Weill Cornell Medicine,
Division Chief
Newborn Medicine
New York Presbyterian Hospital
Komansky Center for Children's Health
New York, NY

Joseph Piccione, DO, MS
Pulmonary Director
Center for Pediatric Airway Disorders
The Children's Hospital of Philadelphia,
Assistant Professor of Clinical Pediatrics
Division of Pediatric Pulmonary Medicine
University of Pennsylvania School of Medicine
Philadelphia, PA

Richard Alan Polin, BA, MD
Director Division of Neonatology
Department of Pediatrics
Morgan Stanley Children's Hospital,
William T Speck Professor of Pediatrics
Columbia University College of Physicians and Surgeons
New York, NY

Yacov Rabi, MD, FRCPC
Assistant Professor
Department of Pediatrics
University of Calgary
Calgary, Alberta, Canada

Aarti Raghavan, MD, FAAP
Assistant Professor Clinical Pediatrics
Attending Neonatologist
Director Quality Improvement, Department of Pediatrics
Program Director, Neonatology Fellowship Program
Department of Pediatrics
University of Illinois Hospital and Health Sciences System
Chicago, Illinois

Matthew A. Rainaldi, MD
Assistant Professor of Pediatrics
Weill Cornell Medicine
New York Presbyterian Hospital
Komansky Center for Children's Health
New York, NY

Tara M. Randis, MD, MS
Assistant Professor of Pediatrics
Division of Neonatology
New York University School of Medicine
New York, NY

Lawrence Rhein, MD
Assistant Professor of Pediatrics
Newborn Medicine and Pediatric Pulmonology
Boston Children's Hospital
Boston, MA

Guilherme Sant'Anna, MD, PhD, FRCPC
Associate Professor of Pediatrics
Department of Pediatrics, Neonatal Division,
Associate Member of the Division of Experimental Medicine
McGill University
Montreal, Quebec, Canada

Edward G. Shepherd, MD
Chief, Section of Neonatology
Nationwide Children's Hospital
Associate Professor of Pediatrics
The Ohio State University
Columbus, OH

Billie Lou Short, MD
Chief, Neonatology
Children's National Health System,
Professor of Pediatrics
The George Washington University School of Medicine
Washington, DC

Nalini Singhal, MBBS, MD, FRCPC
Professor of Pediatrics
Department of Pediatrics
Cumming School of Medicine
University of Calgary
Calgary, Alberta, Canada

Roger F. Soll, MD
Neonatologist
Wallace Professor of Neonatology
University of Vermont College of Medicine
Burlington, VT

Amuchou S. Soraisham, MBBS, MD, DM, MS, FRCPC, FAAP
Associate Professor of Pediatrics
Department of Pediatrics
Cumming School of Medicine
University of Calgary
Calgary, Alberta, Canada

Nishant Srinivasan, MD
Division of Pediatric Surgery, Department of Surgery
Division of Neonatology, Department of Pediatrics
University of Illinois Hospital and Health Sciences Center
Chicago, IL

Daniel Stephens, MD
General Surgery Chief Resident
Department of Surgery
University of Minnesota
Minneapolis, MN

Gautham K. Suresh, MD, DM, MS, FAAP
Section Head and Service Chief of Neonatology
Baylor College of Medicine
Texas Children's Hospital
Houston, TX

Andrea N. Trembath, MD, MPH
Assistant Professor, Pediatrics
Division of Neonatology
UH Rainbow Babies and Children's Hospital
Case Western Reserve University
Cleveland, OH

Anton H. van Kaam, MD, PhD
Professor of Neonatology
Emma Children's Hospital Academic Medical Center
Amsterdam, Netherland

Maximo Vento, MD, PhD
Professor
Division of Neonatology
University and Polytechnic Hospital La Fe,
Professor
Neonatal Research Group
Health Research Institute La Fe,
Valencia, Spain

Michele C. Walsh, MD, MSEpi
Professor, Pediatrics
Division of Neonatology
UH Rainbow Babies and Children's Hospital
Case Western Reserve University
Cleveland, OH

Julie Weiner, MD
Assistant Professor of Pediatrics
Children's Mercy Hospital
University of Missouri - Kansas City
Kansas City, MO

Gary M. Weiner, MD, FAAP
Associate Professor/Director
Neonatal-Perinatal Fellowship Training Program
University of Michigan, C.S. Mott Children's Hospital
Ann Arbor, MI

Dany E. Weisz, BSc, MD, MSc
Assistant Professor of Pediatrics
University of Toronto,
Staff Neonatologist
Newborn and Developmental Paediatrics
Sunnybrook Health Sciences Centre
Toronto, Ontario, Canada

Bradley A. Yoder, MD
Professor of Pediatrics
Medical Director, NICU
University of Utah School of Medicine
Salt Lake City, UT

Huayan Zhang, MD
Attending Neonatologist, Medical Director
The Newborn and Infant Chronic Lung Disease Program
Division of Neonatology
Department of Pediatrics
Children's Hospital of Philadelphia,
Associate Professor of Clinical Pediatrics
Department of Pediatrics
University of Pennsylvania Perelman School of Medicine
Philadelphia, PA

Learn how to exhale, the inhale will take care of itself.

—*Carla Melucci Ardito*

I congratulate Drs. Goldsmith, Karotkin, Keszler, and Suresh on the publication of the sixth edition of their classic text, *Assisted Ventilation of the Neonate*. The first edition was published in 1981, when neonatal ventilation was in its infancy, and long before the availability of surfactant, generalized use of antenatal corticosteroids, and various modern modes of assisted ventilation. Indeed, in the 1970s many units did not have the benefit of neonatal ventilators and were forced to use adult machines that delivered far too great a tidal volume, even with a minimal turn of the knob controlling airflow. Not surprisingly, almost half the babies receiving mechanical ventilation developed air leaks, and the mortality was very high. Respiratory failure in preterm infants was the leading cause of neonatal mortality.

The term *neonatology* was coined in 1960 by Alexander Schaffer to designate the art and science of diagnosis and treatment of disorders of the newborn. Neonatal care was largely anecdote-based, and that era has been designated "the era of benign neglect and disastrous interventions." The all-too-familiar stories of oxygen causing retrolental fibroplasia, prophylactic antibiotics causing death and kernicterus, diethylstilbestrol causing vaginal carcinoma, and the prolonged starvation of extremely preterm infants contributing to their dismal outcome are well documented.

Since 1975 we have witnessed dramatic increases in knowledge and the accumulation of evidence in randomized trials resulting in the transition to evidence-based medicine. This has been progressively documented in each successive edition of this text. There is now extensive science to support the various modalities of assisted ventilation.

The sixth edition documents the new science and the application of translational research from bench to bedside. There have been extensive changes in contributors as well as in the organization of the book. The wide array of authors, well-known experts in their fields, represents many nationalities and points of view. Each mode of ventilation is discussed in detail, yet is easy to comprehend. There is a great balance between physiology, pathophysiology, diagnostic approaches, pulmonary imaging, and the techniques of mechanical ventilation, as well as the short- and long-term outcomes. This edition includes a thoughtful chapter on respiratory care in resource-limited countries and all the latest advances in delivery room management and resuscitation. There are also contributions on quality improvement and ethics and medicolegal aspects of respiratory care, in addition to a very informative chapter on pulmonary imaging. The sections on pharmacologic support provide the reader with all of the novel approaches to respiratory insufficiency and pulmonary hypertension, and the section on neurological outcomes and surgical interventions completes a comprehensive, yet easy-to-read textbook.

Assisted Ventilation of the Neonate, sixth edition, by Drs. Jay P. Goldsmith, Edward H. Karotkin, Martin Keszler, and Gautham K. Suresh, serves as a living, breathing companion, which guides you through the latest innovations in ventilatory assistance. It is a must read for neonatologists, neonatal fellows, neonatal respiratory therapists, and nurses working in the neonatal intensive care unit.

For breath is life, and if you breathe well you will live long on earth.

–*Sanskrit Proverb*

Avroy A. Fanaroff, MD
Emeritus Professor of Pediatrics
Case Western Reserve University
Emeritus Eliza Henry Barnes Professor of Neonatology
Rainbow Babies and Children's Hospital
Cleveland, March 2016

PREFACE

Thirty-nine years ago, before there were exogenous surfactants, inhaled nitric oxide, high-frequency ventilators, and other modern therapies, two young neonatologists (JPG, EHK) were audacious enough to attempt to edit a primer on newborn assisted ventilation for physicians, nurses, and respiratory therapists entrusted with treating respiratory failure in fragile neonates. Because, even in the early days of neonatology, respiratory care was an essential part of neonatal intensive care unit (NICU) care, we thought that such a text could fill a void and provide a reference to the many caretakers in this new and exciting field. We called upon our teachers and mentors to write most of the chapters and they exceeded our expectations in producing a "how to" guide for successful ventilation of the distressed newborn. The first edition, published in 1981, was modeled after the iconic text of Marshall Klaus and Avroy Fanaroff, *Care of the High-Risk Neonate*, which was the "go to" reference for practicing neonatal caregivers at the time. Dr. Klaus wrote the foreword, and *Assisted Ventilation of the Neonate* was born.

The preface to the first edition started with a quotation from Dr. Sydney S. Gellis, then considered the Dean of Pediatrics in the United States:

As far as I am concerned, the whole area of ventilation of infants with respiratory distress syndrome is one of chaos. Claims and counterclaims about the best and least harmful method of ventilating the premature infant make me light-headed. I can't wait for the solution or solutions to premature birth, and I look forward to the day when this gadgetry will come to an end and the neonatologists will be retired.

Year Book of Pediatrics (1977)

Nearly four decades and five editions of the text later, we are still looking for the solutions to premature birth despite decades of research on how to prevent it, and neonatal respiratory support is still an important part of everyday practice in the modern NICU. No doubt, the practice has changed dramatically. Pharmacological, technological, and philosophical advances in the care of newborns, especially the extremely premature, have continued to refine the way we manage neonatal respiratory failure. Microprocessor-based machinery and information technology, the new emphasis on safety, quality improvement, and evidence-based medicine have affected our practice as they have all of medical care.

Mere survival is no longer the only focus; the emphasis of neonatal critical care has changed to improving functional outcomes of even the smallest premature infant. While the threshold of viability has not changed significantly in the past decade, there certainly have been decreases in morbidities, even at the smallest weights and lowest gestational ages. The large institutional variation in morbidities such as bronchopulmonary dysplasia (BPD) can no longer be attributed solely to differences in the populations being treated. The uniform application of evidence-based therapies and quality improvement programs has shown significant improvements in outcomes, albeit not in all centers. We have recognized that much of neonatal lung injury is human-made and occurs predominantly in the most premature infants. Our perception of the ventilator has shifted from that of a lifesaving machine to a tool that can cause harm while it helps—a double-edged sword. However, the causes of this morbidity are multifactorial and its prevention remains controversial and elusive.

Specifically, attempts to decrease the incidence of BPD have concentrated on ventilatory approaches such as noninvasive ventilation, volume guarantee modes, and adjuncts such as caffeine and vitamin A. Yet some of these therapies remain unproven in large clinical trials and the incidence of BPD in national databases for very low birth-weight infants exceeds 30%. Thus, until there are social, pharmacological, and technical solutions to prematurity, neonatal caregivers will continue to be challenged to provide respiratory support to the smallest premature infants without causing lifelong pulmonary or central nervous system injury.

In this, the sixth edition, two new editors have graciously added their expertise to the task of providing the most up-to-date and evidence-based guidelines on providing ventilatory and supportive care to critically ill newborns. Dr. Martin Keszler, Professor of Pediatrics and Medical Director of Respiratory Care at Brown University, is internationally renowned for his work in neonatal ventilation. Dr. Gautham K. Suresh, now the Chief of Neonatology of the Newborn Center at Texas Children's Hospital and a professor at Baylor University, is regarded as one of the foremost authorities on quality improvement in neonatal care. With an infusion of new ideas, the text has been completely rewritten and divided into five sections. The first section covers general principles and concepts and includes new chapters on respiratory diagnostic tests, medical legal aspects of respiratory care, and quality and safety. The second section reviews assessment, diagnosis, and monitoring methods of the newborn in respiratory distress. New chapters include imaging, noninvasive monitoring of gas exchange, and airway evaluation. Therapeutic respiratory interventions are covered in the greatly expanded third section, with all types of ventilator modalities and strategies reviewed in detail. Adjunctive interventions such as pulmonary and nursing care, nutritional support, and pharmacologic therapies are the subjects of the fourth section. Finally, the fifth section of the text reviews special situations and outcomes, including chapters on transport, BPD care, discharge, and transition to home as well as pulmonary and neurologic outcomes.

During the four-decade and six-edition life of this text, neonatology has grown and evolved in the nearly 1000 NICUs in the United States. The two young neonatologists are now near retirement and will be turning over the leadership of future editions of the text to the new editors. We have seen new and unproven therapies come and go, and despite our frustration at not being able to prevent death or morbidity in all of our patients, we continue to advocate for evidence-based care and good clinical trials before the application of new devices and therapies. We hope this text will stimulate its readers to continue to search for better therapies as they use the wisdom of these pages in their clinical practice. We have come full circle, as Dr. Klaus's coeditor of *Care of the High-Risk Neonate*, Dr. Avroy Fanaroff, has favored us with the foreword to this edition. And as we wait for the solution(s) to prematurity, we should heed the wisdom of the old *Lancet* editorial: "The tedious argument about the virtues of respirators not invented over those readily available can be ended, now that it is abundantly clear that the success of such apparatus depends on the skill with which it is used" (*Lancet* 2: 1227, 1965).

Jay P. Goldsmith, MD, FAAP
Edward H. Karotkin, MD, FAAP
Martin Keszler, MD, FAAP
Gautham K. Suresh, MD, DM, MS, FAAP

CONTENTS

Introduction and Historical Aspects

Edward H. Karotkin, MD, FAAP, and Jay P. Goldsmith, MD, FAAP

The past several decades have witnessed a significant reduction in neonatal mortality and morbidity in the industrialized world. A variety of societal changes, improvements in obstetric care, and advances in neonatal medical and surgical care are largely responsible for these dramatic improvements. Many of the advances, in particular those related to respiratory support and monitoring devices, nutrition, pharmacologic agents, and surgical management of congenital anomalies and the airway, which have contributed to improved neonatal outcomes, are discussed in this book.

The results of these advances have made death from respiratory failure relatively infrequent in the neonatal period unless there are significant underlying pathologies such as birth at the margins of viability, sepsis, necrotizing enterocolitis, intraventricular hemorrhage, or pulmonary hypoplasia. However, the consequences of respiratory support continue to be major issues in neonatal intensive care. Morbidities such as chronic lung disease (CLD), also known as bronchopulmonary dysplasia (BPD), oxygen toxicity, and ventilator-induced lung injury (VILI), continue to plague a significant number of babies, particularly those with birth weight less than 1500 g.

The focus today is not only to provide respiratory support, which will improve survival, but also to minimize the complications of these treatments. Quality improvement programs to reduce the unacceptably high rate of CLD are an important part of translating the improvements in our technology to the bedside. However, many key issues in neonatal respiratory support still need to be answered. These include the optimal ventilator strategy for those babies requiring respiratory support; the role of noninvasive ventilation; the best use of pharmacologic adjuncts such as surfactants, inhaled nitric oxide, xanthines, and others; the management of the ductus arteriosus; and many other controversial questions. The potential benefits and risks of many of these therapeutic dilemmas are discussed in subsequent chapters and it is hoped will assist clinicians in their bedside management of newborns requiring respiratory support.

The purpose of this chapter is to provide a brief history of neonatal assisted ventilation with special emphasis on the evolution of the methods devised to support the neonate with respiratory insufficiency. We hope that this introductory chapter will provide the reader with a perspective of how this field has evolved over the past several thousand years.

HISTORY OF NEONATAL VENTILATION: EARLIEST REPORTS

Respiratory failure was recognized as a cause of death in newborns in ancient times. Hwang Ti (2698-2599 BC), the Chinese philosopher and emperor, noted that this occurred more frequently in children born prematurely.[1] Moreover, the medical literature of the past several thousand years contains many references to early attempts to resuscitate infants at birth.

The Old Testament contains the first written reference to providing assisted ventilation to a child (Kings 4:32-35). "And when Elisha was come into the house, behold the child was dead, and laid upon his bed.... He went up, and lay upon the child and put his mouth upon his mouth, and his eyes upon his eyes, and his hands upon his hands: and he stretched himself upon the child; and the flesh of the child waxed warm ... and the child opened his eyes." This passage, describing the first reference to mouth-to-mouth resuscitation, suggests that we have been fascinated with resuscitation for millennia.

The Ebers Papyrus from sixteenth century BC Egypt reported increased mortality in premature infants and the observation that a crying newborn at birth is one who will probably survive but that one with expiratory grunting will die.[2]

Descriptions of artificial breathing for newly born infants and inserting a reed in the trachea of a newborn lamb can be found in the Jewish Talmud (200 BC to 400 AD).[3] Hippocrates (c. 400 BC) was the first investigator to record his experience with intubation of the human trachea to support pulmonary ventilation.[4] Soranus of Ephesus (98-138 AD) described signs to evaluate the vigor of the newborn (which were possibly a precursor to the Apgar score) and criticized the immersion of the newborn in cold water as a technique for resuscitation.

Galen, who lived between 129 and 199 AD, used a bellows to inflate the lungs of dead animals via the trachea and reported that air movement caused chest "arises." The significance of Galen's findings was not appreciated for many centuries thereafter.[5]

Around 1000 AD, the Muslim philosopher and physician Avicenna (980-1037 AD) described the intubation of the trachea with "a cannula of gold or silver." Maimonides (1135-1204 AD), the famous Jewish rabbi and physician, wrote about how to detect respiratory arrest in the newborn infant and proposed a method of manual resuscitation. In 1472 AD, Paulus Bagellardus published the first book on childhood diseases and described mouth-to-mouth resuscitation of newborns.[1]

During the Middle Ages, the care of the neonate rested largely with illiterate midwives and barber surgeons, delaying the next significant advances in respiratory care until 1513, when Eucharius Rosslin's book first outlined standards for treating the newborn infant.[2] Contemporaneous with this publication was the report by Paracelsus (1493-1541), who described using a bellows inserted into the nostrils of drowning victims to attempt lung inflation and using an oral tube in treating an infant requiring resuscitation.[2]

SIXTEENTH AND SEVENTEENTH CENTURIES

In the sixteenth and seventeenth centuries, advances in resuscitation and artificial ventilation proceeded sporadically with various publications of anecdotal short-term successes, especially in animals. Andreas Vesalius (1514-1564 AD), the famous Belgian anatomist, performed a tracheostomy, intubation, and ventilation on a pregnant sow. Perhaps the first documented trial of "long-term" ventilation was performed by the English scientist Robert Hooke, who kept a dog alive for over an hour using a fireside bellows attached to the trachea.

The scientific renaissance in the sixteenth and seventeenth centuries rekindled interest in the physiology of respiration and in techniques for tracheostomy and intubation. By 1667, simple forms of continuous and regular ventilation had been developed.[4] A better understanding of the basic physiology of pulmonary ventilation emerged with the use of these new devices.

Various descriptions of neonatal resuscitation during this period can be found in the medical literature. Unfortunately, these reports were anecdotal and not always appropriate by today's standards. Many of the reports came from midwives who described various interventions to revive the depressed neonate such as giving a small spoonful of wine into the infant's mouth in an attempt to stimulate respirations as well as some more detailed descriptions of mouth-to-mouth resuscitation.[6]

NINETEENTH CENTURY

In the early 1800s interest in resuscitation and mechanical ventilation of the newborn infant flourished. In 1800, the first report describing nasotracheal intubation as an adjunct to mechanical ventilation was published by Fine in Geneva.[7] At about the same time, the principles for mechanical ventilation of adults were established; the rhythmic support of breathing was accomplished with mechanical devices, and on occasion, ventilatory support was carried out with tubes passed into the trachea.

In 1806, Vide Chaussier, professor of obstetrics in the French Academy of Science, described his experiments with the intubation and mouth-to-mouth resuscitation of asphyxiated and stillborn infants.[8] The work of his successors led to the development in 1879 of the Aerophore Pulmonaire (Fig. 1-1), the first device specifically designed for the resuscitation and short-term ventilation of newborn infants.[4] This device was a simple rubber bulb connected to a tube. The tube was inserted into the upper portion of the infant's airway, and the bulb was alternately compressed and released to produce inspiration and passive expiration. Subsequent investigators refined these early attempts by designing devices that were used to ventilate laboratory animals.

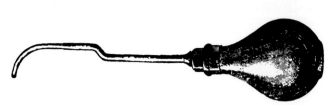

FIG 1-1 Aerophore pulmonaire of Gairal. (From DePaul. *Dictionnaire Encyclopédique*. XIII, 13th series.)

Charles-Michel Billard (1800-1832) wrote one of the finest early medical texts dealing with clinical–pathologic correlations of pulmonary disease in newborn infants. His book, *Traite des maladies des enfans nouveau-nes et a la mamelle*, was published in 1828.[9]

Billard's concern for the fetus and intrauterine injury is evident, as he writes: "During intrauterine life man often suffers many affectations, the fatal consequences of which are brought with him into the world … children may be born healthy, sick, convalescent, or entirely recovered from former diseases."[9]

His understanding of the difficulty newborns may have in establishing normal respiration at delivery is well illustrated in the following passage: "… the air sometimes passes freely into the lungs at the period of birth, but the sanguineous congestion which occurs immediately expels it or hinders it from penetrating in sufficient quantity to effect a complete establishment of life. There exists, as is well known, between the circulation and respiration, an intimate and reciprocal relation, which is evident during life, but more particularly so at the time of birth …. The symptoms of pulmonary engorgement in an infant are, in general, very obscure, and consequently difficult of observation; yet we may point out the following: the respiration is labored; the thoracic parietals are not perfectly develop(ed); the face is purple; the general color indicates a sanguineous plethora in all the organs; the cries are obscure, painful and short; percussion yields a dull sound."[9] It seems remarkable that these astute observations were made almost 200 years ago.

The advances made in the understanding of pulmonary physiology of the newborn and the devices designed to support a newborn's respiration undoubtedly were stimulated by the interest shown in general newborn care that emerged in the latter part of the nineteenth century and continued into the first part of the twentieth century.[10] The reader is directed to multiple references that document the advances made in newborn care in France by Dr. Étienne Tarnier and his colleague Pierre Budin. Budin may well be regarded as the "father of neonatology" because of his contributions to newborn care, including publishing survival data and establishing follow-up programs for high-risk newborn patients.[10]

In Edinburg, Scotland, Dr. John William Ballantyne, an obstetrician working in the latter part of the nineteenth and early twentieth centuries, emphasized the importance of prenatal care and recognized that syphilis, malaria, typhoid, tuberculosis, and maternal ingestion of toxins such as alcohol and opiates were detrimental to the development of the fetus.[10]

O'Dwyer[11] in 1887 reported the first use of long-term positive-pressure ventilation in a series of 50 children with croup. Shortly thereafter, Egon Braun and Alexander Graham Bell independently developed intermittent body-enclosing devices for the negative-pressure/positive-pressure resuscitation of newborns (Fig. 1-2).[12,13] One might consider these seminal reports as the stimulus for the proliferation of work that

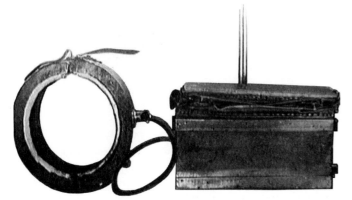

FIG 1-2 Alexander Graham Bell's negative-pressure ventilator, c. 1889. (From Stern L, et al. *Can Med Am J.* 1970.)

followed and the growing interest in mechanically ventilating newborn infants with respiratory failure.

TWENTIETH CENTURY

A variety of events occurred in the early twentieth century in the United States, including most notably the improvement of public health measures, the emergence of obstetrics as a full-fledged surgical specialty, and the assumption of care for all children by pediatricians.[10] In 1914, the use of continuous positive airway pressure for neonatal resuscitation was described by Von Reuss.[1] Henderson advocated positive-pressure ventilation via a mask with a T-piece in 1928.[14] In the same year, Flagg recommended the use of an endotracheal tube with positive-pressure ventilation for neonatal resuscitation.[15] The equipment he described was remarkably similar to that in use today.

Modern neonatology was born with the recognition that premature infants required particular attention with regard to temperature control, administration of fluids and nutrition, and protection from infection. In the 1930s and 1940s premature infants were given new stature, and it was acknowledged that of all of the causes of infant mortality, prematurity was the most common contributor.[10]

The years following World War II were marked by soaring birth rates, the proliferation of labor and delivery services in hospitals, the introduction of antibiotics, positive-pressure resuscitators, miniaturization of laboratory determinations, X-ray capability, and microtechnology that made intravenous therapy available for neonatal patients. These advances and a host of other discoveries heralded the modern era of neonatal medicine and set the groundwork for producing better methods of ventilating neonates with respiratory failure.

Improvements in intermittent negative-pressure and positive-pressure ventilation devices in the early twentieth century led to the development of a variety of techniques and machines for supporting ventilation in infants. In 1929, Drinker and Shaw[16] reported the development of a technique for producing constant thoracic traction to produce an increase in end-expiratory lung volume. In the early 1950s, Bloxsom[17] reported the use of a positive-pressure air lock for resuscitation of infants with respiratory distress in the delivery room. This device was similar to an iron lung; it alternately created positive and negative pressure of 1 to 3 psi at 1-min intervals in a tightly sealed cylindrical steel chamber that was infused with warmed humidified 60% oxygen.[18] Clear plastic versions of the air lock quickly

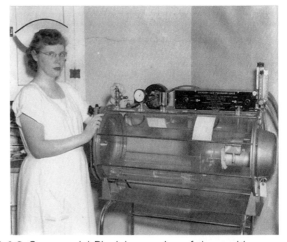

FIG 1-3 Commercial Plexiglas version of the positive-pressure oxygen air lock. Arrival of the unit at the Dansville Memorial Hospital, Dansville, NY, June 1952. (Photo courtesy of James Gross and the *Dansville Breeze.* June 26, 1952.)

became commercially available in the United States in the early 1950s (Fig. 1-3). However, a study by Apgar and Kreiselman in 1953[19] on apneic dogs and another study by Townsend involving 150 premature infants[20] demonstrated that the device could not adequately support the apneic newborn. The linkage of high oxygen administration to retinopathy of prematurity and a randomized controlled trial of the air lock versus care in an Isolette® incubator at Johns Hopkins University[21] revealed no advantage to either study group and heralded the hasty decline in the use of the Bloxsom device.[21]

In the late 1950s, body-tilting devices were designed that shifted the abdominal contents to create more effective movement of the diaphragm. Phrenic nerve stimulation[22] and the use of intragastric oxygen[23] also were reported in the literature but had little clinical success. In the 1950s and early 1960s, many centers also used bag and tightly fitting face mask ventilation to support infants for relatively long periods of time.

The initial aspect of ventilator support for the neonate in respiratory failure was effective resuscitation. Varying techniques in the United States were published from the 1950s to the 1980s, but the first consensus approach was created by Bloom and Cropley in 1987 and adopted by the American Academy of Pediatrics as a standardized teaching program. A synopsis of the major events in the development of neonatal resuscitation is shown as a time line in Box 1-1.

The modern era of automated mechanical ventilation for infants can be dated back to the 1953 report of Donald and Lord,[24] who described their experience with a patient-cycled, servo-controlled respirator in the treatment of several newborn infants with respiratory distress. They claimed that three or possibly four infants were successfully treated with their apparatus.

In the decades following Donald and Lord's pioneering efforts, the field of mechanical ventilation made dramatic advances; however, the gains were accompanied by several temporary setbacks. Because of the epidemic of poliomyelitis in the 1950s, experience was gained with the use of the tank-type negative-pressure ventilators of the Drinker design.[25] The success of these machines with children encouraged physicians to try modifications of them on neonates with some anecdotal success. However, initial efforts to apply intermittent positive-pressure ventilation (IPPV) to premature infants

BOX 1-1   Neonatal Resuscitation Time Line

1300 BC: Hebrew midwives use mouth-to-mouth breathing to resuscitate newborns.

460-380 BC: Hippocrates describes intubation of trachea of humans to support respiration.

200 BC-500 AD: Hebrew text (Talmud) states, "we may hold the young so that it should not fall on the ground, blow into its nostrils and put the teat into its mouth that it should suck."

98-138 AD: Greek physician Soranus describes evaluating neonates with system similar to present-day Apgar scoring, evaluating muscle tone, reflex or irritability, and respiratory effort. He believed that asphyxiated or premature infants and those with multiple congenital anomalies were "not worth saving."

1135-1204: Maimonides describes how to detect respiratory arrest in newborns and describes a method of manual resuscitation.

1667: Robert Hooke presents to the Royal Society of London his experience using fireside bellows attached to the trachea of dogs to provide continuous ventilation.

1774: Joseph Priestley produces oxygen but fails to recognize that it is related to respiration. Royal Humane Society advocates mouth-to-mouth resuscitation for stillborn infants.

1783-1788: Lavoisier terms oxygen "vital air" and shows that respiration is an oxidative process that produces water and carbon dioxide.

1806: Vide Chaussier describes intubation and mouth-to-mouth resuscitation of asphyxiated newborns.

1834: James Blundell describes neonatal intubation.

1874: Open chest cardiac massage reported in an adult.

1879: Report on the Aerophore Pulmonaire, a rubber bulb connected to a tube that is inserted into a neonate's airway and then compressed and released to provide inspiration and passive expiration.

1889: Alexander Graham Bell designs and builds body-type respirator for newborns.

Late 1880s: Bonair administers oxygen to premature "blue baby."

1949: Dr. Julius Hess and Evelyn C. Lundeen, RN, publish *The Premature Infant and Nursing Care*, which ushers in the modern era of neonatal medicine.

1953: Virginia Apgar reports on the system of neonatal assessment that bears her name.

1961: Dr. Jim Sutherland tests negative-pressure infant ventilator.

1971: Dr. George Gregory and colleagues publish results with continuous positive airway pressure in treating newborns with respiratory distress syndrome.

1987: American Academy of Pediatrics publishes the Neonatal Resuscitation Program based on an education program developed by Bloom and Cropley to teach a uniform method of neonatal resuscitation throughout the United States.

1999: The International Liaison Committee on Resuscitation (ILCOR) publishes the first neonatal advisory statement on resuscitation drawn from an evidence-based consensus of the available science. The ILCOR publishes an updated Consensus on Science and Treatment Recommendations for neonatal resuscitation every 5 years thereafter.

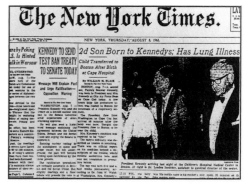

FIG 1-4 Front page of *The New York Times*. August 8, 1963. (Copyright 1963 by The New York Times Co. Reprinted by permission.)

cardiovascular effects, they advocated that the inspiratory phase of a mechanical cycle be limited to one-third of the entire cycle. Some ventilators manufactured in this period were even designed with the inspiratory-to-expiratory ratio fixed at 1:2.

Unfortunately, the findings of Cournand et al. were not applicable to patients with significant parenchymal disease, such as premature infants with RDS. Neonates with pulmonary disease characterized by poor lung compliance and complicated physiologically by increased chest wall compliance and terminal airway and alveolar collapse did not generally respond to IPPV techniques that had worked well in adults and older children. Clinicians were initially disappointed with the outcome of neonates treated with assisted ventilation using these techniques. The important observation of Avery and Mead in 1959 that babies who died from hyaline membrane disease (HMD) lacked a surface-active agent (surfactant), which increased surface tension in lung liquid samples and resulted in diffuse atelectasis, paved the way toward the modern treatment of respiratory failure in premature neonates by the constant maintenance of functional residual capacity and the eventual creation of surfactant replacement therapies.[28]

The birth of a premature son to President John F. Kennedy and Jacqueline Kennedy on August 7, 1963, focused the world's attention on prematurity and the treatment of HMD, then the current appellation for RDS. Patrick Bouvier Kennedy was born by cesarean section at 34 weeks' gestation at Otis Air Force Base Hospital. He weighed 2.1 kg and was transported to Boston's Massachusetts General Hospital, where he died at 39 hours of age (Fig. 1-4). The Kennedy baby was treated with the most advanced therapy of the time, hyperbaric oxygen,[29] but he died of progressive hypoxemia. There was no neonatal-specific ventilator in the United States to treat the young Kennedy at the time. In response to his death, *The New York Times* reported: "About all that can be done for a victim of hyaline membrane disease is to monitor the infant's blood chemistry and try to keep it near normal levels." The Kennedy tragedy, followed only 3 months later by the president's assassination, stimulated further interest and research in neonatal respiratory diseases and resulted in increased federal funding in these areas.

Partially in response to the Kennedy baby's death, several intensive care nurseries around the country (most notably at Yale, Children's Hospital of Philadelphia, Vanderbilt, and the University of California at San Francisco) began programs focused on respiratory care of the premature neonate and the treatment of HMD. Initial success with ventilatory treatment

with respiratory distress syndrome (RDS) were disappointing overall. Mortality was not demonstrably decreased, and the incidence of complications, particularly that of pulmonary air leaks, seemed to increase.[26] During this period, clinicians were hampered by the types of ventilators that were available and by the absence of proven standardized techniques for their use.

In accordance with the findings of Cournand et al.[27] in adult studies conducted in the late 1940s, standard ventilatory technique often required that the inspiratory positive-pressure times be very short. Cournand et al. had demonstrated that the prolongation of the inspiratory phase of the ventilator cycle in patients with normal lung compliance could result in impairment of thoracic venous return, a decrease in cardiac output, and the unacceptable depression of blood pressure. To minimize of HMD was reported by Delivoria-Papadopoulos and colleagues[30] in Toronto, and as a result, modified adult ventilatory devices were soon in use in many medical centers across the United States. However, the initial anecdotal successes were also accompanied by the emergence of a new disease, BPD, first described in a seminal paper by Northway et al.[31] in 1967. Northway initially attributed this disease to the use of high concentrations of inspired oxygen, but subsequent publications demonstrated that the cause of BPD was much more complex that and in addition to high inspired oxygen concentrations, intubation, barotrauma, volutrauma, infection, and other factors were involved. Chapter 35 discusses in great detail the current theories for the multiple causes of BPD or VILI.

BREAKTHROUGHS IN VENTILATION

A major breakthrough in neonatal ventilation occurred in 1971 when Gregory et al.[32] reported on clinical trials with continuous positive airway pressure (CPAP) for the treatment of RDS. Recognizing that the major physiologic problem in RDS was the collapse of alveoli during expiration, they applied continuous positive pressure to the airway via an endotracheal tube or sealed head chamber ("the Gregory box") during both expiration and inspiration; dramatic improvements in oxygenation and ventilation were achieved. Although infants receiving CPAP breathed spontaneously during the initial studies, later combinations of IPPV and CPAP in infants weighing less than 1500 g were not as successful.[32] Nonetheless, the concept of CPAP was a major advance. It was later modified by Bancalari et al.[33] for use in a constant distending negative-pressure chest cuirass and by Kattwinkel et al.,[34] who developed nasal prongs for the application of CPAP without the use of an endotracheal tube.

The observation that administration of antenatal corticosteroids to mothers prior to premature delivery accelerated maturation of the fetal lung was made in 1972 by Liggins and Howie.[35] Their randomized controlled trial demonstrated that the risks of HMD and death were significantly reduced in those premature infants whose mothers received antenatal steroid treatment.

Meanwhile, Reynolds and Taghizadeh,[36,37] working independently in Great Britain, also recognized the unique pathophysiology of neonatal pulmonary disease. Having experienced difficulties with IPPV similar to those noted by clinicians in the United States, Reynolds and Taghizadeh suggested prolongation of the inspiratory phase of the ventilator cycle by delaying the opening of the exhalation valve. The "reversal" of the standard inspiratory-to-expiratory ratio, or "inflation hold," allowed sufficient time for the recruitment of atelectatic alveoli in RDS with lower inflating pressures and gas flows, which, in turn, decreased turbulence and limited the effects on venous return to the heart. The excellent results of Reynolds and Taghizadeh could not be duplicated uniformly in the United States, perhaps because their American colleagues used different ventilators.

Until the early 1970s, ventilators used in neonatal intensive care units (NICUs) were modifications of adult devices; these devices delivered intermittent gas flows, thus generating IPPV. The ventilator initiated every mechanical breath, and clinicians tried to eliminate the infants' attempts to breathe between IPPV breaths ("fighting the ventilator"), which led to rebreathing of dead air. In 1971, a new prototype neonatal ventilator was developed by Kirby and colleagues.[38] This ventilator used continuous gas flow and a timing device to close

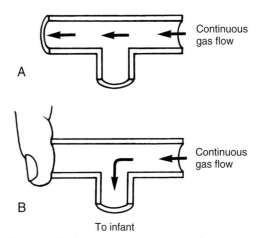

FIG 1-5 Ayre's T-piece forms the mechanical basis of most neonatal ventilators currently in use. **A,** Continuous gas flow from which an infant can breathe spontaneously. **B,** Occlusion of one end of the T-piece diverts gas flow under pressure into an infant's lungs. The mechanical ventilator incorporates a pneumatically or electronically controlled time-cycling mechanism to occlude the expiratory limb of the patient circuit. Between sequential mechanical breaths, the infant can still breathe spontaneously. The combination of mechanical and spontaneous breaths is called intermittent mandatory ventilation. (From Kirby RR. Mechanical ventilation of the newborn. *Perinatol Neonatol.* 5:47, 1981.)

the exhalation valve modeled after Ayre's T-piece used in anesthesia (Fig. 1-5).[24,36,38] Using the T-piece concept, the ventilator provided continuous gas flow and allowed the patient to breathe spontaneously between mechanical breaths. Occlusion of the distal end of the T-piece diverted gas flow under pressure to the infant. In addition, partial occlusion of the distal end generated positive end-expiratory pressure. This combination of mechanical and spontaneous breathing and continuous gas flow was called *intermittent mandatory ventilation* (IMV).

IMV became the standard method of neonatal ventilation and has been incorporated into all infant ventilators since then. One of its advantages was the facilitation of weaning by progressive reduction in the IMV rate, which allowed the patient to gradually increase spontaneous breathing against distending pressure. Clinicians no longer needed to paralyze or hyperventilate patients to prevent them from "fighting the ventilator." Moreover, because patients continued to breathe spontaneously and lower cycling rates were used, mean intrapleural pressure was reduced and venous return was less compromised than with IPPV.[39]

Meanwhile, progress was also being made in the medical treatment and replacement of the cause of RDS, the absence or lack of adequate surfactant in the neonatal lung. Following the 1980 publication of a small series by Fujiwara et al. on the beneficial effect of exogenous surfactant in premature infants with HMD,[40] several large randomized studies of the efficacy of surfactant were conducted. By the end of the decade the use of surfactant was well established. However, for decades there remained many controversies surrounding various treatment regimens (prophylactic vs rescue), types of surfactants, and dosing schedules.[41]

From 1971 to the mid-1990s, a myriad of new ventilators specifically designed for neonates were manufactured and sold.

The first generation of ventilators included the BABYbird 1®, the Bourns BP200®, and a volume ventilator, the Bourns LS 104/150®. All operated on the IMV principle and were capable of incorporating CPAP into the respiratory cycle (known as *positive end-expiratory pressure* [PEEP] when used with IMV).[42]

The BABYbird 1® and the Bourns BP200® used a solenoid-activated switch to occlude the exhalation limb of the gas circuit to deliver a breath. Pneumatic adjustments in the inspiratory-to-expiratory ratio and rate were controlled by inspiratory and expiratory times, which had to be timed with a stopwatch. A spring-loaded pressure manometer monitored peak inspiratory pressure and PEEP. These early mechanics created time delays within the ventilator, resulting in problems in obtaining short inspiratory times (less than 0.5 second).

In the next generation of ventilators, electronic controls, microprocessors, and microcircuitry allowed the addition of light-emitting diode monitors and provided clinicians with faster response times, greater sensitivity, and a wider range of ventilator parameter selection. These advances were incorporated into ventilators such as the Sechrist 100® and Bear Cub® to decrease inspiratory times to as short as 0.1 second and to increase ventilatory rates to 150 inflations per minute. Monitors incorporating microprocessors measured inspiratory and expiratory times and calculated inspiratory-to-expiratory ratios and mean airway pressure. Ventilator strategies abounded, and controversy regarding the best (i.e., least harmful) method for assisting neonatal ventilation arose. High-frequency positive-pressure ventilation using conventional ventilators was also proposed as a beneficial treatment of RDS.[43]

Meanwhile, extracorporeal membrane oxygenation and true high-frequency ventilation (HFV) were being developed at a number of major medical centers.[44,45] These techniques initially were offered as a rescue therapy for infants who did not respond to conventional mechanical ventilation. The favorable physiologic characteristics of HFV led some investigators to promote its use as an initial treatment of respiratory failure, especially when caused by RDS in very low birth-weight (VLBW) infants.[46]

A third generation of neonatal ventilators began to appear in the early 1990s. Advances in microcircuitry and microprocessors, developed as a result of the space program, allowed new dimensions in the development of neonatal assisted ventilation. The use of synchronized IMV, assist/control mode ventilation, and pressure support ventilation—previously used in the ventilation of only older children and adults—became possible in neonates because of the very fast ventilator response times. Although problems with sensing a patient's inspiratory effort sometimes limited the usefulness of these new modalities, the advances gave hope that ventilator complications could be limited and that the need for sedation or paralysis during ventilation could be decreased. Direct measurement of some pulmonary functions at the bedside became a reality and allowed the clinician to make ventilatory adjustments based on physiologic data rather than on a "hunch."

The mortality from HMD, now called RDS, decreased markedly from 1971 to 2007 owing to a multitude of reasons, some of which have been noted above. In the United States, the RDS mortality decreased from 268 per 100,000 live births in 1971 to 98 per 100,000 live births by 1985. From 1985 to 2007, the rate fell to 17 per 100,000 live births. Thus in a 36-year period, the mortality from RDS fell nearly 94%, owing in part to the improvements in ventilator technology, the development of medical adjuncts such as exogenous surfactant, and the skill of the physicians, nurses, and respiratory therapists using these devices while caring for these fragile infants.[47,48]

Since 2005, an even newer generation of ventilators has been developed. These are microprocessor based, with a wide array of technological features including several forms of patient triggering, volume targeting, and pressure support modes and the ability to monitor many pulmonary functions at the bedside with ventilator graphics. As clinicians become more convinced that VILI is secondary to volutrauma more than barotrauma, the emphasis to control tidal volumes especially in the "micro-premie" has resulted in some major changes in the technique of ventilation. Chapters 15 and 18-22 elaborate more fully on these advances.

Concurrent with these advances is an increased complexity related to controlling the ventilator and thus more opportunity for operator error. Some ventilators are extremely versatile and can function for patients of extremely low birth weight (less than 1000 g) to 70-kg adults. Although these ventilators are appealing to administrators who have to purchase these expensive machines for many different categories of patients in the hospital, they add increased complexity and patient safety issues in caring for neonates. Chapter 6 discusses some of these issues.

Respiratory support in the present-day NICU continues to change as new science and new technologies point the way to better outcomes with less morbidity, even for the smallest premature infants. However, as the technology of neonatal ventilators advanced, a concurrent movement away from intubation was gaining popularity in the United States. In 1987, a comparison of eight major centers in the National Institute of Child Health and Human Development group by Avery et al. reviewed oxygen dependency and death in VLBW babies at 28 days of age.[49] Although all centers had comparable mortality, one center (Columbia Presbyterian Medical Center) had the lowest rate by far of CLD among the institutions. Columbia had adopted a unique approach to respiratory support of VLBW infants, emphasizing nasal CPAP as the first choice for respiratory support, whereas the other centers were using intubation and mechanical ventilation. Other centers were slow to adopt the Columbia approach, which used bubble nasal CPAP, but gradually institutions began using noninvasive techniques for at least the larger VLBW infants. A Cochrane review of multiple trials in 2012 concluded that the combined outcomes of death and BPD were lower in infants who had initial stabilization with nasal CPAP, and later rescue surfactant therapy if needed, compared to elective intubation and prophylactic surfactant administration (RR 1.12, 95% CI 1.02 to 1.24).[50] In recent years, "noninvasive" respiratory support with the use of nasal CPAP, synchronized inspiratory positive airway pressure, RAM-assisted ventilation, and neurally adjusted ventilatory assist has become a more widely used technique to support premature infants with respiratory distress in the hope of avoiding the trauma associated with intubation and VILI. Using a noninvasive approach as one potentially better practice, quality improvement programs to lower the rate of BPD have had mixed success. As of this writing, noninvasive ventilation has been supported by a number of retrospective and cohort studies, and there are some recent reports suggesting that the earlier use of noninvasive therapies has a role in treating neonates with respiratory disease and preventing the need for intubation to treat respiratory failure.

See Chapters 17, 19, and 21 for a more in-depth discussion of newer modes of neonatal assisted ventilation.

RECENT ADVANCES AND OUTCOMES

With the advances made in providing assisted ventilation to our most vulnerable patients, survival rates have improved dramatically. For babies born at less than 28 weeks' gestation and less than 1000 g, survival reaches 85 to 90%. However, in recent years the emphasis has shifted from just survival to survival without significant neurologic deficit, CLD, or retinopathy of prematurity. Nonetheless, benchmarking groups such as the Vermont–Oxford Network have shown a wide variance in these untoward outcomes that cannot be explained by variances in the patient population alone. CLD in infants born at <1500 g birth weight (VLBW infants) varies from 6% to over 50% in various NICUs. Thus it appears that overall advances in the morbidity and mortality rates of the VLBW infant group as a whole will be made from more uniform application of technology already available rather than the creation of new devices or medications. Moreover, despite continued technological advances in respiratory support since 2007, there have been only minor improvements in morbidity and mortality rates in high-resource countries. Perhaps entirely new approaches are necessary to produce major leaps forward in the treatment of neonatal respiratory failure. However, in resource-limited areas throughout the world, the use of basic respiratory support technologies (i.e., CPAP, resuscitation techniques) has the potential to have a major impact on the outcomes of newborns (see Chapter 38).

Despite the wide array of technology now available to the clinician treating neonatal respiratory failure, there are still significant limitations and uncertainty about our care. We continue to research and discuss issues such as conventional vs high-frequency ventilation, noninvasive ventilation vs the early administration of surfactant, the best ventilator mode, the best rate, the optimum settings, and the most appropriate approach to weaning and extubation. There are very few randomized controlled trials that demonstrate significant differences in morbidity or mortality related to new ventilator technologies or strategies. This is due to the difficulty in enrolling neonates into clinical trials, the large number of patients needed to detect statistical differences in outcomes, the reluctance of device manufacturers to support expensive studies, and the rapidly changing software, which make it difficult for research to keep up with the technological advances.[51] It is the editors' expectations that this book will provide some more food for thought in these areas and the necessary information for the physician, nurse, or respiratory therapist involved in the care of neonates to provide the best possible care based on the information available in 2016 and beyond.

REFERENCES

A complete reference list is available at https://expertconsult.inkling.com/.

2

Physiologic Principles*

Martin Keszler, MD, FAAP, and Kabir Abubakar, MD

To provide individualized care that optimizes pulmonary and neurodevelopmental outcomes, it is essential to have a good working knowledge of the unique physiology and pathophysiology of the newborn respiratory system.

It is the responsibility of those who care for critically ill infants to have a sound understanding of respiratory physiology, especially the functional limitations and the special vulnerabilities of the immature lung. The first tenet of the Hippocratic Oath states, "Primum non nocere" ("First do no harm"). That admonition cannot be followed without adequate knowledge of physiology. In daily practice, we are faced with the difficult task of supporting adequate gas exchange in an immature respiratory system, using powerful tools that by their very nature can inhibit ongoing developmental processes, often resulting in alterations in end-organ form and function.

In our efforts to provide ventilatory support, the infant's lungs and airways are subjected to forces that may lead to acute and chronic tissue injury. This results in alterations in the way the lungs develop and the way they respond to subsequent noxious stimuli. Alterations in lung development result in alterations in lung function as the infant's body attempts to heal and continue to develop. Superimposed on this is the fact that the ongoing development of the respiratory system is hampered by the healing process itself.

This complexity makes caring for infants with respiratory failure both interesting and challenging. To effectively provide support for these patients, the clinician must have an understanding not only of respiratory physiology but also of respiratory system development, growth, and healing.

Although the lung has a variety of functions, some of which include the immunologic and endocrine systems, the focus of this chapter is its primary function, that of gas exchange.

BASIC BIOCHEMISTRY OF RESPIRATION: OXYGEN AND ENERGY

The energy production required for a newborn infant to sustain his or her metabolic functions depends upon the availability of oxygen and its subsequent metabolism. During the breakdown of carbohydrates, oxygen is consumed and carbon dioxide and water are produced. The energy derived from this process is generated as electrons, which are transferred from electron donors to electron acceptors. Oxygen has a high electron affinity and therefore is a good electron acceptor. The energy produced during this process is stored as high-energy phosphate bonds,

primarily in the form of adenosine triphosphate (ATP). Enzyme systems within the mitochondria couple the transfer of energy to oxidation in a process known as *oxidative phosphorylation*.[1]

For oxidative phosphorylation to occur, an adequate amount of oxygen must be available to the mitochondria. The transfer of oxygen from the air outside the infant to the mitochondria, within the infant's cells, involves a series of steps: (1) convection of fresh air into the lung, (2) diffusion of oxygen into the blood, (3) convective flow of oxygenated blood to the tissues, (4) diffusion of oxygen into the cells, and finally, (5) diffusion into the mitochondria. The driving force for the diffusion processes is an oxygen partial pressure gradient, which, together with the convective processes of ventilation and perfusion, results in a cascade of oxygen tensions from the air outside the body to intracellular mitochondria (Fig. 2-1). The lungs of the newborn infant transfer oxygen to the blood by diffusion, driven by the oxygen partial pressure gradient. For gas exchange to occur efficiently, the infant's lungs must remain expanded, the lungs must be both ventilated and perfused, and the ambient partial pressure of oxygen in the air must be greater than the partial pressure of the oxygen in the blood. The efficiency of the newborn infant's respiratory system is determined by both structural and functional constraints; therefore, the clinician must be mindful of both aspects when caring for the infant.

The infant's cells require energy to function. This energy is obtained from high-energy phosphate bonds (e.g., ATP) formed during oxidative phosphorylation. Only a small amount of ATP is stored within the cells. Muscle cells contain an additional store of ATP, but to meet metabolic needs beyond those that can be provided for by the stored ATP, new ATP must be made by phosphorylation of adenosine diphosphate (ADP).

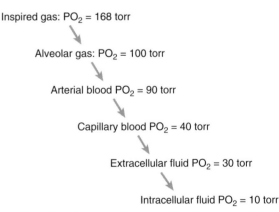

Inspired gas: PO_2 = 168 torr

Alveolar gas: PO_2 = 100 torr

Arterial blood PO_2 = 90 torr

Capillary blood PO_2 = 40 torr

Extracellular fluid PO_2 = 30 torr

Intracellular fluid PO_2 = 10 torr

FIG 2-1 Transfer of oxygen from outside air to intracellular mitochondria via an oxygen pressure gradient: oxygen tension at various levels of the O_2 transport chain.

*We wish to acknowledge gratefully the important contribution of Brian Wood, MD, who was the author of this chapter in the previous editions of this book.

This can be done anaerobically through glycolysis, but this is an inefficient process and leads to the formation of lactic acid. Long-term energy demands must be met aerobically, through ongoing oxidative phosphorylation within the mitochondria, which is a much more efficient process that results in the formation of carbon dioxide and water.

There is a hierarchy of how energy is used by the infant. During periods of high energy demand, tissues initially draw upon the limited stores of ATP, then use glycolysis to make more ATP from ADP, and then use oxidative phosphorylation to supply the infant's ongoing energy requirements. Oxidative phosphorylation and oxygen consumption are so closely linked to the newborn infant's energy requirements that total oxygen consumption is a reasonably good measure of the total energy needs of the infant. When the infant's metabolic workload is in excess of that which can be sustained by oxidative phosphorylation (aerobic metabolism), the tissues will revert to anaerobic glycolysis to produce ATP. This anaerobic metabolism results in the formation of lactic acid, which accumulates in the blood and causes a decrease in pH (acidosis/acidemia). Lactic acid is therefore an important marker of inadequate tissue oxygen delivery.

ONTOGENY RECAPITULATES PHYLOGENY: A BRIEF OVERVIEW OF DEVELOPMENTAL ANATOMY

Lung Development
The tracheobronchial airway system begins as a ventral outpouching of the primitive foregut, which leads to the formation of the embryonic lung bud. The lung bud subsequently divides and branches, penetrating the mesenchyma and progressing toward the periphery. Lung development is divided into five sequential phases.[2] The demarcation of these phases is somewhat arbitrary with some overlap between them. A variety of physical, hormonal, and other factors influence the pace of lung development and maturation. Adequate distending pressure of fetal lung fluid and normal fetal breathing movements are some of the more prominent factors known to affect lung growth and development.

Phases of Lung Development
- Embryonic phase (weeks 3 to 6)
- Pseudoglandular phase (weeks 6 to 16)
- Canalicular phase (weeks 16 to 26)
- Terminal sac phase (weeks 26 to 36)
- Alveolar phase (week 36 to 3 years)

Embryonic Phase (Weeks 3 to 6): Development of Proximal Airways
The lung bud arises from the foregut 21 to 26 days after fertilization.

Aberrant development during the embryonic phase may result in the following:
- Tracheal agenesis
- Tracheal stenosis
- Tracheoesophageal fistula
- Pulmonary sequestration (if an accessory lung bud develops during this period)

Pseudoglandular Phase (Weeks 6 to 16): Development of Lower Conducting Airways
During this phase the first 20 generations of conducting airways develop. The first 8 generations (the bronchi) ultimately acquire cartilaginous walls. Generations 9 to 20 comprise the nonrespiratory bronchioles. Lymph vessels and bronchial capillaries accompany the airways as they grow and develop.

Aberrant development during the pseudoglandular phase may result in the following:
- Bronchogenic cysts
- Congenital lobar emphysema
- Congenital diaphragmatic hernia

Canalicular Phase (Weeks 16 to 26): Formation of Gas-Exchanging Units or Acini
The formation of respiratory bronchioles (generations 21 to 23) occurs during the canalicular phase. The relative proportion of parenchymal connective tissue diminishes. The development of pulmonary capillaries occurs. Gas exchange depends upon the adequacy of acinus–capillary coupling.

Terminal Sac Phase (Weeks 26 to 36): Refinement of Acini
The rudimentary primary saccules subdivide by formation of secondary crests into smaller saccules and alveoli during the terminal sac phase, thus greatly increasing the surface area available for gas exchange. The interstitium continues to thin out, decreasing the distance for diffusion. Capillary invasion leads to an increase in the alveolar–blood barrier surface area. The development and maturation of the surfactant system occurs during this phase.

Birth and initiation of spontaneous or mechanical ventilation during the terminal sac phase may result in the following:
- Pulmonary insufficiency of prematurity (due to reduced surface area, increased diffusion distance, and unfavorable lung mechanics)
- Respiratory distress syndrome (due to surfactant deficiency and/or inactivation)
- Pulmonary interstitial emphysema (due to tissue stretching by uneven aeration, excessive inflating pressure, and increased interstitium that traps air in the perivascular sheath)
- Impairment of secondary crest formation and capillary development, leading to alveolar simplification, decreased surface area for gas exchange, and variable increase in interstitial cellularity and/or fibroproliferation (bronchopulmonary dysplasia [BPD]).

Alveolar Phase (Week 36 to 3 Years): Alveolar Proliferation and Development
Saccules become alveoli as a result of thinning of the acinar walls, dissipation of the interstitium, and invagination of the alveoli by pulmonary capillaries with secondary crest formation during the alveolar phase. The alveoli attain a polyhedral shape.

MECHANICS

The respiratory system is composed of millions of air sacs that are connected to the outside air via airways. The lung behaves like a balloon that is held in an expanded state by the intact thorax and will deflate if the integrity of the system becomes compromised. The interior of the lung is partitioned so as to provide a large surface area to facilitate efficient gas diffusion. The lung is expanded by forces generated by the diaphragm and the intercostal muscles. It recoils secondary to elastic and surface tension forces. This facilitates the inflow and outflow of respiratory gases required to allow the air volume contained within the lung to be ventilated. During inspiration the diaphragm contracts. The diaphragm is a dome-shaped muscle at rest. As it contracts, the diaphragm flattens, and the volume of the chest cavity is enlarged. This causes the intrapleural pressure to decrease and results in gas flow into the lung.[3] During unlabored breathing, the intercostal and accessory muscles serve primarily to stabilize the rib cage as the diaphragm contracts, countering the forces resulting from the decrease in intrapleural pressure during inspiration. This limits the extent to which the infant's chest wall is deformed inward during inspiration.

Although the premature infant's chest is very compliant, the rib cage offers some structural support, serves as an attachment point for the respiratory muscles, and limits lung deflation at end expiration. The elastic elements of the respiratory system—the connective tissue—are stretched during inspiration and recoil during expiration. The air–liquid interface in the terminal air spaces and respiratory bronchioles generates surface tension that opposes lung expansion and promotes lung deflation. The conducting airways, which connect the gas exchange units to the outside air, provide greater resistance during exhalation than during inspiration, because during inspiration, the tethering elements of the surrounding lung tissue increase the airway diameter, relative to expiration. The respiratory system is designed to be adaptable to a wide range of workloads; however, in the newborn infant, several structural and functional limitations make the newborn susceptible to respiratory failure.

Differences between the shape of a newborn infant's chest and that of an adult put the infant at a mechanical disadvantage. Unlike the adult's thorax, which is ellipsoid in shape, the infant's thorax is more cylindrical and the ribs are more horizontal, rather than oblique. Because of these anatomic differences, the intercostal muscles in infants have a shorter course and provide less mechanical advantage for elevating the ribs and increasing intrathoracic volume during inspiration than do those of adults. Also, because the insertion of the infant's diaphragm is more horizontal than in the adult, the lower ribs tend to move inward rather than upward during inspiration. The compliant chest wall of the infant exacerbates this inward deflection with inspiration. This is particularly evident during rapid eye movement (REM) sleep, when phasic changes in intercostal muscle tone are inhibited. Therefore, instead of stabilizing the rib cage during inspiration, the intercostal muscles are relaxed. This results in inefficient respiratory effort, which may be manifested clinically by intercostal and substernal retractions associated with abdominal breathing, especially when lung compliance is decreased. The endurance capacity of the diaphragm is determined primarily by muscle mass and the oxidative capacity of muscle fibers. Infants have low muscle mass and a low percentage of type 1 (slow twitch) muscle fibers compared to those of adults.[4] To sustain the work of breathing, the diaphragm must be provided with a continuous supply of oxygen. The infant with respiratory distress is thus prone to respiratory muscle fatigue leading to respiratory failure.

During expiration the main driving force is elastic recoil, which depends on the surface tension produced by the air–liquid interface, the elastic elements of the lung tissue, and the bony development of the rib cage. Expiration is largely passive. The abdominal muscles can aid in exhalation by active contraction if required, but they make little contribution during unlabored breathing. Because the chest wall of premature infants is compliant, it offers little resistance against expansion upon inspiration and little opposition against collapse upon expiration.

This collapse at end expiration can lead to atelectasis. In premature infants the largest contributor to elastic recoil is surface tension. Pulmonary surfactant serves to reduce surface tension and stabilize the terminal airways. In circumstances in which surfactant is deficient, the terminal air spaces have a tendency to collapse, leading to diffuse atelectasis. Distending airway pressure in the form of positive end-expiratory pressure (PEEP) or continuous positive airway pressure (CPAP) may be applied to the infant's airway to counter the tendency toward collapse and the development of atelectasis. The application of airway-distending pressure also serves to stabilize the chest wall.

Lung compliance and airway resistance are related to lung size. The smaller the lung, the lower the compliance and the greater the resistance. If, however, lung compliance is corrected to lung volume (specific compliance), the values are nearly identical for term infants and adults.[5] In term infants, immediately after delivery, specific compliance is low but normalizes as fetal lung fluid is absorbed and a normal functional residual capacity (FRC) is established. In premature infants, specific compliance remains low, due in part to diffuse microatelectasis and failure to achieve a normal FRC, because the lung recoil forces are incompletely opposed by the excessively compliant chest wall.

The resistance within lung tissue during inflation and deflation is called *viscous resistance*. Viscous resistance is elevated in the newborn. In immature small lungs, there are relatively fewer terminal air spaces and relatively more stroma (cells and interstitial fluid). This is manifested by a low ratio of lung volume to lung weight. Although in absolute terms airway resistance is high in the newborn infant, when corrected to lung volume (specific conductance, which is the reciprocal of resistance per unit lung volume), the relative resistance is lower than in adults. It is important to remember that because of the small diameter of the airways in the lungs of the newborn infant, even a modest further narrowing, will result in a marked increase in resistance. That the newborn's bronchial tree is short and the inspiratory flow velocities are low are teleologic advantages for the newborn because both of these factors decrease airway resistance.

Overcoming the elastic and resistive forces during ventilation requires energy expenditure and accounts for the work of breathing. The normal work of breathing is essentially the same for newborns and adults when corrected for metabolic rates.[5] When the work of breathing increases in response to various disease states, the newborn is at a decided disadvantage. The newborn infant lacks the strength and endurance to cope with a significant increase in ventilatory workload. A large increase in ventilatory workload can lead to respiratory failure.

Elastic and resistive forces of the chest, lungs, abdomen, airways, and ventilator circuit oppose the forces exerted by the respiratory muscles and/or ventilator. The terms *elastic recoil*, *flow resistance*, *viscous resistance*, and *work of breathing* are used to describe these forces. Such forces may also be described as *dissipative* and *nondissipative* forces. The latter refers to the fact that the work needed to overcome elastic recoil is stored like the energy in a coiled spring and will be returned to the system upon exhalation. Resistive and frictional forces, on the other hand, are lost and converted to heat (dissipated). The terms *elasticity, compliance,* and *conductance* characterize the properties of the thorax, lungs, and airways. The static pressure–volume curve illustrates the relationships between these forces at various levels of lung expansion. Dynamic pressure–volume loops illustrate the pressure–volume relationship during inspiration and expiration (Figs. 2-2 to 2-4).

Elastic recoil refers to the tendency of stretched objects to return to their original shape. When the inspiratory muscles relax during exhalation, the elastic elements of the chest wall, diaphragm, and lungs, which were stretched during inspiration, recoil to their original shapes. These elastic elements behave like springs (Fig. 2-5). The surface tension forces at the air–liquid

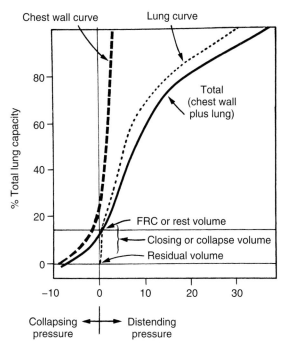

FIG 2-2 Static pressure–volume curves for the chest wall, the lung, and the sum of the two for a normal newborn infant. Functional residual capacity (FRC) or rest volume (less than 20% of total lung capacity) is the point at which collapsing and distending pressures balance out to zero pressure. The lung would empty to residual volume if enough collapsing pressure (forced expiration) was generated to overcome the chest wall elastic recoil in the opposite direction. The premature infant has an even steeper chest wall compliance curve than that shown here, whereas his or her lung compliance curve tends to be flatter and shifted to the right, depending on the degree of surfactant deficiency.

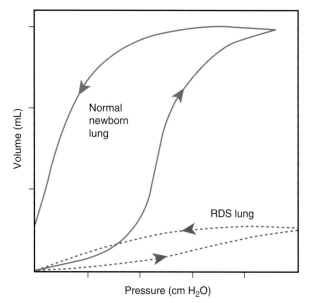

FIG 2-4 Comparison of the pressure–volume curve of a normal infant (*solid line*) with that of a newborn with respiratory distress syndrome (*dotted line*). Note that very little hysteresis (i.e., the difference between the inspiratory and the expiratory limbs) is observed in the respiratory distress syndrome curve because of the lack of surfactant for stabilization of the alveoli after inflation. The wide hysteresis of the normal infant's lung curve reflects changes (reduction) in surface tension once the alveoli are opened and stabilized. *RDS*, Respiratory distress syndrome.

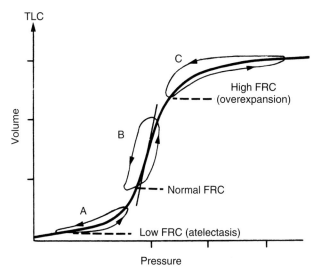

FIG 2-3 Extended compliance or lung expansion curve with "flattened" areas (*A* and *C*) at both ends. Area *A* represents the situation in disease states leading to atelectasis or lung collapse. Area *C* represents the situation in an overexpanded lung, as occurs in diseases involving significant air trapping (e.g., meconium aspiration) or in the excessive application of distending pressure during assisted ventilation. *FRC*, Functional residual capacity.

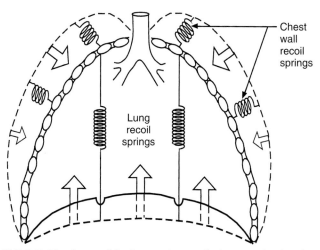

FIG 2-5 Elastic recoil is the tendency of elements in the chest wall and lungs that are stretched during inspiration to snap back or recoil (*arrows*) to their original state at the end of expiration. At this point (functional residual capacity or rest volume), the "springs" are relaxed and the structure of the rib cage allows no further collapse. Opposing forces of the chest wall and elastic recoil balance out, and intrathoracic and airway pressures become equal (this further defines functional residual capacity or rest volume; see also Fig. 2-2).

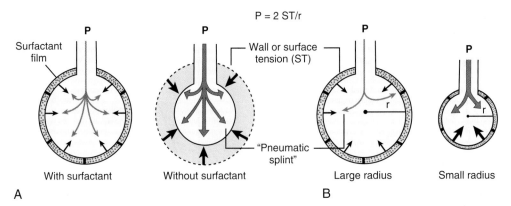

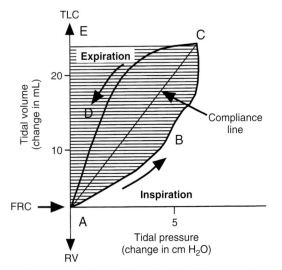

FIG 2-6 Diagrammatic illustration of the Laplace relationship and the effects of (**A**) surfactant film and (**B**) alveolar radius on wall or surface tension. The degree (reflected in the size of the brown arrows) of airway or intra-alveolar pressure (*P*) needed to counteract the tendency of alveoli to collapse (represented by the black arrows) is directly proportional to double the wall or surface tension (*ST*) and inversely proportional to the size of the radius (*r*). Distending airway pressure applied during assisted ventilation can be likened to a "pneumatic splint."

FIG 2-7 Pressure–volume loop showing the compliance line (*AC*, joining points of no flow); work done in overcoming elastic resistance (*ACEA*), which incorporates the frictional resistance encountered during expiration (*ACDA*); work done in overcoming frictional resistance during inspiration (*ABCA*); and total work done during the respiratory cycle (*ABCEA*, or the entire shaded area).

interfaces in the distal bronchioles and terminal airways decrease the surface area of the air–liquid interfaces (Fig. 2-6).

At some point, the forces that tend to collapse are counterbalanced by those that resist further collapse. The point at which these opposing forces balance is called the *resting state of the respiratory system* and corresponds to FRC (Fig. 2-7; see also Fig. 2-2). Because the chest wall of the newborn infant is compliant, it offers little opposition to collapse at end expiration. Thus the newborn, especially the premature newborn, has a relatively low FRC and thoracic gas volume, even when the newborn does not suffer from primary surfactant deficiency. Clinically, this manifests as a mild degree of diffuse microatelectasis and is referred to as *pulmonary insufficiency of prematurity*. This low FRC and the relative underdevelopment of the conducting airway's structural support explain the tendency for

early airway closure and collapse, with resultant gas trapping in premature infants.

The respiratory system's resting volume is very close to the closing volume of the lung (the volume at which dependent lung regions cease to ventilate because the airways leading to them have collapsed). In newborns, closing volume may occur even above FRC (see Fig. 2-2).[6] Gas trapping related to airway closure has been demonstrated experimentally by showing situations in which the thoracic gas volume is greater than the FRC. For this to occur, the total gas volume measured in the chest at end expiration is greater than the amount of gas that is in communication with the upper airway (FRC).

The main contributor to lung elastic recoil in the newborn is surface tension. The pressure required to counteract the tendency of the bronchioles and terminal air spaces to collapse is described by the Laplace relationship:

$$P = \frac{2\,ST}{r}$$

Simply stated, this relationship illustrates that the pressure (*P*) needed to stabilize the system is directly proportional to twice the surface tension (*2 ST*) and inversely proportional to the radius of curvature (*r*). In infants, the relationship should be modified, because, unlike in a soap bubble, there is an air–liquid interface on only one side of the terminal lung unit, so *P = ST/r* probably describes the situation more accurately in the lung.

In reality, alveoli are not spherical but polyhedral and share their walls with adjacent alveolar structures, making strict application of Laplace's law suspect. Nonetheless, the basic concept of the law does apply to both terminal air sacs and small airways, and it provides a crucial framework for the understanding of respiratory physiology. The surface tension in the lung is primarily governed by the presence or absence of surfactant. Surfactant is a surface-active material released by type II pneumocytes. It is composed mainly of dipalmitoyl phosphatidylcholine but contains other essential components, such as surfactant-associated proteins A, B, C, and D, as well.

Surfactant has a variety of unique properties that enable it to decrease surface tension at end expiration and thereby prevent further lung deflation below resting volume and allow an increase in surface tension upon lung expansion that facilitates elastic recoil at end inspiration. In addition, surfactant reduces surface tension when lung volume is decreased.[7] A reduction in the quantity of surfactant results in an increase in surface tension and necessitates the application of more distending pressure to counter the tendency of the bronchioles and terminal air spaces to collapse (see Fig. 2-6, A).

As can be seen from the Laplace relationship, the larger the radius of curvature of the terminal bronchioles or air spaces, the less pressure is needed to hold them open or to expand them further (see Fig. 2-6, B). The smaller the radius of curvature (e.g., in premature infants), the more pressure is required to hold the airways open. Surfactant helps this situation throughout the respiratory cycle. As the radii of the air–liquid interfaces become smaller during exhalation, the effectiveness of surfactant in reducing surface tension increases; as the radii become larger, its effectiveness decreases.

Respiratory distress syndrome (RDS) imposes a significant amount of energy expenditure on the newborn infant, who must generate high negative intrapleural pressures to expand and stabilize his or her distal airways and alveoli (see Fig. 2-4). In untreated RDS, each breath requires significant energy expenditure because lung volumes achieved with the high opening pressures during inspiration are rapidly lost as the surfactant-deficient lung collapses to its original resting volume during expiration. The burden imposed by this large work of breathing may quickly outstrip the infant's ability to maintain this level of output and lead to respiratory failure.

The infant with RDS may need relatively high inflation pressure to open atelectatic alveoli, and provision of adequate end-expiratory pressure will help keep the lung open. However, once the lung is expanded, the radii of the bronchioles and terminal air spaces are larger, and, therefore, less pressure is required to hold them open or to expand them further. Attention should be paid to tidal volume and overall lung volume after initial alveolar recruitment to avoid overdistention and volutrauma, which are major factors in the development of BPD.[8] Failure to reduce inspiratory and distending pressures appropriately and thus avoid lung overdistention once normal lung volume has been achieved may lead to air-leak complications such as pulmonary interstitial emphysema (PIE) and pneumothorax (see Chapter 20).

Compliance

Compliance is a measure of the change in volume resulting from a given change in pressure:

$$C_L = \Delta V / \Delta P$$

where C_L is lung compliance, ΔV is change in volume, and ΔP is change in pressure.

Static Compliance

When measured under static conditions, compliance reflects only the elastic properties of the lung. Static compliance is the reciprocal of elastance, the tendency to recoil toward its original dimensions upon removal of the distending pressure required to stretch the system. Static compliance is measured by determining the transpulmonary pressure change after inflating the lungs with a known volume of gas. Transpulmonary pressure is the pressure difference between alveolar pressure and pleural pressure. It is approximated by measuring pressure at the airway opening and in the esophagus. To generate a pressure–volume curve, pressure measurements are made during static conditions after each incremental volume of gas is introduced into the lungs (see lung curve in Fig. 2-2). If one measures the difference between pleural pressures (esophageal) and atmospheric pressures (transthoracic) at different levels of lung expansion, the plotted curve will be a chest wall compliance curve (see chest wall curve in Fig. 2-2). This kind of plot shows the elastic properties of the chest wall. In the newborn, the chest wall is very compliant; thus large volume changes are achieved with small pressure changes. Taking the lung and chest wall compliance curves together gives the total respiratory system compliance (see the total curve in Fig. 2-2).

Dynamic Compliance

If one measures compliance during continuous breathing, the result is called *dynamic compliance*. Dynamic compliance reflects not only the elastic properties of the lungs but, to some extent, also the resistive component. It measures the change in pressure from the end of exhalation to the end of inspiration for a given volume and is based on the assumption that at zero flow the pressure difference reflects compliance. The steeper the slope of the curve connecting the points of zero flow, the greater the compliance. Dynamic compliance is the compliance that is generally measured in the clinical setting, but its interpretation can be problematic.[9]

At the fairly rapid respiratory rates common in infants, the instant of zero flow may not coincide with the point of lowest pressure. This is because dynamic compliance is rate dependent. For this reason, dynamic compliance may underestimate static compliance, especially in infants who are breathing rapidly and those with obstructive airway disease. Two additional factors further complicate the interpretation of compliance measurements. In premature infants, REM sleep is associated with paradoxical chest wall motion, so pressure changes recorded from the esophagus may correlate poorly with intrathoracic or pleural pressure changes. Chest wall distortion generally results in underestimation of esophageal pressure changes.[10] Also, because lung compliance is related to lung volume, measured compliance is greatly affected by the initial lung volume above which the compliance measurement is made. Ideally, comparisons should be normalized to the degree of lung expansion, for example, to FRC. Lung compliance divided by FRC is called *specific lung compliance.*

Dynamic pressure–volume relationships can be examined by simultaneous recording of pressure and volume changes. The pressure–volume loop allows one to quantify the work done to overcome airway resistance and to determine lung compliance (see Figs. 2-4 and 2-7). Figure 2-3 shows a static lung compliance curve upon which three pressure–volume loops are superimposed. Each of the loops shows a complete respiratory cycle, but each is taken at a different lung volume. The overall compliance curve is sigmoidal. At the lower end of the curve (at low lung volume), the compliance is low, that is, there is a small change in volume for a large change in pressure (see Fig. 2-3, A). This correlates with underinflation. Pressure is required to open up terminal airways and atelectatic terminal air spaces before gas can move into the lung. The lung volume is starting below critical opening pressure. At the center of the curve, the compliance is high; there is a large change in volume for a small change in pressure. This is where normal tidal breathing should occur (see Fig. 2-3, *B*). This is the position of maximum efficiency in a mechanical sense, the best ventilation/perfusion matching and lowest pulmonary vascular resistance. At the upper end of the curve (at high lung volume), the compliance is low; again, there is a small change in volume for a large change in pressure (see Fig. 2-3, *C*). This correlates with a lung that already is overinflated. Applying additional pressure yields little in terms of additional volume but may contribute significantly to airway injury and compromises venous return because of increased transmission of pressure to the pleural space. This is the result of the chest wall compliance rapidly falling with excessive lung inflation. Thus it is important to understand that compliance is reduced at both high and low lung volumes. Low lung volumes are seen in surfactant deficiency states (e.g., RDS), whereas high lung volumes are seen in obstructive lung diseases, such as BPD. Reductions in both specific compliance and thoracic gas volume have been measured in infants with RDS.[11,12]

The rapid respiratory rates of premature infants with surfactant deficiency can compensate for chest wall instability to a certain extent, because the short expiratory time results in gas trapping that tends to normalize their FRC. They also use expiratory grunting as a method of expiratory braking to help maintain FRC. In infants with RDS treated in the pre-surfactant era, serial measurements of FRC and compliance have been shown to be sensitive indicators of illness severity.[13]

Dynamic lung compliance has been shown to decrease as the clinical course worsens and to improve as the recovery phase begins. When mechanical ventilation is used in infants with noncompliant lungs resulting from surfactant deficiency, elevated distending pressures may be required initially to establish a reasonable FRC. Figure 2-4 shows the pressure–volume loop of a normal infant and that of an infant with RDS. A higher pressure is required to establish an appropriate lung volume in the infant with RDS than in the normal infant. However, this lung volume will be lost if the airway pressure is allowed to return to zero without the application of PEEP. Mechanical ventilation without PEEP leads to surfactant inactivation resulting in worsening lung compliance, and the repeated cycling of the terminal airways from below critical opening pressure leads to cellular injury and inflammation (atelectotrauma). This results in alveolar collapse, atelectasis, interstitial edema, and elaboration of inflammatory mediators.

Once atelectasis occurs, lung compliance deteriorates, surfactant turnover is increased, and ventilation/perfusion mismatch with increased intrapulmonary right-to-left shunting develops. A higher distending pressure and higher concentrations of inspired oxygen (FiO_2) will be required to maintain lung volume and adequate gas exchange, resulting in further injury. Early establishment of an appropriate FRC, administration of surfactant, use of CPAP or PEEP to avoid the repeated collapse and reopening of small airways (atelectotrauma), avoidance of overinflation caused by using supraphysiologic tidal volumes (volutrauma), and avoidance of use of more oxygen than is required (oxidative injury) all are important in achieving the best possible outcome and long-term health of patients.[14]

The level of PEEP at which static lung compliance is maximized has been termed the best, or optimum, PEEP. This is the level of PEEP at which O_2 transport (cardiac output and O_2 content) is greatest. If the level of PEEP is raised above the optimal level, dynamic compliance decreases rather than increases.[15] Additionally, venous return and cardiac output are compromised by excessive PEEP. One hypothesis for this reduction in dynamic lung compliance is that some alveoli become overexpanded because of the increase in pressure, which puts them on the "flat" part of the compliance curve (see Fig. 2-3, *C*). Therefore, despite the additional pressure delivered, little additional volume is obtained. The contribution of this "population" of overexpanded alveoli may be sufficient to reduce the total lung compliance. It has been shown that dynamic lung compliance was reduced in patients with congenital diaphragmatic hernia (CDH) even though some of the infants had normal thoracic gas volumes.[11] The reduction in dynamic lung compliance in patients with CDH is attributed to overdistention of the hypoplastic lung into the "empty" hemithorax after surgical repair of the defect. Because CDH infants have a reduced number of alveoli, they develop areas of pulmonary emphysema that persist at least into early childhood.[16]

Based on available evidence, it seems prudent to avoid rapid reexpansion of the lungs in the treatment of CDH. Clinicians must be alert to any sudden improvement in lung compliance in infants receiving assisted ventilation (i.e., immediately after administration of surfactant or recruitment of lung volume). If inspiratory pressure is not reduced as compliance improves, cardiovascular compromise may develop because proportionately more pressure is transmitted to the mediastinal structures as lung compliance improves. The distending pressure that was appropriate prior to the compliance change may become excessive and lead to alveolar overexpansion and ultimately air leak.[17] The use of volume-targeted ventilation would be ideal in these circumstances, because in this mode the ventilator will decrease the inspiratory pressure as lung compliance improves to maintain a set tidal volume.[18]

Because the chest wall is compliant in the premature infant, use of paralytic agents to reduce chest wall impedance is rarely necessary. Little pressure is required to expand the chest wall of a premature infant (see chest wall curve in Fig. 2-2). In studies investigating the use of paralytic agents in premature infants at risk for pneumothoraces, no change in lung compliance or resistance was demonstrated after 24 or 48 hours of paralysis, and many of the infants studied required more rather than less ventilator support after paralysis.[19,20]

In the past, paralysis was often used in larger infants who were "fighting the ventilator" or who were actively expiring against it despite the use of sedation and/or analgesia.[19] It should be noted that poor gas exchange (inadequate support) is usually the cause rather than the result of the infant's "fighting" the ventilator, and heavy sedation or paralysis masks this important clinical sign. The use of synchronized mechanical ventilation modes such as assist/control will obviate the need to paralyze or heavily sedate infants because they will then be breathing in synchrony with the ventilator.[21-23]

During positive-pressure ventilation, the relative compliance of the chest wall and the lungs determines the amount of pressure transmitted to the pleural space. Increased intrapleural pressure leads to impedance of venous return and decreased cardiac output, a well-documented but largely ignored complication of positive-pressure ventilation. The relationship is described by the following equation:

$$P_{PL} = \bar{P}_{aw} \times (C_L / C_L + C_{CW})$$

where P_{PL} is pleural pressure, $\bar{P}_{aw}$ is mean airway pressure, C_L is compliance of the lungs, and C_{CW} is compliance of the chest wall.

Thus it can be seen that in situations of good lung compliance but poor chest wall compliance, transmission of pressure to the pleural space and hemodynamic impairment are increased. This situation commonly arises in cases of increased intra-abdominal pressure with upward pressure on the diaphragm, as may be seen in infants with necrotizing enterocolitis or after surgical reduction of viscera that had developed outside the abdominal cavity—for example, large omphalocele, gastroschisis, or CDH.

Resistance

Resistance is the result of friction. Viscous resistance is the resistance generated by tissue elements moving past one another. Airway resistance is the resistance that occurs between moving molecules in the gas stream and between these moving molecules and the wall of the respiratory system (e.g., trachea, bronchi, bronchioles). The clinician must be aware of both types of resistance, as well as the resistance to flow as gas passes through the ventilator circuit and the endotracheal tube. In infants, viscous resistance may account for as much as 40% of total pulmonary resistance.[24] The relatively high viscous resistance in the newborn is due to relatively high tissue density (i.e., a low ratio of lung volume to lung weight) and the higher amount of pulmonary interstitial fluid. This increase in pulmonary interstitial fluid is especially prevalent after cesarean section delivery[25] and in conditions such as transient tachypnea of the newborn or delayed absorption of fetal lung fluid.

A reduction in tissue and airway resistance has been shown after administration of furosemide.[26] Airway resistance (R) is defined as the pressure gradient ($P1 - P2$) required to move gas through the airways at a constant flow rate ($\dot{V}$ or volume per unit of time). The standard formula is as follows:

$$R = (P1 - P2)/\dot{V}$$

Airway resistance is determined by flow velocity, length of the conducting airways, viscosity and density of the gases, and especially the inside diameter of the airways. This is true for both laminar and turbulent flow conditions.

Although in absolute terms airway resistance is elevated in the newborn infant, when corrected to lung volume (specific conductance, which is the reciprocal of resistance per unit lung volume), the relative resistance is lower than in adults. It is important to remember that because of the small diameter of the airways in the lungs of the newborn infant, even a modest narrowing will result in a marked increase in resistance.

Resistance to flow depends on whether the flow is laminar or turbulent. Turbulent flow results in inefficient use of energy, because the turbulence leads to flow in random directions, unlike with laminar flow, in which molecules move in an orderly fashion parallel to the wall of the tube. Therefore, the pressure gradient necessary to drive a given flow is always greater for turbulent flow but cannot be easily calculated. The Reynolds number is used as an index to determine whether flow is laminar or turbulent.[27] It is a unitless number that is defined as follows:

$$Re = 2 \; r \cdot v \cdot d/\eta$$

where r is the radius, v is the velocity, d is the density, and η is the viscosity. If the Reynolds number is greater than 2000, then turbulent flow is very likely. According to this equation, turbulent flow is likely if the tube has a large radius, a high velocity, a high density, or a low viscosity.

When flow is laminar, resistance to flow of gas through a tube is described by Poiseuille's law:

$$R \propto L \times \eta/r^4$$

where R is the resistance, L is the length of the tube, η is the viscosity of the gas, and r is the radius. In the following paragraphs we will consider each factor in more detail.

Flow Rate

Average values for airway resistance in normal, spontaneously breathing newborn infants are between 20 and 30 cm H_2O/L/s,[28] and these values can increase dramatically in disease states. Nasal airway resistance makes up approximately two-thirds of total upper airway resistance; the glottis and larynx contribute less than 10%; and the trachea and first four or five generations of bronchi account for the remainder.[29] Average peak inspiratory and expiratory flow rates in spontaneously breathing term infants are approximately 2.9 and 2.2 L/min, respectively.[28] Maximal peak inspiratory and expiratory flow rates average about 9.7 and 6.4 L/min, respectively.[30] The range of flow rates generated by spontaneously breathing newborns (including term and premature infants) is approximately 0.6 to 9.9 L/min. Turbulent flow is produced in standard infant endotracheal tubes (ETTs) whenever flow rates exceed approximately 3 L/min through 2.5-mm internal diameter (ID) tubes or 7.5 L/min through 3.0-mm ID tubes.[31] Flow rates that exceed these critical levels produce disproportionately large increases in airway resistance. For example, increasing the rate of flow through a 2.5-mm ID ETT from 5 to 10 L/min raises airway resistance from 32 to 84 cm H_2O/L/s, more than twice its original value.[31]

Flow conditions are likely to be at least partially turbulent ("transitional") when ventilator flow rates exceed 5 L/min in infants intubated with 2.5-mm ID ETTs or when rates exceed 10 L/min in infants with 3.0-mm ID ETTs. With turbulent flow, resistance increases exponentially. The resistance produced by infant ETTs is equal to or higher than that in the upper airway of a normal newborn infant breathing spontaneously. The increased resistance caused by the ETT poses little problem as long as the infant receives appropriate pressure support from the ventilator, because the machine can generate the additional pressure needed to overcome the resistance of the ETT. However, when the infant is being weaned from the ventilator or if the infant is disconnected from the ventilator with the ETT still in place, the infant may not be capable of generating sufficient effort to overcome the increase in upper airway resistance created by the ETT.[32] LeSouef et al.[33] measured a significant reduction in respiratory system expiratory resistance after extubation in premature newborn infants recovering from a variety of respiratory illnesses, including RDS, pneumonia, and transient tachypnea of the newborn.

Airway or Tube Length

Resistance is linearly proportional to tube length. The shorter the tube, the lower the resistance; therefore it is good practice to cut ETTs to the shortest practical length. Shortening a 2.5-mm ID ETT from 14.8 cm (full length) to half its length is feasible, because the depth of insertion in a small preemie is usually about 6 cm. This would reduce the resistance of the tube to half. Cutting the tube to 4.8 cm reduces the flow resistance in vitro to essentially that of a full-length tube of the next size (3.0-mm ID ETT). These relationships are consistent for the range of flows generated by spontaneously breathing newborns.[34]

Airway or Tube Diameter

In a single-tube system, the radius of the tube is the most significant determinant of resistance. As previously described, Poiseuille's law states that resistance is inversely proportional to the fourth power of the radius. Therefore, a reduction in the radius by half results in a 16-fold increase in resistance and thus the pressure drop required to maintain a given flow. It is important to fully appreciate that resistance to flow increases exponentially as ETT diameter decreases. This is one of the reasons extremely low birth-weight infants are difficult to wean from mechanical ventilation. In a multiple tube system, like the human lung, resistance depends on the total cross-sectional area of all of the tubes. Although the individual bronchi decrease in diameter as they extend toward the periphery, the total cross-sectional area of the airway increases exponentially.[35]

Because resistance increases to the fourth power as the airway is narrowed, even mild airway constriction can cause significant increases in resistance to flow. This effect is exaggerated in newborn infants compared to adults because of the narrowness of the infant's airways. Resistance during inspiration is less than resistance during expiration because the airways dilate upon inspiration (Fig. 2-8). This is true even though gas flow during inspiration usually is greater than that during expiration, because as we saw above, the relationship between resistance and flow is linear, whereas that to radius is geometric. There is an inverse, nonlinear relationship between airway resistance and lung volume, because airway size increases as FRC increases. Lung volume recruitment therefore reduces resistance to airflow. Any process that causes a reduction in lung volume, such as atelectasis or restriction of expansion, results in increased airway resistance. At extremely low volumes, resistance approaches infinity because the airways begin to close as residual volume is approached (see Fig. 2-2).

Consistent with the above physiologic principles, the preponderance of evidence indicates that the application of PEEP and CPAP decreases airway resistance.[36-38] ETT resistance is of considerable clinical importance. It has been shown that successful extubation is accomplished more often in infants coming directly off intermittent mandatory ventilation than after a 6-hour preextubation trial of endotracheal CPAP.[32] Nasal CPAP circuit design, specifically its resistance, and the means by which nasal CPAP is attached to the patient are the most important determinants of CPAP success or failure.[39]

Viscosity and Density

Gas viscosity is negligible relative to the viscosity of fluids. However, gas density can be of clinical significance. The relationship between airway resistance and the density of the gas in turbulent flow is directly proportional and linear. Decreasing the density of the gas by two-thirds, such as occurs when heliox, a mixture of 80% helium and 20% O_2, is administered, reduces airway resistance to one-third compared to that when room air is breathed. Heliox can be useful for reducing upper airway resistance (and work of breathing) in patients with obstructive disorders such as laryngeal edema, tracheal stenosis, and BPD.[40] Gas density is influenced by barometric pressure, so airway resistance is slightly decreased at high altitudes, although this has little clinical significance.

Work of Breathing

Breathing requires the expenditure of energy. For gas to be moved into the lungs, force must be exerted to overcome the elastic and resistive forces of the respiratory system. This is mathematically expressed by the following equation:

$$\text{Work of breathing} = \text{Pressure (force)} \times \text{Volume (displacement)}$$

where pressure is the force exerted and the volume is the displacement. Work of breathing is the integrated product of the two, or simply the area under the pressure–volume curve (see Fig. 2-7).

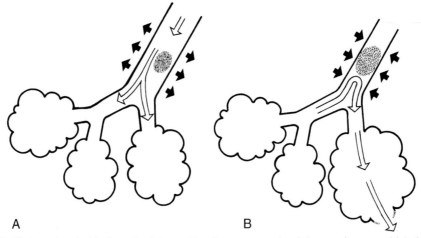

FIG 2-8 Air trapping behind particulate matter (e.g., meconium) in an airway, which leads to alveolar overexpansion and rupture. This illustrates the so-called ball–valve mechanism, in which (**A**) tidal gas passes the particulate matter on inspiration, when the airways naturally dilate but (**B**) does not exit on expiration, when the airways naturally constrict. (From Harris TR, Herrick BR. *Pneumothorax in the Newborn.* Tucson, Ariz., Biomedical Communications, Arizona Health Sciences Center, 1978.)

Work of breathing is the force generated to overcome the frictional resistance and static elastic forces that oppose lung expansion and gas flow into and out of the lungs. The workload depends on the elastic properties of the lung and chest wall, airway resistance, tidal volume (V_T), and respiratory rate. Approximately two-thirds of the work of spontaneous breathing is the effort to overcome the static elastic forces of the lungs and thorax (tissue elasticity and compliance). Approximately one-third of the total work is applied to overcoming the frictional resistance produced by the movement of gas and tissue components (airflow and viscous).[41]

In healthy infants exhalation is passive. A portion of the energy generated by the inspiratory muscles is stored (as potential energy) in the lungs' elastic components; this energy is returned during exhalation, hence it is also referred to as *nondissipative work*, in contrast to the frictional forces that are lost or dissipated as heat. If the energy required to overcome resistance to flow during expiration exceeds the amount of elastic energy stored during the previous inspiration, work must be done not only during inspiration but also during expiration; thus exhalation is no longer entirely passive.

In infants, energy expenditure correlates with oxygen consumption. Resting oxygen consumption is elevated in infants with RDS and BPD.[42] Mechanical ventilation reduces oxygen consumption by decreasing the infant's work of breathing.[13,43] Work of breathing is illustrated in a dynamic pressure–volume loop (see Fig. 2-7). Pressure changes during breathing can be measured with an intraesophageal catheter or balloon, and volume changes can be measured simultaneously with a pneumotachograph. During inspiration (ascending limb of the loop) and expiration (descending limb of the loop), both elastic and frictional resistance must be overcome by work. If only elastic resistance needed to be overcome, the breathing pattern would follow the compliance line; however, because airway resistance and tissue viscous resistance must also be overcome, a loop is formed (hysteresis). The areas *ABCA* and *ACDA* in Figure 2-7 represent the inspiratory work and the expiratory work, respectively, performed to overcome frictional resistance. The area *ABCEA* represents the total work of breathing during a single breath.

The diaphragm is responsible for the majority of the workload of respiration. The most important determinant of the diaphragm's ability to generate force is its initial position and the length of its muscle fibers at the beginning of a contraction. The longer and more curved the muscle fibers of the diaphragm, the greater the force the diaphragm can generate. In situations in which the lung is hyperinflated (overdistended), the diaphragm is flattened and thus at a mechanical disadvantage.

The application of PEEP or CPAP (continuous distending pressure [CDP]) may reduce the work of breathing for an infant whose breathing is on the initial flat part of the compliance curve secondary to atelectasis (see Fig. 2-3, *A*). In this situation, CDP should reduce the work of breathing by increasing FRC and bringing breathing to a higher level on the pressure–volume curve where the compliance is higher (see Fig. 2-3, *B*). Reductions in respiratory work with the application of CDP have been shown in newborns recovering from RDS[44] and in babies after surgery for congenital heart disease.[37]

If the lung already is overinflated, increasing CDP will not result in a decrease in the work of breathing (see Fig. 2-3, *C*). The one exception here is when lung overinflation is the result of airway collapse, as can be seen in infants with BPD. In this unique situation, higher CDP will maintain airway patency and relieve air trapping, reducing lung volume to a more normal level. Alveolar overdistention caused by any reason is often accompanied by an increase in $PaCO_2$ (indicating decreased alveolar ventilation) and a decrease in PaO_2, despite an increase in FRC.[36,45]

Time Constant

The time constant of a patient's respiratory system is a measure of how quickly his or her lungs can inflate or deflate—that is, how long it takes for alveolar and proximal airway pressures to equilibrate. Passive exhalation depends on the elastic recoil of the lungs and chest wall. Because the major force opposing exhalation is airway resistance, the expiratory time constant (K_t) of the respiratory system is directly related to both lung compliance (C_L), which is the inverse of elastic recoil, and airway resistance (R_{aw}):

$$K_t = C_L \times R_{aw}$$

The time constants of the respiratory system are analogous to those of electrical circuits. One time constant of the respiratory system is defined as the time it takes the alveoli (capacitor) to discharge 63% of its V_T (electrical charge) through the airways (resistor) to the mouth or ventilator (electrical) circuit. By the end of three time constants, 95% of the V_T is discharged. When this model is applied to a normal newborn with a compliance of 0.005 L/cm H_2O and a resistance of 30 cm H_2O/L/s, one time constant = 0.15 second and three time constants = 0.45 second.[46] In other words, 95% of the last V_T should be emptied from the lung within 0.45 second of when exhalation begins in a spontaneously breathing infant. In a newborn infant receiving assisted ventilation, the exhalation valve of the ventilator would have to be open for at least that length of time to avoid air trapping. Inspiratory time constants are roughly half as long as expiratory, largely because airway diameter increases during inspiration. This relationship between inspiratory and expiratory time constants accounts for the normal 1:2 inspiratory/expiratory (I:E) ratio with spontaneous breathing.

The concept of time constants is key to understanding the interactions between the elastic and the resistive forces and how the mechanical properties of the respiratory system work together to modulate the volume and distribution of ventilation. A working knowledge of time constants is essential for choosing the safest and most effective ventilator settings for an individual patient at a particular point in the course of a specific disease process that necessitates the use of assisted ventilation. It must be recognized that compliance and resistance change over time and, therefore, the optimal settings need to be reevaluated frequently.

Patients are at risk of incomplete emptying of a previously inspired breath when their lung condition involves an increase in airway resistance with no or only a modest reduction in lung compliance. They also are at risk when the pattern of assisted ventilation does not allow sufficient time for exhalation—that is, the lungs have an abnormally long time constant—or there is a mismatch between the time constant of the respiratory system (time constant of the patient + that of the ETT + that of the ventilator circuit) and the expiratory time setting on the ventilator. In these situations, the end result is gas trapping. This gas trapping is accompanied by an increase in lung volume and a buildup of pressure in the alveoli and distal airways referred to as *inadvertent PEEP* or *auto-PEEP*.[47]

Important clinical and radiographic signs of gas trapping and inadvertent PEEP include (1) radiographic evidence of overexpansion (e.g., increased anteroposterior diameter of the thorax, flattened diaphragm below the ninth posterior ribs, intercostal pleural bulging), (2) decreased chest wall movement during assisted ventilation, (3) hypercarbia that does not respond to an increase in ventilator rate (or even worsens), and (4) signs of cardiovascular compromise, such as mottled skin color, a decrease in arterial blood pressure, an increase in central venous pressure, or the development of a metabolic acidosis. Such late signs of air trapping should never occur today, because all modern ventilators give us the ability to monitor flow waveforms, which allow us to graphically see whether expiration has been completed before the next breath begins.

Time constants are also a function of patient size, because total compliance is proportional to size. The much shorter time constants of an infant are reflected in the more rapid normal respiratory rate, compared to adults. To keep the concept simple, remember that whales and elephants have very large lungs and very long time constants; hence they breathe very slowly. Mice and hummingbirds have tiny lungs with extremely short time constants and have a very rapid respiratory rate to match. Everything else being equal, large infants have longer time constants than "micropreemies." Any decrease in compliance makes the time constant shorter, and therefore tachypnea is the usual clinical sign of any condition leading to decreased compliance.

Extremely low birth-weight infants with RDS have decreased compliance but initially normal airway resistance. This means that the time constants are extremely short. Equilibration of the airway and alveolar pressures occurs very quickly (i.e., early in the inspiratory cycle). Reynolds[48] estimated that the time constant in RDS may be as short as 0.05 second. This means that 95% of the pressure applied to the airway is delivered to the alveoli within 0.15 second, a value consistent with clinical observation. Short time constants make rapid-rate conventional ventilation feasible in these infants and makes them ideal candidates for high-frequency ventilation.

Term infants with meconium aspiration or older growing preterm infants with BPD have elevated airway resistance and correspondingly longer time constants; therefore they are most at risk of inadvertent PEEP. They should be ventilated with slower respiratory rates and longer inspiratory and, especially, expiratory times. Evidence of air trapping should be actively sought by examining ventilator waveforms, before clinical signs of CO_2 retention and hemodynamic impairment develop. It should be noted that the proximal airway PEEP level does not indicate the level of alveolar PEEP nor does it demonstrate the occurrence of alveolar gas trapping. Even under conditions of zero proximal airway PEEP, alveolar PEEP levels and the degree of gas trapping may be dangerously high if the baby has compliant lungs, increased airway resistance, or both (i.e., a prolonged time constant).[49]

Although it is useful clinically to think of the infant's respiratory system as having a single compliance and a single resistance, we know this is not really the case. The resistance and compliance values we obtain from pulmonary function measurements are essentially weighted averages for the respiratory system. There are populations of respiratory subunits with a range of discrete compliance and resistance values, whereas what we measure at the airway are averaged values for those populations of subunits.

GAS TRANSPORT

Mechanisms of Gas Transport

Ventilation or gas transport involves the movement of gas by convection or bulk flow through the conducting airways and then by molecular diffusion into the alveoli and pulmonary capillaries. This makes possible gas exchange (O_2 uptake and CO_2 elimination) that matches the minute-by-minute metabolic needs of the patient. The driving force for gas flow is the difference in pressure at the origin and destination of the gases; for diffusion, it is the difference in the concentrations between gases in contiguous spaces. Gas flows down a pressure gradient and diffuses down a concentration gradient. The predominant mechanism of gas transport by convection is bulk flow, whereas the predominant mechanism of gas transport by diffusion is Brownian motion.

Ventilation of the alveoli is an intermittent process that occurs only during inspiration, whereas gas exchange between alveoli and pulmonary capillaries occurs throughout the respiratory cycle. This is possible because a portion of gas remains in the lungs at the end of exhalation (FRC); the remaining gas provides a source for ongoing gas exchange and maintains approximately equal O_2 and CO_2 tensions in both the alveoli and the blood returning from the lungs.

During spontaneous breathing, inspiration is achieved through active contraction of the respiratory muscles. A negative pressure is produced in the interpleural space, a portion of which is transmitted via the parietal and visceral pleura through the pulmonary interstitial space to the lower airways and alveoli. A pressure gradient between the outside atmospheric pressure and the airway and alveolar pressures results in gas flowing down the pressure gradient into the lungs (Fig. 2-9). Interpleural pressure is more negative than alveolar pressure, which is more negative than mouth and atmospheric pressures.

When an infant receives negative-pressure ventilation, pressure is decreased around the infant's chest and abdomen to supplement the negative-pressure gradient used to move gas into the lungs, mimicking the normal physiologic function. During positive-pressure ventilation, the upper airway of the infant (Fig. 2-10) is connected to a device that generates a positive-pressure gradient down which gas can flow during inspiration. The pressure in the ventilator circuit and in the upper airway is greater than the alveolar pressure, which is greater than the interpleural pressure, which is greater than the atmospheric pressure. The negative intrathoracic pressure during spontaneous or negative pressure respiration facilitates venous return to the heart. Positive-pressure ventilation alters this physiology and inevitably leads to some degree of impedance of venous return, adversely affecting cardiac output.

The amount of gas inspired in a single spontaneous breath or delivered through an ETT during a single cycle of the ventilator is called the *tidal volume*. V_T in milliliters (mL) multiplied by the number of inflations per minute, or respirator frequency (*f*), is called *minute ventilation* (V_E):

$$V_E = V_T \times f$$

The portion of the incoming V_T that fails to arrive at the level of the respiratory bronchioles and alveoli but instead remains in the conducting airways occupies the space known as the *anatomic dead space*. Another portion of V_T may be delivered to unperfused or underperfused alveoli. Because gas

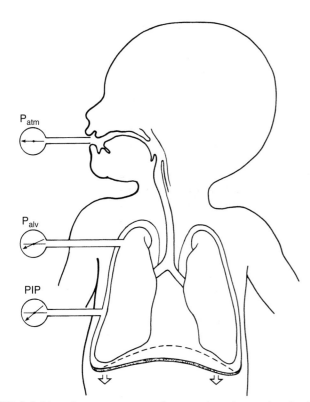

FIG 2-9 Negative-pressure gradient produced upon inspiration by the descent of the diaphragm in a spontaneously breathing infant. Pressures are measured in the interpleural space (PIP), in the alveoli (P_{alv}), and at the opening of the mouth, or atmosphere (P_{atm}). PIP < P_{alv} < P_{atm}.

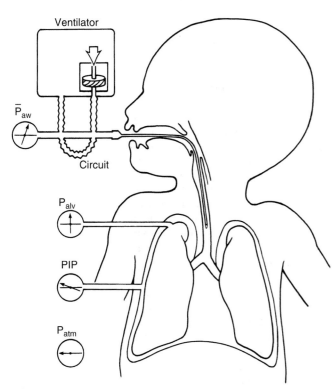

FIG 2-10 Positive-pressure gradient produced by a ventilator. Pressures are measured in the airway ($\bar{P}_{aw}$) and as shown in Figure 2-9. $\bar{P}_{aw}$ > P_{alv} > PIP > P_{atm}. Abbreviations as in Figure 2-9.

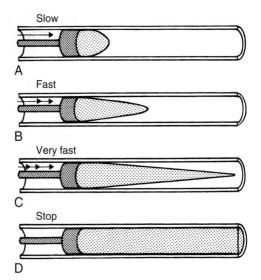

FIG 2-11 Spike theory of panting or high-frequency ventilation. A-C, The quicker or more "energy dense" the puff (or inspiratory pulse), the sharper the spike and the farther it extends into the airway. D, If the pulse is suddenly stopped at end inspiration, mixing occurs instantaneously. (Modified from Henderson Y, Chillingworth FP, Whitney JL. The respiratory dead space. *Am J Physiol.* 1915;38:1.)

exchange does not take place in these units, the volume that they constitute is called *alveolar dead space*. Together, anatomic dead space and alveolar dead space make up *total* or *physiologic dead space* (V_{DS}). The ratio of dead space to V_T (V_{DS}/V_T) defines *wasted ventilation*, which reflects the proportion of tidal gas delivered that is not involved in actual gas exchange. In general, rapid shallow breathing is inefficient because of a high V_{DS} to V_T ratio.

A number of mechanisms of gas transport other than bulk convection and molecular diffusion have been described, particularly as they relate to high-frequency ventilation. They include axial convection, radial diffusive mixing, coaxial flow, viscous shear, asymmetrical velocity profiles, and the pendelluft effect.[50]

The concept of anatomic dead space is a useful one and does apply under conditions of relatively low flow velocities. It assumes that the fresh gas and exhaled gas move as solid blocks without any mixing. However, in small infants, with their rapid respiratory rates and small airways, the concept begins to break down. In 1915, Henderson et al.[51] noted that during rapid shallow breathing or panting in dogs, adequate gas exchange was maintained even though the volume of gas contained in each "breath" was less than that of the anatomic dead space. They hypothesized that low-volume inspiratory pulses of gas moved down the center of the airway as axial spikes and that these spikes dissipated at the end of each "breath" (Fig. 2-11). The faster the inspiratory pulse, the farther it penetrated down the conducting airway and the larger the boundary of mixing between the molecules of the incoming gas (with high O_2 and low CO_2) and the outgoing gas (with high CO_2 and low O_2).

During this kind of breathing, both convection and molecular diffusion are enhanced or facilitated. The provision of a greater interface or boundary area between inspiratory and expiratory gases with their different O_2 and CO_2 partial pressures is known as *radial diffusive mixing*. During high-frequency ventilation (HFV), with each inspiration, gas molecules near the center of the airway flow farther than those adjacent to the walls of the airway, because the gas traveling down the center of the airway is exposed to less resistance. Figure 2-12, *A*, illustrates the velocity profiles using vectors that demonstrate the intra-airway flow patterns of gas molecules in a representation of the airway during inspiration. At the end of the inspiratory phase, the contour of the leading edge of the inspired gas is cone shaped (Fig. 2-12, *B*), having a larger diffusion interface with the preexisting gas than would be present if the leading edge were disk shaped. During exhalation, the velocity profiles are more

uniform across the entire lumen rather than being cone shaped (Fig. 2-12, *C*).[52] The pulse of gas originally occupying the lumen of the airway is displaced to the right (i.e., toward the patient's alveoli), and an equal volume of gas is displaced to the left (Fig. 2-12, *D*). This occurs even though the net displacement of the piston during a cycle of high-frequency oscillatory ventilation (HFOV) is zero.

Although these mechanisms have mostly been recognized to be operative with HFV, evidence suggests that they are present even at conventional respiratory rates in small preterm infants with narrow ETTs.[53,54] The back-and-forth currents of gas through lung units with unequal time constants are called *pendelluft*.[50,55] This gas flow is produced because of local differences in airway resistance and lung compliance that are accentuated under conditions of high-velocity flow. This leads to regional differences in rates of inflation and deflation. "Fast units" with short time constants inflate and deflate more rapidly, emptying out into the conducting airways to be "inhaled" by "slow units" still in the process of filling (Fig. 2-13). Pendelluft thus improves gas mixing and exchange.

Carbon dioxide diffuses more easily across the alveolar/capillary wall, an essential characteristic given the relatively low concentration gradient between the alveoli and the capillary blood. The effectiveness of CO_2 removal is primarily determined by the effectiveness

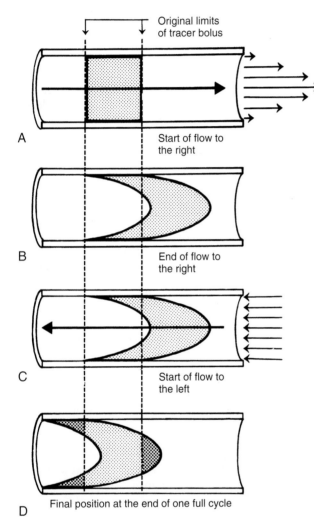

FIG 2-12 Viscous shear and inspiratory-to-expiratory velocity profiles associated with respiratory cycling. **A,** During inspiration or movement toward the right, the gas molecules of a cylindrical tracer bolus that are situated near the center of the tube travel farther and faster than the gas molecules near the wall, as represented by the velocity profile arrows at the right. **B,** At the end of the inspiratory half of the respiratory cycle, a paraboloid front has formed. **C,** During exhalation or movement toward the left, the velocity profiles are essentially uniform across the lumen. **D,** The end result after a complete respiratory cycle (with zero net directional flow) is displacement of axial gas to the right and wall gas to the left. (Modified with permission from Haselton FR, Scherer PW. Bronchial bifurcations and respiratory mass transport. *Science.* 1980;208:69. © 1990 by the American Association for the Advancement of Science.)

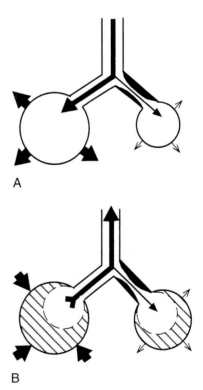

FIG 2-13 Effects of different time constants on the uneven distribution of ventilation and the production of pendelluft. **A,** On inspiration, the fast unit receives the majority of ventilation, whereas the slow unit fills slowly (owing to local increase in airway resistance). **B,** At the beginning of expiration, the slow unit may still be filling and actually "inspires" from the exhaling fast unit. These effects are accentuated at higher frequencies, with gas "pedaling" back and forth between neighboring units with inhomogeneity of time constants. (Modified from Otis AB, McKerrow CB, Bartlett RA, et al. Mechanical factors in distribution of pulmonary ventilation. *J Appl Physiol.* 1956;8:427.)

of ventilation, that is, the process by which CO_2 that has diffused into the alveoli is removed, so that the maximal diffusion gradient is maintained. The movement of any gas across a semipermeable membrane is governed by Fick's equation for diffusion:

$$dQ/dt = k \times A \times dC/dl$$

where dQ/dt is the rate of diffusion in mL/min, k is the diffusion coefficient of the gas, A is the area available for diffusion, dC is the concentration difference of molecules across the membrane, and dl is the length of the diffusion pathway. It is evident from the above that both atelectasis, which will reduce the area available for gas exchange, and pulmonary edema, which will increase the diffusion pathway, will reduce the effectiveness of CO_2 removal. Alveolar minute ventilation is, of course, the most critical element, because it maintains the concentration gradient that drives diffusion.

OXYGENATION

Oxygen transport to the tissues depends on the oxygen-carrying capacity of the blood and the rate of blood flow. The amount of oxygen in arterial blood is called *oxygen content* (CaO_2).

$$CaO_2 = (1.34 \times Hb \times SaO_2) + (0.003 \times PaO_2)$$

where Hb is the hemoglobin concentration and SaO_2 is the arterial oxygen saturation. Oxygen is contained in the blood in two forms: (1) a small quantity dissolved in the plasma and (2) a much larger quantity bound to hemoglobin. The total O_2 content of the blood is the sum of these two quantities. The contribution of hemoglobin to oxygen content is described in the first term of the equation, which states that each gram of hemoglobin will bind 1.34 mL of O_2 when fully saturated with oxygen. The second term of the equation describes the contribution of oxygen dissolved in the plasma.

The dissolved portion of O_2 in blood is linearly related to PO_2, such that an increase in PO_2 is accompanied by an increase in O_2 content. Oxygen content increases 0.003 mL per 100 mL of blood with every 1-mm Hg increase in PO_2. For an infant breathing 21% O_2, the dissolved portion of the blood's O_2 content is only about 2% of the total. However, for a healthy patient breathing 100% O_2, with a very high PaO_2 of 500 mm Hg (not normally recommended because of the dangers of hyperoxia), the dissolved portion of the blood's O_2 content can be as much as 10% of the total. Oxygen binds reversibly to hemoglobin. Each hemoglobin molecule can bind up to four molecules of O_2. The hemoglobin-bound portion of the O_2 content is nonlinear with respect to PO_2. This relationship is illustrated by the oxyhemoglobin dissociation curve, which is sigmoid in shape (Fig. 2-14).

The amount of O_2 that binds to hemoglobin increases quickly at low PO_2 values but begins to level off at PO_2 values greater than 40 mm Hg. After PO_2 exceeds 90 to 100 mm Hg, the curve flattens. Once the hemoglobin is saturated, further increases in PO_2 do not increase the content of bound oxygen. The total amount of O_2 carried by hemoglobin depends on the hemoglobin concentration of the blood and the bloods' oxygen saturation. Several factors affect hemoglobin's affinity for oxygen. These factors include the (1) percentages of fetal and adult hemoglobin present in the patient's blood, (2) amount of 2,3-diphosphoglycerate, (3) pH, and (4) temperature. A greater percentage of fetal hemoglobin (as seen in premature

infants), a decrease in 2,3-diphosphoglycerate content (as occurs in premature infants with RDS), alkalization of the pH (e.g., after infusion of bicarbonate), a reduction in PCO_2 (secondary to hyperventilation), and a decrease in body temperature (as occurs during open heart surgery or therapeutic hypothermia for neuroprotection) all increase the O_2 affinity of hemoglobin (shift the oxyhemoglobin dissociation curve to the left without changing its shape). This means that the same level of hemoglobin saturation can be achieved at lower PO_2 values. In contrast, increased production of 2,3-diphosphoglycerate (as occurs in healthy newborns shortly after birth or with adaptation to high altitudes), a reduction in the percentage of fetal hemoglobin (e.g., after transfusion of adult donor blood to a newborn infant), a more acidic pH, CO_2 retention, and febrile illness each results in a reduction in O_2 affinity (shift of the oxyhemoglobin dissociation curve to the right) (see Fig. 2-14).

Some shifts in the oxyhemoglobin dissociation curve promote O_2 uptake in the lungs, O_2 release at the tissue level, or both. For example, when pulmonary arterial blood (which is rich in CO_2 and poor in O_2) passes through the lung's capillaries, it releases its CO_2; this raises the local pH, which increases O_2 affinity. This allows more of the incoming O_2 to be bound to hemoglobin, while plasma PO_2 is kept low, thus maximizing the concentration gradient down which O_2 diffuses from the alveoli into the pulmonary capillary plasma. Also, when systemic arterial blood (which is rich in O_2 and poor in CO_2) enters the tissue capillaries, it picks up CO_2 (which is in high concentration in the tissues). As a result, pH and O_2 affinity are lowered; this allows the hemoglobin to release its O_2 without significantly

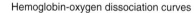

Hemoglobin-oxygen dissociation curves

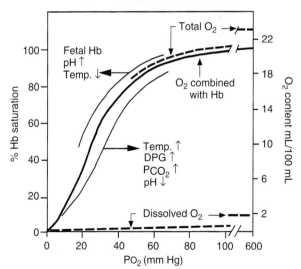

FIG 2-14 Nonlinear or S-shaped oxyhemoglobin curve and the linear or straight-line dissolved O_2 relationships between O_2 saturation (SaO_2) and O_2 tension (PO_2). Total blood O_2 content is shown with division into a portion combined with hemoglobin and a portion physically dissolved at various levels of PO_2. Also shown are the major factors that change the O_2 affinity of hemoglobin and thus shift the oxyhemoglobin dissociation curve to either the left or the right (see also Appendix 12). *DPG,* 2,3 Diphosphoglycerate; *Hb,* Hemoglobin. (Modified from West JB. *Respiratory Physiology: The Essentials.* 2nd ed. Baltimore: Williams & Wilkins, 1979, pp. 71, 73.)

decreasing P_{O_2} and thus helps to maintain the concentration gradient down which O_2 diffuses into the tissues.[56]

SaO_2 as monitored clinically with pulse oximetry (SpO_2) shows the percentage of hemoglobin in arterial blood that is saturated with O_2 and therefore more closely reflects blood oxygen content than does PaO_2, especially in the newborn infant with predominantly fetal hemoglobin. The greater affinity of fetal hemoglobin for oxygen, together with the relative polycythemia normally seen in newborns, allows the fetus to maintain adequate tissue oxygen delivery in the relatively hypoxemic environment in utero. The PaO_2 and SaO_2 in the healthy fetus are only about 25 mm Hg and 60%, respectively. This is, of course, why normal newborn infants emerge from the womb quite cyanotic. It has been demonstrated that SpO_2 in the healthy newborn infant increases gradually after birth and does not normally reach 90% until 5 to 10 minutes of life.[57]

Rapid increases in PaO_2, such as occur when delivery room resuscitation is carried out with 100% oxygen, appear to result in a variety of adverse consequences, including delayed onset of spontaneous breathing and increased mortality.[58] The normal range of SaO_2 in newborn infants is different from that in adults; instead of the SaO_2 levels of 95% or greater in adults, SaO_2 levels of 85% to 92% appear to be adequate for newborns, and higher values may predispose the antioxidant-deficient preterm infant to the dangers of hyperoxia. It has been shown that the O_2 demands of most extremely premature infants can be met by maintaining PaO_2 levels just above 50 mm Hg or SaO_2 levels just above 88%.[59] There is currently insufficient evidence to recommend a definite range of optimal SpO_2 values, but there is mounting evidence that complications of prematurity in which damage from reactive oxygen species is implicated can be reduced by the use of lower SpO_2 targets in the range of 85% to 92%.[60,61a] However, studies have shown a tendency toward increased mortality but less retinopathy with lower oxygen saturation targets between 85% and 89% compared to 91% to 95%.[61b,61c]

Tissue oxygen delivery depends not only on blood oxygen content but also on cardiac output and tissue perfusion. Positive-pressure ventilation impedes venous return to various degrees and therefore can adversely affect cardiac output and pulmonary blood flow. These important cardiorespiratory interactions are often not fully appreciated but nevertheless deserve close attention during mechanical ventilation.

The partial pressure of O_2 in arterial blood (PaO_2) is the tension or partial pressure of O_2 physically dissolved in the arterial blood plasma and is expressed in millimeters of mercury (mm Hg), or torr. This oxygen is in equilibrium with the oxygen that is bound to hemoglobin, which as we saw earlier constitutes the bulk of the total. PaO_2 is measured directly as part of the blood gas analysis. PaO_2 is a useful indicator of the degree of O_2 uptake through the lungs. The fraction of inspired O_2 (FiO_2) is the proportion of O_2 in the inspired gas. FiO_2 is measured directly with an O_2 analyzer and is expressed as a percentage (e.g., 60% O_2) or, preferably, in decimal form (e.g., 0.60 O_2). The FiO_2 in room air is approximately 0.21. The partial pressure of O_2 in alveolar gas (PAO_2) is the tension of O_2 present in the alveoli.

Alveolar gas typically contains oxygen, nitrogen, CO_2, and water vapor. PAO_2 represents the amount of O_2 available for diffusion into the pulmonary capillary blood. The partial pressure of CO_2 in the alveoli, or $PACO_2$, is nearly identical to the amount of CO_2 physically dissolved in the arterial blood, or $PaCO_2$. The partial pressure of water vapor at 100% relative humidity at body temperature and normal atmospheric pressure is 47 mm Hg. One additional correction factor must be used. This is called the *respiratory quotient* (RQ), which is the ratio of CO_2 excretion to O_2 uptake. The respiratory quotient ranges from approximately 0.8 to slightly greater than 1.0, depending on diet. To calculate the partial pressure of O_2 in alveolar gas or PAO_2, we use the alveolar gas equation:

$$PAO_2 = \left[\left(\begin{array}{c} \text{Barometric pressure} - \\ \text{Partial pressure of water vapor} \\ \times FiO_2 - (PaCO_2/RQ) \end{array} \right) \right]$$

At sea level, with normal $PaCO_2$ of 40 mm Hg and respiratory quotient of 0.8, the alveolar gas equation for breathing room air is as follows:

$$PAO_2 = [(760 - 47) \times 0.21] - 40/0.8$$

$$PAO_2 \text{ is approximately } 150 - 50 = 100$$

A high-carbohydrate diet raises the respiratory quotient, thus increasing CO_2 production. It is important to remember that $PACO_2$ is decreased by hyperventilation and that the decrease in $PACO_2$ is matched by an equal increase in PAO_2. Barometric pressure varies with weather conditions and altitude. To demonstrate the effect of altitude on the absolute amount of oxygen available at the alveolar level, let us consider an infant with $PACO_2$ of 40 mm Hg and respiratory quotient of 0.8 who is breathing room air in Denver, Colorado, which is located 5280 feet above sea level and has an average barometric pressure of approximately 600 mm Hg. Subtracting 42 mm Hg (the partial pressure of water vapor is also reduced proportionally at altitude) from 600 mm Hg yields 558 mm Hg, which, when multiplied by 0.21, gives a value of around 117 mm Hg. After subtracting the dividend of 40 mm Hg/0.8, or 50 mm Hg, from 117 mm Hg, a PAO_2 value in Denver of only 67 mm Hg is obtained (instead of the approximately 100 mm Hg that would be expected at sea level). Therefore, the infant has about one-third less available oxygen in the alveoli when breathing room air in Denver compared to when breathing room air at sea level. The alveolar gas equation is useful in calculating a variety of indexes of oxygenation, as well as, for example, the FiO_2 need of an infant with compromised gas exchange who must travel to a home at higher altitude or in a commercial aircraft cabin pressurized to 7000 or 8000 feet above sea level.

Some important values derived from blood gas measurements are useful as clinical indicators of disease severity and are commonly used as criteria for initiation of invasive or costly therapies. They include the following:
1. Arterial–alveolar O_2 tension ratio ($PaO_2:PAO_2$, or the a:A ratio). The a:A ratio should be close to 1 in a healthy infant. A ratio of less than 0.3 indicates severe compromise of oxygen transfer.
2. Alveolar–arterial O_2 gradient or difference ($AaDO_2 = PAO_2 - PaO_2$). In healthy infants $AaDO_2$ is less than 20 in room air. Calculating $AaDO_2$ allows the clinician to estimate disease severity and estimate appropriate FiO_2 change when PaO_2 is high.
3. Oxygenation index $(\bar{P}_{aw} \times FiO_2 \times 100)/PaO_2$

The oxygenation index factors in the pressure cost of achieving a certain level of oxygenation in the form of $\bar{P}_{aw}$. An oxygenation index greater than 15 signifies severe respiratory compromise. An oxygenation index of 40 or more on multiple occasions has historically indicated a mortality risk approaching 80% and continues to be used as an indication for extracorporeal membrane oxygenation (ECMO) in most ECMO centers.[62]

Effects of Altering Ventilator Settings on Oxygenation

Oxygen uptake through the lungs can be increased by (1) increasing PAo_2 via increasing the FiO_2 (increasing the concentration gradient), (2) optimizing lung volume (optimizing ventilation-to-perfusion (V/Q) matching and increasing the surface area for gas exchange), and (3) maximizing pulmonary blood flow (preventing blood from flowing right to left through extrapulmonary shunts). There are functionally two ventilator changes available to the clinician:

1. Alter FiO_2
2. Alter $\bar{P}_{aw}$

Figure 2-15 is a graphic representation of the factors that affect proximal airway pressure for conventional mechanical ventilation. It has been demonstrated that, regardless of how the increase in $\bar{P}_{aw}$ is achieved, it has a roughly equivalent effect on oxygenation.[63] Although increasing each of these variables will increase $\bar{P}_{aw}$, the relative safety and effectiveness of these maneuvers has not been systematically evaluated. Prolongation of the inspiratory time to the point of inverse I:E ratio is potentially the most dangerous measure and is rarely used today. Higher frequency and higher peak inspiratory pressure (PIP) both may result in inadvertent hyperventilation, which is also undesirable. The rate of upstroke has a relatively minor impact. In practice, increasing PEEP appears to be the safest and most effective way to achieve optimal $\bar{P}_{aw}$, in part because normally, the greatest proportion of the respiratory cycle is the expiratory phase.

Control variables for high-frequency jet ventilators (HFJVs) are similar to those for conventional ventilation. However, it should be noted that the I:E ratio of HFJVs is very short (typically 1:6 or even less); therefore, to maintain adequate $\bar{P}_{aw}$, the

PEEP typically needs to be raised by 2 to 4 cm H_2O from the baseline on conventional ventilation. When reducing pressure amplitude in response to improving ventilation, it should be kept in mind that $\bar{P}_{aw}$ comes down as PIP is lowered; therefore, it is necessary to raise the PEEP slightly to maintain $\bar{P}_{aw}$.[64]

The control variables for HFOV allow for direct and independent adjustment of $\bar{P}_{aw}$ and pressure amplitude. This separates the two chief gas exchange functions and makes it relatively easy to understand that ventilation is controlled by pressure amplitude (set as "power") and oxygenation is controlled by $\bar{P}_{aw}$ and FiO_2.[65]

Although general principles and guidelines for ventilator management can be developed, it is important to recognize that individual infants may at times respond differently under apparently similar circumstances. Therefore, individualized care based on these principles is the best approach. To optimize care, the clinician should formulate a hypothesis based on a physiologic rationale, make a ventilator change, and observe the response. This provides the clinician with feedback that either confirms or refutes the hypothesis. The response of biological systems is never entirely predictable and occurs against a background of continuing change in the infant's condition. Additionally, there are complex interactions among the various organ systems. Otherwise appropriate ventilator changes may have adverse hemodynamic effects. Opening of a ductus arteriosus may alter hemodynamics and lung compliance, the infant's own respiratory effort may change because of neurologic alterations, and so on. In addition, it is important to keep in mind that, because ventilators are powerful tools, they can cause significant damage even under the best of circumstances, but especially if they are not used judiciously. We must learn from experience (our own and that of others) and apply that knowledge when making ventilator setting changes during assisted ventilation of the newborn.

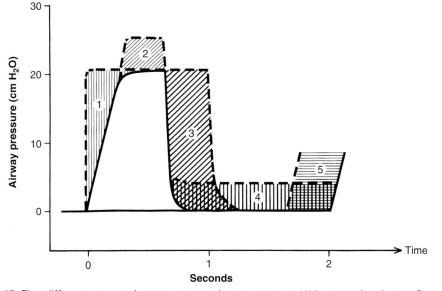

FIG 2-15 Five different ways to increase mean airway pressure: (1) increase inspiratory flow rate, producing a square-wave inspiratory pattern; (2) increase peak inspiratory pressure; (3) reverse the inspiratory-to-expiratory ratio or prolong the inspiratory time (I-time) without changing the rate; (4) increase positive end-expiratory pressure; and (5) increase ventilatory rate by reducing expiratory time without changing the I-time. (Modified from Reynolds EOR. Pressure waveform and ventilator settings for mechanical ventilation in severe hyaline membrane disease. *Int Anesthesiol Clin*. 1974;12:259.)

VENTILATION

For gas exchange to occur efficiently, ventilation and perfusion must be well matched. Gas is distributed through the lung via the airways. The volume of gas moved into and out of the lung with each normal breath is the V_T. The largest volume that can be inhaled after a full exhalation is the vital capacity. The volume of gas that remains in the lung after a normal expiration is the FRC. The volume that remains in the lung after a maximal expiration is the residual volume. Residual volume and vital capacity together are the total lung capacity. The product of V_T and breathing frequency is the minute volume. As previously discussed, only a portion of the minute volume actually reaches the alveoli. The volume of the conducting airways is called the anatomic dead space.

As respiratory rate and/or V_T is increased, minute ventilation increases. When V_T is increased, alveolar ventilation increases even more than minute ventilation because the anatomic dead space remains constant. In contrast, with increases in respiratory rate, alveolar minute ventilation and total minute ventilation increase proportionally. Despite the fact that increasing the V_T has a greater impact on alveolar minute ventilation, increasing the V_T may not always be the optimal choice, because excessive V_T has been shown to be the most important determinant of lung injury, and increasing the V_T appears to be more injurious to the lung than a faster rate.[66,67] The dimensions of the airway system influence ventilation. With progressive dichotomous branching moving toward the lungs' periphery, the overall cross-sectional area of the airways increases, so airflow velocity decreases, as does resistance.

With each breath, inspired gas is distributed by bulk flow to the distal airways, depending on the length of the conducting airways and the rate of flow through them. Gas flow rates are determined by local differences in driving pressure, flow resistance, tissue elasticity, and compliance. For spontaneous breathing, the driving pressure is the interpleural pressure swings generated during inspiration; during assisted ventilation, the transpulmonary pressure swings are produced by the forces exerted by the ventilator (see Figs. 2-9 and 2-10). In practice, with synchronized (assisted) ventilation, the negative inspiratory effort of the infant and the positive pressure generated by the ventilator are additive and together form the *transpulmonary pressure* that determines the V_T. It should be noted that in routine ventilator-based pulmonary mechanics measurement, only the ventilator contribution to the transpulmonary pressure is measured, ignoring the infant's contribution. Therefore, in actively breathing infants, ventilator-based lung mechanics measurements are not accurate.

In the healthy lung, gravity-dependent differences in interpleural or transpulmonary pressure are responsible for most of the regional differences in ventilation. In the sick lung, local differences in compliance and airway resistance (time constants) are the major contributors to uneven distribution of ventilation. Bryan et al.[68] showed that the dependent lung regions in normal subjects have a greater regional volume expansion ratio (change in volume per unit of preinspiratory volume) than do the nondependent regions of lung. When a patient is upright, the basal regions of the lung are ventilated to a greater extent than are the apical regions. When a patient is supine, the basal and apical regions are ventilated to similar extents, but the posterior (lowermost) regions are ventilated to a greater extent than the anterior regions (uppermost).

It is important to remember, however, that at the end of a normal exhalation (at FRC), the volume in the uppermost regions of the lung is greater than that of the dependent regions. This may appear contradictory, but these differences can be explained on the basis of regional interpleural pressure differences (Fig. 2-16). Interpleural pressure at end expiration is more negative in the uppermost portions than in the dependent portions of the lung. Converting the interpleural pressures to transpulmonary pressures, one can plot a pressure–volume curve (lower right of Fig. 2-16). When the lungs are inflated starting from FRC, the dependent lung units will receive proportionally more of the inspired gas, and the nondependent units will receive proportionally less as the height above the dependent units increases. The basilar units are stretched proportionately more than the higher units because they are operating on a steeper slope of the volume–pressure curve. Compliance increases progressively from the highest portion of the lung to the most dependent portion or from high starting lung volumes to lower volumes. At the beginning of a gradual inflation from FRC, the more dependent lung regions operate on a steeper part of the compliance curve than the less dependent regions, so ventilation is greater in the dependent regions. However, because of the small size of newborn infants, the gravity-dependent regional differences are not nearly as large as they are in adults.

Lung units that contain collapsed airways require large pressure changes before the airways open to permit gas transfer. These units are not ventilated as well as units in which the airways are patent from the start. Units with high resistance are ventilated poorly regardless of their position, because these units have low compliance for any given transpulmonary pressure. In newborn infants, airway closure may be present in the resting V_T range, unlike in older individuals in whom pleural surface pressure at FRC is substantially subatmospheric throughout the lung, thus preventing airway closure while the lung is at operational volume.[69] Starting inspiration from a lung volume that is below FRC or rest volume actually reverses the pattern of the distribution of ventilation.[70] If inspiration is started from a low level of lung volume, interpleural pressures are less negative overall (because elastic recoil is minimal at these low lung volumes) and even may be positive in the more dependent regions of the lung.

When regional interpleural pressure exceeds (is more positive than) airway pressure, then airway closure occurs and no gas enters that segment for the first portion of inspiration or until regional interpleural pressure decreases to below airway pressure further along into inspiration. Thus ventilation is reduced in dependent regions and is redirected to the upper lung regions, making them the better ventilated areas; this is a reversal of the usual pattern.

During assisted ventilation, inflation at end inspiration is uniform, as evidenced by the observation of alveoli of equal size throughout the lung.[71] At end expiration or FRC level, however, alveoli in the uppermost regions of the lung are found to have a volume fourfold that of alveoli at the base. Moderate levels of PEEP increase FRC more in dependent regions than in upper regions of the lung because the former are less well expanded initially and are at a lower and more favorable point on their compliance curve. If significant basilar atelectasis preexists, the addition of PEEP or CPAP should help the most in the more dependent areas, opening them for improved regional ventilation. All forms of CDP favor uniformity of ventilation because they expand airways and thus lower resistance and because

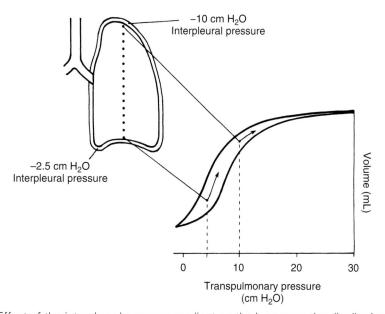

FIG 2-16 Effect of the interpleural pressure gradient up the lung upon the distribution of ventilation. The greatest negative pressure is at the top owing to the gravitational tug (weight) of the lung through its visceral pleura on the parietal pleura. Because the upper and lower areas are on different parts of the pressure–volume curve, different amounts of volume (ventilation) are achieved by the two areas given the same pressure change. The steeper compliance line for the lower area means a greater increase in volume per unit pressure change. (Modified from West JB. *Respiratory Physiology: The Essentials*. 2nd ed. Baltimore: Williams & Wilkins; 1979, p. 96.)

they prevent airway closure and gas trapping during forced exhalation.

Gravitational effects on the distribution of ventilation have been exploited in adult patients with or without ventilatory assistance who have unilateral lung disease[72] or who have undergone thoracotomy.[73] Improved gas exchange in these patients can be accomplished if they are positioned with their "good" side down. This technique increases ventilation to the dependent lung regions, which also receive relatively greater blood flow, resulting in better V/Q matching in the good lung. Body position affects ventilation and gas exchange in infants in the opposite way.

When infants with unilateral lung disease are placed in the lateral decubitus position, the uppermost "good" lung receives a greater portion of ventilation than the dependent lung. This may be the case for infants with restrictive lung disease such as unilateral PIE. In cases of unilateral PIE, one sees ideal circumstances for the occurrence of airway closure in the "bad" lung when it is placed in the dependent position. In patients with unilateral tension PIE, interpleural pressure on the bad side already is elevated secondary to the presence of high (positive) interstitial pressure because of gas trapping outside of the terminal air spaces. Positioning patients with the PIE side down adds the additional weight of the mediastinal structures, which causes the interpleural pressure to exceed local airway pressure and results in airway collapse. This airway closure in the dependent (bad) lung often facilitates resolution of unilateral PIE, while the infant's gas exchange needs are met by the nondependent lung.[74,75]

The pattern of diaphragmatic motion plays a role in the distribution of ventilation in the newborn infant. When the diaphragm is paralyzed and the patient is supine, mechanical ventilation tends to produce greater motion of the superior than of the inferior portion of the diaphragm because the superior portion is less constrained by the abdominal contents and mediastinal structures. Therefore, ventilation of the upper (anterior) segments of the lung is preferential.[76] Because perfusion still is likely to be better in the dependent regions secondary to gravitational effects, paralysis may result in V/Q mismatch with hypoxemia. The improvement in oxygenation achieved after adults with acute respiratory failure[77] or premature infants with respiratory insufficiency[78] are switched from the supine to the prone position is attributable to the enhancement of V/Q matching (or an increase in ventilation to a level that better matches the existing degree of perfusion). In premature infants the prone position affords better distribution of ventilation throughout the lung, especially to the dependent regions that are better perfused.[78]

The most common causes of uneven distribution of ventilation are conditions characterized by local differences in lung compliance, airway resistance, or both. If the patient is receiving assisted ventilation and is faced with local differences in either lung tissue elasticity or airway resistance, the distribution of gas delivered during the inspiratory phase is influenced by the mode of ventilation chosen. Local or regional (lobar) variations in compliance are determined by (1) local tissue water content, (2) presence or absence of surfactant, (3) presence of volume loss, or (4) presence of gas trapping or overexpansion. For example, pneumonia in one lung area makes that lung less compliant than the normal lung; thus the affected lung receives less volume per unit pressure than do the unaffected areas.

Differences in distal airway resistance may be caused by local narrowing secondary to either obstruction or compression. For example, partial obstruction of a bronchus with meconium increases airway resistance and reduces alveolar ventilation in the area distal to the partial obstruction (see Fig. 2-13). Many disease processes common in premature infants involve nonuniform regional compliance and resistance. During conventional mechanical ventilation, distribution of the inspired gas is largely controlled by regional variations in compliance and resistance (i.e., time constants). During HFV, the distribution of inspired gas is dependent more on the mechanical properties of the central airways and chest wall (resistance, inertance) and less so on the compliance of lung tissue. If inspiratory pressure is increased slowly (low inspiratory flow rate), the volume of gas delivered depends mainly on the compliance of the lung. If inspiratory pressure is increased quickly (high inspiratory flow rate), the distribution of gas depends mainly on local airway resistance.

Consequently, the largest volumes are delivered to areas with the least resistance. This information is useful to the clinician trying to decide how best to ventilate a patient with meconium aspiration syndrome or BPD. One would like to be able to ventilate the patient's unobstructed lung regions while minimizing air trapping and overdistention in areas behind partially obstructed airways (see Fig. 2-8). One approach is to use rapid rates (high inspiratory flows) and short inspiration times (T_Is). In this fashion, only regions of the lung with short (or normal) time constants are given sufficient time for pressure equalization (volume delivery); thus these areas are being ventilated while overdistention of lung regions with long time constants is avoided (however, beware of the risk of air trapping if expiratory time is not sufficient for complete exhalation). In cases of pulmonary air leak (pneumothorax or bronchopleural fistula), a strategy incorporating a short T_I and a high rate often is effective in decreasing the magnitude of the leak. Several reports have described the successful application of HFV in adults with airway disruption or bronchopleural fistulae[79,80] and in newborns with persistent air leaks through pneumothoraces[81] or tracheoesophageal fistula.[82]

In cases of PIE, the use of low rates and long T_Is might worsen the clinical situation. Because the lung regions with PIE have long time constants (due to elevated resistance), they could become further overdistended with this mode of ventilation. If ventilated with a conventional ventilator using high rates and short T_Is or if ventilated with an HFV, lung areas with long time constants would be less likely to become overdistended. However, high rates on conventional ventilation increase the likelihood of delivering inadvertent PEEP. HFJV has been shown to be safer and more effective than rapid-rate conventional ventilation in the treatment of newborn infants with PIE.[83] As the PIE resolves and the compression effects on the surrounding lung tissue are alleviated, the distribution of ventilation would become more homogeneous. The clinician's choice of strategy and mode of ventilation can be important determinants of the distribution of ventilation, particularly in situations of nonhomogeneous lung disease.

During assisted ventilation, to minimize risk to the infant, the most minimal amount of pressure required to achieve adequate gas flow and alveolar ventilation should be used. Enough distending pressure should be applied to optimize lung volume and homogeneity of lung expansion and prevent airway collapse. Enough driving pressure should be applied so as to achieve an appropriate V_T.

Effects of Altering Ventilator Settings on Ventilation

During conventional ventilation, increasing V_T or increasing the ventilator rate are the two primary methods for increasing ventilation (enhancing CO_2 removal). The ventilator rate is controlled either directly or by altering the inspiratory and/or expiratory time. V_T is controlled in different ways depending on the type of ventilator. With volume-controlled ventilators, V_T can be manipulated directly. However, the volume that is controlled is the volume injected into the ventilator circuit, not directly into the patient's lungs. A significant but variable portion of that volume is lost to compression of gas in the circuit or to leaks around uncuffed ETTs.[84] Consequently, the ability to directly control effective V_T is greatly limited. With time-cycled pressure-limited devices, adjustments that increase ΔP (pressure amplitude or difference between PIP and PEEP) will increase V_T, provided the compliance remains the same. To control ventilation or CO_2 elimination during HFJV, the operator manipulates basically the same parameters in the same direction as during conventional ventilation.[64] Ventilation during HFOV is generally controlled by altering the power setting, which controls the stroke length of the piston and therefore pressure amplitude. The larger the amplitude, the greater the V_T and thus the greater the CO_2 removal. With both HFJV and HFOV, minute ventilation is more closely related to frequency $\times V_T^2$ and thus even small changes in amplitude result in substantial changes in PCO_2.[65] V_T delivered during HFOV is frequency-dependent and decreases as the operating frequency increases.[85] This means that in the unusual clinical setting in which amplitude settings are maximized, frequency may need to be reduced if an improvement in ventilation is desired. It is important for the clinician to remember the passive change in amplitude that occurs with changes in frequency. At the other extreme, on the rare occasions when V_T or power settings are at minimum levels and the infant is not yet ready for extubation, operating frequency may have to be increased to decrease CO_2 removal.[86]

PERFUSION

Before delivery, only 8% to 10% of cardiac output flows to the lungs. In the fetus, pulmonary vascular resistance is high and systemic vascular resistance is low.[87] Most of the blood coming from the fetal inferior vena cava flows from right to left through the foramen ovale and much of the right-ventricular output shunts through the ductus arteriosus, thus bypassing the lungs. Under normal circumstances after delivery, a relatively rapid transition to the adult pattern of circulation occurs, after which virtually all right-heart output goes through the lungs, then through the left side of the heart, and out the aorta.

Key to this transition is a decrease in pulmonary vascular resistance and an increase in pulmonary blood flow preceding closure of the fetal shunts. Experiments carried out on fetal lambs and investigations into the actions of certain mediators, including nitric oxide (NO) (Table 2-1), have demonstrated a number of factors that contribute to the decrease in pulmonary vascular resistance that occurs at birth. These include (1) expansion of the lung with a gas,[88] (2) increase in PAo_2,[89] (3) increase in PaO_2,[90] (4) increase in pH,[91] and (5) elaboration of vasoactive substances such as bradykinin,[92] the prostaglandins (PGE$_1$, PGA$_1$, PGI$_2$ [prostacyclin],[93,94] and PGD$_2$[95]), and endothelium-derived relaxing factor,[96] which subsequently was shown to be the gas NO.[97] Blood flow through the pulmonary circuit is directly proportional to the pressure gradient across the pulmonary vessels and the total cross-sectional area of the vessels that make up the pulmonary vascular bed. Blood flow is inversely proportional to the blood's viscosity.

TABLE 2-1 Factors Affecting Pulmonary Blood Flow

Increasing Flow	Decreasing Flow
Optimization of lung volume	Lung atelectasis
Increase in PAo2	Decrease in PAo2
Increase in PaO_2	Hypoxemia (reduction in PaO_2)
Alkalosis (respiratory or metabolic)	Acidosis (respiratory or metabolic)
Release of mediator substances (e.g., bradykinin, prostaglandins)	Mast cell degranulation with release of histamine
Left-to-right shunting (intracardiac or ductal)	Right-to-left shunting (intracardiac or ductal)
Endogenous production of NO	Systemic hypotension (when right-to-left shunting is already present)
Inhalation of exogenous NO	Lung overexpansion

NO, Nitric oxide; *PaO₂,* partial pressure of oxygen in arterial blood; *PAo₂,* partial pressure of oxygen in the alveoli.

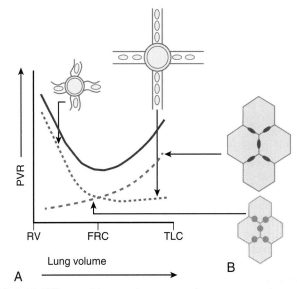

FIG 2-17 Effects of lung volume on pulmonary vascular resistance (*PVR, solid curved line*). **A,** "Extra-alveolar" vessels pose high resistance (*dotted curved line*) at low and high lung volumes, at the former because they become narrow and at the latter because they become stretched. **B,** "Alveolar" vessels pose the least resistance (*dashed curved line*) when they are open widest at the functional residual capacity (FRC) lung volume level, but they become compressed under conditions of lung overinflation. *RV,* Residual volume; *TLC,* total lung capacity. (Modified from West JB. *Respiratory Physiology: The Essentials.* 2nd ed. Baltimore: Williams & Wilkins; 1979, p. 39.)

Increased blood viscosity interferes with gas exchange by reducing pulmonary perfusion.

As the lung expands after birth, pulmonary vascular resistance decreases and pulmonary blood flow increases.[88] With inflation of the lungs, some "straightening out" of pulmonary vessels occurs. The larger vessels are pulled open by traction of the lung parenchyma that surrounds them. The perialveolar capillary lumens enlarge because of the action of surface tension produced by the newly established air–fluid interfaces. There are two types of pulmonary blood vessels: alveolar vessels, which are composed of capillaries and the slightly larger vessels in the alveolar walls (these vessels are exposed to alveolar pressure), and extra-alveolar vessels, which include the arteries and veins that run through the lung parenchyma but are surrounded by interstitial tissue rather than alveoli (Fig. 2-17).[98]

The diameter of alveolar vessels is determined by the balance between the alveolar pressure and the hydrostatic pressure within the vessel. The vessel walls contain little elastic tissue and virtually no muscle fibers. Alveolar vessels collapse if alveolar pressure exceeds pulmonary venous pressure. Extra-alveolar vessels have structural support in their walls and are not significantly influenced by alveolar pressure. The vessel diameter of extra-alveolar vessels is affected by lung volume, because expanding the lung tends to pull these vessels open. If an airless lung is inflated to total lung capacity, pulmonary vascular resistance shows a U-shaped response, with high resistance at the low and high ends of inflation and low resistance in the middle (see Fig. 2-17). Resistance is high at low lung volumes because the extra-alveolar vessels are narrowed (they are not being pulled open). Resistance is high at high inflation volumes because the alveolar vessels are narrowed by compression (they may even collapse). The lowest pulmonary vascular resistance, as well as the best lung compliance, is found when the lung is neither underinflated nor overinflated.

The rapid rise in oxygen tension in the alveoli (PAO_2) and in the arterial blood (PaO_2) perfusing the pulmonary vessels plays a major role in the circulatory adaptation that occurs during transition to extrauterine life. It is the influence of PaO_2 on adjacent arteries that exerts the greatest effect on decreasing pulmonary vascular resistance with the initiation of breathing air.[90] With the initiation of breathing air, the lung is exposed to a PO_2 of approximately 100 mm Hg. PaO_2 in the central circulation of the newborn infant rises from the fetal range between 25 and 30 mm Hg to greater than 60 mm Hg within the first hours after birth.

Many mediator substances have been implicated in the pulmonary vasodilation seen in the newborn infant. Bradykinin is a vasoactive peptide that produces pulmonary vasodilation in fetal lambs.[92] Bradykinin concentration increases transiently in blood that has passed through the lungs of fetal lambs ventilated with oxygen, but it does not increase if the lungs are ventilated with nitrogen. Bradykinin stimulates the local production of prostacyclin, which is also a potent pulmonary vasodilator.[93] PGA_1, PGE_1, and prostacyclin decrease pulmonary vascular resistance by dilating both pulmonary veins and arteries.[93,94,99] Prostacyclin production is stimulated by lung expansion with air and by mechanical ventilation.

The decrease in pulmonary vascular resistance associated with mechanical ventilation can be attenuated by prior administration of a prostaglandin synthesis inhibitor (indomethacin).[94] PGD_2, another prostaglandin, is a semiselective pulmonary vasodilator. It promotes pulmonary vasodilation without causing the systemic vasodilatory effect produced by other prostaglandins.[95] The pulmonary vasodilatory effect of PGD_2 is present only during the first few days after birth; thereafter, it becomes a pulmonary vasoconstrictor. This observation suggests that PGD_2 plays a role in the transition from fetal to adult-type circulation after birth. PGD_2, like histamine, is released through mast cell degranulation. The number of mast cells in the lungs increases just before birth and then declines after delivery.[100] Mast cells play an important role in the pulmonary vasoconstrictive response to hypoxia.[101] Mast cells are abundant in the lung and are ideally located for modulation of vascular tone. Mast cell degranulation has been demonstrated to occur after acute alveolar hypoxia.[102] Pretreatment with cromolyn sodium (a mast cell degranulation blocking agent) prevents the pulmonary vasoconstriction normally induced by alveolar hypoxia.[103]

NO, previously known as endothelium-derived relaxing factor, plays an important role in regulating pulmonary vascular resistance. Its action reduces pulmonary vasoconstriction, thereby increasing pulmonary blood flow.[104-106] Endogenous NO is generated in vascular endothelial cells by enzymatic cleavage of the terminal nitrogen from L-arginine; production is accelerated at birth owing to the increase in Po_2. NO diffuses into the vascular smooth muscle cells and stimulates the production of cyclic guanosine monophosphate, which causes smooth muscle relaxation.

The primary factor keeping pulmonary vascular resistance high in the fetus is relative hypoxia. Because of the preferential perfusion of the pulmonary circuit with the most desaturated blood (venous blood returning from the fetus's head), the PaO_2 of blood perfusing the lungs of a fetal lamb is around 18 to 21 mm Hg. Profound fetal hypoxia causes further pulmonary vasoconstriction. A decrease in pulmonary arterial Po_2 to about 14 mm Hg diminishes pulmonary blood flow in the fetus to approximately 50%, its base level.[107] Hypoxemic stress produces progressively greater increases in pulmonary vascular resistance as the gestational age of a fetus advances.[108] Chronic hypoxia in the fetus produces an increase in the medial smooth muscle of the pulmonary arterioles, which may lead to pulmonary hypertension and increased pulmonary vasoreactivity.[109] This may contribute to the development of persistent pulmonary hypertension of the newborn (PPHN) in some newborn infants and may explain why infants born through meconium-stained fluid are at high risk for PPHN. Passage of meconium is thought to be a sign of fetal intolerance of labor, which is more likely to occur in infants whose placental function is compromised and who may have had prolonged fetal hypoxia.

For these same reasons, infants living at high altitudes have an increase in pulmonary vascular resistance that persists into childhood. They have relative pulmonary hypertension and are at increased risk for developing cor pulmonale.[110] Infants with cyanotic congenital heart disease and chronic hypoxemia are also at risk for developing pulmonary hypertension and cor pulmonale, as are oxygen-dependent infants with BPD. The vasoconstriction response to alveolar and arterial hypoxemia is potentiated by acidosis.[91]

PPHN is a clinical syndrome, peculiar to the early neonatal period, characterized by severe arterial hypoxemia caused by increased pulmonary vascular resistance with resultant right-to-left shunting through fetal channels (at the atrial and ductal levels). PPHN is associated with a variety of conditions, including RDS, pneumonia, meconium aspiration syndrome, and congenital heart disease, and is also seen in infants with chronic fetal distress or peripartum stress.[111,112]

Infants with PPHN exhibit hypoxemia secondary to extrapulmonary right-to-left shunting, near-systemic or supra-systemic pulmonary artery pressures, and lability in pulmonary artery pressure secondary to pulmonary vasoreactivity

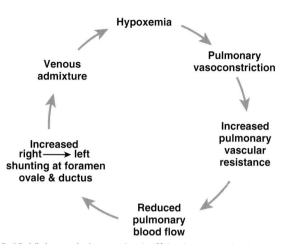

FIG 2-18 Vicious circle touched off by hypoxemia that reverts transitional circulation back to the fetal type, as seen in persistent pulmonary hypertension.

(Fig. 2-18). Hyperventilation of infants with PPHN has been shown to decrease pulmonary artery pressure.[113] However, hyperventilation with resultant hypocarbia has been shown also to be associated with poor pulmonary and neurologic outcomes.[114-116] As such, hyperventilation is no longer advocated as a treatment modality in infants with PPHN.

Inhaled NO causes a decrease in pulmonary vascular resistance and an increase in pulmonary blood flow, without affecting systemic arterial pressure.[117-119] It is a selective pulmonary vasodilator, because it is inactivated by being bound to hemoglobin upon entering the systemic circulation.[120] When used at low concentrations, inhaled NO also improves ventilation–perfusion matching by selectively vasodilating the well-ventilated areas of the lung (see Chapter 32).[121]

The pulmonary arteries, like the airways, form a treelike structure. The pulmonary circulation is perfused by the entire cardiac output. Blood flow is determined by the pressure difference between pulmonary arteries and veins and by the vascular resistance. The pulmonary circulation is a low-pressure low-resistance system. The distribution of blood flow to the gas exchange units depends on the distribution of resistances, which are affected by contraction of the smooth muscle walls of the arteries. In hypoxia, resistance increases, owing to hypoxic pulmonary vasoconstriction.[122]

There are regional differences in ventilation and perfusion. The dependent portions of the lung are better ventilated and better perfused than the upper portions. Hypoxic vasoconstriction shunts blood away from poorly ventilated acini, which helps preserve V/Q matching. Ideally, ventilation and perfusion are evenly matched, with a V/Q ratio of 1. When a lung or lung unit is relatively underventilated but normally perfused or is normally ventilated but overperfused, it is said to have a low V/Q (less than 1). When a lung unit is overventilated and normally perfused or is normally ventilated and underperfused, the resultant V/Q is high (greater than 1).

The more dependent the lung region, the greater its perfusion.[123] The vessels in dependent regions of the lung are more distended and thus present less resistance to flow because their transmural pressure is greater. Transmural pressure is the difference between the pressure inside and the pressure outside the vessel wall. Inside "hydrostatic" pressure increases the more dependent a vessel's position is in the lung. Outside interstitial

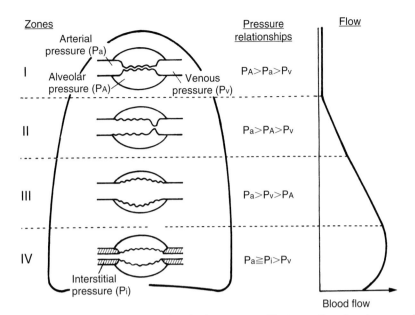

FIG 2-19 Various intraluminal and extraluminal pressure effects on the alveolar vessels of the lung in relation to blood flow in the four perfusion zones. Alveolar vessels represent "Starling resistors," which consist of collapsible tubes in pressure chambers. Note the situation in zone II, where there is a constriction in the "downstream end" of the collapsible vessel. Here, chamber (alveolar) pressure exceeds intraluminal downstream (venous) pressure and the vessel collapses; pressure inside the tube at the constriction is equal to the chamber (alveolar) pressure. Flow is thus determined by the arterial–alveolar pressure difference rather than by the usual arterial–venous pressure difference. (Modified from West JB, Dollery CT, Naimark A. Distribution of blood flow in isolated lung: relation to vascular and alveolar pressures. *J Appl Physiol.* 1964;19:713.)

pressure reflects interpleural pressure (see Fig. 2-15). Interpleural pressure decreases the more dependent the lung region is. Because the hydrostatic pressure increase (inside the vessel) is greater than the interpleural pressure decrease (outside the vessel), the transmural pressure increase is greater the more dependent the lung region.

In the upright adult, the lung is divided into four perfusion zones (Fig. 2-19) based on up-and-down distance and specific pressure differences.[123] Zone I is the least dependent (uppermost) region and has almost no blood flow because alveolar pressure exceeds pulmonary capillary pressure. This causes collapse of the capillaries around the alveoli. Zone II is the upper middle region and has some flow because pulmonary artery pressure exceeds alveolar pressure. Zone III is the lower middle region, where flow is determined by the difference in pressure between the pulmonary arteries and pulmonary veins. Zone IV is the most dependent region, where interstitial pressure is great enough to cause narrowing of extra-alveolar vessels and thus reduce blood flow as a result of increased pulmonary vascular resistance.

In infants, under normal circumstances the entire lung is considered to have zone III characteristics from a physiologic standpoint. In some situations, as in the presence of air trapping or alveolar overdistention, a portion of the lung may behave as zone I or II, with a decrease in pulmonary blood flow. In other conditions such as interstitial edema (fluid overload; left-sided heart failure, as in congenital heart disease or significant patent ductus arteriosus; capillary leakage following hypoxic insult or asphyxia; BPD), much of the dependent portion of the lung behaves like zone IV, with increased vascular resistance and decreased pulmonary blood flow. In this clinical situation, fluid restriction, administration of a diuretic, or both may result in significant improvements in gas exchange because of an improvement in pulmonary blood flow (as well as an improvement in lung compliance and a decrease in airway resistance). Conditions in which significant left-to-right shunting and pulmonary hyperperfusion occur tend to abolish the unevenness of blood flow in the lungs.[68]

Regional hypoventilation produces local pulmonary vasoconstriction that diverts blood flow away from underventilated areas. This is a protective mechanism that decreases the perfusion of nonventilated or poorly ventilated areas of the lung. Term newborn and premature lambs are capable of redirecting blood flow away from hypoxic regions produced by atelectasis or bronchial obstruction.[122,124] The flow directed away from atelectatic and hypoxic lung segments is directly proportional to the amount of lung volume loss.[125] Lung scans in infants have identified perfusion deficits in areas of atelectasis.[126] Alveolar overdistention secondary to air trapping may reduce area blood flow by collapsing surrounding capillaries.

When CPAP or positive-pressure ventilation is used to recruit atelectatic lung units, improvement in both local ventilation and perfusion may result in those regions. However, those areas of the lung, which already are well expanded, may be further inflated, which can increase rather than decrease pulmonary vascular resistance in those areas. The overall effect on pulmonary blood flow produced by positive-pressure ventilation depends on the initial lung volume status of the various functional lung regions and the net result of the therapy on global pulmonary blood flow.

CONTROL OF VENTILATION

The respiratory control center in the newborn infant is immature compared to that of adults and therefore more easily influenced by changes in acid–base status, temperature, sleep state, hypoxia, medications, and other variables. Because of this relative immaturity, the central and peripheral chemoreceptors that respond to changes in arterial O_2 and CO_2 tensions act both quantitatively and qualitatively differently compared to those in adults. Additionally, a set of chest wall stretch proprioceptors is able to reflexively inhibit or drive respiration.[127-130] REM sleep also has a significant effect on the control of respiration in the newborn infant. During REM sleep, the normal phasic tone changes in the intercostal muscles, which are important for stabilizing the rib cage during inspiration, are inhibited. Because the intercostal muscles fail to tighten with inspiration, the infant's chest wall deforms during inspiration. Contraction of the diaphragm worsens the paradoxical movement, increases its O_2 consumption measured during REM sleep, and may lead to fatigue-induced apnea.[129]

Application of CPAP or PEEP causes the infant's respiratory rate to slow and his or her respiratory efforts to become more regular with a reduction in periodic breathing and apneic episodes.[131,132] The distending pressure stabilizes the infant's compliant chest wall by providing a "pneumatic splint" that counters the tendency of the chest wall to collapse during inspiration. The application of CDP shortens and intensifies inspiratory effort while prolonging expiration. Methylxanthines such as caffeine and aminophylline (or theophylline) increase alveolar ventilation through central stimulation.[133] Methylxanthines cause an increase in diaphragmatic contractility and resistance to fatigue with a shift of the CO_2 response curve to the left so that an increase in V_T occurs in response to an increase in CO_2.[134,135] A more detailed discussion on the control of ventilation can be found in Chapter 3.

CONCLUSION

Based on an understanding of the physiologic principles of assisted ventilation, we know that ventilation strategies must be individualized for each patient. It is also clear that the use of the appropriate strategy to provide mechanical ventilatory support and the skill with which this is done are more important than the specific type of device used to deliver that support. Each time we encounter an infant in respiratory distress, we must determine the specific pathophysiology of the infant's condition and then decide what level of support is required, addressing the infant's specific condition. The least invasive level of support that is adequate to accomplish the task should be selected, and the infant's response to therapy must be closely monitored.[136] We must be cognizant of how our strategies and techniques of providing assisted ventilation to infants influence their long-term outcomes. Repeated cycling of the terminal airways from below critical opening pressure leads to cellular injury and inflammation (atelectotrauma). This results in alveolar collapse, atelectasis, interstitial edema, and elaboration of inflammatory mediators. The resulting atelectasis leads to a further reduction in lung compliance that necessitates higher inspiratory pressures, which further compromises surfactant production. Atelectotrauma leads to further lung injury, which necessitates increased levels of distending airway pressure and/or increased levels of inspired oxygen. The increase in FiO_2 may lead to oxidative injury and further cellular dysfunction. Despite many years of diligent research, there are still more questions than answers. However, we do know that mechanical ventilation causes lung injury that leads to inflammatory response[137]; oxygen exposure is harmful[138,139]; lung overdistention (volutrauma) causes lung injury[140]; lung injury and inflammation exacerbate the deleterious effects of oxygen toxicity and volutrauma[141]; and finally, atelectotrauma is a source of lung injury.[142]

Establishment of an appropriate FRC (optimization of lung volume), administration of surfactant, avoidance of mechanical ventilation (if possible), use of adequate PEEP to avoid the repeated collapse and reopening of small airways, avoidance of lung overinflation caused by using excessive distending airway pressure or supraphysiologic V_Ts, and avoidance of the use of more oxygen than is necessary all are important in achieving the best possible outcomes and long-term health of our patients.[84,143] While caring for your patients, always remember the words of the Hippocratic Oath, "First do no harm."

REFERENCES

A complete reference list is available at https://expertconsult.inkling.com/.

3

Control of Ventilation

Richard J. Martin, MBBS

INTRODUCTION

The transition from fetal to neonatal life requires a rapid conversion from intermittent fetal respiratory activity not associated with gas exchange to continuous breathing upon which gas exchange is dependent once the baby is born. This encompasses the development of neural circuitry that regulates respiratory control and serves as a unique link between the maturing lung and the brain. The frequent apneic events exhibited by preterm infants may be akin to the episodic pauses in respiratory movements that characterize fetal breathing. However, after birth, frequent apnea—often associated with bradycardia and oxygen desaturation events—may be one of the most troublesome problems in neonatal intensive care. The problem of vulnerable neonatal respiratory control is typically enhanced by the mechanical disadvantages of a compliant chest wall and unfavorable lung mechanics. This is compounded by the clinical observation that neonatal respiratory control is vulnerable to a diversity of pathophysiologic conditions (Fig. 3-1). Understanding the maturation of neonatal respiratory control is essential to providing a rational approach to ventilatory support for neonates.

PATHOGENESIS OF APNEA OF PREMATURITY

Our understanding of the pathogenesis of apnea of prematurity is hampered by our limited understanding of the integration of chemo- and mechanosensitive inputs to the autonomic control circuitry of the developing human brainstem. Neonatal animal models, such as rodents, are immature at birth compared to the human trajectory but do not typically exhibit apnea. Nonetheless, we are clearly dependent on animal models to characterize the maturation of neuroanatomic architecture and neurochemical transmitter changes in the brain-stem. Undoubtedly there are significant changes in adenosine, γ-aminobutyric acid (GABA), and serotonin content and corresponding receptor subtypes in respiratory-related brain-stem regions.[1]

Central (CO_2) Chemosensitivity

CO_2 is sensed primarily at or near the ventral medullary surface, but also by the carotid bodies, and is the major chemical driver of respiration at all ages. It has been recognized for several decades that preterm infants exhibit a diminished ventilatory response to CO_2 compared to more mature infants.[2] The response to CO_2 in preterm neonates results in an increase in tidal volume with little, if any, increase in frequency.[3] Furthermore, apneic preterm infants have a diminished CO_2 response compared to nonapneic preterm controls.[4] In preterm and term infants, the baseline $PaCO_2$ has been shown to be only up to 1.5 mm Hg above the apneic threshold; this narrow margin might predispose these children to apnea in the face of only minor oscillations in $PaCO_2$.[5] Breathing patterns tend to be more irregular in rapid eye movement (REM) than in quiet sleep, and it is possible that the closeness of the eupneic and apneic CO_2 thresholds may contribute to greater breath-to-breath respiratory irregularity in REM sleep. Unfortunately, REM sleep, quiet sleep, transitional sleep, and even wakefulness are often difficult to distinguish in preterm infants. This complicates the ability to draw conclusions about sleep state and respiratory control in the preterm population.

Peripheral (Hypoxic) Chemosensitivity

The peripheral chemoreceptors are located primarily in the carotid body and are responsible for stimulating breathing in response to hypoxia. Both enhanced and reduced peripheral chemoreceptor functions have been proposed as contributors to apnea of prematurity.[6] In utero, carotid chemoreceptor oxygen sensitivity is adapted to the normally low PaO_2 of the mammalian fetal environment (~23 to 27 mm Hg). After birth, in response to the increase in PaO_2 with the establishment of breathing, the peripheral chemoreceptors are silenced, followed by a gradual increase in hypoxic chemosensitivity. Once peripheral chemosensitivity is established, hyperoxic resuscitation rapidly elicits apnea, as clearly shown in rat pups.[7] It follows that inappropriate hyperoxic ventilatory support of an apneic infant may hinder recovery of the respiratory drive. Interestingly, infants with bronchopulmonary dysplasia seem to exhibit blunted peripheral chemoreceptor responses compared to controls,[8] which may increase their vulnerability to apnea.

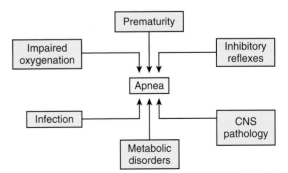

FIG 3-1 Specific contributory causes of apnea. *CNS*, Central nervous system.

Excessive peripheral chemoreceptor sensitivity in response to repeated hypoxia may also destabilize breathing patterns in the face of significantly fluctuating levels of oxygenation. This is consistent with an earlier finding in preterm infants that a greater hypoxia-induced increase in ventilation correlates with a higher number of apneic episodes.[9] Data from rat pups indicate that conditioning with intermittent hypoxic exposures results in facilitation of carotid body sensory discharge in response to subsequent hypoxic exposure. This effect appears to persist into adult life, raising questions about a longer lasting effect of early apnea in human respiratory control.[10]

In the neonatal period, it is well known that the ventilatory response to hypoxia, an initial increase in minute ventilation, is followed by a posthypoxia decline in frequency of breathing. This so-called hypoxic ventilatory depression is seen in less dramatic form in later life, and may be an appropriate response to sustained hypoxia when coupled with a decrease in metabolic rate. Descending inhibition from the midbrain and other structures appears to cause this hypoxic depression rather than a decline in peripheral chemoreceptor firing, although a contribution from the latter cannot be excluded. The role of hypoxic depression in contributing to apnea of prematurity is unclear; however, low baseline oxygenation is associated with more episodic desaturation in preterm infants.[11]

Role of Mechanoreceptor (Laryngeal) Afferents

Activation of the laryngeal mucosa elicits a potent airway-protective reflex, which, in preterm and term neonates and immature animals of various species, results in a host of autonomic perturbations including apnea, bradycardia, hypotension, closure of upper airways, and swallowing movements. While this strong inhibitory reflex, termed the *laryngeal chemoreflex*, is thought to be an important contributor to apnea and bradycardia associated with excessive suctioning or aspiration, its relationship to apnea of prematurity is less clear. The pronounced inhibitory effect on ventilation in early life may be the result of enhanced central inhibitory pathways, and GABA has been proposed to mediate this effect.[12] Despite the physiologic rationale for a relationship between stimulation of laryngeal afferents and apnea of prematurity, a temporal relationship between apnea of prematurity and gastroesophageal reflux is rare in preterm infants, as discussed later. Of interest are the data from piglets, confirmed in infants, showing that respiratory inhibition may precede a loss of lower esophageal sphincter tone and theoretically predispose to reflux.[13,14]

GENESIS OF CENTRAL, MIXED, AND OBSTRUCTIVE APNEA

Apnea is classified into three categories traditionally, each based upon the absence or presence of upper airway obstruction: (1) central, (2) obstructive, and (3) mixed. Central apnea is characterized by total cessation of inspiratory efforts with no evidence of obstruction. In obstructive apnea, the infant tries to breathe against an obstructed upper airway, resulting in chest wall motion without airflow throughout the entire apneic episode. Mixed apnea consists of obstructed respiratory efforts, usually following central pauses. The site of obstruction in the upper airways is primarily in the pharynx, although it also may occur at the larynx and possibly at both sites. Interestingly, upper airway closure may also occur during central apnea.

Unlike adult sleep apnea, which is primarily obstructive, apnea of prematurity has a predominantly central etiology with loss of respiratory drive initiated in the brainstem. During mixed apnea it has been assumed that there is an initial loss of central respiratory drive and the resumption of inspiration is accompanied by a delay in activation of the upper airway muscles superimposed upon a closed upper airway.[15] This may be due to a lower CO_2 threshold for activation of chest wall vs upper airway muscles. Mixed apnea typically accounts for more than 50% of long apneic episodes, followed in decreasing frequency by central and obstructive apnea.[16] Purely obstructive spontaneous apnea in the absence of a positional problem is probably uncommon. As standard impedance monitoring of respiratory efforts via chest wall motion cannot recognize obstructed respiratory efforts, mixed (or obstructive) apnea is frequently identified by the accompanying bradycardia or desaturation, although these are not the initiating events.

RELATIONSHIP BETWEEN APNEA, BRADYCARDIA, AND DESATURATION

Cessation of respiration or hypoventilation is almost invariably the event that initiates various patterns of apnea, bradycardia, and desaturation in preterm infants. There is no clear consensus as to when a respiratory pause, which is universal in preterm infants, can be defined as an apneic episode. It has been proposed that apnea may be defined by its duration (e.g., >15 seconds) or by accompanying bradycardia and/or desaturations. However, even the 5- to 10-second pauses that occur in periodic breathing may be associated with bradycardia or desaturation. Periodic breathing—ventilatory cycles of 10- to 15-second duration with pauses of 5- to10-second duration—is considered a "normal" breathing pattern in infants who should not require therapeutic intervention, as discussed earlier. Periodic breathing is speculated to be the result of dominant peripheral chemoreceptor activity responding to fluctuations in arterial oxygen tension. The rapidity of the fall in oxygen saturation after a respiratory pause is directly proportional to baseline oxygenation, and this, in turn, is related to lung volume and severity of lung disease.

Bradycardia is a prominent feature in preterm infants with apnea. The mechanism underlying bradycardia associated with apnea in preterm infants is not entirely clear. A significant correlation between decrease in oxygen saturation and heart rate has been noted, and the bradycardia during apnea might be related to hypoxic stimulation of the carotid body chemoreceptors, especially in the absence of lung inflation. On the other hand, bradycardia may occur simultaneously with apnea during stimulation of laryngeal receptors, suggesting a vagally mediated central mechanism for the production of both. Data in preterm infants indicate that isolated bradycardic events (<70/min) in the absence of accompanying hypoxemia are unlikely to significantly affect tissue oxygenation measured by near-infrared spectroscopy.[17]

CARDIORESPIRATORY EVENTS IN INTUBATED INFANTS

If apnea is the precipitant of episodic bradycardia and desaturation in spontaneously breathing events, what is the etiology of such events in intubated and ventilated infants? The likely answer is that mechanical ventilation does not always result in effective ventilation in intubated infants. Loss of lung volume and excessive abdominal expiratory muscle activity have been shown to accompany desaturation events in such infants.[18] Loss of spontaneous ventilatory effects may also occur under these conditions. The presence of episodic desaturation and bradycardia in ventilated infants reinforces the need to synchronize spontaneous and ventilator-delivered breaths in infants. Extubation, if feasible, may effectively decrease the frequency of such events.

THERAPEUTIC APPROACHES

Impaired respiratory control is clearly a major contributor to the need for neonatal assisted ventilation. Our ability to enhance neonatal respiratory control will, therefore, probably diminish potential morbidity induced by ventilation. Aggressive therapy for apnea may be beneficial in avoiding intubation, enhancing extubation, and decreasing any adverse effects of apnea or gas exchange. To achieve these goals we have both nonpharmacologic and pharmacologic and ventilatory strategies. Many of the latter are addressed elsewhere in this book.

Optimization of Mechanosensory Inputs

The respiratory rhythm-generating circuitry within the central nervous system depends on intrinsic rhythmic activity and sensory afferent inputs to generate breathing movement. Bloch-Salisbury et al. have demonstrated that their novel technique of stochastic mechanosensory stimulation, using a mattress with embedded actuators, is able to stabilize respiratory patterns in preterm infants as manifest by a decrease in apnea and an almost threefold decrease in percentage of time with oxygen saturations <85%.[19] Interestingly, the level of stimulation employed was below the minimum threshold for behavioral arousal to wakefulness, thus inducing no apparent state change in the infants, and the effect could probably not be attributed to the minimal increase in sound level associated with stimulation. Such an approach is clearly still a research tool but worthy of future study. It points to the important consideration that environmental stimulation of the infant must be optimized. Similarly, skin-to-skin care is a highly desirable practice in the neonatal intensive care unit (NICU) to encourage parental attachment and potentially influence respiratory control.[20] Data have shown that this practice is not only safe but also associated with decreased electrical diaphragm activity, potentially benefiting energy expended on respiratory efforts.[21]

Optimization of Blood Gas Status

Intermittent hypoxic episodes are almost always the result of respiratory pauses, apnea, or ineffective ventilation, aggravated by poor respiratory function (Fig. 3-2). Targeting lower baseline oxygen saturation has been associated with persistence of intermittent hypoxic episodes.[11] It is unclear whether this lower baseline oxygen saturation increases the incidence of apnea with resultant hypoxemia (via hypoxic depression of breathing) or whether the incidence of apnea is comparable between oxygen targets, but the lower oxygen saturation baseline predisposes to more frequent or profound intermittent hypoxemia. Regardless of mechanism, a low baseline oxygen saturation (e.g., <90%) should be avoided in the face of immature respiratory control superimposed upon poor respiratory function. It is also unclear whether the beneficial effect of packed red cell transfusion is

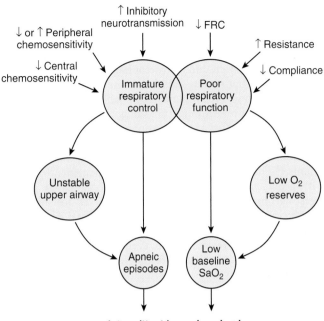

Intermittent hypoxic episodes

FIG 3-2 Mechanisms whereby immature respiratory control superimposed upon poor respiratory function contributes to episodic desaturation. *FRC*, Functional residual capacity.

secondary to improved respiratory control or decreased vulnerability to hypoxia in the face of apnea.[22,23] These studies demonstrate that improvement in intermittent hypoxic episodes after red cell transfusion is manifest only after the first weeks of postnatal life and that nursing reports significantly underestimate the frequency of such cardiorespiratory events.[22,23] Obviously any benefit of packed cell transfusion on apnea, bradycardia, and desaturation must be balanced against potential hazards of transfusion.

Automated control of inspired oxygen is under study. This automated technique has been compared to routine adjustments of inspired oxygen as performed by clinical personnel in infants of 24 to 27 weeks' gestation.[24] During the automated period, time with oxygen saturation within the intended range of 87% to 93% increased significantly, and times in the hyperoxic range were significantly reduced. This was not associated with a clear benefit for hypoxic episodes; nonetheless, future refinement of this technology may prove useful to minimize intermittent hypoxia. Finally, a novel approach is supplementation of inspired air with a very low concentration of supplemental CO_2 to increase respiratory drive.[25] While of interest from a physiologic perspective, and likely to be successful in decreasing apnea, it is doubtful that this would gain widespread clinical acceptance as most preterm infants have residual lung disease and are prone to baseline hypercarbia, which may make clinicians reluctant to administer supplemental inspired CO_2.

Role of Gastroesophageal Reflux

While pharyngeal and laryngeal stimulation may trigger apnea, caution should be exercised before apnea is attributed to gastroesophageal reflux. Despite the frequent coexistence of apnea and gastroesophageal reflux in preterm infants, investigations into the timing of reflux in relation to apneic events indicate that they are not commonly temporally related.[26] Monitoring studies demonstrate that when a relationship between reflux and apnea is observed, apnea may precede rather than follow reflux.[14] This finding suggests that loss of respiratory neural output during apnea may be accompanied by a decrease in lower esophageal tone and gastroesophageal reflux. Such a phenomenon is supported by data from a newborn piglet model, in which apnea was accompanied by a fall in lower esophageal sphincter pressure. Although physiologic experiments in animals reveal that reflux of gastric contents to the larynx induces reflex apnea, no clear evidence is available showing that treatment of reflux will affect frequency of apnea in most preterm infants.[27] Therefore the pharmacologic management of reflux with agents that decrease gastric acidity or enhance gastrointestinal motility generally should be reserved for infants at specific risk, e.g., those with neurodevelopmental disability or following surgical repair of gastrointestinal anomalies. Caution is advised in preterm infants, even those who exhibit signs of emesis or regurgitation of feedings, regardless of whether apnea is present, as acid suppression therapy is associated with increased risk of neonatal sepsis. Once initiated, such treatment should be discontinued in the absence of clear clinical benefit.

Xanthine Therapy

Xanthine therapy has had a remarkable impact on neonatal care over the past 40 years. Questions remain about its mode of action in enhancing neonatal respiratory control, but its efficacy and safety are widely accepted. Of interest is its remarkable ability to decrease apnea of prematurity, which is probably not the case for apnea in later life when the generalized stimulating effect of caffeine would not be well tolerated. It appears that the neonate exhibits a selective caffeine (or theophylline)-induced stimulation of respiratory neural output without a generalized stimulant effect.

Both caffeine and theophylline can be used to treat apnea of prematurity. They have multiple physiologic and pharmacologic mechanisms of action. The ability of xanthine therapy to enhance respiratory neural output in early life is manifested by an increase in minute ventilation, improved CO_2 sensitivity, and decreased hypoxic depression of breathing. The precise pharmacologic basis for this increase in respiratory neural output is still under investigation; however, competitive antagonism of adenosine receptors is a well-documented effect of xanthines.[28] While adenosine acts as an inhibitory neuroregulator in the central nervous system via activation of adenosine A_1 receptors, activation of adenosine A_{2A} receptors appears to excite GABAergic interneurons, and released GABA may contribute to the respiratory inhibition induced by adenosine.[29] The xanthines also inhibit phosphodiesterase, which normally breaks down cyclic adenosine monophosphate (cAMP), although the relationship of cAMP accumulation with relief of apnea in infants is questionable.

These complex neurotransmitter interactions elicited by caffeine led to concerns regarding its safety, and a large multicenter trial was undertaken. The results of this study have demonstrated that caffeine treatment (used to treat apnea or enhance extubation) is effective in decreasing the rate of bronchopulmonary dysplasia (BPD) and improving the neurodevelopmental outcome at 18 to 21 months, especially in those receiving respiratory support.[30,31] There is also evidence for a reduction in developmental coordination disorder in the caffeine-treated cohort at 5 years of age.[32] It is possible that

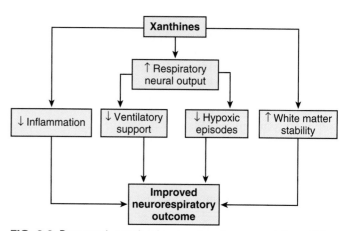

FIG 3-3 Proposed mechanisms whereby neonatal xanthine therapy benefits later outcomes.

this benefit is secondary to a decrease in apnea and resultant intermittent hypoxic episodes; however, this is speculative (Fig. 3-3).

Data in neonatal rodents demonstrate an antiinflammatory effect of caffeine in proinflammatory states elicited by postnatal hyperoxia or antenatal endotoxin exposure.[33,34] In these studies improved lung pathology and respiratory system mechanics were observed after caffeine treatment. In contrast, other data raise concerns about potential adverse effects of neonatal caffeine exposure in various animal models. Data on the effects of caffeine on the developing brain are also in conflict and include no effect in an ovine model, a protective effect in hypoxia-induced perinatal white matter injury, and an adverse effect on brain imaging.

Caffeine is traditionally administered at a 10- to 12.5-mg/kg caffeine base loading dose followed by 2.5- to 5-mg/kg caffeine base maintenance dose every 24 hours. Changes in dosing that deviate from proven beneficial protocols should proceed with caution and be the subject of prospective clinical trials. The timing of xanthine administration has already changed, and caffeine use is now widespread in a prophylactic mode.[22] Initial studies suggest that very early initiation of caffeine therapy results in improved outcome; however, these findings are based on retrospective review with potential confounders.[35] Finally, the extended use of caffeine to 40 weeks' postmenstrual age was associated with a decrease in intermittent hypoxia among a cohort of preterm infants.[36] Clearly more work is needed to further optimize caffeine therapy.

Continuous Positive Airway Pressure

Continuous positive airway pressure (CPAP) has also proven to be a relatively safe and effective therapy for over 40 years and, together with caffeine, has revolutionized apnea management in infants. It has a dual function to stabilize lung volume and improve airway patency by limiting upper airway closure. Because longer episodes of apnea frequently involve an obstructive component, CPAP appears to be effective by "splinting" the upper airway with positive pressure and decreasing the risk of pharyngeal or laryngeal obstruction.[37] At the lower functional residual capacity that accompanies many preterm infants with residual lung disease, pulmonary oxygen stores are probably reduced, and there is a very short time from cessation of breathing to onset of desaturation and bradycardia. Therefore, CPAP is likely to reduce this vulnerability to episodic desaturation.

Nasal CPAP is well tolerated in most preterm infants; however, as discussed elsewhere in this book, low- or high-flow nasal cannula therapies are being increasingly used as an equivalent treatment modality that may allow CPAP delivery while enhancing the mobility of the infant.

LONGER TERM CONSEQUENCES OF NEONATAL APNEA

Fortunately, apnea of prematurity generally resolves by about 36 to 40 weeks' postconceptional age, although in more immature infants, apnea can persist beyond this time. This is of particular relevance in those who develop BPD. Available data indicate that cardiorespiratory events in most infants return to the baseline normal level at about 43 to 44 weeks' postconceptional age.[38] In other words, beyond 43 to 44 weeks' postconceptional age, the incidence of cardiorespiratory events in preterm infants does not significantly exceed that in term babies. For a subset of infants, the persistence of cardiorespiratory events may delay hospital discharge. For a few of these infants home cardiorespiratory monitoring, until 43 to 44 weeks' postconceptional age, is offered in the United States as an alternative to a prolonged hospital stay. The absence of an obvious relationship between persistent apnea of prematurity and sudden infant death syndrome (SIDS) has significantly decreased the practice of home monitoring, with no increase in the SIDS rate.

Infants born prematurely experience multiple problems during their time in the NICU, and many of these conditions, such as apnea and resultant intermittent hypoxia, may contribute to poor neurodevelopmental outcomes. The problem of correlating apnea with outcome is compounded by the fact that nursing reports of apnea severity may be unreliable, and impedance monitoring techniques often fail to identify mixed and obstructive events. Despite these reservations, available data suggest a link between the number of days apnea and assisted ventilation were recorded during hospitalization and the impaired neurodevelopmental outcome.[39] A relationship has also been shown between a delay in resolution of apnea and bradycardia beyond 36 weeks' corrected age and a higher incidence of unfavorable neurodevelopmental outcome.[40]

Studies might better focus on the incidence and severity of desaturation events, as techniques for long-term collection of pulse oximetry data are now advanced and can provide higher

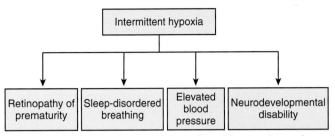

FIG 3-4 Proposed morbidities attributable to intermittent hypoxia in the neonatal period, childhood, or adolescence.

resolution of desaturations in monitored patients. Furthermore, it is likely that recurrent hypoxia is the detrimental feature of the potential longer term abnormalities exhibited by preterm infants. The incidence of intermittent hypoxic episodes in preterm infants is relatively low during the first week of life and then increases rapidly and is sustained over several weeks.[41] This time course may correspond to a postnatal rise in peripheral chemosensitivity and resultant respiratory instability as discussed earlier. Figure 3-4 summarizes proposed morbidities that might be attributable to intermittent hypoxic episodes in early life.[42] These proposed clinical consequences of neonatal intermittent hypoxia need to be correlated with physiology studies that document any modulatory effects upon neuronal plasticity related to peripheral and/or central respiratory control mechanisms. We are currently learning a lot from ongoing studies in cohorts of former preterm infants. For example, the incidence of sleep-disordered breathing is exceedingly high in children born prematurely regardless of whether they were randomized to caffeine vs placebo therapy.[43] Elevated blood pressure is seen in prematurely born adolescents.[44] Is this the result of intermittent hypoxia-induced inflammatory changes in the vasculature[45]? Much work remains to be done to elicit the biological basis for the sequelae we observe in preterm infants and the roles of both respiratory control and ventilatory management in their pathogenesis.

REFERENCES

A complete reference list is available at https://expertconsult .inkling.com/.

4

Ethical Issues in Assisted Ventilation of the Neonate

Julie Weiner, MD, Jessica Brunkhorst, MD, and John D. Lantos, MD

INTRODUCTION

For over half a century doctors have struggled with the ethical dilemmas surrounding assisted ventilation. The biggest controversies have been around the groups of babies who have very high predicted mortality and morbidity. There are three relatively distinct groups of babies who meet these criteria: (1) babies born at the threshold of viability; (2) babies born with severe and life-limiting anomalies; and (3) babies who develop severe neurologic injury during the first days and weeks of life or who develop irreversible pulmonary failure as a result of prolonged assisted ventilation. There is some overlap between these groups. These infants have been the subject of many legal cases over the years. Some of the more famous cases were those involving Baby Doe, a baby with Down syndrome and esophageal atresia who was born in Indiana in 1982;[1] Baby K, a baby born with anencephaly who developed respiratory distress;[2] and Baby Miller, a baby born at the borderline of viability whose parents objected to life-sustaining treatment.[3] These cases, in turn, led to federal legislation, more court cases, and ongoing ethical debates.

Over time, these debates and discussions have led to changes in the acceptable norms for initiating and for withdrawing mechanical ventilation (and other forms of life support). The fundamental question, however, has remained the same: "Which neonates should be provided life support (i.e., assisted ventilation)?"

This question can be divided into two types of questions. The first is procedural rather than substantive. Who is empowered to decide for the neonate? Neonates are unable to make these decisions for themselves. Therefore, the decisions are more complicated than comparable decisions for competent adults. In those cases, the adult (if competent) can decide for himself or herself. In neonates, the decision always needs to be made by another person.

The second type of question is substantive, rather than procedural. Under what circumstances should such decisions be considered legally acceptable and ethically justifiable? There is now a strong consensus in the medical, legal, and ethical literature that such decisions should be guided by considerations of what is in the best interests of the infant. That is, neither parents nor physicians should make decisions that violate the interests of the infant.[4] This is a historical shift from the days when infants were seen as the property of the parents without any independent rights of their own. Today, they are patients (and human beings) in their own right.[5] The implication is that, although parents should continue to be involved in decision making for their children, they do not have an absolute right to refuse or require medical treatment for their infant. The child's best interest, and that alone, should direct medical care.

Of note, this discussion will focus on assisted ventilation, but the reasoning process and the ethical considerations that we will discuss could easily be applied to situations involving any other life-support device or life-saving therapy.

Regarding neonatal resuscitation, the American Heart Association and the American Academy of Pediatrics jointly issued guidelines about when mechanical ventilation and resuscitation are not medically indicated. They state that treatment should be withheld when the likely outcome is almost certain early death or survival with unacceptably high morbidity.[6] They further specify the situations in which these conditions are met as follows: "Extreme prematurity (gestational age <23 weeks or birth weight <400 g), anencephaly, and some major chromosomal abnormalities, such as trisomy 13." They also discuss "conditions associated with uncertain prognosis in which survival is borderline, the morbidity rate is relatively high, and the anticipated burden to the child is high." In such situations, they recommend that parents should be allowed to decide whether to provide resuscitation and mechanical ventilation.

Translated into practice, that standard means that if the burden on the infant is overwhelming or the prospects are extremely bleak—as is true, for example, in the presence of a lethal abnormality or the birth of an extremely premature very low birth-weight infant—there is no obligation to subject the child to further procedures.[7] In such cases, the parents' decision to omit further treatment is to be respected. Alternatively, if out of ignorance, fear, misguided pessimism, or simple refusal to accept a compromised infant, parents were to decline relatively low-level, high-benefit interventions that would save the life of a child, even if the child were likely to survive with some permanent but not devastating neurocognitive impairment, there is no question that the physicians should treat.

Understanding the historical viewpoints and the past half-century of shifting practice patterns is important in developing the ethical considerations in assisted ventilation of the neonate. This is best done by reviewing some of the landmark medical–legal cases and pivotal research studies over the past 50 years that have not only shaped our present model of care but also, at times, challenged our perspective on how best to care for seriously compromised infants.

HISTORICAL BACKGROUND

Initiating Ventilator Support

Deciding to initiate ventilator support and other life-sustaining therapies in the neonate presents unique challenges unparalleled elsewhere in medicine. Often, the discussion begins and prognostication occurs before the health care provider can even lay eyes on the patient. If the mother presents in advanced labor, there may not be the luxury of time before a decision must be made. Additionally, the emotions, pain, and exhaustion of childbirth can cloud logic and reasoning for all parties involved. Sometimes the decision is clear cut and easy; a full-term infant with meconium aspiration will clearly benefit from assisted ventilation, should he or she develop respiratory failure. Other situations quickly challenge the principles of beneficence and nonmaleficence. Are we doing more harm or good by intubating an extremely preterm infant born at 23 weeks? Will we cause undue suffering by initiating assisted ventilation in an infant with trisomy 13 and multiple congenital anomalies? Would comfort care be more appropriate in these situations? As John Paris and colleagues state, "society's role is to assure that the patient is not undertreated by the omission of beneficial therapies or overtreated with unwanted or unwarranted interventions."[8]

Whenever possible, discussions should occur with the family prior to the time of delivery. This is more easily accomplished in the case of prenatally diagnosed congenital anomalies and genetic disorders than with an unanticipated preterm delivery. It may be beneficial for all the parties who will be involved in the care of the child to meet with the family and on multiple occasions, when possible. For example, in the case of a complex congenital heart lesion, meeting with cardiology, cardiovascular surgery, neonatology, genetics, feeding specialists, etc., may provide the parents with a more complete picture and help them to make an educated and informed choice about their wishes for their child. In all prenatal counseling the caveat must be included that all information will not be available until after the infant is born and even the best laid out plans may change.

For the extremely preterm infant, right or wrong, decisions and discussions about initiating ventilator support usually begin with gestational age. But it should be noted that even under the best circumstances, dating via ultrasound is accurate only at ±7 to 10 days.[9,10] Nonetheless, above 25 weeks' gestation, most clinicians will provide resuscitation and life-sustaining therapies. Below 22 weeks, few would intervene aggressively and comfort care would be provided. The "gray zone" of 22 to 24 weeks is where ethical dilemmas typically occur. Other factors, such as antenatal corticosteroid exposure, sex, weight, and multiples, have also been shown to significantly influence outcomes for extremely preterm infants in addition to gestational age.[11] The National Institute of Child Health and Human Development has developed a website with an online calculator to estimate mortality/morbidity risks for extremely preterm infants and assist providers in counseling parents.[12] While this tool provides a useful starting point, it is only a report of population statistics derived from major academic centers and does not estimate the outcome for an individual infant. Outcome data also vary widely from country to country and from hospital to hospital and may be affected by publication time lag.[13]

If the decision is made to initiate ventilator support, it is important to recognize that the discussion does not stop there. Communication between the medical team and the family must be ongoing. The infant's condition and best interests must be constantly reassessed. If assisted ventilation is deemed to be no longer in the infant's best interest, withdrawal of ventilator support is an ethically justifiable option.

Withdrawal (Nonescalation) of Ventilator Support

Withdrawal of care, specifically removal of assisted ventilation, has become the most frequent mode of death for neonates in the neonatal intensive care unit (NICU).[14] But that was not always the case. In a landmark article in the *New England Journal of Medicine*, Duff and Campbell first described the rare practice of withdrawal of care in 1973.[15] Since that time the practice has become a common occurrence that health care providers face in the NICU. At the time, the courts had not addressed the issue of whether it was legally permissible to withhold or withdraw life-sustaining treatment. Nevertheless, Duff and Campbell recommended that such decisions were permissible and that they should be made privately by parents and doctors together. That recommendation has been adopted by most bioethicists and professional societies, within limits. Two publications, the Nuffield Council on Bioethics' extensive report in Britain on "Critical Care Decisions in Fetal and Neonatal Medicine"[16] and the 2007 policy statement of the American Academy of Pediatrics (AAP) on "Noninitiation or withdrawal of intensive care for high-risk newborns,"[17] take the position that there are times when withdrawal of care is appropriate. Generally, two driving themes guide decisions regarding withdrawal of care. One is the anticipated quality of life of potential survivors. The other is the perception that treatment is medically futile. The same principles apply to nonescalation of ventilator support as to withdrawal. Nonescalation is generally applied to situations in which parents do not want to withdraw life support but they recognize that further escalation of treatment may simply prolong the dying process.[18] In such situations, doctors may continue ventilation but not monitor blood gases, adjust ventilator settings, or change to more aggressive approaches such as high-frequency or jet ventilation.

Quality of Life

There are two issues in any discussion about quality of life (QoL) in neonates. The first is about prognostication. Generally, we make decisions based not upon the infants' current QoL but based on our best prediction of what their QoL is likely to be in the future. Such predictions have well-described margins of error. For example, in a study, many infants who had an Apgar score of 0 at 10 min not only survived, but when they were of school age, they had no disability.[19]

The second issue related to QoL focuses on the ways in which we define and assess an individual's QoL. Again, the issues for young children are quite different from those for adults. For adults, we can simply ask them. For young children, others must make a determination based on objectively measurable or observable factors. Payot and Barrington reviewed the sorts of scales that are available to measure QoL.[20] They write, "The scales that are available to measure quality of life make comparisons between different health states, evaluate the effectiveness of medical interventions, and describe the life trajectories of individuals or groups." They go on to note that any assessment of QoL necessarily requires many different types of data, including objective facts, social relationships, family structure, physical health, mental abilities, and many other factors. In some cases, a divergence between objective measures of disability or impairment and a subjective measure of self-assessed well-being has, in adults, led to what has been described as "the disability paradox."[21] By this paradox, a life with severe functional limitations may be considered of high quality by the individual him- or herself but of very limited quality to external observers. Of this phenomenon, Payot and Barrington write,

> The fact that even impaired survivors can view their lives in a positive light has been dismissed as "making lemonade" by some commenters. We feel, in contrast, that it is a cause for celebration that individuals with impairments (lemons) can nevertheless find value and meaning in their lives (and make lemonade). Such resilience should not be dismissed, but should not at the same time impede our efforts to investigate methods to reduce such impairments .... We can illustrate the gulf which sometimes may exist between subjective and objective evaluations of QoL with studies regarding the QoL of infants with meningomyelocele, who have multiple functional problems in the long term, but have a QoL which they themselves find to be good or very good, including those who are wheelchair bound and incontinent.

Medical Futility

The concept of futile care is hard to define and is controversial. Efforts to prolong life, once considered an outcome of healing, may now be viewed by some as harmful acts of prolonging suffering. The early literature on medical futility challenged the "life at all cost" stance. In the now classic 1974 *JAMA* article by Richard McCormick, a renowned Jesuit moral theologian, entitled "To Save or Let Die: The Dilemma of Modern Medicine,"[22] McCormick argued there was no moral obligation to force treatment on a patient who was dying or who was totally dependent on intrusive measures to sustain life, and there was no obligation to do so for a patient who had no possibility for meaningful relationships. That stance has continued to prevail and has influenced nearly every group that has attempted to set standards and guidelines directed at the care of the dying neonate.

An increasingly difficult conundrum in medicine has arisen owing to a shift to a consumer-driven model: what does a physician do when a request for treatment is believed to be futile, ineffective, or inappropriate. This issue first appeared in the literature when Paris and colleagues wrote of a case in which the physicians at Boston Children's Hospital who had cared for a profoundly compromised baby for some 23 months refused a mother's request to put her child once again on a ventilator.[23] This case was one of the first cases in the literature to highlight a growing issue in which physicians were being requested to provide medical therapies believed to be futile. Prior to this the demand for certain treatments had been viewed as simply requests, such as antibiotics for viral infections or a computed tomography scan for routine headaches. Most physicians agree that such treatment ought not to be given, but with increasing practice constraints and parental demands, many found it easier to just go along with the requests that were perceived as harmless. However, that approach is flawed. The role of the physician was changed from one with knowledge and expertise to one that responded to whatever the patient preferred. Over time, the requests escalated into demands for more and more exotic and inappropriate treatments. With the shift to a consumer-driven model for health care came the belief that informed consent and patient autonomy implied not only that patients had the

right to accept or reject certain therapies, but also that patients had the right to choose whatever treatment they desire. In the minds of some bioethicists, such as Veatch and Spicer,[24] patient autonomy, or the right of self-determination, dictates that families have a right to demand whatever life-prolonging therapies they want, and that physicians are obligated to provide it, even if the request "deviates intolerably" from established standards or is, from the physician's perspective, "grossly inappropriate." Veatch and Spicer's position would require the physician to unrelentingly inflict aggressive procedures and treatments on infants if requested to do so by the parents despite the overwhelming evidence that the interventions cannot relieve or change the child's devastating condition. Robert Truog, the director of clinical ethics at Harvard Medical School, also supports this position. In an essay, he states that doctors should honor the family's choices on end-of-life care "even when we believe their decisions are wrong."[25] However, these approaches create great moral distress, when families seek treatments that are not in the best interest of the child or are seen as prolonging suffering.

Since 2005, physicians have lashed out against such stances and the notion that patients have the right to demand inappropriate care. Even for simple requests, the medical community has pushed for and educated against antibiotic use for viral infections, with success. This has led some physicians to ask if they are, in fact, obligated to do what they believe to be futile or ineffective. The Nuffield Council on Bioethics[26] and the AAP[16] make it very clear that newborns are to be treated as any other patient—on the basis of their best interest. This position implies that although parents may and should continue to be involved in decision making for their children, they do not have the exclusive right to refuse—or to demand—medical treatment for the child. To avoid clashes between parents and physicians on treatment choices, it is advisable, whenever possible, that there be a joint discussion that involves the parents and the medical care team with regard to survival rates, outcomes, and severity of potential disabilities. It is important that the family receive consistent information from all providers.

The "futility" debate has mainly centered around end-of-life treatments, specifically cardiopulmonary resuscitation (CPR) and the need for "do not resuscitate" orders.[27] It is now well understood that for certain patient populations there is near 100% mortality.[28] Blackhall[29] states that, even if the family requests CPR, the physician should decline to provide it in these situations. Futility is generally applied to an acute setting, when the medical condition has deteriorated to a point at which further increase in aggressive medical treatment, such as CPR, would not change the impending death. In cases in which death is imminent, there has been an increased emphasis on providing a "peaceful death." A study by Wall and Partridge[30] reveals that in the face of imminent death, most neonatologists recommend the withdrawal or withholding of treatment. A study found that, even though withdrawal of care at the end of life had remained constant over 10 years, withholding treatment had increased while the use of CPR in an unstable, dying neonate had decreased.[31] Most of the change seen in management of death seemed likely to be due to a change in physicians' practice. In 2000 and 2003, statements from the AAP and the Institute of Medicine called for improvement in care for the dying neonate, creating greater awareness among caregivers regarding the end-of-life process.[32,33] More recently, the AAP Committee on Fetus and Newborn[17] again noted there is no ethical difference between withdrawal and withholding of an intervention. When death is imminent or medical care is considered futile, the goal is to provide a peaceful, controlled setting for the infant and family.

Are These Debates Resolvable?

The medical literature regarding "medical futility" and "quality of life" continues to grow. But disagreements persist about what these terms mean or what implications they convey. For medical futility, Younger[34] has asked: Does it signify absolute impossibility? Is it purely physiologic? Does it include the ability to achieve only a heartbeat but not to achieve discharge from the hospital? For QoL, Younger and others colleagues[17] questioned whether it is ever possible to assess another person's QoL. All assessments seem to incorporate problematic considerations about social value and cultural values. Lantos et al. noted that even among physicians there is no consensus on these terms.[34] Physicians disagree on the chances of success, the goals of therapies, and the prediction of long-term outcomes. Some declare a treatment futile only if the chance of success is 0%, whereas others view a treatment as futile if the success rate is <10%, and even others view it so if the success rate is as high as 18%. Others consider a treatment futile if all it can hope to provide is a couple of days in an intensive care unit. On the other hand, "[s]uch a goal can be of supreme value to a dying patient or the patient's family."[35]

There are similar disagreements about QoL. Many doctors, for example, consider the QoL that is associated with trisomy 18 to be so terrible that death is preferable.[36] Many parents disagree.[37] The lack of agreement on the meaning of medical futility and QoL, along with the varied use of both terms, makes it increasingly difficult to develop guidelines to assist the clinician in deciding to remove assisted ventilation in a particular neonate. Hackler and Hiller, in their article about a devastated child who was forced to undergo repeated resuscitation attempts because of parental requests pleaded for a better approach and compassion for treating the dying child.[38] It is not the aggressive intervention at all costs approach but the patient's response to treatment and continued best interests of the newborn that should direct our care.

Chronic Ventilation

As technology and survival for some of the most fragile neonatal patients improve, so do the ability and need for chronic ventilation. The prevalence of home mechanical ventilation for children is 5-6.3/100,000.[39] The 2005 pediatric census in Massachusetts showed a threefold increase in the number of children needing chronic respiratory ventilation compared to the previous 15-year interval census.[40] The number needing long-term ventilation can only be expected to rise in the future as technologies improve and are applied to a broader patient population. In the neonate, it is no longer only infants with complications related to prematurity, such as severe bronchopulmonary dysplasia (BPD), needing tracheostomy and prolonged mechanical ventilation, but those with a host of neonatal conditions that can lead to the final common pathway of ventilator dependence. Children with congenital anomalies, neuromuscular diseases, congenital or perinatal acquired neurologic disorders, and craniofacial anomalies now compose the majority of those with tracheostomy and long-term ventilation needs.[41-44] Chronic lung disease due to prematurity represents only 7% to 29% of children needing long-term ventilation in

recent population studies.[38,39,45] However, a study showed that, in ~58% of the infants who needed tracheostomy for prolonged mechanical ventilation in the NICU, the underlying disease was BPD.[46] Long-term ventilation consumes a large allocation of resources both for hospitals and for communities.[47] These fragile infants require prolonged hospitalization, home equipment, home nursing, and frequent readmissions, and up to one-third of patients live in acute or long-term care facilities.[39,40,43]

Infants needing long-term ventilation are at a high risk for morbidities and mortality. There is uncertainty in the prognosis, length of therapy, and outcomes of these infants. The 5-year survival rate for infants with tracheostomy and chronic ventilation is approximately 80%.[48,49] Reports show that half of the deaths are unexpected, acute events, such as dislodged or plugged tracheostomy tube, and were not related to an underlying disease process.[48,50] The 5-year decannulation rate reported is ~25%.[48,50] Children with chronic lung disease had the highest rate of successful decannulation.[50] Of the children able to be decannulated, the mean time needing ventilation was 24 to 39 months.[38,47] However, reports suggest that if a child is not off of positive-pressure ventilation by 5 years and decannulated by 6 years of age, there is little chance of tolerating removal of the ventilator after that age (<10%).[47] These children also face developmental impairments, with 14% having extremely delayed neurocognition.[49]

Uncertain prognosis, unknown length of treatment, and high risk of death for infants needing long-term ventilation can pose many ethical dilemmas for both providers and families. Performing a tracheostomy and providing long-term ventilation from infancy, with the potential for lifelong ventilator dependency, can cause great moral distress. Other ethical dilemmas surround which patient population to offer chronic ventilation and should family dynamics factor in the decision. It may seem more acceptable to offer long-term ventilation to patients who have a chance of decannulation versus patients with life-limiting conditions, such as trisomy 13. However, it is hard to state that diagnosis alone should drive the decision on which patients receive chronic ventilation. Family wishes should also be factored into the decision, but how does that work when there is a difficult family structure with limited resources? Does that mean the child is placed in medical foster care when families are unable to provide care for their medically complex child or a child is placed in a long-term care facility? These are difficult decisions that families and medical care providers face.

Appropriate Care after Withdrawal of Life Support

One of the other moral issues facing physicians involved in the withdrawal of medical treatments is to assure the patient and family that the withdrawal will not produce suffering for the patient and ensuring the medical team will not abandon them.[51] As Civet[52] notes, pain during the end of life is of particular concern. With regard to the withdrawal of mechanical ventilation, care should be directed toward avoiding air hunger or dyspnea. This may present as gasping or struggle in the patient. To prevent these events physicians should be willing to provide analgesic and/or antianxiety medication. The goal of these medications is symptom relief, not death, and the physician should provide the appropriate dose to relieve the symptoms but not to cause apnea.

Families have described the feeling of abandonment[53] by the health care team once the decision was made to withdraw care. The death of a child is the most difficult thing a family may experience; the health care team can have an impact on the lasting memories of their child's final moments, both positively and negatively. It should always be the goal to provide the support the family needs during this difficult time. Chaplains, palliative care teams, and bereavement programs can help provide comfort to the families. In making a decision, what is called for is not rigid rules but a realistic assessment of the infant's physical prospects based on current data from the medical literature, as well as outcome data. Acknowledging different cultural norms and family values is also important. As in all medical decision making, the primary consideration in treatment decisions for newborns is and continues to be a commitment to act in the best interests of the patient.

Finally, doctors should always be aware of the possibility that a child will not die after "life support" has been withdrawn. This was famously true of Karen Ann Quinlan, a case that led to a landmark legal decision.[54] In that case, the doctors testified in court that the withdrawal of mechanical ventilation would lead to Ms. Quinlan's death. After the ventilator was withdrawn, she survived for 7 years.[55] This has happened in pediatric cases as well and can lead to moral distress, distrust, and communication problems.[56]

CONCLUSION

Despite most literature and legal cases, highlighting the ethical challenges when families and health care providers disagree about the needed treatment or the withdrawal of treatment, most decisions are faced together. The parents and providers, together, face the difficult ethical dilemmas that arise daily for fragile, medically complex neonates. In every situation open, honest communication should take place among all caregivers, including the family. Starting the dialog early in the course helps facilitate trust and respect between the medical care team and the family. Other impartial groups, such as ethics committees or palliative care teams, provide useful tools to help guide and support the medical team and families when making tough medical decisions. Pediatric studies looking at the parents' perspective in end-of-life care have identified six common priorities during the dying process, which are honest information, empowered decision making, parental care, faith, pain control, and emotional expression and support from staff.[16-18,57,58] Parents need to know the health care team will not abandon them in the final moments of their child's life. Parents are not asking physicians to perform miracles but simply to show that their child has worth and value regardless of diagnosis. Whether it is the noninitiation, nonescalation, or active withdrawal of mechanical ventilation, the most we can do as physicians is keep the infant comfortable, comfort and support the family, and be present with them in the last moments of their child's life.

REFERENCES

A complete reference list is available at https://expertconsult.inkling.com.

5

Evidence-Based Respiratory Care

Krithika Lingappan, MD, MS, FAAP, and Gautham K. Suresh, MD, DM, MS, FAAP

BACKGROUND

Clinicians caring for infants with respiratory disease should make diagnoses, choose treatments, and counsel parents based on the best evidence available (preferably from high-quality research studies) while still using clinical judgment, patient values, and knowledge of the local circumstances. This approach, known as evidence-based medicine (EBM), discourages the sole use of less reliable "sources of truth" such as reasoning based on anatomy or pathophysiology, extrapolation from animal data, expert opinion that is not based on evidence, or adoption of a practice because peers and colleagues use it. Although the principles and steps of evidence-based practice are well described, it is common for diagnostic tests and treatments to be overused, underused, or misused. Therefore clinicians providing respiratory care should become proficient in using the tools and skills of evidence-based practice. The technical skills for EBM, listed in the order they are used, are framing a question; searching for evidence; assessing its quality; weighing risks, benefits, and costs; and implementation. In addition to these technical skills, several cognitive tools are also required to practice EBM, such as critical thinking, clinical reasoning, and decision making, particularly decision making in the face of uncertainty. EBM can be used to make decisions about the care of an individual patient, or for creating a guideline or protocol for the care of a defined category of patients (such as preterm infants with respiratory distress syndrome).

THE TECHNICAL STEPS OF EBM

Formulating the Question

The first step in practicing EBM is to clearly delineate the clinical question. The components of a well-formulated question are patients, population, or problem (P); the intervention (I); the control or comparison (C); the outcomes of interest (O); and the type of study or Time frame (T). These can be remembered with the acronym PICOT.[1] An example of a PICOT question is "In preterm infants of less than 28 weeks' gestation with respiratory distress syndrome (P), does the prophylactic use of vitamin A (I) compared to placebo (C) reduce the risk of bronchopulmonary dysplasia (O) *at 36 weeks post-menstrual age (T)*? The best type of study (T) to answer this question is a randomized controlled trial."

Searching for the Evidence

Once a clear question is formulated, the clinician should then perform a search for all the relevant evidence. Collaborating with a medical librarian can ensure that the search is efficient and comprehensive, identifying all key published articles, abstracts, and reviews. The search can be performed using

several electronic databases. The best known of these is MEDLINE (a bibliographic database of life sciences with a concentration on biomedicine), which can be accessed either using the free interface, PubMed (www.pubmed.gov), or through a proprietary interface such as Ovid. A particularly useful feature in PubMed is the "Clinical Queries" tab, which allows a user-friendly, quick, and focused search on a given topic that can help the clinician make informed decisions. There are three search filters available in Clinical Queries: clinical study categories (etiology, diagnosis, therapy, prognosis, and clinical prediction guides), systematic reviews, and medical genetics. Although MEDLINE contains millions of articles, it may still not contain all the relevant articles, and if an exhaustive search is essential, other databases such as CINAHL (an index of journal articles in nursing, allied health, biomedicine, and health care) and EMBASE (a biomedical and pharmacologic database of published literature) should also be searched. To identify unpublished abstracts (an important but often overlooked source of evidence), the proceedings and published abstracts (usually available online) of pediatric or neonatology conferences such as the Pediatric Academic Societies Meeting or the American Academy of Pediatrics National Conference and Exhibition should also be searched. Google Scholar is another Web-based search tool that searches the World Wide Web. In addition to published articles, it also identifies conference proceedings, books, and institutional repositories. It may serve as an adjunct but cannot replace a systematic search of a more comprehensive database such as MEDLINE.[2] Other online sources of information include TRIP (tripdatabase.com), which is a clinical search engine designed to allow users to quickly find high-quality relevant evidence. Finally, the reference lists of full-text articles obtained from the electronic search should also be hand-searched to identify additional relevant articles.

Evidence identified through the search may fall into one of two categories: primary sources (i.e., original articles and abstracts) and reviews or summaries ("predigested sources") of existing evidence on a given topic or question. Among such reviews, conventional narrative reviews (similar to textbook chapters) can provide useful background information about the topic but are subject to the biases and viewpoints of the authors. Therefore systematic reviews are preferred because their explicit methodology and transparency allow readers to replicate the methods and draw their own conclusions and inferences. The Cochrane Database of Systematic Reviews is a particularly useful source of high-quality systematic reviews in neonatology, and the full text of these reviews is available freely on the website of the National Institute of Child Health and

Human Development (www.nichd.nih.gov/Cochrane). Only human studies/trials are included in Cochrane reviews—they do not cover studies in animal or mechanical models. For other primary articles and reviews, the full text of each article can be obtained from the journal's website, without a fee in some cases, and in other cases by an individual subscription or an institutional library subscription.

The search is typically performed by entering keywords (e.g., using the Medical Subject Headings—MeSH—database in PubMed) and using Boolean operators ("OR," "AND," and "NOT") to restrict the results to the most relevant articles. Custom search filters can be used to narrow the search by criteria such as study type, publication period, or type of journal.

In addition to performing searches for the evidence around specific clinical questions, clinicians should also develop good habits of keeping up-to-date with emerging evidence. With several thousand medical articles published each year, it is impossible for any clinician to read or even skim each published article or its abstract. Clinicians can keep up-to-date by subscribing to periodic updates from databases such as PubMed, RSS feeds, listservs managed by universities or scientific organizations, and table of content (TOC) alerts from journals. They can also regularly peruse websites such as www.neoknowledge.com and www.ebneo.org.

Once the search is completed and the relevant articles have been obtained, the next task is to evaluate the evidence to determine whether and how it can be used in decision making.

Evaluating Evidence about Therapy
Evaluating the Quality of Evidence

Determining the quality of evidence requires each article or abstract to be critically appraised, and to do this the clinician should be aware of the strengths and weaknesses of different study designs. Table 5-1 summarizes the most common types of study designs and the advantages and disadvantages of each. Observational studies are useful for hypothesis generation, and randomized trials are best for hypothesis testing. Most of our current knowledge about risk factors and exposures that result in disease or poor outcomes comes from observational studies. Most of our current knowledge about therapies comes from trials.

Earlier systems of grading the quality of evidence relied almost exclusively on overall study design and ranked the evidence in a pyramid based on study design, with systematic

TABLE 5-1   Study Designs

Type of Study	Description	Advantages	Disadvantages
Intervention Studies (Trials)			
Randomized controlled trial	Subjects are allocated to either the intervention (experimental) group or a comparison (control) group by a pure chance process. The two groups are followed prospectively for a specified period of time and then compared in terms of outcome measures specified at the outset. Can be a parallel group trial or crossover trial. Useful to study the efficacy of an intervention in preventing or altering the course of a disease and to identify causes or risk factors or subjects at high risk.	Controls for major biases. Likely to yield valid results. Useful to detect small differences between groups.	Results may sometimes not be generalizable. Complex and expensive to conduct.
Cluster randomized trial	Instead of individual subjects, an entire group or a neonatal unit or a community is randomly assigned to intervention and control groups.	Avoids inadvertent exposure of control subjects to intervention ("contamination").	Usually unblinded. Potential for recruitment bias. Can generate difficult ethical challenges. Requires statistical analysis that adjusts for nonindependence of observations within a cluster.
Non-randomized trial	Allocation of subjects to experimental intervention and control group occurs by nonrandom methods. Useful to study the efficacy of an intervention in preventing or altering the course of a disease and to identify causes or risk factors or subjects at high risk. However, can be subject to bias.		Can suffer from selection bias.
Observational Studies			
Cohort study	The course of a group of individuals is followed forward over time to monitor the natural history of a disease, to determine prognosis, or to identify causes of disease. Can be prospective or retrospective. The researcher does not influence the exposure of the subjects to treatment or other interventions; exposure is not intentional. Good design to determine the natural history of the disease and to identify causes or risk factors or subjects at high risk	Can establish causation, determines incidence. Can match for known confounders.	Needs considerable time and resources (although less expensive than randomized trials), controls may be difficult to find, difficult to study rare disorders, subject to bias.
Case–control study	Subjects with the disease or outcome of interest (cases) are compared to a group of subjects without the disease (controls). The frequency of causal or risk factors (exposures) in cases relative to controls is determined and expressed as the odds ratio. Always retrospective. Careful selection of controls is required to avoid bias. Useful to identify causes or risk factors or subjects at high risk.	Less expensive, can be performed quickly, requires fewer patients, useful for rare diseases and when interval between exposure and outcome is long, can study multiple exposures.	Improper selection of controls can introduce bias, inefficient for rare exposures, temporal relationship may be difficulty to establish, cannot derive incidence, subject to recall bias.

TABLE 5-1	Study Designs—cont'd		
Type of Study	Description	Advantages	Disadvantages
Cross-sectional study	Individuals with a defined disease, risk factor, or other condition of interest are identified at a point in time (a "snapshot"). Exposure and outcome are determined simultaneously. Good design to estimate prevalence of the condition, which is calculated as the number of individuals with the condition divided by the total number in the sample. Useful to identify causes or risk factors or subjects at high risk.	Inexpensive and easy to perform.	Cannot establish causation. Exposure and outcome may depend on recall. Sample sizes or groups could be unequal.
Ecologic study	An observational study is conducted at a population level rather than an individual level. Differences in outcome between populations or over time are related to population characteristics that could be risk (or preventive) factors.	Inexpensive. Can potentially use data from existing databases.	Unable to assess how many exposed subjects actually develop the outcome. Tends to overestimate the degree of correlation.
Case series	Description of features of a coherent/consecutive set of cases.	Provides useful description of rare conditions. May be followed by clinical trials.	In the absence of controls, cannot assess risk factors and exposures or draw inferences about efficacy of treatments.
Case report	Reports a rare or interesting finding in a single patient.	Useful to raise awareness of a potential complication of treatment or an unusual presentation or course of a disease.	Does not provide generalizable knowledge.

reviews occupying the apex of the pyramid (and comprising the best evidence) and reasoning from physiology or expert opinion occupying the base of the pyramid (the least reliable form of evidence).

Currently, the quality of evidence is best evaluated using the criteria of the GRADE (grading of recommendations, assessment, development, and evaluation) system (Table 5-2). In this system, study design remains a critical, but not the sole, factor in judging the quality of evidence. Additional criteria are incorporated into a judgment of the quality of the evidence. Also, the quality of evidence is assigned for each outcome, not for each study.

Applying the GRADE method to the evidence from therapeutic interventions involves five distinct steps[3]:

Step 1: Assign an a priori ranking of "high quality" to randomized controlled trials (RCTs) and "low quality" to observational studies.

Step 2: Downgrade or upgrade initial ranking.

Reasons to downgrade the quality of evidence for RCTs include:

- Risk of bias—due to lack of clearly randomized allocation sequence, lack of blinding, lack of allocation concealment, failure to adhere to intention-to-treat analysis, large losses to follow-up, early cessation of the trial, or selective outcome reporting.
- Imprecision—wide confidence intervals.
- Indirectness—extrapolation of results from a different population, outcome, or intervention or indirect comparison of two interventions (i.e., not a head-to-head comparison).
- Inconsistency of results—when the results vary significantly across trials without explanation.
- Publication bias—when studies with negative results are not published (this can bias the results of the review).

The quality of evidence for an observational study can be upgraded if there was a large magnitude of effect, a dose–response relationship is noted, and all plausible biases would only reduce the treatment effect noted in the study (suggesting that the actual effect is likely to be larger than the study results suggest).

TABLE 5-2	GRADE (Grading of Recommendations, Assessment, Development, and Evaluations) System
Quality of Evidence	Definition
High	Further research is very unlikely to change our confidence in the estimate of effect. • Several high-quality studies with consistent results • In special cases: one large, high-quality multicenter trial
Moderate	Further research is likely to have an important impact on our confidence in the estimate of effect and may change the estimate. • One high-quality study • Several studies with some limitations
Low	Further research is very likely to have an important impact on our confidence in the estimate of effect and is likely to change the estimate. • One or more studies with severe limitations
Very low	Any estimate of effect is very uncertain. • Expert opinion • No direct research evidence • One or more studies with very severe limitations

Step 3: Assign a final grade for the quality of evidence as high, moderate, low, or very low.

Step 4: Consider other factors, such as side effects of therapy, patient preference, and cost-effectiveness, that affect the strength of recommendation.

Step 5: Make the recommendation for the actual implementation of the therapy in the form of a strong or weak recommendation to either use or not use the therapy.

Determining the Quantitative Effects of a Therapy

The *p* value: Clinical studies that use hypothesis testing rely on tests of statistical significance and often derive a *p* value to answer the question "Are the observed results purely due to chance?" The *p* value indicates the probability of obtaining a result as extreme as or more extreme than the result noted in the study, if the null hypothesis were true. If the *p* value is smaller than the threshold set by the investigators (conventionally chosen to be 0.05 or 5%) the null hypothesis is rejected in favor of the alternate hypothesis, and the result is said to be "statistically significant." A large *p* value indicates that the null hypothesis cannot be rejected.

Statistical versus clinical significance: Even if the results in a study are *statistically* significant, they may not necessarily be *clinically* significant. For example, in trials with a large sample size, statistical testing may show significance, but the results may not be clinically significant—the overall impact may be minuscule, the benefits may not outweigh the risks, and the costs of intervention may not be justifiable. Conversely, a lack of statistical significance (a high *p* value) could be the result of an inadequate sample size that led to a true effect not being detected in the study.

Confidence intervals: The confidence interval (CI) represents the degree of uncertainty in estimating the population parameter owing to sampling error. Because the results of almost all studies are derived from sample data (and not from the entire population), the sample parameter may vary from the true population parameter and may vary in its degree of precision. The CI quantifies this imprecision. It indicates the range of values that is likely to include the "true" result of a study. It is most commonly reported as 95% CI. The values for the 95% CI imply that if a study were repeated 100 times, the measured statistical parameter would fall within the interval 95 of 100 times. Narrow CIs indicate greater precision in the results. If the CI is wide, it implies that the "true value" lies somewhere within a large range of values. Therefore if a study found no differences in outcomes between groups being compared, examination of the CIs can help clinicians assess whether there was indeed no true difference between the two groups or whether the lack of difference noted was the result of a small sample size. The value that shows "no effect" for ratios (odds ratio, relative risk) is 1 and for differences (risk difference, etc.) is 0. If the value of the measured outcome that signifies "no effect" (1 for ratio and 0 for absolute difference) lies outside the CI, then it represents statistical significance.

Composite endpoints: Composite endpoints (in which multiple types of undesirable outcomes are combined into a single measurement) are commonly used in neonatology, either to jointly measure multiple negative outcomes or because one negative outcome such as death does not allow the other adverse outcome to occur (also known as a competing outcome, as when a baby dies before 36 weeks' postmenstrual age and cannot be assessed for the presence or absence of bronchopulmonary dysplasia). The results of trials reporting composite outcomes can sometimes be confusing to interpret and apply in clinical decision making, particularly when one of the included negative outcomes is increased and the other is decreased. In such a case the clinician has to weigh the severity of each of the outcomes and estimate the net benefit or harm before making clinical decisions.

Example: In an RCT, Bassler et al.[4] evaluated the effects of early inhaled budesonide compared to placebo in neonates at 23 0/7 to 27 6/7 weeks of gestation with a primary outcome of death or bronchopulmonary dysplasia (BPD).

For the primary outcome (death or BPD), the control event rate (placebo group) was 46.3%, and the experimental

(budesonide group) event rate was 40%. The relative risk for inhaled budesonide was 40/46.3 = 0.86, with a 95% CI of 0.75-1 and a *p* value = 0.05. This is an example of a composite primary outcome with two components. However, when the investigators looked at the incidences of death and BPD individually, the effects were in opposite directions. For BPD the control event rate (placebo group) was 38%, and the experimental event rate (budesonide group) was 27.8%. The relative risk for BPD was therefore 27.8/38 = 0.73, with a 95% CI of 0.6-0.91 and a *p* value of 0.004. This was a statistically significant reduction in BPD. For death, the control event rate (placebo group) was 13.6%, and the experimental (budesonide group) event rate was 16.9%. The relative risk for inhaled budesonide was therefore 16.9/13.6 = 1.24, with a 95% CI of 0.91-1.69 and a *p* value of 0.17. In other words, there was an increased incidence of death in the budesonide group but this was not statistically significant. These results suggest that the risks of budesonide therapy (a possible increase in mortality up to 1.69 times higher, based on the upper limit of the CI) may outweigh the benefit (a reduction in BPD).

Once the clinician is satisfied with the internal validity of a study, the next step is to analyze the quantitative results of the study and assess the effect size.

Measures of treatment effect (effect size): The following measures of association are commonly reported in therapeutic trials that use dichotomous measures of outcome (examples are yes/no outcomes such as mortality, retinopathy of prematurity, or intraventricular hemorrhage):

Control event rate (CER): The incidence of the outcome in the control group (e.g., the placebo group in an RCT).

Experimental event rate (EER): The incidence of the outcome in the experimental group.

Relative risk (RR): EER/CER.

RR reduction: 1 − RR.

Absolute risk reduction (ARR): CER − EER, the absolute difference in the incidence of the outcome in the control and experimental groups.

Number needed to treat (NNT): 1/ARR, the number of patients who need to be treated to achieve one therapeutic success. The lower the NNT, the stronger the therapeutic effect and the fewer nonresponders who need to be exposed to the therapeutic intervention and to its risks and costs. When the outcome is an undesirable one, the term used is number needed to harm (NNH).

RR and RR reduction measure the strength of the association. To determine the actual number of patients affected, the absolute risk difference and NNT are more useful.

Example: The SUPPORT (Surfactant, Positive Airway Pressure, and Pulse Oximetry) study group compared outcomes in extremely preterm infants[5] (infants born between 24 0/7 and 27 6/7 weeks of gestation) maintained in a lower target range of oxygen saturation (85%-89%) versus a higher (91%-95%) range. In this study, for the primary outcome (severe retinopathy or death before discharge), the event rate was 28.3% in the lower saturation group and 32.1% in the higher saturation group. The RR with lower saturation was 28.3/32.1 = 0.9 with a 95% CI of 0.76-1.06 (which crossed 1, the value of no effect) and the *p* value was 0.21; hence, the null hypothesis could not be rejected. For death alone, the event rate was 19.9% in the lower saturation group and 16.2% in the higher saturation group. The RR with lower saturation was 19.9/16.2 = 1.23 with a 95% CI of 1.01-1.60 (not crossing 1) and the *p* value was 0.04. This was a statistically significant result, raising the concern that there was increased mortality in the babies in the lower saturation group. The relative risk reduction (actually an increase in this case) was 1-1.23 = 0.23. This meant there was a 23% increased risk of death in the lower saturation group. The ARR, also known as absolute risk difference (ARD; a more appropriate term because the risk actually increased) was 19.9 − 16.2 = 3.7, or 0.037. The NNH in this case was (1/ARD) = (1/0.037) = 27. This would mean that of 27 babies maintained in the lower saturation range as opposed to the high range, there would be one additional death. For severe retinopathy, the event rate was 8.6% in the lower saturation group and 17.9% in the higher saturation group. The RR was 8.6/17.9 = 0.48 with a 95% CI of 0.37-0.73 (not crossing 1) and a p value of less than 0.001. This was a statistically significant result, showing that the risk of severe retinopathy was lower among babies in the lower saturation group. The RR reduction was $1 - RR = 1 - 0.48 = 0.52$. This meant that there was 52% lesser risk of developing severe retinopathy in the lower saturation group. The ARR, also known as ARD, was 8.6 − 17.9 = 9.3, or 0.093 (absolute value). The NNH in this case therefore was (1/ARD) = (1/0.093) = 11. This would mean that of 11 babies maintained in the lower saturation range as opposed to the high range, one additional case of severe retinopathy would be prevented.

Odds ratio: The odds ratio is a measure of association between an exposure and an outcome. In a cohort study, the odds ratio is the ratio of the odds of an event in exposed subjects to the odds of the same event in unexposed subjects. In a case–control study, the odds ratio is the ratio of the odds that a case (a subject experiencing an event) was exposed to a factor to the odds that a control (a subject not experiencing an event) was exposed to the same factor.

Null value: The "no effect" value (null value) for ratios (odds ratio, RR) is 1 and for risk difference is 0. In practice, the 95% CI is often used as a proxy for the presence of statistical significance if it does not overlap the null value. Specifically, when the control and experimental groups are compared, if the CI of the estimate of the difference between the two groups excludes 1 for RR and 0 for ARD, then the result is considered statistically significant.

All the above measures are useful in describing dichotomous measures of outcome. In studies measuring continuous data (like duration of ventilation, length of hospital stayf, FiO_2, etc.) the groups are compared using mean differences.

Systematic Reviews of Therapeutic Interventions and Meta-analyses

A systematic review is a review of a clearly formulated question that uses systematic, explicit, and transparent methods to identify, select, and critically appraise relevant research and to collect, pool, and analyze data from the studies that are included in the review. A well-performed, up-to-date systematic review is a quick, reliable source of evidence for a clinician. However, not all systematic reviews are of high quality and systematic reviews also require critical appraisal.

Ideally, the systematic review should address a clearly formulated question (in the PICOT format), use multiple bibliographic databases, specify the search terms used (text and MeSH), include published as well as unpublished studies in all languages (not just English), specify a priori, the criteria to include and exclude studies, and use objective criteria to assess the quality of studies. Including all available studies avoids

publication bias (negative studies tend not to get published and require special effort to be identified). The quantitative results of different studies may then be combined using a meta-analysis to derive the pooled effect size after assigning weights to each study based on its sample size. The results are displayed in the form of a Forest plot. Before applying the findings of a systematic review in practice, the clinician should critically appraise it. The results of a systematic review should be trusted only if the review asked a focused research question, performed a comprehensive search to include all relevant studies, assessed the quality of the studies included, included only valid studies, combined studies only if there were reasonably similar, and included all important outcomes. A meta-analysis within a systematic review, for example, should not pool the results of studies with different devices, ventilator modes, populations or studies that span different epochs during which there were major changes in clinical practice (e.g. antenatal steroids, surfactant administration). The Neonatal Review Group of the Cochrane Collaboration creates and maintains a collection of high-quality systematic reviews, available at www.nichd.nih.gov/Cochrane.

Example: A good example of a systematic review related to ventilation is the analysis of volume-targeted ventilation versus pressure-limited ventilation in preterm infants. Peng et al. approached this question with a systematic review and meta-analysis.[6] The authors included 18 trials and concluded that the use of volume-targeted ventilation reduces the incidence of BPD with an RR for volume-targeted ventilation of 0.61 with a 95% CI of 0.46-0.82. They also concluded that volume-targeted ventilation decreased the length of mechanical ventilation (by 2 days), intraventricular hemorrhage (IVH), grade 3/4 IVH, pneumothorax, and periventricular leukomalacia compared with preterm infants who received pressure-limited ventilation.

Weighing Risks, Benefits, and Costs

After evaluating the quality of evidence and determining the quantitative results, the clinician has to evaluate the risks, benefits, and costs of various therapeutic strategies. To weigh benefits against risks for a therapy, a simple method is the NNT/NNH ratio, or the use of a balance sheet.[7] The balance sheet format underlies the summary of findings tables that are included in most Cochrane reviews now, and these tables allow an easy quantitative comparison of important benefits and risks. More elaborate and detailed estimation of benefits and risks can also be derived using decision analysis. Formal descriptions of decision analysis, cost-effectiveness, and cost–benefit analyses are provided in other publications and are outside the scope of this chapter. Finally, when weighing benefits against risks, the values that parents of infants place on various health outcomes should be incorporated, because different families may value the same health outcome differently and this can affect the relative weight of benefits and risks.

Evaluating Evidence about Diagnostic Tests
Evaluating the Quality of Evidence for Diagnostic Tests

To assess the evidence for a diagnostic test the first question to address is whether the results of the study are valid (Can you believe the results of the study?). The answer to this question depends on the risk of bias in the study used to evaluate the diagnostic test, which is a function of the design of the study, and on how well the study was actually conducted. The study should be evaluated for the possibilities of bias from the way patients were selected, index tests were performed and interpreted, reference standards were applied and interpreted, and patients were recruited to the study groups. Ideally, a study used to assess a diagnostic test should include a wide spectrum of patients selected in an unbiased manner (this avoids "spectrum bias"), not exclude patients inappropriately, enroll consecutive patients or randomly selected ones, include all patients in the final analysis, and avoid a case–control design. The diagnostic test (index test) results should have clear prespecified criteria for abnormality and should be interpreted without knowledge of the results of the reference standard (gold standard). The reference standard used should correctly classify the target condition, be applied to all included patients irrespective of the results of the index test, be applied at an appropriate interval after the index test, and ideally be interpreted without knowledge of the results of the index test. The items listed above can be formally assessed using a tool known as QUADAS 2 (Quality Assessment of Diagnostic Accuracy Studies).[8] This tool is applied in four phases: summarize the review question, tailor the tool and produce review-specific guidance, construct a flow diagram for the primary study, and judge bias and applicability. Specific GRADE criteria for diagnostic tests can also be applied to assign the quality of evidence.

Determining Diagnostic Test Accuracy

Traditionally, the results of diagnostic tests are depicted in a 2×2 table that is used to calculate sensitivity, specificity, positive predictive value, and negative predictive value.

Sensitivity is the proportion of persons with a disease who have a positive diagnostic test. It is a measure of the true positives. A test with a high sensitivity is useful in ruling out a disease if the test result is negative.

Specificity is the proportion of persons without a disease in whom the diagnostic test is negative. It measures the true negatives. The false positive rate of the test is $1 -$ specificity. A test with a high specificity is useful in ruling in a disease if the test result is positive.

By themselves sensitivity and specificity cannot be used to estimate the probability of a disease in an individual patient.

Positive predictive value is the proportion of persons with a positive test who have the disease.

Negative predictive value is the proportion of persons with a negative test who do not have the disease.

Both the positive and the negative predictive values are dependent on the disease prevalence. Therefore if published predictive values for a diagnostic test are available from one sample of patients, a clinician should not apply these values to patients in whom the prevalence of disease might be different from that of the sample of patients in the published study.

The calculations discussed above describe the accuracy of a diagnostic test. However, when faced with a patient, the task of the clinician is not to determine how well the test performs but to determine the probability that the patient does or does not have the disease, given a positive or negative diagnostic test. This can be determined using the likelihood ratio, which is independent of the disease prevalence and can be used to calculate the probability of disease for individual patients.

Likelihood ratio: The likelihood ratio (LR) is the ratio of the likelihood (probability) of a given result in patients with the disease to the probability in patients without the disease. It indicates how many times more (or less) likely patients with the disease are to have that particular result than patients

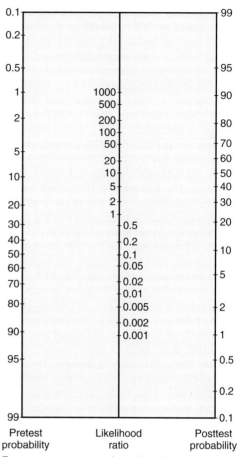

FIG 5-1 Fagan nomogram. A straight line drawn through the pretest probability (*first column*) and the likelihood ratio (*second column*) provides the posttest probability (*third column*) of the disease or condition.

without the disease, A positive LR (LR+) indicates how many times more likely persons with the disease are to have a positive diagnostic test than persons without the disease. A negative LR (LR-) indicates how many times more likely persons with the disease are to have a negative diagnostic test than persons without the disease.

Bayesian Reasoning in Diagnostic Testing

Using the estimated probability of the presence of a disease or condition before a diagnostic test is ordered (pretest probability) and the LR of a diagnostic test once a positive or negative result is obtained, we can calculate the posttest probability of the condition in question. To calculate the posttest probability, the pretest probability is converted to pretest odds, which is then multiplied by the LR to derive the posttest odds. This is then converted to posttest probability. Alternately, a nomogram (the Fagan nomogram)[9] can be used to derive posttest probability (Fig. 5-1).

If the LR is 1, then the posttest probability is exactly the same as the pretest probability. An LR much lower than 1 makes the posttest probability much lower (the disease is unlikely to be present in the patient). A very low LR of 0.1 or less virtually rules out the disease. An LR much higher than 1 makes the posttest probability much higher (the disease is much more likely to be present in the patient). A very high LR of 10 or greater virtually confirms ("rules in") the disease.

The posttest probability of disease is the most useful estimate and helps the clinician decide whether to order additional diagnostic tests, to reassure the parents of an infant that the disease is unlikely to be present, or to initiate treatment for the disease. The posttest probability of a disease after one test becomes the pretest probability for the next diagnostic test, if one is performed.

Example: Brat et al.[10] determined the diagnostic accuracy of a neonatal-adapted lung ultrasonography score (LUS) to predict the need for surfactant administration. The authors included all inborn neonates admitted to the neonatal intensive care unit with respiratory distress in the study and avoided a case–control design. The reference standard in this study for surfactant administration was according to the 2013 European guidelines. The criteria for abnormality were prespecified for the LUS. Neonatologists who were blinded to the clinical condition analyzed the results from the LUS. The authors reported that an LUS score cutoff of 4 predicted surfactant administration with 100% sensitivity and 61% specificity in babies of less than 34 weeks' gestation. The positive LR in this group of patients was 2.6, and the posttest probability was 72%.

Special Considerations in Applying Evidence to Respiratory Interventions

1. Respiratory interventions are often device-based (ventilator, CPAP, high flow nasal cannula) and are thus difficult to blind. Inability to blind interventions may allow other biases (e.g., performance bias) to creep in and adversely affect the internal validity of the study.
2. The technology in the devices used for providing respiratory care constantly evolves with the development of better models/modes of ventilation, etc. The comparison between these various devices/modes may be difficult.
3. Trials with respiratory intervention usually have short-term physiological outcomes (e.g., oxygen saturation) or short-term predischarge outcomes such as BPD as the primary outcome. Long-term outcomes such as lung function at school age and adolescence may be better outcome measures, but they are difficult to gather due to logistic challenges and lack of resources for prolonged follow-up. Also, the commonly used outcome measure of BPD has multiple definitions and makes the comparison of trials challenging.
4. The effectiveness of a respiratory intervention depends on many other factors apart from the device itself, such as the clinical expertise and skills of physicians, nursing staff, and respiratory therapists using the device; consistency of care; presence of a champion; and closeness of monitoring. These subcomponents are often difficult to tease out in trials and may affect the external validity of the study.

COGNITIVE SKILLS FOR EVIDENCE-BASED PRACTICE

Critical Thinking

At its core, EBM is an application of critical thinking in medicine, which is defined as the ability to apply higher order cognitive skills (conceptualization, analysis, evaluation) and the disposition to be deliberate about thinking (being open-minded or intellectually honest) that lead to action that is logical and appropriate.[11] Critical thinking allows a clinician to frame a problem appropriately; focus thinking around relevant issues; proceed systematically through analysis, evaluation, and decision making; and be self-aware of his or her own cognitive processes. Papp et al. postulate that milestones in critical thinking range from being an unreflective thinker (stage 1) to being an accomplished critical thinker (stage 5). As a developing critical thinker, the clinician should openly acknowledge his or her assumptions and accept uncertainty as the reason for further questions and research.[11] Instead of accepting established practices, the clinician should be able to ask appropriate questions and modify his or her practice based on new/emerging evidence. Good critical thinkers are open-minded, are fair-minded, search for the evidence, try to be well informed, are attentive to others' views and their reasons, hold beliefs in proportion to the evidence, and are willing to consider alternatives and revise beliefs.[12]

Clinical Reasoning and Decision Making

Knowledge of the available evidence, its quality, and the quantitative estimates of benefits, harms, and costs as described above should all be incorporated into a formal and explicit process of clinical reasoning that leads to a clinical decision or clinical guideline or protocol. In the GRADE method, either a strong or a weak recommendation to use or not use a diagnostic test or treatment can be generated. In reality, many decisions faced by clinicians have to be made under conditions of uncertainty. Uncertainty in decision making arises when:

- The evidence available is sparse,
- The available evidence lacks internal validity (poor study design or conduct),
- Study results are not important (small effect size or when a positive effect cannot be ruled out), or
- The study lacks external validity or applicability (different population or methodology from that in the clinician's practice).

In clinical situations there is often pressure to act in the face of insufficient evidence. "Doing something" in such situations may not always be appropriate, and watchful waiting may be better than intervening. Acknowledging uncertainty of evidence in these situations is important, and involving colleagues (for brainstorming) and parents may be helpful for decision making. The clinician should also be clear about the distinction between a situation where sufficient evidence exists that proves an intervention is ineffective (i.e., there are multiple high-quality studies showing lack of efficacy) and one where insufficient or low quality evidence exists for an intervention (i.e., the intervention is inadequately studied, and the possibility still exists that the intervention may be efficacious) – *'absence of evidence of effect is not evidence of absence of effect.'*

TRANSLATING EVIDENCE INTO PRACTICE

Once the process of finding, appraising, and analyzing the evidence is completed, the clinician is now faced with the daunting task of converting this knowledge into practice. Knowledge translation is a dynamic and iterative process that includes synthesis, dissemination, exchange, and ethically sound application of knowledge to improve health, provide more effective health services and products, and strengthen the health care system.[13] The process of translating knowledge into action is not linear; considering the local context (policy and work culture) is an integral part of making this

TABLE 5-3   Definitions

CER: This is the control event rate, the rate or incidence of event or disease in the control group

EER: This is the experimental event rate, the rate or incidence of event or disease in the experimental group

Relative risk (RR) = EER/CER. If RR < 1, then the therapy decreased the risk of outcome; if RR = 1, then the treatment had no effect; if RR > 1, then the treatment increased the risk of outcome.

Absolute risk reduction (ARR) or risk difference = CER − EER. An ARR of 0 signifies no treatment effect.

Relative risk reduction = 1 − RR.

Number needed to treat (NNT) = 1/ARR.

Odds ratio (OR): If a is the number of exposed cases, b is the number of exposed noncases, c is the number of unexposed cases, and d is the number of unexposed noncases, then:

OR = $(a/c)/(b/d)$ = ad/bc.

Disease Test	Present	Absent
Positive	a	c
Negative	b	d

Sensitivity (true positives): $a/a+b$

Specificity (true negatives): $d/c+d$

Positive predictive value: $a/a+c$

Negative predictive value: $d/b+d$

Positive likelihood ratio (LR+) = sensitivity/(1 − specificity)

Negative likelihood ratio = (1 − sensitivity)/specificity

Posttest odds = pretest odds × LR

happen. Engaging stakeholders (leadership, bedside nurses, respiratory therapists) is important and it may entail education and training of all the team members involved in patient care before the research knowledge can be translated to clinical practice. The use of quality improvement methods allows systematic yet adaptive implementation of evidence-based practices.

SUMMARY

EBM encompasses both technical and cognitive skills that help the clinician to convert knowledge into practice and provide the best care to the neonate requiring respiratory care.

REFERENCES

A complete reference list is available at https://expertconsult.inkling.com.

6

Quality and Safety in Respiratory Care

Gautham K. Suresh, MD, DM ,MS, FAAP, and Aarti Raghavan, MD, FAAP

QUALITY AND SAFETY: TERMINOLOGY AND FRAMEWORKS

The quality of health care is defined as "the degree to which health services for individuals and populations increase the likelihood of desired health outcomes and are consistent with current professional knowledge."[1,2] Many publications and expert reports[1,3-5] have emphasized that, in addition to widespread deficiencies of quality in health care, preventable harm to hospitalized patients from medical errors is frequent. A medical error is defined as the failure of a planned action to be completed as intended or the use of a wrong plan to achieve an aim.[5] An adverse event is defined as an injury resulting from a medical intervention.[5]

Institutions providing care for neonates with respiratory and pulmonary illness should ideally monitor and continually improve the quality and safety of care provided to ensure that their patients receive the best care possible and that they attain the best clinical outcomes possible. To ensure this, each neonatal intensive care unit should have a framework and approach for assessing, monitoring, and improving the quality of care in general and for neonates with respiratory illness in particular. Two frameworks in particular are useful—Donabedian's triad and the six domains of quality described by the Institute of Medicine.

Donabedian's Triad

An important framework for quality of care was proposed in the 1960s by Donabedian, who proposed that the domains of quality are structure, process, and outcomes.[6-8] *Structure* denotes the facilities, equipment, services, and labor available for care; the environment in which care is provided; the qualifications, skills, and experience of the health care professionals in that institution; and other characteristics of the hospital or system providing care. Therefore, for a neonatal unit it encompasses aspects of quality such as space per patient, the layout of the unit, the nurse/patient ratio, the availability of radiology facilities around the clock, the types of respiratory equipment used, and the neonatology training and skills of the personnel. *Process* is defined as a "set of activities that go on between practitioners and patients." It refers to the content of care, i.e., how the patient was moved into, through, and out of the health care system and the services that were provided during the care episode. Process is what physicians and other health care professionals do to and for patients. For a neonatal unit, process can include aspects of quality such as the percentage of personnel washing their hands prior to patient contact, the duration of time between birth and the first dose of surfactant, the percentage of infants in whom the examination for retinopathy of prematurity is performed on time, the efficiency with which a neonate is transported from a referring hospital, the frequency of medical errors, and so on. Finally, *outcomes* are the end results of care. They are the consequences to the health and welfare of individuals and society or, alternatively, the measured health status of the individual or community. Outcomes of care have also been defined as "the results of care ... [which] can encompass biologic changes in disease, comfort, ability for self-care, physical function and mobility, emotional and intellectual performance, patient satisfaction and self-perception of health, health knowledge and compliance with medical care, and viability of family, job and social role functioning."[9] For neonatal intensive care unit (NICU) patients and their parents, examples of outcome measures are mortality rate, the frequency of chronic lung disease, the number of nosocomial bloodstream infections per 1000 patient days, the percentage of NICU survivors who are developmentally normal, and parental satisfaction with the care of their baby. Table 6-1 demonstrates common quality measures in the field of neonatal respiratory care.

The Institute of Medicine's Domains of Quality

Six domains of quality were described by the Institute of Medicine in its 2001 report *Crossing the Quality Chasm*[1]—safety, timeliness, effectiveness, efficiency, equity, and patient-centeredness (these can be remembered by the acronym STEEEP). A neonatal unit should try to provide respiratory care optimally in all these domains. *Safety* in particular is a high-priority domain that deserves separate emphasis and is defined as freedom from accidental injury (avoiding harm to patients from the care that is intended to help them). *Timeliness* is the reduction of delays and unnecessary waits for patients, their families, and health professionals. *Effectiveness* is the provision of health care interventions supported by high-quality evidence to all eligible patients and avoidance of those that are unlikely to be beneficial. *Efficiency* is avoiding waste, including waste of equipment, supplies, ideas, and energy. *Equity* is the provision of care that does not vary based on a patient's personal characteristics such as gender, ethnicity, geographic location, and socioeconomic status. *Patient-centered care* is the provision of care that is respectful of, and responsive to, an individual neonate's family preferences, needs, and values and ensuring that the family's values guide all clinical decisions.

TABLE 6-1   Errors and Adverse Events Related to Mechanical Ventilation

Endotracheal Intubation

Use of wrong size of endotracheal tube

Right main stem bronchus intubation

Unplanned extubation

Obstruction of endotracheal tube due to inadequate suction

Airway injury leading to subglottic stenosis

Tracheal perforation from endotracheal tube suction catheter

Kinking of endotracheal tube

Initiation of Mechanical Ventilation

Improper setup of ventilator and accessories

    Failure to add water to humidifier

    Misconnection of ventilator tubing

    Omission of safety limits on ventilator settings

    Omission of alarm settings

Use of Mechanical Ventilation

Delay in changing ventilator settings in response to blood gas results

Inadvertent delivery of high or low ventilator pressures (e.g., auto-positive end-expiratory pressure)

Failure to wean inhaled oxygen when oxygen saturation is high

Ventilator-associated pneumonia

Inadequate drainage of condensate in ventilator tubing leading to inadvertent pulmonary lavage

Ventilator failure due to poor maintenance by biomedical engineering

Overriding ventilator alarms

Ignoring ventilator alarms

ASSESSING AND MONITORING THE QUALITY OF CARE

The quality of respiratory care can be assessed and monitored using a set of quality indicators that measure different domains of quality. Individual units should choose the exact indicators to monitor based on local priorities, previously identified deficiencies of care, local patterns of practice, and ease of access to data and resources required to collect, analyze, and display data. Quality indicators should be collected both for (1) comparison and (2) improvement.

QUALITY INDICATORS FOR COMPARATIVE PERFORMANCE MEASURES

Such indicators are typically used to compare a unit's clinical performance (and not process measures) against comparators. Comparators can be the quality indicators of other similar units, national benchmarks, or targets. Ideally these data should be risk adjusted to make the comparisons valid. Risk adjustment applies statistical methods to differentiate intrinsic heterogeneity among patients (e.g., comorbid conditions) and institutions (e.g., available hospital personnel and resources). With risk adjustment, an outcome can be better ascribed to the quality of clinical care provided by health professionals and institutions. Several models of risk adjustment have been developed for the NICU setting and used to evaluate interinstitutional variation.

When quality indicators are monitored, although there is often a long time lag between the events being measured and the analysis, display, and comparison of the data, the discrepancy between an individual unit's performance and the comparators can be used to motivate change and launch improvement projects around specific topics. Quality indicators for such judgment may also be used by regulators and payers to rank neonatal units (sometimes publicly) according to the quality of care they provide (their performance), withhold payments, and provide incentive payments. They may also be used by families of patients, when choice is feasible (e.g., in an antenatally diagnosed fetal anomaly), to choose the neonatal unit where their infant will receive care. Many neonatal networks such as the Vermont Oxford Network (VON), the Pediatrix neonatal database, and the Canadian Neonatal Network, collect predefined data items from member neonatal units and provide reports to these units that include quality indicators. For example, the VON provides member units quarterly and annually with a report that includes their rates of ventilation, use of postnatal steroids, use of surfactant, use of inhaled nitric oxide, pulmonary air leak, bronchopulmonary dysplasia, and mortality.

Published data from several neonatal networks reveal the existence of wide variations in neonatal process measures and neonatal outcomes (including respiratory outcomes) that persist after risk adjustment.[10-14] This suggests that the observed differences in outcomes are the result of the quality of care provided to the patients and that the units with the poorer clinical outcomes have room to improve their quality of care.

A particularly important subset of quality indicators is that of patient safety events. Each neonatal unit should monitor medical errors and adverse events (patient safety events) related to respiratory care. These events are most commonly identified through reporting by health professionals involved in or witnessing the event, a method that is convenient and requires few resources.[14] Other methods to identify patient safety events[15] are the use of trigger tools, chart review, random safety audits, mortality and morbidity meetings, autopsies, and review of patient family complaints or medical–legal cases. These methods do not yield a true rate of these events and therefore cannot be used to evaluate a unit's performance against comparators. The ideal method to identify these events is prospective surveillance.[16] This system yields accurate rates and can be used for comparison but is not widely used because it is laborious and requires many resources. A variety of medical errors and adverse events related to neonatal respiratory care have been described in the literature (see Table 6-1).[17,18] In one study of 10 Dutch neonatal intensive care units, 9% of patient safety incidents were related to mechanical ventilation. Of all recorded incidents, those related to mechanical ventilation and to blood products had the highest risk scores (an indicator of the likelihood of recurrence and likelihood of severe consequences).[19]

QUALITY INDICATORS FOR IMPROVEMENT

These indicators are used to monitor the progress of a specific quality improvement project. These usually are a combination of outcome measures and process measures. They are collected in real time and used by quality improvement teams (see below) to monitor the progress of the project, identify unintended consequences, and draw inferences about the effects of their attempts to make change. Ideally these data are disaggregated as much as possible (not lumped together) and displayed over

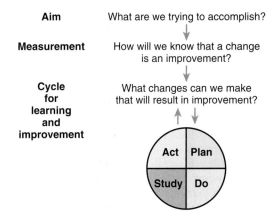

Aim What are we trying to accomplish?

Measurement How will we know that a change is an improvement?

Cycle for learning and improvement What changes can we make that will result in improvement?

Act | Plan
Study | Do

FIG 6-1 The model for improvement.

time (with time on the *x* axis and the indicator on the *y* axis) in the form of either run charts or statistical process control charts as displayed in Figure 6-1.

IMPROVING THE QUALITY OF CARE

Since 1995 quality improvement (QI) has emerged as a strong movement in the health care systems of developed countries. It reflects the effort to import into health care principles, tools, and techniques from other industries for improving product quality to meet their customers' needs and expectations. The basic premise of QI in health care is that improvements in patient care can be achieved by making a focused, conscious effort, using a defined set of scientific methods and by constant reflection on the results of our attempts to improve care. It is based heavily on systems thinking and therefore emphasizes the organization and systems of care. Many approaches to QI have been described (IMPROVE, Model for Improvement, Lean or Lean-Six-Sigma (Define, Measure, Analyse, Improve, Control [DMAIC]) or Toyota Production System, Rapid Cycle Improvement, Four Key Habits (VON), Advanced Training Program of Intermountain Healthcare, Microsystems approach) and all are broadly similar in their approaches. Of these, one simple and effective approach that can be used to improve the quality of care is the Model for Improvement (see Fig. 6-1) that was formalized by Langley et al.[20] The use of the Institute for Healthcare Improvement model and the Plan–Do–Study–Act cycles to achieve improvement are discussed below.

THE IMPROVEMENT TEAM

To successfully carry out QI projects, it is important to have a core team of people in each unit. This is usually a multidisciplinary team composed of physicians, nurses, and others who are directly or indirectly involved in aspects of the topic that is targeted for improvement. The more disciplines represented, the better the QI efforts will be. The members of this team have to become skilled in several techniques, such as how to have productive meetings, how to work together as a team, how to bring about change in a unit, how to deal with barriers to improvement, and how to collect, analyze, and display data. The involvement of the entire NICU team in QI efforts should increase "buy-in" and heighten awareness of a problem, thereby possibly creating a Hawthorne effect, which is beneficial.

COLLABORATION

Improvement in patient care is impossible without cooperation—working together to produce mutual benefit or attain a common purpose. Collaboration and cooperation have to occur within each unit. Collaboration is a powerful force in motivating people toward improvement and in sustaining the momentum for change in each unit. The improvement team has to get buy-in from other members in their unit and get them to participate in the improvement effort. Collaboration and cooperation among units is also helpful. Different units can work together, share ideas, and help one another to improve care. Clemmer et al.[21] suggest five methods to foster cooperation: (1) develop a shared purpose; (2) create an open, safe environment; (3) include all those who share the common purpose and encourage diverse viewpoints; (4) learn how to negotiate agreement; and (5) insist on fairness and equity in applying rules.

AIM: WHAT ARE WE TRYING TO ACCOMPLISH?

The first step in any improvement project is to set a clear aim. This can be done in three stages. First, a list of problems faced by the unit or opportunities for change is made. The existence of quality indicators as described above will assist the compilation of such a list. Second, the problems or opportunities for change that are listed are then prioritized using criteria such as the resources available, the probability of achieving change, emotional appeal, the importance to stakeholders (including patients and their families), and practicality. Third, one item is finally selected from this list as the aim for improvement. For those unfamiliar with QI, it is best to choose for the initial project a small and well-focused topic on which data are easy to obtain that will be more likely to generate interest among clinicians and nurses. Very low birth-weight (VLBW) neonates have been the obvious target for QI in many QI initiatives. VLBW neonates contribute significantly to the mortality and morbidity burden in the neonatal units, consume the largest proportion of resources, are easily identified, and develop potentially preventable outcomes like nosocomial infections, intraventricular hemorrhage, bronchopulmonary dysplasia (BPD), and retinopathy of prematurity (ROP). When an aim is selected, it should be specified as a SMART aim—that is, it should be specific, measurable, achievable, realistic, and time-bound.

MEASUREMENT: HOW WILL WE KNOW THAT A CHANGE IS AN IMPROVEMENT?

Measurement is key to QI. Measuring the quality of care serves three purposes: (1) It indicates the current status of the unit or practice. This is called assessing "current reality." Without objective measurement, clinicians will be left guessing or relying on subjective impressions. Objective measurement of structures, processes, and outcomes provides strong motivation for a unit to embark on an improvement project. (2) Measurement of quality will inform QI teams whether they are actually making an improvement, without having to rely on subjective impressions or opinions, with the attendant risk of being misguided. (3) Measuring quality helps teams learn from attempts to make improvements and also learn from their successes as well as failures. Fig. 6-2 represents a statistical control chart - a common way of displaying measured metrics over time.

WHAT CHANGES CAN WE MAKE THAT WILL RESULT IN AN IMPROVEMENT?

The answers to this question come from many sources. Some of these include:

1. A detailed analysis and mapping of the process by which care is provided (process mapping). For medical errors and adverse events a detailed systems analysis[22] is recommended. Such an analysis (the most extensive form of which is a root cause analysis (RCA),[23] which attempts to identify workplace-related, human-related, and organizational factors[24] that contributed to the occurrence and propagation of the event. Table 6-2 details the steps involved in the RCA process. It is critical for the leader of the RCA process to be well versed in RCA methodology and also be focused on identifying system-related challenges rather than assignment of individual blame.

2. A review of published literature and using the principles of evidence-based medicine.

3. Benchmarking—that is, learning from superior performers in the area chosen for improvement.

4. Advice from experts or others who have attempted improvement in similar topics.

5. Brainstorming, critical thinking, and hunches about the current system of care.

6. Use of "change concepts," a set of principles of redesign of process or work flow (such as "change the sequence of steps" or "eliminate unnecessary steps").[20]

7. Particularly for patient safety projects, use of knowledge of human psychology, the science of human factors engineering.

Through the use of one or a combination of these approaches, one or more interventions are identified that, if implemented, have the potential to result in improvements in patient care and outcomes. These interventions are variously known as "change concepts" or "potentially better practices"[25] or "key clinical activities"[26] or, for patient safety events, "safety practices." They are sometimes grouped into a set of synergistic or complementary interventions that are known as "bundles."

The well-known Swiss cheese model[27] depicts how an error reaches a patient despite a series of existing safety mechanisms because the "holes in the Swiss cheese line up" (multiple safety mechanisms fail concurrently or serially and allow propagation of the error). A key principle of improving patient safety and reducing medical errors is to focus not on individual health care providers as the cause of errors (the "person approach") but more broadly on the system of care (in which the provider is embedded) as the desired locus of prevention (the "system approach"). Ensuring patient safety involves the establishment of operational systems and processes that minimize the likelihood of errors and maximize the likelihood of intercepting them when they occur.[5] Optimal design of equipment, tasks, and the work environment can enhance error-free human performance, and the use of principles of human factors engineering can successfully guide such optimal design.

After the changes or potentially better practices or safety practices are selected it is not sufficient to implement them and assume that patient outcomes will improve. The next step in the improvement process is to carry out a series of Plan–Do–Study–Act cycles.

PLAN–DO–STUDY–ACT CYCLES

No matter what the sources of our ideas for improvement are, there is no guarantee that these changes will improve the quality of care. The results of the implementation of these changes have to be studied, using the measures that have previously been set up when answering the question "How will we know that a

TABLE 6-2 **Steps in a Root Cause Analysis**
Step 1: Identify a sentinel event.
Step 2: Assemble a multidisciplinary team including executive and operational leadership, quality improvement coaches, and providers who come into contact with the system.
Step 3: Verify facts surrounding the event and collect associated data.
Step 4: Chart causal factors using process maps, brainstorming, Pareto charts, fishbone diagrams, etc.
Step 5: Identify root causes by asking why five times for each issue, to get to the bottom of the cause.
Step 6: Develop strategies and make recommendations for process change.
Step 7: Present results to all stakeholders.
Step 8: Perform "tests of change."

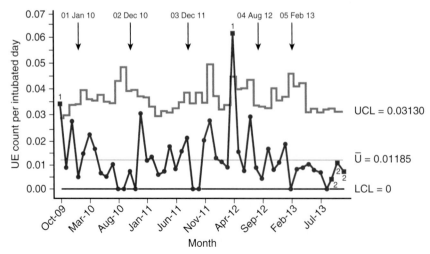

FIG 6-2 Example of a statistical process control chart.

change is an improvement?" In other words, the change has to be tested. This process also allows process-related obstacles to be identified and resolved. This process of testing a change is called a Plan–Do–Study–Act (PDSA) cycle. This is a critical step in the process of QI, because it allows troubleshooting prior to widespread implementation. The PDSA cycles include planning an intervention (e.g., steps to enhance adherence to handwashing), carrying out the intervention, studying its effect (e.g., handwashing compliance rate, hospital-acquired infection rate), and finally implementing the intervention in day-to-day practice. Common questions the QI team should ask itself are, Why did we succeed? Why did we fail? What further changes do we now need to make to succeed? By doing a series of PDSA cycles and thus learning from each effort at improvement, the team can achieve lasting improvements in the way they provide patient care and in patient outcomes. The apparent simplicity of the PDSA cycle is deceptive. The cycle is a sophisticated, demanding way to achieve learning and change in complex systems.[28]

Table 6-3 demonstrates the steps of the QI process using an example of a project designed to modify oxygen saturation guidelines in VLBW infants in a single tertiary NICU.

ENSURING THE SUCCESS OF QUALITY IMPROVEMENT PROJECTS

QI projects often are not completed as intended, are unsuccessful in achieving the desired results, or are unable to achieve sustained results. The following 10 tips can contribute to successful completion and sustained results:

1. Gain a deep understanding of the problem first using systems thinking[29] ("formulate the mess") before trying to implement solutions and resist quick "off-the-shelf" solutions.
2. Avoid using solely a research mentality, especially with measurement. Successful QI requires a combination of rigorous scientific thinking and pragmatism. Particularly with measurement, seek usefulness, not perfection.[30]
3. Focus on sustainability from the beginning and not just on short-term wins.
4. Develop a consensus-based approach to decision making when the evidence for interventions is sparse, incomplete, or flawed.
5. Manage change carefully using published expert recommendations.[31,32]

TABLE 6-3   Steps in the Improvement Process with Example of a Project to Improve Compliance with New Oxygen Saturation Guidelines to Reduce Retinopathy of Prematurity*

Steps in Improvement Process	Example
Evaluate indicators for improvement	Review of VON quality indicators for VLBW infants
Identify "problem"	1. Poor compliance with oxygen saturation guidelines (based on sampling by volunteers) 2. New evidence regarding oxygen saturation goals from SUPPORT trial
Develop a multidisciplinary improvement team	Team comprising physician, nursing respiratory therapy leadership, and end providers—physician, nursing RTs, QI coaches, trainees (medical residents, neonatal fellows, nursing students)
Develop a SMART aim	Increase compliance with O_2 saturation guidelines to >95% in 6 months in the NICU
Create process maps, brainstorming and key driver diagrams	OWL task force met every week for a month to review the evidence surrounding oxygen saturation goals, create process maps, identify potential obstacles (e.g., tight staffing), brainstorm for potential solutions (e.g., use of an OWL nurse "buddy system") to help a nurse with a labile patient
Identify process, outcome, and balance measures	Process: Implement new oxygen saturation guidelines Outcome: Compliance with saturation guidelines Balance: BPD and ROP rates, staff satisfaction, alarm fatigue
Start continuous data collection immediately	Compliance audited by RTs during every shift for all patients on respiratory support
Plan and conduct PDSA cycles	Multiple cycles conducted on one to three patients, e.g., slight variations in alarm limits, the nurse OWL buddy system
Receive and incorporate feedback regarding PDSA cycle	Verbal/written feedback (feedback forms provided at the bedside with space for open comments, option to stay anonymous) obtained from staff. Recommendations through feedback incorporated: change in saturation cycling time, change in amount of oxygen delivered by manual breaths through ventilator
Implement changes	Once providers were satisfied with new process, training was provided to staff through group sessions, one-on-one feedback, and newsletters
Monitor sustainability of process and outcomes	Initial compliance monitored through data collected by RTs on every shift and reviewed by task force weekly Ongoing random audits four or five times per week in random shifts
Share data continuously with providers	Data shared with providers through posters and staff meetings
Identify breaks in new process/system	Two-week time period when compliance was noted to drop below 90%
Perform RCA and modify system according to findings	RCA performed: outliers noted to be in cases with specific oxygen saturation compliance (complex heart disease)—staff noted confusion regarding guidelines because bedside sign was for regular alarm limits. Space was introduced on signs for special cases, which was to be approved by physician providers on a case-by-case basis

*Oxygen with Love (OWL).

BPD, Bronchopulmonary dysplasia; *NICU*, neonatal intensive care unit; *PDSA*, plan–do–study–act; *QI*, quality improvement; *RCA*, root cause analysis; *ROP*, retinopathy of prematurity; *RT*, respiratory therapist; *SMART*, specific, measurable, achievable, realistic, and time-bound; *SUPPORT*, Surfactant, Positive Airway Pressure, and Pulse Oximetry; *VLBW*, very low birth weight; *VON*, Vermont Oxford Network.

6. Learn from "failure" through multiple PDSA cycles. Understanding the reasons for failure can guide future refinements of the changes implemented, with eventual success.
7. Use the principles and methods of project management,[33] including good meeting skills.
8. Go beyond just using jargon such as "silo," "low-hanging fruit," and "checklist."
9. Use a QI coach if possible. Coaching can enhance the success of QI teams.[34]
10. Do not feel compelled to adhere rigidly to any one approach to QI.

LEADERSHIP AND UNIT CULTURE

Finally, the involvement, support, and encouragement of the leaders of the organization or the clinical unit, as well as a favorable organizational culture, are crucial elements for the success of quality and safety improvement efforts. Without such support many improvement efforts will be doomed to failure. Leaders of neonatal units must focus on the quality of care as an important part of the mission of their units and must actively work to create an organizational culture in the unit that will encourage efforts to improve the quality of care. For patient safety in particular this involves fostering a culture in which staff members feel safe (i.e., not intimidated) in pointing out safety hazards, challenging authority, and stopping a work process or procedure if they feel it is unsafe ("stopping the line"[35]). One useful method to promote safety culture is "executive walk rounds,"[36] in which senior organizational leaders periodically walk through the neonatal unit and talk to frontline staff about their perceptions of patient safety problems, hazards, and requirements.

WHY IS QUALITY IMPROVEMENT IMPORTANT IN NEONATAL RESPIRATORY CARE?

Published literature on a wide variety of respiratory process measures and respiratory morbidity that persists after risk adjustment[10-14] suggests that the observed differences in outcomes are the results of the quality of care provided to the patients. That is to say that a significant proportion of neonates managed in NICUs suffer from preventable respiratory morbidity and that the units with the poorer clinical outcomes have room to improve their quality of care. A particular concern is the high incidence in VLBW infants of chronic lung disease (CLD), a condition that has a major impact on long-term pulmonary function and is associated with high health care and societal costs and neurodevelopmental morbidity. Despite significant advances in neonatal pulmonary care since 1985, the rates of CLD in infants weighing <1500 g have remained relatively unchanged since 2005 and also vary significantly across centers in the United States (despite adjustment for confounding factors). Neonatal health outcomes are influenced by a variety of endogenous and exogenous factors like birth weight, gestation, obstetric management during delivery, resuscitation practices, initial respiratory support, nutritional management, and measures to prevent nosocomial infections. Application of systematic QI efforts has the potential to reduce CLD and other forms of respiratory morbidity through reliable and consistent application of existing high-level evidence, without depending on new medications, technology, or innovations to be developed. Such efforts are described below.

EXAMPLES OF QUALITY AND SAFETY IMPROVEMENT IN NEONATAL RESPIRATORY CARE

Quality Improvement Projects in Individual Units

Birenbaum et al. reported a significant reduction in the rate of CLD as a result of a QI project in their unit.[37] The rate of BPD in VLBW neonates was reduced by more than half by avoidance of intubation, adoption of new pulse oximeter limits, and early use of nasal continuous positive airway pressure therapy (CPAP).

Nowadzky et al.[38] used QI methods to reduce CLD by implementing nasal bubble CPAP to reduce mechanical ventilation. Although the group was successful in implementing the use of bubble CPAP, the rate of CLD was unchanged and a concomitant increase in ROP rate was noted.

Merkel et al.[39] reduced unplanned extubations from 2.38 to 0.41 per 100 patient-intubated days by having at least two staff members participate in procedures such as retaping and securing endotracheal tubes; weighing and transferring the patient out of the bed; placement of alert cards at the bedside indicating the risk level for an unplanned extubation, the security of the endotracheal tube, the depth of placement at the gums, and the proper care of the endotracheal tube. In addition to these measures a commercial product was used to secure the endotracheal tube, education of staff by staff experts was initiated ("champions"), the use of a real-time analysis form to identify causes of unplanned extubations was started, the use of a centrally located display of the days since last unplanned extubation was begun, and the nurses placed mittens or socks on the hands of intubated patients greater than 34 weeks' postmenstrual age. They suggest that the benchmark for unplanned extubation should be a rate of less than 1 per 100 patient-intubated days.

Collaborative Quality Improvement Projects

One successful approach that has been used in neonatology by the VON is that of collaborative QI in which a group of neonatal units collaborate for the purpose of improving the quality of neonatal care.[11,40] With this approach, a team of personnel from each hospital (from multiple disciplines involved in neonatal care, such as neonatologists, nurses, respiratory therapists, and others) meets periodically, with ongoing collaboration in between meetings carried on by the use of e-mail and telephone calls among these team members. The network acts as a coordinator, facilitator, and motivator of this collaborative effort and provides expert faculty members who work with individual sets of teams to facilitate their improvement efforts.

The VON has implemented a number of such collaborative projects called the Neonatal Intensive Care Quality (NICQ) projects. The major components of NICQ projects included multidisciplinary collaboration within and among hospitals, feedback of information from the network database regarding clinical practice and patient outcome, training and QI methods, site visits to project NICUs, benchmarking visits to superior performers within the network, identification and implementation of potentially better practices, and evaluation of the results. In the first NICQ project, teams from the 10 hospitals worked together in cross-institutional improvement groups.[11] Six NICUs focused on reducing nosocomial infections, and four units focused on reducing CLD. The potentially best practices that were proposed were based on an evidence review and careful analysis of other practices at best-performing centers. During the project period from 1994 to 1996, the rate of infection with coagulase-negative

Staphylococcus decreased from 22.0% to 16.6% at the six project NICUs in the infection group; the rate of supplemental oxygen at 36 weeks' adjusted gestational age decreased from 43.5% to 31.5% at the four NICUs in the CLD group. Another NICQ project evaluated how the adoption of "best practices" in 16 centers of the VON during 2001-2003 might reduce the incidence of BPD among VLBW neonates.[41] BPD rates dropped significantly in 2003 compared with the baseline year. In addition, severe ROP, severe intraventricular hemorrhage, and supplemental oxygen at discharge dropped significantly. The VON reported another QI project with an objective of promoting evidence-based surfactant treatment of preterm neonates.[42] Participating centers were randomized to a control or an intervention arm. Hospitals in the intervention arm received QI advice including audit and feedback, evidence reviews, an interactive training workshop, and ongoing faculty support via conference calls and e-mail. Although there was no significant difference in the incidence of pneumothorax or mortality, neonates born in intervention hospitals were more likely to receive surfactant in the delivery room or within 2 hours of birth.

Payne et al.[43] reported the results over 9 years from eight NICUs that participated in a VON collaborative to reduce lung injury (the ReLI group). This group successfully decreased delivery room intubation, conventional ventilation, and the use of postnatal steroids for BPD. They increased the use of nasal CPAP, and survival to discharge increased. Nosocomial infections decreased. However, BPD-free survival remained unchanged, and the BPD rate increased.

In a cluster randomized trial done by the Canadian Neonatal Network[44] six neonatal intensive care units were identified to adopt practices to reduce nosocomial infections (infection group) and six units to reduce BPD (pulmonary group). Practice change interventions were implemented using rapid-change cycles for 2 years. The incidence of BPD decreased in the pulmonary group, and the incidence of nosocomial infections decreased significantly in both the infection and the pulmonary groups.

In a cluster randomized QI trial, 14 centers of the National Institute of Child Health and Human Development Neonatal Research Network were randomized to intervention or control clusters.[45] Intervention centers implemented practices of the three best performing centers of the network to reduce the rate of BPD. Although the intervention centers successfully implemented practices of the best performing centers, the rate of BPD was not reduced in intervention or control centers. Explanations given for the failure to reduce the rate of BPD were choosing interventions that were not evidence based and targeting a multifactorial disease with a single-prong strategy of reducing oxygen exposure.

More recently, statewide collaboratives have been developed in multiple U.S. states where some or all NICUs in the state work collaboratively on the same clinical topics using QI methods, share data, and learn from one another to make improvements in clinical outcomes and processes. Such statewide collaboratives[46-49] have reported significant decreases in central-line-associated bloodstream infections and are targeting other clinical outcomes as well.

CONCLUSION

Every neonatal unit providing respiratory care should monitor the quality of respiratory care provided and continuously try to improve the process measures and outcomes of infants in their unit. It is important to recognize that QI methods do not replace formal randomized controlled trials (RCTs) as a research method; rather they complement RCTs in ensuring the implementation of evidence-based practices to improve outcome. The complex multifactorial nature of respiratory outcomes such as CLD often raises challenges in implementation of potentially better practices that have been successful elsewhere. It is thus imperative that changes be based on a review of the evidence when possible, to mitigate the possibility of perceived improvement ideas. By using evidence-based practices adapted to local context within structured QI projects, neonatal units can reduce unplanned extubations, prevent BPD, and improve other respiratory outcomes. Participation in a multicenter collaborative project may enhance such improvements.

REFERENCES

A complete reference list is available at https://expertconsult .inkling.com.

7

Medical and Legal Aspects of Respiratory Care

Jonathan M. Fanaroff, MD, JD

Caring for critically ill newborns takes years of training in which the clinician learns both the art and the science of the field. Relatively little time is spent learning about the legal system related to this discipline. The myriad regulations, unfamiliar language, and multimillion-dollar malpractice verdicts are hard to understand and comprehend. Consequently, most clinicians view the legal system with great mistrust and trepidation. Yet it is essential that physicians, nurses, and other health care providers understand their rights, duties, and liabilities while practicing health care. Additionally, modern neonatal medicine is a team endeavor and is built on a number of relationships. Physicians must understand the legal relationship they have with their patients and families and must also understand the legal relationships they have with employers, the hospital and nurses, referring physicians, respiratory therapists, neonatal nurse practitioners, and physician assistants.

This chapter provides an overview of the legal system in the United States, including the way it is structured as well as basic vocabulary and concepts. The goal is to provide the clinician with a better comprehension of the legal principles that affect neonatal respiratory care on a daily basis. While this chapter will center on the U.S. legal system, legal issues and medical malpractice affect clinicians globally. In fact, some European countries are experiencing triple-digit increases in the number of cases presumed "malpractice or bad health care."[1] Accordingly, physicians who practice in any country must understand the particular laws and regulations where they practice.

DISCLAIMER

The purpose of this chapter is to provide an overview of legal issues to educate clinicians. This chapter does not create an attorney–client relationship and should not be taken as substantive legal advice. Medicine is regulated at both the state and the federal levels, and laws vary significantly from state to state. The outcome of a legal case is based upon a particular set of facts, witnesses, attorneys, judges, and juries. A clinician should never assume that his or her situation is exactly the same as that of any case mentioned in this chapter. For specific questions, the reader should consult a qualified attorney.

GENERAL LEGAL PRINCIPLES

If law is the system of rules upon which we live, then the U.S. Constitution is the highest law of the land. Dating back to 1789, the Constitution sets up the framework of the federal and state governments. The federal government is divided into three separate but equal branches. Congress, composed of the Senate and House of Representatives, forms the legislative branch and is charged with making laws. The executive branch, led by the president and by far the largest branch, with approximately 5 million employed, carries out the laws. The judicial branch, which includes the U.S. Supreme Court, reviews the ways in which laws are applied and mediates between the other two branches. State governments have the same organization as the federal government except the executive branch is led by the governor instead of the president.

Both the state and the federal government court systems have hierarchies that are shown in Figure 7-1. While both federal and state laws affect the practice of medicine, medicine is primarily regulated by the states. Thus, for example, a physician or respiratory therapist licensed in one state cannot practice in another state without obtaining an additional license to practice in that state. Similarly, the majority of legal cases involving medicine are adjudicated in the state court system. For this reason it is important for a clinician to understand the relevant laws affecting practice in the states in which he or she has a medical license.

SUPERVISION OF OTHERS

Modern neonatology is a team effort. The attending physician is generally considered to be the leader of the team and as such has traditionally been held responsible for the acts of other team members. This can even include situations in which the physician has had no contact, direct or indirect, with the patient filing the lawsuit. There have been a number of legal theories to justify this position. One analogy has held physicians, especially surgeons, to be analogous to the "captain of the ship" and thus responsible for all of the crew under his or her command.[2] As care models have evolved and health care systems expanded, courts have increasingly rejected the captain of the ship doctrine, recognizing that the "theory" that the attending "directly controls *all* activities of whatever nature … is not realistic in present day medical care."[3]

While the attending neonatologist is no longer held responsible for all activities that occur in the neonatal intensive care unit (NICU), he or she still has authority over the actions of others in the unit. Consequently he or she may still be held liable under the legal theory of respondeat superior, which is Latin for "let the master answer."[4] When there is negligence by a nurse practitioner or resident who is within the legitimate scope of authority of the attending neonatologist, such as during an intubation, the attending may be held liable.

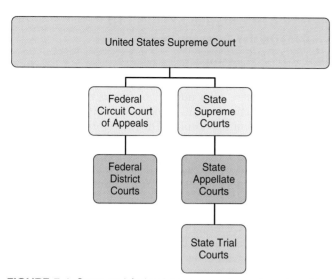

FIGURE 7-1 State and federal government court system hierarchies.

Attending physicians are also expected to provide appropriate supervision of residents and other health professionals and can be held liable for "negligent supervision." In one high-profile lawsuit, an attending anesthesiologist failed to respond to a resident physician's request to assist in an emergent cesarean section. The plaintiff alleged that the delay in timely supervision was the cause of permanent brain damage to the fetus, and the case settled for $35 million.[5]

MALPRACTICE

The cost of medical malpractice in the United States has been estimated at $55.6 billion per year.[6] Indeed several presidents have addressed the issue, including President Obama during his 2011 State of the Union Address, in which he lent support for "medical malpractice reform to rein in frivolous lawsuits."[7] These lawsuits have an impact on a large number of physicians. A study released by the American Medical Association (AMA) contained staggering numbers, including the fact that 95 liability claims were filed for every 100 physicians and that 61% of physicians 55 and older have been sued.[8] The AMA report found that the majority of cases (65%) were dropped, dismissed, or withdrawn and another 26% settled, but when the case did go to trial the physician prevailed 90% of the time. In the United States, however, each side pays its own costs, and the average defense costs were over $40,000 per claim and over $100,000 when the case went to trial.

Most medical malpractice cases are filed with the plaintiff claiming that the physician was negligent. Negligence lawsuits are part of the broader category of law known as *torts*, which is French for "wrong." Other broad legal categories include contracts, real property, and criminal law. Tort law is generally divided into intentional and unintentional torts. Most malpractice cases are considered unintentional torts, which is preferable as intentional torts such as defamation often carry broader penalties.

To prevail in a malpractice lawsuit the plaintiff must prove that the clinician has failed to act as a reasonably prudent physician in the same or similar circumstances.[9] In practice, this requires the plaintiff to prove four elements: that the physician had a *duty* to the patient that was *breached* and that in turn *caused* measurable *damages*.[10]

Duty

The first element that must be shown in a malpractice case is that the physician had a duty or physician–patient relationship with the patient. If there is no duty to the plaintiff, then the physician has no obligation toward the patient and there is no negligence. For example, if a physician practices only at hospital A, he or she cannot be held liable for refusing to attend a delivery at hospital B. The existence of a duty, however, is usually not in dispute in most neonatal malpractice cases. Furthermore, it is possible for a physician who has cared for a pregnant woman to have a duty toward the newborn even if the baby is cared for by a separate physician. This was shown in the case of *Nold v Binyon*, in which a newborn became a chronic carrier of hepatitis B and the obstetrician had failed to inform the woman of her hepatitis B status.[11] The obstetrician claimed that there was no duty toward the newborn but the Kansas Supreme Court disagreed, stating that "A physician who has a doctor–patient relationship with a pregnant woman who intends to carry her fetus to term and deliver a healthy baby also has a doctor–patient relationship with the fetus." As discussed earlier, another situation in which a duty may attach even when the physician never saw the patient is in the context of supervising other clinicians such as residents and nurse practitioners.

Breach

Once a duty has been established the plaintiff must next show that the clinician breached his or her duty by violating the "standard of care." There are misconceptions about "standard of care" that are important to clarify. First, physicians are not expected to be perfect but rather are expected to act as a "reasonably prudent" physician exercising "reasonable care and diligence." Second, "standard of care" is a legal concept that must be applied to a specific fact pattern of a case in litigation. The plaintiff's attorneys claim that the defendant has departed from an acceptable standard of care. The defense counters that the clinician has met the standard of care. Third, traditionally physicians were compared to other physicians in their local community. With changes in communication (i.e., national meetings, national journals) and a move toward national board certification, physicians in specialties such as neonatology have increasingly been compared to other specialists nationally. Thus a neonatologist in California can testify as an expert witness about the standard of care in Ohio.

The Expert Witness

In most areas of negligence a jury can understand "reasonably prudent" behavior using common sense. A driver speeding 85 miles an hour in a snowstorm is obviously not using "due care." In most medical malpractice cases, however, lay juries do not know what a reasonably prudent practitioner would have done. So expert witnesses are used to explain it to a jury. Each state decides what "qualifies" an individual to serve as an expert witness. Expert witnesses testify under oath, and the American Academy of Pediatrics expects pediatricians who serve as experts to provide "thorough, fair, objective, and impartial" testimony for reasonable compensation.[12] Nevertheless, concerns remain that "hired gun" experts "fuel inappropriate litigation through testimony that is not well grounded in prevailing clinical standards or science."[13] Many states are taking proactive steps in an attempt to improve the quality of expert testimony. Florida, for example, now requires physician experts from out of state to obtain an expert witness certificate issued by the state.[14] By obtaining the certificate the expert physician is then subject to discipline by the Florida Medical Board.

Causation

In addition to showing that the clinician breached his or her duty to the patient, the plaintiff must show that the breach in question was actually the cause of the injury for which the patient is suing for damages. It can be difficult to determine whether it was the breach of care rather than the underlying medical condition that led to the injury, especially in neonatal cases. Normal healthy newborns, for example, do not require resuscitation. So when an infant is born depressed and requires significant resuscitation it may be difficult to prove that it was the delay in intubation, for example, rather than the underlying pathology requiring intubation that led to a poor outcome. As with the element of breach, expert witnesses testify before the lay jury about causation issues.

Damages

The ultimate purpose of tort law is to "make whole" a party who has been injured through negligence. Accordingly, the final element a plaintiff must prove is that the injury led to measurable damages. There are two broad categories of damages: economic and noneconomic. Economic damages include items such as medical expenses, lost wages, home accommodations, and education expenses. Noneconomic damages include claims that are subjective and often more difficult to quantify, such as pain and suffering, emotional distress, or loss of the parent–child relationship. "Runaway jury" awards are often associated with noneconomic damages, and thus many state legislatures have placed limits on them as part of tort reform efforts. California, for example, has a $250,000 damage cap on noneconomic damages. The California Supreme Court ruled that such a cap was constitutional.[15] However, other states, including Georgia and Illinois, have decided that state caps on noneconomic damages are in violation of their state constitutions.[16,17]

If behavior is particularly egregious, courts may sometimes award punitive damages to the injured party. These are relatively rare in medical malpractice cases, but can occur, for example, in cases in which the physician has behaved in a particularly reckless manner. An example would be if a physician practiced while under the influence of drugs or alcohol or intentionally altered or destroyed pertinent medical records in an effort to avoid liability.

Burden of Proof

The burden of proof refers to the "degree of belief" that the judge or jury must have to decide that a particular fact is true and find for one side over the other. In criminal cases, because of the injustice of jailing an innocent person, there is a very high burden of proof known as "beyond a reasonable doubt." Medical malpractice cases, on the other hand, have a much lower burden of proof. In general the plaintiff must show for each element that it is "more likely than not," otherwise known as the preponderance of the evidence or the "51% test."

MALPRACTICE ISSUES SPECIFIC TO NEONATOLOGY AND NEONATAL RESPIRATORY CARE

Caring for sick newborns can be extremely rewarding, but unfortunately there are a number of factors that increase the risk of a malpractice lawsuit. Babies in the NICU have among the longest stays in the hospital. During that time they receive multiple medications that are individually dosed and, in fact, the same baby will have multiple dosages of the same medication over time owing to changes in weight. The requirement for a round-the-clock care increases the number of caregivers involved and increases the risk of communication/hand-off errors. Additionally, many personal injury attorneys specialize in birth injury cases for a number of reasons. Economic damages for a brain-damaged infant can easily reach several million dollars and juries tend to be very sympathetic toward the infant and his or her family.

Box 7-1 lists common malpractice suits in neonatology. A number of areas specifically relate to neonatal respiratory care.

Resuscitation

Resuscitation of the depressed newborn is a relatively rare event that requires a combination of knowledge, teamwork, and technical skill. The Neonatal Resuscitation Program (NRP) provider course has been revised to incorporate teamwork and communication skills and an increasing emphasis on simulation.[18] Particular areas of medicolegal risk include timely attendance at delivery, giving medications without delay when indicated, and timely recognition of when the endotracheal tube is placed incorrectly. Additionally, as recognized by the NRP, prompt evaluation and referral for therapeutic hypothermia may help avoid a delay in establishing cooling within the 6-h therapeutic window.

Prematurity/Periventricular Leukomalacia

Prematurity has not traditionally been a focus of medical malpractice litigation, and when lawsuits were filed they usually were directed at obstetricians. As outcomes have improved,

---

BOX 7-1   Common Malpractice Lawsuits in Neonatology

Delivery Room Management/Resuscitation
- Delay in resuscitation
- Unrecognized esophageal intubation
- Failure to appropriately monitor after resuscitation

Hypoxic–Ischemic Encephalopathy (HIE)
- Failure to recognize HIE and initiate therapeutic hypothermia
- Delayed transfer of a candidate for therapeutic hypothermia

Late Preterm Infants
- Treated as term with unrecognized complications in well-baby nursery
- Early discharge with complications occurring at home
- Lack of proper follow-up after discharge

Neonatal Jaundice
- Failure to recognize risk factors for jaundice
- Lack of proper follow-up after discharge
- Delay in performing an exchange transfusion when indicated

Patient Safety
- Medication errors
- Poor communication
- Failure to adequately monitor/delayed treatment (hypoglycemia, electrolytes)

however, expectations have increased and prematurity has become a burgeoning area of malpractice lawsuits. Obstetricians remain at risk, as one recent case illustrates. A pregnant woman presented to the hospital with premature rupture of the membranes at just over 24 weeks' gestation. When the baby was born a few hours later in distress, the obstetrician and hospital were sued for failing to perform a cesarean section in a timely manner. The jury subsequently awarded the plaintiffs $14.5 million dollars.[19]

The vast majority of extremely premature infants have a period of time during which their blood sugar, blood pressure, blood count, or blood gas is out of the "normal" range. When an adverse outcome occurs, the abnormal value can be cited as the proximate cause of the injury. Hypocarbia, for example, has been shown to be an independent predictor of periventricular leukomalacia.[20] As periventricular leukomalacia has in turn been associated with poor long-term neurodevelopmental outcomes (particularly cerebral palsy), it is advisable to respond to low CO_2 levels in a mechanically ventilated infant and document that response.

RESPIRATORY FAILURE/MECHANICAL VENTILATION

While there is an increasing emphasis in neonatology on non-invasive ventilation there are still situations in which surfactant is an appropriate therapy. Consequently, delay in giving surfactant leading to worsened respiratory failure with subsequent acidosis and potentially poor long-term neurodevelopmental outcomes can be an area of malpractice risk. Similar allegations can occur when there is delayed recognition and response to a pneumothorax, particularly tension pneumothorax, while an infant is mechanically ventilated. Clinicians should be vigilant and responsive to a number of complications associated with mechanical ventilation, including a plugged or displaced endotracheal tube, kinked ventilator tubing, and mechanical problems with the ventilator itself.

Patient Safety/Culture of Safety

Critically ill neonates require 24-h care in a rapidly changing, complex, and technologically oriented environment. As in the delivery room, communication and teamwork are required to provide high-quality safe care. There has been an increasing focus on patient safety since a 1999 Institute of Medicine report estimated that preventable errors cause up to 98,000 patient deaths annually.[21] Efforts to improve patient safety have focused on adaptation of techniques from high-reliability industries including aviation and nuclear power. High-reliability organizations share a number of characteristics, including:

- Preoccupation with failure
- Reluctance to simplify interpretations
- Sensitivity to operations
- Commitment to resilience
- Deference to expertise[22]

Efforts to create a safer health care environment require more than updated policies and standards. Ultimately there must be a culture of safety as opposed to a culture of finger pointing and blame. Traditionally when, for example, a medication error occurred, the "solution" would be to fire the clinician who gave the medicine rather than look at potential system causes of the error. An institutional culture in which health care providers feel supported in efforts both to point out vulnerabilities in safe care delivery and to respond appropriately when an error occurs is much more likely to meet the World Health Organization vision of patient safety: Every patient receives safe health care, every time, everywhere.[23]

DECREASING THE RISK OF A MALPRACTICE LAWSUIT

Being sued is an incredibly stressful experience. Unfortunately the litigation can stretch out for years and cost thousands of dollars in defense costs alone. Additionally, it is common for physician defendants to suffer from a number of physical and emotional effects known as *medical malpractice stress syndrome*.[24] Just as adverse outcomes are not always preventable, physicians are always at risk of being named in a malpractice lawsuit. It is important to involve risk management proactively when an unexpected adverse outcome occurs. A number of strategies (Box 7-2), however, may be helpful to avoid tort litigation.

Competency

Neonatology is a rapidly changing specialty, and it is important for clinicians to remain up-to-date in the field. There are a number of ways to achieve this goal, including attending local, regional, and national conferences and reading journals and textbooks. An example of the changing recommendations for the practice of neonatology is seen in the postnatal use of steroids in ventilator-dependent babies. Dexamethasone was widely used on ventilated preemies in the 1990s to enhance rapid weaning and extubation from ventilator support. In 2002 the American Academy of Pediatrics Committee on Fetus and Newborn recommended against the routine use of the drug owing to concerns over long-term neurologic effects. This position was reaffirmed in 2010 and again in 2014 with the advice that high-dose dexamethasone or other steroid use should be an "individualized decision … made in conjunction with the infant's parents."[25]

Communication

Communication is an important skill in providing safe and effective medical care. As The Joint Commission notes, "When communication is effective, it can help improve the care an organization provides. When it is poor it can lead to inconvenience, frustration, error, and sometimes tragedy."[26] Additionally, poor communication with patients and families is cited in more than 40% of malpractice cases.[27]

BOX 7-2 Strategies to Avoid Tort Litigation

Stay current in the field
- Conference attendance
- Literature
- Textbooks

Communicate
- With other members of the team
- With the parents

Document
- Factually
- Professionally

Be aware of state laws that affect your practice.

Documentation

There is an old saying that "if it is was not documented, it was not done." This is not, of course, strictly correct. It may be several years, however, between the time care is provided and when a lawsuit is filed. The amount of time available to file a lawsuit, known as the *statute of limitations*, is determined by state law, and in many states it can be as long as 20 or more years for minors. Accordingly, documenting the care provided in a factual and professional manner is important. It is important not to speculate or attribute causation when this is uncertain. Communication with other team members as well as the family should also be documented, but the chart should not be used as a battleground between caretakers.

THE FUTURE OF MALPRACTICE LITIGATION

Few would disagree that the current malpractice system is expensive and inefficient. Malpractice premiums for obstetricians in Miami are more than $190,000 per year,[28] yet one study found that for every dollar spent on malpractice compensation, 54 cents went to administrative expenses such as lawyers, expert witnesses, and the courts.[29] For this reason, as well as increased efforts by health care in general to become both safer and more transparent, there are a number of "nontraditional" reform approaches that show some promise.[30] The University of Michigan Health System, for example, instituted a communication and resolution program in which they perform active surveillance for medical errors, fully disclose found errors to patients, and offer compensation when they are at fault.[31] Since implementing the program they experienced fewer lawsuits, which were resolved more quickly and with dramatically lower legal costs. The states of Florida and Virginia have initiated Neurologic Injury Compensation Acts (or NICA laws), which allow newborns who are injured at birth to receive compensation through a "no fault"-type system.[32]

CONCLUSION

The field of neonatology has made tremendous progress over the past decades. With this progress have come greater expectations. Additionally, there is an increasing emphasis on transparency and creating a culture of safety with the goal of learning from both mistakes and near misses. The current adversarial malpractice system has been described as "prolonged, expensive, and inconsistent."[30] Nontraditional approaches to malpractice liability reform show promise but are mainly still in the testing phase. Clinicians will benefit from a greater understanding of the medical malpractice system, common areas of malpractice risk, and strategies to minimize the risk of being named in a malpractice lawsuit.

REFERENCES

A complete reference list is available at https://expertconsult .inkling.com/.

Physical Examination

Edward G. Shepherd, MD, and Leif D. Nelin, MD

HISTORICAL ASPECTS

The physical examination, along with the history, is the oldest tool available to the physician to diagnose and assess response to treatment. Hippocrates and his contemporaries wrote about the importance of the physical examination including inspection, palpation, and direct auscultation nearly 2500 years ago.[1] Leopold Auenbrugger first described the technique of percussion in 1761 and has been credited with the beginning of the modern physical examination. René Laennec invented the stethoscope and in 1819 published *On Mediate Auscultation*, which was essentially a manual on the stethoscope and included many terms still used today. The development of all components of the physical examination continued during the nineteenth century such that by the beginning of the twentieth century the physical exam we perform today was fully established.[2]

The last half of the twentieth century saw a rapid development of diagnostic technology, which continues today. However, none of the currently available technologies has entirely supplanted the physical exam. Indeed, a study by Paley et al.[3] published in 2011 found that more than 80% of newly admitted internal medicine patients could be correctly diagnosed on admission based on the history and physical examination, and that basic clinical skills remain a powerful tool, sufficient for achieving an accurate diagnosis in most cases. In a study in a general medicine inpatient service it was found that 26% of patients had physical findings by the attending physician that led to important changes in clinical management.[4] Thus, the physical exam remains the foundation upon which diagnosis and therapy are based.

IMPORTANCE OF THE PHYSICAL EXAMINATION

The physical examination is central to the care of the neonate, especially those requiring assisted ventilation. It provides immediate information on each patient's status and how he or she is responding to therapy without the delays inherent in any diagnostic test. Further, neonatal intensive care unit (NICU) patients are unique in that they are conscious and not routinely sedated while on intermittent positive pressure ventilation (IPPV).[5] Thus, the physical exam remains accurate in assessing both current status and immediate responses to changes in support. The physical examination must guide the care that the patient receives; especially any subsequent diagnostic workup and therapies. In patients with evolving pathophysiology, physical exams should be frequently repeated as responses to therapy may be rapid. Indeed, the most reliable, most cost-effective, and least invasive way to determine the success or failure of a change in therapy for any patient is to observe his or her response.

TECHNIQUE OF THE PHYSICAL EXAMINATION

Overview

The examiner should obtain the permission of the bedside nurse before the hands-on assessment, and the entire examination of the baby (including exposure to ambient light) should be done as gently and noninvasively as possible. Ideally the examination should be clustered with other cares so that the baby is disturbed as little as possible. Physical examination of newborn infants is uniquely challenging as "normal" findings are dependent on a number of variables influenced by gestational age, age at examination, size, mode of respiratory support, and other factors.[6-8] In addition to these, a number of other exam findings change predictably with time and age. Skin color is blue or pale at birth but rapidly turns pink if transition occurs properly. Normal respiratory rates depend on gestational age, size, and mode of respiratory support, whereas normative goals for blood pressures depend on gestational age at birth and corrected gestational age at time of obtainment.[9-11] Blood pressure is low at the time of birth and gradually increases with each day and month until pediatric norms are achieved, whereas respiratory rate typically starts fast and slows until pediatric norms are achieved. In particular, physical examination findings in a newly born infant should be interpreted in light of the unique anatomic and physiologic changes that occur during transition from the intrauterine to the extrauterine environment. The following sections will therefore focus on the unique physiologic factors that influence the newborn respiratory physical exam and the specific exam techniques and findings most helpful in neonates at different ages and with specific conditions.

Performing the Neonatal Respiratory Physical Examination

The newborn respiratory exam begins with observation followed by auscultation and palpation. Optimal physical examination of the respiratory system in the newborn requires both observation and hands-on assessment. Observation is focused on obtaining an overall impression of the infant's comfort, color, perfusion, movement patterns, respiratory effort, respiratory rate, and level of interaction with the environment. Hands-on assessment includes auscultation and palpation. Ideally, observation occurs prior to any hands-on assessment to obtain steady-state information, as hands-on assessments are likely to disturb the infant.

The respiratory physical exam can be divided into the following questions the examiner should answer sequentially:
- How does the baby look?
- What am I hearing?
- What am I feeling?

The examination begins with an overall assessment of the baby's status and a rapid assessment of vital signs, keeping in mind that normal vital signs depend on gestational age at delivery and time in minutes and/or days of life.[11] The respiratory rate should be normal for age and gestation, and respiratory effort should be unlabored. For a period of time after birth up to 12 to 24 hours of age, mild retractions and tachypnea may be present as respiratory compliance improves (particularly in premature infants). The infant should be pink and resting comfortably, although acrocyanosis may persist well after delivery. The infant should be well perfused with brisk capillary refill and should have normal tone with a vigorous response to external stimuli. Respirations should be quiet, without stridor or stertor, and the infant must be able to breathe comfortably with a closed mouth. The thorax and abdomen should be normally shaped. The presence of a "barrel chest" suggests lung hyperinflation, a bell-shaped chest may indicate poorly inflated lungs, whereas a scaphoid abdomen may suggest displacement of abdominal contents into the thorax. The rib cage and abdomen should move in synchrony during the respiratory cycle, but in the presence of lung disease thoracoabdominal asynchrony may be marked. Specifically, movement of the rib cage lags behind movement of the abdomen on inhalation, so-called paradoxic movement, suggesting increased respiratory resistance or decreased compliance.[12]

A brief inspection of the infant should determine that the facies are normal in appearance, ears are properly placed and rotated, abdomen and chest are normal in appearance, and that the extremities are supple with a full range of motion. Abnormalities in any of these observations should guide the subsequent examination and evaluation. For example, cyanosis out of proportion to respiratory distress should prompt a thorough cardiac evaluation, whereas contractures or other signs of Potter syndrome should prompt a careful respiratory, neurologic, and renal evaluation. This is followed by a detailed examination of the airway that includes examination of the palate and lip for possible clefts, the chin and tongue for possible airway obstruction, the neck for possible tracheal deviation or goiter, the nares for atresia or stenosis, the ear canals, and the eyes.

The initial observation should be followed by auscultation. This and all subsequent portions of the examination should be informed by any findings on initial observation; however, the examiner must ensure that a complete and thorough examination is performed on every newborn regardless of initial findings. Auscultation should begin with careful evaluation of heart and lung sounds although the presence or absence of a murmur does not definitively include or exclude congenital heart disease, especially in the immediate postpartum period.

Breath sounds both anteriorly and posteriorly should be clear and equal without wheezing or rhonchi; crackles are occasionally heard in the immediate postpartum period but should resolve quickly as lung water is resorbed. Audible bowel sounds in the chest suggest a congenital diaphragmatic hernia. The abdomen should be auscultated for the presence of bowel sounds, and the liver and head should be auscultated for the presence of bruits. In addition to auscultation with a stethoscope, the clinician should also listen for the presence of stridor (suggestive of upper airway obstruction) or audible wheezing (suggestive of bronchial constriction).

Once auscultation is completed, the examiner should palpate for determination of the presence or absence of crepitus; fractured clavicles, femurs, or humeri; hepatosplenomegaly; any intra-abdominal masses; hernias; or abdominal tenderness. The chest should be palpated to determine heart position, as well as the presence of thrills or heaves. The abdomen should be soft and nondistended, and the liver edge should be even with the costal margin.

INTERPRETATION OF THE FINDINGS OF PHYSICAL EXAMINATION

General Physical Examination Findings

In the neonate with respiratory distress, hypoxemia, and/or respiratory failure the physical examination may change with disease progression. The neonate often comes to the attention of the clinician with evidence of tachypnea, nasal flaring, retractions, and/or grunting. These signs on physical examination relate to pulmonary problems but are not pathognomonic for any particular neonatal respiratory disease. Thus, the spectrum of neonatal respiratory disease must be considered, and frequent reassessment of the patient is needed because the evolution of these symptoms can help to differentiate particular causes (Fig. 8-1). For example, if the symptoms improve within hours then it is likely the patient had transient tachypnea of the newborn (TTN). On the other hand, if the symptoms continue to worsen and the patient is a preterm infant, then surfactant deficiency (respiratory distress syndrome, or RDS) is the more likely diagnosis. It should be kept in mind that none of the currently available laboratory testing or imaging definitively differentiates the underlying causes of neonatal respiratory diseases. For example, a low lung volume diffusely hazy chest X-ray in a preterm infant is likely to be RDS; however, other common causes of respiratory distress like neonatal pneumonia, TTN, and congestive heart failure cannot be ruled out. Thus, physical examination on admission and frequent reassessment are likely to be the best way to diagnose neonatal respiratory diseases. Furthermore, when a patient is improving and respiratory support is weaned, the first indication that a patient is not tolerating that wean is likely to come from the physical examination, particularly new findings of head bobbing, tachypnea, and nasal flaring.

There is a huge variety of potential abnormal findings on newborn examination, each of which may reflect a number of potential pathologies or normal variants. Asymmetric breath sounds, for example, may reflect pneumothorax, pneumonia, congenital diaphragmatic hernia, atelectasis, or malpositioned endotracheal tube or may be an artifact of the listener. Hepatosplenomegaly may reflect venous congestion, intrinsic liver disease, infection, platelet aggregation, or lung hyperinflation. Abdominal distention may reflect obstruction, atresia, malrotation, or swallowed air. The presence of abnormal findings,

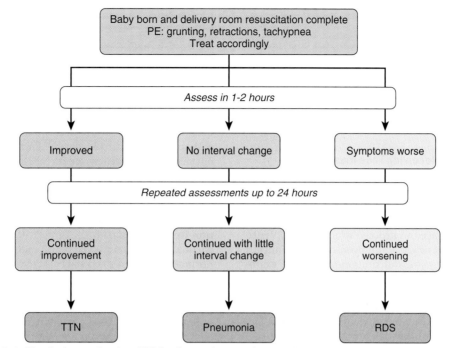

FIG 8-1 Physical examination (PE) in diagnosing respiratory distress in the newborn. Babies born with transient tachypnea of the newborn (TTN) are sick at birth, but their signs and symptoms begin to resolve nearly immediately. Babies born with pneumonia will be sick at birth and show little improvement until the pneumonia begins to clear; with bacterial pneumonia this can take 2-3 days. Babies born with respiratory distress syndrome (RDS), otherwise known as *surfactant deficiency*, continue to have worsening of symptoms until treated with exogenous surfactant or after about 48 hours of age. The key for physical examination of these infants is frequently repeated assessments.

or the lack of normal findings, on physical examination should prompt and direct the ensuing laboratory and/or imaging diagnostic workup.

Although many of these exam findings will be static (e.g., once it is determined that the infant does not have a cleft palate this portion of the exam may not need to be repeated daily), other aspects of an infant's exam will change with time, disease progression, and age. Retractions, for instance, may be significant in the initial stages of both TTN and RDS, but they will improve steadily in the former and probably worsen in the latter if exogenous surfactant has not been given. Similarly, initial tachypnea by definition resolves in TTN but may not in RDS or pneumonia. Conversely, once compliance is improved after the administration of exogenous surfactant in RDS, both retractions and tachypnea tend to improve rapidly.

Special Technique of Examination: Transillumination

Pneumothorax is a potentially life-threatening complication in neonates and may be difficult to diagnose emergently; the chest X-ray remains the gold standard of diagnosis if time permits. Unfortunately, infants suffering this complication may require therapy well before a chest X-ray can be obtained. In such situations, transillumination may be helpful. The examiner places a cool, bright light source against the chest wall on the potentially involved side, and if a pneumothorax is present the light will typically radiate across the chest and illuminate the entire hemithorax. While this test can be helpful in emergent situations, it is prone to false positive or negative results and thus must be

carefully considered in the context of all other available diagnostic information.

Physical Examination Findings in Specific Clinical Situations

Examination at Birth

The physiology of the newborn is uniquely adapted to the transition from intrauterine to extrauterine life. This transition leads to many of the physical exam findings noted at birth and is also the basis for a number of normal physical findings in neonates that would be atypical for older children and adults. Specifically, newborn infants are exiting a fluid-filled environment in which blood with relatively low oxygen tension (Po_2) is supplied by the placenta to one in which blood with relatively high Po_2 is supplied by the newly air-filled lungs; thus the neonate's skin color is often cyanotic even in the absence of deranged respiration. In addition, there are numerous hormonal surges associated with labor and delivery, such as antidiuretic hormone, that have an impact on the hypothalamic–pituitary axis, which can lead to the signs of hypoperfusion such as delayed capillary refill even in the absence of shock. Moreover, the newborn infant has a relatively compliant chest wall, especially if he or she is born prematurely. This increased chest wall elasticity may lead to decreased functional residual capacity, resulting in tachypnea and increased work of breathing even in the absence of pulmonary disease. Finally, newborn infants, especially those born prematurely, are at high risk for deranged control of breathing leading to apnea and bradycardia. Immediate observation at birth is well described in the Neonatal Resuscitation Program

(NRP) and consists of a quick assessment of tone and respiratory effort followed by color. Subsequent assessments follow based on the results of this initial survey. Current NRP recommendations require placement of a pulse oximeter in the delivery room to follow oxygenation (SpO_2). Of note, during the immediate postpartum period, SpO_2 will typically take more than 5 min to reach 80% and 10 minutes to reach 90%.[6] Once the infant is stabilized, a thorough respiratory exam should follow.

Examination of an Infant Receiving Face Mask or Laryngeal Mask Ventilation

Noninvasive ventilation may be provided to neonates via face mask or laryngeal mask airway (LMA) application. In most cases, such ventilation is adequate for neonatal resuscitation, and relatively few babies will need to proceed to intubation. Ventilation via either face mask or LMA, however, can be technically difficult, especially during stressful situations, and the examiner must be well attuned to the signs of proper noninvasive ventilation. Specifically, if ventilation is applied effectively the baby should have a rapidly improving heart rate, tone should improve (unless the baby is hypotonic owing to extrinsic factors such as medication administration), color should improve, and, most important, the baby should have good chest rise with each bagged ventilation. If poor chest rise is noted, the patient's position should be readjusted to ensure the proper "sniffing" position, the seal between mask and face should be ensured, and the pressure applied via the bag should be evaluated to ensure adequacy. In those relatively few newborns and infants with highly significant lung disease, high pressures may be required to achieve adequate chest excursion.

Examination of a Ventilated Infant

The neonatal respiratory examination is further complicated because it is heavily influenced by the medical therapies and support many of these infants require as part of their care. Extremely low birth-weight infants with very compliant chest walls, for instance, will all require positive pressure (nasal constant positive airway pressure (nCPAP), IPPV, or high-frequency ventilation) in the first few weeks of life. Each mode of positive pressure support will interact with the infant's respiratory system in different ways and will create unique respiratory findings. Once the infant is stabilized on properly applied positive pressure, the physical examination should improve markedly, and failure to improve should conversely be taken as a warning that the infant may not be receiving adequate support. Typical signs of improvement include decreased respiratory rate; significant reduction in retractions; reduction in nasal flaring, grunting, and/or head bobbing; improved color; improvements in tone; and less agitation.

Conventional Ventilation. This section focuses on the essentials of the physical examination in ventilated neonates and how to interpret changes in the physical examination. Some key concepts to consider include (1) infants requiring IPPV will have both spontaneous and ventilator-assisted respirations, each of which will manifest distinctively; (2) infants with a large leak around the endotracheal tube will often have an audible air leak around the tube with each ventilator-delivered inflation; and (3) a patient on IPPV whose delivered minute ventilation is too small (i.e., the patient is undersupported) will exhibit worsening physical exam findings as the patient "fights" the ventilator to try to improve minute ventilation.

The NICU is a unique environment for caring for patients with respiratory distress. Many of our patients remain on IPPV for long periods of time. A report from the Eunice Kennedy Shriver National Institute of Child Health and Human Development Neonatal Research Network (NRN) found that, in a cohort of appropriate-for-gestational-age infants born at <27 weeks admitted to NRN centers, the average duration of IPPV was 26 ± 26 days.[13] In a population cohort of infants born at <27 weeks in Sweden the median IPPV days were 11 with a range of 1 to 134 days.[14] Therefore, it is no longer recommended to routinely sedate NICU patients on IPPV, as this has been found to result in negative outcomes related to duration of IPPV and neurodevelopment.[5] The majority of NICU patients on the ventilator for pulmonary disease will then be awake and alert, which allows the use of the physical examination to assess adequacy of support. If the ventilator support is adequate the patient is likely to breathe comfortably and have normal awake and sleep states (Fig. 8-2). On the other hand, if the respiratory support is inadequate (i.e., the patient's needs are undersupported) the patient will exhibit signs of air hunger including tachypnea, retractions, nasal flaring, and/or head bobbing, as well as being irritable, tachycardic, and difficult to console. Undersupported neonates often are given sedatives to try to control their irritability and movements, and yet what the undersupported patient really needs is an increase in respiratory support. It must also be kept in mind that our patients will do what they can via spontaneous respiratory effort to compensate when they are undersupported, such that at least initially the blood gases may not reflect the fact that the patient is undersupported. That is to say, if a patient has too low a minute ventilation (tidal volume times frequency), then the patient will compensate by tachypnea and an increased work of breathing such that the irritable, tachypneic, retracting patient may actually have a normal carbon dioxide tension (Pco_2) on the blood gas, until such time that the patient can no longer maintain those spontaneous breaths (Fig. 8-3). Thus, it is likely that at least for some patients the physical exam may be a better indicator of acute patient status than the blood gases.

High-Frequency Ventilation: Oscillation. A patient placed on high-frequency oscillatory ventilation (HFOV) may not breathe regularly, and auscultation of the chest may not reveal

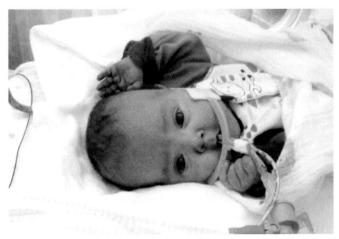

FIG 8-2 A typical awake and alert baby on intermittent positive pressure ventilation. The patient is interactive with the environment, which allows for developmentally appropriate care to be successfully done.

breath sounds in a patient who is adequately supported. Properly applied HFOV will create a "wiggle" in the infant's chest that will be accompanied by vibratory sounds on auscultation. The presence of an adequate wiggle is a good sign, indicating that the ventilator is able to enhance gas exchange. A poor chest wiggle is a sign of low lung compliance (and is often associated with a wiggle of the abdomen that is more prominent than that of the chest). It will usually be impossible to hear typical breath sounds on a patient undergoing HFOV, so additional examination findings necessarily must be substituted to ensure proper placement of the endotracheal tube, symmetry of breath sounds, and so forth. Asymmetric oscillator sounds can indicate asymmetric lung expansion, which may be due to a main stem bronchus intubation (in which the right is most likely, given the anatomy) or a unilateral pneumothorax.

High-Frequency Ventilation: Jet Ventilation. A patient placed on the jet ventilator will have findings and interpretations similar to those on HFOV in terms of chest wiggle. One difference with high-frequency jet ventilation (HFJV) is that it is used with a conventional ventilator to apply positive end-expiratory pressure and often to supply sigh breaths. Thus, during HFJV when conventional sigh breaths are used, auscultation can determine air entry and chest rise during the sigh breaths.

Examination of an Infant on CPAP

Infants requiring nCPAP will typically have either "bubbling" breath sounds, if they are on properly applied bubble nCPAP, or a CPAP "roar" if on properly applied infant-flow nCPAP. A preterm infant who has severe retractions, nasal flaring, and grunting and who is placed on nCPAP may quickly exhibit improvement or even resolution of symptoms.

SUMMARY

The physical examination has been used in its current form for over a century. Despite the rapid proliferation of various laboratory and imaging modalities, the physical examination remains the cornerstone of medical care. Ventilated patients in the NICU are not routinely sedated, and modern ventilators allow for sensing of spontaneous breaths; therefore the physical examination can be used as a rapid determinant of the adequacy of the support provided by the ventilator. Patients on IPPV who are adequately supported should have normal sleep/wake cycles,

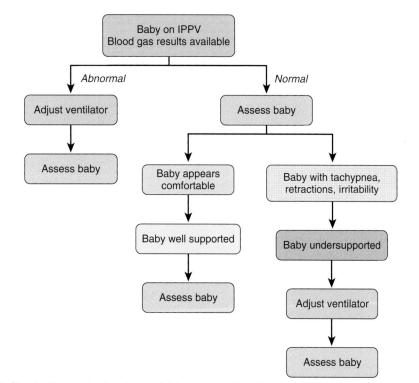

FIG 8-3 Physical examination is useful in determining the adequacy of ventilator support for babies on intermittent positive pressure ventilation (IPPV). Steady-state blood gases (i.e., those obtained from an indwelling vascular catheter) are often followed on these babies, particularly those with acute lung diseases in the first few days of life. When a blood gas is done on a baby on IPPV and it is abnormal, then the ventilator has to be adjusted accordingly. If the blood gas is normal it is imperative to look at the baby. If the baby is well supported then the baby will look comfortable on the ventilator—that is, breathing easily with minimal retractions, no tachypnea, and little evidence of "fighting" the ventilator. On the other hand, if the baby is undersupported and tachypneic with increased work of breathing, then the baby is likely to be compensating for the lack of adequate support such that the blood gas is normal but clearly the ventilator needs to be adjusted to improve the level of support. Once adjustments have been made it is important to continue to frequently assess the baby on IPPV as this will be the first evidence of changes in the patient's respiratory status.

should breathe comfortably while being supported, and should not be irritable. One should consider adjusting the ventilator of any patient in the NICU on IPPV who is irritable, is tachypneic, or manifests increased work of breathing, rather than assuming that the patient requires sedation and/or paralysis. Although steady-state blood gases remain a mainstay of assessing adequacy of ventilator support, the physical examination remains the gold standard for assessing the neonate requiring mechanical ventilation.

REFERENCES

A complete reference list is available at https://expertconsult .inkling.com/.

9

Imaging: Radiography, Lung Ultrasound, and Other Imaging Modalities

Erik A. Jensen, MD, D. Andrew Mong, MD, David M. Biko, MD, Kathryn L. Maschhoff, MD, PhD, and Haresh Kirpalani, BM, MRCP, FRCP, MSc

INTRODUCTION

Respiratory illnesses are among the most common and potentially life-threatening conditions encountered in the newborn. This makes the radiologic examination of the infant chest a common and essential tool to guide the diagnosis and treatment of neonatal lung disease. Using and interpreting imaging studies well requires teamwork and open lines of communication between clinicians (including obstetricians, surgeons, and pediatric subspecialists as appropriate) and radiologists. This is particularly true now, as digital radiology and point-of-care ultrasound make direct interaction between clinicians and radiologists less common. Although the plain radiograph remains the mainstay of neonatal chest imaging, other modalities such as ultrasound and computed tomography are increasingly used in the evaluation of acutely ill neonates. Technologic advances in fetal imaging also now permit improved prenatal diagnosis and in some cases fetal treatment of congenital chest lesions.

To provide high-quality care to the ill neonate, clinicians must understand the capabilities and limitations of common imaging tools and learn to identify the radiographic findings of common neonatal respiratory conditions. Although written materials aid in this process, pattern recognition can be gained only through regular review of films. This chapter highlights important aspects of neonatal chest imaging and provides specific clinical examples directed toward trainees and practicing clinicians. More in-depth discussions of neonatal chest imaging can be found in other reviews.[1,2]

RADIATION EXPOSURE

Several common imaging modalities including plain radiography, computed tomography (CT), fluoroscopy, and nuclear medicine use ionizing radiation to produce images. As radiation dose exposure is cumulative and even low total exposure in infancy is associated with slightly increased risk of later malignancy, clinicians must weigh the diagnostic advantage of an imaging modality with its expected radiation dose.[3,4] The typical dose from a single chest X-ray is approximately 0.008 to 0.03 millisieverts (mSv) depending on the technique and equipment.[5,6] When combined with an abdominal radiograph, the dose is 1.5 to 2 times higher.[5,6] By comparison, the total natural radiation exposure from sources such as the sun and radioactive materials in the air and soil amounts to about 3 mSv per year at sea level and 5 to 6 mSv at an elevation of 5000 feet.[7]

The dose from a continuous digital fluoroscopic voiding cystourethrogram is approximately 0.45 to 0.59 mSv.[8] The use of pulsed fluoroscopy optimized for children reduces the dose to 0.05 to 0.07 mSv.[8] The effective dose received from an upper gastrointestinal series is 1.2 to 6.5 mSv.[9] For a chest CT taken without consideration of a patient's weight or dose-lowering techniques, the radiation dose is approximately 4 to 7 mSv.[7,10] With low-dose, high-resolution CT, the dose is reduced to about 1 mSv with negligible loss in image quality.[10]

To minimize radiation exposure, clinicians and radiologists should adhere to the practice of as low as reasonably achievable (ALARA), which requires weight-based protocols, limiting the number of studies performed, and the use of non-radiation modalities such as ultrasound (US) and magnetic resonance imaging (MRI) when appropriate.[11] The use of collimation (restriction of the X-ray beam to the desired anatomic area) and shielding of adjacent structures, particularly the gonads, is essential to reduce unnecessary radiation exposure. Health care workers also need to be aware of the potential risks to themselves and take appropriate precautions to minimize exposure.

IMAGING MODALITIES

Chest Radiograph

The plain chest radiograph or X-ray (CXR) is the most widely used imaging modality in the neonatal intensive care unit (NICU). The CXR utilizes the natural contrast between air (dark or black on a standard radiograph) and fluid or tissue (white or gray). Appropriate positioning of the infant is essential to produce a high-quality radiograph. A "rotated" CXR may lead to a false diagnosis of cardiomegaly, mediastinal shift, atelectasis, or abnormal central line location (Fig. 9-1). When possible, the infant's arms should be extended away from the chest to prevent the scapulae from obscuring the upper lung fields.

In most cases, a single anterior–posterior (AP) view with the infant in a supine position is adequate to assess the chest wall, heart, airway, and lungs, and any invasive lines or tubes. Lateral radiographs of the chest are not routinely necessary but can aid in specific circumstances such as assessment of the retrocardiac lung fields, diagnosis of air-leak syndromes, and evaluation of pleural drain location. A systematic approach is recommended when describing a CXR to avoid missing potentially important findings. The "alphabet" approach reminds clinicians to assess the Airway (trachea and its branches), Bones (clavicles, ribs,

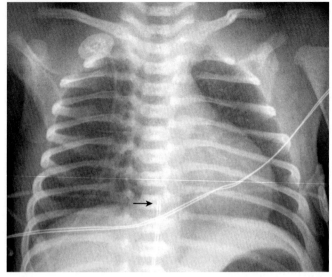

FIG 9-1 Rotated anterior–posterior chest radiograph in a 4-day-old full-term infant. The right-sided ribs are foreshortened and the left are elongated. The mediastinum appears shifted to the left. An appropriately positioned umbilical venous catheter projects over the left of the spine, just above the diaphragm (*arrow*).

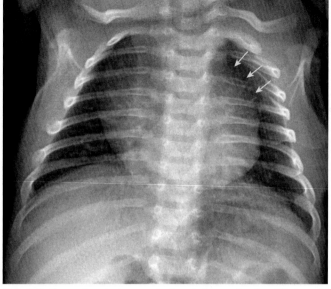

FIG 9-2 Normal anterior–posterior radiograph of a 26-day-old full-term female. The lungs are clear. There is a left-sided aortic arch and the heart is normal in size. The prominent superior mediastinal contour with wavy borders (*arrows*) is compatible with a normal thymus.

scapulae, vertebrae, and humeri), Cardiac structures (heart site, size, shape, and border and great vessels), Diaphragm, Effusions (small effusions blunt the costophrenic angle), Fields and fissures (adequacy and symmetry of lung field expansion and thick or fluid-filled fissures), Gastric fundus (stomach bubble and other visible intra-abdominal structures), and Hilum and mediastinum.

In a normal, correctly positioned AP CXR the neonatal chest is trapezoid in shape with horizontal ribs (Fig. 9-2). The diaphragm is domed bilaterally and lies at the level of the sixth to the eighth ribs. Both lungs should be symmetrically aerated with uniform radiolucency soon after birth. Air bronchograms in the lung bases, particularly in the lower left lobe behind the cardiac border, are normal. Pulmonary vascular markings are visualized centrally and become less prominent toward the periphery. The transverse cardiothoracic ratio should not exceed 60% to 65%.[12] Elimination of the normal border between the radiopaque thoracic structures (e.g., heart, great vessels) and the radiolucent lung, commonly referred to as the "loss of the silhouette" sign, suggests lobar atelectasis or pneumonia, a localized fluid collection, or intrathoracic mass. The thymus is often prominent after birth and may occupy the majority of the upper chest. It can involute during the first days of life, particularly in stressed infants. If a thymic shadow is not visualized on CXR, a US may help evaluate for thymic aplasia.[13]

Ultrasound

US is an oscillating sound wave with a frequency outside the human hearing range. The most common form of US used in diagnostic imaging is the pulse-echo technique with a brightness-mode (B-mode) display. B-mode involves transmission of a US pulse into the body. The depth of penetration of the pulse depends on the acoustic impedance of the tissue. The reflection of the pulse ("echo") by the tissue back to the US transducer generates the image. Doppler and motion mode are additional US modes that facilitate visualization of blood flow and motion of tissue over time (Fig. 9-3).

The use of US to examine the airway and lungs of neonates is gaining popularity; however, further studies are needed to define its diagnostic accuracy and interrater reliability. The advantages of US include its relative ease of use, "real-time" imaging capabilities, and lack of ionizing radiation. In the NICU, lung US is most commonly used to diagnose pleural effusion and to assess diaphragmatic movement. US can also be used to evaluate for suspected congenital lung lesions and for point-of-care diagnosis of air-leak syndromes and assessment of endotracheal tube and vascular catheter location.[14-18] The use of US to differentiate between common respiratory conditions such as respiratory distress syndrome, transient tachypnea of the newborn, and meconium aspiration has been reported but requires further study.[19-22]

In the healthy neonate, the normal pleural–lung interface appears on lung US as "A-lines," echogenic horizontal lines that move continuously with respiration (Fig. 9-4). The remaining lung is air filled and appears black. The presence of fluid or consolidation of the interstitial or alveolar compartments produces "B-lines," white projections that extend from the pleural line to the edge of the screen and obscure A-lines (see Fig. 9-4). B-lines are often present in the first few days of life even in infants without respiratory distress and indicate the presence of unabsorbed fetal lung fluid.

Computed Tomography

CT combines a series of X-rays performed helically around an axis of rotation to generate high-quality cross-sectional images of the body. Chest CT is useful for the identification and diagnosis of space-occupying lesions such as congenital pulmonary airway malformation (CPAM), bronchopulmonary sequestration (BPS), and congenital lobar emphysema. CT and CT angiography (CTA) are also increasingly used in the diagnosis and management of severe bronchopulmonary dysplasia (BPD) and pulmonary hypertension.[23-26] Although low-dose CT substantially

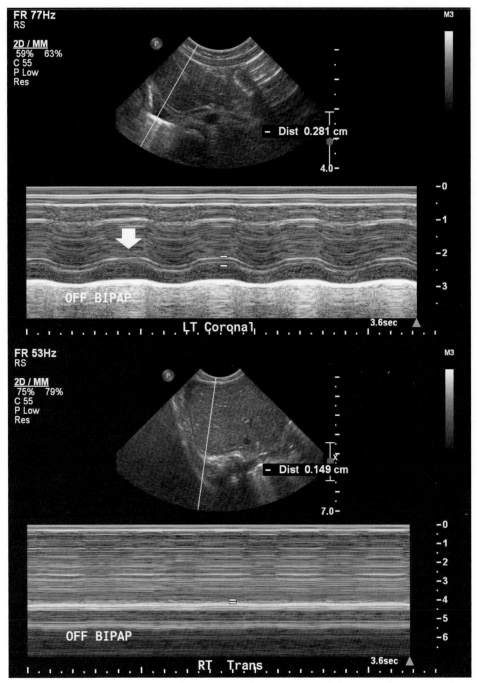

FIG 9-3 Motion-mode ultrasound of the chest of a 1-month-old female whose status is post repair of coarctation of the aorta. The top image demonstrates normal sinusoidal motion (*arrow*) of the left leaflet of the diaphragm. In the bottom image, there is no motion of the right leaflet of the diaphragm, compatible with paralysis.

reduces the effective radiation dose compared to previous techniques, clinicians should carefully assess the risks and benefits of this imaging modality prior to ordering any study.

Fluoroscopy

Fluoroscopy produces real-time, dynamic images using rapid, sequential X-rays. Fluoroscopy is most commonly used in neonates and infants to image the gastrointestinal and genitourinary tracts. In infants with respiratory distress of unclear etiology, fluoroscopy may aid in the identification of a tracheoesophageal fistula or occult aspiration. Fluoroscopy can also assess diaphragmatic excursion and diagnose large-airway disease such as tracheobronchomalacia. As described earlier, fluoroscopy can result in substantial radiation exposure if dose-limiting procedures such as pulsed fluoroscopy, reduced pulse widths and pulse rates, appropriate beam filtration, increased source-to-skin distance, and proper collimation are not used appropriately.[27]

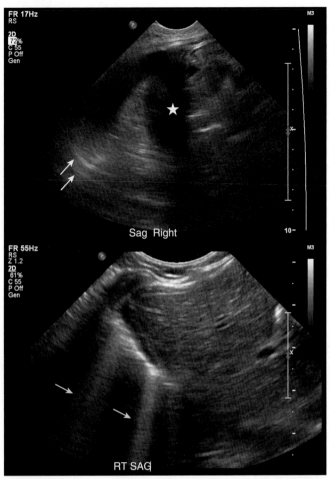

FIG 9-4 Sagittal ultrasound images of the right lung. In the top image, A-lines (*white arrows*) are the horizontal lines inferior to the atelectatic lung, which is compressed by a surrounding pleural effusion (*star*). In the bottom image, vertical B-lines are seen (*yellow arrows*) projecting from the diaphragm.

Magnetic Resonance Imaging

MRI utilizes the energy emitted by magnetically aligned protons to image anatomic structures within the body.[28] MRI does not require exposure to ionizing radiation; however, its use is limited by its lack of availability, its expense, and the frequent need to administer anesthesia to infants to acquire high-quality images of the lung. The primary role of MRI in the neonate is to image the brain and heart. It can also evaluate mediastinal structures, osseous lesions, and vascular malformations. At present the utility of MRI to assess the lung parenchyma is limited. The introduction of arterial spin labeling and hyperpolarized gas imaging, which provide information about lung perfusion and regional ventilation, may expand the role of MRI in the future.[29]

INVASIVE SUPPORT DEVICES

There is no evidence to support daily use of CXRs to evaluate the position of invasive support devices, but if malposition is suspected, imaging is warranted to prevent or ameliorate iatrogenic complications. In ventilated infants, the endotracheal tube (ETT) should be placed in the mid trachea between the second and fourth thoracic vertebral bodies and at least 1 cm above the

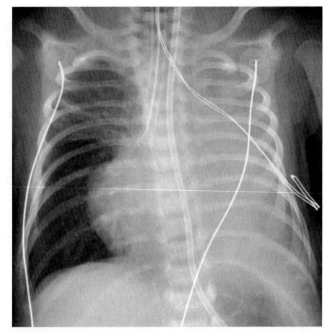

FIG 9-5 Deep positioning of an endotracheal tube (ETT) in a 19-day-old male with truncus arteriosus. The ETT terminates in the right main stem bronchus, and there is resultant "white-out" from atelectasis of the left lung. The streaky atelectasis seen in the right upper lobe suggests this lobe is also underventilated secondary to the malpositioned ETT.

carina. Deep positioning, typically into in the right main stem bronchus, can result in unilateral baro- and volutrauma, pneumothorax, and collapse of the contralateral lung (Fig. 9-5). When performing a radiograph to determine ETT location, care should be taken to position the infant without rotation and with the neck in neutral position. Extension of the neck will misleadingly suggest high placement of the ETT, and flexion the opposite.

The umbilical artery and vein are commonly used to gain vascular access during the first days of life in preterm and ill neonates. On radiograph, an umbilical vein catheter (UVC) should lie above the liver and diaphragm near the junction of the inferior vena cava and the right atrium. Lateral CXR and thoracic vertebral level on AP CXR do not accurately identify UVC tip location.[30] Echocardiogram is a more reliable, but costlier means to determine UVC location.[30,31] An umbilical artery catheter (UAC) can be placed in a "high" position, with the tip above the abdominal visceral arteries between the T7 and the T9 vertebral bodies, or in a "low" position with the tip between the L3 and the L5 vertebral bodies (Fig. 9-6). Data from a small number of randomized infants suggest that "high" placement of UACs is associated with a lower incidence of vascular complications (e.g., ischemic injury, aortic thrombosis).[32]

Peripherally inserted central venous catheters (PICCs) are optimally placed in an upper or lower extremity with the terminal end in a major vein near the heart (Fig. 9-7).[33,34] As a reference, the cavoatrial junction is located approximately two vertebral bodies below the carina on AP CXR.[35] US can identify peripheral veins during PICC placement and assess line position.[15,36] As PICCs are prone to migration, periodic surveillance is recommended to prevent iatrogenic complications such as pleural effusion or cardiac tamponade (Fig. 9-8).[37,38] In particular, sudden worsening of respiratory status when an upper extremity PICC is

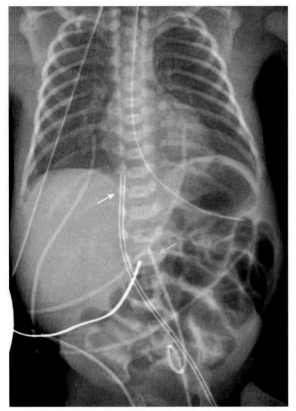

FIG 9-6 Combined chest and abdominal radiograph of a preterm infant with acceptably positioned umbilical catheters. The tip of the umbilical venous line (*white arrow*) is in the inferior vena cava just above the diaphragm and the tip of a "low"-lying umbilical arterial line (*yellow arrow*) is just above the L3 vertebral body.

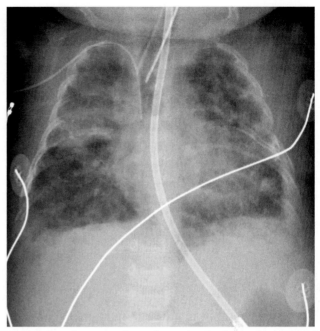

FIG 9-7 Anterior–posterior radiograph of a 3-month-old female with severe diffuse chronic lung disease. Patchy coarse opacities from atelectasis are present throughout the lung and are especially prominent and confluent in the right middle lobe. The right-sided peripherally inserted central venous catheter is appropriately placed with the tip just proximal to the superior caval–atrial junction.

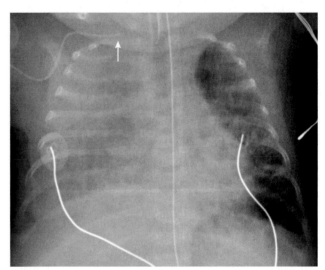

FIG 9-8 Anterior–posterior radiograph of a 5-month-old male with severe bronchopulmonary dysplasia (BPD) who developed a large pleural effusion from extravasation of parenteral nutrition after inadvertent migration of a peripherally inserted central venous catheter (*arrow*). The scattered coarse opacities characteristic of severe BPD are seen throughout the right lung. The tip of the endotracheal tube is just below the thoracic inlet.

present and new onset limb swelling warrant prompt evaluation of the catheter's location and function. Arm positioning during placement and surveillance of upper extremity PICCs also requires specific attention as movement (flexion/extension at the elbow and abduction/adduction at the shoulder) can alter tip location.[39]

Infants with gestational ages greater than 34 weeks with early, severe, and reversible cardiorespiratory failure who do not respond to conventional therapy may require extracorporeal membrane oxygenation (ECMO). Venoarterial (VA) and venovenous (VV) ECMO are both utilized in neonates. In VA ECMO, catheters are inserted into the internal jugular vein and common carotid artery. The tip of the venous cannula is most commonly placed in the mid-right atrium and the tip of the arterial cannula is placed at the junction of the common carotid artery and the aortic arch (Fig. 9-9).[40,41] In VV ECMO, blood is drained and reinfused though a dual-lumen catheter inserted though the internal jugular vein into the right atrium.[40,41] CXR can confirm correct placement of ECMO catheters, but echocardiography is a more reliable technique.[16]

COMMON ETIOLOGIES OF RESPIRATORY DISTRESS IN INFANTS

Respiratory Distress Syndrome

Primary respiratory distress syndrome (RDS) results from surfactant deficiency in the premature neonate and is the most common respiratory disorder among infants born at less than 32 weeks' gestation.[42] Lower gestational age and birth weight, lack of exposure to antenatal corticosteroids, perinatal asphyxia, and maternal diabetes are important risk factors for RDS.[43,44] Clinical signs of RDS often present at or soon after birth and include tachypnea, grunting, chest wall retractions, nasal flaring, and hypoxia.[44] Importantly, these signs may be

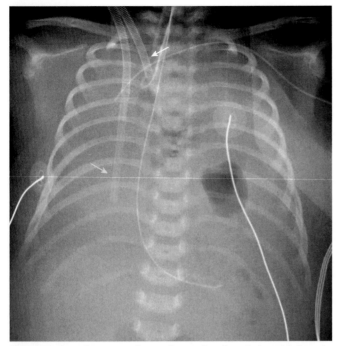

FIG 9-9 Anterior–posterior radiograph of a 6-day-old female with left-sided congenital diaphragmatic hernia who was placed on venoarterial extracorporeal membrane oxygenation (ECMO). The venous ECMO catheter overlies the right atrium (*yellow arrow*), which is shifted to the right because of the bowel in the left hemithorax. The arterial catheter (*white arrow*) overlies the right carotid artery. The lungs are completely opacified with the exception of an aerated loop of bowel located in the left hemithorax. This "white-out" appearance is common during the first week of an ECMO run and should be resolved prior to decannulation.

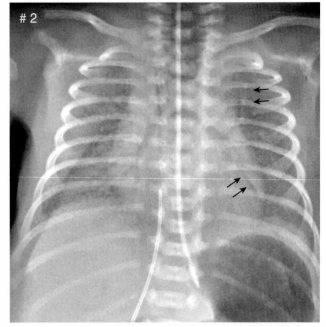

FIG 9-10 Anterior–posterior radiograph of a newborn 26-week-gestation female infant with respiratory distress syndrome. There are diffuse ground-glass opacities throughout the lung fields with prominent air bronchograms (*arrows*). A nasogastric tube and a large stomach bubble are seen. The umbilical venous catheter is in good position.

indistinguishable from other causes of early respiratory failure such as congenital pneumonia (especially secondary to group B *Streptococcus*), sepsis, and persistent pulmonary hypertension of the newborn (PPHN) in more mature infants. Secondary surfactant deficiency may also occur later in the neonatal period concomitant with episodes of hypoxemia, pulmonary edema, or infection (e.g., respiratory syncytial virus, bacterial pneumonia).

The CXR appearance in RDS depends on the severity of the disease. The classic findings are low lung volumes with a fine granular or "ground-glass" appearance with air bronchograms (Fig. 9-10). In mild RDS, a diffuse, linear granular pattern is most common. Air bronchograms become more prominent as the disease worsens and in severe cases the lungs are opaque and the cardiac border is often difficult to identify (eFig. 9-1). These CXR findings are modified by the administration of positive airway pressure and exogenous surfactant. Exogenous surfactant typically distributes throughout the lung in a non-uniform way and can result in a heterogeneous radiographic appearance with asymmetric multifocal opacities. This pattern may mimic the appearance of pneumonia and can be difficult to differentiate if earlier imaging is not available. When severe "RDS" is observed in more mature infants and fails to respond to conventional management, clinicians should consider congenital etiologies such as surfactant deficiencies and alveolar capillary dysplasia.

Transient Tachypnea of the Newborn

Transient tachypnea of the newborn (TTN) is characterized by mild to moderate respiratory distress that gradually improves during the first 48 to 72 hours of life. TTN results from the delayed clearance of fetal lung fluid and is more commonly observed in infants with a history of maternal diabetes and those born via cesarean section.[45-47] The CXR shows normal to mildly overexpanded lungs with a diffuse hazy appearance and increased interstitial streaky shadowing extending to the periphery. Small pleural effusions, typically seen as prominence of the interlobar fissures, are common (Fig. 9-11). Early CXRs in TTN can appear similar to those of more serious conditions such as infection, surfactant deficiency, or cardiac failure.

Meconium Aspiration Syndrome

Meconium is a viscous, hyperosmolar substance composed of water, mucus, gastrointestinal secretions, bile acids, pancreatic enzymes, lanugo, vernix caseosa, and blood.[48,49] Meconium-stained fluid is present in approximately 10% to 15% of live births, but only 1% to 2% suffer significant respiratory compromise due to aspiration of meconium.[50,51] Fetal stress (e.g., hypoxemia, acidosis, infection) is a common antecedent of in utero passage of meconium, and most infants with meconium aspiration syndrome (MAS) are born at or near full term.[52] Severe respiratory distress and hypoxia are characteristic of MAS, and ventilation perfusion mismatch and acidosis can worsen PPHN.

The CXR findings in MAS range from lung hyperexpansion with or without heterogeneous patchy infiltrates to complete opacification of the thorax (Fig. 9-12). Pleural effusion can also develop and air trapping due to a "ball–valve" phenomenon may lead to pneumothorax. Exogenous surfactant therapy is

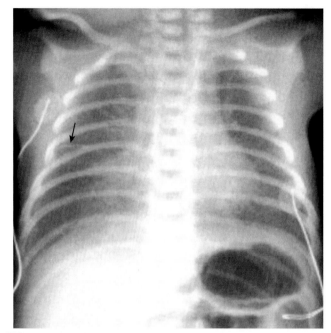

FIG 9-11 Anterior–posterior radiograph of a 1-day-old full-term male born via cesarean section with moderate respiratory distress secondary to transient tachypnea of the newborn (TTN). Fine granular opacities, similar to respiratory distress syndrome, are seen throughout. The prominent perihilar streaking and small pleural effusion observed in the interlobar fissure on the right (*arrow*) are common findings in TTN.

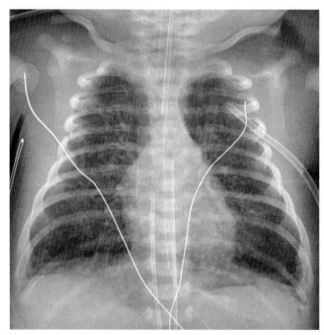

FIG 9-12 Anterior–posterior radiograph of a 1-day-old full-term male with meconium aspiration syndrome (MAS). The lungs are hyperinflated (flattened diaphragms and 10–11 rib lung expansion) with patchy, rope-like opacities projecting from the hilum to the periphery. A "high"-lying umbilical arterial catheter is seen at T6 and a malpositioned umbilical venous catheter is seen close to the right atrium. The percutaneous chest tube present on the left was placed to drain a large pneumothorax, a common complication in severe MAS.

often beneficial, but similar to RDS, it can transiently increase the heterogeneous appearance of the lung parenchyma.[53]

Pneumonia

Pneumonia is an important cause of neonatal morbidity and mortality. The estimated incidence ranges from 1.5 to 5 cases per 1000 live births.[54] Neonatal pneumonia is generally classified as early or late in onset. Early-onset pneumonia presents within the first week of life with respiratory distress and systemic signs of sepsis including poor perfusion, lethargy, and jaundice. Most early-onset pneumonias are acquired congenitally from transplacental inoculation or perinatally from the maternal vaginal tract. The presentation of early-onset pneumonia is similar to RDS, but a history of prolonged rupture of membranes, chorioamnionitis, or elevated inflammatory markers may help distinguish between the two. Pleural effusion is also more common in pneumonia than in RDS (Fig. 9-13). The most common pathogens associated with early pneumonias are group B *Streptococcus* and gram-negative rods. Congenital viral infections and occasionally atypical bacterial (e.g., *Chlamydia trachomatis*) and fungal infections can also present as early pneumonia.

Late-onset pneumonia presents after the first week of life and is often a nosocomial complication of mechanical ventilation. Common pathogens include coagulase-negative *Staphylococcus*, *Staphylococcus aureus*, gram-negative rods (e.g., *Pseudomonas*), and *Candida*.[55] Viral infections such as rhinovirus, respiratory syncytial virus, and influenza can also cause late-onset pneumonia. The CXR in late-onset pneumonia is diffusely hazy, similar to RDS, but in contrast to early-onset pneumonia, the lungs often exhibit normal or hyperexpansion with heterogeneously distributed densities (eFig. 9-2). Localized lobar pneumonias are uncommon in neonates but can develop in older infants and, when severe, result in lung necrosis and empyema. A chest CT can help confirm the diagnosis in these cases (eFig. 9-3).

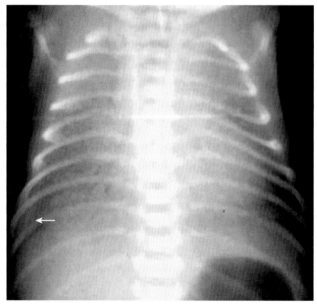

FIG 9-13 Anterior–posterior radiograph of a late preterm infant diagnosed with early-onset pneumonia secondary to group B *Streptococcus*. The low lung volumes, diffuse granular opacities, and air bronchograms are indistinguishable from those seen in respiratory distress syndrome (RDS). A small pleural effusion (*arrow*) can help distinguish between RDS and pneumonia but is not pathognomonic.

Air-Leak Syndromes

The application of positive airway pressure to poorly compliant or "stiff" lungs can result in leakage of air from the alveoli into the extra-alveolar space. The most common conditions that arise from alveolar air leak are pneumothorax, pneumomediastinum, pneumopericardium, and pulmonary interstitial emphysema (PIE). Rarely, pneumoperitoneum and subcutaneous emphysema can also develop.

Pneumothorax

Pneumothorax is the most common air-leak syndrome in infants and occurs in approximately 2% to 10% of those with birth weights between 500 and 1500 g.[56-58] The clinical presentation of pneumothorax varies from an incidental finding on CXR to severe respiratory distress and cardiovascular collapse. A large pneumothorax is easily detected on AP CXR. The characteristic findings are air in the pleural space with compression of the affected lung, flattening of the diaphragm, and shift of the mediastinum to the contralateral side (Fig. 9-14, eFig. 9-4). In contrast, small pneumothoraces can be difficult to appreciate. In the supine infant, free air collects anterior to the lung and a collapsed edge may not be visible. Increased lucency on the affected side or a tiny lucent rim along the diaphragm may be the only findings. A lateral decubitus X-ray with the affected side up is often helpful in this situation. Large pneumothoraces generally require percutaneous decompression, whereas smaller ones that do not cause cardiorespiratory compromise may resorb spontaneously.[59]

Two findings on lung US that indicate pneumothorax are absence of "pleural sliding" seen as movement of the visceral pleura on the parietal pleura with respiration and the "lung point" sign.[17] Lung point occurs at the border of the pneumothorax where there is intermittent contact of the lung with the chest wall.[18]

Pneumomediastinum

Pneumomediastinum results from leakage of air into the mediastinal space. In most cases, affected infants are asymptomatic, but large collections of air may lead to respiratory or cardiac compromise. Similar to pneumothorax, pneumomediastinum most commonly occurs during positive-pressure ventilation. On radiograph, a pneumomediastinum is most commonly seen as air surrounding the thymus above the cardiac shadow (Fig. 9-15). When large, it appears as a halo around the heart on AP view and as a retrosternal or superior mediastinal lucency on the lateral view.[60,61] The characteristic "spinnaker sail" sign is best appreciated on a left anterior oblique view, in which air is seen surrounding the thymus above the cardiac shadow (Fig. 9-16).[61]

Pneumopericardium

Pneumopericardium results from entrapment of air in the pericardial space and typically occurs only in the infants with severe RDS who also have a pneumothorax or other air leak. Although it can be insidious in onset, the most common presentation is abrupt hemodynamic compromise due to cardiac tamponade. Pneumopericardium and pneumomediastinum share similar findings on AP CXR. A characteristic feature in pneumopericardium is air surrounding the cardiac border that does not extend beyond the reflection of the aorta or the pulmonary artery.[62] The presence of air under the heart is also diagnostic.[63] US detection of pneumopericardium is especially rapid and can be life-saving.[64]

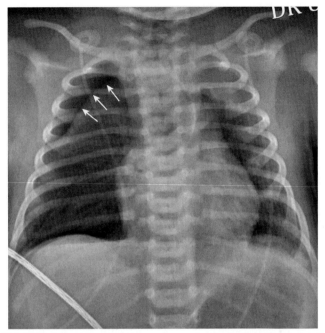

FIG 9-14 Anterior–posterior radiograph of a 1-day-old 41-week-gestation female infant who developed a right-sided pneumothorax after receiving positive-pressure bag–mask ventilation in the delivery room. The lateral edge of the right lung is displaced from the chest wall (*arrows*), and air within the pleural cavity outlines the right diaphragm.

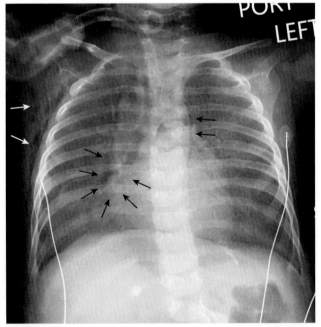

FIG 9-15 Anterior–posterior radiograph of a 6-month-old female with pneumomediastinum. Streaky lucencies are seen along the upper mediastinum, outlining the thymus and descending thoracic aorta (*black arrows*). There is extension of air into the neck, and subcutaneous emphysema is present along the right lateral chest wall (*white arrows*). The diffuse ground-glass opacification of the lungs is from surfactant C protein deficiency.

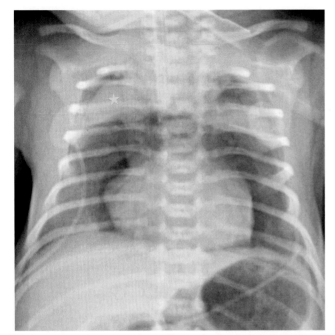

FIG 9-16 Anterior–posterior radiograph of a 1-day-old 34-week-gestation male infant with pneumomediastinum. The lungs are diffusely hazy bilaterally with ground-glass opacities consistent with respiratory distress syndrome. The thymus (*star*) is outlined by air and elevated away from the cardiac borders, creating a spinnaker sail sign. An anterior right-sided pneumothorax is also probably present.

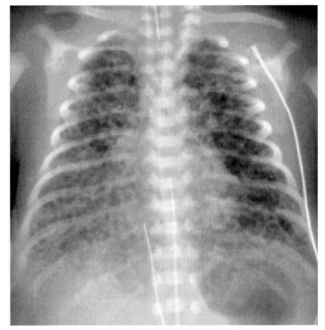

FIG 9-17 Anterior–posterior radiograph of a 7-day-old 26-week-gestation male infant with bilateral pulmonary interstitial emphysema. The lungs are hyperinflated (flattened diaphragm and prominent posterior lung fields) with streaky lucencies throughout. The tip of the endotracheal tube is at the thoracic inlet and should be advanced. An umbilical venous catheter and "high"-lying umbilical arterial catheter are appropriately positioned.

Pulmonary Interstitial Emphysema

PIE is a consequence of alveolar rupture into the peribronchial space with subsequent spreading of air through the lymphatic vessels within the lung interstitium. PIE most commonly develops during the first week of life in preterm infants with moderate to severe RDS who are treated with high-pressure mechanical ventilation. The clinical presentation typically includes worsening hypoxemia and hypercarbia, which may trigger clinicians to increase ventilator settings and potentially exacerbate the disease. There is no definitive treatment for PIE; however, minimization of further baro- or volutrauma may help prevent additional air leak. Subsequent development of BPD is common in preterm infants with PIE.[65]

On CXR, PIE appears as small cystic or linear translucencies extending from the hilum to the periphery (Fig. 9-17, eFig. 9-5). Generally both lungs are diffusely affected but unilateral and unilobar disease is also possible. Lung volume usually appears increased in PIE and as a result may be mistaken for improvement in RDS, as the lungs commonly appear darker and better aerated in both cases.[66] Subpleural cysts can also develop and rupture, causing a pneumothorax.

Pulmonary Hemorrhage

Pulmonary hemorrhage is an acute, often severe form of pulmonary edema that ranges in clinical presentation from a small amount of fresh, frothy blood from the airway to catastrophic bleeding and cardiopulmonary collapse. Prematurity is the most common risk factor. Other predisposing factors are asphyxia, patent ductus arteriosus, coagulopathy, infection, and severe respiratory distress. The findings on CXR range from patchy infiltrates to complete opacification of one or more lung fields

(eFig. 9-6). Using a "splint" of high mean airway pressure may decrease bleeding in pulmonary hemorrhage while attempts are made to correct the underlying etiology. Mortality is 30% to 40%.

Pleural Effusion

Pleural effusion results from an excess of fluid between the visceral and the parietal pleura. Pleural effusions are defined based on the timing of onset (congenital or acquired) and the content of the fluid (hydrothorax, chylothorax, or hemothorax). When sufficiently large, pleural effusions cause respiratory distress and hypoxemia due to impaired lung expansion. Congenital pleural effusions can also cause pulmonary hypoplasia.

Congenital hydrothorax is often associated with hydrops fetalis. Congenital chylothorax results from malformation of the thoracic lymphatic vessels and may be syndromic (e.g., Turner, Down, or Noonan syndrome). Newborns with large congenital effusions present with severe respiratory distress at birth, and emergent drainage is often necessary. Acquired hydrothorax is categorized as infectious or noninfectious in etiology. Common infectious organisms include Group B *Streptococcus*, *S. aureus*, and *Bacteroides fragilis*.[67] Noninfectious etiologies include RDS, TTN, MAS, congenital heart disease, and renal failure. Hydrothorax may also result from extravasation of parenteral nutrition from a central venous catheter (see Fig. 9-8). Acquired chylo- and hemothorax are potential complications of thoracic surgery or misplacement of pleural drains.

On CXR, small pleural effusions blunt the costophrenic angle (Fig. 9-18). As the volume of pleural fluid increases, there is progressive opacification of the hemithorax (see Fig. 9-8). US can confirm the presence and size of a pleural effusion and may help

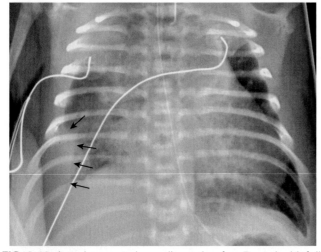

FIG 9-18 Anterior–posterior radiograph of a 5-week-old full-term male with trisomy 21 with a moderate right-sided pleural effusion (*black arrows*). The appearance of cardiomegaly and diffuse vascular congestion is consistent with the complete atrioventricular canal defect.

identify an optimal site for drainage (see Fig. 9-4). MR lymphangiography may aid in the diagnosis of congenital or acquired lymphatic abnormalities and permit simultaneous treatment with ethiodized oil embolization (Fig. 9-19, eFig. 9-7).[68]

Bronchopulmonary Dysplasia

BPD is the most common chronic respiratory complication associated with preterm birth.[42] Affected infants suffer higher rates of neonatal and childhood mortality, and survivors are predisposed to long-term respiratory and cardiovascular impairments, growth failure, and neurodevelopmental delay.[42,69] BPD was first described by radiologists, who noted the classic pattern of lung scarring and fibrosis with interspersed areas of hyperinflation and atelectasis on the CXRs of surviving moderate- and late-preterm infants exposed to prolonged mechanical ventilation.[70] These radiographic findings accompanied by 28 days of supplemental oxygen exposure formed the original National Heart, Lung, and Blood Institute consensus conference definition of BPD.[71] As neonatal care improved and survival rates for extremely preterm infants increased over the subsequent decades, the burden of BPD shifted to the smallest, and least mature, babies.[72] To reflect this change, the definition of BPD was revised to the more appropriate supplemental oxygen requirement at 36 weeks, postmenstrual age.[73,74] Although specific radiographic findings were not included in this updated definition, imaging remains an essential component of the assessment and management of BPD.

The CXR findings in infants with or at risk for BPD vary throughout the neonatal period and depend on the age of the infant and the severity of lung disease. Many infants born at less than 1000 g display minimal lung disease right after birth and can have an initial clear CXR. If atelectasis develops and there is a need for supplemental oxygen, the CXR becomes diffusely hazy. Once positive airway pressure is applied, the CXR will show a more heterogeneous pattern of lung collapse (Fig. 9-20, *A*). If lung disease persists, coarse interstitial densities and small cyst-like areas can develop. This may progress over the subsequent weeks and months into generalized hyperinflation with larger cystic areas and increased linear densities (Fig. 9-20, *B*).[75] Acquired lobar emphysema can develop as a sequela of severe BPD and

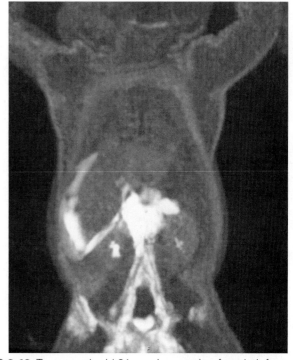

FIG 9-19 Two-month-old 31-week-gestation female infant with lymphangiomatosis. The coronal T1-weighted image was taken after bilateral inguinal lymph node Magnevist injection. Contrast opacifies the lymphatic system overlying the iliac vessels and abdominal aorta, draining into the lymphatic malformation present in the upper abdomen. Contrast is also seen leaking into the right upper quadrant of the abdomen. Photo courtesy of Dr. Yoav Dori, The Children's Hospital of Philadelphia.

may require surgical resection if the emphysematous lobe prevents adequate aeration of the remaining lung (eFig. 9-8).[76] Right ventricular enlargement from cor pulmonale may also become apparent. The radiographic abnormalities seen in surviving infants with BPD often improve over time as new alveoli develop, but this process may take years in the most severely affected infants and residual scarring is seen even into adulthood.[77-79]

Chest CT is more sensitive for detecting pulmonary lesions than CXR and is increasingly utilized to assess lung disease in BPD.[29] Ochiai et al. developed a CT scoring system for BPD based on the presence and severity of the following three findings: hyperexpansion, emphysema, and fibrous/interstitial abnormalities.[25] CT is also useful for identification of occult complications of BPD such as acquired lobar emphysema and focal atelectatic or infectious consolidations. Comparison of inspiratory and expiratory CT images allows for the diagnosis of dynamic airway disease such as tracheobronchomalacia.[80,81] CTA may complement echocardiography and cardiac catheterization detection of pulmonary hypertension (Fig. 9-21).[23,24] As of this writing, lung US and MRI have limited roles in BPD, although this may change in the future, particularly for MRI, as new techniques are developed.

CONGENITAL AND SURGICAL CAUSES OF RESPIRATORY DISTRESS

Congenital Lung Lesions

The terms *congenital lung lesion* (CLL) and *congenital lung malformation* refer to a broad range of developmental pulmonary

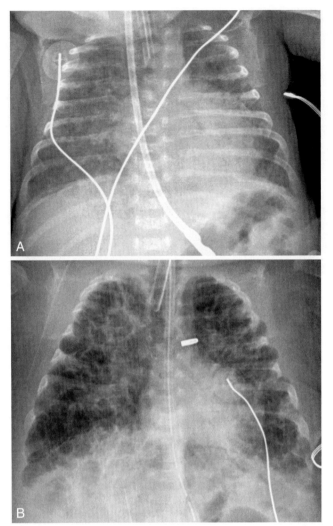

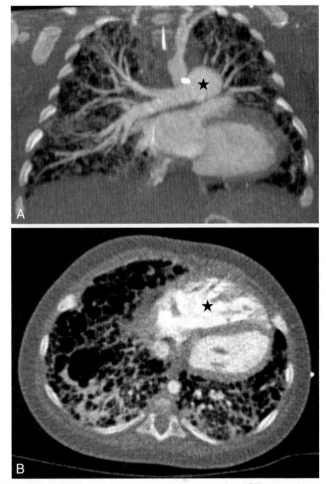

FIG 9-20 Anterior–posterior radiographs of a male infant born at 23 weeks' gestation and 590 g who developed severe bronchopulmonary dysplasia. **A,** At 6 weeks of age there are coarse, diffuse interstitial markings consistent with subsegmental atelectasis and early chronic lung disease. **B,** At 3 months of age the lungs are hyperinflated with diffuse cystic disease in a "honeycomb" pattern. The heart appears small in comparison to the earlier radiograph (**A**) probably because of high intrathoracic pressure. A surgical clip from a patent ductus arteriosus closure is also seen in the later radiograph.

FIG 9-21 **A,** Coronal computed tomography (CT) reconstruction of an infant with severe bronchopulmonary dysplasia and pulmonary hypertension. Engorgement of the pulmonary arterial branches is seen centrally (*star*) with thinning and tapering ("pruning") of the vessels peripherally. **B,** Axial image of a CT angiogram in an infant with pulmonary hypertension. The right ventricle is enlarged (*star*) and the intraventricular septum is bowed abnormally away from the right ventricle into the left ventricle. Although this is not a lung window, findings of chronic lung disease are noted throughout the parenchyma with cystic formation and areas of architectural distortion.

abnormalities. The nomenclature of these lesions has evolved in recent years, with the recognition that many share similar developmental origins and have overlapping radiographic and histologic features.[82] The most common CLLs diagnosed in infancy are bronchial atresia (BA), CPAM, and BPS.[83] Other less common CLLs include congenital lobar emphysema (or infantile lobar hyperinflation), bronchogenic cysts, pulmonary arteriovenous malformations, pulmonary agenesis/aplasia/hypoplasia, and tracheal bronchus.[83]

Pulmonary Agenesis, Aplasia, and Hypoplasia

Pulmonary agenesis is a rare congenital anomaly that results from failure of the primitive lung bud to develop and results in unilateral or bilateral absence of lung tissue. The lung parenchyma is also absent in pulmonary aplasia, but in contrast

to pulmonary agenesis, there is a short, blind-ending bronchus. Pulmonary hypoplasia is a condition of underdeveloped lungs and most often occurs secondary to another underlying abnormality. These secondary causes are categorized as malformations of the chest wall, space-occupying lesions within the chest cavity (e.g., congenital diaphragmatic hernia (CDH), CPAM, pleural effusion), oligohydramnios due to renal or urologic abnormalities or prolonged rupture of membranes (particularly with rupture before 20 weeks' gestation), and neuromuscular disorders that prevent normal fetal breathing. Primary pulmonary hypoplasia is rare. It occurs in congenital acinar dysplasia and can be a feature of Down syndrome.[84] PPHN is a common complication of both primary and secondary pulmonary hypoplasia and usually portends a poor prognosis.

The radiographic findings in pulmonary hypoplasia depend on the underlying etiology and severity of the disease. The typical features are small or absent lungs, crowded ribs, and an elevated diaphragm (eFig. 9-9). If unaffected, the contralateral lung may be overexpanded and the mediastinum shifted toward the affected side. A space-occupying lesion is often visible on CXR, but lung US or CT may be necessary to identify the specific etiology. CTA may also show a reduction in the size, number, and branching patterns of the pulmonary vessels.[85]

Bronchial Atresia or Stenosis

Congenital BA results from focal interruption of a lobar, segmental, or subsegmental bronchus and may represent the underlying developmental abnormality in several CLLs including CPAM, BPS, and congenital lobar emphysema.[86,87] BA typically affects a single segment although multisegmental disease is possible. The left followed by the right upper lobes are the most common sites.[88] Postnatally, mucus collects in the distal portion of the affected bronchus and forms a mucocele (impacted mucus). There is no ball–valve effect, however, due to a lack of communication with the central airways.[89] The affected segment is aerated through collateral channels and is often only mildly overdistended.[89] Acquired bronchial stenosis can also develop from baro- and volutrauma to the cartilaginous airway and is associated with BPD.[90] BA appears on CXR as a tubular or nodular mass sometimes with an air–fluid level and an adjacent overinflated or cystic-appearing lung. Small lesions may be difficult to detect on plain radiograph, and chest CT is often necessary to distinguish between BA and other cystic lesions.[91]

Congenital Pulmonary Airway Malformation

CPAMs, previously known as congenital cystic adenomatoid malformations, are the most common form of CLL. The estimated incidence ranges from 1 in 10,000 to 1 in 30,000 live births.[92] Several classification schemes exist based on the embryologic origin, the appearance on prenatal imaging, and the size and epithelial lining of the resected cysts.[93-95] "Hybrid" lesions with histologic features of both CPAM and BPS are also possible.[96] The most common CPAMs have multiple air-filled cysts that are greater than 2 cm in diameter. A CXR taken soon after birth may show a dense mass that is indistinguishable from other CLLs. Later radiographs show air-filled cysts and collapse of the surrounding parenchyma (Fig. 9-22). Microcystic and solid forms also exist and generally carry a poorer prognosis (eFig. 9-10). Overall, CXR has a low sensitivity for detecting CPAMs, and other imaging modalities such as CTA or MRI with angiography are recommended to define the anatomy and blood supply of the lesion (eFig. 9-11).[97]

Bronchopulmonary Sequestration

BPS is an isolated portion of lung tissue that does not communicate with the bronchial tree. Most sequestrations receive blood supply from a systemic artery, often the aorta, although this is not uniformly true. Venous drainage may be through pulmonary or systemic veins or both. Up to 50% of BPS cases contain histologic areas of cystic adenomatous malformation.[98]

BPS is divided into two categories: intralobar and extralobar. Intralobar sequestrations are found within the normal lung tissue, predominantly in basal segments of the lower lungs. Extralobar sequestrations are contained within a pleural covering distinct from the surrounding lung tissue. Most are located in the thoracic cavity but can also be found below the diaphragm. BPS appears on CXR as a dense mass, usually in the medial basal segment of the left lower lobe. Similar to CPAMs,

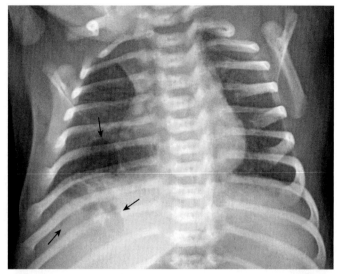

FIG 9-22 Initial anterior–posterior radiograph of a full-term female infant with prenatally diagnosed right lower lobe macrocystic congenital pulmonary airway malformation (*arrows*). Consistent with retained fetal lung fluid, the remaining lung is diffusely hazy with air bronchograms, and there is a small pleural effusion in the interlobar fissure on the right.

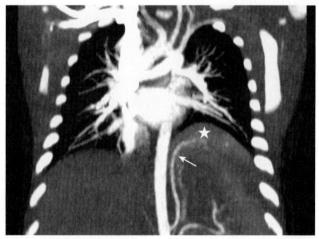

FIG 9-23 Postnatal computed tomography with angiography of a full-term infant with a bronchopulmonary sequestration. Coronal reconstructed image demonstrates the feeding vessel (*arrow*) arising from the abdominal aorta to supply the lesion at the left lung base (*star*).

identification of the blood supply can be done by US, CTA, or MRI with angiography (Fig. 9-23, eFig. 9-12). Additional congenital anomalies including diaphragmatic hernia and heart abnormalities can occur in infants with BPS, and chest imaging in these infants should be reviewed to assess for other lesions.

Congenital Lobar Emphysema

CLE results from air-filled distention of one or more lobes of the lung. CLE most commonly affects the left upper lobe (50%), followed by the right middle lobe (30%) and the right upper lobe (20%).[99] Lower lobe involvement is rare. The etiology of CLE is idiopathic in approximately half of cases.[100] The remaining cases are divided into intrinsic and extrinsic causes.[100] Intrinsic mechanisms include dysplasia of the

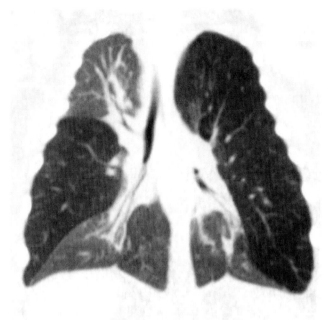

FIG 9-24 Coronal reconstructed image of a chest computed tomography of a 6-month-old female (for the plain radiograph of the same infant see eFig. 9-13) with congenital lobar emphysema of the left upper and right middle lobes. There is marked hyperexpansion of the affected lobes with compression of the right upper lobe and bilateral lower lobes.

bronchial cartilage, bronchial torsion or atresia, or extensive proliferation of the mucosa. Extrinsic etiologies usually result from bronchial compression or hypoplasia of the adjacent lung tissue. A CXR obtained soon after birth may show opacification of the affected lobe as air more rapidly fills the surrounding, healthy lung. Once filled, however, the affected lung is overexpanded and hyperlucent and the adjacent lung appears dense and compressed (Fig. 9-24, eFig. 9-13). Mediastinal shift can also occur, and large lesions may be confused with pneumothorax. CT may be necessary to identify which lobe is involved as unaffected structures are often too distorted to discern clearly on plain radiograph.

Congenital Diaphragmatic Hernia

CDH affects approximately 1 in 2500 infants and results from a failure of the pleural–peritoneal fold to close early in gestation. The diaphragmatic defect permits the abdominal contents to herniate into the thorax and creates a mass effect that impedes lung development. Greater than 95% of CDHs result from a posterolateral diaphragmatic defect (Bochdalek hernias). Most (80% to 85%) occur on the left side.[101] Morgagni hernias (anterior parasternal defect), septum transverse defects, and hiatal hernias are rare types of CDHs. Common abdominal organs that herniate into the chest include the small and large bowel, stomach, spleen, pancreas, and liver. Greater lung hypoplasia and presence of the liver in the thorax are associated with decreased survival rates.[102] In addition to underdevelopment of the lungs, the peripheral pulmonary vasculature is also abnormal and hypermuscular.[101] As a result, pulmonary arterial hypertension complicates most CDH cases and may require treatment

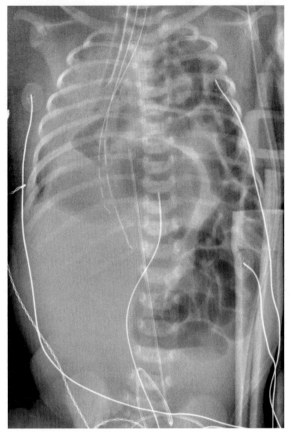

FIG 9-25 Anterior–posterior radiograph of a full-term infant with left-sided congenital diaphragmatic hernia. Aerated loops of bowel are seen extending from the abdomen into the left hemithorax. The mediastinum is shifted to the right demonstrated by the cardiothymic silhouette, endotracheal tube, and gastric sump coursing through the esophagus, all overly shifted to the right hemithorax. This results in the visible compressive atelectasis of the right lung. A "high"-lying umbilical arterial catheter terminates at T7 and umbilical venous catheter at T9.

with ECMO. Other congenital anomalies are present in 20% of infants with CDH. These include abnormalities of the central nervous system (e.g., neural tube defects), lungs (e.g., BPS), gastrointestinal tract (e.g., malrotation, omphalocele), and cardiovascular and genitourinary systems. The typical postnatal CXR shows air-filled loops of bowel within the hemithorax, compression of the lung on the affected size, and contralateral displacement of the mediastinum (Fig. 9-25). The X-ray findings in diaphragmatic eventration, a disorder in which all or part of the diaphragm is replaced by fibroelastic tissue, can mimic those of a CDH if the weakened diaphragm is displaced into the thoracic cavity. US can help distinguish between these two entities and also determine what organs are herniated into the chest if not established prenatally. CT can also confirm the diagnosis of CDH if other imaging modalities are inconclusive.

REFERENCES

A complete reference list is available at https://expertconsult
.inkling.com/.

10

Blood Gases: Technical Aspects and Interpretation

Yacov Rabi, MD, FRCPC, Derek Kowal, RRT, and Namasivayam Ambalavanan, MBBS, MD

Arterial blood gas measurements are the gold standard by which the adequacy of oxygenation and ventilation is assessed in sick neonates. In modern intensive care, blood gas measurements are used concurrently with continuous noninvasive monitoring devices, particularly pulse oximeters and transcutaneous carbon dioxide monitors, that provide real-time estimates of blood gas values.

The measurement of blood gases is invaluable for management of patients with respiratory difficulty, for such measurements not only enable the diagnosis of respiratory failure by estimation of the magnitude of respiratory illness severity but also provide crucial information required by the clinician to guide adjustments to the mechanical ventilator or other form of respiratory support. In this chapter, we first discuss the physiology of gas transport in the blood, followed by a description of techniques of measurement of blood gases commonly used in the neonatal intensive care unit (NICU). Next, we will describe the technical aspects of blood gas estimation by commercially available devices. Finally, we will discuss the interpretation of blood gases, as well as some perils and pitfalls of blood gas measurement in clinical practice.

BLOOD GAS PHYSIOLOGY

Gas exchange occurs primarily in lung saccules in extremely preterm infants and in alveoli in more mature preterm and term infants, although some gas exchange occurs through immature skin soon after birth.[1–3] In the postnatal period after transition, systemic venous blood travels to the right atrium and on to the right ventricle, which pumps the deoxygenated blood to the pulmonary arterial system. This blood travels through the pulmonary vasculature until reaching the capillaries, which are contiguous to alveoli, thereby facilitating gas exchange. Gas exchange occurs in ventilated alveoli, with absorption of oxygen from alveoli into the alveolar capillaries and removal of carbon dioxide from the circulation into the alveoli. In general, the oxygen concentration of arterial blood exiting the left ventricle reflects the matching of ventilation and perfusion. A decrease in oxygen content would occur if perfusion (blood) is not matched with ventilation (aerated alveoli), either because blood passes from the right side of the heart to the left side of the heart without traversing the pulmonary circulation (e.g., extrapulmonary shunt) or because blood is traversing parts of the lung that are atelectatic and/or underventilated (intrapulmonary shunt).

Carbon dioxide (CO_2) elimination is primarily dependent upon the magnitude of alveolar ventilation. As alveolar ventilation increases, the partial pressure of carbon dioxide in alveolar gas (P_{ACO_2}) decreases, and more CO_2 is removed from the blood flowing through the lungs, and the partial pressure of carbon dioxide in blood ($PaCO_2$) leaving the left heart decreases. Conversely, a decrease in alveolar ventilation will increase the $PaCO_2$ in systemic arterial blood. An important concept is that while arterial PaO_2 and $PaCO_2$ provide important information about ventilation–perfusion matching and adequacy of alveolar ventilation, they do not provide direct information about the adequacy of oxygen delivery to the systemic vascular bed and peripheral tissues.

Aerobic metabolism of glucose for the production of adenosine triphosphate (ATP) is responsible for the consumption of oxygen and the production of CO_2. Aerobic metabolism produces approximately 38 ATP molecules for each molecule of glucose consumed, although some of the ATP is consumed in the process, yielding a net of 30 ATP.[4]

During conditions of insufficient oxygen delivery to cells, tissue hypoxia occurs, characterized by anaerobic metabolism of glucose to pyruvate for ATP production. This process is less efficient than aerobic metabolism and yields two molecules of ATP for each molecule of glucose consumed. Pyruvate is metabolized to lactic acid, which increases the base deficit (or decreases base excess) of arterial blood. Base excess is defined as the difference between the actual buffer capacity and the ideal buffer capacity. To more accurately estimate if adequate oxygen has been delivered to tissues, blood returning from the systemic circulation to the heart (mixed venous blood) can be evaluated. Blood sampling from the right atrium, which can be done using an umbilical venous catheter with its tip in the low right atrium, closely approximates mixed venous blood. Monitoring of mixed venous oxygenation is extremely helpful in assessing the adequacy of tissue oxygen delivery and is widely used in adult ICUs and in neonatal extracorporeal membrane oxygenation (ECMO).

Oxygen Transport

Oxygen delivery to tissues depends upon the oxygen content of the blood as well as the cardiac output and its distribution to the tissues. In most neonates, cardiac output ranges from 120 to 150 mL/kg/min, although objective assessment of cardiac output is not easy or accurate, generally depending upon functional echocardiography and Doppler methods or alternative methods such as pulse contour analysis, bioimpedance, or indicator dilution techniques (generally in larger and older infants).[5a]

The oxygen content of arterial blood (C_aO_2) consists of oxygen bound to hemoglobin and free dissolved oxygen. Hence,

$$C_aO_2 = (HbO_2) + (\text{dissolved } O_2),$$

where C_aO_2 is the oxygen content, HbO_2 is the oxygen bound to hemoglobin, and dissolved O_2 is the oxygen in solution.

The relationship between the PaO_2 and the hemoglobin saturation is sigmoidal over the physiologic range. Hemoglobin is almost fully saturated at a PaO_2 of 80 to 100 mm Hg (Fig. 10-1, *curve A*). This sigmoidal oxyhemoglobin dissociation curve (ODC) describes the percent of hemoglobin saturated with oxygen at a given PaO_2. The concentration of red blood cell diphosphoglycerate (DPG) and the ratio of adult hemoglobin (A) to fetal hemoglobin (F) can shift the position of the dissociation curve. With increasing postnatal age, the concentration of DPG and the proportion of hemoglobin A increase, shifting the curve to the right (Fig. 10-2). DPG has a greater effect on oxygen binding for adult hemoglobin, as compared to fetal hemoglobin.[5b,5c] Increases in temperature, $PaCO_2$, and hydrogen ion concentration (acidosis) also shift the curve to the right. As the curve shifts to the right, hemoglobin can bind less oxygen at a given PaO_2 and therefore releases oxygen more easily to the tissues (Fig. 10-3). The fetus has a lower red blood cell DPG concentration and more hemoglobin F, and the dissociation curve is hence shifted to the left, which helps maintain a higher oxygen saturation at a lower PaO_2. Conditions such as respiratory alkalosis or therapeutic hypothermia will also shift the dissociation curve to the left, resulting in a higher hemoglobin oxygen saturation for a given PaO_2.

All gases dissolved in the blood exert pressure proportional to the amount of the gas. The pressure exerted by dissolved oxygen in the blood is represented by the PaO_2. Normally, only a small amount of oxygen is dissolved in the plasma, unless the PaO_2 is extremely high (e.g., exposure to high FiO_2 or hyperbaric oxygen therapy). At 38°C, 0.3 mL of oxygen is dissolved in 100 mL of plasma (0.003 mL/dL/mm Hg of PaO_2, at an assumed PaO_2 of 100 mm Hg). This relationship is linear over the entire range of PaO_2 (see Fig. 10-1, *curve B*). Because the amount of oxygen that is dissolved in the blood is much less than the amount that is bound to hemoglobin, the oxygen content of blood is approximately equal to the amount of oxygen bound to hemoglobin, as represented by the equation:

$$C_aO_2 \approx (HbO_2).$$

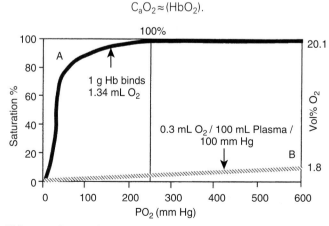

FIG 10-1 Comparison between the dissociation curve of hemoglobin (*curve A*) and the amount of oxygen dissolved in plasma (*curve B*). Note that the hemoglobin is almost 100% saturated at Po_2 80 mm Hg. When fully saturated, 15 g Hb will bind 20.1 mL O_2. (From Duc G. Assessment of hypoxia in the newborn. Pediatrics. 1971;48:469.)

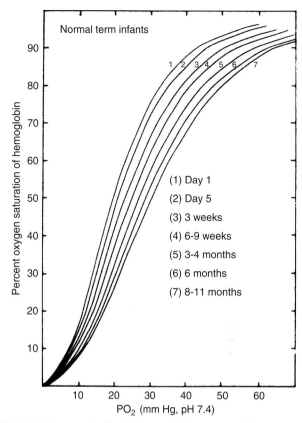

FIG 10-2 Oxygen dissociation curves from term infants at various postnatal ages. (From Delivoria-Popadopoulos M, Roncevic NP, Oski FA. Postnatal changes in oxygen transport of term, premature and sick infants. Ped Res. 1971;5:235.)

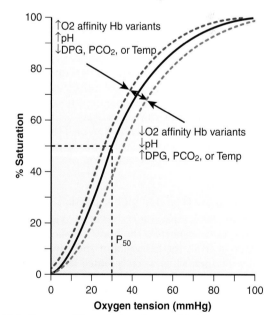

FIG 10-3 Oxygen Dissociation Curve Of Hemoglobin. The percent saturation of hemoglobin with oxygen at different oxygen tensions is depicted by the sigmoidal curves. The P50, indicated by the dashed lines, is about 27 mm Hg in normal erythrocytes. Modifications of hemoglobin function that increase oxygen affinity shift the curve to the left, whereas those that decrease oxygen affinity shift the curve to the right. (From Kelley's Textbook of Internal Medicine, 4th ed. Philadelphia, Lippincott Williams & Wilkins, 2000.)

The amount of oxygen bound to hemoglobin depends on the hemoglobin concentration, the percentage saturation of the hemoglobin, and the oxygen-carrying capacity of hemoglobin, which can be expressed mathematically as:

$$C_aO_2 \approx (HbO_2) = (\text{grams of Hb}) \times (O_2 \text{ capacity}) \times (\% \text{ saturation}).$$

O_2 capacity represents the maximum amount of oxygen that can be carried by a gram of hemoglobin that is fully saturated. This value is 1.34 mL of O_2 per gram of 100% saturated hemoglobin.[6]

Assuming a hemoglobin level of 15 g/100 mL blood, and 100% saturation of arterial blood, and ignoring the small amount of dissolved oxygen in blood, the oxygen content of normal arterial blood is approximately:

$$C_aO_2 = 15 \times 1.34 \times 1.0 = 20 \text{ mL } O_2 \text{ per 100 mL arterial blood or} \\ 0.2 \text{ mL per milliliter of blood.}$$

Using the same assumptions, and with the additional assumption that the normal cardiac output in a newborn is approximately 120 mL/kg/min, the amount of O_2 that can be delivered to the systemic circulation can be calculated as follows:

$$O_2 \text{ delivered} = (\text{Cardiac Output}) \times (C_aO_2) \\ = (120 \text{ mL blood/kg/min}) \times (0.2 \text{ mL } O_2/\text{mL blood}) \\ = 24 \text{ mL } O_2/\text{kg/min}.$$

Oxygen consumption for a neonate is approximately 6 mL/kg/min under normal circumstances.[7,8] Therefore, the body extracts 6 mL/kg/min of oxygen from the approximately 24 mL/kg/min that is delivered via the systemic circulation. The amount of oxygen delivered is usually much higher than the amount required by tissues, providing a natural reserve. The tissues become hypoxic and switch to anaerobic metabolism only when the oxygen delivery falls below the threshold at which the delivered amount of oxygen is less than the amount required by the tissues. Because only about 25% of the oxygen has been removed from the blood by the time it returns to the heart, the mixed venous blood is approximately 75% saturated. In general, a mixed venous saturation of 70% to 75% represents adequate tissue oxygen delivery. Therefore, mixed venous saturations are usually maintained in the normal physiologic range of 70% to 75% in patients in whom mixed venous saturations can be directly monitored (e.g., patients on ECMO).

Understanding the Oxyhemoglobin Dissociation Curve

One of hemoglobin's main roles is binding oxygen in the lungs to allow oxygen transport to the body's tissues. The oxygen is then released from the hemoglobin and enters a dissolved phase in the plasma, which is represented by the partial pressure of oxygen (PaO_2). Without hemoglobin, the cardiac output would have to increase tremendously to meet the body's metabolic demands as the amount of dissolved oxygen in blood is minimal. The relationship between oxygen saturation and the PaO_2 is described by the sigmoidal ODC. The steep portion of the curve demonstrates that oxygen saturations change quickly during the loading and unloading of hemoglobin with oxygen. This reflects the relaxation of the hemoglobin structure that occurs with oxygen binding. As oxygen binds to heme, the hemoglobin molecule relaxes, thereby exposing further heme molecules, facilitating subsequent binding

of oxygen. This process of relaxation is called *allosteric modification* and is governed by the Haldane effect. The reverse process occurs with oxygen unloading from the hemoglobin molecule. As the oxygen binding sites on the hemoglobin molecule approach full saturation with oxygen, the ODC begins to flatten. Therefore, at higher oxygen saturations it becomes increasingly difficult to predict the PaO_2 from the oxygen saturation. An oxygen saturation of 100% can correspond to a PaO_2 ranging from 80 to over 300 mm Hg.

While the PaO_2 contributes very little to the overall oxygen content of blood, its physiologic importance cannot be overstated as it is the dissolved oxygen in plasma that is available to enter cells. The oxygen that is bound to hemoglobin is not readily available to tissues until it has been released from heme and can dissolve in plasma. Under normal circumstances (e.g., euthermia, normoxemia), 100 mL of blood contains approximately 20 mL of oxygen. The vast majority of this oxygen is bound to hemoglobin with only approximately 0.31 mL of oxygen dissolved in plasma.

The position of the ODC is described by the P50, which represents the PaO_2 at an oxygen saturation of 50%. The position of the ODC, and hence the P50, is dependent on several factors. An increase in body temperature, hydrogen ion concentration (decreased pH), $PaCO_2$, 2,3-DPG, or adult hemoglobin concentration will each independently shift the ODC to the right, whereas a decrease in any of these factors will shift the curve to the left. Therefore, the PaO_2 for any given oxygen saturation will vary within an individual over time as these factors change. For example, in the presence of a fever, the rightward shift of the curve results in a higher PaO_2 for the P50 value. Both adult hemoglobin concentrations and 2,3-DPG concentrations increase over the first year, causing a shift in the ODC position to the right.[9]

Considerations Regarding Fetal Hemoglobin

As all neonates generally have mostly fetal hemoglobin, it is worth expanding on its importance further. Babies born at <30 weeks' gestation have nearly 100% fetal hemoglobin. The ratio of fetal to adult hemoglobin gradually diminishes so that by 40 weeks' gestation, fetal hemoglobin accounts for approximately 70% of all hemoglobin species, with adult hemoglobin accounting for the remaining 30%.[10] This shift to producing adult hemoglobin and away from producing fetal hemoglobin is related to postmenstrual age and not to chronological age.[11] Therefore, premature delivery does not affect the rate of transitioning away from fetal hemoglobin production. A baby born at 24 weeks with nearly 100% fetal hemoglobin would be expected to have approximately 70% fetal hemoglobin at 16 weeks of age (40 weeks' corrected gestational age), similar to a baby born at 40 weeks' gestation, although the ratio will change more quickly following transfusion with adult blood.

The first observation that fetal hemoglobin has different oxygen binding properties than adult hemoglobin was reported in 1930.[12] Fetal hemoglobin is composed of two α chains and two γ chains, in contrast to adult hemoglobin, which contains two α and two β chains. This difference results in fetal hemoglobin having a higher oxygen affinity than adult hemoglobin. This promotes the movement of oxygen from the maternal side of the placental circulation to the fetal side because fetal hemoglobin will hold onto oxygen "more tightly" than adult hemoglobin, and this is reflected in the position of the ODC. The P50 observed in a term newborn is approximately 21 mm Hg compared to a P50 of 27 mm Hg observed in adults (see Fig 10-2).[13,14] In preterm babies the P50 may be as low as 18 mm Hg because of the presence of higher fetal hemoglobin and lower 2,3-DPG concentrations.[15]

It is important to consider how therapies can alter the position of the ODC curve. Perhaps most important in this regard is the influence of transfusions of packed red blood cells. Because the packed red blood cells administered to patients are donated by adults, the transfused blood essentially contains 100% adult hemoglobin. The result is a shifting of the ODC to the right after a transfusion. As preterm babies have higher concentrations of fetal hemoglobin, blood transfusions in this population will have an even greater effect in shifting the ODC compared to babies at term. Preterm babies are more likely to receive blood transfusions, which further highlights the importance of this practice in this vulnerable population.[16] There are other important factors to consider regarding the effects of blood transfusions on the ODC, such as the 2,3-DPG concentration, temperature, and type of preservative used in the packed red blood cells. However, a detailed discussion of these factors is beyond the scope of this text.

Is this clinically important? Wimberley and colleagues state that based on the position of the ODC, the oxygen saturation limits for hypoxemia and hyperoxemia can vary between 85% and 94% and between 96% and 98%, respectively.[17] This demonstrates the importance of considering how oxygen saturation targets are related to the PaO_2 as described by the ODC. In practice, clinicians target specific oxygen saturation ranges to help guide oxygen titration and avoid the dangers of both hyperoxemia and hypoxemia. However, oxygen saturation targets are not routinely changed when the position of the ODC shifts, such as following a blood transfusion, which may result in a higher PaO_2 for any given oxygen saturation compared to pretransfusion. Arguably, this is appropriate, because it is the oxyhemoglobin saturation rather than PaO_2 that directly affects oxygen content of blood and tissue delivery of oxygen.

Modern blood gas analyzers have two presets for fetal hemoglobin: 0% and 80%. While not exact, using the preset for 80% fetal hemoglobin is preferable for newborn blood gas testing. For example, consider a blood gas sample corrected to 80% fetal hemoglobin with a P50 of 15 mm Hg and an oxygen saturation of 92% to 97%. The same blood gas sample run on a blood gas analyzer not corrected for fetal hemoglobin would give a P50 of 20 mm Hg, corresponding to an oxygen saturation of 86% to 95%.[15]

On occasion, errors in reporting uncorrected blood gas values are not obvious to the clinician. A blood gas result giving an oxygen saturation of 100% that was corrected for fetal hemoglobin corresponds to an uncorrected oxygen saturation of 105%.[18] However, because blood gas machines do not report oxygen saturations >100%, this would not be apparent to the clinician.

Hypoxemia and Hypoxia

Although hypoxemia and hypoxia often occur together, they are not synonymous. Hypoxemia is generally defined as low arterial blood oxygen content, whereas hypoxia refers to inadequate delivery of oxygen to tissue. Hypoxemia occurs in any situation in which blood enters the systemic circulation without perfusing adequately ventilated alveoli (reduction in ventilation–perfusion matching). Blood can bypass adequately ventilated alveoli by extrapulmonary shunts, by

intrapulmonary shunts, or by some combination of the two. With cyanotic congenital heart disease, a structurally abnormal heart leads to some blood entering the aorta without passing through the pulmonary circulation (extrapulmonary shunt). Similarly, infants with persistent pulmonary hypertension of the newborn can also have extrapulmonary shunting through the foramen ovale and/or ductus arteriosus. A right-to-left shunt across the ductus arteriosus can often be detected by comparing the PaO_2 or oxygen saturation of preductal and postductal blood (Fig. 10-4). If the saturation of the preductal blood is significantly higher (≥5% to 10% difference) than the saturation of the postductal blood, a clinically significant right-to-left shunt exists. However, equal pre- and postductal saturations do not exclude the possibility of pulmonary hypertension with a shunt through the foramen ovale. Hypoxemia associated with lung diseases that are characterized by atelectasis (e.g., respiratory distress syndrome, pneumonia) are caused primarily by intrapulmonary shunting. Whenever alveoli are inadequately ventilated, the blood flowing to those alveoli may not become fully saturated. Thus, the greater the degree of atelectasis, the greater the intrapulmonary shunt, and the greater the degree of hypoxemia.

Tissue hypoxia results when the amount of oxygen delivered to the tissues decreases below the critical threshold of oxygen consumption. Hypoxia can occur despite adequate PaO_2. It is helpful to conceptualize hypoxia in terms of imbalances in supply, delivery and demand for oxygen. Decreased 'supply'

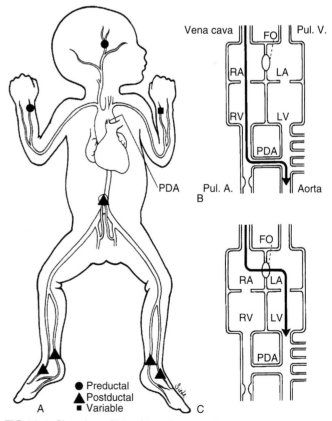

FIG 10-4 Shunting of blood in pulmonary hypertension. A, Sampling sites. B, Right-to-left shunt across the ductus arteriosus. C, Right-to-left shunt across the foramen ovale. *FO*, foramen ovale; *LA*, left atrium; *LV*, left ventricle; *PDA*, patent ductus arteriosus; *RA*, right atrium; *RV*, right ventricle.

of oxygen is observed at high altitude due to a lower partial pressure of oxygen in the atmosphere. 'Delivery' of oxygen is impaired in the settings of inadequate tissue perfusion (e.g., reduced cardiac output), anemia and abnormal hemoglobin species (e.g., methemoglobin) where the unloading of oxygen to the tissues is negatively affected. The 'demand' for oxygen will increase as tissue oxygen requirements rise in response to illness such as fever or sepsis.

Carbon Dioxide Transport

Carbon dioxide transport is significantly less complicated than oxygen transport. Carbon dioxide is produced in tissues during the aerobic metabolism of glucose and is transported in the blood to the lungs, where it is exhaled. Eighty-five percent of the carbon dioxide in blood is transported as carbonic acid, 10% is carried by hemoglobin as carbamate, and 5% is transported as either dissolved gas or carbonic acid.[19,20] Owing to the equilibrium between dissolved carbon dioxide and the bicarbonate ion, the relationship between the partial pressure of carbon dioxide in the blood ($PaCO_2$) and the total CO_2 content of blood is essentially linear over the physiologic range (Fig. 10-5).

Because carbon dioxide diffuses rapidly from blood into alveolar gas, the partial pressure of CO_2 in blood ($PaCO_2$) leaving the lungs is essentially the same as the partial pressure of CO_2 in alveolar gas ($PACO_2$). Thus increasing minute alveolar ventilation decreases the $PACO_2$ and thereby decreases the $PaCO_2$. This is the reason $PaCO_2$ is dependent on the magnitude of alveolar ventilation.

Metabolic Acidosis

Anaerobic metabolism of glucose leads to the accumulation of lactic acid, resulting in metabolic acidosis. Lactic acid reacts with bicarbonate (a base), causing the serum bicarbonate to fall, resulting in a base deficit. This is usually caused by inadequate tissue oxygen delivery as a result of some combination of hypoxemia, anemia, and inadequate cardiac output. Other causes of metabolic acidosis in the newborn include sepsis, inborn errors of metabolism, and renal bicarbonate wasting. Iatrogenic causes, such as a large protein load in parenteral nutrition, especially when extra cysteine is added, are also a frequent cause of metabolic acidosis in very preterm infants.

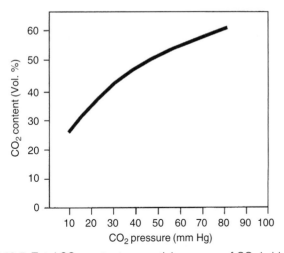

FIG 10-5 Total CO_2 content vs. partial pressure of CO_2 in blood. (From Comroe JH. The Lung. Chicago, Year Book Medical Publishers; 1962, 44–49.)

In most healthy newborns, the base deficit is usually between +3 and −1. Although it is logical to provide base to infants who have a metabolic acidosis from bicarbonate loss, there is essentially no evidence that acute bicarbonate therapy is beneficial in patients with metabolic acidosis from tissue hypoxia. In contrast, there is much evidence indicating that bicarbonate administration may be deleterious to the patient with hypoxia and metabolic acidosis, and it should not be used routinely.[21-23] In patients with metabolic acidosis, restoring tissue oxygen delivery by correcting the underlying problem is far more important than administering exogenous base. Sodium bicarbonate is no longer recommended during cardiopulmonary resuscitation.[21]

If metabolic acidosis is to be treated with exogenous base, the most commonly used drug is sodium bicarbonate. The number of milliequivalents of bicarbonate needed to half correct a base deficit can be approximated from the following equation:

$$\text{Bicarbonate (mEq) to be administered} = (\text{base deficit}) \times (\text{body weight in kg}) \times 0.3.$$

Owing to its hypertonicity, sodium bicarbonate (1 mEq/mL) should be diluted 1:1 with sterile water and administered slowly, preferably over 30 to 60 minutes.[24] Bicarbonate should be administered with care, if at all, in the infant with a combined respiratory and metabolic acidosis, because as the bicarbonate is metabolized, the $PaCO_2$ will further increase, unless there is also an increase in minute ventilation. Thus, the use of sodium bicarbonate should be limited to the few cases of severe renal tubular wasting or certain rare causes of congenital lactic acidosis.

Metabolic Alkalosis

By far the most common cause of relative metabolic alkalosis in neonates is a chronic compensation for respiratory acidosis. If a compensated respiratory acidosis is corrected by rapidly lowering the $PaCO_2$, an absolute metabolic alkalosis will result. Other causes of metabolic alkalosis in the newborn include hypochloremia from chronic diuretic therapy, or chronic drainage of gastric secretions (or frequent vomiting), and the administration of excess acetate in parenteral nutrition. Mild metabolic alkalosis can also occur following an exchange transfusion, when the citrate in the anticoagulant is metabolized. It is rarely necessary to aggressively correct metabolic alkalosis with administration of acidic compounds such as ammonium chloride or arginine hydrochloride or with bicarbonate-wasting diuretics such as acetazolamide. In most cases, treating a relative metabolic alkalosis with these agents merely results in an uncompensated respiratory acidosis.[25]

TECHNIQUES FOR OBTAINING BLOOD SAMPLES

Although it is possible to manage a sick newborn without arterial access, the presence of an arterial catheter often simplifies care significantly. It not only allows the accurate measurement of arterial blood gases without disturbing the patient but also allows direct measurement of arterial blood pressure and provides a route for obtaining other blood samples. Although valuable, umbilical catheters may be overused and are not without risk; therefore, standardization of their usage is preferred.[26]

Umbilical Artery Catheters

Umbilical artery catheters are the preferred route for arterial access in most intensive care nurseries, particularly for infants in the first few days of life. They usually can be quickly and easily placed with small risk of complications. The umbilical arteries are readily accessible during the first several days of life. Though successful cannulation is considerably less likely after a few days, it is still possible in some patients up to 2 weeks of age. Blood gas measurements performed on blood drawn from an umbilical catheter reflect postductal blood.

An umbilical catheter should be flexible, nonkinking, radiopaque, transparent, and nonthrombogenic and should have an end hole but no side hole.[27] There are two common catheter sizes, 3.5 and 5.0 F. Some clinicians feel that the larger catheter should be used whenever possible to minimize problems with thrombus formation within the catheter, making it less prone to "clotting off." Others feel that the smaller catheter is better because it minimizes the changes in aortic blood flow that occur when a catheter is in place.[28] Because almost no published evidence is available about the relative merits of the two catheter sizes, the decision about which catheter size to use is usually based on personal preference and patient size. Our usual approach is to use a 3.5-F single-lumen catheter in infants weighing less than 1500 or 2000 g and a 5.0-F single-lumen catheter in infants who weigh more than 1500 or 2000 g. We only use single lumen catheters when cannulating the umbilical artery.

The procedure for cannulation of the umbilical vessels can be seen in a video by Anderson et al. in the *New England Journal of Medicine*.[29] Additional videos describing the method are also available through Pedialink, the American Academy of Pediatrics Online Learning Center (https://vimeo.com/57453941).

Prior to insertion, the catheter is attached to a three-way stopcock and syringe containing a heparinized saline solution and then flushed thoroughly. When the catheter has been inserted and is functioning adequately, the stopcock should be attached to a continuous infusion of heparinized fluid and to a pressure transducer. Care should be taken in stabilizing stopcock connections to minimize the possibility of accidental disconnection.

The catheter is inserted while the infant is under a radiant warmer or in a heated incubator where the infant's temperature can be maintained and the vital signs monitored. The infant's legs should be loosely restrained, and it may be helpful to also loosely restrain the arms. The insertion of the catheter should be done under sterile conditions, after the umbilical cord is cleaned with povidone iodine or chlorhexidine, which should be removed after cleaning as these agents may cause skin injury if allowed to remain on the skin. A sterile umbilical tie is then placed around the lower portion of the cord and tied loosely with a single knot. The tie is placed so it can be either tightened, if bleeding occurs when the cord is cut, or loosened, if it prevents passage of the catheter. Next, the cord is cut approximately 0.5 cm above the skin. Leaving too long of an umbilical stump makes insertion of the catheters more difficult as it becomes harder to immobilize the vessels that are being cannulated. Cutting the cord with a scalpel in a single cut, rather than with a sawing motion, results in a flat umbilical surface from which the umbilical arteries usually protrude. The two thick-walled arteries and the single, larger, patulous thin-walled vein can easily be identified.

One of the more important steps in the insertion of an umbilical arterial catheter (in addition to maintaining sterile techniques) is dilation of the arterial lumen. Failure to carefully dilate the artery is one of the most common causes of catheter insertion failure. The goal of dilation is to open the lumen enough to allow smooth catheter passage without tearing the intima of the vessel. If the catheter tip tears the intima and creates a "false lumen" within the vessel, it will not reenter the lumen and successful catheter passage is nearly impossible. The dilation of the vessel should begin by placing one arm tip of a small forceps into the lumen. Forceps with teeth should be avoided as great care should be used to avoid shearing the intima. If done gently, the vessel will dilate, allowing both arms of the forceps to be placed into the lumen (Fig. 10-6). Once both arms have been placed, they can be slowly spread, gradually dilating the vessel to the caliber of the catheter. As the vessel lumen dilates, the forceps should be advanced with the goal of dilating at least 5 to 8 mm. Once the vessel has been adequately dilated, the catheter can be inserted. It is easier to pass the catheter if the vessel is stabilized with one or two small curved forceps. Usually, the catheter passes smoothly. When the catheter meets significant resistance, it usually means that the catheter has dissected through the intima and has created a false lumen within the wall of the vessel. When this occurs, the catheter should be removed. Forcing the catheter at this point is more likely to result in damage to the vessel or perforation of the peritoneum than to success.

On occasion, a catheter will travel down into the external iliac artery, which becomes the femoral artery that perfuses the lower limb, rather than up into the aorta. If this occurs, a second catheter can sometimes be inserted into the same umbilical artery without removing the first catheter. With the first catheter lodged in the external iliac artery, the second is often directed into the aorta.[30]

Once the catheter enters the aorta, it should be advanced to either "high position" or "low position." The goal of both positions is to place the tip of the catheter so that it is not adjacent to the origin of the renal, mesenteric, or celiac vessels originating from the descending aorta. If a low position is chosen, the catheter tip should be between the levels of the third and fourth lumbar vertebrae on a radiograph, safely below the renal and mesenteric arteries. If a high position is chosen, the catheter tip should be between the sixth and the tenth thoracic vertebrae, above the origin of the celiac vessels. Although both positions are commonly used, several prospective randomized studies and a subsequent meta-analysis comparing low versus high catheter placement have found a greater rate of peripheral vascular complications in infants

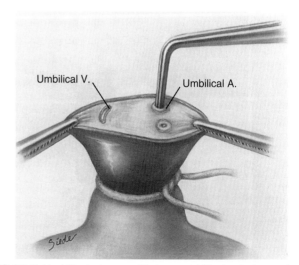

FIG 10-6 Umbilical stump with two umbilical arteries and one vein. A small forceps is used to gently dilate one artery.

with catheters in the low position; however, most of these complications were minor.[31]

Several published graphs are available for estimating the distance a catheter must be inserted to correctly place it in the lower position.[32,33] The simplest method is based on the infant's weight.[34] When a low position is targeted, for a 1-kg infant, the catheter should be inserted approximately 7 cm; for a 2-kg infant, it should be inserted approximately 8 cm; and for a 3-kg infant, it should be inserted approximately 9 cm. For a catheter to be placed in the high position, the formula "3 times the weight plus 9" gives a rough estimate of the required catheter insertion length in centimeters. A 2008 study suggests that the formula "4 times the weight plus 7" for very preterm infants gives a better estimate of the required catheter insertion length.[35] Gupta et al. indicate that surface measurements (umbilicus–nipple length minus 1 cm plus twice the distance from umbilicus to symphysis pubis) are useful for estimating correct insertion length.[36] Regardless of the method used for calculating the depth of insertion, the length of the umbilical stump must be added to determine the final intended depth of insertion. Following insertion, the catheter position should be confirmed radiographically (Fig. 10-7), as these methods are not always accurate.[37] Ultrasound can also be used to check for catheter tip position.[38] Once correct positioning is confirmed, the catheter should be fixed in place using sutures and tape. Generally, one uses a 3-0 silk suture tied to the circumference of the umbilical cord and then tied to the catheter. Special care must be taken not to puncture the catheter with the suture needle. The catheter is then secured with a tape bridge. Commercially sold "bridge" fixation devices are now commonly available.

Subumbilical Cutdown

If attempts to cannulate both umbilical arteries and peripheral arteries are unsuccessful, and the patient cannot be adequately managed without an arterial catheter, the umbilical arteries can sometimes be cannulated via subumbilical cutdown.[39] This is a surgical procedure and should not be attempted by anyone other than a physician who has previous experience with the technique, as several complications can result, including entering the peritoneal cavity and subumbilical hernia.

Complications of Umbilical Artery Catheterization

Although umbilical artery catheterization is safe and well tolerated in most patients, it is important to remember that it is not without risks. Complications related to umbilical arterial catheters include vascular compromise, complications related to malposition, infection, bleeding, and catheter-related accidents (accidental disconnection, rupture, etc.). Occasionally, catheter placement is associated with severe thrombotic complications, including frank gangrene and necrosis of the buttocks or leg. Studies indicate that umbilical artery catheters in the first 5 days are not associated with a high risk of thrombosis, although animal evidence suggests that even short-term umbilical arterial catheter use is associated with histological evidence of aortic thrombi and neointimal proliferation of the vascular wall that may not be clinically evident.[40,41]

Infants with umbilical artery catheters in place will occasionally develop dusky or purple discoloration of their toes, presumably from microemboli or vasospasm. In some cases, warming of the contralateral leg may cause reflex vasodilation and increased perfusion in the compromised extremity. Although this is a common practice, a study in normal infants without vasospasm showed that local warming has no effect on peripheral blood flow to the contralateral heel.[42] Regardless of whether there is any value in warming the contralateral foot, the compromised leg should not be warmed because of the possibility that this might increase the metabolic rate of the warmed tissues, leading to increased hypoxic tissue injury. Although the majority of patients with dusky toes have adequate perfusion and suffer no

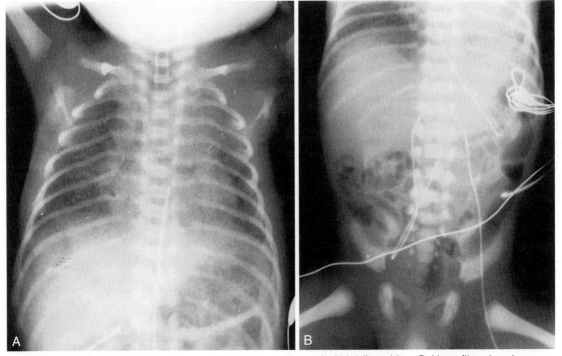

FIG 10-7   A, X-ray film showing umbilical artery catheter in "high" position. **B,** X-ray film showing umbilical artery catheter in "low" position.

ill effects, one must always be aware that this may represent a potentially significant vascular compromise. Failure to recognize worsening perfusion may result in necrosis and loss of a portion of the foot. If the toes remain dusky, with poor capillary filling, the catheter should be removed. Similarly, if the dusky discoloration involves more of the foot or leg, the catheter should be removed.

In rare instances, an infant with an umbilical catheter will develop blanching of the foot or part of the leg. Because blanching represents severely compromised arterial blood flow, the catheter should be immediately removed.

If perfusion to the limb does not immediately improve with withdrawal of the catheter, the infant should be evaluated for possible severe thrombotic complications. Evaluation in this case usually includes some combination of ultrasound or Doppler assessment, or even angiography. Both systemic vasodilators and topical vasodilators have been described as having some efficacy in this situation, but definitive evidence for efficacy is lacking.[43,44] When a significant clot is identified, thrombolysis with tissue plasminogen activator, infused either directly into the affected vessel or systemically, has been attempted.[45,46] The potential advantages of thrombolytic therapy must be weighed against the risks of such therapy, particularly in the infant with a preexisting intracranial hemorrhage that could potentially extend. Unfortunately, there is little literature available regarding the optimal approach to infants with severe vascular obstruction.

The incidence of infection associated with umbilical artery catheters appears to be lower than the incidence of infections associated with central venous catheters. However, as with all central catheters, meticulous care must be taken to maintain sterility during catheter insertion and during subsequent withdrawal of blood from the catheter. We recommend minimizing line "breaks" to reduce the risk of central line infection. A Cochrane review suggests that there is inadequate evidence to recommend either for or against routine antibiotic use in infants with umbilical catheters in place, and it is recommended to not use prolonged empiric antimicrobial therapy with negative cultures in infants.[47]

A concern of umbilical artery catheters is the effect of blood sampling on cerebral blood flow. Ultrasonographic and near-infrared spectroscopy studies have shown that routine blood sampling from an umbilical catheter alters cerebral hemodynamics and oxygenation.[48,49] While reducing the volume of blood withdrawn may reduce these changes, it is unclear whether a slower withdrawal is also beneficial.[50,51] Although it is unknown whether these changes in cerebral hemodynamics increase the risk of any complications such as intraventricular hemorrhage, it is reasonable to avoid rapidly withdrawing from or infusing into any umbilical catheter and to reduce the volumes withdrawn.

Concomitant enteral nutrition with umbilical artery catheters in place is generally considered safe, with most clinicians continuing to feed with umbilical catheters.[52] Superior mesenteric arterial flow is not affected by the presence of an umbilical catheter during trophic feeding.[53]

There is little published literature on which to base decisions about how long an umbilical artery catheter can remain safely in place. In most institutions, they are usually removed within several days, when the infant no longer requires significant respiratory support or frequent blood sampling. As with all therapies, the potential risks of umbilical artery catheterization must be balanced against the potential advantages for each infant.

Other Indwelling Catheter Sites

In some infants, umbilical artery catheterization is unsuccessful. In these cases, percutaneous cannulation of a peripheral artery may be the best alternative. Percutaneous arterial cannulation is also the best option for infants who no longer have an umbilical artery cannula but still require arterial access. Other techniques, such as umbilical artery or peripheral artery cutdown, are more difficult to perform and involve more risk to the patient. Although percutaneous cannulation of a peripheral artery is technically challenging, especially in infants weighing less than 1 kg, cannulation of the radial, dorsalis pedis, or posterior tibial artery is often possible. One should avoid cannulating the temporal artery because cerebral emboli and stroke have been reported in patients with temporal artery catheters.[54,55]

If the radial artery is to be cannulated, an Allen's test may be performed to ensure ulnar artery patency. However, the reliability of this test has been questioned.[56] Conversely, if the ulnar artery is to be cannulated, radial artery patency should be assessed. Begin the Allen's test by gently squeezing the hand to empty it of blood. Apply pressure to both the radial and the ulnar arteries and then remove pressure from the hand and the artery that will not be cannulated. If the entire hand flushes and fills with blood, it is safe to proceed with cannulation.[19] Doppler evaluation may also be used to document collateral circulation.

The artery can be localized by either palpation or transillumination. If the radial or ulnar artery is to be cannulated, the hand should be restrained in mild hyperextension. We usually administer an analgesic dose of morphine or fentanyl to the infant before beginning the cannulation. Local anesthesia with lidocaine is sometimes used, and the resulting wheal may require gentle massage and waiting a few minutes.

The insertion site should be cleaned prior to proceeding with a povidone–iodine or chlorhexidine solution. The radial artery is usually most easily cannulated at the point of maximal pulsation over the distal portion of the radius, proximal to the superficial palmar branch of the artery. In this position, the artery lies between two tendons, superficial and lateral to the median nerve (Fig. 10-8).

The catheter can be used either dry or flushed with a heparinized saline solution to facilitate flashback of blood. The catheter and needle are advanced at an angle of approximately 30 degrees until the vessel is entered and a pulsatile blood return is encountered. The needle is held stationary and the catheter is threaded into the artery. The needle is then withdrawn.

An alternative technique is to puncture the artery through both the anterior and the posterior walls and then withdraw the needle. The catheter is then withdrawn until its tip reenters the vessel lumen and a brisk blood return is obtained, at which point it is threaded into the vessel. However, in our experience, this method is frequently less successful than the previous technique.

Once in place, the catheter should be taped securely and connected to an infusion of heparinized saline with a T-connector and a three-way stopcock. The tape securing the catheter must allow for unobstructed view of all five digits because hypoperfusion, potentially leading to ischemic necrosis, is the major complication of peripheral arterial catheters. It is important to appreciate that the limb chosen for insertion of the peripheral artery catheter will determine whether blood gas testing reflects pre- or postductal values.

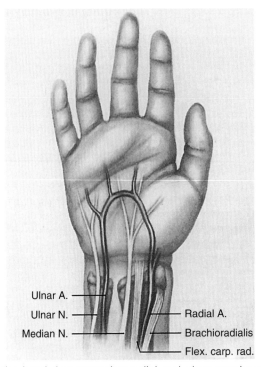

FIG 10-8 Anatomy of the hand demonstrating radial and ulnar arteries and surrounding structures. *A.,* artery; *Flex. carp. rad.,* flexor carpi radialis; *N.,* nerve.

In the figure: Ulnar A., Ulnar N., Median N., Radial A., Brachioradialis, Flex. carp. rad.

Infusion of Fluids through Arterial Catheters

The patency of both central and peripheral arterial catheters should be maintained with a heparinized solution. In most centers, the heparin concentrations range from 0.25 to 1.0 unit/mL. Heparinization of the infusate decreases the incidence of catheter occlusion but does not affect the frequency of aortic thrombosis, intracranial hemorrhage, death, or clinical ischemic phenomena.[57] Although there is no published evidence on safe rates at which to run fluids through arterial catheters, most clinicians use a minimal rate of 1 mL/hr.

Saline, glucose, and hyperalimentation solutions can all be infused into an umbilical artery catheter, and it has been shown that infusing an amino acid–containing solution of normal osmolarity causes less hemolysis than does a quarter normal saline solution, while improving nutrition.[58] In contrast to umbilical arteries through which one can infuse a wide range of solutions, there is concern about the irritant effects of anything other than a physiologic saline solution infused into a peripheral artery. In very preterm infants for whom 1 mL/hr of a physiologic saline solution provides an excessive sodium load, clinicians often infuse 0.45% saline. In cases in which extra base is required, we infuse sodium acetate rather than sodium chloride. Medications or blood products are never administered through a peripheral arterial catheter.

Arterial Puncture

Blood gas samples can be obtained from intermittent puncture of the radial, ulnar, temporal, posterior tibial, or dorsalis pedis arteries. In general, the femoral and brachial arteries should not be used for arterial puncture because significant thrombus formation could lead to loss of the extremity, and median nerve damage has been reported with brachial puncture.[59] As noted above, an Allen's test may be performed before puncture of the radial or ulnar artery.

After the exact location of the desired artery has been determined by transillumination or by palpation, the skin should be prepared with a povidone–iodine or chlorhexidine solution. A small gauge needle (e.g., 22 to 25 gauge) is inserted in the bevel-up position at an angle through the skin, against the direction of the arterial flow. Blood should flow into the tubing spontaneously or with gentle suction. After the needle is removed, continuous pressure should be applied to the artery for 5 minutes. If hematoma formation is prevented, the same artery can be reaccessed several times.

The main drawback to arterial puncture is that the procedure can rarely be done without disturbing the patient. One study showed that venipuncture, generally regarded as less traumatic than arterial puncture, caused a 6-mm Hg decrease in $PaCO_2$ and a 17-mm Hg decrease in PaO_2.[60] Although subcutaneous administration of lidocaine (without epinephrine) over the artery before arterial puncture will provide partial analgesia, most infants still become agitated during the puncture. For this reason, arterial puncture to obtain blood gases is used infrequently.

Arterialized Capillary Blood

Arterialized capillary blood can provide a crude estimate of arterial blood values. In theory, blood flowing through a dilated peripheral capillary bed has little time for O_2 and CO_2 exchange to occur, making capillary blood gas values approximate those in the arterial blood.

Capillary samples can be obtained from a warmed heel. To arterialize the capillary blood, the extremity should be warmed for several minutes. Warming should be performed with exothermic chemical packs specifically designed for arterializing capillary blood, rather than with warm compresses, which provide poor control over temperature. The site should be carefully cleaned, and a small lancet should be used to puncture the skin.

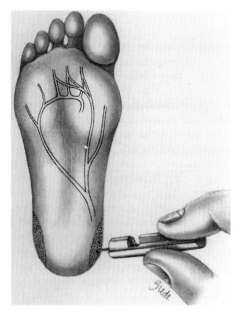

FIG 10-9 Technique for obtaining an arterialized capillary heel sample. Stippled sections denote the correct areas for sampling.

When obtaining blood from the heel, the puncture should be made on the medial or lateral aspect of the plantar surface. The posterior curvature should not be used (Fig. 10-9).

There are multiple technical challenges to obtaining optimal capillary blood samples. Inadequate warming of the site will result in inadequate arterialization of the blood. Excessive squeezing will cause contamination of the "arterialized" blood with venous blood or interstitial fluid. Exposure of blood to air during collection will skew the Po_2 (falsely increased) and PCO_2 (falsely decreased) values. Low peripheral perfusion states lead to stasis and often result in falsely elevated PCO_2 values. For this reason, obtaining a capillary specimen in a 2-hour-old infant with obvious acrocyanosis seldom yields useful information and risks unnecessary intubation for apparent respiratory acidosis due to stasis. Longer term problems associated with capillary samples include calcaneal osteochondritis and calcified heel nodules.[61] These calcified nodules may persist for several months to years but do not seem to cause permanent problems for the infant.

Capillary puncture can be done only rarely without disturbing the infant. This, plus the fact that arterialized capillary blood is not the same as true arterial blood, means that a capillary blood gas represents only an approximation of the infant's baseline arterial blood gas status. Blood obtained simultaneously from the umbilical artery catheter and warmed heels of infants demonstrated poor predictability of arterial values from arterialized capillary pH and $PaCO_2$ as well as for PaO_2.[62] Arterialized capillary samples are probably most useful in chronically ventilated infants as they are moderately useful for tracking gross changes in pH and $PaCO_2$.

Continuous Invasive Monitoring

Since 1995, a number of devices have been developed for the direct intravascular or "inline" measurement of hemoglobin saturation, PaO_2, and $PaCO_2$.[63,64] However, despite their apparent advantages, these devices still have not made it into common use in most North American NICUs, both because of

their cost and complexity and because of the ease of use of noninvasive technology. One study demonstrated a reduction in the need for blood transfusions in premature infants using an inline blood gas analyzer.[65]

Noninvasive Estimation of Blood Gases

The development of techniques for simply and safely obtaining continuous noninvasive estimates of blood gases is one of the most important advances in neonatal care since 1985. Pulse oximeters are so ubiquitous in intensive care nurseries that many think oxygen saturation is as important a vital sign as heart rate or blood pressure. Although less widely used than pulse oximeters, with recent technologic advances, both transcutaneous monitoring and end-tidal CO_2 monitoring have an important role in the management of neonates. Near-infrared spectroscopy (NIRS) is another technology that is gradually moving from research to routine clinical use in selected infants.

Pulse Oximetry

Oxygen saturation monitoring via pulse oximetry is standard practice in NICUs. While it has reduced the frequency of blood gas testing, it has important limitations. Pulse oximeters work on the principle that saturated hemoglobin (oxyhemoglobin) is a different color from desaturated hemoglobin (deoxyhemoglobin) and thus absorbs light of a different frequency.[66–68] Oxyhemoglobin demonstrates higher absorbance of infrared light at a wavelength of 940 nm compared to deoxyhemoglobin, which demonstrates a higher absorbance of red light at a wavelength of 660 nm. The ratio of light absorbance at these two wavelengths is used to derive the transcutaneous oxygen saturation.

A probe consisting of a light source and a photosensor is placed so that the light source and photosensor are on opposite sides of each other with tissue in between. As light passes through the tissues, the saturated and desaturated hemoglobin absorb different frequencies of light. By measuring the difference between the ratio of the different frequencies of light absorbed during systole and diastole, the amount of light absorbed due to arterial flow can be calculated. Then, by comparing the absorption at the two appropriate frequencies, the percentage of saturated hemoglobin can be calculated. Refinements of this system include complex algorithms for calculating more exact saturation and for separating arterial pulsations from motion artifact. The calculation of saturation is dependent on sensing light so that ambient light striking the sensor can lead to a false reading.

The so-called functional oxygen saturation measured by pulse oximeters is represented by the equation $100 \times$ OxyHb/(OxyHb + DeoxyHb), where OxyHb is oxyhemoglobin and DeoxyHb is deoxyhemoglobin. With advancing technology, the number of wavelengths of light employed by some pulse oximeter manufacturers has increased, allowing the pulse oximeter to measure total hemoglobin and other hemoglobin species such as methemoglobin and carboxyhemoglobin.[69] However, this technology is quite new and is still undergoing validation in the newborn population.

By focusing only on oxyhemoglobin and deoxyhemoglobin, traditional pulse oximetry may provide misleading values in the setting of elevated levels of other hemoglobin species. In the setting of elevated carboxyhemoglobin levels, pulse oximetry will overestimate oxygen saturation by 1% for every 1% increase in carboxyhemoglobin.[70] This occurs because carboxyhemoglobin absorbs light similar to oxyhemoglobin (Fig. 10-10). In

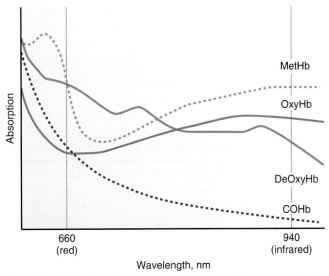

FIG 10-10 Light absorption. *COHb*, carboxyhemoglobin; *DeOxyHb*, deoxyhemoglobin; *MetHb*, methemoglobin; *OxyHb*, oxyhemoglobin.

contrast, methemoglobin absorbs equal amounts of red and infrared light (see Fig. 10-10). As the amount of methemoglobin increases, the ratio of light absorbance at both wavelengths approaches 1, which corresponds to an oxygen saturation of 85%.[71,72]

Co-oximetry is utilized in modern blood gas analyzers and differs from pulse oximetry in that is uses spectrophotometry to determine the relative concentrations of hemoglobin derivatives by measuring their absorbances of different wavelengths of light. Modern co-oximeters utilize over 100 different wavelengths of light.[73] In this manner, they directly measure several hemoglobin species including oxyhemoglobin, deoxyhemoglobin, carboxyhemoglobin, methemoglobin, and sulfhemoglobin. Therefore, they are less prone to error in reporting oxygen saturations compared to pulse oximetry in the presence of different hemoglobin species. The "fractional" oxygen saturation measured by blood gas analyzers is represented by the equation 100 × OxyHb/(OxyHb + DeoxyHb + COHb + MetHb), where OxyHb is oxyhemoglobin, DeoxyHb is deoxyhemoglobin, COHb is carboxyhemoglobin, and MetHb is methemoglobin. In the setting of elevated concentrations of abnormal hemoglobin species, blood gas testing should guide therapy, and pulse oximetry results should be critically examined to determine if they are accurate.

Several factors commonly observed in the newborn patient population do not adversely affect the accuracy of pulse oximetry, however. The presence of fetal hemoglobin, anemia, or hyperbilirubinemia has negligible effects on the accuracy of pulse oximetry.[74–76]

In general, pulse oximeters provide excellent data about oxygenation in the physiologic range. However, the values they provide must be interpreted with care. Poor perfusion, ambient light, and motion all interfere with an adequate signal. Also, different manufacturers use different algorithms for calculating saturation and so may give slightly different results. It is important to know that manufacturers are constantly updating the software in their devices, making many published articles on the limitations of specific devices out of date.

Pulse oximeters are dependent on adequate pulsatile blood flow. In situations such as shock, or if severe edema obscures pulsatile flow, the oximeter may not function reliably. Similarly, in patients on total support from venoarterial ECMO, who have minimal arterial pulsations, many pulse oximeters do not function well if the pulse pressure is less than 10 mm Hg.

The flat upper part of the S-shaped oxygen–hemoglobin dissociation curve (see Fig. 10-1) makes it difficult for pulse oximeters to differentiate between degrees of hyperoxemia. For example, a PaO_2 of 80 and a PaO_2 of 180 mm Hg both represent essentially 100% saturation in a preterm neonate. Some clinicians suggest that this is a significant limitation of pulse oximetry compared with transcutaneous oxygen monitoring, particularly as avoiding hyperoxemia to decrease the risk of retinopathy of prematurity is an important priority in neonates.[77] Pulse oximeters are also less accurate in the low end of the saturation range (e.g., less than 70% saturation) than in the normal physiologic range. Fortunately, this does not usually pose a clinically significant problem because the exact degree of severe desaturation is usually less important for clinical decision making than the occurrence of the desaturation itself.

One major advantage of pulse oximetry is that oxygen saturation is a better indicator of oxygen content than is PaO_2, as saturation is a variable in calculating oxygen carried by hemoglobin (the major contributor to oxygen content in blood), whereas PaO_2 represents dissolved oxygen, which is only a minor, yet important, component of oxygen transport.

Transcutaneous Monitoring

Transcutaneous oxygen and carbon dioxide electrodes allow continuous indirect estimation of PaO_2 and $PaCO_2$. Although pulse oximetry has largely replaced transcutaneous oxygen monitoring as a tool for estimating oxygenation, many centers find an important role for transcutaneous CO_2 monitoring. Current transcutaneous CO_2 monitoring devices can be run at lower temperatures than previous generations of monitors and are therefore less likely to cause thermal injury to immature skin.[78,79] There are several good reviews of the theory and practice of transcutaneous monitoring.[68,79–81]

Transcutaneous Po_2 ($tcPo_2$) essentially measures the Po_2 of skin. Although the Po_2 of skin is usually lower than the PaO_2, heating of the skin directly under the $tcPo_2$ electrode causes local cutaneous vasodilation resulting in the skin Po_2 approaching PaO_2. Although heating the skin causes several effects other than vasodilation, these effects on the oxygen dissociation curve, tissue oxygen consumption, and electrode oxygen consumption cancel out for most patients. Studies have shown that $tcPo_2$ approximates PaO_2 even in patients with poor perfusion; however, in older infants with chronic lung disease, $tcPo_2$ underestimates PaO_2.[82]

The relationship between $PaCO_2$ and transcutaneous Pco_2 ($tcPco_2$) is more complex than between PaO_2 and $tcPo_2$. $TcPco_2$ is always greater than $PaCO_2$ because of the combination of several effects. Among these effects is the fact that heating causes increased production of CO_2 by blood and skin cells, there is a significant arterial–cellular CO_2 gradient, and the skin has a cooling effect on the electrode. These effects are fairly uniform at a given temperature and combine to create a linear relationship between $tcPco_2$ and $PaCO_2$.[83]

Despite its limitations, transcutaneous CO_2 measurement is helpful for trending $PaCO_2$ values, particularly in the absence of reliable clinical indicators of adequacy of ventilation. It may be particularly helpful in the management of infants on high-frequency ventilation in which it is difficult to assess tidal volume and in cases in which the patient's work of breathing may be difficult to assess.

Many clinicians consider $tcPco_2$ monitoring essential when initiating high-frequency ventilation because both jet and oscillatory ventilation often change $PaCO_2$ rapidly when transitioning from conventional ventilation.

Capnography

Capnography, also known as *end-tidal CO_2 monitoring*, is the measurement of exhaled CO_2. This is a technique that has found widespread use in adult and pediatric intensive care units, as well as in the operating room, and may be helpful in larger neonatal patients. It is an attractive technology because it is relatively inexpensive, portable, noninvasive, and easy to use. However, it has not been as widely accepted into intensive care nurseries, primarily because it gives only a rough estimate of $PaCO_2$ in patients with significant lung disease. End-tidal CO_2 monitoring can be done using mainstream, sidestream, or microstream techniques.[84–86]

Because alveolar Pco_2 approximates $PaCO_2$, a sample of pure alveolar gas will provide an estimate of $PaCO_2$. Capnography measures the concentration of CO_2 in exhaled gas and displays this concentration as a function of time. If there is a good end-tidal plateau in exhaled Pco_2, this usually represents the alveolar Pco_2. In adult and pediatric patients with relatively large tidal volumes and relatively low respiratory rates, this alveolar plateau is readily measured. In sick neonates, the limitation of capnography is the difficulty in obtaining a sample of alveolar gas that is not mixed with gas from the airways. Ill newborns are usually too tachypneic and have tidal volumes that are too small to obtain an adequate end-tidal sample of alveolar gas. In addition, animal studies suggest that alveolar disease interferes with the relationship of end-tidal CO_2 compared to $PaCO_2$, independent of respiratory rate and tidal volume.[87] Studies in newborns demonstrate that capnography is an accurate method of estimating $PaCO_2$ in healthy infants, or in ventilated postsurgical infants with normal lungs, but provides only a rough estimate of $PaCO_2$, which is usually underestimated, in infants with significant lung disease.[85,88–91] One study of capnography during transport of infants found that the end-tidal Pco_2 significantly underestimated $PaCO_2$ but that the degree of underestimation was independent of either the $PaCO_2$ or the severity of lung disease.[92] In addition to using capnography to estimate $PaCO_2$, quantitative curve analysis of capnographic curves may indicate the magnitude of spontaneous compared to ventilator-assisted breaths.[93]

One of the most useful applications of exhaled CO_2 monitoring is in rapidly confirming proper endotracheal tube placement.[94,95] Small, disposable colorimetric devices can be attached to the hub of an endotracheal tube immediately after intubation to ensure that exhaled CO_2 is being detected. This approach is extremely useful for determining successful intubation. Moreover, the Neonatal Resuscitation Program suggests that during resuscitation, if the baby's heart rate does not respond to intubation and ventilation, a colorimetric CO_2 detector should be used to verify the placement of the endotracheal tube. Babies with very poor cardiac output may not exhale sufficient CO_2 to be detected reliably by CO_2 detectors. Although qualitative (colorimetric) detection is useful to confirm endotracheal tube placement, there is no strong evidence supporting the need for quantitative monitoring of end-tidal CO_2 in the delivery room or during resuscitation.[96–98] Many of the newer generations of bedside monitors now have built-in end-tidal CO_2 monitoring as an option, making continuous monitoring of exhaled CO_2 a realistic option for ventilated infants, with the caveat that some end-tidal CO_2 monitors may themselves increase dead space to a substantial proportion of delivered tidal volume in very preterm infants.

Near-Infrared Spectroscopy

The light-absorbing characteristics of oxygenated and deoxygenated hemoglobin can be used for techniques other than pulse oximetry. NIRS is a technique that relies on this differential absorption of light and also on the relatively transparent nature of tissue to infrared light to give an estimation of tissue oxygenation. Although this technique has been intermittently studied in infants since the 1980s and has been gaining acceptance (primarily in cardiac intensive care units), its true value in caring for patients remains largely unknown, as improvement in outcomes with NIRS monitoring have not yet been demonstrated.[99–101] NIRS monitoring is different from pulse oximetry in many aspects as the tissue saturation measured by NIRS represents a weighted average of arterial and venous saturation wherein the weighting factor cannot be precisely determined and varies from tissue to tissue and over time.[102]

CHOICE OF MONITORING METHODS

Since 2005 several factors have led to a gradual decline in the reliance on arterial blood gas samples. The heightened awareness of blood transfusion risks has resulted in a general decrease in the number of blood tests, including blood gases, in an effort to reduce the volume of iatrogenic blood loss. "Permissive hypercarbia" has led to a wider range of accepted $PaCO_2$ values and therefore less frequent blood gas measurements. The increased use of patient-triggered ventilator modes such as assist control and pressure support, whereby the patients control their respiratory rate and minute ventilation, and even more so the use of volume-targeted ventilation, which is capable of maintaining stable ventilation despite changes in lung compliance, have led many neonatologists to further decrease the frequency of blood gas sampling.

Despite these trends, there remains the need for reliable arterial blood gas sampling in unstable infants. Our approach is to place an umbilical catheter into any newborn with respiratory distress that is significant enough to require relatively frequent arterial blood sampling. We routinely place an umbilical artery catheter in infants who require intubation or nasal continuous positive airway pressure with significant oxygen requirements and in most infants who weigh less than 1 kg. We usually remove umbilical artery catheters after a few days when frequent blood gas or continuous blood pressure measurements are no longer needed, although we will sometimes leave them in for as long as 2 to 3 weeks (and accept the potential risks, including aortic thrombosis) in extremely unstable infants who weigh less than 1 kg. For other infants who are critically ill and need arterial monitoring, peripheral arterial catheters are placed.

We monitor all but the most stable infants with continuous pulse oximetry. Infants requiring significant respiratory support are usually followed with transcutaneous CO_2 monitoring in addition to pulse oximetry. Capnography as a method of estimating $PaCO_2$ has gradually become more widely used in the NICU, particularly for large infants with minimal lung disease such as postoperative infants. NIRS monitoring, although intriguing and potentially useful, has not yet become routine in many NICUs.

Continuous monitoring of ventilated infants is supplemented with intermittent measurements of blood gases. In our NICU, stable ventilated infants without arterial access usually have capillary blood gases performed every 24 to 48 hours, whereas less stable infants have them performed as frequently as two to four times per day. In critically ill infants without arterial access, we sometimes use samples drawn from an umbilical venous catheter to provide a crude estimate of pH and P_{CO_2}. Although venous P_{CO_2} is at least several millimeters of mercury higher than arterial (and may be significantly higher), we believe it is sometimes preferable to use this crude measure than to perform repeated arterialized capillary blood gas samples or intermittent arterial punctures.[103,104]

BLOOD GAS ANALYZERS

Blood gas analyzers continue to evolve, offering more than basic blood gas measurement of pH, $PaCO_2$, and PaO_2. Modern blood gas analyzers are capable of measuring various forms of hemoglobin, serum electrolytes, and metabolites. Point-of-care blood gas analyzers facilitate analyzing of the blood sample near the bedside (and especially in the delivery room), which can accelerate clinical decision making versus the hospital central laboratory.[105,106] Arterial, venous, and capillary blood gas samples may be analyzed in the NICU, reducing pre- and post-sample collection errors and reducing time to results.[105,106] Analyzers come in a variety of sizes from hand-held to portable desktop systems, which are more user friendly, more automated, and require less technical expertise and maintenance by the end user compared with earlier analyzers.

Measuring Principle of a Blood Gas Analyzer

Traditional blood gas electrodes for pH, $PaCO_2$, and PaO_2 measure changes in electrical current or voltage and are linked to a chemical measurement. Electrodes are constructed of a permeable membrane and are bathed in a solution that allows H^+, CO_2, or O_2 to pass through the membrane, react with the solution, and cause a current or voltage change that equates to the measurement of pH, $PaCO_2$, or PaO_2. Today, given the variety of analyzers, many technologies such as potentiometry, amperometry, fluorescence, and ion-selective electrodes are utilized to measure blood gases, electrolytes, and metabolites.[106] The analyzer will derive or calculate other variables from the pH, $PaCO_2$, and PaO_2 measured values through algorithms and nomograms. Plasma bicarbonate, or actual bicarbonate, is calculated from the pH and $PaCO_2$ measured values. Calculated values may be customized and can include base excess/deficit, bicarbonate, oxygen saturation of hemoglobin, and other indicators of oxygenation such as the oxygenation index. One must keep in mind that derived values are calculated and therefore may not be accurate compared with measured values. The oxygen saturation of hemoglobin calculation fails to account for dyshemoglobins. A co-oximeter is preferable in this instance as it can directly measure different hemoglobin species. For this reason, most modern blood gas analyzers also incorporate a co-oximeter. Sample volumes required for capillary and arterial blood gas measurements are analyzer dependent and may range from 65 to 150 μL. Smaller sample volumes may provide fewer analytes or no co-oximeter values. The validity of blood gas results is dependent on analyzer function, sample collection and sample handling techniques (pre- and post-analytical factors). Blood samples introduced into the analyzer must be collected in an appropriate syringe or capillary tube containing the correct anticoagulant.

Blood Gas Analyzer Quality Assurance

To ensure consistent reliable results, the blood gas analyzer should be part of a quality assurance program that monitors, documents, and regulates the accuracy of the analyzer. Internal quality control measures may consist of calibration, quality control and maintenance schedules, comparing samples to lab equipment, and external proficiency testing.[107] The newest generation of point-of-care analyzers contains disposable sealed packs that include sensors, electrodes, quality control solutions, cleaning solutions, and waste containment. These self-contained packs may decrease the chance of error while handling sensitive electrodes, quality control solutions, and biohazard material. The analyzers will autocalibrate, analyze quality control samples, and detect errors. Advantages of these systems are less maintenance, better error detection, and consistent quality control.[108,109] Traditional analyzers are still in use today and require more maintenance, manual care of electrodes, quality control solutions, and waste management.[106,109]

A comparison of different analytical methods for measuring oxygen saturation is presented in Table 10-1.

CLINICAL INTERPRETATION OF BLOOD GASES

Understanding the physiology of gas exchange makes the interpretation of blood gases a relatively straightforward process. Hypoxemia is the result of ventilation–perfusion mismatch or shunting, usually resulting from atelectasis and/or extrapulmonary shunting. In these instances, hypoxemia can be treated by reversing atelectasis and/or decreasing pulmonary vascular resistance or, in infants with cyanotic congenital heart disease, improving pulmonary blood flow by promoting ductal patency, invasive cardiovascular interventions, or surgical methods. Our goal in all infants should be to ensure optimal oxygen delivery to the tissues by maintaining proper oxygenation, as well as hemoglobin level and cardiac output, at levels that avoid tissue hypoxia while minimizing the risks of hyperoxia.

Hypercarbia is the result of inadequate alveolar minute ventilation and is treated by increasing minute ventilation, usually by increasing tidal volume and/or respiratory rate. However, it is uncertain what "normal" and "acceptable" ranges are, particularly in the premature infant.

In this section we review the physiology that is relevant to interpreting the core elements of a blood gas analysis—the pH, $PaCO_2$, PaO_2, bicarbonate HCO_3^-, and base excess. The blood gas analyzer directly measures the pH, $PaCO_2$, and PaO_2. Normally, these results are collected on either arterial blood or an arterialized capillary sample. pH and $PaCO_2$ can be evaluated on venous blood samples too, although, as described above, the values will differ from those of arterial blood.

COMPONENTS OF BLOOD GAS TESTING THAT ARE MEASURED DIRECTLY

pH

When reviewing blood gas results, the pH is a good place to start for an overall acid–base assessment. Current technology is not able to measure intracellular acid–base status for clinical purposes. The pH reported on a blood gas result reflects the concentration of extracellular hydrogen ions: $pH = -\log[H^+]$.

TABLE 10-1 Analytical Methods for Measuring Oxygen Saturation

Device	Specimen	Measurement	Reported Data	Advantages	Disadvantages
Arterial Blood Gas (ABG) Analyzer	Blood	Partial pressure of oxygen dissolved in whole blood at an electrode	PaO_2, SO_2 (oxygen saturation) Some models available with CO-oximetry capabilities	Also measures pH and $PaCO_2$	Invasive, SaO_2 may be inaccurate if abnormal hemoglobin species present
CO-oximeter	Blood	Absorption of Hb derivatives using multiple wavelengths of light	SaO_2, FO_2Hb^*, $FHHb^*$, $FMetHb^*$, $FCOHb^*$, $FSHb^*$, total hemoglobin concentration	Measures the concentration of Hb species	Invasive, performed in laboratory
Pulse oximeter	Transcutaneous	Absorption at two wavelengths (660 nm and 940 nm) in blood	SpO_2	Non-invasive, continuous bedside monitoring	Inaccurate when interfering substances are present: MetHb, certain dyes

*The 'F' preceding each acronym refers to 'fractional' referring the fractional concentration of each hemoglobin species.
Reproduced with modifications from Haymond S, Oxygen Saturation, A Guide to Laboratory Assessment, Clinical Laboratory News, 10-12, 2006 February.

More accurately, the pH is equal to the negative log of the hydronium ion (H_3O^+), though we make reference to hydrogen ions by convention. Higher concentrations of these hydrogen ions result in a low pH, and vice versa. Because pH is equal to the negative log of the hydrogen ion concentration, large changes in the concentration of hydrogen result in just small changes in the pH.

The concentration of hydrogen ions in the blood is surprisingly low compared to other common ions. For example, the concentration of serum sodium is over 3 million times greater than the concentration of hydrogen ions.[110] Maintaining the pH within a normal range is important for maintaining normal cellular function throughout the body as pH affects the function of proteins and cell membranes. For this reason, the body maintains very tight control of hydrogen ion concentrations. Chemoreceptors in our arteries and the medulla adjust ventilation based on the pH (and also the PaO_2 and $PaCO_2$).[111–113]

Berend and colleagues state that across the entire range of pH compatible with life (6.9 to 7.6) the observed difference in hydrogen ion concentration is less than 0.13 mmol/L.[110] This tight control is achieved through a series of buffering systems and compensatory mechanisms within the body. The most important buffering system is the carbonic acid–bicarbonate buffer in which H^+ and HCO_3^- combine to form H_2CO_3, which is in equilibrium with water and carbon dioxide. The normal ratio of bicarbonate to dissolved CO_2 is 20:1. Hemoglobin, proteins such as albumin and globulin, and phosphate also have important acid-buffering functions. When the body's ability to manage acid–base disturbances is inadequate, the result is either an acidosis (low pH) or an alkalosis (high pH). The normal pH range is 7.35 to 7.45. Even in states of significant "acidosis" (e.g., pH 7.10), the blood is still relatively alkaline, as acid–base neutrality is defined as a pH of 7.0.

In addition to buffering, or neutralizing acids, volatile acids can be removed from the body via the lungs, whereas the kidneys can excrete fixed acids and regulate the concentration of bicarbonate. Hasselbalch introduced the use of the term *compensation* to describe the means to correct acid–base disturbances in 1915.[114] Compensatory mechanisms operate to restore the pH toward normal levels but usually do not result in the pH returning to the middle of the normal range or overshooting to reach abnormal levels on the opposite side, because the stimulus driving the compensation is lost as the pH approaches normal levels.

For example, a baby with metabolic acidosis and a pH of 7.30 may increase its minute ventilation to remove carbon dioxide from the body with a resulting increase in pH to 7.35 but not higher. However, there is more recent evidence citing correction of pH to >7.40 in adult patients with chronic respiratory acidosis, which raises questions about our understanding of this topic.[115–117]

Some clinicians believe that the term *compensation* is misleading and recommend referring to this process as a *secondary response*.[118] The respiratory secondary response to acid–base derangements begins nearly immediately and affects the pH within minutes, whereas the renal response begins within 6 to 12 hours and takes 3 to 5 days.[111,112,119]

The first step in assessing the acid–base status of the body is evaluating the pH to determine if it is normal. In the setting of an abnormal pH, the next step is to determine if the derangement is respiratory or metabolic in nature.

Carbon Dioxide

Whereas the pH is the first variable to evaluate, the $PaCO_2$ is usually the next variable examined, especially in the ventilated patient, as it is the single best indicator of respiratory sufficiency. Carbon dioxide is a normal by-product of cellular aerobic metabolism. It is produced when pyruvate is oxidized via the Krebs cycle to ultimately produce ATP in the mitochondrion. $PaCO_2$ represents the partial pressure of carbon dioxide that is dissolved in the blood. Carbon dioxide is over 20 times more soluble than oxygen in blood. $PaCO_2$ is the best indicator of the respiratory contribution to acid–base control. The normal range of $PaCO_2$ is 35 to 45 mm Hg.[111,112,120]

The body removes carbon dioxide via the lungs. Most of the CO_2 in blood is transported to the lungs in the form of bicarbonate, before converting it back to CO_2, which is exhaled.[121] Hence, any maneuvers that increase alveolar ventilation in a properly inflated lung will reduce the $PaCO_2$. Alveolar ventilation is represented by the following equation: respiratory rate × (tidal volume − dead space volume). Increasing the ventilator rate, increasing the tidal volume, and/or decreasing the dead space volume will lead to a decrease in $PaCO_2$ in a properly inflated lung. Traditional teaching that $PaCO_2$ is related to the minute ventilation (equal to respiratory rate × tidal volume) does not account for the important contribution of the dead space, which can be up to 20% of tidal volume in an intubated extremely low birth-weight neonate. Maintenance of $PaCO_2$ within physiologic ranges is dependent both on alveolar ventilation and on the rate of CO_2 production.

PaO₂

The PaO_2 represents the oxygen dissolved within the plasma of the blood and offers an assessment of the patient's oxygenation status. By examining the equation for the oxygen content of the blood (oxygen content = 1.34 × hemoglobin concentration × oxygen saturation/100 + 0.003 × PaO_2), it is clear that the PaO_2 contributes very little to the total amount of oxygen in the body. However, it is critically important, as it is this dissolved form of oxygen that is readily available to enter cells.

The PaO_2 can be accurately measured only from arterial blood. The site of arterial blood testing is important to consider in the newborn with a patent ductus arteriosus, especially in the setting of pulmonary hypertension in which preductal blood will have a higher PaO_2 than postductal blood. Blood drawn from the right radial or ulnar artery is preductal, whereas blood drawn from the posterior tibial artery or from an umbilical artery catheter is postductal. While the origin of the left subclavian artery is more likely to be preductal than postductal in location, the clinician cannot be certain about its location unless he or she obtains an echocardiogram.[122] Therefore, it is not recommended to use blood drawn from the left radial or ulnar artery if possible.

Hypoxia is a qualitative term that refers to inadequate tissue oxygenation. It should not be confused with hypoxemia, which refers to a below "normal" PaO_2 in the blood. The definitions of normoxemia, hypoxemia, and hyperoxemia will depend on what is considered "normal" for PaO_2. Rather than selecting a number as representative of hypoxemia, the clinician should evaluate the presence of lactic acid, base deficit, and other clinical signs to determine if the patient is truly metabolizing anaerobically.

Changing therapy in response to hypoxemia requires careful evaluation of the patient, as there are a wide variety of causes for hypoxemia and several organ systems that may be involved. For example, simply increasing the oxygen concentration for a hypoxemic patient who has inadequately inflated or overinflated lungs and a ventilation–perfusion mismatch is not the optimal approach. It is vital to direct therapy toward correcting the underlying cause before simply adjusting the oxygen concentration.

COMPONENTS OF BLOOD GAS TESTING THAT ARE NOT MEASURED DIRECTLY

The following values commonly reported on blood gas results are derived from other measured values or calculated using nomograms or algorithms.

HCO_3^-

Bicarbonate is a base, meaning that it is an acceptor of hydrogen ($HCO_3^- + H^+ \leftrightarrow H_2O + CO_2$). It is therefore "consumed" when neutralizing acids, resulting in a lower bicarbonate serum concentration in the setting of a metabolic acidosis. A chronic increase in $PaCO_2$ will eventually lead to an increased HCO_3^- as the body attempts to maintain a 20:1 ratio of bicarbonate to dissolved CO_2. The kidneys play an important role in acid–base homeostasis through reabsorption of HCO_3^-, urinary excretion of ammonium, and titratable acid formation. Similarly, giving a patient sodium bicarbonate can transiently elevate the $PaCO_2$ levels until the lungs can correct them. Sodium bicarbonate was once commonly administered for the treatment of lactic acidosis.[123] However, this practice has more recently been called into serious question and probably should be abandoned.[21] The search for the underlying cause and its correction should instead be the focus. The normal concentration of bicarbonate in blood is 22 to 24 mEq/L.

The HCO_3^- concentration reported on a blood gas result is not directly measured but rather calculated from the pH and $PaCO_2$. It reflects the inferred metabolic status of the acid–base balance. Various methods have been reported over the years to calculate the HCO_3^- level in a blood gas sample given a certain level of pH and $PaCO_2$. Standard bicarbonate is calculated with blood equilibrated to a $PaCO_2$ of 40 mm Hg at 37° C. Calculated HCO_3^- values may not reflect a pure metabolic index during hypo and hypercapnea and the clinicians should learn which method their own institution uses to calculate HCO_3^- values. We encourage the reader to explore publications that describe in greater detail the relationship between $PaCO_2$ and HCO_3^-.[110]

Base Excess

Base excess (BE) refers to the difference between the observed and the normal buffer base concentration or, expressed differently, the amount of acid or base required to return the pH to 7.4 in the setting of a normal $PaCO_2$.[124] The BE is commonly derived from nomograms. Because different models of blood gas analyzers use different methods of calculating the BE, the results may differ among manufacturers.[125]

Although the name implies an excess of base, a deficit can occur when the observed base concentration is below normal. Some clinicians prefer to use the term *base deficit* to refer to levels of base that are below normal and to use the term *BE* for the opposite scenario. Base excess/deficit is another indicator of the metabolic acid–base status. Some centers may measure standard BE or BE of extracellular fluid. The standard BE is calculated differently from BE and was developed as a $PaCO_2$-independent index.[110]

Normal BE values in newborns range from −3 to +1.[126] A negative BE, or a base deficit, is observed in the setting of a metabolic acidosis, whereas a positive BE occurs in metabolic alkalosis. The BE is interpreted along with the bicarbonate concentration.

Oxygen Saturation

A broader discussion of oxygen saturation is provided earlier in this chapter. The arterial oxygen saturation (SaO_2) reported by a standard blood gas machine is a calculated value. Because the calculation does not consider nonstandard hemoglobin species (e.g., carboxyhemoglobin, methemoglobin), it may provide an inaccurate estimate.

Blood gas machines that utilize co-oximetry measure multiple hemoglobin species directly and therefore provide a more accurate SaO_2. Co-oximetry directly measures the following types of hemoglobin:
1. Oxyhemoglobin—hemoglobin that is bound to oxygen
2. Deoxyhemoglobin—hemoglobin that is not bound to oxygen
3. Carboxyhemoglobin–hemoglobin that is bound to carbon monoxide
4. Methemoglobin—an oxidized form of hemoglobin
5. Sulfhemoglobin—an abnormal form of hemoglobin that cannot bind oxygen

Lactate

Lactate is not a traditional blood gas value. However lactate is routinely measured by many blood gas analyzers, so a brief basic discussion of its value is warranted. Analyzers equipped to measure lactate will directly measure the blood with a biosensor utilizing amperometric principles.[106] Lactate is the result of the metabolism of glucose during tissue hypoxia whereby lactate, ATP, and water are produced.[127] Tissue hypoxia and poor tissue perfusion can lead to hyperlactatemia, which can also result from other mechanisms.[128] Blood lactate levels are a reflection of the difference between production and elimination, with the liver being responsible for the majority of lactate clearance.[128] Normal blood lactate levels for the term infant depend on local established values and have been reported at <2.0 mmol/L.[129] Arterial, venous, and capillary values for lactate levels have been used clinically, with most reporting good correlation between the sample types.[127,130] Samples should be run within 15 minutes to prevent lactate levels from increasing prior to testing.[127] Lactate values have a useful role in the assessment of the newborn. Lactate measured in umbilical cord blood was shown to agree with pH and BE and has similar predictive value for short-term morbidities compared to pH and BE.[131] A retrospective study of term infants with intrapartum asphyxia comparing the predictive value of pH, base deficit, and lactate for the incidence of moderate to severe hypoxic encephalopathy (HIE) showed that the highest lactate levels in the first hours of life are important predictors of moderate to severe HIE.[127] Measurement of serum lactate is very helpful in differentiating increased acid production (e.g., due to inadequate tissue oxygen delivery) from loss of bicarbonate, such as occurs in renal tubular acidosis.

ERRORS IN BLOOD GAS MEASUREMENTS

Even small air bubbles in a blood gas sample can cause significant errors. The air bubbles contain room air, which has four main components: nitrogen (78%), oxygen (21%), argon (1%), and carbon dioxide (0.04%). Room air has a $PaCO_2$ that is nearly zero and a PaO_2 of approximately 150 mm Hg. If air bubbles contaminate a blood gas sample, they lower the $PaCO_2$ and can either raise or lower the PaO_2, depending on whether the PaO_2 is below or above 150 mm Hg.[132] The amount of air that comes in contact with arterial blood drawn through a butterfly (scalp vein) infusion set is enough to alter the PaO_2 measurement.[133] Therefore it is very important to expel air bubbles from the blood sample before placing it in the blood gas analyzer.

Dilution of a blood sample with intravenous fluids will typically lower the $PaCO_2$ and increase the base deficit without affecting the pH. This is probably due to the diffusion of CO_2 from blood into the intravenous fluid, which contains no CO_2.[132,134,135] Because of the buffering capacity of the blood, the pH changes little, despite the decrease in $PaCO_2$, giving the appearance of a combined metabolic acidosis and respiratory alkalosis. Dilution of a blood gas sample with a lipid emulsion does not appear to have any effect on the blood gas measurements.[136] Dry heparin also does not affect blood gas results.[134]

Blood gas results may be inaccurate if the specimen is not processed promptly, as the cells continue to consume oxygen and produce carbon dioxide after sampling. Therefore, samples are often placed on ice to slow down the metabolism of the cells in the sample. However, a bench study found that samples were stable for PaO_2 and SaO_2 for up to 30 minutes either at room temperature or when kept in iced water, and that changes after 60 minutes were small and unlikely to be clinically significant.[137] $PaCO_2$ showed a statistically significant increase after 20 minutes at room temperature, but the changes were not clinically significant.[137]

Most blood gas analyzers measure PaO_2 and then calculate the saturation with the assumption that the blood sample is from an adult. However, if the sample contains a significant amount of fetal hemoglobin, the calculated saturation will be inappropriately low (because of the leftward shift of the hemoglobin dissociation curve with fetal hemoglobin). If it is important to exactly measure the patient's saturation, this should be done with a co-oximeter rather than with a standard blood gas analyzer.

ASSESSING THE ACCURACY OF A BLOOD GAS RESULT

Determining if a blood gas result is valid requires critical thinking on the part of the clinician. There are several potential errors that can adversely affect the accuracy of blood gas results. Broadly, the timing of these errors can be divided into preanalytical and analytical phases.

Preanalytical errors refer to errors that occur during the period of time before testing the sample in the blood gas analyzer. They include errors in sample collection and handling. The discussion below focuses on preanalytical errors as these are the errors that the clinician is most likely to encounter.

A note on temperature: Modern blood gas analyzers correct samples to 37°C. While this is standard in modern NICUs, there are situations in which the clinician may wish to test a non-temperature-corrected sample. For example, infants with hypoxic–ischemic encephalopathy are treated with therapeutic hypothermia for a period of 72 hours. The target core body temperature is usually in the range of 33.5 to 34.5°C. Should we correct this sample to 37°C? Doing so may not reflect the true acid–base status of the patient as it will change the reported PaO_2 ($\approx$15 mm Hg higher) and $PaCO_2$ ($\approx$6 mm Hg lower).[138,139] There is confusion regarding the best approach to temperature correction in these situations. Many clinicians in adult intensive care units do not correct blood gases to 37°C for this reason. The

evidence in the pediatric population is less clear, leading some centers to advocate providing both temperature-corrected and non-temperature-corrected blood gas results for patients with body temperatures significantly outside the normal range.[139,140]

Clinicians are encouraged to critically evaluate blood gas results to determine their level of confidence in their accuracy. There are several accepted approaches. Below is a brief discussion of a few of these approaches:

1. Review the relationship between pH and acute changes in $PaCO_2$. Assuming a normal and constant metabolic rate, an acute increase in $PaCO_2$ of 1 mm Hg causes a corresponding decrease in pH of 0.006, whereas an acute decrease in $PaCO_2$ of 1 mm Hg leads to a 0.01 increase in pH. Understanding this relationship allows the clinician to compare the expected and measured pH. For example, following an acute increase in $PaCO_2$ of 15 mm Hg, the pH should decrease by 0.09 ($15 \times 0.006 = 0.09$), leading to an expected pH of 7.31 ($7.40 - 0.09 = 7.31$). If the measured pH differs from the expected pH by ± 0.03 units, a nonrespiratory or metabolic disorder must be present.
   a. In hypocarbia, expected pH
      $= 7.40 + (40 \text{ mm Hg} - PaCO_2) \, 0.01$
   b. In hypercarbia, expected pH
      $= 7.40 - (PaCO_2 - 40 \text{ mm Hg}) \, 0.006$
   This independent accuracy check aids the clinician in assessing the patient's metabolic condition without the need to refer to the HCO_3^- or BE values.[19]
2. Utilize formulas, nomograms, or a blood gas map to calculate or plot the acid–base variables.[19]
3. Compare the calculated plasma bicarbonate to total CO_2.
   a. Total CO_2 is a measure of CO_2 in all states, is measured with venous blood during lab electrolyte testing, and is an indicator of plasma bicarbonate.
   b. The total CO_2 value will be slightly higher than plasma bicarbonate because of the venous blood; however, it can be another check for blood gas accuracy.

Regardless of the methods used, it is critical to consider the patient's clinical status when interpreting the blood gas result.

FINAL THOUGHTS

Although arterial blood gas values are frequently invaluable in managing patients with respiratory distress, they should not be interpreted in the absence of other clinical data. A blood gas result that is significantly different from previous results may indicate a major change in the patient's status or may represent an error in blood gas measurement. Neither a blood gas laboratory nor sophisticated noninvasive monitors can replace careful clinical observation.

There are several useful online and mobile-friendly tools for interpreting blood gases.

See Appendix 19 for a few apps related to blood gas evaluations in the newborn developed by a neonatologist from India, Dr. Satish Deopujari.

ACKNOWLEDGEMENT:

The authors acknowledge the contributions of Drs David Durand and Nick Mickas, previous authors of this chapter.

REFERENCES

A complete reference list is available at https://expertconsult.inkling.com/.

11

Noninvasive Monitoring of Gas Exchange

Bobby Mathew, MD, and Satyan Lakshminrusimha, MBBS, MD

Gas exchange is a dynamic process that is dependent on complex interactions between the respiratory, cardiovascular, and central nervous systems. In a healthy individual breathing room air, the arterial blood levels of oxygen and carbon dioxide are maintained within a narrow normal range. In neonates receiving assisted ventilation or supplemental oxygen or suffering from impaired respiratory control, gas exchange may be compromised and close monitoring of blood gases becomes imperative to maintain homeostasis. Analysis of an arterial blood gas (ABG) sample is the gold standard for assessment of gas exchange. However, inherent risks associated with arterial access such as vasospasm, thrombosis, ischemia, and blood loss with resulting anemia necessitate alternate noninvasive methods to assess gas exchange. Blood gas analysis provides only a snapshot of a very dynamic process and results are frequently delayed (unless performed using a point-of-care device). The deleterious effects of hypoxia, hyperoxia, hypocarbia, and hypercarbia on morbidity, mortality, and neurodevelopmental outcomes have been well documented, and the importance of close frequent monitoring of these parameters cannot be overemphasized. This chapter briefly describes the techniques, indications, strengths, and limitations of the common noninvasive modalities used to monitor gas exchange (Fig. 11-1) in the neonatal intensive care unit (NICU). These monitors provide a large amount of data that, with careful interpretation, can guide therapeutic strategy and achieve the best possible outcome.[1]

NONINVASIVE MONITORING OF OXYGENATION

Pulse Oximetry

Oxygen has been widely used in the NICU since the mid-twentieth century. The misadventures with oxygen therapy and retinopathy of prematurity are well documented in the neonatal literature. There is controversy surrounding the target saturations during intensive care of preterm infants despite multiple large randomized controlled trials.[2-6] In the premature infant, the amount and type of hemoglobin and the percentage of arterial oxygen saturation of hemoglobin (SaO_2) are the major determinants of tissue oxygen delivery (Fig. 11-2). Clinically cyanosis is detectable by visual observation only when deoxyhemoglobin (DeoxyHb) is above 5 g/dL and is an unreliable assessment of oxygenation.[7] Hence continuous monitoring of saturation by pulse oximetry (SpO_2) is crucial to provide optimal care.

Pulse oximetry measures the percentage of hemoglobin saturated with oxygen. It provides a transcutaneous, noninvasive estimate of SaO_2 and displays a plethysmographic waveform with a heart rate. The monitoring of hemoglobin saturation is possible by pulse oximetry because of the transparency of tissue to light in the near-infrared spectrum and the distinct absorption spectra of the chromophores such as oxyhemoglobin (HbO_2) and DeoxyHb (Fig. 11-3). Pulse oximetry is based on the Beer-Lambert law, which states that absorption of light of a given wavelength is proportional to the concentration of the light-absorbing substance (chromophore) and the light path length.[8,9] Pulse oximetry is based on two principles: (1) spectrophotometry—HbO_2 and reduced DeoxyHb have different absorption spectra at different wavelengths of light (red and near infrared)—and (2) photoplethysmography—the amount of light absorbed by blood in the tissue changes with the arterial pulse (see Fig. 11-3). The pulse oximeter probe consists of two light-emitting diodes and a photodetector that are positioned facing each other with the light passing intermittently at very high frequency through the interposed tissue. Saturation is estimated from the relative absorption of the two wavelengths during pulsatile flow (due to arterial blood—referred to as AC by convention) versus nonpulsatile flow (venous and tissue absorption—referred to as DC):

$$SpO_2 = f(AC_{red}/DC_{red})/(AC_{infrared}/DC_{infrared}),$$

where f is the calibration constant.

The calibration algorithm for pulse oximetry is generated by subjecting healthy volunteers to varying inspired oxygen concentrations and correlating the arterial gas SaO_2 with the ratio of absorption (shown in the formula above) over a range of saturation values.[10] As it is unethical to expose healthy volunteers to hazardously low saturations, readings below 75% are based on data extrapolated from calibration values obtained between 100% and 75%. Values obtained by pulse oximetry are within ±2% to 3% of the true SaO_2 value between 70% and 100%. Recently, "Blue" sensors (Masimo, Irvine, CA) calibrated for the 60% to 80% range are being used in neonates with cyanotic congenital heart disease (CHD) (http://www.masimo.com/sensors/specialty.htm). Harris et al reported that these sensors have better accuracy in the 75-85% SpO_2 range with 86% of the samples demonstrating <5% difference compared to co-oximetry (compared to only 69% of samples with <5% difference from co-oximetry values from standard pulse oximetry sensors). However, there was a further increase in differences for SaO_2 values <75% and neonates <3 kg were not tested.[11]

Although pulse oximetry is now the standard of care in the NICU, there are no clearly established normal values in neonates. Pulse oximetry studies in normal healthy term infants and preterm infants breathing room air have shown average saturations to be 97% and 95%, respectively.[12,13] However, defining a target range of SpO_2 in preterm infants on oxygen therapy or mechanical respiratory support as well as in term infants with persistent pulmonary hypertension of the newborn (PPHN) remains a topic of controversy.[14,15]

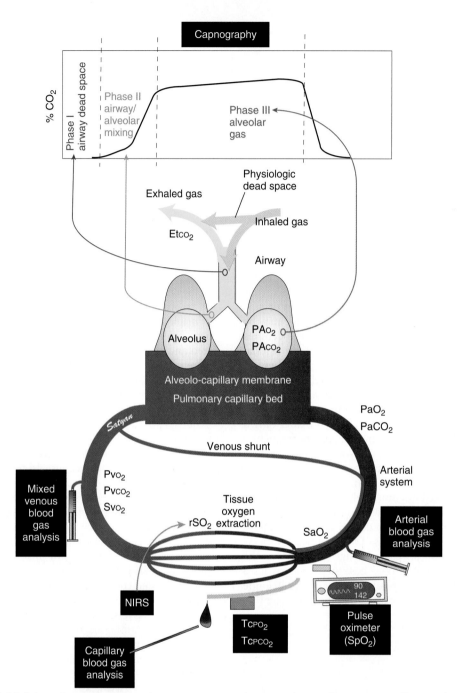

FIG 11-1 Invasive and noninvasive assessment of gas exchange in neonates. Gas exchange in the lung occurs at the alveolocapillary membrane. Oxygen and CO_2 diffuse from and to the alveolus. The alveolar tension of CO_2 and O_2 ($PAco_2$ and PAo_2) is in equilibration with pulmonary blood. During exhalation, the initial part of exhaled gas (phase I) is predominantly from the airway and has minimal CO_2. During phase II, a mixture of airway and alveolar gas is exhaled, resulting in an increase in CO_2. During phase III, alveolar gas is exhaled and the end-tidal CO_2 ($Etco_2$) evaluated by capnography. The physiologic dead space "dilutes" exhaled gas, and increased dead space increases the difference between $PAco_2$ and $Etco_2$. Arterial blood gas analysis is the gold standard invasive assessment of gas exchange and measures partial pressure of arterial oxygen, CO_2, and arterial oxygen saturation (PaO_2, $PaCO_2$, and SaO_2). Increasing venous shunt (because of pulmonary hypertension, congenital heart disease, or ventilation–perfusion mismatch) can decrease PaO_2. A pulse oximeter measures oxygen saturation (SpO_2) and is a reliable estimate of SaO_2. Transcutaneous sensors heat the cutaneous capillary bed and measure CO_2 and O_2 tension ($TcPco_2$ and $TcPo_2$). A capillary blood sample obtained after warming the heel ("arterialized" sample) is commonly used in neonates. Near-infrared spectroscopy (*NIRS*) can measure tissue (regional) oxygen saturation (rSO_2). Mixed venous blood gas analysis provides partial pressure of CO_2 and O_2 and oxygen saturation ($Pvco_2$, Pvo_2, and Svo_2).

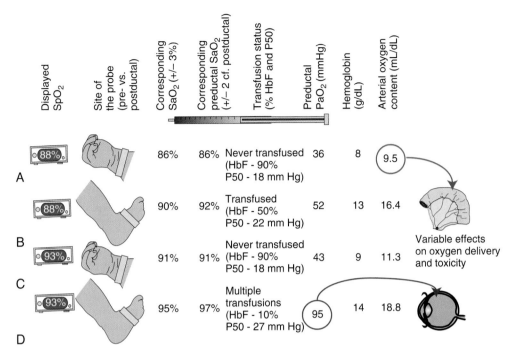

FIG 11-2 Variables that influence oxygen delivery (based on arterial oxygen content) and oxygen toxicity (based on PaO_2). The variation in arterial oxygen content compared to pulse oximetry based on factors such as site of probe placement, hemoglobin type, and content is illustrated. Each row represents an infant with a specific combination of variables. The oxygen content can vary twofold with a 5% difference in displayed oxygen saturation (SpO_2) on the pulse oximeter, and an infant with a lower SpO_2 (88%) can actually have a higher oxygen content than one with a higher SpO_2 (93%). Infant A has a preductal SpO_2 of 88%, which can correspond to an arterial oxygen saturation (SaO_2) of 85% to 91% in approximately two-thirds of subjects (±3% variation with pulse oximeters). If the corresponding preductal SaO_2 is assumed to be 86% and she has never received a transfusion, her hemoglobin F (HbF) concentration is ~90%. The corresponding preductal PaO_2 is 36 mm Hg. If this infant has a hemoglobin (Hb) concentration of 8 g/dL, her arterial oxygen content will be approximately 9.5 mL/dL. Infant B has a postductal SpO_2 of 88%, which can correspond to an SaO_2 of 85% to 91% in approximately two-thirds of subjects. If postductal SaO_2 is assumed to be 90%, the corresponding preductal SaO_2 may be 92%. If this baby has received two transfusions, her HbF concentration is approximately 50% and the corresponding preductal PaO_2 is 52 mm Hg. If this infant's Hb concentration is 13 g/dL, her arterial oxygen content will be approximately 16.4 mL/dL. Infant C, who has never been transfused with blood and has a preductal SpO_2 of 93% and a PaO_2 of 43 mm Hg, is at significantly reduced risk of oxygen toxicity compared with infant B despite a higher displayed SpO_2. Infant D has the same displayed SpO_2 as infant C (93%). However, his pulse oximeter is located on his left foot (postductal), and he has received blood transfusions. His PaO_2 is considerably higher (95 mm Hg) compared with infant C (43 mm Hg), placing him at risk for oxygen toxicity. A higher Hb concentration results in higher arterial oxygen content.

Indications for Pulse Oximetry

In the NICU, pulse oximetry has become the standard of care and is considered the fifth vital sign. Estimation of SpO_2 by continuous pulse oximetry is used to (1) titrate inspired oxygen concentration in infants receiving supplemental oxygen, (2) define bronchopulmonary dysplasia (BPD) with the oxygen-reduction test,[16] (3) monitor stable growing premature infants for bradycardia and desaturation spells, (4) titrate supplemental oxygen therapy during delivery room resuscitation and stabilization, (5) screen for critical CHD in the newborn period,[17,18] (6) monitor an infant's status during transport, (7) diagnose PPHN with ductal shunt by dual-pulse oximetry (postductal lower limb SpO_2 >5% to 10% lower than right upper limb value), and (8) perform car seat testing prior to discharge of at-risk infants.

Delivery Room Resuscitation

With the recognition of the dangers of oxidative stress associated with hyperoxia in the immediate newborn period, the use of oxygen blenders and pulse oximetry has been recommended for resuscitation and stabilization of newborn infants in the delivery room.[19] Pulse oximetry assists in monitoring response to resuscitation (improvement in heart rate) and titration of supplemental oxygen therapy. The Neonatal Resuscitation Program (NRP) 2016 guidelines define target saturations based on time after birth to guide optimal use of oxygen in the delivery room.[20-23] The use of pulse oximetry in the delivery room presents unique challenges. Delay in obtaining a stable tracing and readout of SpO_2 and heart rate is common. The average time to detect reliable signal on pulse oximetry has been estimated to be between 1 and 2 minutes.[21,24,25] Using the correct order of

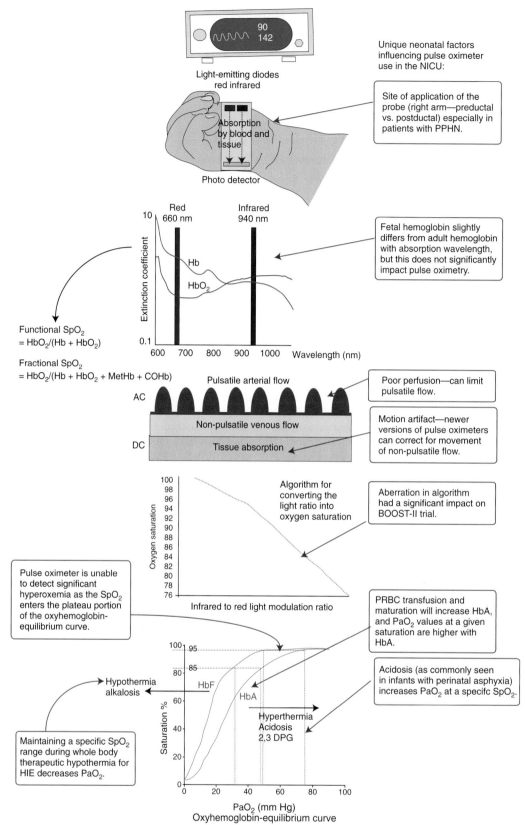

FIG 11-3 Infographic showing the basic principles of pulse oximetry and its limitations in neonates. The pulse oximeter probe has diodes that emit light in the red and infrared spectra. After absorption of this light by pulsatile arterial blood, venous blood, and tissue, it is detected by photodetectors in the pulse oximeter probe. The extinction coefficients for deoxyhemoglobin (*Hb*) and oxyhemoglobin (*HbO₂*) are different at red and infrared spectra. The infrared-to-red light modulation ratio is converted to an SpO_2 number using an algorithm. The SpO_2 is usually within ±3% of the SaO_2. The relationship between PaO_2 and SaO_2 is the oxyhemoglobin-equilibrium curve. Limitations of pulse oximetry are shown in red boxes. *COHb*, carboxyhemoglobin; *2,3 DPG*, diphosphoglycerate; *HbA*, adult hemoglobin; *HbF*, fetal hemoglobin; *HIE*, hypoxic–ischemic encephalopathy; *MetHb*, methemoglobin; *NICU*, neonatal intensive care unit; *PPHN*, persistent pulmonary hypertension of the newborn; *PRBC, packed red blood cells.*

connection minimizes time to obtaining a stable signal. (1) First, connect the oximeter cable to the pulse oximeter monitor; (2) turn on the pulse oximeter monitor; (3) apply the probe to the baby; and (4) connect the probe to the oximeter cable. The average difference in time with this optimized sequence has been shown to be 7 seconds as compared to connecting the sensor to the cable first and then applying the sensor to the infant.[26a] However, a more recent study performed in the delivery room with infants >/= 28 weeks gestation questioned this approach and suggested that applying pulse oximetry sensor to the oximeter first and then to the infant resulted in an earlier detection of a reliable signal.[26b] Preductal pulse oximetry should be recorded from the right upper limb as there is a substantial pre/postductal SpO_2 difference in the immediate newborn period. The NRP guidelines for delivery room SpO_2 were created using preductal SpO_2. In addition, signal detection has been demonstrated to be faster with the pulse oximetry probe applied to the hand compared to the foot.[27] Movement, poor perfusion, difficulties with probe placement, and high ambient light can all interfere with obtaining a reliable pulse oximetry signal.

Limitations of Pulse Oximetry

1. Hyperoxia, hypoxia, and hypercarbia: Owing to the sigmoid shape of the oxyhemoglobin equilibration curve (see Fig. 11-3), pulse oximetry is unable to detect significant hyperoxia and is slow to detect acute hypoxemia. In infants receiving supplemental oxygen even large changes in PaO_2 result in little change in SpO_2 if the saturation is close to 100%. Alveolar hypoventilation may also be missed in infants on supplemental oxygen monitored solely with pulse oximetry and can lead to significant hypercarbia without an appreciable change in SpO_2. Hence patients on supplemental oxygen at risk of hyperoxia/hypoxia/hypercarbia should have intermittent PO_2 and PCO_2 measured by blood gases. Anemia (unless very severe) and polycythemia do not affect pulse oximetry readings.[28]
2. Hypoperfusion and hypothermia: Pulse oximetry relies on normal pulsatile flow for its signal and hence can be falsely low in the setting of impaired perfusion or vasoconstriction associated with hypothermia, vasopressor treatment for hypotension, tourniquet effect from blood pressure cuff, etc.[29] When applying the sensor circumferentially to the finger, hand, or foot, it should not be applied too tightly.[30]
3. Movement artifact: Conventional pulse oximetry is based on pulsatile flow of blood and calculates SpO_2 based on the assumption that arterial blood is the only component that moves at the site of measurement. During periods of body movement the blood in the venous and tissue compartment also moves and interferes with the SpO_2 reading or causes a signal dropout. This can disrupt monitoring during transport or during periods of spontaneous activity. Newer pulse oximeters with signal extraction technology use adaptive filtering to separate the components of data and filter noise from the signal to limit motion artifact.[31,32]

Functional vs Fractional Saturation

Functional saturation refers to the percentage of hemoglobin that is saturated with oxygen in relation to the amount of hemoglobin that is capable of transporting oxygen—that is, HbO_2/(HbO_2 + DeoxyHb). In contrast, fractional saturation is the percentage of oxygenated hemoglobin to the total hemoglobin, which includes variant hemoglobin molecules such as methemoglobin (MetHb) and carboxyhemoglobin (COHb) that are incapable of binding oxygen. Conventional oximeters display functional

saturation and do not distinguish the variant hemoglobins from HbO_2 and provide saturation readings that are higher than the fractional saturation in patients with dyshemoglobinemias. High levels of COHb cause an increase in the SpO_2 approximately equal to the amount of COHb that is present.[33] The presence of MetHb will bias the functional SpO_2 reading towards 85%, which will result in over- or underestimation of saturation for %HbO_2 values below and above 85% respectively. In normoxic subjects, high levels of MetHb decrease the SpO_2 reading by about half of the MetHb percentage concentration.[34] New-generation oximeters are capable of detecting COHb and MetHb by using additional wavelengths of light and provide saturation readings that are more accurate in the clinical setting. When oxygen saturation determination by co-oximetry on a blood gas sample is discrepant by 5% or greater than the saturation measured by pulse oximetry, the presence of a variant hemoglobin has to be considered.

Additional Considerations

Fetal hemoglobin has light absorption characteristics similar to those of adult hemoglobin and does not affect pulse oximetry readings.[35] However, one has to keep in mind its effect on the oxygen dissociation curve and tissue oxygenation at the displayed SpO_2 values (see Fig. 11-3). Indirect bilirubin has a different light absorption spectrum at 450 nm and typically will not affect SpO_2 readings.[36,37] However, interference from ambient light with phototherapy and elevated COHb with hemolysis can alter SpO_2 in neonates. Discoloration from bronze-baby syndrome (due to phototherapy in the presence of direct hyperbilirubinemia) has also been reported to interfere with pulse oximetry readings.[38]

Various indices have been derived from the data provided by oximetry and are of potential use in interpreting clinical status and guiding clinical care. These include the following:

The **oxygen saturation index (OSI)**: The oxygenation index (OI = $FiO_2 \times 100 \times$ mean airway pressure [MAP in cm H_2O] $\div PaO_2$ [in mm Hg]) has been used to monitor the severity of hypoxemic respiratory failure (HRF) and response to treatment. Because the calculation of OI requires PaO_2 obtained by an ABG, OSI has been suggested as an alternative. Rawat et al. have shown that in newborn infants with HRF, the OSI ($FiO_2 \times 100 \times$ MAP $\div$ preductal SpO_2) correlated closely with the OI.[39] The relationship of OSI with OI in the saturation range of 70% to 99% is OI = $2 \times$ OSI. The use of OSI will allow continuous assessment of the severity of HRF.

The **perfusion index (PI)** is a measure derived from pulse oximetry[40] and compares the pulsatile to the nonpulsatile signal [(pulsatile signal (AC)/nonpulsatile signal (DC)) $\times 100$] and gives an indication of the perfusion at the monitored site[41] (Fig. 11-4). The value of PI as an indicator of a patient's circulatory status is being investigated for identification of CHD (left obstructive heart disease is not typically identified on routine pulse oximetry screening for critical congenital heart disease [CCHD]), subclinical chorioamnionitis, severity of illness, and intravascular volume status.[41] The value can range from 0.02% (very weak pulse strength) to 20% (very strong pulse strength) and is influenced by stroke volume, vasoactive drugs, temperature, and vasoconstriction at the site of probe placement.[40]

The **plethysmographic variability index (PVI)** is also derived from pulse oximetry. The arterial pulse volume changes during phases of the respiratory cycle, and this is more pronounced when the preload is inadequate (see Fig. 11-4). PVI measures the change in PI during a respiratory cycle and is expressed as a percentage as shown in the following equation: PVI = [($PI_{max} - PI_{min}$)/PI_{max}] $\times 100$%.[42] Early studies suggest that PVI may prove helpful

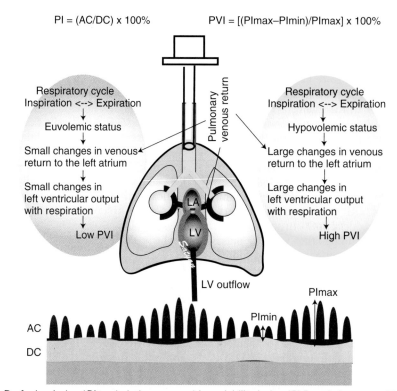

$$PI = (AC/DC) \times 100\%$$

$$PVI = [(PImax-PImin)/PImax] \times 100\%$$

FIG 11-4 Perfusion index (*PI*) and plethysmographic variability index (*PVI*) and changes with hypovolemia. Changes in intrathoracic pressure with respiration alter venous return to the left atrium (*LA*) and influence left ventricular (*LV*) preload and LV output and PI. These changes in LV output and PI with respiration (*PVI*) are more marked in the presence of hypovolemia and can predict response to a fluid bolus.

in assessing the hemodynamic significance of patent ductus arteriosus in preterm infants[43] and intravascular volume status in neonatal patients.[44] A high PVI in the presence of hypotension may be an indication for a fluid bolus to increase intravascular volume.[1] Cannesson et al. showed that a PVI of >14% before volume expansion identified response to a fluid load in adults with a sensitivity of 81% and specificity of 100%.[45] PVI can also predict fluid responsiveness in infants undergoing congenital heart surgery, with a threshold of 13% helping to discriminate between responders and nonresponders with a sensitivity of 84% and specificity of 64%.[46]

Transcutaneous Oxygen Monitoring

Transcutaneous oxygen ($TcPo_2$) is occasionally used in NICUs as an alternative to arterial PaO_2 measurements in infants without arterial access but in need of continuous monitoring of PaO_2. The sensor consists of a platinum cathode and a silver reference anode. The electrode is separated from the skin surface by a thin membrane through which the oxygen diffuses. The reduction of oxygen at the platinum sensor cathode generates a current that is processed to a PO_2 readout. Studies comparing PaO_2 with $TcPo_2$ in infants show good correlation.[47] However, sensors need frequent repositioning and recalibration with ABGs, and the need for higher operating temperature is associated with a risk of thermal burns in preterm infants. With oxygenation being routinely monitored by pulse oximetry, transcutaneous monitoring of oxygen is becoming less common.

NONINVASIVE ASSESSMENT OF PaCO₂

Arterial PCO_2 is a reflection of the interaction of CO_2 production in the body (metabolism), transport (systemic and pulmonary

perfusion), and elimination (ventilation). Capnography provides instantaneous breath-to-breath analysis of exhaled CO_2 and has become an integral part of monitoring in the operating room. $PaCO_2$ in normal healthy infants ranges between 35 and 45 mm Hg. Cerebral blood flow is dependent on the arterial $PaCO_2$[48] and increases with hypercarbia and decreases with hypocarbia. In mechanically ventilated extremely preterm infants fluctuations of $PaCO_2$ are common and predispose the infants to intraventricular hemorrhage, periventricular leukomalacia, and BPD.[49-51] Approaches to ventilation strategy (high frequency vs conventional) and adjustment of ventilator settings are frequently based on $PaCO_2$. Assessment of $PaCO_2$ with intermittent ABGs can lead to unrecognized periods of hypercarbia and hypocarbia and missed opportunities for ventilator weaning. The continuous noninvasive assessment of $PaCO_2$ may be achieved using end-tidal CO_2 ($Etco_2$) or transcutaneous CO_2 ($TcPco_2$).

Capnography and End-Tidal CO₂ Monitoring

Capnography, the measurement of $Etco_2$ levels in exhaled breath, is based on the principle that the CO_2 diffuses easily from the pulmonary capillary into the alveolus and rapidly equilibrates with alveolar CO_2 ($PAco_2$). The capnogram is a graphic display of the levels of CO_2 during a respiratory cycle. During inspiration, PCO_2 on the capnogram is zero as the atmospheric air contains very little CO_2. At the beginning of exhalation the gas from the anatomic dead space is expired first and has minimal CO_2 (phase I, see Fig. 11-1). In phase II, gas from the alveoli mixes with gas in the dead space, resulting in a sharp increase in the CO_2 concentration, and this reaches a peak and then plateaus as all of the expired gas is derived from the alveoli (phase III). The CO_2 level

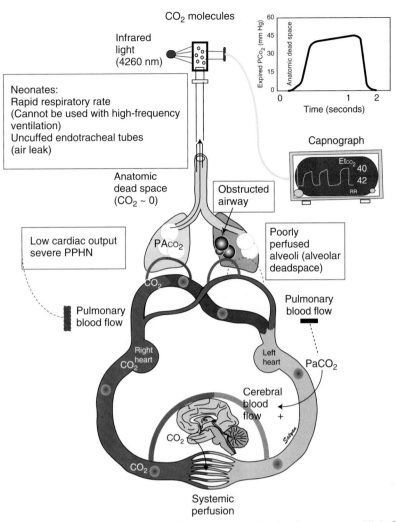

FIG 11-5 Uses and limitations of end-tidal CO_2 (Etco$_2$) monitoring in neonates. High CO_2 levels increase cerebral blood flow and decrease pulmonary blood flow. Increased dead space (anatomic and alveolar, often due to ventilation–perfusion mismatch as shown in the left lung) contributes to inaccuracy with Etco$_2$ monitoring. Limitations for Etco$_2$ monitoring are shown in red boxes. *PPHN*, persistent pulmonary hypertension of the newborn.

in the sampled gas is measured using infrared spectroscopy. CO_2 absorbs infrared light of a specific wavelength ($4.26\,\mu m$), and this is used to calculate the amount of CO_2 in the sample (Fig. 11-5).

Mainstream and Sidestream Capnography

Etco$_2$ monitors fall into two categories based on the position of the measurement device with respect to the infant's airway. In mainstream capnography, the sensor is in line with the ventilator circuit, and all of the inhaled and exhaled gas passes directly over the infrared bench. In the sidestream devices the sensor is located away from the airway, and the gas sample is continuously aspirated from the breathing circuit (via a microstream of ~50 mL/min) and delivered to the sensor for analysis. Mainstream sensors have the advantages of faster response time and reliable single-breath capnometry measurements and are less affected by high ventilator rates. The disadvantage of mainstream capnography is that it adds respiratory dead space and can cause rebreathing of exhaled CO_2. Sidestream devices add minimal dead space and can be used for long-term monitoring; however, their accuracy is less than that of mainstream devices. At low expiratory gas flow rates, dilution of the sampled gas

with the surrounding air can affect the accuracy of measurements. Sidestream measurements also tend to be less accurate in infants with high respiratory rates.

CO_2 Monitoring in the NICU

Studies on capnography in the NICU have focused largely on the correlation between Etco$_2$ and PaCO$_2$. Capnography can be used to monitor rate, rhythm, and effectiveness of respiration (spontaneous or assisted); evaluate pulmonary and systemic perfusion and metabolism; and guide ventilator management. Capnography is valuable in monitoring infants with hypoxic–ischemic encephalopathy (HIE), as hyperventilation secondary to metabolic acidosis in these patients can lead to hypocarbia and impaired cerebral blood flow. Infants with HIE receiving therapeutic hypothermia have decreased metabolism, which may be reflected as a decrease in Etco$_2$. A widening gap between PaCO$_2$ and Etco$_2$ in a patient with lung disease indicates a mismatch between ventilation and perfusion and increasing alveolar dead space. Etco$_2$ monitoring has been shown to be useful in cardiopulmonary resuscitation to guide the effectiveness of chest compressions and for detection of return of spontaneous circulation.[52-54]

Capnography during Neonatal Anesthesia

$Etco_2$ monitoring is the standard of care for monitoring infants in the operating room as it provides rapid and reliable (breath by breath) assessment of the adequacy of the airway in an intubated patient. Loss of the capnogram signal or a sudden fall in $Etco_2$ would indicate accidental extubation or plugging of the tracheal tube. Alternatively, a rapid rise in $Etco_2$ level may indicate inadequate ventilation as commonly occurs with decreased tidal volume during surgical procedures. Examples of this include abdominal surgery, in which pressure on the diaphragm decreases tidal excursion, accidental or procedural lung collapse and migration of tracheal tube associated with patient repositioning during surgery. Changes in $Etco_2$ are rapid and precede changes in SpO_2, and hence capnography is able to detect airway/ventilator compromise early and may avert hypoxia and related injury.

Colorimetric CO_2 Detectors

Colorimetric CO_2 detectors are the standard of care for ensuring correct placement of tracheal tubes. A colorimetric CO_2 detector uses a modified form of litmus paper in which metacresol purple changes color depending on pH. Carbon dioxide reacts with water to form carbonic acid vapor in exhaled breath. A graded change in color from purple to yellow occurs with increasing concentration of $Etco_2$. Lack of a color change (to yellow) after six respiratory cycles indicates esophageal intubation. False negatives (lack of color change with correct tracheal tube placement) may occur with (1) low cardiac output state even in the presence of severe hypercarbia or (2) impaired gas exchange in the presence of fetal lung fluid. False-positive colorimetric CO_2 may occur with accidental contamination of the sensor with gastric acid and resuscitation drugs such as epinephrine.[55] A mnemonic for confirmation of intubation using a colorimetric capnogram is Yellow—Yes and Purple—Problem.

$Etco_2$ in nonintubated patients can be assessed by sidestream capnography using a nasal cannula or mask. Studies by Lopez et al. and Tai et al. have shown good correlation and minimal bias between $PaCO_2$ and $Etco_2$ by sidestream capnography. However, in both studies, the $PaCO_2$–$Etco_2$ gap widened in the presence of lung disease and in infants with BPD,[56,57] suggesting that $Etco_2$ monitoring may be less reliable with the diseased lung.

Optimizing Ventilation Settings with Capnography

Volumetric capnography can assist in optimizing ventilator settings and weaning from mechanical ventilation. Hubble et al. have shown that in ventilated infants and children, capnogram-derived parameters of the ratio of physiologic dead space to tidal volume can reliably predict success of extubation.[58] Excessive positive end-expiratory pressure causes increase in the dead space and decreased pulmonary perfusion through increased intrathoracic pressure. This can be seen as a prolongation of phase I and a decline in the slope of phase II with a decrease in the volume of CO_2 eliminated through breaths per minute in the capnogram.[59]

Limitations of Capnography

Errors in estimation of $PaCO_2$ using $Etco_2$ may occur because of ventilation–perfusion mismatch, airway obstruction as with meconium aspiration syndrome, or severe parenchymal lung disease (see Fig. 11-5). In infants with PPHN, the decreased pulmonary blood flow causes $Etco_2$ to decrease despite elevated $PaCO_2$. Whereas impaired ventilation may elevate $Etco_2$, a coexisting perfusion problem is likely to decrease $Etco_2$. In infants with cyanotic CHD, decreased pulmonary blood flow and increased right-to-left shunting (e.g., during a spell in a patient with tetralogy of Fallot) cause an increase in $PaCO_2$. However, the right-to-left shunt causes a decrease in $PAco_2$ and the $Etco_2$–$PaCO_2$ gap is widened. Rapid respiratory rates and low tidal volumes compromise the ability of sampled gas to adequately reflect alveolar gas. As tachypnea and hypoventilation are common in premature infants, this is a major limitation to $Etco_2$ monitoring in neonatology. Gas mixing proximal to the uncuffed tracheal tube due to air leaks and malfunction of the sensor that often occurs with condensation of water from the respiratory tree can also contribute to poor correlation between $PaCO_2$ and $Etco_2$.

Transcutaneous CO_2 Monitoring

Severinghaus in 1960 first described the method for transcutaneous measurement of CO_2 in skin capillaries that are arterialized by application of heat.[60] The sensor unit consists of a glass pH electrode and a silver chloride reference electrode, a heating element, a temperature sensor, and an electrolyte reservoir (Fig. 11-6). The electrodes are separated from the surface of the skin by a membrane. When the sensor is attached to the skin, the generated heat causes local vasodilation and increases the permeability of the skin to CO_2. The CO_2 diffuses through the membrane and reacts with water to form carbonic acid, which dissociates to hydrogen and bicarbonate ions. The change in pH causes a potential difference between the electrodes. This change in pH is converted to a PCO_2 reading based on the linear relationship between pH and $\log PCO_2$. Johns et al. have shown a linear correlation of $TcPco_2$ with $PaCO_2$ in the range of 20 to 74 mm Hg.[61] It is important to recognize that the measured value is the gas tension in the cutaneous tissue. Under stable hemodynamic conditions these correlate closely with ABG values. As the electrodes operate at an elevated temperature, increased tissue metabolism at the site may increase the local CO_2 production. Hence the value is corrected to the body temperature. Calibration of a $TcPco_2$ monitor can be performed by gas calibration using mixtures of known CO_2 concentration or by using the patient's ABG sample. The in vivo calibration has been shown to align more closely with the $PaCO_2$ tension as it eliminates many of the patient-related factors that influence $TcPco_2$ measurements. The commercially available monitors have a measurement range of $TcPco_2$ between 0 and 200 mm Hg and accuracy within ±4.5 mm Hg. Following application of the sensor, it takes approximately 20 minutes for stabilization and to obtain a reliable measurement of the $TcPco_2$. Therefore transcutaneous monitoring is used more for following $TcPco_2$ over periods of time. In settings such as anesthesia or intubation in which a more rapid response time is needed, capnography and $Etco_2$ monitoring may be more appropriate.

A good correlation between $TcPco_2$ and $PaCO_2$ has been established in preterm and ill neonates.[62-64] However, a prospective study of infants of less than 28 weeks' gestation by Aliwalas et al. showed only moderate correlation.[65] This discrepancy may be due to differences in monitors, methodologies, and patient characteristics between studies. Both patient- and instrument-related factors can cause erroneous estimation of $TcPco_2$ levels. Improper placement, trapped air bubbles, membrane, and calibration errors can lead to inaccurate readings.

There are many commercially available monitors that combine electrodes for $TcPco_2$/$TcPo_2$ into a single sensor. Sensors with electrodes measuring PO_2 require a higher temperature at the site than PCO_2 sensors, and this may be a drawback of combined sensors, especially in preterm infants. Manufacturers recommend changing the position of the sensors every 4 to 12 hours, depending on the operating temperature of the

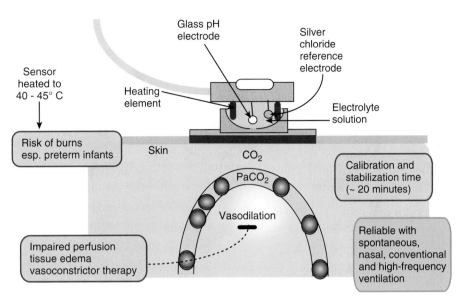

FIG 11-6 Transcutaneous CO_2 monitoring. The benefits are shown in the green box, and limitations are shown in the red boxes. See text for details.

TABLE 11-1 Comparison of End-Tidal and Transcutaneous Monitoring of CO_2	
Capnography/Etco$_2$	**Transcutaneous CO_2**
Measures CO_2 in expired gas	Measures CO_2 at the cutaneous capillaries
Does not need frequent calibration	Needs frequent calibration
Responds instantaneously to change in PAco$_2$	Slower response to change in PaCO$_2$
Reads instantaneously	Stabilization time of approximately 20 min prior to obtaining reading
Often lower than PaCO$_2$ (based on physiologic dead space)	Better correlation to PaCO$_2$
Unreliable in infants with lung disease, shunts, or ventilation–perfusion mismatch or with large leak around the tracheal tube	Unreliable in infants with impaired perfusion, acidosis, or edema or on vasoconstrictors
May increase dead space in extremely preterm infants	Risk of skin burns, need for changing sensor position to avoid thermal injury
Cannot be used with high-frequency ventilation	Can be used with any mode of ventilation: spontaneous, conventional, or high frequency
Limited use with spontaneous breathing	

electrode and the condition of the infant's skin. A comparison between transcutaneous and end-tidal CO_2 monitoring is shown in Table 11-1.

TISSUE OXYGEN SATURATION MONITORING USING NEAR-INFRARED SPECTROSCOPY

Near-infrared spectroscopy (NIRS) is an indirect assessment of tissue oxygen utilization. However, this technology is not currently widely used in clinical care of newborn infants. Limited published data on normal values based on the site of application, intervention thresholds and impact on long-term outcomes of monitored infants may explain the reluctance among practitioners towards adopting this technology. NIRS may be regarded at this time as an emerging technology and needs

further study before adoption into routine clinical practice. The cost of these probes and space required to apply them on the head and abdomen have limited their use among preterm infants. Oxygen delivery to the tissue is dependent on the hemoglobin content, oxygen saturation, and cardiac output. When oxygen demand exceeds the oxygen delivery, a state of oxygen debt is created, and energy is derived from the inefficient anaerobic metabolic pathway. The parameters currently in use for cardiovascular monitoring, such as blood pressure, capillary refill time, urine output, and lactate levels, lack sensitivity and specificity and are late indicators of hypoperfusion. As of this writing there is no reliable way of monitoring the oxygenation status of the tissue in newborns unless simultaneous arterial and mixed venous (such as umbilical venous) blood gases are evaluated (see Fig. 11-1).

Franz Jobosis in 1977 first described the use of near-infrared spectroscopy (NIRS) in the human brain. Much like pulse oximetry, NIRS is based on the modified Beer-Lambert law. Light of specific wavelengths is generated by light-emitting diodes and passed through the interposed tissue in an arclike configuration (Fig. 11-7). The depth of penetration of the transmitted light is proportional to the distance between the transmitting optode and the receiving optode. The reflected light is detected by the receiving optode and is measured and processed to estimate the amount of HbO_2 and DeoxyHb in the interposed tissue. NIRS oximetry measures a weighted average of arterial capillary and venous compartments, and a fixed ratio of venous-to-arterial blood volume is assumed, usually 70:30. There are different methodologies used by manufacturers of NIRS devices, but the most commonly used in commercially available devices is the spatially resolved spectroscopy. The following measurements are obtained through NIRS:

Tissue (regional) oxygen saturation $(rSO_2) = SaO_2 - VO_2/DO_2$,

where VO_2 is the oxygen consumption and DO_2 is the oxygen delivery

Arteriovenous oxygen saturation difference $= SpO_2 - rSO_2$

Fractional oxygen extraction $(fOE) = (SpO_2 - rSO_2)/SpO_2$

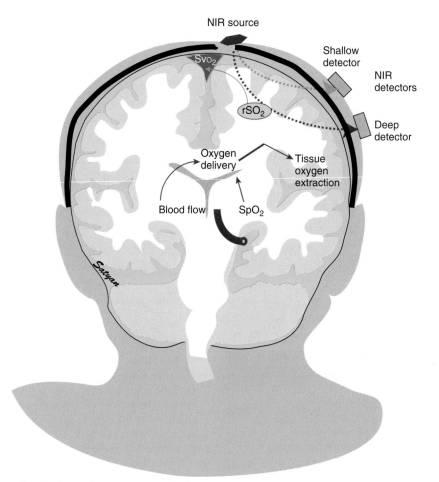

FIG 11-7 Cerebral monitoring with near-infrared (*NIR*) spectroscopy. The light-emitting optode is placed over the scalp. Two detectors, a shallow detector and a deep detector, are placed a short distance from the emitting optode. The regional oxygen saturation (*rSO₂*) depends on oxygen delivery and tissue oxygen extraction. Low oxygen delivery or high oxygen extraction can decrease the rSO₂.

NIRS can be considered the pulse oximetry equivalent for the circulatory system. It provides continuous noninvasive monitoring of the venous side of the vascular beds of various organs and provides information in real time of the balance between oxygen supply and demand. NIRS is very well suited to application in newborns and infants because of the decreased thickness of the scalp and skull and smaller amount of fat in the abdominal wall. NIRS has been applied mainly in assessing regional cerebral and splanchnic saturation in the neonatal population. There have been many studies that have demonstrated good correlation between cerebral oxygenation measured by NIRS and jugular venous oxygen saturation.[66] Cerebral oximetry has also been validated using correlation with levels of tissue adenosine triphosphate and phosphocreatine in the brain.[67] Studies of gastric tonometry (mucosal pH) have been shown to correlate with splanchnic/mesenteric rSO₂.[68]

Normal Values

In infants breathing room air the cerebral rSO₂ is around 60% to 70% and the splanchnic rSO₂ is about 80%. The rSO₂ also depends on the metabolic state of the tissue and is elevated in brain tissue following ischemic damage and during treatment with therapeutic hypothermia. It is decreased during increased metabolic activity, for example, during seizures, despite normal oxygen delivery.

The utility of tissue oximetry at this time is in monitoring trends with determination of a baseline for each individual patient and a percentage below this baseline chosen for intervention.

Application of Near-Infrared Spectroscopy in Newborns

The clinical utility of NIRS monitoring in infants and newborns has been studied mainly in cardiac surgery. In infants undergoing surgery for CHD, low cerebral oximetry during surgery and in the postoperative period has been associated with abnormalities on neuroimaging, seizures, prolonged length of stay, need for extracorporeal membrane oxygenation, and death.[69-71]

Management of Hypotension

In hypotensive newborns impaired cerebral autoregulation increases the risk of adverse neurodevelopmental outcomes. Autoregulation can be presumed to be intact when low blood pressure is not associated with a decrease in cerebral oxygenation by NIRS. NIRS can provide information on the oxygen supply and demand and guide the need for and choice of inotropes/vasopressors as well as the response to use of therapies.[72,73]

Patent Ductus Arteriosus

Impairment of cerebral blood flow and oxygenation due to diastolic runoff occurs in hemodynamically significant patent ductus arteriosus (PDA). Recent evidence suggests that changes in rSO_2 and fOE by NIRS in combination with echocardiography may be used to monitor the status of the ductus arteriosus and response to pharmacological treatment for PDA.[74a,74b]

Cerebral Perfusion with Changes in Mean Airway Pressure and Ventilation

Preterm infants who are mechanically ventilated for respiratory distress syndrome are at high risk for intraventricular hemorrhage. Increased intrathoracic pressure associated with high mean airway pressure may decrease preload and cardiac output and cause impairment of cerebral blood flow.[75] Changes in cerebral rSO_2 and fOE by NIRS can lead to early recognition and timely intervention to prevent related complications. Cerebral blood flow is very sensitive to changes in $PaCO_2$, and rapid fluctuations in $PaCO_2$ may occur especially in infants on high-frequency ventilation. NIRS, by providing real-time information on changes in cerebral oxygenation, can alert the clinician of the need for closer monitoring of $PaCO_2$ by ABG in these infants.

Mesenteric Ischemia and Risk of Necrotizing Enterocolitis

The cerebrosplanchnic oxygenation ratio (CSOR) is the ratio of splanchnic rSO_2 to cerebral rSO_2. Values less than 0.75 are indicative of splanchnic ischemia. Low CSOR values may identify infants at risk for necrotizing enterocolitis.[76,77] A body of literature on transfusion-associated necrotizing enterocolitis and mesenteric blood flow and oxygenation during transfusion of packed red blood cells and changes associated with feeding is emerging in neonatology.[78-80]

Limitations of Near-Infrared Spectroscopy

NIRS is still an emerging technology that requires further study before adoption into practice. There are no well-established normative values for rSO_2 or thresholds for intervention. Further, there is wide intra- and interpatient variability in rSO_2 values with a coefficient of variation for absolute baseline values of approximately 10%. The reading obtained is site specific and does not exclude abnormalities in other areas of the brain or other organ being monitored. To be able to obtain reliable readings, nursing and medical staff require training and experience in the correct placement and fixation of optodes and shielding from ambient light. The response to an abnormal reading should include, in addition to clinical assessment, evaluation of gas exchange, oxygen transport, hemodynamics, and regional perfusion.

CONCLUSION

Timely, reliable, easy-to-use, comprehensive, and accurate monitoring is absolutely essential for the management of a critically ill neonate. Significant progress has been made in neonatology largely through advances in respiratory care. Survival of extremely preterm infants has improved, but morbidity remains high among survivors. Innovations in microprocessor technology and miniaturization of devices have made it possible to apply technology developed for monitoring and treatment of adults to NICU patients. In the NICU, noninvasive monitoring can decrease, but does not completely replace, the need for invasive blood gas monitoring. Noninvasive monitoring of respiratory and cardiovascular interactions has been possible through pulse oximeters, capnographs, transcutaneous monitors, and NIRS. Modern respiratory monitors offer the capability to monitor and quantify changes in respiratory mechanics and carbon dioxide elimination continuously and noninvasively using volumetric capnography. As neonatal providers, we are challenged to apply these innovations by defining the normal for our patient population and formulating interventions to rectify the abnormal. The dynamic physiology of the neonate results in rapid changes.[81] Noninvasive monitors must be capable of detecting these changes instantly so that the neonatal provider may respond promptly. Advances in our ability to monitor noninvasively should lead to better patient care, less iatrogenic blood loss, improved patient safety, and decreased need for and duration of mechanical ventilation. The cost-effectiveness and impact of these advances on clinical outcomes require validation with rigorous controlled studies. Interpretation of data from continuous noninvasive monitoring can complement clinical observations, leading to rapid diagnosis and intervention to stabilize and improve the outcomes of critically ill neonates.

ACKNOWLEDGMENTS

We thank Drs. Corinne L. Leach and Sara Berkelhamer for their critical review of the chapter.

REFERENCES

A complete reference list us available at https://expertconsult.inkling.com/.

12

Pulmonary Function and Graphics*

Donald Morely Null Jr., MD, and Gautham K. Suresh, MD, DM, MS, FAAP

Understanding the physiology of the normal lung, the pathophysiology of the diseased lung, and how various forms of respiratory support affect lung physiology and function are key to achieving the goals of neonatal respiratory support—optimizing pulmonary gas exchange while minimizing lung injury. Modern conventional ventilators are always used along with monitors that display real-time breath-to-breath pulmonary function measurements at the bedside and also store the data, enabling a better assessment of the patient's overall pulmonary mechanics.[1] The accuracy of these measurements has improved dramatically so that one can assess pulmonary function even in extremely low birth-weight patients (Tables 12-1 and 12-2). Unfortunately this rich source of information is often ignored by clinicians when adjusting ventilator settings. This chapter discusses the use and limitations of pulmonary function assessment and specifically graphics in the management of ventilated neonates, so that clinicians may learn to use these bedside displays along with the results of other bedside monitoring devices, laboratory tests, and, most importantly, physical examination findings, in adjusting ventilator settings. Despite the wealth of electronic data now available at the bedside, appropriate "hands-on" evaluation is still the most important aspect of care, allowing clinicians to interpret and use these data wisely in decision making, particularly if the various data are conflicting: "If all else fails, try examining the patient."

Using this multimodal approach, clinicians can determine an individual infant's pathophysiology, select the appropriate ventilator mode and settings, and assess the infant's responses to changes in ventilator settings.

TECHNICAL ASPECTS

Bedside pulmonary function assessment and graphics as of this writing are available only with conventional ventilators employing flow sensors and not with high-frequency ventilation or with less invasive forms of support such as continuous positive airway pressure (CPAP), noninvasive positive pressure ventilation (NIPPV), high-flow nasal ventilation (HFNV), and bilevel positive airway pressure (BIPAP).

There are multiple flow measuring technologies that are effective for use in bedside pulmonary function assessment and graphics in term and preterm neonates.[2-4]

Pneumotachometers

These are resistive-type devices utilizing either a fine mesh screen or a group of small capillaries (Fleisch type). Gas flowing through a fixed resistance creates a pressure differential, which is measured with a differential pressure transducer. This is linear for a specific range of flow. Conventional pneumotachometers for flow measurement, when appropriately calibrated, have linear input and output characteristics. They generally have a dead space that is excessive for neonates, especially preterm neonates. One can use this device for single measurement pulmonary function tests but not for continuous monitoring.

Alternative Sensors

Alternatives to pneumotachometers include the following: (1) nonlinear flow resistive sensors, which measure a pressure difference produced by gas flowing through a tube but which are not linear; (2) flow sensors that use a piezoelectric film for detecting flow, in which vibration of the film results in an electrical output proportional to the flow; and (3) hot wire anemometers, which measure the electrical current needed to maintain a specific temperature in a heated wire placed across the airflow. The relationship is nonlinear and not inherently direction sensitive (but can be modified to sense direction).

These alternative devices all have the limitations of being nonlinear, nondirectional, or potentially both. Because of these characteristics, they are more difficult to calibrate. These devices have the advantages of being much smaller, having significantly less dead space, and being light enough to be placed in the ventilator circuit near the endotracheal tube (ETT). These features make them suitable for continuous monitoring and their accuracy is sufficient for clinical use. The sensors typically have a heated wire to negate the condensation of water, which will create inaccurate measurements. Volumes should be measured only near or at the ETT, as this avoids inaccurate patient tidal volumes due to circuit tubing distention.

Although these sensors are typically used in intubated patients, they can be used with a mask as well. The mask must fit snugly without a leak. Whereas most newborns breathe primarily through their nose, some mouth breathing does take place.[5] Because of this, the use of tight nasal prongs or a nasal mask may result in inaccurate measurements.

The requirement to maintain accuracy of measurements entails regular assessment of the flow sensor. Cleaning and calibration must be regularly accomplished, and one must recognize that temperature, humidity, and gas consumption may significantly affect the accuracy of the flow sensor.[6-8]

Signal Calibration

The sensors should be adequately calibrated and recalibrated periodically. Calibration should be performed under both static

---

* This chapter uses a number of figures and tables from the same chapter in the previous edition of the book, written by Drs. Bhutani and Benitz. The section on resistive properties is unaltered from the previous edition's chapter.

TABLE 12-1   Basic Respiratory Parameters Observed in Spontaneously Breathing Neonates in Several Weight Ranges

Weight Range (g) Percentiles	PEAK INSPIRATORY FLOW (L/MIN)			PEAK EXPIRATORY FLOW (L/MIN)			TIDAL VOLUME (ML/KG)			MINUTE VENTILATION (ML/MIN)		
	10th	50th	90th	10th	50th	90th	10th	50th	90th	10th	50th	90th
500-1000	0.8	1.3	2.1	0.5	0.9	1.6	3.2	5.4	8.3	230	400	600
1001-2500	1.3	2.3	3.5	1.0	1.8	3.0	3.4	5.7	8.1	250	400	600
2501-5000	1.8	3.2	5.2	1.6	2.9	4.8	2.4	4.7	7.2	170	300	500
5001-15,000	4.1	5.9	9.9	3.4	4.9	8.6	5.2	6.9	8.9	180	240	400

TABLE 12-2   Predicted Probability of Bronchopulmonary Dysplasia Based on Pulmonary Mechanics and Gestational Age Based on a Predictive Model for the Study Infants with Respiratory Distress Syndrome Categorized by Birth Weight*

Birth Weight (g)	Gestational Age (weeks)	Pulmonary Compliance (mL/cm H$_2$O/kg)	Pulmonary Resistance (cm H$_2$O/L/s)	Likelihood Ratio for BPD	Percentage Predicted Probability
500-750	26 ± 0.4	0.3 ± 0.03	102 ± 16	537 ± 171	93% ± 3%
751-1000	28 ± 0.3	0.5 ± 0.05	176 ± 24	76 ± 35	73% ± 5%
1001-1250	29 ± 0.3	1.0 ± 0.2	96 ± 1.1	5.5 ± 1.8	42% ± 7%
1251-1500	31 ± 0.3	1.5 ± 0.2	69 ± 8	0.8 ± 0.3	15% ± 5%
1501-2000	32 ± 0.3	1.8 ± 0.3	69 ± 11	0.3 ± 0.1	8% ± 3%

*Predicted probability and likelihood ratio (LR) of BPD evaluated on the previously reported predictive model based on gestational age (GA) and pulmonary mechanics: LR = exp(33.6 – 1.13 GA – 0.93 Cl/kg – 0.001 Rt), where Cl is compliance and Rt is resistance.
Data from Bhutani VK, Bowen FW, Sivieri E. Biol Neonate. 2005;87:323-331.

BPD, Bronchopulmonary dysplasia.

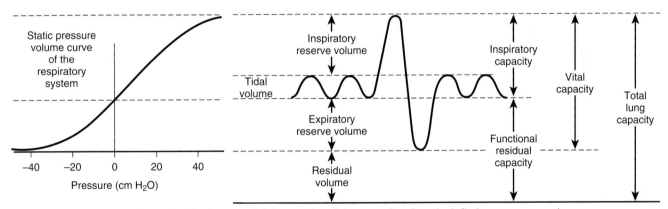

FIG 12-1 Traditional spirometry (*right panel*) and the associated static deflation pressure–volume relationship measured for a vital capacity maneuver (*left panel*).

and dynamic conditions. Typically this is accomplished by using the following appropriate devices: calibrated syringes, precise ball-in-tube flowmeters, water column manometers, and reference transducers. To maintain accuracy of measurements, the devices must be operated in their linear calibration range.

RESPIRATORY PHYSIOLOGY AND PATHOPHYSIOLOGY

A detailed description of respiratory physiology is provided in Chapter 2. Here, a brief recap of aspects relevant to bedside pulmonary monitoring is provided.

Figure 12-1 demonstrates typical spirometry findings. It shows the various measurements of tidal volume, inspiratory

and expiratory reserve, functional residual capacity (FRC), residual volume (RV), vital capacity, and total lung capacity.

Normal spontaneous respiration takes place by fixing the diaphragm and expanding the thorax with the respiratory muscles. This creates flow into the lung by decreasing the intrapulmonary pressure compared to the pressure at the mouth. Expiration occurs passively, driven by the elastic recoil of the lungs, which increases intrathoracic pressures to a level greater than the pressure at the mouth (Fig. 12-2). The inspiratory driving pressure, either by the ventilator or by the respiratory muscles, must be great enough to overcome the elastic, resistive, and inertial properties of the respiratory system.

Rohrer[9] described this relationship with the equation $P = P_e + P_r + P_i$, where P_e is the elastic, P_r the resistive, and P_i

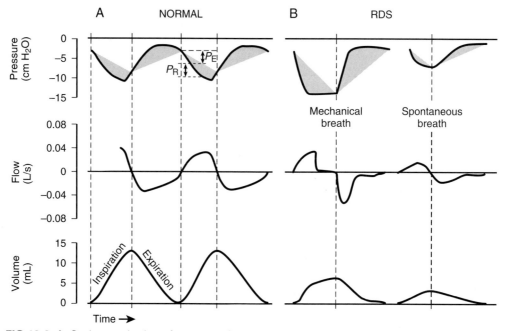

FIG 12-2 A, Scalar monitoring of pressure, flow, and volume signals during spontaneous breathing. The pressure signal has been divided (as demarcated by a *straight line* connecting points of zero flow) to differentiate the elastic pressure from the resistive pressure (*shaded portion*). **B,** Scalar monitoring of pressure, flow, and volume signals during mechanical ventilation. Driving pressure can be approximated as peak inflating pressure minus positive end-expiratory pressure. *RDS,* respiratory distress syndrome; P_E, elastic pressure; P_R, resistive pressure.

the inertial pressure. In this relationship, the elastic pressure is assumed to be proportional to volume change by a constant (E) representing the elastance (or elastic resistance) of the system. The resistive pressure component is assumed proportional to airflow ($\dot{V}$) by a constant (R) representing inelastic airway and tissue resistance. The inertial component of pressure is assumed to be proportional to gas and tissue acceleration ($\ddot{V}$) by an inertial constant (I) and is usually negligible during conventional ventilation; thus $P = EV + R\dot{V} + I\ddot{V}$. This model is based on a single component and assumes linearity between pressure and volume and pressure and flow with the coefficients E, R, and I remaining constant during the ventilatory cycle. However, sick lungs, especially those mechanically ventilated, do not fit this model.[10-12]

MEASUREMENTS DISPLAYED ON PULMONARY GRAPHICS

Pressure Measurement

The appropriate pressure needed is that pressure necessary to overcome the elastic, resistive, and inertial properties of the respiratory system and delivering an adequate volume to the exchange areas of the lung. Figure 12-2 shows the pressure generated with spontaneous breathing. For mechanical breaths the driving pressure is the difference between the peak inspiratory pressure (PIP) and the positive end-expiratory pressure (PEEP)—that is, $\Delta P = (\text{PIP} - \text{PEEP})$.

The mean airway pressure is a function of inspiratory time, flow, PIP, PEEP, and respiratory rate. In general, mean airway pressure reflects oxygenation and driving pressure reflects ventilation. However, as noted they do have an interrelationship, especially in nonhomogeneous lung disease.

Instrumentation for Pressure Measurement

Pressure is measured by pulmonary graphics devices at the bedside at the attachment of the circuit to the ETT or CPAP device. This measures PIP and PEEP/CPAP. This provides adequate monitoring for the pressure–volume (PV) loops displayed in the ventilator graphics. True pulmonary function testing, however, requires more sophisticated pressure measurements. This would be the differential pressure between the ETT and the pleural space. The pleural space pressure is typically estimated using an esophageal catheter. Such a catheter can be used if a chest tube is in place, is patent, and has no ongoing air leak. Esophageal pressure measurement may be used for pleural pressure in the larger preterm and term infant. In the extremely and very low birth-weight preterm infant, the esophageal pressure has been shown to correlate poorly with pleural pressure. Using this technique to determine pulmonary function tests for these infants would yield suspect results.

Volume Measurement

Volume is the area under the curve of the flow signal. Inspiratory and expiratory volumes will differ somewhat because of the change in temperature, water vapor, viscosity, and gas consumption ($O_2 + CO_2$). However, a difference of more than 10% is likely to be due to a faulty flow sensor or a leak, either around the ETT or out of a chest tube, and should be investigated.

Pulmonary Graphic Representation of Tidal Volume

Tidal volume is measured separately for inspiration and expiration. Many modern ventilators have a feature that allows the patient's weight to be entered through the ventilator interface, and many have a default weight included. This weight is then used to calculate parameters such as tidal volume per kilogram body weight. If the entered weight is inaccurate or only the default weight is being used, the displayed "per-kilogram" values will be inaccurate and misleading. Therefore clinicians should look at the total values for such parameters (e.g., total tidal volume) and also examine the infant for inconsistencies between the values displayed on the pulmonary graphics and the clinical examination. For example, a baby with a poor chest expansion in response to a ventilator inflation but a high tidal volume per kilogram displayed on the ventilator may have an inaccurately low weight entered into the ventilator.

The presence of a leak around the ETT makes the exhaled tidal volume a more accurate reflection of true tidal volume, because the leak is always greater during a mechanical inflation. Normal volumes in healthy spontaneously breathing neonates have been shown to be 5 to 8 mL/kg.[13-17] Table 12-1 shows parameters of tidal volumes at the 10th, 50th, and 90th percentiles.

Tidal volumes delivered are dependent on the ventilator settings and the pathophysiology of the lung. The use of 4- to 6-mL/kg tidal volume breaths has been espoused as avoiding volutrauma. Volumes greater than 8.5 mL/kg are considered to cause overdistention. However, if the lung is at the upper end of the PV curve because of excessive PEEP, the 4- to 6-mL/kg tidal volume will excessively distend the lung, resulting in volutrauma. Thus, what is thought to be lung protective will instead be injurious. Conversely if the lung resides at the lower end of the PV curve because of inadequate PEEP a 4- to 6-mL/kg tidal volume will allow portions of the lung to remain atelectatic, causing atelectrauma. The nonhomogeneous lung is more complicated. To recruit atelectatic areas the inflated portion of the lung must become overinflated to a point at which its compliance is less than the atelectatic areas, subsequently allowing for these areas to inflate. Thus a combination of atelectrauma and volutrauma occurs. Maintaining an optimal lung volume by monitoring pulmonary graphics can help avoid these issues.

Flow Measurement (Inspiratory and Expiratory Airflow)

Figure 12-2 demonstrates visually how airflow occurs during inspiration and expiration. Airflow is measured at its peak because of its dependence on airway resistance. Peak flow ranges for various weight infants are shown in Table 12-1. Ventilator circuit airflow is different from the flow that traverses the ETT. Airflow during normal respiration is determined by the tidal volumes and peak inspiratory and expiratory flow. The expiratory flow pattern will demonstrate the natural expiratory airflow limitations in normal newborns, but this may be exaggerated by airway disease (Figs. 12-3 and 12-4). Typically inspiratory airflow peaks at midinspiration and peak expiratory flow values precede midexpiration (Fig. 12-5).

Figure 12-6 demonstrates the various causes of inspiratory and expiratory flow limitations. Severe expiratory flow limitation (flow–volume loop E in Fig. 12-6) is seen frequently in preterm and some term infants owing to malacic airways. Higher PEEP/CPAP will often alleviate this. However, bronchodilators will often worsen it. Hence, examination of the flow–volume loop allows the PEEP/CPAP to be increased or decreased and the expiratory time to be lengthened or shortened. In some ventilators, the speed with which expiration gets to baseline can also be adjusted. These changes may have positive or negative effects on pulmonary mechanics and ultimately on blood gases. The neonate obviously cannot be asked to exhale rapidly as an adult patient can. However, in the neonate this can be simulated using a rapid thoracic compression technique.[13,18-21]

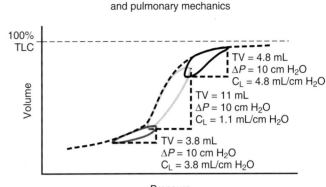

FIG 12-3 Deflation limb of the respiratory pressure–volume (PV) curve (*dashed sigmoid line*, defined from total lung capacity to residual volume) is shown on an *x–y* plot. In this simulated example, tidal volume ventilation is occurring at the functional residual capacity (or the lung volume at end expiration) that is governed by the positive end-expiratory pressure (PEEP). Thus, for a baby (birth weight 1190 g and gestational age 28 weeks) who is being administered a peak inspiratory pressure (PIP) of 15 cm H_2O and PEEP of 5 cm H_2O and has a recorded tidal volume of 11 mL, the estimated compliance is 11 divided by 10 (difference of 15 and 5), which is 1.1 mL/cm H_2O. Thus two inferences may be calculated: (1) tidal volume = 9.2 mL/kg and (2) for a change in driving pressure (either PIP or PEEP), the tidal volume should change by 1.1 mL per 1 cm H_2O. For example, a decrease in PIP from 15 to 14 cm H_2O or PEEP from 5 to 4 cm H_2O should linearly decrease the tidal volume from 11 to 9.9 mL. If the infant was being ventilated with the PIP close to the "flattened" segment of the overdistended PV relationship, the decrease in tidal volume would be nonlinear and weaning from PEEP would result in an improvement of the tidal volume. On the other hand, if the baby is being ventilated at the flattened portion of the atelectatic lung, the change in tidal volume will be nonlinear and the tidal volume will fail to improve upon weaning from the PEEP. *TLC*, Total lung capacity; *TV*, tidal volume; *CL*, compliance of lung.

Minute Ventilation

Minute ventilation is the total sum of volume delivered over a minute, with spontaneous as well as mechanical inflations. Typical minute ventilation for term infants is 240 to 360 mL/kg/min. Alveolar ventilation is calculated by subtracting dead-space ventilation from total minute ventilation. Alveolar/saccular ventilation in the absence of intrapulmonary shunts determines $PaCO_2$. Neonates with respiratory distress syndrome (RDS) typically breathe over 100 times a minute, with smaller tidal volumes and unchanged dead space volume resulting in decreased alveolar minute ventilation. Their increased respiratory rate in a noncompliant lung is due to the lower work of breathing required with small rapid breaths rather than with larger breaths.

Pressure–Volume Curve

The shape of the PV curve describes the pattern of tidal volume as a function of driving pressure. Figure 12-3 demonstrates the effect of the PV curve residing at the atelectatic, midportion, and overdistended portion of the PV curve. This will assist one

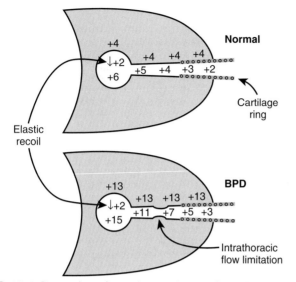

FIG 12-4 Dynamics of passive expiratory flow during spontaneous breathing in a normal term infant (*upper panel*) compared to an infant with bronchopulmonary dysplasia (*BPD*). Intrathoracic pressures are shown in the shaded areas. Gradient of intratracheobronchial pressures is estimated based on likely elastic recoil pressure of the lung and its final equilibration with atmospheric pressure at end expiration. The elevated intrathoracic pressure at end inspiration and at the onset of expiration is a reflection of the increased work of breathing and the higher peak inflating pressure generated in an infant with a moderate degree of BPD. The lower panel illustrates the mechanism of intrathoracic expiratory flow obstruction by external compression of the compliant airways.

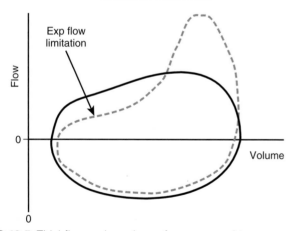

FIG 12-5 Tidal flow–volume loops from a normal term neonate ("lemon-shaped") and a preterm neonate with high expiratory resistance (or compliant airways), which illustrates a "ski-slope" effect during expiration.

in understanding the nonlinearity of pressure changes as they relate to volume changes depending on the area of the PV curve on which they are operating. Figure 12-7 demonstrates the various conditions of increased airflow resistance, overdistention (pressure or volume), low compliance, and low, normal, and high FRC.

Pulmonary Mechanics

Lung Compliance

Inflation of the lung follows a curve when pressure is applied. The deflation curve is different and is dependent on the compliance of the lungs and on airway resistance (see Fig. 12-7, A). The compliance of the lung, represented by slope of the $\Delta V/\Delta P$ curve, is linear over the midportion of the PV curve, from the level of the FRC through the normal tidal volume. A given change in driving pressure will increase tidal volume by the equation $\Delta V = C \times \Delta P$. A decrease in lung compliance causes the lung to become stiffer, whereas an increase in lung compliance causes the lung to become more expandable. The compliance is determined by alveolar surface tension and lung elasticity. The typical value for a healthy newborn is 1.5 to 2 mL/cm H_2O/kg. Total respiratory compliance (chest + lungs) is the tidal volume/change in driving pressure. In patients who are being ventilated, the driving pressure is equal to the difference between the PIP and the PEEP.

Dynamic Compliance

Dynamic compliance, which is the tidal volume/change in driving pressure, is likely to be overestimated when there is poor alveolar/saccular inflation as seen in patients with RDS. Infants who have bronchopulmonary dysplasia (BPD) due to an increased resistive load may have an underestimation of tidal volume and therefore underestimation of lung compliance. However, for the clinician, it still provides a measure of volume change that can be expected for each 1 cm H_2O change in driving pressure as long as the patient is maintained at optimal FRC.

Using the primary variables measured by bedside pulmonary graphics devices, compliance can be calculated from the driving pressure required and the volume delivered. The change in volume for a given change in pressure will be relatively linear but only when the lung is being ventilated on the midportion of the PV curve (see Fig. 12-3). This knowledge allows one to understand the anticipated change in volume for a driving pressure change. This will allow the clinician to anticipate appropriate inflation, overinflation, or underinflation as driving pressure changes are occurring.

Resistive Properties

Nonelastic properties of the respiratory system characterize its resistance to motion. Because motion between two surfaces in contact usually involves friction or loss of energy, resistance to breathing occurs in any moving part of the respiratory system. These resistances include frictional resistance to airflow, tissue resistance, and inertial forces. Lung resistance is predominantly (80%) attributed to frictional resistance to inspiratory and expiratory airflow in the larger airways. Tissue resistance (19%) and inertial forces (1%) also influence long resistance. Airflow through the airway requires a driving pressure resulting from changes in alveolar pressure. When alveolar pressure is less than atmospheric pressure (during spontaneous inspiration), air flows into the lung. When alveolar pressure is greater than atmospheric pressure, air flows out of the lung. By definition, resistance to airflow is equal to the resistive component of driving pressure (P_R) divided by airflow ($\dot{V}$). Thus:

$$\text{Resistance} - (P_R)/\dot{V}$$

When determining lung resistance, the resistive component of the measured transpulmonary pressure is used as the driving pressure (see Fig. 12-2). To measure airway resistance, the differential between alveolar pressure and atmospheric pressure is used as the driving pressure. Under normal tidal breathing conditions, there is a linear relationship between airflow and

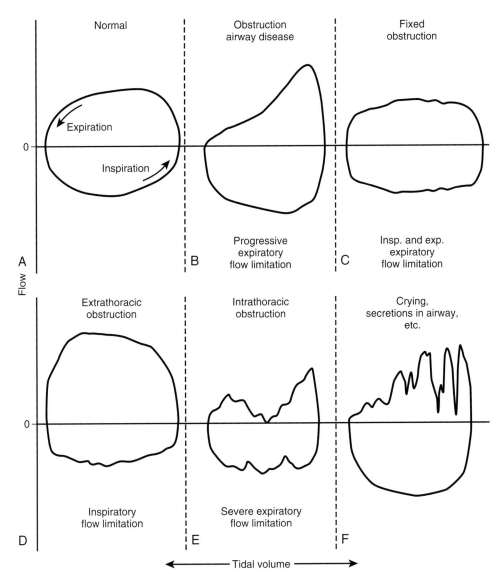

FIG 12-6 Tidal flow–volume loops illustrating various manifestations of flow limitation that results from heterogeneity in airway resistance. **A,** Normal loop. **B,** "Ski-slope" loop observed with expiratory airflow limitation as seen in babies with bronchopulmonary dysplasia. **C,** Extrathoracic airway obstruction with inspiratory and expiratory airflow limitation as seen in babies with subglottic stenosis or narrow ETT. **D,** Intrathoracic inspiratory airflow limitation as seen in babies with intraluminal obstruction (close to the carina) or an aberrant vessel compressing the trachea. **E,** Unstable airways or tracheomalacia. **F,** This type of loop usually is suggestive of an erratic airflow limitation, as seen with airway secretions.

driving pressure. The slope of the flow versus pressure curve changes as the airways narrow, indicating that the patient with airway obstruction has a greater resistance to airflow. The resistance to airflow is greatly dependent on the size of the airway lumen. According to Poiseuille's law, the resistive pressure (ΔP) required to achieve a given flow ($\dot{V}$) for a gas of viscosity and flowing through a rigid and smooth cylindrical tube of specific length (L) and radius (r) is given as follows:

$$\Delta P = 8\eta L\dot{V}/\pi r^4$$

According to this relationship, resistance to airflow increases by a power of 4 with any decrease in airway radius. Because the newborn airway lumen is approximately half that of the adult, the neonatal airway resistance is about 16-fold that of the adult.

Normal airway resistance in a term newborn is approximately 20 to 40 cm H_2O/L/s, which is about 16-fold the value observed in adults (1 to 2 cm H_2O/L/s). Also, the hysteresis of the PV relationship represents the resistive work of breathing and can be separated into inspiratory and expiratory components.

In babies with obstructive airway disease, the expiratory component of resistive work of breathing is increased (see Fig. 12-7, B and C). Nearly 80% of the total resistance to airflow occurs in large airways up to about the fourth to fifth generation of bronchial branching. The patient usually has large airway disease when resistance to airflow is increased. Because the smaller airways contribute a small proportion of total airway resistance, they are sometimes known as the "silent zone" of the lung in which airway obstruction can occur without being readily detected. Unlike babies with RDS, babies with BPD (because of the associated

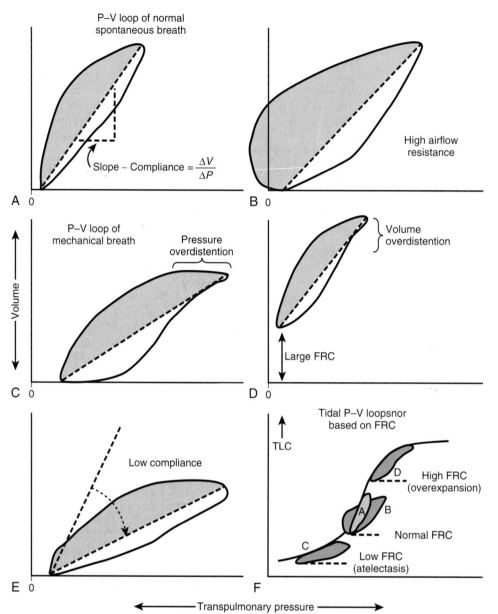

FIG 12-7 Pressure–volume (*P–V*) relationship illustrations show components of inspiratory elastic work and inspiratory elastic and resistive work. **A,** A normal P–V relationship. **B,** Increased expiratory resistive work (such as obstructive airway disease, meconium aspiration syndrome, or bronchopulmonary dysplasia). **C,** Increased expiratory resistive work with excessive inspiratory pressure (such as overdistention due to high positive inspiratory pressure or high tidal volume). **D,** Increased expiratory resistive work due excessive functional residual capacity (such as overdistention due to air trapping, shortened expiratory time, etc.). **E,** Decreased inspiratory elastic work (such as respiratory distress syndrome, pneumonia, atelectasis, etc.). **F,** Comparison of P–V relationships affected by the functional residual capacity. *FRC,* function residual capacity; *TLC,* total lung capacity.

airway barotrauma) have higher values of airway resistance with an associated increased resistive work of breathing.

Synchronous and Asynchronous Breathing

Real-time evaluation of synchronous respiratory cycles allows for visualization of successive PV and flow–volume (*V̇–V*) loops as they superimpose neatly over each preceding loop. Asynchrony of respiratory cycles may be evident during airway obstruction (secretions, bronchospasm), "bucking" (during mechanical ventilation or involuntary Valsalva maneuvers),

and agitation (pain, excessive handling, impaired gas exchange). Objective evaluation of asynchrony is difficult to quantify. On the other hand, synchronous ventilation is easily observed.

ROLE OF PULMONARY GRAPHICS IN VENTILATOR MANAGEMENT

Pulmonary graphics along with numeric estimates of pulmonary function constitute important tools to help manage significant pulmonary and airway problems. To effectively use

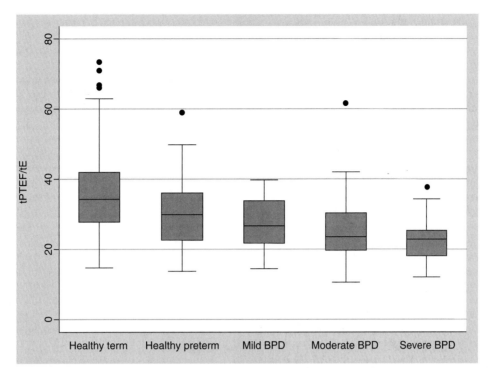

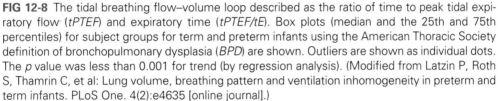

FIG 12-8 The tidal breathing flow–volume loop described as the ratio of time to peak tidal expiratory flow (*tPTEF*) and expiratory time (*tPTEF/tE*). Box plots (median and the 25th and 75th percentiles) for subject groups for term and preterm infants using the American Thoracic Society definition of bronchopulmonary dysplasia (*BPD*) are shown. Outliers are shown as individual dots. The *p* value was less than 0.001 for trend (by regression analysis). (Modified from Latzin P, Roth S, Thamrin C, et al: Lung volume, breathing pattern and ventilation inhomogeneity in preterm and term infants. PLoS One. 4(2):e4635 [online journal].)

this tool, one must understand how a given ventilator works, interpret the displayed graphics, and determine the underlying pulmonary pathophysiology. Bedside pulmonary graphics can assist the clinician in determining the many factors involved in a given patient's abnormal pulmonary function. These factors include (1) compliance, (2) resistance, (3) tidal volume, (4) under- or overinflation, (5) effect of end-expiratory pressure, and (6) the patient's own support (positive or negative). When ventilator parameters are changed, graphics will help determine if the alterations improve or worsen the patient's status.

Optimizing Peak Inspiratory Pressure

On occasion, patients will be managed on pressure-controlled ventilation. A PIP that delivers a tidal volume of 4 to 6 mL/kg should be sufficient. Looking at the PV curve will also assist in determining the appropriate PIP.

Optimizing End-Expiratory Pressure

End-respiratory pressure has been a critical feature that allowed assisted ventilation to actually work in the neonate with surfactant-deficient respiratory distress.[22,23] However, choosing the optimal PEEP/CPAP has become somewhat more difficult especially with the use of surfactant. Responders to surfactant need less end-expiratory pressure, and nonresponders need more. In the pre-surfactant era, PEEP/CPAPs of 10 to 12 cm H$_2$O were often needed and in some patients who have not responded to surfactant, this level may still be needed. However, maintaining a PEEP/CPAP that is too high after surfactant will probably increase complications such as air leak and intraventricular hemorrhage. Also, if end-expiratory pressure is inadequate, the

lung will not be managed in the midportion of the PV curve. Graphics help determine if the lung at end expiration is collapsing. To ensure optimal PEEP levels that allow lung functioning in the midportion of the PV curve, a skilled clinician standing at the bedside should observe the changes in pulmonary graphics with PEEP/CPAP adjustments. The skill required becomes more important as the lung pathophysiology becomes more severe. There is no place for being just a "dial twiddler."

Optimizing Expiratory Airflow

The goal of assisted respiratory support, whether invasive (ETT) or less invasive (nasal CPAP, high-flow nasal cannula, NIPPV, BIPAP, or HFNV), is to keep the lung ventilation in the midportion of the PV curve. Expiratory flow is dependent on the elastic and resistive properties of the lung. On assisted ventilation, the slope of the expiratory waveform plays a role also. A too rapid (steep slope) decline of the expiratory wave may lead to air-trapping and movement away from the midportion of the PV curve. This can be especially true of the patient with established BPD or evolving BPD. Latzin et al. used time of peak tidal expiratory flow (tPTEF) divided by expiratory time (tE) to measure compliance (Fig. 12-8). Patients with BPD had decreased tPTEF/tE suggestive of poorer lung compliance.

Optimizing Inspiratory Time

Increasing or decreasing inspiratory time will change delivered volume and mean airway pressure. It obviously will also affect expiratory time. One must understand the physiology of the lung disease being treated and also the properties of the preterm lung. Very short I-times in the preterm infant with a poorly compliant lung generally result in airway dilatation and poor delivery of gas to the saccules/alveoli. One can see this in graphics as poor lung expansion. As previously mentioned, the preterm lung has a high dead space-to-tidal volume ratio. Therefore, longer I-times may be needed in some patients, especially those who did not respond well to surfactant, for recruiting lung volume. In the early 1970s, I-times of 0.6 to 1 second were used to help recruit the lung, but once the lung was adequately recruited, the I-time would be decreased to 0.35 to 0.45 seconds. Because this maneuver decreases the mean airway pressure, an increase in the rate, PIP, or PEEP might be required to maintain the mean airway pressure. Because the effects of changing these parameters are not predictable, the clinician must be prepared to individualize settings for specific patients.

Optimizing Synchrony and Rate of Ventilatory Support

The use of patient-triggered ventilation has been available for more than 30 years. Early on it was not very effective for the very low birth-weight neonate as the triggering devices were not sensitive enough for these patients. Today, devices associated with pressure support ventilation have helped assisted ventilation be more effective. Patients who continue to not synchronize with the ventilator will probably require sedation or paralysis. This will depend on the overall negative effect of the asynchrony on the pulmonary status.

Optimizing Tidal Volume

The finding that large tidal volumes were more likely to produce lung injury (volutrauma) compared to specific PIPs causing injury (barotrauma) has resulted in more clinicians using tidal volume-oriented ventilation. An effect of this finding has been to keep the tidal volume in the 4- to 6-mL/kg range. This may or may not be lung protective. If the lung has not been adequately recruited and only 50% of the lung is open, then that portion of the lung may be experiencing 8 to 12 mL/kg per breath. If the lung is not adequately inflated with poor alveolar/saccular compliance then the volume is distending the airways and not inflating the saccular/alveoli, leading to atelectrauma. Pulmonary graphics can help guide the clinician in selecting the required tidal volume, but physical examination of the patient is also required, as tidal volume thought to be adequate may only be dilating the airways rather than ventilating the gas-exchanging part of the lung.

Optimizing Inspiratory Oxygen

Avoidance of high inspired oxygen greater than 40% is critical to reducing oxidative stress. This critical level is almost certainly lower in the extremely low birth-weight newborn. The most efficient way to minimize FiO_2 requirement is to keep the lung on the midpoint of the PV curve and ensure uniform inflation. Patients with significant pulmonary hypertension should be managed with medications such as inhaled nitric oxide as opposed to high inspired oxygen levels.

Permissive Hypercarbia

The goal of allowing the neonate to have a $PaCO_2$ in the high 50s or 60s was to avoid ventilator-induced lung injury (volutrauma/barotrauma). However, to accomplish this safely, the occurrence of volutrauma because the lung is overinflated or atelectrauma because the lung is underinflated should be recognized. Graphics can help with this by assessing the appropriate placement of the lung on the PV curve.

LIMITATIONS OF BEDSIDE PULMONARY GRAPHICS

Understanding the neonatal lung will help in determining the limitations of the use of pulmonary function and graphics. For these to make sense, the neonatal lung needs to be uniformly inflated. This is often a difficult task. Furthermore, it is important to appreciate that with synchronized ventilation, the patient and the ventilator work together; the transpulmonary pressure that generates a tidal volume is the sum of the positive inflation pressure from the ventilator and the negative inspiratory pressure generated by the infant. The latter is not measured by standard ventilator pulmonary mechanics and thus in actively breathing infants, the values will not be accurate. When a substantial leak exists around the endotracheal tube, the graphics will be distorted and the measured values will be inaccurate.

There are structural issues of the preterm lung that complicate assessment. A major issue is the distensibility of the airways. The dead space-to-tidal volume ratio is high. This can result in a measured tidal volume that should be adequate at 4 to 6 mL/kg, but because of the distensibility of the airways with associated alveolar/saccular collapse, the volume merely inflates the airways and never gets to the saccule or alveolus to exchange gas. This phenomenon explains the patient whose chest is moving well but does not ventilate or oxygenate well.

A nonhomogeneous lung results in areas of the lung being adequately inflated with other areas poorly inflated. With positive-pressure breaths, the normally inflated areas will overdistend before the poorly inflated (low compliance) areas will expand. Nonhomogeneous lung disease, distensible airways, malacic airways (common in the preterm infant), partial airway obstruction (pneumonia, evolving BPD, etc.) all make the use of graphics for decision making challenging. Understanding the pathophysiology of the lung disease one is treating assists in understanding the limitations of these measurements.

The clinician should have an expectation of what an adjustment in the ventilator should do to the respiratory parameters (PaO_2, $PaCO_2$, and HCO_3). If that occurs then one can continue to manage the ventilator in that mode. However, if that expectation does not occur, one must rethink the physiology of the lungs that are being treated. The complicated patient needs someone at the bedside making adjustments, observing for expected results, and reassessing if they do not occur. Accuracy and reproducibility of graphics measurements are critical to their use. In particular, accuracy in extremely low birth weight has been poorly studied.[24] The American Thoracic Society and European Respiratory Joint Committee have published guidelines for standardization.[25]

NEWER TECHNIQUES

Recent publications[25,26] have discussed techniques that are likely over the next several years to help refine ventilator settings for patients with various pulmonary pathophysiologies. These include surfactant deficiency (low lung compliance), meconium aspiration (nonhomogeneous with partial airway obstruction), pulmonary hypoplasia (uniform bilateral) nonuniform (diaphragmatic hernia), pneumonia (combination of normal lung and saccular/alveolar infiltrates), bronchiolitis, predominantly high airway resistance creating air trapping, and BPD (combination of airway disease, atelectasis, hyperinflation, and pulmonary hypertension).

As of this writing those techniques are not built into a ventilator and require stand-alone devices that may be used short term for measurements or longer term for assessing multiple treatments provided to the patients (e.g., surfactant, bronchodilators, steroids, diuretics, nitric oxide, other pulmonary vasodilators such as sildenafil, prostacyclin (PGI2), and milrinone).

The techniques that may provide significant help are the following: respiratory plethysmography and electrical impedance tomography. Respiratory inductance plethysmography can be used to evaluate asynchronous breathing. It can also be used to assess lung volume and its changes with adjustments of noninvasive support.

Electrical impedance tomography uses a belt of multiple electrical signal transmitters and receivers that assess the impedance of the lung. This allows for an assessminant of lung volume as air-filled areas are the major determinant of impedance in the lung. It will assess volume changes but does not give actual volume results. The benefit is determining ventilator adjustments that will keep the lung at an appropriate mean lung volume, avoiding volutrauma and atelectrauma, which make up most if not all of ventilator-induced lung injury. Unlike most techniques of pulmonary function measurements this technique is not subject to difficulties with leak around the ETT.

Two additional techniques that offer promise are capnography and inert gas washout. However, in the neonate both of these are not accurate if ETT leak is >10%.

Once appropriate reference values have been established for these newer modalities, and their effectiveness in guiding invasive and noninvasive respiratory support has been established, they have the potential to improve our ability to adjust assisted respiratory support so that pulmonary gas exchange is optimized while minimizing lung injury.

SUMMARY

Graphics offer the clinician:
1. The ability to look at how an individual patient's pulmonary status is changing over time.

2. The ability to follow basic lung function parameters. Using these findings, the clinician can make ventilator adjustments that will avoid volutrauma or atelectrauma, which may help avoid ventilator-induced lung injury. It is now recognized that even being on appropriate ventilator support still appears to carry the risk of lung injury.[27]
3. The ability to make ventilator adjustments and assess their usefulness in improving lung function of the patient.
4. The ability to assess how the patient's lung function is handling weaning, which may help earlier extubation to a less invasive support.
5. The ability to assess the effects of medications such as surfactant, bronchodilators, diuretics, steroids, etc., on lung function. This will allow for more appropriate use of these medications.

CAVEATS

1. Pulmonary graphics may suggest the lung is quite stable, but the clinician should be cognizant of the ventilator support being provided. A patient on a PIP of 28 cm H_2O and a PEEP of 8 cm H_2O may well be on the midportion of the PV curve, but if the PEEP is reduced to 5 cm H_2O, the lung will steadily derecruit.
2. For graphics to be useful, a dedicated respiratory therapy staff, nursing staff, residents, nurse practitioners, and, most of all, attending physicians who understand graphics and utilize this information to manage their patients are all required.
3. Understanding the device being used, its limitations, and how to troubleshoot it are critical to successful management.
4. Nothing supplants the continued physical assessment of the patient by all individuals involved in care.

REFERENCES

A complete reference list is available at https://expertconsult.inkling.com/.

13

Airway Evaluation: Bronchoscopy, Laryngoscopy, and Tracheal Aspirates

Clarice Clemmens, MD, and Joseph Piccione, DO, MS

INTRODUCTION

Over the past few decades the instruments available for examining the airway have evolved to become increasingly smaller while providing better optical resolution. It is now possible to directly evaluate the airway of even the smallest premature infant. The optimal approach to airway evaluation depends upon the indication for the procedure, the risk of adverse effects, and the magnitude of potential benefit. This chapter will assist those caring for critically ill neonates in determining which diagnostic modalities will obtain the most relevant information while minimizing risk to the patient.

FLEXIBLE NASOPHARYNGOLARYNGOSCOPY IN THE NEONATE

Indications

Flexible laryngoscopy is utilized as a diagnostic tool to assess pathology at or superior to the glottis. This procedure may be performed at the bedside during wakefulness or sleep. It is non-invasive with relatively low risk to the patient as sedation is not necessary.

Flexible laryngoscopy is valuable for narrowing the differential diagnosis in infants with noisy breathing. The evaluation begins at the nares and proceeds through the nasal turbinates to the choana. Because neonates are obligate nasal breathers, severe nasal obstruction can lead to significant respiratory distress with cyclical cyanosis and feeding difficulties. Narrowing of the pyriform aperture, known as congenital nasal pyriform aperture stenosis, is a rare cause of severe nasal obstruction in the neonate. Choanal atresia is a congenital anomaly representing complete obstruction of the nasal airway with an incidence of 1 in 10,000 live births.[1] Infants typically experience severe respiratory distress, especially when it is bilateral (50% of cases). It can be bony or membranous or have features of both.[2]

After the laryngoscope is passed through the nasopharynx, the oropharynx and larynx can be examined. Obstruction at the level of the supraglottic or glottic structures results in inspiratory stridor. The most common cause of stridor in infants is laryngomalacia, which in severe cases presents with dyspnea, feeding difficulties, failure to thrive, dysphagia, and obstructive sleep apnea. It is the result of a congenital abnormality of the laryngeal cartilage or its supportive muscle tone resulting in dynamic collapse of the supraglottic structures during inspiration. Severity initially worsens with growth, but in most cases it resolves between 6 and 18 months of age.[3] Treatment of laryngomalacia is dependent upon the severity of symptoms. Those with mild to moderate laryngomalacia may be managed by observation. Medical therapies can improve symptoms in those with concurrent gastroesophageal reflux disease (GERD). Surgical management with supraglottoplasty can resolve the associated respiratory and feeding problems.[4]

Vocal cord paralysis (VCP) is the second most common laryngeal anomaly identified in neonates. Unilateral VCP often results from iatrogenic injury during cardiothoracic surgery or ligation of a patent ductus arteriosus. It may also be idiopathic or result from neurologic disorders. Iatrogenic unilateral VCP frequently resolves with time, and regular follow-up with repeated endoscopic examinations is recommended prior to considering surgical interventions.[5,6] Bilateral VCP is less common, usually congenital, and associated with other anomalies in 50% of cases.[7] It presents at birth with respiratory compromise and either inspiratory or biphasic stridor. Infants with unilateral VCP typically have a hoarse cry, whereas those with bilateral VCP vocalize well.

Flexible laryngoscopy is also helpful in differentiating the etiology of hoarse cry in neonates. Hoarse cry may develop following endotracheal intubation as a consequence of glottic edema or granulomata. In the majority of cases, these problems resolve spontaneously or with management of coincident GERD.

Risks, Contraindications, and Limitations

Flexible laryngoscopy, when performed correctly, is a relatively low-risk procedure. Minor risks include vasovagal reactions resulting in bradycardia and laryngospasm. They generally resolve with the removal of the laryngoscope. Maintaining a superior location of the scope and avoiding contact with the glottic structures helps prevent laryngospasm. Coagulopathies are considered a relative contraindication, as the risk of mucosal bleeding from the nose must be weighed against the anticipated benefit of the procedure. The presence of an endotracheal tube substantially limits the value of this procedure. While the nasal airway can still be visualized well, useful information about the larynx is rarely obtained.

Equipment

Necessary equipment required for flexible nasopharyngolaryngoscopy (NPL) includes only a light source and the scope itself. At our institution, the 2.2-mm flexible nasopharyngolaryngoscope is used most often in neonates. Use of "antifog" solutions or alcohol swabs minimizes condensation on the objective lens of the scope and improves visualization.

DIRECT MICROLARYNGOSCOPY AND RIGID BRONCHOSCOPY IN THE NEONATE

Indications

Direct rigid telescope microlaryngoscopy and rigid bronchoscopy (ML&B) can be useful as a diagnostic and therapeutic tool for upper airway and subglottic pathology (Fig. 13-1). In contrast to bedside flexible laryngoscopy, general anesthesia is required. Evaluation with ML&B should be considered when a need for surgical intervention is determined based on findings during NPL or when better visualization of the airway is required.

If vocal cord immobility has been established, arytenoid mobility should be assessed by palpation during microlaryngoscopy to determine if the cord mobility is impaired as a result of recurrent laryngeal nerve pathology or arytenoid fixation resulting from fibrosis or atresia of the posterior glottis. In cases of severe laryngomalacia (Fig. 13-2), ML&B can be used to perform cold surgical or laser supraglottoplasty.

Laryngeal webs, cysts, clefts, and laryngoceles are rare congenital anomalies of the larynx that are difficult to visualize on bedside examination. Laryngeal webs are caused by incomplete recanalization of the laryngotracheal tube during the third month of gestation.[8] Laryngoceles are air-filled dilations of the laryngeal saccule that communicate with the laryngeal ventricle, whereas saccular cysts are fluid-filled dilations of the saccule that do not communicate with the airway. Rigid microlaryngoscopy is also used in the diagnosis and treatment of submucosal lesions, such as venolymphatic malformations. Laryngeal and subglottic infantile hemangiomas may cause progressive, biphasic stridor within the first few months of life. They are sometimes associated with cutaneous hemangiomas and often respond well to chronic propranolol therapy, which is used until the growth phase has subsided and involution has occurred.[9]

Laryngeal clefts are rare anomalies that present with stridor and aspiration. A type I laryngeal cleft is confined to the interarytenoid space, a type II cleft extends through part of the cricoid, a type III cleft extends completely through the cricoid, and a type IV cleft extends beyond the cricoid into the trachea.[10]

When the etiology of noisy breathing in the neonate is not apparent based on NPL examination, it is important to visualize the subglottis with ML&B. Subglottic cysts can cause obstruction of the subglottic airway, resulting in stridor. They are almost always associated with a history of endotracheal intubation and often occur in association with subglottic stenosis (Fig. 13-3). Subglottic stenosis is an important cause of stridor in neonates. In most cases it is acquired, but 5% of cases represent congenital forms of this condition.[11] It should be considered in the differential diagnosis when an age-appropriate endotracheal tube cannot be passed during attempts at intubation. Acquired subglottic stenosis results when subglottic edema associated with the presence of an endotracheal tube impairs capillary perfusion of the subglottic mucosa. Necrosis and chondritis ensue and a fibrocartilaginous scar is formed.[12] Risks are increased with larger endotracheal tubes, prolonged intubation, repeated or traumatic intubations, and infection.

The severity of subglottic stenosis is graded using the Cotton-Myer grading system. A stenosis is grade 1 when 0% to 50% of the lumen is obstructed, grade 2 with 50% to 75% obstruction, grade 3 with 75% to 99% obstruction, and grade 4 when the airway lumen is completely obstructed.[13] Based upon the etiology, grade, and thickness of obstruction, various surgical techniques have been developed for the management of subglottic stenosis including laryngotracheal reconstruction with costal cartilage grafting, cricoid split, and cricotracheal resection. In neonates with severe stenosis, a tracheostomy may be required until definitive surgical management can be performed.

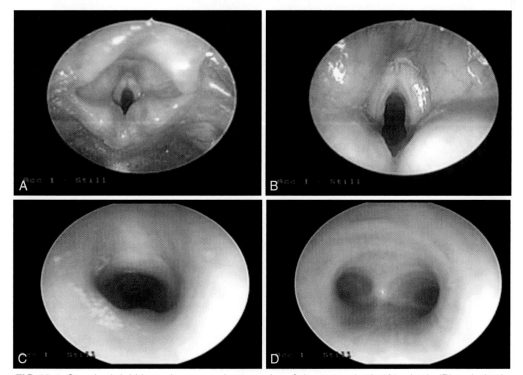

FIG 13-1 Standard rigid bronchoscopy photographs of the supraglottis (**A**), glottis (**B**), subglottis (**C**), and main stem bronchi (**D**).

Another important cause of stridor in the neonate is congenital tracheal stenosis due to complete cartilaginous tracheal rings. In these infants, the membranous posterior wall of the trachea is replaced by cartilage. The number of rings varies, and the diameter tends to narrow with each subsequent ring, giving a funneled appearance on radiographic images.[14] The airway of a neonate with complete tracheal rings is tenuous and must be treated with caution because of the risk of obstructive mucous plugs and limited options for endotracheal intubation. Irritation of the mucosa in the stenotic segment by rigid bronchoscopy or an endotracheal tube can result in airway edema and exacerbate airflow obstruction in the trachea.

Tracheoesophageal fistulae (TEF) are well visualized with rigid bronchoscopy. A TEF results from failed closure of the tracheoesophageal septum during embryologic development. There are five types of TEF, the most common of which is

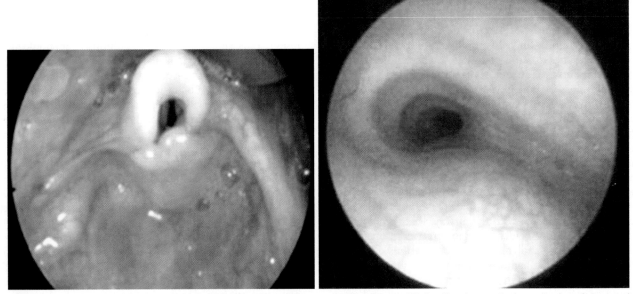

FIG 13-2 **Left,** Laryngomalacia: omega-shaped epiglottis with arytenoid prolapse. **Right,** Tracheomalacia: collapse of the trachea.

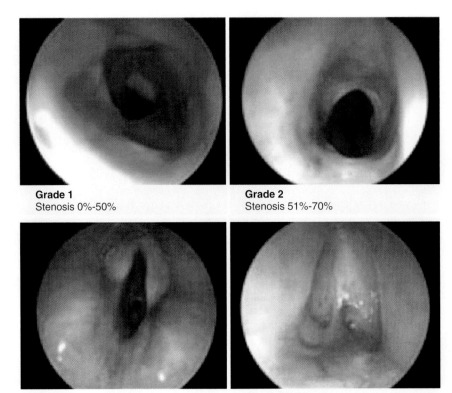

Grade 1
Stenosis 0%-50%

Grade 2
Stenosis 51%-70%

Grade 3
Stenosis 71%-99%

Grade 4
Stenosis 100%

FIG 13-3 Examples of subglottic stenosis.

associated with proximal esophageal atresia and the distal esophagus arising from the lower trachea or carina. Some degree of associated tracheomalacia is inherent to this disorder.[15]

Risks, Contraindications, and Limitations

The requirement of general anesthesia for ML&B make it a higher risk procedure than NPL; however, the risk of serious complications remains low. Common adverse events include cough, oxyhemoglobin desaturation, hypoventilation, and laryngospasm. Bleeding and damage to the lips, gums, and maxillary alveolus are uncommon when appropriate precautions are taken.

Equipment

The procedure requires a light source; a rigid laryngoscope, telescope, or microscope; and a suspension arm if interventions are to be performed. Laryngoscopes are available in a variety of lengths, diameters, and angles. Selection is based upon surgeon preference, indications for the procedure, and which interventions need to be performed (Figs. 13-4 and 13-5).

The setup should also include antifog solutions for the telescope and a topical anesthetic (1% to 2% lidocaine) to prevent laryngospasm. Care must be taken to avoid lidocaine toxicity in neonatal populations. The maximum safe dose of lidocaine (without epinephrine) is 4 mg/kg.

FIBER-OPTIC FLEXIBLE BRONCHOSCOPY

Indications

Flexible bronchoscopy may be considered for both diagnostic and therapeutic purposes. A comparison with ML&B is shown in Table 13-1. One of the most common indications for flexible bronchoscopy is sampling the contents of the airways and alveoli by obtaining bronchoalveolar lavage (BAL) fluid. Another important role of flexible bronchoscopy is to assist endotracheal intubation in neonates with difficult airway access. The bronchoscope may be inserted through an endotracheal tube and, after navigating through the airway to a suitable position, the tube is advanced into place along the shaft of the bronchoscope.[16]

Infants with artificial airways (endotracheal intubation/tracheostomy) may require inspection of the tube lumen when obstruction is suspected.[17] When the tube diameter is sufficient to accommodate a bronchoscope with an internal suction channel, mucous plugs[18] and blood clots can be evacuated from the airway (see below). Similarly, in those with persistent or recurrent chest radiographic opacities, flexible bronchoscopy can help differentiate between anatomic, infectious, hemorrhagic, and mechanical etiologies. An important anatomic consideration for infants with recurrent or persistent right upper lobe opacities is the possibility of a tracheal bronchus, in which the right upper lobe bronchus originates from the distal trachea. A seemingly appropriate placement of the endotracheal tube can occlude the right upper lobe orifice, resulting in localized atelectasis when this common anatomic variant is present.[19]

When recurrent opacities are observed in varied locations and aspiration of gastroesophageal refluxate is suspected, flexible bronchoscopy can be performed to identify TEF. The more common distal-type TEF is easily seen at the posterior wall of the carina, whereas the H-type TEF is located more proximally in the trachea beneath a mound of mucosa on the posterior tracheal wall.[20] In the case of known or suspected pulmonary hemorrhage, flexible bronchoscopy can be utilized to evacuate clots from the lower airways and identify mucosal and endoluminal sources of bleeding. This may be particularly useful in neonates requiring extracorporeal membrane oxygenation.

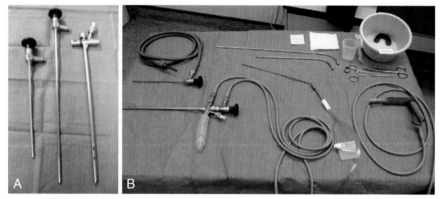

FIG 13-4 Bronchoscopy setup. (Courtesy of Joanne Stow, CRNP.)

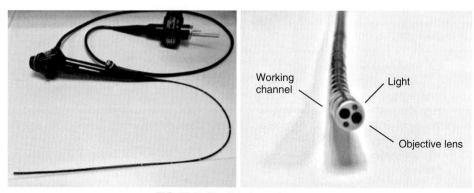

FIG 13-5 Flexible bronchoscope.

TABLE 13-1   Flexible Bronchoscopy in Comparison with Direct Rigid Telescope Microlaryngoscopy and Rigid Bronchoscopy

Indication	Rigid Instruments	Flexible Instruments
Stridor	May alter airway dynamics	Preferred
Persistent wheeze (not responsive, or poorly responsive, to bronchodilator therapy)		Preferred, especially to evaluate distal airway structure and dynamics
Atelectasis (persistent, recurrent, or massive)	May be needed to remove airway obstruction (e.g., foreign body)	
Localized hyperinflation		Preferred
Pneumonia • Recurrent • Persistent • Patients unable to produce sputum • Atypical or in unusual circumstances (e.g., immunocompromised patients)		Preferred (much better to obtain BAL specimens)
Hemoptysis	May be best if there is brisk bleeding	Preferred to evaluate distal airways
Foreign body aspiration • Known • Suspected	Mandatory for removal of foreign bodies	May be useful to examine for possibility of foreign body; rarely useful for removal
Cough (persistent)		Preferred
Suspected aspiration	Preferred to evaluate posterior larynx and cervical trachea	• Preferred to obtain BAL • Combined use of both instruments very useful
Evaluation of patients with tracheostomies	Preferred to evaluate posterior larynx and subglottic space	Preferred to evaluate tube position and airway dynamics
Suspected mass or tumor	Preferred for laryngeal or tracheal lesions	Preferred for lesions in distal airways
Suspected airway anomalies		
Complications of artificial airways		

BAL, bronchoalveolar lavage.

In children with persistent pneumothoraces or suspected bronchopleural fistulae, flexible bronchoscopy can assist in identifying the anatomic location of the air leak.[21] Using an inflatable balloon-tipped catheter advanced sequentially into each bronchial segment in the affected lung, the source of the air leak will become evident when the chest tube output ceases.

When attempts at extubation fail in association with noisy breathing (stridor, stertor, or wheezing), flexible fiber-optic evaluation of the airway is critical to uncovering the etiology. Techniques for evaluating obstruction in the upper airway are described in the section on flexible laryngoscopy; however, as lower airway obstruction commonly occurs concomitant with these abnormalities, careful inspection from nose to bronchi may be prudent. Evaluation of dynamic obstruction in the airway requires the presence of spontaneous respiratory effort and careful modulation of the level of sedation.[22] The presence and severity of airway pathology are likely to be masked by positive-pressure ventilation, inadequate respiratory effort, or the stenting effect of an endotracheal tube.

Tracheomalacia and bronchomalacia result from inherent weakness in the airway cartilage, reduced large-airway smooth muscle tone, or both.[23] During exhalation, the diameter of the airway lumen can be reduced by transluminal pressure differences. In some cases, cartilaginous weakness is further exacerbated by compression from the heart and great vessels. Vascular compression may result from a right-sided or double aortic arch, pulmonary artery sling, aberrant innominate artery, or anomalous subclavian artery. If pulsatile tracheal compression is noted during bronchoscopy, further vascular imaging may be warranted. Symptoms of tracheomalacia typically include homophonous wheezing, barking-quality cough, and hypoxemic spells resulting from end-expiratory airway collapse. Treatment options range from supportive care (supplemental oxygen, continuous positive airway pressure) and medical therapies (inhaled ipratropium bromide, bethanechol)[24] in moderate cases to surgical intervention (tracheostomy, aortopexy) in severe cases. In some children, inhaled β agonists may exacerbate symptoms; however, coexisting small-airways bronchial constriction is common in these infants, and the potential benefit of inhaled bronchodilators may greatly exceed the risk.

Risks, Contraindications, and Limitations

Flexible bronchoscopy can be safe and well tolerated in critically ill neonates,[25,26] provided that a skilled and experienced team is available to perform the procedure, administer sedation with careful hemodynamic monitoring, and provide adequate respiratory support. Clear and effective communication between team members is of utmost importance, because a stable situation can quickly deteriorate in neonates with minimal cardiorespiratory reserve. Situational awareness is critical, and failure to recognize impending problems can result in resuscitation delay and poor outcomes. Resuscitation equipment and medications should be readily available.

Common side effects include fever, cough, hemoglobin desaturation, hypoventilation, and, in spontaneously breathing infants, laryngospasm.[27] Fever is observed in approximately 25% of cases when BAL is performed. It is typically low grade (<102°F), develops within 12 hours, and resolves within 24 hours. Persistent fever should warrant consideration of infectious etiologies. Cough and laryngospasm can be mitigated by topical anesthesia such as lidocaine, sedation, or neuromuscular blockade (when dynamic examination is not indicated). Hypoxemia and hypoventilation may develop as a consequence of anesthesia, bronchospasm, and obstruction of the airway lumen by the bronchoscope. In mechanically ventilated infants, positive airway pressures may need to be increased to accommodate for the increased resistance attributable to the presence of the bronchoscope in the endotracheal or tracheostomy tube. Likewise, higher fractions of inspired oxygen administered during the procedure will also reduce the risk of hypoxemia. Serious complications such as bleeding and pneumothorax are rare.

Often the most serious complications of flexible bronchoscopy are the result of cognitive errors. Clinically significant diagnostic findings may be quite subtle, and misinterpretation could delay appropriate treatment or lead to more invasive interventions without benefit to the patient. Another type of error is the failure to perform a bronchoscopy when the results of the procedure can lead to significant therapeutic benefit. A careful assessment of probability and magnitude of potential risks and benefits should be considered in the context of the team's experience and abilities. An experienced bronchoscopist can be a critical asset for an advanced neonatal critical care program.

Equipment

Flexible bronchoscopes are available from several manufacturers in a variety of sizes. They may be inserted via an endotracheal tube or a laryngeal mask airway in the mechanically ventilated neonate or through the nares when a better assessment of airway dynamics in desired and mechanical ventilation is not required. Flexible bronchoscopes require a light source, which transmits light through thin glass fibers to the tip of the instrument. An objective lens in the tip transmits the image back to the eyepiece or into a video processor for viewing on the monitor. Recording devices can be utilized and allow for review of the procedure findings at a later time.

The 2.2-mm external diameter bronchoscope allows airway evaluation in neonates of virtually any size or gestational age but lacks a channel for suction or saline administration needed to perform BAL. It can be accommodated through tracheostomy and endotracheal tubes of 3.0 mm or larger. The 2.7- and 2.8-mm bronchoscopes contain a 1.2-mm suction channel. They can be used to assist endotracheal intubation in tubes as small as 3.0 mm; however, a 3.5-mm tube is required to allow for adequate ventilation and maneuverability during diagnostic and therapeutic bronchoscopy. They are also available as a hybrid bronchovideoscope with which a magnified video image can be displayed on a monitor. The standard bronchoscope requires direct visualization via an eyepiece. A camera adapter can be attached to the eyepiece and displayed on a monitor; however, clarity and brightness of the image are reduced.

A lever positioned on the bronchoscope handle allows the user to flex or extend the tip of the bronchoscope when navigating the airway. Bronchoscopes with suction capability offer a suction valve and biopsy/injection port for instrumentation and lavage. Biopsy forceps and brushes can prove useful for obtaining diagnostic samples as well as aiding in evacuation of mucous plugs and clots from the airway.

At the conclusion of the procedure, careful handling and cleaning of the bronchoscope will reduce the risk of infection via contamination in future patients and ensure longevity of the equipment.

BRONCHOALVEOLAR LAVAGE AND TRACHEAL ASPIRATES

BAL refers to the sampling of airway and alveolar spaces by washing a segment or subsegment of the lung with saline and recovering the contents of the epithelial fluid lining (EFL).[28] It is best performed with bronchoscopic guidance in which the tip of the bronchoscope is wedged into the desired location. This effectively isolates the region to be lavaged and reduces spillover into other parts of the lung. Simple tracheal aspirates and nonbronchoscopic lavage can be performed by blindly inserting a catheter via the endotracheal tube. These options may be useful for obtaining cultures but are more likely to sample the contents of the large airways as opposed to the EFL.

Factors to be considered in selecting the location for BAL include physical exam findings, chest radiography, endoscopic findings, and the relative ease or difficulty in fluid recovery. The right middle lobe and lingula provide the greatest potential yield of fluid return because of their anterior position in the supine patient. Lavage aliquot volumes of 5 to 20 mL of body temperature saline are usually sufficient. A sterile collection container is attached to the suction valve of the bronchoscope, and the sample can be distributed into additional containers for a variety of laboratory analyses.

The BAL fluid will contain both cellular and noncellular elements. Cytologic analysis can be useful in determining the presence of infection. Whereas macrophages typically represent >90% of the alveolar white blood cell count, an abundance of neutrophils suggests the presence of bacterial infection. Lymphocyte predominance may prompt further evaluation for fungal or viral infections. Eosinophils are rarely recovered from the BAL fluid.

Microbial studies include bacterial, fungal, acid-fast and viral cultures, immunoassays, viral polymerase chain reaction tests, and organism-specific stains. Gomori methenamine silver stain can detect pneumocystis and fungal infection, whereas acid-fast stains identify tuberculous and nontuberculous mycobacterial infection. Other special stains can be used in cases of suspected pulmonary hemorrhage or chronic pulmonary aspiration. Iron stains can identify hemosiderin-laden macrophages, which are found in abundance approximately 72 hours following a pulmonary bleed. The lipid-laden macrophage index can be calculated as a marker for chronic aspiration. Unfortunately, this procedure is relatively time-intensive and limited by a degree of subjectivity in its interpretation. Published reports demonstrate a wide range of sensitivity and specificity.[29] Pepsin content is another potential marker of chronic aspiration; however, evidence to support this is still limited at the time of writing.[30]

SUMMARY

Flexible and rigid endoscopic examination of the neonatal airway provides valuable diagnostic information and can be safely performed in even the smallest neonates. Identifying the most appropriate diagnostic modalities requires understanding the strengths and limitations of each approach. This will allow the neonatal care team to communicate effectively with collaborating otolaryngology and pulmonary specialists and deliver the highest standard of care.

REFERENCES

A complete reference list is available at https://expertconsult .inkling.com/.

14

Cardiovascular Assessment

Dany E. Weisz, BSc, MD, MSc, and Patrick Joseph McNamara, MD, MRCPCH, MSc

INTRODUCTION

The goals of neonatal intensive care include the preservation of cardiorespiratory function and optimal tissue oxygen delivery, prevention of cerebral injury, and ensuring survival with normal neurodevelopment. While respiratory distress and the need for assisted ventilation are common in neonates and often appear pulmonary in origin, clinicians should remember that the heart and lungs are interdependent. Disturbance in one system may rapidly spread to the other, disrupting the balance between tissue oxygen supply and demand, and leading to hypoxia and cell death. Interventions aimed at improving one system may have paradoxically detrimental effects on the other or on the developing brain.

Cardiorespiratory maladaptation in the perinatal period and during postnatal critical illness is dependent on both gestational age at birth and the cascade of subsequent end-organ maldevelopment that follows disturbed preterm or term delivery. Physiologic and technological advances have facilitated the near-routine survival of infants previously considered to be at the limit of viability, though frequently with significant morbidity. However, the optimal approach to hemodynamic monitoring and cardiovascular decision making in critically ill neonates remains inadequately understood. The primary challenge is a lack of knowledge about the influence and pathophysiology of neonatal cardiovascular health on acute and chronic end-organ function. It is further complicated by the dynamic relationship between systemic and pulmonary hemodynamics and cellular metabolism. This chapter provides a pathophysiologic approach to the hemodynamic assessment and management of circulatory disorders of the ventilated neonate, incorporating high-quality evidence and highlighting areas for further research. In addition to the material in this chapter, the management of cardiovascular problems and pulmonary hypertension is also described in Chapters 32 and 33.

CARDIOVASCULAR CARE IN THE DELIVERY ROOM

Transitional Cardiovascular Physiology

At birth, dramatic and rapid changes in cardiovascular function and blood flow occur because of the initiation of lung aeration and removal of the placental circuit. Immediate neonatal hemodynamic and metabolic stability requires three critical adaptations.

Lung aeration triggers an increase in pulmonary blood flow (PBF): Lung aeration results in a rapid decrease in pulmonary vascular resistance (PVR) and increase in PBF to 10 to 20 times resting fetal levels. Pulmonary vasodilation occurs via several mechanisms, including increased oxygenation, enhanced activity of vasodilator agents, and changes in surface tension at the alveolar air–liquid interface that reduce perivascular tissue pressures and facilitate lung recoil.[1,2]

Central blood flow patterns are significantly altered: At birth, the increases in PBF and arterial oxygen tension, concomitant with clamping of the umbilical cord, result in major alterations in the blood flow across fetal channels. Ductus venosus flow, which is of placental origin via the umbilical vein, decreases markedly after umbilical cord clamping (UCC). Removal of the low-resistance placental circuit results in increased systemic vascular resistance and reduced systemic venous return to the right heart. Simultaneously, increased PBF results in increased pulmonary venous return to the left atrium. Increased left atrial pressure and decreased right atrial pressure displaces the flap of the foramen ovale over the fossa, abolishing the right-to-left atrial flow, although a residual left-to-right atrial shunt may transiently persist.

The postnatal reduction in PVR and increase in systemic vascular resistance (SVR) result in reversal of the fetal right-to-left ductus arteriosus shunt, which becomes balanced by 5 min of age, mostly left to right by 10 to 20 minutes, and entirely left to right by 24 hours of age in healthy term neonates.[3,4]

Increase in combined ventricular output: Right ventricular output (RVO) increases as the reduction in PVR and abolition of the right-to-left foramen ovale shunt lead to all systemic venous return moving through the right ventricle. The obligatory respiratory work and thermoregulation after delivery result in a tripling in oxygen demand in newborns relative to fetal levels. In addition, the left ventricle, which supplied oxygen to the brain, heart, and upper body during fetal life, must now supply oxygen to the entire body. The result is a near tripling of left ventricular output, which occurs because of increased heart rate and stroke volume. In contrast to the fetal left ventricle, which has a limited capacity to increase output, the left ventricle at birth is able to dramatically increase output because of increased β-adrenergic receptor activity and because it is no longer constrained by a pressure-loaded right ventricle.[5]

Delayed Cord Clamping

The shared fetal–placental circulation is abruptly divided at the time of UCC. Compared with delayed UCC, immediate UCC prior to the onset of ventilation results in a 30% to 50%

reduction in cardiac output due to the combined effects of decreased systemic venous return and increased left ventricular afterload.[6] Establishing ventilation prior to UCC maintains cardiac output by preserving systemic venous return and ventricular preload while allowing PBF to increase.

Very preterm infants, in whom low left ventricular output in the first hours of life is associated with increased intraventricular hemorrhage (IVH), may benefit from placental transfusion strategies.[7] Delayed UCC and umbilical cord milking reduce mortality, IVH, hypotension, and the need for blood transfusion in this population, with a limited number of studies supporting its use in extremely low birth-weight infants.[8,9] The optimal duration of delayed UCC in very preterm infants is unknown, although clinical trials have utilized durations of 30 to 120 seconds.

APPROACH TO THE CARE OF THE NEONATE WITH COMPROMISED OXYGENATION

Physiology

Impaired oxygenation occurs as a result of hypoventilation, ventilation–perfusion mismatch, impairment in the diffusion of oxygen across the alveolar–capillary membrane, or intra- or extrapulmonary vascular shunts that either reduce pulmonary arterial blood flow or permit mixing of deoxygenated blood into the systemic circulation. The etiologies of compromised systemic oxygenation can be broadly classified as cardiac or pulmonary in origin. Congenital heart lesions include ductal-dependent PBF (e.g., tricuspid atresia) or obligate mixing lesions (e.g., total anomalous pulmonary venous return). Pulmonary disease comprises lesions of both the airways and parenchyma (e.g., pneumonia, pneumothorax, pleural effusion) and the vasculature (pulmonary hypertension).

Pulmonary Hypertension

Pulmonary hypertension (PH) is characterized by a sustained elevation of pulmonary artery pressure (PAP), defined as a mean PAP >25 mm Hg when measured by right-heart catheterization or pulmonary artery peak systolic pressure >35 mm Hg when measured by echocardiography. Mean PAP is influenced by PBF, PVR, and pulmonary capillary wedge pressure (PCWP):

$$mPAP = [PVR \times PBF] + PCWP$$

PVR represents the net resistance to PBF and is influenced primarily by the number and diameter of pulmonary arterioles and blood viscosity. PCWP is the "back pressure" mitigating pulmonary venous return. It is typically analogous to left atrial pressure, except in cases of pulmonary vein stenosis, in which PCWP is elevated in the setting of normal left atrial pressure.[10] PH may therefore be due to increased PBF, PVR, or PCWP (Fig. 14-1). PBF is increased in systemic-to-pulmonary shunt lesions, which may be cardiac (ventricular or atrial septal defect, patent ductus arteriosus) or extracardiac (arteriovenous malformation, twin-to-twin transfusion) in origin. Elevated PCWP occurs with left-heart obstructive lesions (e.g., pulmonary vein or mitral valve stenosis) or impairment in left ventricular (LV) filling (e.g., related to ischemia or hypertrophic cardiomyopathy). PVR may remain elevated in infants with impaired transition and

congenital or acquired lesions, which may be pulmonary or extrapulmonary in origin.

Persistent Pulmonary Hypertension of the Newborn

Persistent pulmonary hypertension of the newborn (PPHN) is characterized by severe hypoxemic respiratory failure presenting shortly after birth because of inadequate postnatal reduction in PVR. Persistently elevated PVR may be due to neonatal maladaptation (e.g., asphyxia, meconium aspiration syndrome, sepsis), pulmonary maldevelopment (e.g., chronic fetal hypoxia, premature closure of the ductus arteriosus), or pulmonary underdevelopment (e.g., pulmonary hypoplasia, congenital diaphragmatic hernia). The pathophysiology of circulatory derangements in PPHN represents the common final pathway of the effects of excessive right ventricular (RV) afterload (of which PVR is the primary contributor), irrespective of the etiology of PPHN.

Decreased PBF and RV function are the interrelated primary aberrations that culminate in hemodynamic instability (Fig. 14-2). Unlike the thicker-walled and elliptical left ventricle, which is well-equipped to overcome increased afterload, the right ventricle is thin-walled and crescent-shaped, designed to function as a flow generator accommodating the entire systemic venous return to the heart.[11] High PVR results in decreased RV systolic ejection time, stroke volume, and PBF. The right ventricle may adapt by increasing myocardial contractility (known as a homeometric adaptation),[12] but if this adaptation fails, RV dilatation occurs, causing bowing of the interventricular septum into the left ventricle, impairing LV filling, and reducing LV function by disrupting the elliptical configuration that is optimal for LV myocardial performance. The resulting decrease in LV preload, stroke volume, and systemic blood pressure potentiates further negative systolic interaction and right ventricle–arterial uncoupling. Contractile dysfunction of the right ventricle further impairs LV function by virtue of their shared myocardial fibers, a phenomenon termed "ventricular interdependence." As systemic blood pressure decreases and right atrial pressure (RAP) increases (secondary to elevated RV pressure), right coronary perfusion pressure decreases, resulting in RV ischemia.[13]

PPHN, in its severe form, is called *persistent fetal circulation*, reflecting a very high PVR state that is associated with elevated RV and RA pressures, very low PBF, and reduced left-heart and aortic volume and pressure. In this setting, pure pulmonary-to-systemic (i.e., "right-to-left") shunts occur across the foramen ovale and patent ductus arteriosus (PDA), culminating in the systemic delivery of deoxygenated blood. While a right-to-left shunt across the patent foramen ovale (PFO) and PDA may help offload the pulmonary circulation, prevent RV failure, and support systemic blood flow (albeit with deoxygenated blood), it may also potentiate ongoing hypoxemia by perpetuating the low PBF state.

Comorbid neonatal lung disease, such as pneumonia or meconium aspiration syndrome, is negatively synergistic. The reduced PBF exacerbates preexisting V/Q mismatch, hypoxemia, and acidosis, which induces further pulmonary vasoconstriction and may impair the response to pulmonary vasodilator therapies.

Chronic Pulmonary Hypertension

Chronic PH is a clinically and pathophysiologically distinct entity from acute PH, developing later in life and representing a secondary rise in PVR that is driven by either acquired disease or the residual effects of symptomatic congenital pulmonary disease (e.g.,

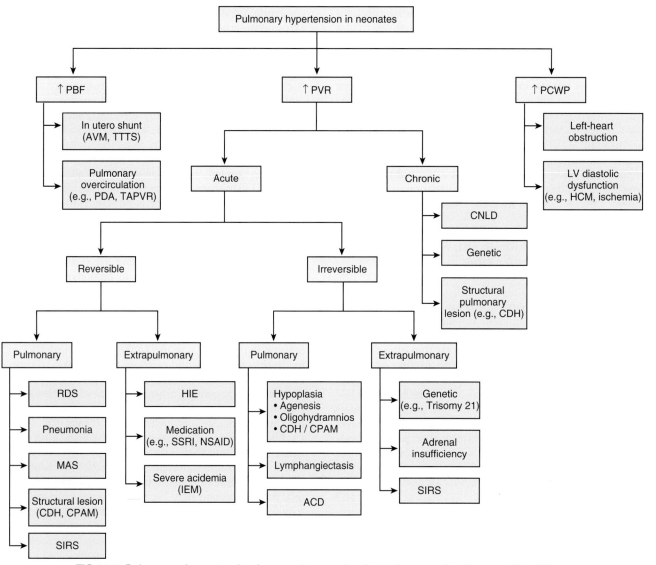

FIG 14-1 Pulmonary hypertension in neonates may be due to increased pulmonary blood flow (*PBF*), pulmonary vascular resistance (*PVR*), or pulmonary capillary wedge pressure (*PCWP*). Increased PVR may be classified as acute or chronic and may arise from a variety of underlying disorders. *ACD*, alveolar capillary dysplasia; *AVM*, arteriovenous malformation; *CDH*, congenital diaphragmatic hernia; *CNLD*, chronic neonatal lung disease of prematurity; *CPAM*, cystic pulmonary adenomatoid malformation; *HCM*, hypertrophic cardiomyopathy; *HIE*, hypoxic–ischemic encephalopathy; *IEM*, inborn error of metabolism; *LV*, left ventricle; *MAS*, meconium aspiration syndrome; *NSAID*, nonsteroidal antiinflammatory drug; *PDA*, patent ductus arteriosus; *RDS*, respiratory distress syndrome; *SIRS*, systemic inflammatory response syndrome; *SSRI*, selective serotonin reuptake inhibitor; *TAPVR*, total anomalous pulmonary venous return; *TTTS*, twin-to-twin transfusion.

congenital diaphragmatic hernia). Chronic lung disease of prematurity is a common complication among extremely preterm infants and is the most common cause of chronic PH in preterm infants.

Clinical Assessment

The diagnosis and evaluation of acute PPHN has been reviewed in previous chapters, and this section will focus on the circulatory assessment and support of infants with PPHN.

Cyanotic Congenital Heart Disease versus PPHN

In infants with suspected PPHN, alternate diagnoses such as cyanotic congenital heart disease (CHD) should be

considered and excluded early. Several clinical signs should raise suspicion of CHD in the setting of severe hypoxemia (Table 14-1). An abnormally shaped cardiac silhouette on a chest radiograph, and a markedly abnormal electrical axis of conduction on an electrocardiogram, may be suggestive of CHD (e.g., extreme right-axis deviation in Ebstein's anomaly). Echocardiography is the only routinely available method of definitive evaluation, and assessment is mandatory when infants with presumed PPHN fail to demonstrate improvement in hypoxemia as would be expected with resuscitative measures and pulmonary vasodilator therapies, or if extracorporeal membrane oxygenation is being considered.

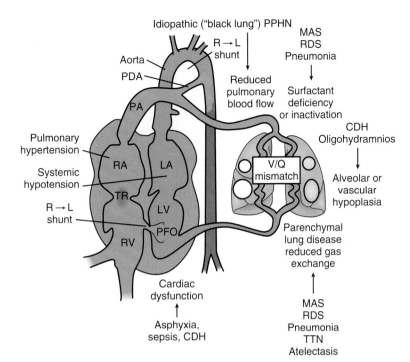

FIG 14-2 Circulatory pathophysiology in persistent pulmonary hypertension of the newborn (*PPHN*). Increased pulmonary vascular resistance results in RV dysfunction, reduced pulmonary blood flow (PBF), and right-to-left shunt through PDA and/or PFO. Pulmonary hypertension is often associated with septal deviation to the left and impaired LV filling and function. Cardiac dysfunction secondary to asphyxia, sepsis, or congenital diaphragmatic hernia (*CDH*) may complicate hypoxemic respiratory failure. Parenchymal lung disease secondary to respiratory distress syndrome (*RDS*), pneumonia, or meconium aspiration syndrome (*MAS*) can result in V/Q mismatch and hypoxemia that exacerbates LV dysfunction. Together, decreased LV preload (due to low PBF) and LV function manifest as systemic hypoperfusion and shock. Pulmonary hypoplasia secondary to CDH or due to oligohydramnios (prolonged leakage of fluid or reduced production due to renal compromise) causes alveolar and vascular hypoplasia and PPHN. *LA*, left atrium; *LV*, left ventricle; *PA*, pulmonary artery; *PDA*, patent ductus arteriosus; *PFO*, patent foramen ovale; *RA*, right atrium; *RV*, right ventricle; *TR*, tricuspid regurgitation; *TTN*, transient tachypnea of the newborn. (From Nair J, Lakshminrusimha S. Update on PPHN: mechanisms and treatment. *Semin Perinatol.* 38(2):78–91, 2014.)

TABLE 14-1 **Clinical Signs Suggestive of Congenital Heart Disease in the Setting of Hypoxemia**	
Clinical Sign	**Significance and Physiology**
Reverse differential cyanosis (preductal oxygen saturation is >10% lower than postductal)	Indicates right-to-left shunt of oxygenated blood across PDA (e.g., TGA, TAPVD)
Murmur	Critical valvular obstruction or coarctation
Oxygen saturation that is minimally variable with increases/decreases in FiO₂	Indicates reduced or relatively fixed PBF and the absence of a labile pulmonary vascular bed
Onset of severe hypoxemia after the first 12 h of life	Ductal-dependent PBF lesions presenting at time of closure of the ductus arteriosus
Diminished amplitude of lower limb pulses OR blood pressure in the lower limbs (postductal) >10-20 mm Hg lower than in the right arm (preductal)	Critical coarctation of the aorta

PBF, pulmonary blood flow; *PDA,* patent ductus arteriosus; *TAPVD,* total anomalous pulmonary venous return; *TGA,* transposition of the great arteries.

Delayed diagnosis of cyanotic CHD presenting with cardiovascular collapse and end-organ dysfunction is associated with increased mortality.[14]

The hyperoxia test may be helpful to distinguish between PPHN and cyanotic CHD in neonates with hypoxemic respiratory failure. A rise in PaO₂ >80 to 120 mm Hg above baseline after 100% oxygen administration, or an absolute PaO₂ >150 mm Hg in 100% oxygen, suggests that cyanotic CHD is unlikely. PaO₂ <50 mm Hg in 100% oxygen is highly suggestive of cyanotic CHD and should prompt the initiation of intravenous prostaglandin E₂ and referral to a pediatric cardiology center.[15] PaO₂ 50 to 150 mm Hg in 100% oxygen is equivocal and necessitates further evaluation.

Management

PPHN is a common, challenging clinical scenario that requires management in a tertiary-level neonatal intensive care unit (NICU). The management of PPHN comprises resuscitative measures and general management strategies aimed at optimizing cardiopulmonary status and targeted, judicious use of pulmonary vasodilators and vasoactive medications to optimize PBF and systemic oxygen delivery.

Resuscitation and General Management

In infants with mild hypoxic respiratory failure, stabilization and amelioration may frequently be achieved by the timely initiation of optimal intensive care support, without the need for inotropes or pulmonary vasodilator therapies. Some infants with mild PPHN secondary to hypoxic–ischemic encephalopathy, respiratory distress syndrome, or sepsis may achieve stability with noninvasive ventilation. However, infants with more significant disease typically require endotracheal intubation and invasive mechanical ventilation, which permits the administration of higher peak and mean airway pressures to facilitate alveolar recruitment and ventilation.

Several physiologic and therapeutic targets for ventilated infants with PPHN may lower PVR and should be employed when the etiology of PPHN is suspected or proven to be due to elevated PVR and unrelated to increased PCWP or PBF. Mean airway pressure should be titrated to achieve alveolar recruitment and maintain lung volumes at functional residual capacity, which is the point of maximum pulmonary compliance and minimal PVR (Fig. 14-3). Acidemia should be corrected, initially by targeting normal (but not low) $PaCO_2$ and by optimizing the systemic delivery of oxygen to minimize ischemia and associated lactic acidosis, with the goal of achieving a normal serum pH. In neonates with adequate assisted ventilation (defined as a near-normal $PaCO_2$) the administration of a slow intravenous infusion of sodium bicarbonate may augment serum pH and reduce PVR, though the clinical benefits of exogenous alkali administration remain unproven. Oxygen supplementation should be titrated to target PaO_2 of 60 to 80 mm Hg, which minimizes PVR and avoids the deleterious effects of hyperoxia. Agitation and work of breathing precipitate an acute rise in PVR and therefore adequate sedation/analgesia should be administered, with neuromuscular blockade for severely affected infants.

Specific Pulmonary Vasodilator Therapies and the Role of Targeted Neonatal Echocardiography

Infants with severe hypoxemic respiratory failure (HRF) may have insufficient improvement after the initiation of invasive mechanical ventilation, and the oxygen index (OI) should be calculated to quantify the derangement in oxygenation.

$$\text{Oxygen Index} = \frac{\text{Mean Airway Pressure} * \text{FiO}_2 * 100}{\text{PaO}_2}$$

Infants with HRF and OI>25 may benefit from inhaled nitric oxide (iNO), which has been demonstrated to reduce the composite outcome of death or extracorporeal membrane oxygenation (ECMO).[16] The earlier initiation of iNO for OI 15 to 25 improves oxygenation but without improvement in mortality or the need for ECMO.[17] In units in which access to iNO and high-frequency ventilation is limited, oral sildenafil improves oxygenation and reduces mortality in term infants with HRF.[18]

For preterm infants with HRF, the potential benefits of routine iNO are less clear and a targeted approach to administration is required. A recent meta-analysis of individual patient data from international trials found that iNO conferred no improvement in mortality, bronchopulmonary dysplasia (BPD), or severe neurologic events compared with placebo.[19-21] The lack of benefit of iNO in preterm infants may reflect the heterogeneity of clinical disease in the study

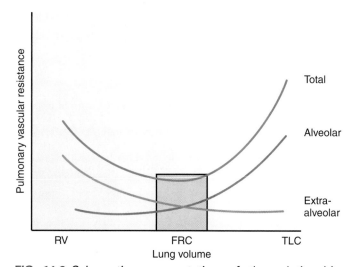

FIG 14-3 Schematic representation of the relationship between pulmonary vascular resistance (PVR) and lung volume. As lung volume increases from residual volume (*RV*) to total lung capacity (*TLC*), the alveolar vessels become increasingly compressed by the distending alveoli, resulting in increased resistance in the intra-alveolar vessels. The resistance of extra-alveolar vessels decreases with increasing lung volumes because they become less tortuous. The net effect of increasing lung volumes on the pulmonary vasculature produces the typical "U-shaped" curve, with its nadir (representing lowest PVR) at functional residual capacity (*FRC*). (Data from Shekerdemian L, Bohn D. *Archives of Disease in Childhood.* 80:475–480, 1999.)

population, in which pulmonary parenchymal disease and less reversible etiologies of increased PVR are more common. Nitric oxide may be beneficial in highly selected preterm infants with refractory HRF and echocardiography-proven PH. Observational studies have associated iNO with improvement in oxygenation and neonatal outcomes in preterm infants with pulmonary hypoplasia from prolonged exposure to oligohydramnios after second-trimester premature rupture of the fetal membranes.[22-24]

Echocardiography should be performed in any infant with severe HRF with a suboptimal response to iNO, both to exclude CHD and to characterize the hemodynamic derangement (Tables 14-2 and 14-3). First, the severity of PH should be assessed, using quantitative and qualitative measures and assessment of the ductal and atrial shunts. Second, the effects of elevated PVR on ventricular (RV and LV) myocardial performance, outputs, and dilatation should be evaluated. Targeted neonatal echocardiography (TNE) may help guide the administration of second-line pulmonary vasodilators whose use is primarily supported by physiologic principles.

Vasopressin may improve oxygenation in infants with refractory severe HRF and hypotension despite iNO therapy, especially in infants with decreased PBF as evidenced by exclusively right-to-left shunts across the foramen ovale and ductus arteriosus.[25] The mechanism of action of vasopressin has not been fully elucidated, but may involve a reduction in PVR/SVR ratio and improved LV filling, resulting in improved PBF, myocardial performance, and LV output (LVO).[26] Vasopressin administration should be avoided in infants with cardiogenic shock due to primary LV dysfunction, as its potent systemic vasoconstrictive

TABLE 14-2 Targeted Neonatal Echocardiographic Assessment in Persistent Pulmonary Hypertension of the Newborn

Pulmonary Artery Resistance and Pressure	Left-Heart Function and Systemic Circulation	Right-Heart Function and Pulmonary Blood Flow
Quantitative: Estimation of RVSp from peak velocity of TR jet or PDA Doppler	*LV preload:* Subjective assessment of LV chamber size and Doppler of pulmonary venous inflow and mitral valve inflow in diastole	*RV contractility:* Quantitative assessment • Tricuspid annular plane systolic excursion • Tissue Doppler-derived peak systolic velocity of base of RV • Fractional area change
Semiquantitative: Monitor progress using serial measurements of Doppler-derived time intervals characteristic of systolic blood flow in MPA—pulmonary artery ejection time to pulmonary artery acceleration time.	*LV contractility:* Quantitative assessment • Fractional shortening • Ejection fraction (Simpson biplane method) • mVCFC • Tissue Doppler-derived peak systolic velocity of LV free wall	Qualitative assessment of RV contractility and dilatation *Pulmonary blood flow:* Quantitative measurement of RVO and stroke distance in the MPA
Qualitative: Estimation of RVSp relative to systemic systolic pressure—interventricular septal curvature and pattern of blood flow across PDA and PFO	Qualitative assessment of LV contractility *Systemic blood flow:* Quantitative measurement of LVO and stroke distance in the ascending aorta	

LV, left ventricle; *LVO*, left ventricular output; *MPA*, main pulmonary artery; *mVCFC*, mean velocity of circumferential fiber shortening corrected for heart rate; *PDA*, patent ductus arteriosus; *PFO*, patent foramen ovale; *RV*, right ventricle; *RVO*, right ventricular output; *RVSp*, right ventricular systolic pressure; *TR*, tricuspid regurgitation.
(Data from MacDonald MG, Seshia MMK, *Avery's Neonatology: Pathophysiology and Management of the Newborn.* Lippincott Williams and Wilkins/Wolters Kluwer Health; 2015.)

TABLE 14-3 Progression of Clinical and Echocardiographic Indices by Severity of Persistent Pulmonary Hypertension of the Newborn

PPHN Severity		MILD ➤ SEVERE		
		Isolated HRF	**HRF, Low Systemic Output**	**HRF, Low Systemic Output, RV Failure**
Clinical		• Increased WOB • High FiO$_2$ • Normal end-organ function	• Mild pre/post-SpO$_2$ gradient • ↓ SBP/normal DBP • ± ↓ End-organ function	• Pre/post-SpO$_2$ gradient >10% • ↓↓ SBP/↓DBP • Shock (e.g., ↑ lactate, acidosis)
Echocardiography	RVSp	Systemic (approx.)	Systemic/suprasystemic	Suprasystemic
	IVS	Flat	Flat	Paradoxical (bows into LV)
	PDA	Bidirectional	Mostly R to L	Pure R to L
	PFO	Bidirectional/L to R	Bidirectional	Pure R to L
	LV	Normal	• ↓ Preload • ↓/Low–normal LVO • ± Reduced function	• ↓↓ Preload • ↓↓ LVO • ± Reduced function
	RV	Normal	• ↓ PBF (low RVO) • ↓ Function • None/mild dilatation	• ↓↓ PBF • ↓↓ Function • Moderate/severe dilatation

DBP, diastolic blood pressure; *FiO$_2$*, fraction of inspired oxygen; *HRF*, hypoxic respiratory failure; *IVS*, interventricular septum; *LV*, left ventricle; *LVO*, left ventricular output; *PBF*, pulmonary blood flow; *PDA*, patent ductus arteriosus; *PFO*, patent foramen ovale; *PPHN*, persistent pulmonary hypertension of the newborn; *RV*, right ventricle; *RVO*, right ventricular output; *RVSp*, right ventricular systolic pressure; *SBP*, systolic blood pressure; *WOB*, work of breathing.

effects (and increased LV afterload) may result in reduced LVO.[27] Although vasopressin administration results in increased renal blood flow, its use may be associated with hyponatremia due to free water retention, an effect that resolves upon discontinuation.

Intravenous low-dose epinephrine is an alternative to vasopressin and provides inotropic support for infants with myocardial dysfunction; however, its effect on the PVR/SVR ratio is unpredictable and it has been associated with lactic acidosis.

Infants with severe RV dysfunction and dilatation whose ductus arteriosus is closed or restricted may benefit from an intravenous infusion of prostaglandin E$_2$ (PGE$_2$) to restore ductal patency and reduce RV afterload. However, PGE$_2$ should be used cautiously in the setting of diastolic hypotension because of its systemic vasodilatory effects, which may decrease systemic venous return, exacerbate coronary hypoperfusion, and precipitate acute circulatory collapse.

Intravenous milrinone, a phosphodiesterase-3 inhibitor with lusitropic, inotropic, and systemic vasodilatory effects, has been associated, in case series and nonrandomized studies, with improved oxygenation in term and preterm infants with PH and RV dysfunction.[28-30] Use of milrinone should be avoided in infants with diastolic hypotension and with hypoxic–ischemic encephalopathy undergoing therapeutic hypothermia, in whom reduced milrinone metabolism may result in profound hypotension.

APPROACH TO THE INFANTS WITH COMPROMISED SYSTEMIC HEMODYNAMICS

Physiology

A low systemic blood flow (SBF) state is defined as having inadequate ventricular output to meet tissue oxygen consumption. Delivery of oxygen (DO$_2$) also comprises measures of oxyhemoglobin saturation and the arterial tension of oxygen; however, cardiac output is the most important contributor to DO_2 in neonates in the absence of profound anemia or severe hypoxemia.

$$DO_2 = \text{Cardiac output} \times \text{Arterial } O_2 \text{ concentration}$$
$$[SV \times HR] \; [1.34 \times Hb \times SaO_2] + [PaO_2 \times 0.003]$$

The clinical relevance of low SBF is emphasized by its high incidence and association with cerebral injury. In preterm infants, low SBF (commonly estimated as LVO or superior vena cava (SVC) flow) occurs in one-third of very low birth-weight (VLBW) infants in the first days of life and is associated with increased mortality, IVH, abnormal cerebral electrical activity, and neurodevelopmental impairment in early childhood.[7,31,32]

Blood pressure is frequently used as a surrogate for SBF, and serial monitoring of blood pressure may be performed using oscillometry or direct catheter measurement (via the umbilical artery or a peripheral artery). Oscillometric devices (i.e., cuff) have varying reliability in blood pressure measurement compared with invasive catheters, with cuff pressures tending to overestimate blood pressure in critically ill, hypotensive infants, though studies are prone to selection bias by the inclusion of infants with indwelling arterial catheters.[33-35]

The natural history of systemic arterial pressure has been described in large cohorts of infants. Systolic blood pressure (SBP) changes rapidly in the immediate transitional period, with a nadir at 4 to 6 hours of age in preterm infants.[36] Younger gestation is associated with lower blood pressure, and values rise with increasing gestational age, with normative data available for both term and preterm infants[37,38] (Tables 14-4 and 14-5). Delayed cord clamping and umbilical cord milking reduce the risk of early hypotension in preterm infants and support a causal role of decreased circulating blood volume in the pathogenesis of low blood pressure during the transitional period.[39]

While the use of mean blood pressure (MBP) to define hypotension (often as MBP less than gestational age) approximates published normative data, the individual components of SBP and diastolic blood pressure (DBP) may provide additional insight into the etiology of the hypotension. Low SBP is suggestive of reduced LV stroke volume, which may be due to reduced preload, decreased contractility, or increased afterload (Table 14-6). Low DBP reflects reduced intravascular volume status and/or SVR (Table 14-7). Combined systolic and diastolic hypotension represents the final common endpoint at which the circulatory system is unable to compensate for ongoing hemodynamic stress. The evolution of events and blood pressure measurements preceding the onset of combined hypotension may provide an indication of the underlying etiology.

In neonates, and, in particular, the transitional circulation of preterm infants, the correlation between blood pressure and SBF is weak. Blood pressure demonstrates poor correlation with LVO or RVO, SVC flow, and descending aorta blood flow in moderate and extremely preterm infants.[40,41] Although older studies reported a significant association between hypotension and adverse neurodevelopmental outcome, more recent large cohort studies have reported mixed results. In a prospective cohort study of 945 extremely preterm infants, hypotension in the first 24 hours of life was not associated with sonographic cerebral white matter injury or neurodevelopmental outcome at 24 months corrected gestational age.[42,43] Management of hypotension in preterm infants without the integration of measures of SBF and cerebral perfusion

TABLE 14-4 Blood Pressure Thresholds (3rd Percentile) According to Postconceptual Age in Preterm Infants

Postconceptual Age (weeks)	Systolic (3rd Percentile)	Mean (3rd Percentile)	Diastolic (3rd Percentile)
24	32	26	15
25	34	26	16
26	36	27	17
27	38	27	17
28	40	28	18
29	42	28	19
30	43	29	20
31	45	30	20
32	46	30	21
33	47	30	22
34	48	31	23
35	49	32	24
36	50	32	25

Blood pressure presented as mm Hg.
(Adapted from Systolic blood pressure in babies of less than 32 weeks gestation in the first year of life; Data from Northern Neonatal Nursing Initiative. *Arch Dis Child Fetal Neonatal Ed.* 1999;80:F38–42.)

TABLE 14-5 Blood Pressure Thresholds According to Postnatal Age in Healthy Term Neonates

Threshold		Day 1	Day 2	Day 3	Day 4
95th percentile	Systolic	78	83	86	88
	Mean	57	62	64	65
50th percentile	Systolic	65	69	70	71
	Mean	48	51	53	55
5th percentile	Systolic	54	57	59	63
	Mean	39	41	41	43

Blood pressure presented as mm Hg.
(Data from Kent AL, Kecskes Z, Shadbolt B, et al. Normative blood pressure data in the early neonatal period. *Pediatr Nephrol.* 2007;22:1335–41.)

may result in the misidentification of at-risk infants and the subsequent inappropriate administration or withholding of treatment.

Central venous pressure (CVP) monitoring may provide additional information to help guide management in the neonate with low SBF. CVP represents RAP averaged over the entire cardiac cycle and provides an invasive measure of RV preload in infants without PH or obstructive shock. Monitoring in the NICU is not routinely performed and requires the placement of a venous catheter with its tip entering the right atrium. Healthy (nonventilated) term neonates have CVP ranging from −2 to 4 mm Hg. There is a shortage of data for the ventilated neonate, though a small case series of ventilated preterm infants with hyaline membrane disease reported a mean CVP of 2.6 to 7.0 mm Hg.[44]

Low CVP (<1 mm Hg) in the ventilated neonate may be indicative of hypovolemia.[44] Higher CVP values may reflect greater cardiac preload, but may also represent higher right-heart pressures from PH, myocardial dysfunction, or elevated intrathoracic pressure (e.g., tension pneumothorax). As a result, serial measurements of CVP are necessary and must be interpreted within the clinical context.

TABLE 14-6   Systolic Hypotension in Neonates: Pathophysiology and Common Etiologies

Primary Pathophysiology	Secondary Pathophysiology	Clinical Examples
Decreased LV preload	Impaired systemic and pulmonary venous return due to increased intrathoracic/intracardiac pressure (obstructive shock)	• Pulmonary overdistension due to excess mean airway pressure • Tension pneumothorax • Pericardial effusion with tamponade
	Decreased pulmonary blood flow and pulmonary venous return	• Pulmonary arterial hypertension
	Impaired LV filling due to diastolic dysfunction	• Hypertrophic obstructive cardiomyopathy (e.g., IDM)
Cardiogenic shock	Myocardial ischemia	• Hypoxic–ischemic encephalopathy • Acute coronary syndrome • Tachyarrhythmia
	Intrinsic/congenital defects	• Cardiomyopathy
Excess LV afterload	Failure of adaptation after change in loading conditions	• Transitional loss of low-resistance placental circuit after birth • Ligation of patent ductus arteriosus
	Cold shock	• Sepsis with peripheral vasoconstriction due to redistribution of blood to vital organs
	Iatrogenically elevated SVR	• Exogenous vasopressor administration

IDM, infant of diabetic mother; *LV*, left ventricular; *SVR*, systemic vascular resistance.

TABLE 14-7   Diastolic Hypotension in Neonates: Pathophysiology and Common Etiologies

Primary Pathophysiology	Secondary Pathophysiology	Clinical Examples
Intravascular volume depletion	Hemorrhage	• Perinatal (e.g., placental abruption, acute TTTS) • Postnatal (e.g., adrenal, intraventricular)
	Capillary leak	• Systemic inflammatory response syndrome (e.g., sepsis, NEC) • Hypoalbuminemia (e.g., hepatic failure)
	Dehydration or insensible water loss	• Prematurity (transepidermal water loss, polyuria due to inadequate renal concentrating ability) • Gastrointestinal (gastric suctioning, diarrhea)
Decreased systemic vascular tone	Autonomic dysregulation	• Extremely preterm infant
	Warm shock	• Sepsis with peripheral vasodilation
	Inadequate stress response	• Primary or secondary adrenocortical insufficiency
	Iatrogenically lowered SVR	• Exogenous vasodilator administration • Sedative/narcotic administration
Enlarged vascular bed	Low resistance circuit in parallel with systemic circulation	• Patent ductus arteriosus • Arteriovenous connection (e.g., vein of Galen aneurysmal malformation)

NEC, necrotizing enterocolitis; *SVR*, systemic vascular resistance; *TTTS*, twin-to-twin transfusion.

Clinical Evaluation

A low SBF state should be suspected when clinical or biochemical parameters suggest reduced end-organ perfusion (Table 14-8). Therapy should be directed at the underlying etiology, which may be difficult to identify. The clinical history may identify risk factors for various causes of a low output state, such as perinatal hypoxia–ischemia, dehydration, risk factors for sepsis, and respiratory status such as mean airway pressure and oxygenation.

In the setting of acute hemodynamic collapse in previously stable neonates, several diagnoses should be rapidly considered and treated. Reversible causes of acute obstructive shock such as tension pneumothorax and pericardial tamponade should be excluded. Ductal-dependent SBF lesions, such as critical aortic stenosis, should also be considered, with pediatric cardiology consultation sought early. If sepsis is suspected, broad-spectrum antimicrobial and/or antiviral agents should be administered.

In the unwell infant with clinical evidence of inadequate systemic perfusion, the finding of a systemic blood pressure in the normal range should not delay the initiation of therapy, as this may reflect a state of compensated shock. In the hypotensive infant, the presence of isolated systolic or diastolic hypotension may provide insight into the underlying pathophysiology and etiology. Infants with a rapidly progressive process, such as overwhelming septic shock, benefit from aggressive therapy and early echocardiography.

VLBW (<1500 g) preterm infants with early postnatal hypotension represent a unique diagnostic and therapeutic challenge. The prevention of early IVH and periventricular hemorrhagic infarction (PVHI), both associated with neurodevelopmental impairment, is an important management goal. These infants frequently require positive-pressure ventilatory support for respiratory distress syndrome and the unfavorable pulmonary mechanics of small airway size and a compliant chest wall. While

TABLE 14-8   Clinical and Biochemical Parameters of Reduced End-Organ Function

Organ System	Physical Examination	Laboratory Tests and Radiographs	Other Tests
Central nervous system	Abnormal mental status/lethargy Seizures	• CT/MRI brain: hypoxia–ischemia, AVM, hemorrhage, increased ICP	• aEEG: seizures, abnormal background
Cardiovascular	Tachy/bradycardia Hypotension Abnormal heart sounds/murmur Capillary refill time (vasoconstriction/ dilation) Pulse amplitude (stroke volume)	• Chest radiograph: cardiac silhouette size (underfilled, volume loaded, pericardial effusion, abnormal shape suggestive of congenital heart disease) • Troponin/creatinine kinase: myocardial ischemia • Blood gas (base deficit >5) and arterial lactate (>2) • Systemic venous O_2 saturation	• ECG • 2D echo
Airway and pulmonary	Reduced air entry Tachypnea Hypoxemia	• Chest radiograph: air leak, pleural effusion, parenchymal infection or inflammation, edema, overdistension, mediastinal mass, diaphragmatic hernia • Arterial blood gas: respiratory acidosis	• Pressure–volume graph (invasive mechanical ventilation)
Renal	Low urine output Urine microscopy: active urine sediment or inflammation	• Serum urea, creatinine, cystatin-C	

Gastrointestinal	Emesis or gastric residuals
	Abdominal distension and discoloration, tenderness
		• Abdominal radiograph/sonography
		  – NEC: pneumatosis intestinalis, bowel wall edema, pneumobilia, sentinel loop
		  – Perforation: intra-abdominal free air
		  – Intestinal dilatation: obstruction/impaired transit	

Hepatic	Jaundice Petechiae/purpura (coagulopathy)	• Coagulation profile (PT/PTT, D-dimer, fibrinogen): DIC • Other hepatic function (glucose, albumin, bilirubin) • Hepatocellular injury (AST, ALT, ALP, GGT)	

aEEG, amplitude-integrated electroencephalography; *ALP*, alkaline phosphatase; *ALT*, alanine aminotransferase; *AST*, aspartate aminotransferase; *AVM*, arteriovenous malformation; *CT*, computed tomography; *DIC*, disseminated intravascular coagulation; *ECG*, electrocardiogram; *GGT*, γ-glutamyl transferase; *ICP*, intracranial pressure; *MRI*, magnetic resonance imaging; *NEC*, necrotizing enterocolitis; *PT*, prothrombin time; *PTT*, partial thromboplastin time; *2D echo*, two-dimensional echocardiography.

hypotension frequently co-occurs with respiratory failure, there is a current lack of understanding regarding the etiologies and long-term sequelae of this physiologic event. The discordance between hypotension and low SBF, a weak association between hypotension and neurodevelopmental outcome, and the lack of improvement in outcomes with treatment of early hypotension have resulted in uncertainty regarding which infants may benefit from treatment.[40,42,43,45]

In ventilated VLBW preterm infants with borderline hypotension in the first day of life who demonstrate no clinical or echocardiographic indicators of a low SBF state, the risk of developing sonographic brain injury is low and a period of close clinical observation may be warranted.[7] However, in infants with hypotension and clinical, laboratory, or echocardiographic indicators of a low SBF state, treatment should be considered, targeting the suspected underlying etiology.

Role of Targeted Neonatal Echocardiography

Echocardiography provides direct visualization and evaluation of ventricular preload, myocardial performance, and the effect of shunt lesions, which may be clinically identified only with a very high index of suspicion. Early identification of ductal-dependent SBF lesions or pericardial tamponade may be lifesaving. In addition, echocardiography may confirm the hemodynamic profile suspected based on the clinical history, such as poor LV filling due to hypertrophic cardiomyopathy in infants born to mothers with diabetes mellitus. Hypotensive infants with hypoxic–ischemic encephalopathy and concomitant PPHN are a complex population in which echocardiography is paramount in identifying the relative

contributions of myocardial dysfunction and low PBF to the systemic low-flow state.

Infants with refractory septic shock are a high-risk population in which TNE may provide critical hemodynamic insight to guide therapy. Direct assessment of ventricular filling assists in determining the need for additional intravascular volume expansion in the face of evolving capillary leak. Empirical vasopressor use is common, and verifying the presence or absence of LV dysfunction assists the clinician in the decision to respectively reduce or augment the dose. Finally, TNE may determine whether the infant is in a high or low CO state and direct the need for vasopressors or inotropes/inodilators, respectively.

TNE may be especially illuminating in the management of the hypotensive VLBW preterm infant. In the setting of systolic hypotension, echocardiography may differentiate between a low LV preload state (e.g., due to low systemic venous return from pulmonary hyperinflation) or reduced myocardial function secondary to high postnatal afterload. Common etiologies for early diastolic hypotension in this population include sepsis, intravascular volume loss, adrenocortical insufficiency, autonomic dysregulation, and PDA, the last of which is often clinically silent in the first days of life and detectable only by echocardiography.

Echocardiography may also identify a systemic low-flow state in VLBW preterm infants at risk of IVH/PVHI, by estimating ventricular output or SVC flow. In observational studies of extremely preterm infants, IVH/PVHI is associated with low LVO (<175 mL/kg/min) and SVC flow (<30 mL/kg/min at 6 hours or <34 mL/kg/min at 12 hours) in the first 6 to 18 hours of life followed by rapid increases to normal levels at 24 to 48 hours of life.[7,31]

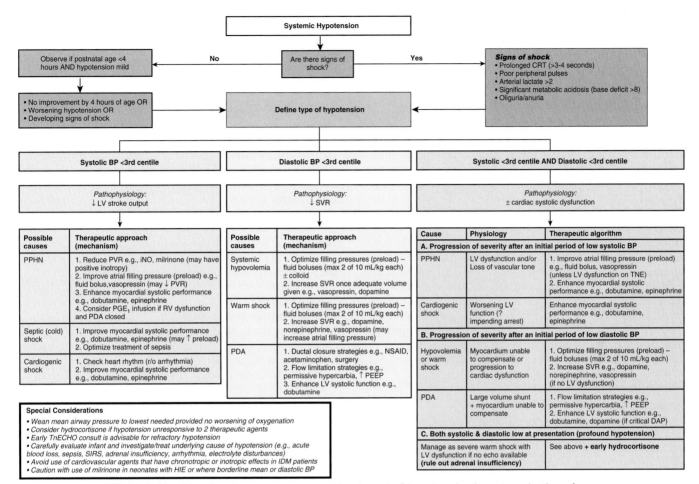

FIG 14-4 Algorithm for the assessment and treatment of hypotension by categorization of systolic, diastolic, or combined systolic and diastolic hypotension. *BP*, blood pressure; *CRT*, capillary refill time; *DAP*, diastolic arterial pressure; *iNO*, inhaled nitric oxide; *LV*, left ventricle; *NSAID*, nonsteroidal antiinflammatory drug; *PDA*, patent ductus arteriosus; *PEEP*, positive end-expiratory pressure; *PGE₁*, prostaglandin E₁; *PPHN*, persistent pulmonary hypertension of the newborn; *PVR*, pulmonary vascular resistance; *RV*, right ventricle; *SVR*, systemic vascular resistance; *TNE*, targeted neonatal echocardiography. (Data from MacDonald MG, Seshia MMK. *Avery's Neonatology: Pathophysiology and Management of the Newborn.* Lippincott Williams and Wilkins/Wolters Kluwer Health; 2015.)

Management

There is considerable uncertainty regarding the optimal timing, patient selection, and pharmacotherapeutic agent for the treatment of hypotension in ventilated term and preterm infants. For clinical scenarios in which there is a dearth of studies to guide management, patient evaluation and treatment should follow a pathophysiologic approach guided by the known or presumed etiology. Distinguishing between systolic and diastolic hypotension may aid in identifying the underlying pathology (Fig. 14-4). While the therapeutic approach described in the sections below provides a physiologic framework for the management of infants with hypotension, most of the interventions described are not supported by high-quality evidence and research is required to investigate their efficacy and safety.

Systolic Hypotension

Systolic hypotension reflects diminished LV stroke volume, and management should be directed at augmenting LV performance. Obstruction to LV filling due to pneumothorax or pericardial tamponade should be rapidly alleviated. In hypotensive infants of mothers with poorly controlled diabetes mellitus, biventricular hypertrophy may impair LV filling and should be treated with fluid resuscitation and weaning of inotropic medications that exacerbate impaired diastolic relaxation. LV preload may be optimized by rationalizing the positive end-expiratory pressure (PEEP) or mean airway pressure (MAP) in invasively ventilated infants to improve systemic venous return. A bolus of 10 to 20 mL/kg of 0.9% sodium chloride (normal saline) may be administered to augment preload in infants who are suspected to have MAP-associated decreased systemic venous return but in whom ventilatory pressures cannot be weaned.[46] In the setting of hypoxic respiratory failure, systolic hypotension may be secondary to decreased PBF from PH, and therapies aimed at reducing PVR should be considered (see section on Persistent Pulmonary Hypertension of the Newborn).

Dobutamine, a synthetic catecholamine with predominantly β-adrenergic activity, may be used in neonates with systolic hypotension due to impaired LV function. Epinephrine, a predominantly β-adrenergic agonist at lower doses (0.01 to 0.05 mcg/kg/min) and α-adrenergic agonist at higher doses (0.1 to 0.5 mcg/kg/min), should be considered a second-line agent in the setting of myocardial dysfunction. Epinephrine increases myocardial oxygen demand, and long-term use may be associated with myocardial strain. Infants with myocardial dysfunction related to high LV afterload (e.g., cold septic shock, post-PDA ligation), characterized clinically by a normal/high DBP and narrow pulse pressure, may benefit from the combined lusitropic, inotropic, and afterload-reducing effects of an intravenous infusion of milrinone.

For very preterm newborns on the first day of life, systolic hypotension may be uniquely related to myocardial dysfunction from increased afterload after removal of the low-resistance placental circuit. Although milrinone is a therapeutic option supported by physiologic rationale, a randomized placebo-controlled trial of prophylactic intravenous milrinone on day 1 demonstrated no improvement in SVC flow or IVH.[47] Dobutamine is an alternative therapeutic option for preterm infants with low SVC flow or suspected or proven mild-to-moderate LV dysfunction and may reduce the risk of late IVH/PVHI.[32]

Diastolic Hypotension

Low DBP generally reflects reduced SVR or intravascular volume depletion, and treatment should target the underlying etiology (see Table 14-7). Intravascular volume expansion with a 10 to 20 mL/kg bolus of 0.9% sodium chloride is a first-line therapy in the setting of dehydration, capillary leak, or warm septic shock. Additional volume may be administered based on clinical evaluation and the biochemical and echocardiographic response to the initial bolus. Diastolic hypotension due to reduced SVR but refractory to fluid resuscitation may be treated with intravenous vasopressor infusions such as dopamine (5 to 15 mcg/kg/min), which has been consistently demonstrated to be superior to dobutamine at increasing blood pressure. Epinephrine may be considered in the setting of diastolic hypotension and concomitant LV dysfunction. Norepinephrine is a potent β1- and α-adrenergic agonist, which increases systolic and DBP and SVR, with limited evidence in term neonates that it may be effective in septic shock refractory to fluid resuscitation, dopamine, and dobutamine.[48]

Glucocorticoids have been demonstrated to increase blood pressure in neonates with refractory hypotension by upregulating catecholamine production and adrenergic receptor expression and should be considered in cases of refractory hypotension. Hydrocortisone has been well studied in neonates and is typically administered at a dose of 0.5 to 1 mg every 6 hours.

Identifying the etiology of diastolic hypotension in very preterm infants on the first day of life is challenging. A combined clinical–echocardiographic evaluation is important to define and manage the relative contributions of intravascular volume depletion, reduced SVR, and PDA, which all merit different therapeutic approaches. Diastolic hypotension due to a large PDA may be supportively managed with strategies to judiciously increase PVR (see next section) or with intravenous dobutamine. Adrenocortical insufficiency is common in extremely preterm infants and intravenous hydrocortisone is

effective in the treatment of refractory hypotension without an increase in short-term adverse effects.[49]

APPROACH TO THE INFANT WITH PATENT DUCTUS ARTERIOSUS

Pathophysiologic Continuum of the Ductal Shunt in Neonates

In ventilated neonates, the ductal shunt may be conceptualized as residing on a continuum between lifesaving conduit, innocent bystander, and prime pathologic contributor. For infants with critical CHD, patency of the ductus arteriosus may be necessary for adequate PBF or SBF. In severe PPHN, the right-to-left ductal shunt may support postductal SBF and reduce RV afterload. A bidirectional shunt in milder cases of PPHN may play a neutral role, merely permitting the noninvasive estimation of the systemic–pulmonary pressure gradient.

Persistent PDA may become pathologic in infants with low PVR and a large systemic-to-pulmonary (left-to-right) shunt. Blood flows across the PDA continuously in both systole and diastole, resulting in volume overload of the pulmonary artery, pulmonary veins, and left heart. Shunt volume is proportional to ductal diameter and length, the aortopulmonary pressure gradient, and blood viscosity. Increased PBF may lead to alveolar edema, reduced pulmonary compliance, and increased need for respiratory support. Left-heart volume loading manifests as LV and left-atrial dilatation and elevated end-diastolic pressure. Ductal diastolic "steal" from the descending aorta, shorter diastolic (and coronary perfusion) times due to tachycardia, and increased myocardial oxygen demand may result in subendocardial ischemia.

Clinical Importance of the Patent Ductus Arteriosus

The clinical importance of the PDA in preterm infants is highlighted by its high incidence (up to 65%) in extremely preterm infants and its consistent association with adverse neonatal outcomes, including death, IVH, BPD, necrotizing enterocolitis, and retinopathy of prematurity (ROP).[50] While a causal link between PDA and adverse outcomes has not been firmly established, the prevention of IVH by the administration of prophylactic indomethacin, which causes ductal constriction, provides some support for a causal role of the PDA.[51]

The natural history of the PDA is toward closure. In a study of 70 extremely preterm infants (mean gestational age 26 weeks) with PDA on day 3 who were closely followed but not medically or surgically treated, ductal closure occurred prior to discharge in 73% of infants. Importantly, the clinical outcomes of this cohort were characterized by above-average rates of severe IVH, BPD, and death.[52] However, decades of clinical trials aimed at facilitating late (after day 7 of life) ductal closure have failed to demonstrate improvement in outcomes. This may be due to a true lack of treatment benefit (i.e., that preterm infants with PDA are "programmed" for increased morbidity), suboptimal patient selection upon trial entry, or the ubiquitous use of open-label treatment. Studies have demonstrated that infants with longer exposure to high-volume PDA shunts, as staged by echocardiography, are at increased risk of BPD.[53] Further correlation with clinical outcomes is required to refine the definition of which PDA shunts are "pathologic" and may benefit from treatment.

Determining the Hemodynamic Significance of the Ductus Arteriosus

The evaluation of the hemodynamic significance of the PDA in preterm infants requires an estimation of the volume of ductal shunting (by clinical examination, echocardiography, and ancillary tests) and a clinical interpretation of the relative impact of the shunt in the context of the severity of prematurity and coexisting multisystem morbidity, such as respiratory distress syndrome, enteral feeding intolerance, or a low SBF state.

The classical clinical and radiologic signs of a hemodynamically significant PDA in preterm infants are related to the physiologic effects of pulmonary overcirculation, left-heart volume loading, and systemic steal. Alveolar edema and impaired pulmonary compliance lead to oxygenation and ventilation failure and an increased need for ventilatory support. The precordium is active and a systolic or continuous murmur may be audible at the upper-left sternal border, often radiating to the entire precordium. The manifestations of systemic steal are variable and range from the common findings of a wide pulse pressure and bounding peripheral pulses to diastolic hypotension, metabolic acidosis, and renal insufficiency. The clinical signs of a hemodynamically significant PDA are insensitive in the first week of life and lag behind the echocardiographic diagnosis by approximately 2 days.[54,55]

Imaging and plasma biomarkers may assist in the diagnosis of a hemodynamically significant PDA. Electrocardiography may demonstrate LV hypertrophy and left-atrial dilatation, but has poor sensitivity. Chest radiography may reveal left-heart dilatation and pulmonary edema. Plasma brain natriuretic peptide (BNP) and amino-terminal pro-BNP, two biomarkers of cardiac pressure and volume loading, are predictive of hemodynamically significant PDA after the second day of life. Chen et al. reported that BNP <40 pg/mL excluded a moderate or large PDA shunt with high sensitivity (92%) and BNP >200 pg/mL was highly specific (91%),

but that results within the 40 to 200 pg/mL range are inadequately discriminatory and necessitate echocardiographic evaluation.[56] Although these biomarkers have been repeatedly shown to have high sensitivity and specificity for a significant PDA, the heterogeneity in various testing kits, study methodologies, and populations used to assess diagnostic validity limits the broad use of these biomarkers in clinical practice.[57]

Echocardiography

Echocardiography is the most reliable and available method for diagnosis of PDA in preterm infants. Evaluation and staging of severity requires assessment of ductus arteriosus size and transductal flow pattern, indices of pulmonary overcirculation and left-heart volume loading, and systemic arterial diastolic flow reversal (Table 14-9).

Assessment of Patent Ductus Arteriosus Size and Transductal Flow Pattern. A ductal diameter ≥1.5 mm on the first day of life predicts a subsequently symptomatic PDA.[58] The transductal flow pattern permits a simultaneous evaluation of the systemic–pulmonary pressure gradient and the degree of restriction to ductal blood flow[59] (Fig. 14-5). A hemodynamically significant PDA is characterized by an "unrestrictive" or "pulsatile" arterial left-to-right flow pattern. Whereas a peak systolic velocity <1.5 m/s has been described as unrestrictive, an elevated peak systolic velocity is not, in isolation, pathognomonic of a restrictive PDA. Higher peak systolic velocities (2.0 to 3.5 m/s) may be seen in infants with a very high volume shunt and low PVR. Peak PDA systolic velocity should therefore be interpreted in the context of the "pulsatility" of the ductal shunt Doppler pattern, which can be quantified using the peak PDA systolic velocity/end-diastolic velocity ratio, which correlates with prolonged ductal patency.[60] The restricted or "closing" pattern of a PDA depicts a high-velocity ductal shunt throughout systole and diastole, due to ductal narrowing and associated flow acceleration.

TABLE 14-9 Echocardiography Parameters of Ductal Hemodynamic Significance

Parameter		HEMODYNAMIC SIGNIFICANCE		
		Mild	**Moderate**	**Severe**
Ductus arteriosus size and flow pattern	PDA diameter			
	2D diameter	<1.5 mm	1.5-3 mm	>3 mm
	PDA/LPA ratio	<0.5	0.5-1	>1
	PDA Doppler			
	Peak systolic velocity*	>2.5	1.5-2.5	<1.5
	Peak systolic velocity: minimum diastolic velocity	<2	2-4	>4
Pulmonary overcirculation/ left-heart loading	LV output (mL/kg/min)	<300	300-450	>450
	LV dilatation	None ($Z < +1.5$)	Mild–moderate ($+1.5 < Z < +2.5$)	Marked ($Z > +2.5$)
	LA hypertension			
	LA/Ao	<1.5	1.5-2.0	>2.0
	Mitral valve E/A ratio	<1	<1	>1
	IVRT	>45 ms	30-45 ms	<30 ms
	LPA V_{max} diastole	<0.3 m/s	0.3-0.5 m/s	>0.5 m/s
Systemic steal	Abdominal aorta	No diastolic reversal	Diastolic reversal	Diastolic reversal
	Celiac/aorta VTI ratio	—	—	<0.10

*Very large left-to-right ductal shunts may have higher peak systolic velocities (>1.5 m/s), indicating high shunt volume rather than flow restriction.
Ao, aorta; *IVRT*, isovolumic relaxation time; *LA*, left atrium; *LPA*, left pulmonary artery; *LV*, left ventricle; *PDA*, patent ductus arteriosus; V_{max}, maximum velocity; *VTI*, velocity–time integral.
(Data from MacDonald MG, Seshia MMK. *Avery's Neonatology: Pathophysiology and Management of the Newborn.* Lippincott Williams and Wilkins/Wolters Kluwer Health; 2015.)

Assessment of Pulmonary Overcirculation and Left-Heart Volume Loading. Left-heart dimensions and output, pulmonary artery diastolic velocities, and transmitral Doppler flow patterns are surrogate estimates of the pulmonary-to-systemic flow ratio (Q_p/Q_s), though they may underestimate Q_p/Q_s in the presence of a large left-to-right transatrial shunt. Infants with a hemodynamically significant PDA have elevated LVO and left-heart dilatation. Normal LVO is 200 to 300 mL/kg/min. LVO >300 mL/kg/min on the first day of life predicts later symptomatic PDA, and LVO >450 mL/kg/min suggests a large shunt.[58]

LV end-diastolic dimension (LVEDD) is a surrogate for LV end-diastolic volume. LVEDD may be compared to published normative data in healthy preterm infants, and LVEDD >15 mm typically indicates significant LV dilatation in infants with weight <1250 g.[61,62]

Left-atrial dilatation occurs because of volume loading from excessive pulmonary venous return and may be quantified using the left atrium-to-transaortic root ratio (LA/Ao). LA/Ao ≥1.5 has high sensitivity for a hemodynamically significant PDA after the first day of life.[63]

Left-atrial pressure loading occurs because of LV diastolic dysfunction and impaired LV filling in the setting of excessive pulmonary venous return and may be estimated using mitral valve inflow Doppler indices and isovolumic relaxation time[64] (Fig. 14-6).

Assessment of Systemic Steal. Diastolic flow reversal in the abdominal aorta is a reliable indicator of a hemodynamically significant PDA, which correlates best with MRI-derived estimates of shunt volume and resolves after ductal closure.[65,66] Reduced celiac artery flow (CAF), as quantified by a CAF/LVO ratio <0.1, is also a sensitive marker of a large ductal

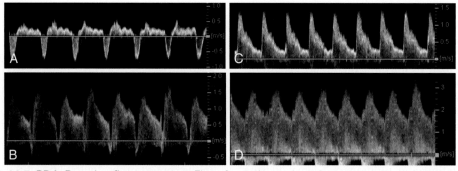

FIG 14-5 PDA Doppler flow patterns. Flow from the main pulmonary artery to the aorta is depicted as a Doppler signal below the baseline and flow from the aorta to the pulmonary artery is depicted as a Doppler signal above the baseline. **A,** Pulmonary hypertension pattern, characterized by a right-to-left or bidirectional shunt (as shown here) with significant right-to-left component in systole. **B,** Growing pattern, characterized by almost entirely left-to-right shunting with a small right-to-left component in early systole. **C,** Pulsatile or unrestrictive pattern, characterized by a left-to-right shunt with an arterial waveform and high peak systolic velocity/end-diastolic velocity ratio. **D,** Restrictive pattern, characterized by high systolic and diastolic velocity and low peak systolic velocity/end-diastolic velocity ratio. (From Weisz DE, Jain A, McNamara PJ. *Patent Ductus Arteriosus.* Ediciones Journal SA; 2016.)

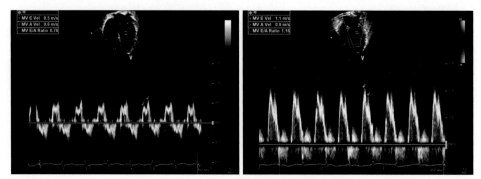

FIG 14-6 Pulse-wave Doppler of left ventricular (LV) inflow across the mitral valve, demonstrating the early (*E*) and late (*A,* during atrial contraction) ventricular filling velocities. Transmitral LV filling in normal term infants is characterized by a predominance of *E* diastolic filling, with limited *A* LV filling occurring during atrial contraction, resulting in an *E/A* ratio of >1. *Left,* healthy preterm infants without a patent ductus arteriosus (PDA) have intrinsically decreased LV diastolic function, relying more on *A* atrial filling, and *E/A* of <1. *Right,* preterm infants with a large PDA have increased left-atrial pressure, which results in earlier mitral valve opening and drives early passive filling, resulting in shortened isovolumic relaxation time (<45 ms) and a "pseudonormalized" *E/A* of >1. (From Weisz DE, Jain A, McNamara PJ. *Patent Ductus Arteriosus.* Ediciones Journal SA; 2016.)

shunt.[67] Although PDA is associated with altered flow in the superior mesenteric and middle cerebral arteries, the clinical consequences of this are unknown.

Management of a Hemodynamically Significant PDA
Conservative Management: Strategies to Limit Shunt Volume

Supportive measures are strategies aimed to reduce shunt volume or improve an infant's physiologic tolerance of the ductal shunt, without targeting ductal closure. Administration of PEEP may reduce systemic and pulmonary venous return, unloading the LV toward a more favorable position on the Frank–Starling curve and improving left-heart dilatation. It may also reduce left-to-right ductal shunting through MAP-associated increases in PVR. In infants with large PDA receiving mechanical ventilation, an increase in PEEP from 5 to 8 cm H_2O reduces echocardiographic indices of ductal shunting without adversely affecting cerebral perfusion or oxygenation.[68]

The rationale for other commonly used strategies are based primarily on physiologic principles or extrapolation of clinical studies in term infants. Maintaining a higher hematocrit may mitigate ductal shunting by increasing PVR, without adversely affecting systemic oxygen delivery or LV stroke work.[69] Although targeting a lower, instead of higher, oxygen saturation range (85% to 90% vs 90% to 95%) may reduce ductal shunting by increasing PVR, this strategy of relative hypoxemia is associated with higher mortality in broader populations of extremely low birth-weight infants and should be used with caution.[70] Diuretics, such as furosemide, may reduce pulmonary edema and left-heart dilatation, though its use in preterm infants with PDA is extrapolated from term infants with other acyanotic shunts. However, furosemide increases renal prostaglandin synthesis, which may impair ductal constriction, and long-term use is associated with nephrocalcinosis.

Fluid restriction has been reportedly used to reduce left-heart volume loading and pulmonary edema in infants with a large ductal shunt. However, total fluid intake (TFI) would have to be severely restricted (beyond renal concentrating ability) to reduce ventricular preload, which may affect nutritional intake and growth. Moderate fluid restriction has not been demonstrated to mitigate ductal shunting. In a study of 18 extremely preterm infants with large PDA, moderate fluid restriction (restriction of TFI from 145 to 108 mL/kg/day) was associated with reduced SBF without any improvement in left-heart volume loading.[71]

Ductal Closure Strategies

Pharmacotherapy: Inhibition of Circulating Prostaglandins. Early postnatal ductal patency is promoted by circulating PGE_2, whose production from membrane phospholipids is catalyzed by several enzymes, including prostaglandin H_2 synthase (PGHS). PGHS complex comprises both cyclooxygenase and peroxidase (POX) moieties, which are potential pharmacotherapeutic targets to reduce PGE_2 and facilitate ductal closure (Fig. 14-7). Nonsteroidal antiinflammatory drugs (NSAIDs), such as indomethacin and ibuprofen, are potent cyclooxygenase inhibitors and have been reliably demonstrated to facilitate ductal closure in preterm infants. Efficacy of NSAIDs for ductal closure decreases with advanced postnatal age as vasodilators other than prostaglandins become more prominent regulators of ductal patency. More recently, acetaminophen, an inhibitor of the POX moiety of PGHS, has been demonstrated to result in ductal constriction.

Prophylaxis. The administration of intravenous prophylactic indomethacin to extremely preterm infants after birth reduces the risk of intraventricular and pulmonary hemorrhage, symptomatic PDA, surgical PDA ligation, and periventricular leukomalacia, compared with later symptomatic treatment only, but without improvement in mortality or neurodevelopmental outcomes at 2 years.[51] Although the broad usage of prophylactic indomethacin has declined, evidence of improved childhood language development in boys, coupled with the clear short-term benefits, has led to its continued use in some centers.[72] Prophylactic ibuprofen similarly prevents the development of symptomatic PDA and the need for surgical ligation, but increases the risk of gastrointestinal bleeding, without improvement in IVH or other neonatal outcomes.

Early (Day 1 to 3) Treatment of Asymptomatic Patent Ductus Arteriosus. Early treatment of infants with echocardiographically diagnosed but clinically asymptomatic PDA prevents the administration of universal prophylaxis to the 30% to 40% of extremely preterm infants who would not develop PDA. A placebo-controlled randomized trial demonstrated that treatment

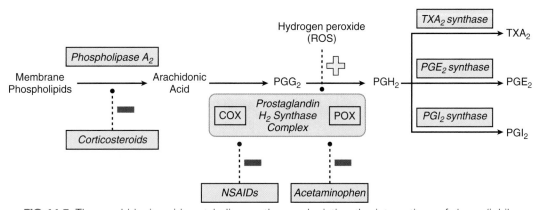

FIG 14-7 The arachidonic acid metabolism pathway, depicting the interactions of drugs (inhibitory, such as corticosteroids, NSAIDs, or acetaminophen/paracetamol) and endogenous compounds (stimulating, such as hydrogen peroxide and reactive oxygen species) with the enzymes involved in this pathway that regulate the production of prostaglandins. *COX,* cyclooxygenase; *PG,* prostaglandin; *POX,* peroxidase; *ROS,* reactive oxygen species; *TXA2,* thromboxane A2. (From Weisz DE, Jain A, McNamara PJ. *Patent Ductus Arteriosus.* Ediciones Journal SA; 2016.)

with indomethacin for infants with PDA ≥1.5 mm in the first 6 hours of life reduced the risk of pulmonary hemorrhage.[73] Other trials have demonstrated that early treatment of asymptomatic PDA reduces the risk of later symptomatic PDA but without improvement in neonatal outcomes.[74,75]

Treatment of Symptomatic Patent Ductus Arteriosus. Contemporary randomized controlled trials have compared the efficacy of early (day 3) vs late (after day 7 to 10) treatment of symptomatic PDA in mixed populations of moderately and extremely preterm infants. Early treatment reduces the incidence of later symptomatic PDA but without improvement in neonatal outcomes, suggesting that moderately delayed PDA closure (at 10 to 14 days) may be tolerated, reducing the need for NSAID treatment without increased morbidity.[76,77] However, the potential detriment of prolonged exposure to a large ductal shunt in the most fragile babies is unknown. Ibuprofen is as effective as indomethacin for PDA closure, but with lower risk of necrotizing enterocolitis and transient renal insufficiency.[78] Compared with intravenous ibuprofen, oral ibuprofen reduces the failure rate of PDA closure, with a similar adverse effects profile. Oral acetaminophen has been demonstrated to have efficacy similar to that of oral ibuprofen for ductal closure in a trial of 90 preterm infants with birth weight ≤1250 g with PDA at 48 to 96 hours of life.[79]

Surgical Ligation. Surgical PDA ligation is reserved as rescue therapy after failure or contraindication to pharmacologic treatment, often for infants with persistent dependence on mechanical ventilation. Immediate surgical mortality is very low (<1%) but complications are not uncommon and include bleeding, pneumothorax, chylothorax, left vocal cord paresis, and inadvertent ligation of an adjacent bronchus or branch pulmonary artery.

Compared with medically treated infants, surgical ligation has been associated with increased BPD, severe ROP, and neurodevelopmental impairment in early childhood.[80] Despite the presence of residual bias due to confounding by indication, these studies have been accompanied by a secular trend toward avoiding surgical ligation, with mixed results. In a single-center study comparing outcomes in an epoch of delayed selective ligation compared with early routine ligation after failure of medical PDA closure, the strategy of delayed selective ligation was associated with a reduced need for surgical ligation and improved neurodevelopmental outcomes.[81] Other observational studies have associated a conservative approach to the PDA, including avoidance of surgical ligation, with increased mortality and BPD.[82,83] The possibility of spontaneous PDA closure after failure of medical treatment appears to safely permit a limited period of conservative management prior to surgical ligation. However, the association of persistent symptomatic PDA with adverse outcomes suggests the ductal shunt is potentially hazardous and that surgical ligation remains an important treatment option.

Percutaneous (transcatheter) occlusion of PDA is an emerging alternative to transthoracic surgical ligation. Case series have reported successful PDA device closure in preterm infants using either a femoral venous or an arterial approach.[84-86] Although successful device occlusion occurs in most (>85%) infants, small infant size at surgery remains the primary limitation to the percutaneous approach, because of the physical size of the device, stiffness of the device delivery system, protrusion risk of the device into the left pulmonary artery or aorta, and technical difficulties in device retrieval if misplaced or embolized. A retrospective case series of 52 very preterm infants with median

procedural weight of 2.9 kg reported adverse events in 33% of infants, with the most common being acute arterial injury.[85] No clinical trials have compared the efficacy and safety of surgical ligation vs percutaneous occlusion of the PDA in preterm infants.

Perioperative Physiology and Management. Adrenocortical insufficiency is common in preterm infants undergoing PDA ligation, and infants should undergo a preoperative adrenocorticotropic hormone (ACTH) stimulation test. A post-ACTH serum cortisol level of <750 nmol/L is associated with increased postoperative cardiorespiratory instability.[87] Intraoperatively, the administration of high-dose fentanyl (≥10 mcg/kg) at the time of induction anesthesia is associated with reduced postoperative respiratory instability.[88]

Ligation of the PDA results in an instantaneous reduction in LV preload and increase in afterload, which places up to half of infants at risk of postoperative respiratory insufficiency and hypotension, termed *postligation cardiac syndrome (PLCS)*. PLCS is characterized by a decline in LV performance and output, which clinically manifests as systolic hypotension and ventilation/oxygenation failure beginning 4 to 12 hours after surgery. Weight <1 kg and postnatal age <28 days are preoperative risk factors for PLCS.[89] The administration of targeted intravenous milrinone prophylaxis to infants with a 1-hour postoperative LVO <200 mL/kg/min has been associated with a reduced risk of PLCS.[90] Infants who develop PLCS may benefit from treatment with dobutamine or milrinone to augment LV systolic performance and reduce afterload, though milrinone monotherapy should be avoided in infants with concomitant diastolic hypotension. Immediate postoperative diastolic hypotension is unlikely to be related to PLCS, and an alternate etiology (e.g., pneumothorax, hemorrhage, adrenocortical insufficiency) should be sought. Infants who fail to mount a postoperative surge in serum cortisol are at increased risk of catecholamine-resistant hypotension. Early postoperative estimation of cortisol levels in hypotensive patients and hydrocortisone administration may be helpful.[91]

HEART–LUNG INTERACTIONS IN THE INTENSIVE CARE UNIT: THE EFFECTS OF MECHANICAL VENTILATION ON HEMODYNAMICS

The heart and lungs work closely together to provide sufficient tissue oxygen delivery, and interventions implemented to assist one system may have beneficial or detrimental effects on the other. Mechanical ventilation induces changes in lung volumes and intrathoracic pressures that may dramatically affect preload, contractility, and afterload in the critically ill neonate.

Atrial Preload

Blood flow to the right atrium is dependent on a driving gradient between the extrathoracic great veins and the right atrium. In healthy infants, thoracic expansion during inspiration generates a negative intrathoracic and intrapleural pressure and ultimately a reduced RAP, increasing this gradient and enhancing systemic venous return. Diaphragmatic descent during inspiration further enhances the driving gradient by increasing intra-abdominal pressure, facilitating venous return from the lower extremities and abdomen.

Increased RAP may diminish ventricular preload and may be due to intrinsic factors (e.g., PH) or extrinsic factors, such as pericardial tamponade, tension pneumothorax, or positive airway pressure. Positive airway pressure during invasive mechanical ventilation is transmitted to the right atrium, reducing the extrathoracic great vein–right atrium gradient and compromising atrial preload. Excessive MAP may impair CO throughout the respiratory cycle, though this is partially offset by an increase in systemic arterial pressure that occurs in response to increased intrathoracic pressure. Intravascular volume expansion may improve CO when high MAP is needed.[46]

Initiation and Augmentation of Mechanical Ventilation, Premedication, and Intravascular Volume

Clinicians should consider the potential adverse effect of MAP in reducing atrial preload and CO when initiating or augmenting invasive mechanical ventilation. Premedication, commonly an opioid analgesic and neuromuscular blocker, is commonly administered to optimize the conditions for successful and timely endotracheal tube placement. However, these medications may result in a decrease in systemic vascular tone, peripheral blood pooling, and reduced atrial preload. For infants with intravascular volume depletion (e.g., hemorrhage, dehydration, capillary leak due to systemic inflammatory response syndrome) or pressure-passive pulmonary circulation (e.g., Fontan circulation), the combined negative effects of positive-pressure ventilation and premedication on right-atrial preload and CO may precipitate acute circulatory collapse at the time of the endotracheal intubation.

The initiation of high-frequency (HF) modes of ventilation may have a significant impact on systemic venous return and CO compared with intermittent positive-pressure ventilation (IPPV). The effect of mechanical ventilation on CO is ultimately dependent on MAP, as demonstrated by similar outputs when IPPV or HF modes utilize the same MAP.[92] However, when an HF mode is initiated as "rescue" after inadequate ventilation and oxygenation on IPPV, it is common practice to use a higher MAP, which may be associated with reduced CO.[93] Compared with HF oscillatory ventilation, HF jet ventilation may facilitate similar gas exchange using a lower MAP because of its use of passive exhalation.[94] MAP should be titrated to optimize alveolar inflation and systemic venous return.

Left Ventricular Function and Afterload: The Effects of Intrathoracic Pressure

Aortic valve opening and ejection of blood from the left ventricle into the aorta occurs when LV end-diastolic pressure (P_{LVED}) exceeds aortic pressure. At end diastole, P_{LVED} equals the sum of the pressure across the LV wall (known as the LV transmural pressure, P_{LVTM}) and any forces applied to the ventricular wall by the surrounding tissues, namely transpericardial and pleural pressures ($P_{TRANSPERICARDIAL}$ and $P_{PLEURAL}$, respectively). Pleural pressure represents the aggregate of forces arising from the interaction between the chest wall and the lung.

$$P_{LVED} = P_{LVTM} + P_{TRANSPERICARDIAL} + P_{PLEURAL}$$

During spontaneous, negative-pressure inspiration, both intravascular aortic and pleural pressures fall, but the decrease in pleural pressure is relatively greater than the fall in aortic pressure. Consequently, LV transmural pressure increases (to generate adequate end-diastolic LV pressure), resulting in increased LV afterload and reduced stroke volume.

For infants with LV dysfunction, the administration of PEEP during invasive mechanical ventilation may have several beneficial effects. First, the reduction in right-atrial preload associated with PEEP decreases PBF and LV preload, which may optimize LV position on the Starling curve. Second, pleural pressure is positive in infants receiving PEEP, reducing the LV transmural pressure gradient and decreasing LV afterload.[95] Finally, PEEP may improve alveolar patency and ventilation–perfusion mismatch caused by secondary pulmonary edema.

Pulmonary Hypertension and Overcirculation: Lung Volumes and Pulmonary Vascular Resistance

PVR, the main determinant of RV afterload, is influenced by lung volumes. PVR is minimized when lung volumes are at functional residual capacity (FRC), which reflects the optimal balance of vascular resistance in alveolar and extra-alveolar pulmonary vessels (see Fig. 14-3). Neonates with pulmonary arterial hypertension due to high PVR benefit from the titration of lung volumes to achieve FRC, both to facilitate ventilation (and optimize the delivery of inhaled pulmonary vasodilators such as nitric oxide) and to minimize PVR.

Targeting changes in lung volume to modulate PVR may be helpful in the intensive care management of infants with structural heart disease. Excessive PBF in acyanotic shunt lesions (e.g., PDA) may be modulated by modest augmentation in PEEP, presumably because of increased pulmonary arterial pressure and a decreased systemic–pulmonary pressure gradient.[68] Targeting higher lung volumes to increase PVR may also be a useful adjunct in the neonate with univentricular physiology and excessive PBF (e.g., hypoplastic left-heart syndrome) to improve SBF.

REFERENCES

A complete reference list is available at https://expertconsult.inkling.com/.

15

Overview of Assisted Ventilation

Martin Keszler, MD, FAAP, and Robert L. Chatburn, MHHS, RRT-NPS, FAARC

Effective mechanical ventilation of newborn infants is a relatively late phenomenon in the care of newborn infants, having evolved within the lifetime of many practitioners active today. The death in 1963 of the late preterm son of a president of the United States from respiratory failure is a stark reminder of how inadequate respiratory care was only 50 years ago. Today, few babies die as a result of primary respiratory failure; mortality is more often from complications of extreme prematurity and infection. However, while mechanical ventilation has greatly reduced mortality from pulmonary causes, morbidity, including bronchopulmonary dysplasia, remains high.

As discussed in Chapter 17, avoidance of mechanical ventilation may be the best way of avoiding ventilator-induced lung injury. With increased use of antenatal steroids and improved delivery room stabilization approaches, most moderately preterm and many very preterm infants are able to be supported noninvasively. In contrast, a substantial proportion of extremely low gestational-age neonates (ELGANs) continue to require mechanical ventilation. Almost 90% of extremely low birth-weight infants (ELBW) cared for in the Neonatal Research Network centers in 2005 were treated with mechanical ventilation during the first day of life, and 95% of survivors were invasively ventilated at some point during their hospital stay.[1] In the Surfactant, Positive Pressure, and Oxygenation Randomized Trial (SUPPORT), 83% of the ELBW infants initially assigned to noninvasive support received endotracheal intubation and mechanical ventilation at some point during their neonatal intensive care unit (NICU) stay.[2] Thus invasive ventilation is largely reserved for the relatively small number of the most immature or very sick infants. Because fewer infants now receive mechanical ventilation, there is a decreased level of experience for trainees and practitioners. Infants who receive mechanical ventilation today tend to be smaller and more immature than those ventilated in an earlier era and may remain ventilator-dependent for extended periods, sometimes for reasons not related to their lung disease. The spectrum of lung disease that neonatologists treat has expanded into more chronic conditions that we are less accustomed to treating. Furthermore, today's patients may be uniquely susceptible to lung injury because of the very early stages of lung development at which they are born.

All these issues make it important to optimize the way mechanical ventilation is managed so that preventable mortality and morbidity can be avoided. Some degree of lung injury is probably inevitable in mechanically ventilated ELGANs even with optimal respiratory support. However, the wide range of the incidence of bronchopulmonary dysplasia in the individual NICUs within the U.S. Neonatal Research and Vermont–Oxford Networks suggests that mechanical ventilation may be a potentially modifiable risk factor.[3] Although the evidence to guide respiratory support strategies remains incomplete, the potentially best practices and the rationale for them will be outlined in this and subsequent chapters.

UNIQUE CHALLENGES IN MECHANICAL VENTILATION OF NEWBORN INFANTS

Individuals involved in the care of critically ill newborn infants should be keenly aware that newborns are not simply small children, any more than children are simply small adults. Sophisticated microprocessor-based ventilators with advanced features enabling effective synchronized ventilation are now widely available. However, it is essential to recognize that better technology alone will not improve outcomes. Unless used with care and with optimal ventilation strategies that are appropriate for the specific condition being treated, these machines cannot materially influence outcomes. To optimally utilize the complex devices at our disposal, we need to be aware of the many unique aspects of a newborn infant's respiratory physiology. These are reviewed in detail in Chapter 2, but key aspects that directly affect the provision of invasive mechanical ventilation are summarized below.

Lung Mechanics

Small infants with poorly compliant lungs have very short time constants and normally have rapid respiratory rates with very short inspiratory times to match their lung mechanics. They have limited muscle strength and a very compliant chest wall so they struggle to develop adequate inspiratory flow or pressure. This situation imposes great technological challenges on device design, especially in terms of triggering ventilator inflations in synchrony with the onset of inspiratory effort, inflation termination, and tidal volume measurement. Suboptimal ventilator design for neonatal applications may lead to excessive trigger delay with asynchrony, failure to trigger or terminate inflation, and errors in tidal volume measurement or delivery. These technological challenges have largely been overcome in modern ventilators but remain a problem in some older devices still in use.

Uncuffed Endotracheal Tubes

Uncuffed endotracheal tubes (ETTs) have traditionally been used in newborn infants, because of concern about pressure necrosis of the tracheal mucosa. The small size of the tubes also makes inflatable cuffs difficult to incorporate without compromising lumen size. For this reason, some degree of gas leak around the ETT is present in most infants. Despite the lack of supporting evidence, some practitioners believe that it is important to have an audible leak around the tube to ensure the fit is not too tight. Unfortunately, substantial leak makes tidal volume estimation increasingly inaccurate, an issue that has become more relevant with increasing use of volume-targeted ventilation. Increasing leak around the ETT develops over time in infants who require prolonged ventilation, because the larynx and trachea progressively dilate from the cyclic stretch of many thousands of inflations per day. Leak is greater during inflation, because the pressure gradient driving the leak is greater and because the airways distend with the higher inflation pressure. Therefore, it is important to measure both inspiratory and expiratory tidal volume (V_T), with the latter more closely approximating the volume of gas that had entered the lungs. The leak varies from moment to moment because the ETT is inserted only a short distance beyond the larynx and thus the leak will change with any change in the infant's head position and movement of the ETT up and down in the trachea. Because of these difficulties, a reconsideration of the prohibition of cuffed tubes has been proposed.[4]

Measurement of Tidal Volume

The importance of very accurate V_T measurement in any sort of volume-controlled/volume-targeted ventilation of extremely small infants is obvious, considering that infants weighing 400 to 1000 g require V_T in the range of 2 to 5 mL. Unfortunately, most so-called universal ventilators designed primarily for adult patients, but capable of supporting the full range of ages, measure flow and calculate V_T at the output of the flow control valve within the ventilator rather than at the input to the patient (i.e., the airway opening). This approach is convenient and avoids extra wires and the added instrumental dead space of a flow sensor. However, in neonates, this remote placement of flow measurement introduces a high degree of inaccuracy of V_T data. When the V_T is measured at the ventilator end of the circuit, the value does not account for compression of gas in the circuit, distention of the circuit, or leak around the ETT and is subject to inaccuracies related to approximate corrections for heat and humidification of the cold dry air from the control valve. The loss of delivered V_T in the circuit is proportional to the compliance of the ventilator circuit and humidifier (and the compressibility of the volume of gas they contain), relative to the compliance of the patient's lungs. In large patients with a cuffed ETT, the volume measured at the ventilator correlates reasonably well (using appropriate corrections) with the actual V_T entering the lungs. In tiny infants, whose lungs are very small and noncompliant, the loss of volume to the circuit is proportionally much larger and not easily corrected, especially in the presence of significant ETT leak.

PRINCIPLES OF VENTILATOR DESIGN, FUNCTION, AND NOMENCLATURE

A mechanical ventilator is simply a device designed to augment or replace a patient's own respiratory effort and ensure adequate entry of fresh gas into the lungs to satisfy the body's respiratory needs. There is a wide variety of ventilator designs, but they all offer most of the basic modes of ventilation. To understand how ventilators work, the clinician should focus on how the specific modes work and on understanding the sometimes complex interactions between an awake, breathing infant and the particular mode on the specific device. This is important, because with today's confusing terminology, ventilation modes with identical names may function differently on different devices. Thus the question of interest is, "How does this specific mode work on this device and how can I best use this tool to support my patient?"

A mode of ventilation is defined as a predetermined pattern of interaction between a patient and a ventilator. Unfortunately, there is no standardization in the industry regarding either naming modes or explaining their operation. Because different manufacturers employ different nomenclature to describe often closely related modes of ventilation, communication among users of different devices has become increasingly difficult.

For example, one ventilator commonly used for infants (the CareFusion Avea) offers the clinician the choice of 44 different modes. To better understand ventilator function and improve communication among clinicians, we need a ventilator mode taxonomy, or classification system.[5,6] This taxonomy is not as intimidating as it may sound. It is based on a small set of specifically defined terms (known as a standardized vocabulary) and is organized as a hierarchical structure, similar to the order, family, genus, and species outline used in biology.

To better appreciate the need for a systematic approach, consider that at last count we have identified 290 names of modes on 33 ventilators in the United States alone. Can you imagine having to use that many drugs by trade name only without any generic or chemical names and no classification system? That is the situation with ventilator modes today. Additionally, many ventilators used around the world today are designed to span the entire age range from preterm newborn to adult and have a variety of modes that have never been evaluated in newborn infants. The importance of having a classification system is to be able to identify, on different ventilators, which modes are the same and which are different. Then we can identify the technological capabilities of different ventilators for both purchasing decisions[7] and clinical application. Indeed, having identified the modes themselves, we can then compare and contrast their specific features to determine which modes best meet the clinical goals of mechanical ventilation for a particular patient at a particular time. Whereas there are many indications for initiating mechanical ventilation, we must provide mechanical ventilation with three key goals in mind[8]: (1) safety—optimize gas exchange with a minimum of hemodynamic adverse effects and minimize ventilator-associated lung and brain injury,[9] (2) comfort—minimize asynchrony between the ventilator and spontaneous breathing, and (3) liberation—minimize the duration of ventilation and incidence of adverse events. Thus, three basic skills (mode classification, goal selection, and mode selection) make up a rational framework for mastering the art and science of mechanical ventilation.[10]

The following paragraphs will focus on conventional mechanical ventilation. Classification of high-frequency ventilation modes and indications for high-frequency ventilation use are addressed in detail in Chapters 22 and 23.

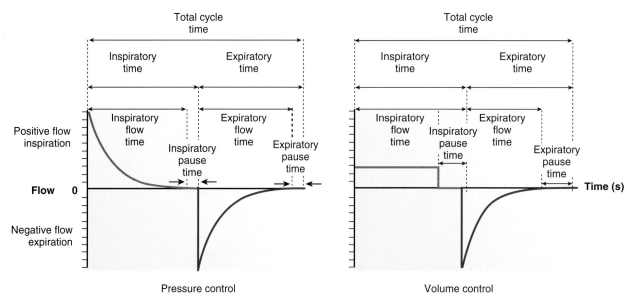

FIG 15-1 A ventilator cycle is defined in terms of the flow–time curve. Important timing parameters related to ventilator settings are labeled. (Modified from Mandu Press Ltd., with permission.)

TEN MAXIMS FOR UNDERSTANDING MODES OF CONVENTIONAL VENTILATION

In this section some basic terms related to mechanical ventilation will be defined in general, with specific applications to neonatal ventilation highlighted along the way. To understand these terms in context, 10 basic technological concepts (maxims) that underlie all modes of ventilation will be described. These concepts are each fairly simple and intuitively obvious. But taken together, they result in a classification system applicable to any mode on any ventilator.

Defining a Ventilator Cycle

A ventilator cycle is defined as one cycle of positive flow (inflation) and negative flow (expiration) defined in terms of the flow–time curve (Fig. 15-1). As pointed out in an editorial, ventilators do not breathe, and so they do not deliver breaths, they deliver inflations.[11] Only living people and animals breathe. We will therefore use terminology that avoids confusion between patient breaths and ventilator inflations.

Defining the Assisted Breath

A breath is assisted if the ventilator inflation provides some or all of the work of breathing. Graphically, this corresponds to airway pressure increasing above baseline during inspiration.

Assistance with Volume or Pressure Control

A ventilator assists breathing using either "pressure control" or "volume control" based on the equation of motion for the respiratory system:

$$P(t) = EV(t) + R\dot{V}(t)$$

This equation relates pressure (P), V_T (V), and flow in the ETT ($\dot{V}$) as continuous functions of time (t) with the parameters of elastance (E) and resistance (R). If any one of the functions (P, V, or ($\dot{V}$)) are predetermined, the other two may be derived.

The term *control variable* refers to the function that is controlled (predetermined or preset) during a ventilator cycle.

This form of the equation assumes that the patient makes no inspiratory effort and that expiration is complete (no auto-positive end-expiratory pressure [PEEP]) at the end of each cycle.

Volume control (VC) means that both V_T and ETT flow (variables on the right-hand side of the equation) are preset. In journal articles on neonatal and pediatric mechanical ventilation, you will often see the following terms used interchangeably to mean VC: *volume targeted*, *volume limited*, and *volume preset*. *Pressure control* (PC) means that inflation pressure (the variable on the left-hand side of the equation) is preset. In practice, this means one of two things: (1) the peak inflation pressure is preset (i.e., airway pressure rises to some target value and remains there until inflation time is complete; this is the traditional approach in neonates) or (2) inflation pressure is controlled by the ventilator so that it is proportional to the patient's inspiratory effort; this is a newer method represented by the modes called *proportional assist ventilation* and *neurally adjusted ventilatory assist*. In journal articles on neonatal and pediatric mechanical ventilation, you will often see the following terms used interchangeably to mean PC: *pressure controlled*, *pressure limited*, and *pressure preset*.

Time control (TC) is a general category of ventilator modes for which flow, volume, and pressure are all dependent on respiratory system mechanics. As no parameters of the pressure, volume, or flow waveforms are preset, the only control of the cycle is the timing. Examples of this category are high-frequency oscillatory ventilation (CareFusion 3100 ventilator) and volumetric diffusive respiration (Percussionaire ventilator). Characteristic waveforms for VC and PC are shown in Figure 15-2.

Trigger and Cycle Events

Inflations are classified according to the criteria that trigger (start) and cycle (stop) an inflation. The most basic trigger variable during ventilation of the neonate is time, as in the case of a preset inflation frequency (the period between inflations is $1/f$). Other trigger variables include a preset apnea interval or various indicators of inspiratory effort (e.g., changes in baseline pressure or flow or electrical signals derived from diaphragm

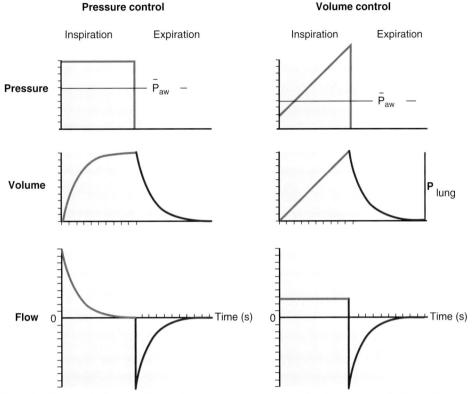

FIG 15-2 Characteristic waveforms for pressure control and volume control. Note that mean airway pressure ($\bar{P}_{aw}$) is less for volume control than for pressure control given the same tidal volume and inspiratory time. (Modified from Mandu Press Ltd., with permission.)

movement). The most common cycle variable is a preset inflation time (time-cycled ventilation). Other cycle variables include pressure (e.g., peak airway pressure), volume (volume cycled), flow (e.g., percentage of peak inflation flow, i.e., flow cycled), and electrical signals derived from diaphragm movement. A more detailed discussion of common neonatal modes of synchronized ventilation can be found in Chapter 18.

Machine versus Patient Trigger and Cycle Events

Trigger and cycle events can be either patient or ventilator initiated. Inflation can be patient triggered or patient cycled by a signal representing inspiratory effort (e.g., changes in baseline airway pressure, or changes in baseline bias flow, or the electrical signal derived from diaphragm activity as with neurally adjusted ventilatory assist (NAVA)).[12]

Patient triggering means starting inflation based on a patient signal independent of a ventilator-generated trigger signal.

Ventilator triggering means starting inflation based on a signal (usually time) from the ventilator, independent of a patient trigger signal.

Patient cycling means ending the inflation based on signals representing the patient-determined components of the equation of motion (i.e., elastance or resistance and including effects due to inspiratory effort). Note that flow cycling (as used in the mode called *pressure support*) is a form of patient cycling because the rate of flow decay to the cycle threshold, and hence the inflation time, is determined by patient mechanics (i.e., the time constant and effort).

Ventilator cycling means ending inflation independent of signals representing the patient-determined components of the equation of motion.

Spontaneous versus Mandatory "Breaths"

Traditional terminology uses the term *breath* to describe both ventilator inflations and spontaneous breaths (inspirations). Describing spontaneous or mandatory inflations as breaths can be confusing.

A *spontaneous breath* is made by the patient. It may or may not be assisted by the ventilator. A spontaneous breath is both triggered and cycled by the patient.

A *mandatory breath* (better termed an *inflation*) is triggered either by the baby or by the ventilator. Inflations may be mandatory or triggered by the patient and may be cycled by the ventilator or by the patient.

Breath/Inflation Sequences

A breath/inflation sequence is a particular pattern of spontaneous breaths and/or mandatory inflations. The three possible sequences are continuous mandatory ventilation (CMV), intermittent mandatory ventilation (IMV), and continuous spontaneous ventilation (CSV). In CMV, commonly known as "assist/control" (AC), every inspiratory effort triggers a ventilator inflation and unassisted spontaneous breaths are not possible. IMV is a breath sequence in which unassisted spontaneous breaths are possible between mandatory inflations. The mandatory inflations may or may not be triggered by the baby; thus we have IMV or synchronized IMV (SIMV). CSV means the patient is breathing spontaneously with continuous positive airway pressure, with or without volume or pressure support. CSV with pressure support is commonly referred to as *pressure support ventilation* (PSV). However, CSV with pressure support as implemented on universal ventilators differs from PSV as implemented on purpose-designed neonatal ventilators.

On universal ventilators it is a true CSV mode that requires a mature respiratory control center with apnea ventilation kicking in after a user-preset delay. In the neonatal ventilators, PSV is much like AC in that every spontaneous effort is supported, but each inflation is flow, rather than time, cycled; different from universal ventilators, there is a backup rate that continuously maintains a minimum respiratory rate preset by the user (see Chapter 18).

Ventilatory Patterns

A ventilatory pattern is a sequence of inflations and/or spontaneous breaths (CMV, IMV, or CSV) with a particular control variable (volume or pressure) for the ventilator inflations. Thus, with two control variables and three breath sequences there are five basic ventilatory patterns: VC-CMV (commonly known as VC-AC), VC-IMV, PC-CMV (commonly known as PC-AC), PC-IMV, and PC-CSV. In principle, the combination VC-CSV is not possible because VC implies ventilator cycling, and ventilator cycling makes every inflation mandatory, not spontaneous (see Maxim 6). A pattern of time-controlled IMV (TC-IMV) is possible but rare and as of this writing available only on some high-frequency ventilators.

Targeting Schemes

Within each ventilatory pattern there are several types that can be distinguished by their targeting schemes. A targeting scheme is a model of the relationship between operator inputs and ventilator outputs to achieve a specific ventilatory pattern, usually in the form of a feedback control system.[8] Targets can be set for parameters during an inflation (within-inflation targets).

These parameters relate to the pressure, volume, and flow waveforms. Examples of such targets include peak inflation flow and V_T or inflation pressure and rise time, that is, slope of the pressure wave (set-point targeting); pressure, volume, and flow (dual targeting); and constant of proportionality between inflation pressure and patient effort (servo targeting), as in proportional assist ventilation (PAV)[13] and NAVA.[14]

Targets can be set between inflations to modify the within-inflation targets and/or the overall ventilatory pattern (between-inflation targets). These are used with more advanced targeting schemes, in which targets act over multiple inflations. In neonatal ventilation, the between-inflation target is typically V_T (for PC using adaptive targeting).

The targeting scheme (or combination of targeting schemes) is what distinguishes one ventilatory pattern from another. There are currently seven basic targeting schemes that account for the wide variety of ventilator patterns seen in different modes of ventilation (Table 15-1). However, only three of them are commonly used in neonatal ventilation and are described as follows:

Set-point: This is a targeting scheme in which the operator sets all the parameters of the pressure waveform (PC modes) or volume and flow waveforms (VC modes). The ventilator does not adjust any targets automatically. This is how the mode called *time cycled, pressure limited* works.

Servo: This is a targeting scheme in which the output of the ventilator (e.g., inflation pressure) automatically follows a varying input (e.g., inspiratory effort). Current examples for neonatal ventilation are NAVA and PAV.

TABLE 15-1   Summary of Targeting Schemes for Mechanical Ventilation

Name	Abbreviation	Description	Advantage	Disadvantage	Example Mode Name	Ventilator	Manufacturer
Set-point	s	The operator sets all parameters of the pressure waveform (pressure control modes) or volume and flow waveforms (volume control modes).	Simplicity	Changing patient condition may make settings inappropriate.	Volume control continuous mandatory ventilation	Evita infinity V500	Dräger
Dual	d	The ventilator can automatically switch between volume control and pressure control during a single inspiration. Inspiration may start as either volume or pressure control and then switch to the other.	Can adjust to changing patient condition and ensure either a preset tidal volume or a peak inspiratory pressure.	Complicated to set correctly on some ventilators. Loss of control over size of tidal volume with large patient effort.	Volume control	SERVO-i	Maquet
Servo	r	The output of the ventilator (pressure/ volume/flow) automatically follows a varying input. Implemented as inspiratory pressure proportional to inspiratory effort.	Proportion of total work of breathing supported by the ventilator is constant regardless of inspiratory effort.	Requires estimates of artificial airway and/or respiratory system mechanical properties.	Proportional assist ventilation plus	Puritan Bennett 840	Covidien

TABLE 15-1	Summary of Targeting Schemes for Mechanical Ventilation—cont'd						
Name	Abbreviation	Description	Advantage	Disadvantage	Example Mode Name	Ventilator	Manufacturer
Adaptive	a	The ventilator automatically sets target(s) between breaths in response to varying patient conditions.	Can maintain stable tidal volume delivery with pressure control for changing lung mechanics or patient inspiratory effort.	Automatic adjustment may be inappropriate if algorithm assumptions are violated or they do not match physiology.	Pressure-regulated volume control	SERVO-i	Maquet
Bio-variable	b	The ventilator automatically adjusts the inspiratory pressure or tidal volume randomly.	Simulates the variability observed during normal breathing and may improve oxygenation or mechanics.	Manually set range of variability may be inappropriate to achieve goals.	Variable pressure support	Evita infinity V500	Dräger
Optimal	o	The ventilator automatically adjusts the targets of the ventilatory pattern to either minimize or maximize some overall performance characteristic (e.g., work rate of breathing).	Can adjust to changing lung mechanics or patient inspiratory effort.	Automatic adjustment may be inappropriate if algorithm assumptions are violated or they do not match physiology.	Adaptive support ventilation	G5	Hamilton Medical
Intelligent	i	Targeting scheme that uses artificial intelligence programs such as fuzzy logic, rule-based expert systems, and artificial neural networks.	Can adjust to changing lung mechanics or patient inspiratory effort.	Automatic adjustment may be inappropriate if algorithm assumptions are violated or they do not match physiology.	SmartCare/PS	Evita infinity V500	Dräger

Targeting schemes are models of the relationship between operator inputs and ventilator outputs to achieve a specific ventilatory pattern.

Adaptive: This is a targeting scheme that allows the ventilator to automatically set one target (e.g., pressure within an inflation) to achieve another target (e.g., V_T). Modes that use PC with adaptive targeting are often referred to in the literature as *volume targeted* or *volume guarantee* modes.

Mode Classification

A mode of ventilation is classified according to its control variable, breath/inflation sequence, and targeting scheme(s). Thus, the ventilator mode taxonomy has four hierarchical levels:
Control variable (pressure or volume, for the primary inflation)
    Breath/inflation sequence (CMV, IMV, or CSV)
        Primary targeting scheme (for CMV or CSV)
            Secondary targeting scheme (for IMV)
The primary inflation is either the only inflation there is (mandatory inflations for CMV and spontaneous breaths for CSV) or the mandatory inflation in (S)IMV. We consider it primary because if the patient becomes apneic, it is the only thing keeping the patient alive. The targeting schemes can be represented by single, lowercase letters: s, set-point; d, dual; r, servo; b, bio-variable; a, adaptive; o, optimal; i, intelligent.

Translating a name of a mode into a mode classification using the taxonomy is a simple three-step procedure:

Step 1: Identify the primary control variable. If the inflation pressure is preset, or if pressure is proportional to inspiratory effort, then the control variable is pressure. On the other hand, if the operator sets both V_T and flow, then the control variable is volume.

Step 2: Identify the breath/inflation sequence.

Step 3: Identify the targeting schemes for the primary and (if applicable) secondary inflations.

For example, the mode that is commonly called *time cycled, pressure limited* in the neonatal literature is classified as follows: (1) inflation pressure is preset, so the control variable is pressure; (2) inflation time is preset, indicating machine cycling and thus the presence of mandatory inflations, plus the allowance for spontaneous breaths between mandatory inflations, indicating the sequence is IMV; (3) all targets are operator preset so the targeting scheme is set-point. The "tag" (classification abbreviation) for this mode is hence PC-IMVs. In contrast, for a mode called *volume support*, the operator sets a target V_T but flow is not preset; hence the control variable is pressure. Every inflation is both patient triggered (pressure or flow) and patient cycled (at a certain percentage of peak flow) and hence the breath sequence is CSV. Finally, the ventilator automatically adjusts the inflation pressure between inflations to achieve (on average) the operator-set target expired V_T. Hence the classification would be PC-CSVa.

INITIATION OF MECHANICAL VENTILATION

Indications for Mechanical Ventilation

The goal of mechanical ventilation is to maintain acceptable gas exchange with a minimum of adverse effects and to wean from invasive support at the earliest opportunity. Adverse effects of positive pressure ventilation include acute lung injury, air-leak syndrome, hemodynamic impairment, nosocomial infection, and brain injury; these are discussed in detail in Chapters 30 and 42. Secondary goals include comfort (reducing asynchrony), reducing the work of breathing, and minimizing oxygen consumption. Because of the wide range of clinical conditions, weights, and gestational ages of neonatal patients, no simple formula exists to define indications for intubation and mechanical ventilation. In general, reasonable indications include inadequate or absent respiratory effort, clinical signs of impending respiratory failure, a high and rising Pco_2 level, persistent high oxygen requirement ($FiO_2 > 0.40$-0.60), and excessive work of breathing despite optimized noninvasive support (Table 15-2).

Optimal respiratory support of the neonate requires a careful consideration of the context in which it is being applied. The range of situations in which mechanical ventilation is used in the newborn infant is broad, with a variety of pathophysiologic disturbances. Table 15-3 provides a list of the common situations in which mechanical ventilation is used and includes some key considerations regarding ventilator modes and initial settings for each situation.

Choosing the Ventilator Mode

The clinician's choice of ventilator modes may be limited by the equipment available in his or her NICU. Although most modern ventilators are capable of providing the basic modes of synchronized ventilation, there are a variety of hybrid modes and combinations that may be unique to each device, as discussed earlier and reviewed in detail in Chapter 25. Ventilators designed primarily for adult/pediatric patients, but capable of also supporting neonates (so-called universal ventilators), have a greater variety of modes, including volume-controlled ventilation. Some of these modes have never been evaluated in newborn infants. Therefore, when ventilating newborns with these devices, the clinician must be aware of the pitfalls of applying various "adult" or novel

TABLE 15-2 Suggested Indications for Mechanical Ventilation	
Category	**Specific Findings or Values**
Inadequate/absent respiratory effort	Absent, weak, or intermittent spontaneous effort
	Frequent (>6 events/hr) or severe apnea requiring PPV
Excessive work of breathing (relative)	Marked retractions, severe tachypnea >100/min
High oxygen requirement	$FiO_2 > 0.40$-0.60; labile SpO_2 if PPHN is suspected
Severe respiratory acidosis	pH <7.2 and not improving, Pco_2 >65 on days 0-3, >70 beyond day 3
Moderate or severe respiratory distress *and* contraindications for noninvasive support	Intestinal obstruction; intestinal perforation; recent gastrointestinal surgery; ileus; CDH
Postoperative period	Residual effect of anesthetic agents; fresh abdominal incision; need for continued muscle relaxation (e.g., fresh tracheostomy)

PPV, Positive pressure ventilation; *SpO₂*, arterial oxygen saturation on pulse oximetry; *PPHN*, persistent pulmonary hypertension of the newborn; *CDH*, congenital diaphragmatic hernia.

TABLE 15-3 Common Situations When Mechanical Ventilation Is Employed and Key Considerations in Choosing Support					
Situation	**Example**	**Predominant Pathophysiologic Disturbance**	**Suggested PEEP**	**V_T Range***	**Considerations Regarding Ventilator Mode and Settings**
Apnea	• Preterm infant with apnea of prematurity	Poor respiratory drive, relatively normal lung function	4-5 cm H_2O	4-5 mL/kg	Should need only minimal ventilator support. Lungs often relatively compliant, care must be taken to avoid lung injury, excessive V_T
	• Preterm infant with RDS apnea because of impending respiratory failure	Support should address the underlying RDS (see below)			Same as for RDS (see below)
Lung disease					
Diffuse alveolar disease	• Preterm infant with RDS	Low lung compliance, compliant chest wall, microatelectasis, ventilation:perfusion mismatch, very prone to ventilator-associated lung injury	6-8 cm H_2O, transiently may be higher	4-5 mL/kg	Recruitment using PEEP with CMV or MAP increments with HFOV. Short T_I and fast rate well tolerated. Optimizing lung inflation and avoiding volutrauma are key considerations
	• Term or preterm infant with hemorrhagic pulmonary edema	Poor lung compliance, surfactant inactivation, pulmonary edema, fluid in the airways	8-10 cm H_2O during acute event	4-6 mL/kg	Acutely increase PEEP and PIP to tamponade edema fluid. Recruitment using PEEP increments and fixed V_T may be helpful. Longer T_I needed to help recruitment

TABLE 15-3 Common Situations When Mechanical Ventilation Is Employed and Key Considerations in Choosing Support—cont'd

Situation	Example	Predominant Pathophysiologic Disturbance	Suggested PEEP	V_T Range*	Considerations Regarding Ventilator Mode and Settings
Obstructive and/or heterogeneous disease	• Term infant with meconium aspiration syndrome	High airway resistance, low compliance, heterogeneous inflation, prolonged time constants. With thin meconium, surfactant inactivation predominates and mimics diffuse alveolar disease	4-6 cm H_2O	5-6 mL/kg	Potential for overdistention of relatively normal lung regions. Need for lower ventilator rate to avoid air trapping. Higher V_T/kg is needed owing to increased alveolar dead space. When surfactant dysfunction predominates, treat like RDS
Pulmonary hypoplasia	• Preterm infant born after prolonged oligohydramnios • Term infant with congenital diaphragmatic hernia	Low lung compliance related to small total lung volume. Prone to overdistention, air leak, and pulmonary hypertension	4-6 cm H_2O	4-5 mL/kg	Avoid high V_T/PIP, avoid overexpansion. Consider high-frequency ventilation if PIP >25 cm H_2O or if there is refractory hypoxic respiratory failure
Air leak	• Preterm infant with pulmonary interstitial emphysema	Compression of normal airspaces by interstitial gas, poor compliance, and high airway resistance	4-6 cm H_2O	4-5 mL/kg	Accept higher Pco_2, avoid large V_T, maintain lung volume with moderate PEEP. Low PEEP leads to atelectasis resulting in need for higher PIP. Selective single bronchus intubation if unilateral. High-frequency ventilation (especially HFJV) is preferable
	• Pneumothorax	Continued leak of gas into the pleural space			
Persistent pulmonary hypertension (PPHN)	• PPHN with parenchymal lung disease	Reduced pulmonary blood flow secondary to increased pulmonary vascular resistance superimposed on underlying lung disease	6-8 cm H_2O	4-6 mL/kg	V_T and PEEP requirements depend on associated parenchymal disease. Optimize lung inflation, correct acidosis, avoid overexpansion, avoid lung injury
Pulmonary arterial hypertension	• PPHN with normal lung parenchyma	Reduced pulmonary blood flow secondary to increased pulmonary vascular resistance. Pulmonary vascular remodeling	4-5 cm H_2O	4-5 mL/kg	Avoid overexpansion, excessive V_T. Avoid increasing airway pressure to improve oxygenation. Early use of iNO may be beneficial
	• Severe chronic lung disease (BPD)	Reduced pulmonary vascular bed, pulmonary vascular remodeling, increased pulmonary vasoreactivity	6-8 cm H_2O	6-8 mL/kg	Optimize treatment of BPD, maintain high SpO_2. Consider long-term pulmonary vasodilator therapy
Severe chronic lung disease (BPD)	• Former preterm infant with established chronic lung disease	Multicompartmental lung with regions of low compliance and increased resistance, poorly supported airways prone to collapse. Decreased alveolarization with less gas-exchanging surface and fewer pulmonary capillaries. Increased pulmonary vascular resistance	6-10 cm H_2O, sometimes higher	6-8 mL/kg, sometimes higher	Slow rate, longer T_I and T_E to allow ventilation of the diseased lung regions with long time constants. Sufficient PEEP is needed to prevent expiratory flow limitation at low lung volumes. Larger V_T is needed because of increased alveolar and anatomic dead space

Continued

TABLE 15-3   Common Situations When Mechanical Ventilation Is Employed and Key Considerations in Choosing Support—cont'd

Situation	Example	Predominant Pathophysiologic Disturbance	Suggested PEEP	V_T Range*	Considerations Regarding Ventilator Mode and Settings
Cardiac disease					
Left to right shunts	• Preterm infant with patent ductus arteriosus • Term infant with large ventricular septal defect	Pulmonary overcirculation with decreased lung compliance from pulmonary engorgement and edema	5-8 cm H_2O	5-6 mL/kg	High PEEP mitigates left to right shunt. Increasing CO_2 can help limit blood flow to some degree
Vulnerable pulmonary circulation	• Pulmonary atresia with duct-dependent pulmonary circulation • Hypoplastic left heart syndrome, post Norwood operation	Pulmonary blood flow highly variable and under the influence of intra-alveolar pressure	3-5 cm H_2O	5-7 mL/kg	Lung overdistention with high pressure settings will impede pulmonary blood flow. Manipulation of Pco_2 can help to control pulmonary blood flow: lower CO_2 to encourage blood flow, increase CO_2 to restrict blood flow
Neuromuscular disease	• Term infant with myopathy	Poor muscle strength, low FRC and V_T secondary to compromised respiratory muscle function	3-5 cm H_2O	4-5 mL/kg	Pressure support for each spontaneous breath is optimal
Airway obstruction					
Large airway obstruction	• Tracheobronchomalacia	Increased airway obstruction with crying or increased respiratory effort due to airway collapse	6-10 cm H_2O	4-6 mL/kg	Titrate PEEP upward until obstruction is relieved by splinting airway open
Small airway obstruction	• Former preterm infant with BPD	Inflammation, secretions, smooth muscle hypertrophy lead to mostly fixed airway obstruction. There may be a variable bronchospastic component. Prolongation of T_E and gas trapping. Expiratory flow limitation at low lung volumes	6-8 cm H_2O, sometimes higher	4-6 mL/kg	Slower rate, longer T_I and T_E to accommodate long time constants. Titrate PEEP upward until obstruction is relieved by splinting airway open. Antiinflammatory agents and bronchodilators may be of some value
Postoperative support					
General aspects	• Any infant with a painful surgical incision	Suppression of respiratory drive due to sedation. Limitation of respiratory excursion due to pain	4-6 cm H_2O	4-5 mL/kg	Heavy sedation may predispose to atelectasis by suppressing sighs. Adequate set rate needed as the infant may not breathe above set rate or trigger adequately
Abdominal surgery	• Term infant with gastroschisis repair • Preterm infant s/p laparotomy for necrotizing enterocolitis	Raised intra-abdominal pressure and diaphragmatic splinting	6-8 cm H_2O	4-5 mL/kg	High PEEP needed to maintain EELV and recruitment but may compromise venous return if lung compliance is normal. Adequate V_T may be difficult to achieve without very high PIP. HFOV or HFJV preferred

*V_T refers to exhaled tidal volume measured at the airway opening. V_T need is also affected by size. Very small infants need a larger V_T/kg. V_T may be controlled directly when using volume-targeted ventilation modes or be a target value achieved by adjusting PIP when using pressure-controlled modes.

BPD, Bronchopulmonary dysplasia; *CMV*, conventional mechanical ventilation; *EELV*, end-expiratory lung volume; *FRC*, functional residual capacity; *HFOV*, high-frequency oscillatory ventilation; *HFJV*, high-frequency jet ventilation; *iNO*, inhaled nitric oxide; *MAP*, mean airway pressure; *PEEP*, positive end-expiratory pressure; *PIP*, peak inflation pressure; *PPHN*, persistent pulmonary hypertension of the newborn; *RDS*, respiratory distress syndrome; *s/p*, status post; T_I, inflation time; T_E, expiratory time; V_T, tidal volume.

modes to this unique population. Unlike the specialty neonatal ventilators, PSV on these devices does not have a continuous backup rate and thus requires a reliable respiratory effort, seldom present in preterm infants. Volume-controlled ventilation controls the volume delivered into the proximal (ventilator) end of the circuit (known as V_{del}), not the V_T entering the patient's lungs. Because of compression of gas and stretching of the circuit, as well as a variable leak around ETTs, there is only a very indirect relationship between V_{del} and the volume of gas that enters the patient's lungs. For this reason, pressure-controlled ventilation (commonly referred to as time-cycled, pressure-limited ventilation in the neonatal literature) became the standard ventilation mode in the NICU, more recently with modifications that allow volume targeting. These are discussed in detail in Chapter 20. Despite decades of routine use, uncertainty remains regarding the relative merits of the commonly used modes of synchronized ventilation, discussed in detail in Chapter 18.

Initial Settings for Pressure-Controlled Ventilation

Immediately after intubation, a period of manual ventilation using a portable ventilation device is usually required until the ETT is secured, the nasogastric tube inserted, and the baby properly positioned for ventilation. If intubation occurred in the delivery suite, bolus surfactant may be given at this time, and some distance of in-house transport may be needed until initiation of mechanical ventilation. Use of adequate PEEP is strongly recommended during this period. If the manual ventilation device does not allow for delivery of PEEP (e.g., self-inflating bag lacking a PEEP valve), the infant should be connected to the ventilator as quickly as possible.

The initial ventilator settings should take into account the gestational age, underlying pulmonary pathology, and clinical response to settings used during ventilation with a portable device. There should be a logical approach to choosing ventilator settings and an immediate assessment of their effectiveness, guided by a combination of careful clinical evaluation and observation of waveforms and other displayed parameters on the ventilator screen. The PEEP level is a key determinant of end-expiratory lung volume (EELV) and therefore of adequacy of oxygenation. An initial level of 5 to 6 cm H_2O is a reasonable starting point for most infants, with titration upward if FiO_2 remains above 0.30. Adequate PEEP is a key factor in lung-protective ventilator strategies. PEEP optimization schemes and approaches to lung-protective ventilation strategies are discussed in detail in Chapter 19.

The key considerations to guide PEEP settings are (1) There is no universal PEEP setting that is appropriate for all patients and all lung diseases. Even for an individual patient the PEEP requirement evolves over time. Mandating a standard PEEP level for reasons of simplicity misses opportunities to manage respiratory support optimally and according to sound physiologic reasoning. Suggested ranges for PEEP are given in Table 15-3, but these should be considered in the context of the individual circumstances, with further adjustment according to the physiologic response and the course of the disease. See also Chapter 23 for discussion of appropriate settings for various lung pathologies. The PEEP setting should be reevaluated whenever there is an alteration to pulmonary mechanics, for example, after surfactant administration. (2) Very low PEEP (<4 cm H_2O) is inappropriate in the diseased lung, predisposing to low EELV, poor oxygenation, impaired pulmonary mechanics, greater turnover of surfactant, and a risk of greater lung injury. (3) Conversely, a PEEP level that is set too high, or

becomes too high when PEEP is not reduced as lung compliance improves, leads to overdistention of the lung, incomplete exhalation with hypercarbia, increased pulmonary vascular resistance, and impairment of venous return with decreased cardiac output. (4) PEEP is not, by itself, a recruitment tool; PEEP increments will not recruit the lung optimally without an adequate inflating pressure that must reach the critical opening pressure to reinflate nonaerated lung units. Once the lung is recruited it becomes more compliant and the PEEP and peak inflation pressure (PIP) must then be reduced to avoid overventilation and lung injury.

Choice of the inflation time (T_I) should be based on the time constant of the infant's respiratory system (how quickly gas gets in and out; see Chapter 2 for a detailed explanation of the concept of time constant). It should be set at around 0.4 to 0.5 second for term infants and 0.25 to 0.35 second for a preterm infant and quickly adjusted if needed based on the analysis of the flow–time curve displayed on most modern neonatal ventilators. T_I should be long enough to allow completion of inspiratory flow before the ventilator cycles off but should avoid a long inspiratory hold that increases patient–ventilator asynchrony and risk of air leak. For flow-cycled modes (e.g., pressure support or volume support), the T_I set value is really the upper limit that comes into play only if flow cycling fails to occur; it should be set long enough to permit flow cycling to occur. In some devices the breath termination criterion is adjustable by the user (typically at 10-25% of peak flow); in neonatal ventilators with effective leak compensation, this value is fixed at 15%. Setting PIP should be guided by a visual appreciation of a just adequate chest rise, audible breath sounds, and preferably the measured exhaled V_T, which should range between 4 and 6 mL/kg, depending on the patient size, age, and diagnosis. There is no optimal PIP for all infants and the PIP required to achieve adequate V_T is not a function of the size of the infant. Very small infants may have very poor lung compliance and transiently need quite high PIP. The reason larger infants often need higher PIP than small ones is that they cope better with the increased load imposed by lung disease and thus develop signs of respiratory failure with more severe disease than tiny infants. Peak pressure by itself is not injurious to the lungs without generating a correspondingly high V_T (see Chapter 20). Finally, expiratory time (T_E) (determined by direct setting or indirectly by preset ventilator rate) is adjusted to achieve a sufficient level of support to reduce the work of breathing and produce adequate minute ventilation, a value also usually available on the ventilator display. Depending on the ventilator mode, the ventilator rate may be a minimum value with the actual rate determined by the infant, as in CMV (AC or PSV) or may directly determine the actual ventilator cycling frequency (apneic infant, IMV or SIMV). Please see Chapter 18 for further discussion of various modes of synchronized ventilation.

Assessment after Starting Ventilation

A thorough clinical evaluation after initiation of ventilation is essential, recognizing that further adjustments to ventilator settings may be indicated after evaluating the patient's response to the initial choices (Table 15-4). Relying solely on blood gas measurement potentially exposes the patient to a period of suboptimal support, something that can usually be discerned clinically and corrected before obtaining a blood gas. Careful note of the rate of spontaneous breathing and the effectiveness of triggering should be made as the infant recovers from the intubation and the effects of any sedative and muscle relaxant

TABLE 15-4   Clinical Evaluation after Initiation of Mechanical Ventilation

Observation	• Color and activity
	• Patient–ventilator interaction
	  • Triggering
	  • Autocycling
	• Chest rise and diaphragmatic excursion
	• Work of breathing
	• Respiratory rate
	• Circulation
	• Gastric distention

Auscultation	• Breath sounds to all lung areas
	  • Adequacy of air entry
	  • Symmetry of air entry
	• Adventitial sounds
	• Large airway sounds
	  • ETT leak
	  • Obstruction on carina
	• Heart sounds

Ventilator monitor display	• Exhaled tidal volume of
	  • Mechanical inflations
	  • Spontaneous breaths (if applicable)
	• Working (measured) PIP (if applicable)
	• Percentage leak
	• Flow–time curve—evidence of sufficient inspiratory and expiratory time
	• Excessive inspiratory hold
	• Evidence of triggering/autocycling

PIP, Peak inflation pressure; *ETT,* Endotracheal tube.

drugs used during the procedure. Adequacy of breath sounds and exhaled V_T should be evaluated. FiO_2 should be coming down with adequate support and if it remains high, an increase in PEEP (and perhaps PIP) should be seriously considered.

Observation of the chest rise and abdominal motion gives a rough estimate of the adequacy of V_T, although this clinical skill requires some time to master and often underestimates the actual V_T.[15] For this reason, the chest rise should be only just perceptible; a large, easily seen chest rise indicates excessive V_T. Auscultation of both sides of the chest is essential to detect mainstem bronchus intubation, atelectasis, or pneumothorax. Low-pitched sounds may indicate a large ETT leak or partial tube obstruction against the carina. Listening over the larynx or the open mouth will help confirm the source of the upper airway noise. Slight tension on the ETT may confirm ETT position as the source of the noise. Persistent increased work of breathing may reflect inadequate V_T, inadequate minute ventilation, or tube obstruction or malposition, which must be corrected promptly. In the immediate postintubation period, respiratory system compliance may be transiently decreased because of gastric distention, especially after prolonged face mask ventilation. Venting of the stomach with an adequately sized nasogastric tube should be routine to avoid this problem.

A key component of the clinical assessment after initiating ventilation is a careful appraisal of the data available on the ventilator display. In actively breathing infants, the displayed values will fluctuate; therefore observations should be made over a number of cycles. The exhaled V_T for a set PIP, or, conversely, the PIP required to deliver a set V_T, should be evaluated and adjustments made if necessary. In a volume-targeted mode, the PIP limit may need to be increased if the desired V_T cannot be delivered.

An estimate of minute ventilation can be made using the product of measured V_T and respiratory rate, with a value of 200 to 300 mL/kg/min usually indicating adequate ventilation before the first Pco_2 reading is obtained. Immediate assessment of the flow waveform is essential to detect insufficient T_E, which is recognized by failure of the expiratory flow to return to zero before the next inflation. A detailed discussion of ventilator waveforms is available in Chapter 12. Avoidance of inadvertent PEEP can be difficult when an infant has a rapid spontaneous breathing rate and each breath is being supported by the ventilator. Tachypnea is sometimes due to pain or agitation, which should be recognized and treated if present, but more commonly reflects inadequate ventilator support. Increasing PEEP and/or PIP will typically achieve more adequate support and allow the infant's respiratory rate to return to more physiologic values, thus allowing adequate T_E.

Trigger sensitivity may need to be adjusted to optimize patient–ventilator interaction. In general, the trigger threshold should be as low as possible without causing auto-triggering, because a higher trigger threshold is associated with increased work of breathing and longer trigger delay. If a patient remains tachypneic despite apparently good support, an attempt should be made to confirm whether the ventilator is auto-triggering. This situation is more likely when there is a significant ETT leak,[16] or with condensed water collecting in the ventilator tubing, and can lead to hyperventilation and air-trapping, especially in modes that support every spontaneous breath (AC and PSV). Specialized neonatal ventilators, such as the Dräger VN 500, have effective leak compensation and are much less susceptible to auto-triggering due to ETT leak but may still be affected by water in the circuit. The use of heated patient circuits and modern ventilator circuits with a semipermeable expiratory limb, which effectively eliminates water condensation (Evaqua™, Fisher & Paykel, Auckland, New Zealand), has virtually eliminated auto-triggering. Therefore, when using specialty neonatal ventilators with effective leak compensation and these circuits, the trigger sensitivity should normally remain at the most sensitive value with no concern about auto-triggering.

A chest radiograph should always be performed to confirm the position of the ETT, evaluate the lung parenchyma, and assess lung inflation. Because radiographs are theoretically taken at peak inflation, the apparent lung volume reflects $EELV + V_T$, and thus the chest radiograph is not very helpful for titrating PEEP. Adequacy of PEEP is better determined on the basis of oxygen requirement, because PEEP is the key determinant of ventilation/perfusion matching.

The need for further sedation/analgesia should be assessed. Muscle relaxation is rarely indicated in the era of effective synchronized ventilation. Narcotic analgesia should be used judiciously, if at all. Evidence from a large randomized trial indicates that while morphine administration relieves pain in ventilated neonates, it may increase the risk of adverse neurologic outcomes and prolongs the duration of ventilation.[17] When an infant is "fighting the ventilator," it is tempting to prescribe sedation. However, it must be clearly understood that this sign typically means that support is inadequate, even if gas exchange as measured by a blood gas is satisfactory. When gas exchange is inadequate, sedation will only mask the clinical signs of inadequate support. The infant is, in fact, struggling to breathe and the blood gas is not bad because the infant is fighting the ventilator; the infant is fighting the ventilator because the blood gas is bad! Finding the optimal level of support along with physical means of comfort will allow most infants to settle down without pharmacotherapy.

Subsequent Ventilator Adjustments

The therapeutic goals of mechanical ventilation include adequate oxygenation, sufficient alveolar minute ventilation to achieve an acceptable range of pH and Pco_2, and reduction in the work of breathing.

Oxygenation

In the absence of right to left shunting through fetal channels, oxygenation is a reflection of ventilation/perfusion matching and is most effectively addressed by manipulation of the EELV, commonly referred to as *functional residual capacity*. The most effective way of optimizing EELV during conventional ventilation and high-frequency jet ventilation is adjustment in PEEP. With high-frequency oscillatory ventilation, changes in mean airway pressure are used to optimize lung volume and ventilation:perfusion matching. Increased PIP and T_I also increase mean airway pressure and thus can affect oxygenation, but these steps are less effective and should not be used primarily to control oxygenation.[18] End-expiratory pressure is critical in maintaining end-expiratory alveolar stability. Increased PIP without adequate PEEP is likely to overdistend already expanded lung units and increase lung injury.

There is no easy direct way of visualizing lung volume. Chest radiographs are of limited value in assessing lung inflation/EELV,[19] and more precise techniques, such as electrical impedance tomography, remain research tools at this time.[20] Under most circumstances, the best assessment of EELV is the oxygen requirement. Oxygenation-guided lung volume recruitment strategies have been described with both high-frequency oscillatory ventilation[21] and conventional ventilation.[22] The approach with conventional ventilation is to increase PEEP in increments of 0.5 to 1 cm H_2O until FiO_2 is <0.30 or until there is no further improvement in oxygenation for two consecutive steps. This is probably best accomplished while keeping V_T stable with volume-targeted ventilation, thus increasing PIP in the process, which will serve to achieve the critical opening pressure. While an attempt at lung volume recruitment is indicated in most neonates with significant oxygen requirements, it must be recognized that not all causes of hypoxemia are due to atelectasis. If the hypoxemia is due to diffuse severe pneumonia or right to left shunting, lung volume recruitment may not be feasible or helpful. However, low lung volume and/or severe lung disease in and of themselves will increase pulmonary vascular resistance. If an echocardiogram indicates elevated pulmonary arterial pressure and the lungs are diffusely opacified, lung recruitment should still be attempted and will often mitigate the pulmonary hypertension when lung volume is improved. Optimizing lung volume is not only important in improving oxygenation and thus reducing oxygen toxicity from lung exposure to high FiO_2 but is also a critical component of lung-protective ventilation strategies.[23] Please see Chapter 16 for a discussion of target PaO_2 and SpO_2 ranges and Chapter 19 for a discussion of lung-protective ventilation strategies.

Ventilation/CO₂ Elimination

Ventilation, that is, CO_2 elimination, is primarily determined by alveolar minute ventilation, which maintains the partial pressure gradient between blood and alveolar gas. Alveolar minute ventilation is the product of inflation rate and the difference between V_T and dead-space volume. Increasing either will increase alveolar minute ventilation, but increasing V_T has a greater impact than increasing rate, because of the effect of dead space. If we assume dead space to be 2 mL and we are ventilating with a V_T of 4 mL, the alveolar V_T is 2 mL. Increasing V_T by 1 to 5 mL, a 25% increase, will increase alveolar V_T from 2 to 3 mL and thus increase alveolar minute ventilation by 50%. Note that the minute ventilation displayed on the ventilator screen does not account for alveolar or instrumental dead space, which may be substantial in some circumstances. The benefit of improved ventilation with larger V_T must be weighed against the potential for volutrauma. However, rapid shallow breathing, such as may occur with an insufficient level of inflation pressure or low IMV rate, leads to high dead space to V_T ratio and reduced alveolar ventilation. The V_T therefore needs to be sufficiently large to overcome dead space. End-tidal CO_2 monitors should be avoided in the small preterm infants because of the added dead space. The flow sensor that is essential to measure V_T and to provide synchronized ventilation also adds some dead space but is essential for state-of-the-art care; it has been demonstrated that some of the dead space is effectively bypassed in small infants ventilated through narrow ETTs.[24,25]

MONITORING AND DOCUMENTATION DURING MECHANICAL VENTILATION

Infants receiving mechanical ventilation are critically ill and are receiving life support. Thus they require intensive monitoring and careful documentation of physiologic and ventilatory parameters. All mechanically ventilated infants should have, at a minimum, cardiorespiratory monitoring, continuous measurement of oxygen saturation (SpO_2) via a transcutaneous pulse oximetry probe, and temperature monitoring. An indwelling arterial catheter for continuous monitoring of blood pressure and periodic arterial blood gas sampling is essential in the unstable and critically ill infant and helpful during the acute phase of invasive respiratory support of all infants. Continuous transcutaneous Pco_2 monitoring is desirable when using PC ventilation or high-frequency ventilation, less necessary when volume-targeted ventilation is used. End-tidal CO_2 monitoring adds significantly to the instrumental dead space and is often inaccurate in small infants whose rapid respiratory rates do not allow for an end-tidal plateau to be reached. Thus transcutaneous monitoring is preferred in most ventilated neonates when continuous monitoring of carbon dioxide is desirable.

Ventilation settings and measured variables should be recorded at regular intervals. Most modern ventilators provide the ability to trend key variables over time, allowing the user to see the evolution of the disease process and patient–ventilator interactions at a glance. The specific variables to be recorded depend on the mode that is in use but should include ventilator set and measured pressures, set and observed inflation rate, exhaled V_T (and the target V_T, if using volume-targeted ventilation), and the proportion of leak. To be accurate, V_T must be measured at the airway opening, not at the ventilator end of the circuit. The humidifier temperature should be regularly checked and recorded. Most modern ventilators also provide continuous display of waveforms and/or tidal ventilation loops, and these can be very helpful in fine-tuning ventilator settings, as described in this and other chapters in this text. Most modern ventilators allow for screen capture of waveforms, which can be a useful tool for subsequent evaluation/consultation when something unusual or unexplained appears to be happening.

VENTILATION PROTOCOLS

Mechanical ventilation is one of the most common therapies in the NICU and is associated with substantial morbidity and mortality. Mechanical ventilation is a complex and highly specialized area of neonatology, made more complicated by the availability of many different modes, techniques, and devices. Yet the management of infants receiving mechanical ventilation remains largely dependent on individual preferences and an individual's training, rather than scientific evidence. Thus it comes as no surprise that mechanical ventilation has been identified as one of the major risk factors for iatrogenic errors in the NICU.[26] While the preceding considerations argue in favor of developing ventilation protocols for management of mechanically ventilated infants,[27] there is a danger of oversimplifying a very complex procedure and failing to provide optimal support for individual patients. For this reason, while establishing a common and standard basic approach to mechanical ventilation is important, such unit protocols must take into account the need to tailor ventilation strategies to the underlying pathophysiology and its evolution over time and allow for reassessment of the strategy/settings based on the patient's response to the initially chosen ventilation approach. Table 15-3 provides a brief outline of the approach to various clinical scenarios when mechanical ventilation may be employed. A detailed discussion of common neonatal respiratory conditions and approaches to mechanical ventilation best suited to these patients is provided in Chapter 23. It is hoped that the information in this book will produce a sound basis for establishing such unit-based protocols.

REFERENCES

A complete reference list is available at https://expertconsult .inkling.com/.

16

Oxygen Therapy

Maximo Vento, MD, PhD

HISTORY OF THE USE OF OXYGEN IN CLINICAL MEDICINE

Although anecdotal information indicates that oxygen was already known by the Chinese in the thirteenth century, our present knowledge of its chemical and biological characteristics and its clinical application derives from the discoveries made almost simultaneously by C.W. Scheele (Sweden), Joseph Priestley (Britain), and Antoine-Laurent de Lavoisier (France). By heating mercury oxide, silver carbonate, magnesium nitrate, and potassium nitrate, they all produced the same gas previously known as *phlogiston* and that later was identified as a source of life because it allowed the survival of a mouse in a sealed jar, while without addition of this gas the mouse would die. Moreover, Priestley showed that plants were capable of producing it, and thus he opened the path for further studies on photosynthesis. The name *oxygen* comes from the Greek words *oxys* (acrid) and *gene* (something that produces something), meaning a substance that produces acids. Still today, in German oxygen is known as *Sauerstoff*, or acidic substance.[1]

Oxygen was first used in neonatology in the eighteenth century for the resuscitation of newborn infants. At the beginning of the twentieth century, oxygen was infused in the umbilical vessels of asphyxiated infants or directly given into the pharynx or via a gastric catheter.[2] In the 1930s oxygen started to be used liberally in the treatment of preterm infants suffering respiratory distress. With the ongoing use of oxygen, clinical scientists started to describe its positive and negative effects undoubtedly associated with its restricted or liberal use in the treatment of neonatal patients. Oxygen when liberally used was identified as the agent that caused what was initially called *retrolental fibroplasia* (RLF), characterized by the formation of a thick membrane in the retrolental space that resulted in damage and detachment of the retina and frequently blindness. This severe ophthalmologic condition had already caused blindness in about 10,000 infants in the early 1950s. Randomized trials performed in 1954-1956 clearly showed that the liberal use of oxygen was a major cause of RLF. It is important to note that at that time the level of oxygenation of the patients could be monitored only by taking into account variables such as respiratory rate, heart rate, and/or color. Beginning in the 1960s, objective oxygen monitoring, such as blood gas analysis, transcutaneous oxygen monitoring, and later on pulse oximetry, was incorporated into the routine of care of preterm infants, allowing a more precise means of supervising oxygen status and supplementation.

On the other hand, the establishment of a causative relationship between excessive oxygen and RLF pushed the pendulum to the opposite extreme, and oxygen was drastically limited even in the most severe cases of respiratory distress. Prolonged and extreme hypoxemia resulted in an exponential increase in cerebral palsy and mortality from respiratory failure; thus for every baby saved from RLF, 16 died from respiratory insufficiency.

Since 1995, experimental and clinical research has exponentially increased our knowledge of oxygen metabolism and its toxic consequences in the neonatal period. The front line of neonatal research is directed especially at three different stages during the perinatal period when oxygen is most frequently needed: (1) the fetal-to-neonatal transition and postnatal adaptation—that is, the need for oxygen in the delivery room; (2) the oxygen saturation target ranges when oxygen is supplemented in the neonatal intensive care unit (NICU); and (3) the need for oxygen at home after hospital discharge of patients with chronic conditions.[3,4]

This chapter is meant to provide a comprehensive approach to the relevant basic, metabolic, and clinical aspects related to oxygen therapy in the newborn period.

BASIC PRINCIPLES OF OXYGEN PHYSIOLOGY

Aerobic Metabolism

Oxygen (O_2) is one of the most abundant elements in nature; the second most abundant component of breathing air, constituting 21% of its composition; and probably the most widely used drug in neonatology.[5] The presence of oxygen will allow the complete combustion of glucose, amino acids, and free fatty acids in a highly efficient process that produces approximately 20 times more energy than anaerobic combustion. This process takes place within the mitochondria, which act as the energy factories of the cell (Fig. 16-1). Substrates are metabolized into acetyl coenzyme A, which enters the tricarboxylic acid cycle (Krebs cycle) where energy in the form of highly energized electrons is liberated and transported by specific proteins (NADH, NADPH, FADH) to the electron transport chain (ETC) located in the inner mitochondrial membrane. Electrons, considered reducing equivalents, provide the energy necessary to maintain the electrochemical gradient that drives adenosine triphosphate (ATP) synthesis. Components of the ETC pump protons across the inner mitochondrial membrane against an electrochemical gradient, and the protons are taken in again by ATP synthase. In this process, energy is recovered and employed to transform adenosine diphosphate into ATP. Electrons are captured by oxygen thus permitting the formation of water and avoiding electron leakage and formation of free radicals; thus, each molecule of dioxygen will be completely reduced by four electrons.[6] Metabolic substrates used to provide energy are highly organ specific; thus, the central nervous system and erythrocytes almost exclusively depend on glucose, whereas cardiac contraction uses energy provided

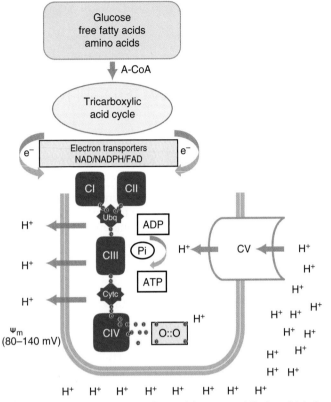

FIG 16-1 Nutrients are transformed into acetyl-CoA, which is metabolized in the inner mitochondrial space along the tricarboxylic acid cycle. During this process energized electrons are liberated and transported to the electron transport chain, creating a mitochondrial transmembrane potential (Ψ_m). Energy is used to first extrude protons (H$^+$) that are thereafter taken in again by adenosine triphosphate (ATP) synthase, and liberated energy is employed to resynthesize ATP from adenosine diphosphate (ADP). Oxygen will be reduced with four electrons. This process is known as *oxidative phosphorylation.*

from the combustion mainly of free fatty acids.[7] Oxidative phosphorylation provides most of the ATP needed by the body and is especially relevant in aerobic-dependent tissues known as oxyregulators, such as brain. These organs cannot adapt for even short periods of time in the absence of oxygen without undergoing necrosis and/or apoptosis.[8]

Reactive Oxygen Species, Redox Regulation, and Antioxidant Enzymes

The term *reactive oxygen species* (ROS) refers to a series of molecules derived from incomplete reduction of molecular dioxygen (Fig. 16-2). Even under physiologic conditions, a small percentage of electrons will "leak," causing a "partial" reduction of oxygen (oxygen with fewer than four electrons). The incomplete reduction of oxygen with one electron elicits the production of anion superoxide ($\cdot O_2^-$), [$\cdot O_2^-$] with the addition of two electrons will lead to the generation of hydrogen peroxide (H_2O_2), and with a third electron, the highly reactive hydroxyl radical (OH) will be produced.[9] ROS are also relevant in the regulation of nitric oxide (NO) metabolism and availability and therefore indirectly have an important influence on airway and vascular reactivity. Hence, when superoxide anion binds to NO, peroxynitrite ($ONOO^-$) will

be produced. Peroxynitrite is a highly reactive nitrogen species but also influences vascular reactivity in such areas as the lung, where its production can lead to increased vasoconstriction, causing pulmonary hypertension.[10] The production of ROS under physiologic and also pathologic conditions is highly dependent on the concentration of oxygen in the tissue. ROS are produced in hypoxic and hyperoxic situations and especially when the oxygen concentration fluctuates from hyperoxia to hypoxia and vice versa. ROS can be extremely aggressive when acting as free radicals, causing direct structural and/or functional damage and/or interfering with essential redox-regulatory elements. In other circumstances, ROS can be relatively stable and act as signaling molecules in physiologic processes.[11]

The term *free radical* refers to any molecule capable of independent existence with one or more unpaired electrons in the outer shell (e.g., anion superoxide, hydroxyl radical). Free radicals form covalent bonds to share one electron with other molecules; however, the resulting molecule easily decomposes, leading to the formation of toxic products. Free radicals may also react with nonradical molecules in typical chain reactions, causing damage to DNA, proteins, and lipids or promoting the formation of adducts with DNA. Under very stressful conditions (ischemia–reperfusion, inflammation, or hyperoxia) damage caused by free radicals can lead to cell death by necrosis or apoptosis or marked cellular dysfunction.[12] In addition to mitochondrial respiration, ROS are produced also by the cytochrome P450 monooxygenase system, xanthine oxidoreductase, nitric oxide synthases, heme oxygenases, and other enzymes involved in inflammatory processes. Moreover, in the presence of transition metals such as iron, copper, zinc, and manganese, the generation of ROS can be exponentially increased.[8]

ROS also have a relevant role in cell physiology. At low/moderate concentrations, especially those ROS that are not free radicals (e.g., hydrogen peroxide) elicit an ample array of cellular responses acting as signaling molecules. Thus, ROS-mediated actions can be protective against ROS-induced oxidative stress and reestablish or maintain redox homeostasis. One of the most important roles of ROS is the regulation of NO production, the oxidative burst produced as a response to infectious agents by phagocytic NAD(P)H oxidase, or acting as sensing elements for regulating tissue oxygen needs, cell adhesion, immune responses, or induced apoptosis.[13]

Redox Regulation

The concept of oxidative stress as a global imbalance affecting the entire economy no longer adequately explains redox biology. Central sulfur–disulfide couples, which include reduced and oxidized glutathione (GSH/GSSG), cysteine/cystine, and reduced and oxidized thioredoxin, function as reducing counterparts of H_2O_2 and other oxidants in controlling the redox state of oxidizable thiols in proteins. These sulfur switches in which hydrogen peroxide has a relevant role are used for cell signaling, protein structure, protein trafficking, and regulation of enzyme, transporter, receptor, and transcription factor activity. Redox mechanisms control proinflammatory and profibrotic signaling, cell proliferation, apoptosis, and a range of other biologic processes by modifying the protein structure without involving oxidative structural or functional changes. This concept differs from previous thinking in which the importance of free radical mechanisms and

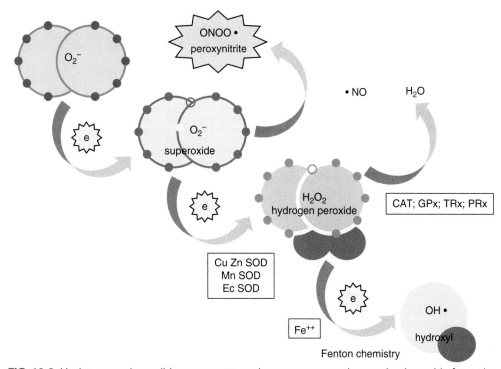

FIG 16-2 Under normal conditions, oxygen undergoes a tetravalent reduction with four electrons. However, under certain circumstances, oxygen is reduced stepwise by one electron at a time. This leads to the formation of reactive oxygen species, some of which are free radicals (e.g., superoxide anion from monovalent reduction and hydroxyl radical from trivalent reduction), whereas others are not (hydrogen peroxide from divalent reduction). Hydrogen peroxide acts as a signaling molecule. Hydroxyl radical formation is enhanced in the presence of transition metals such as iron, copper, and manganese by the so-called Fenton chemistry. The antioxidant system neutralizes the chemical reactivity of free radicals. *CAT*, Catalase; *GPx*, glutathione peroxidase; *TRx*, thioredoxin; *PRx*, peroxiredoxin; *SOD*, superoxide dismutase.

macromolecular damage as an underlying mechanism was overemphasized.[14]

Antioxidant Defenses

The redox balance at various sites in our organism requires the intervention of antioxidant defenses to counterbalance the generation of ROS. These mechanisms include both enzymatic and nonenzymatic processes. Antioxidant enzymes, through catalytic reactions, remove ROS and protect proteins through the use of chaperones, transition metal-containing proteins (transferrin, ferritin, ceruloplasmin), and low-molecular-weight compounds that function as oxidizing or reducing agents. Superoxide dismutases (SODs) constitute a family of enzymes located in the cytoplasm (Cu/Zn SOD), in the mitochondria (Mn/Cu SOD), or extracellularly (Zn/Cu SOD), which convert or dismutate superoxide anions to H_2O_2. Catalases and glutathione peroxidases (GPx) convert H_2O_2 into H_2O and O_2. GPx couples H_2O_2 reduction to water with the oxidation of GSH to GSSG. GSSG is again reduced to GSH by the activity of the pentose shunt. Other systems that detoxify hydrogen peroxide in mitochondria and other organelles include glutaredoxin, thioredoxin, thioredoxin reductase, and the peroxiredoxins. Other enzymes with antioxidant and signaling functions are heme oxygenases (HO-1 and HO-2). HO-1 removes heme, a prooxidant, and generates biliverdin, an antioxidant-releasing iron, and carbon monoxide. Finally, nonenzymatic antioxidants such as GSH, vitamin C, vitamin E, and β-carotene also function to protect cells from the damaging effects of ROS.[9] The ontogeny of enzymatic antioxidant expression progresses gradually during gestation. Compared to full-term infants, preterm infants have immature antioxidant defenses, which are more susceptible to ROS-associated conditions derived from hypoxia–reoxygenation, inflammation, or infection. In addition, transplacental passage of antioxidants also occurs late in gestation. In assays performed in human abortus materials, it has been shown that antioxidant enzyme activities in response to oxidant insults increase with advancing gestation. As a consequence, conditions occurring during pregnancy such as preeclampsia significantly alter placental antioxidant enzyme expression, causing a prooxidant burden for the fetus.[15]

Biomarkers of Oxidative Stress

Oxidative stress can be assessed by various means. Direct damage to molecules such as proteins, lipids, and DNA can be measured, determining the results of the interaction with free radicals on their chemical structure. However, oxidative stress can also be indirectly measured by increased activity of antioxidant enzymes or increment in the concentration of oxidized antioxidants such as the GSH/GSSG ratio. In clinical research, determination of the concentration derived from free radical aggregation in biofluids such as blood, plasma, serum, urine, or cerebrospinal fluid has gained popularity. Table 16-1 summarizes the most widely employed biomarkers of oxidative

TABLE 16-1   Main Oxidative Biomarkers Used in the Clinical Setting and Human Research and the Most Reliable Techniques to Measure Them

Biomarker	Target Molecule	Biologic Effect	Biofluid Determination	Analytical Method
Glutathione (GSH/GSSG ratio)	Antioxidants	General redox status	Total blood	LC-MS/MS
MDA	Lipids	PUFA peroxidation	Plasma	HPLC (UV detection)
HNE	Lipids	PUFA peroxidation	Plasma	HPLC
o-Tyrosine (o-Tyr/Phe ratio)	Proteins	Tyrosine hydroxylation	Urine	LC-MS/MS
m-Tyrosine (m-Tyr/Phe ratio)	Proteins	Tyrosine hydroxylation	Urine	LC-MS/MS
3N2-Tyrosine	Proteins	Tyrosine nitration	Urine	LC-MS/MS
8OHdG (8OHdG/2dG ratio)	Lipids	AA peroxidation	Urine/plasma	LC-MS/MS
F2-IsoPs	Lipids	AA peroxidation	Urine/plasma	GC-MS/MS; LC-MS/MS
D2/F2-IsoPs	Lipids	AA peroxidation	Urine/plasma	GC-MS/MS; LC-MS/MS
IsoFs	Lipids	AA peroxidation	Urine/plasma	GC-MS/MS; LC-MS/MS
NeuPs	Lipids	DHA peroxidation	Urine/plasma	GC-MS/MS; LC-MS/MS
NeuFs	Lipids	DHA peroxidation	Urine/plasma	GC-MS/MS; LC-MS/MS

GSH, Reduced glutathione; *GSSG*, oxidized glutathione; *MDA*, malondialdehyde; *HNE*, 4-hydroxy-2-nonenal; *o-Tyr*, *ortho*-tyrosine; *m-Tyr*, *meta*-tyrosine; *3N2-Tyrosine*, 3-nitrotyrosine; *8OHdG*, 8-hydroxy-2'-deoxyguanosine; *2dG*, 2'-deoxyguanosine; *IsoPs*, isoprostanes; *IsoFs*, isofurans; *NeuPs*, neuroprostanes; *NeuFs*, neurofurans; *PUFA*, polyunsaturated fatty acid; *AA*, arachidonic acid; *DHA*, docosahexaenoic acid; *HPLC*, high-performance liquid chromatography; *LC*, liquid chromatography; *GC*, gas chromatography; *MS/MS*, tandem mass spectrometry.

stress. The GSH/GSSG ratio is a comprehensive indicator of redox status and can be determined in whole blood. Lipid peroxidation is determined by measuring malondialdehyde in blood or urine. However, isoprostanes, reflecting non-cyclooxygenase oxidation of arachidonic acid, are now widely employed because they are very stable and not influenced by diet, parenteral nutrition, or gestational age. The preferred method is liquid chromatography coupled to mass spectrometry. Isofurans, which reflect the oxidation of arachidonic acid under hyperoxic conditions, have been very satisfactorily employed in neonatal studies involving the use of oxygen. Other similar biomarkers are neuroprostanes and neurofurans. Neurofurans reflect the oxidation of docosahexaenoic acid specifically present in the brain and therefore may reflect damage caused by oxidative stress to brain tissue. Damage to proteins can be assessed by mass spectrometry determining *ortho-* or *meta*-tyrosine, which reflects the oxidation of circulating phenylalanine in a nonphysiologic metabolic pathway. Finally, determining the oxidation of the guanidine bases in urine or plasma assesses DNA damage, reflecting oxidation of the cell nucleus. There are many other biomarkers (RNA, glycoproteins, exhaled compounds, etc.) under evaluation, but these are still applicable only in more basic research.[16]

Oxygen-Sensing Mechanisms and Physiologic Response

The following is a brief description of oxygen and hypoxia-inducible factor (HIF-1) interaction and erythropoietin (EPO) expression. Oxygen homeostasis is critical for the survival and function of cells and organisms. On one hand, oxygen in excess (hyperoxia) inevitably causes an excessive production of ROS, causing cell damage. On the other hand, the complete absence of oxygen (anoxia) is lethal. Physiologic systems are, therefore, adapted to achieve the proper equilibrium between oxygen demand and availability to ensure correct cellular functioning. A number of redox-sensitive transcription factors such as HIF-1, cAMP response element-binding protein, nuclear factor κB, activator protein 1, and p53 regulate gene expression in response to changes in the concentration of ROS.[17]

Variations in oxygen concentration in the body elicit two types of responses. During acute hypoxia, pulmonary vasoconstriction and carotid body neurosecretion dependent on increased intracellular calcium levels mediated by ROS are essential for survival. If hypoxia is prolonged, activation of the HIF transcription factors will be triggered.[18] The oxygen level in utero at the time of implantation is around 15 to 20 mm Hg and remains at this low level until the end of the first trimester, providing an adequate environment (reductive) for fetal and placental development.[19-21] Angiogenesis is stimulated by low oxygen concentrations in tissue through transcriptional and posttranscriptional regulation of growth factors such as vascular endothelial growth factor (VEGF), EPO, placental growth factor, and angiopoietins 1 and 2.[17] The master regulator of the cell's adaptive response to hypoxia is HIF-1, a heterodimeric transcription factor comprising HIF-1α and HIF-1β subunits. HIF-1α protein is continuously synthesized; however, if the O_2 concentration in tissue is normal or high, it will undergo proteasomal degradation. Under conditions below the specific critical oxygen threshold, HIF-1α protein will be stabilized and will bind to the hypoxia-responsive element of DNA and elicit the expression of numerous genes (Fig. 16-3). HIF-1β is constitutively present in the cell nucleus. Activated genes, and especially VEGF and EPO, are meant to enhance O_2 delivery to tissues.[21]

OXYGEN IN THE FETAL-TO-NEONATAL TRANSITION AND POSTNATAL ADAPTATION

Fetal-to-Neonatal Transition

The fetal arterial partial pressure of oxygen (PaO_2) is 25 to 35 mm Hg (3.5 to 4.5 kPa), reaching even lower values of 17 to 19 mm Hg (2.2 to 2.5 kPa) in the pulmonary circulation.[22] Although apparently isolated by the fetal membranes, the fetus is highly susceptible to changes in the mother's oxygenation status. Therefore, maternal hypoxia and/or hyperoxia will rapidly induce changes in the oxygen metabolism of the fetus. Hence, maternal hyperoxia induced by oxygen supplementation during anesthesia will cause an oxidative stress in the fetus with increased concentrations of malondialdehyde and F2-isoprostanes in the

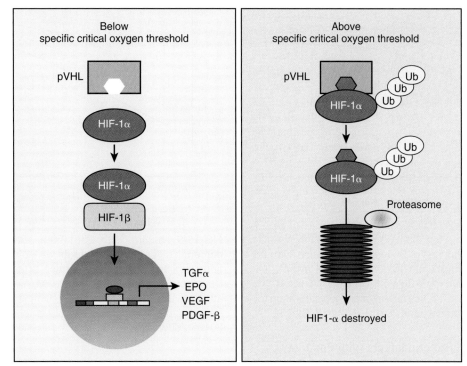

FIG 16-3 HIF-1α protein is predominantly regulated posttranscriptionally by the O_2-dependent hydroxylation of two proline residues by the prolyl-hydroxylase enzymes, leading to ubiquitination and proteasomal degradation. HIF-1α is stabilized when the concentrations of oxygen are below the specific critical oxygen threshold, thus accumulating in the hypoxic cell. When oxygen overcomes metabolic needs, HIF-1α binds to the von Hippel-Lindau (pVHL) protein, which recruits a ubiquitin (Ub) ligase that targets HIF-1α for proteasomal degradation. HIF-1β is constitutively present in the cell nucleus. *TGFα*, Transforming growth factor α; *EPO*, erythropoietin; *VEGF*, vascular endothelial growth factor; *PDGF-β*, platelet-derived growth factor β. (Modified from Vento M, Teramo K. Evaluating the fetus at risk for cardiopulmonary compromise. Semin Fetal Neonatal Med. December 2013;18(6):324-329.)

cord blood.[23] With the initiation of air respiration and the cardiopulmonary circulatory changes that characterize postnatal adaptation after cord clamping, PaO_2 will rise to approximately 65 to 75 mm Hg in the first 5 to 10 minutes after birth in the healthy full-term infant. Increased oxygen availability will cause physiologic oxidative stress and trigger specific gene expression to ensure postnatal adaptation. Term newborn infants reach stable arterial oxygen saturation (SpO_2) values around 85% to 90% by 5 minutes after birth. However, some healthy normal newborn infants need even more time, especially if they are born by cesarean section. Remarkably, preterm infants, especially extremely preterm, those with gestational ages ≤28 weeks, need almost 10 minutes to reach preductal SpO_2 of around 85%. Postnatal oxygenation is highly dependent on gestational age, type of delivery, and whether the baby is breathing spontaneously or requires some type of respiratory support.[4]

Arterial Oxygen Saturation Nomogram

By collecting data prospectively using preductal pulse oximetry with identical methodology in 468 newly born infants with gestational ages ranging from 25 to 42 weeks who did not receive oxygen at birth, it was possible to build an oxygen saturation nomogram reflecting the first 10 minutes after birth. The data were represented in a smoothed graph that included mean and ±3 standard deviations of preductal SpO_2 minute by minute for the first 10 minutes after birth. Data collected by Dawson and coworkers in term and preterm

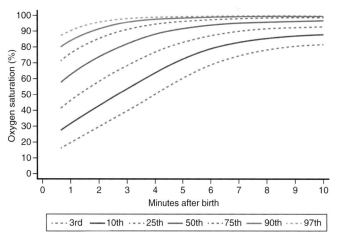

FIG 16-4 The 3rd, 10th, 25th, 50th, 75th, 90th, and 97th SpO_2 percentiles for all infants with no medical intervention after birth. (Modified from Dawson JA, Kamlin CO, Vento M, Wong C, Cole TJ, Donath SM, Davis PG, Morley CJ. Defining the reference range for oxygen saturation for infants after birth. Pediatrics. June 2010;125(6):e1340-e1347.)

infants are shown in Figures 16-4 and 16-5. As of this writing, Dawson's oxygen saturation nomogram represents the best estimate of the physiologic oxygenation that occurs in normal term or well-adapted preterm infants in the first minutes after birth.[24]

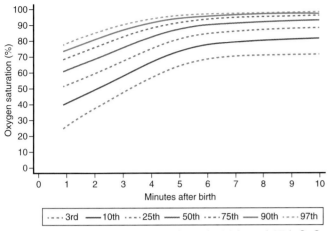

FIG 16-5 The 3rd, 10th, 25th, 50th, 75th, 90th, and 97th SpO$_2$ percentiles for term infants at >37 weeks of gestation with no medical intervention after birth. (Modified from Dawson JA, Kamlin CO, Vento M, Wong C, Cole TJ, Donath SM, Davis PG, Morley CJ. Defining the reference range for oxygen saturation for infants after birth. Pediatrics. June 2010;125(6):e1340-e1347.)

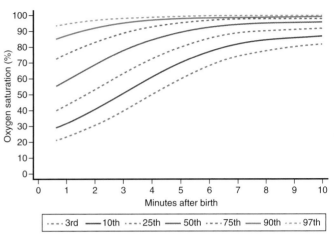

FIG 16-6 The 3rd, 10th, 25th, 50th, 75th, 90th, and 97th SpO$_2$ percentiles for preterm infants at 32 to 36 weeks of gestation with no medical intervention after birth. (Modified from Dawson JA, Kamlin CO, Vento M, Wong C, Cole TJ, Donath SM, Davis PG, Morley CJ. Defining the reference range for oxygen saturation for infants after birth. Pediatrics. June 2010;125(6):e1340-e1347.)

Oxygen Saturation in Preterm Infants with Positive Pressure Ventilation and Air

Continuous positive airway pressure (CPAP) applied immediately after birth with a pressure of 5 to 6 cm H$_2$O facilitates the achievement of a functional residual capacity (FRC) in preterm babies immediately, thereby improving oxygenation and decreasing work of breathing[25] (Fig. 16-6). Very preterm babies with gestational ages ≤28 weeks receiving CPAP and inspiratory fraction of oxygen (FiO$_2$) of 0.21 achieved stable preductal SpO$_2$ values significantly earlier than babies of similar gestational ages who were breathing spontaneously without CPAP (Fig. 16-7). It was intriguing that female premature infants achieved saturation targets significantly more rapidly than males.[26] These data indicate that the use of CPAP facilitates lung volume recruitment and the establishment of an adequate FRC, which in turn reduces the need for supplemental oxygen during postnatal stabilization, consistent with numerous experimental studies that have shown the benefit of positive end expiratory pressure in the fetal-to-neonatal transition.[27,28]

Oxygen Administration in the Delivery Room

The use of room air (21% oxygen) in the resuscitation of asphyxiated term newborn infants reduces the time needed to achieve a spontaneous respiration, improves Apgar score at 1 minute, reduces the oxygen load and oxidative stress, reduces damage to the heart and kidney, and, most importantly, significantly reduces mortality compared to the initial use of 100% oxygen.[4,29] Based on these studies, the International Liaison Committee on Resuscitation 2010 guidelines recommend the use of air as the initial gas mixture for the depressed neonate. Moreover, both pulse oximetry monitoring of SpO$_2$ and titration of the FiO$_2$ to avoid hyperoxic or hypoxic damage are also encouraged.[30]

Initial FiO$_2$ for preterm infants in the delivery room remains a matter of debate. Meta-analyses have shown no significant differences in relevant outcomes such as mortality, bronchopulmonary dysplasia (BPD), combined outcome of death or BDP, retinopathy of prematurity (ROP), intra/periventricular hemorrhage (IPVH), or necrotizing enterocolitis (NEC) when

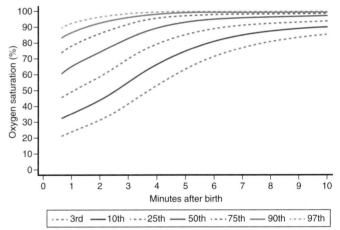

FIG 16-7 The 3rd, 10th, 25th, 50th, 75th, 90th, and 97th SpO$_2$ percentiles for preterm infants at <32 weeks of gestation with no medical intervention after birth. (Modified from Dawson JA, Kamlin CO, Vento M, Wong C, Cole TJ, Donath SM, Davis PG, Morley CJ. Defining the reference range for oxygen saturation for infants after birth. Pediatrics. June 2010;125(6):e1340-e1347.)

using an initial FiO$_2$ of <50% vs >50%.[31] The use of lower initial FiO$_2$ could have the advantage of reducing the oxygen load received during initial stabilization and thus reduce oxidative stress. In two studies, initiation of resuscitation with very high initial FiO$_2$ (90% or 100%) with subsequent titration resulted in increased oxidant stress and BPD incidence compared to starting with 21% or 30%.[32,33] In contrast, no differences in clinical outcomes or biomarkers of oxidative stress were found when an initial FiO$_2$ of 30% was compared to 60% or 65%.[34] Therefore, at present it can be stated that it is feasible to start resuscitation, even in very preterm infants, with an initial FiO$_2$ of 21% to 30% as long as the inspiratory fraction of oxygen is titrated against SpO$_2$ and heart rate is kept within normal limits.[33] However, because many very preterm infants resuscitated with 21% oxygen experience an initial fall in SpO$_2$,[36] most clinicians prefer to initiate resuscitation with FiO_2 of 30% to 40% with subsequent titration to achieve target SpO_2.

The use of pulse oximetry has become an essential tool in the delivery room. Preductal pulse oximetry reflects oxygenation of blood going to the brain and therefore is preferred during postnatal stabilization. Reliable preductal readings within 1 to 2 minutes of birth can be rapidly obtained with adequate training. Data are rapidly displayed if these steps are followed: (1) turn on the oximeter, (2) apply the sensor to the infant's right hand or wrist, (3) connect the sensor to the oximeter cable, and (4) shield the sensor from light. By attaching the sensor to the baby before connecting the oximeter cable to the monitor, the response time to reliable readings is shortened. Once reliable readings of the pulse oximeter are achieved and the baby is being ventilated, FiO_2 should be titrated against pulse oximeter readings of the heart rate and saturation. The air/oxygen blender should be adjusted accordingly to avoid hyper- and hypoxia. Hence, if SpO_2 is below the 10th percentile, then FiO_2 should be increased in 10% increments every 30 seconds until SpO_2 reaches its 10th to 50th percentile, always avoiding going above the 90th percentile of SpO_2.[25] These recommendations are based on experts' opinions; there is no evidence-based information as of this writing regarding the best way of adjusting the oxygen concentration according to the pulse oximeter readings. The American Heart Association has defined the target ranges for 1, 2, 3, 4, 5, and 10 minutes after birth at 60% to 65%, 65% to 70%, 70% to 75%, 75% to 80%, 80% to 85%, and 85% to 90%, respectively.[30] Hence, until sufficiently powered studies are available, our aim should be to reduce the oxygen load during resuscitation in the first minutes of life, trying to adjust SpO_2 to the reference charts, which at present are our best estimate of the best oxygenation targets in preterm infants. It is unknown whether the optimal target should be near the top, middle, or bottom of the published reference ranges. Additionally, the practitioner should take into account not only the value currently displayed but also the direction of change. Although the pulse oximeter should always be set for a short averaging interval, there is still a substantial lag time between the time an FiO_2 adjustment is made and the response seen on the oximeter. Taking into account the direction and rate of change in SpO_2, as well as allowing sufficient time for changes to be reflected, should minimize overshoot and undershoot of the target range.

Oxygen During Neonatal Care in the Neonatal Intensive Care Unit

The establishment of optimal oxygen saturation targets for preterm infants needing oxygen supplementation in the NICU remains elusive. Preterm infants are very sensitive to hyperoxia, which may lead to lung and retinal damage and also to hypoxia, which may cause increased mortality, NEC, or white matter injury.[5] The lung of the extremely preterm infant has a tendency to suffer oxidative stress and inflammation because it lacks an adequately developed antioxidant defense system, is structurally and functionally immature, and frequently requires mechanical ventilation and supplemental oxygen. Additionally, the lungs are prone to infection and are exposed to increased circulating free iron.[37,38] A connection between oxygen, oxidative stress, mechanical ventilation, and genetic factors and later appearance of BPD has been substantiated in various studies.[39] Thus, preterm neonates who later

developed BPD exhibited elevated concentrations in blood and tracheal aspirates of carbonyl adducts, which represent by-products of the attack of oxygen free radicals upon structural and functional proteins of the lung.[40-42] Similarly, elevated plasma isofurans immediately after birth with higher oxygen load and F2α-isoprostanes in the first week after birth have also been associated with later development of BPD and periventricular leukomalacia, indicating an important role for oxidative injury.[34,35,43] In addition to the acute and direct effects of free radicals upon the lung tissue, evidence reveals that specific oxygen species such as hydroperoxides may act as signaling molecules inducing the expression of transcription factors that may alter cell growth, differentiation, chemotaxis, inflammatory response, and/or apoptosis.[44]

Exposure to elevated oxygen concentration leads to the release of specific mediators such as VEGF and angiopoietin 2 capable of disrupting the alveolar–capillary membrane and thus causing pulmonary edema and subsequent lung injury. Other cytokines are also released from lung cells and attract inflammatory cells to the lung. These inflammatory cells, as well as hyperoxia per se, release ROS, which can initiate the mitochondrial-dependent cell death pathway.[45]

A series of randomized controlled trials has tried to assess the optimal SpO_2 range for preterm infants needing oxygen supplementation after postnatal stabilization. In the BOOST I trial, the effect of higher (95% to 98%) versus lower (91% to 94%) targeted saturations for babies of <30 weeks, gestation was compared. The use of higher SpO_2 limits was associated with an increased length of oxygen therapy, increased incidence of chronic lung disease, and increased frequency of babies discharged on home oxygen therapy, whereas it did not improve neurodevelopment or somatic growth.[46] In another randomized controlled trial (STOP-ROP, or Supplemental Therapeutic Oxygen for Prethreshold Retinopathy of Prematurity), a group of preterm infants with prethreshold ROP was randomized to SpO_2 limits set between 89% and 94% or between 95% and 99% for a minimum of 2 weeks. The beneficial effect of higher SpO_2 on the evolution of eye disease was minimal, whereas the negative effects such as prolonged hospitalization, respiratory morbidity, and prolonged need for oxygen supplementation were significantly higher.[47]

Five large multicenter, international, masked, randomized controlled trials, the NeOProM studies, have been conducted. These trials enrolled nearly 5000 extremely low birth-weight (ELBW) infants of <28 weeks' gestation and sought to identify the optimal saturation target while following almost identical designs to allow for subsequent individual-level patient meta-analysis. All of these studies compared low-target SpO_2 (85% to 89%) with high-target (91% to 95%).[48] The SUPPORT trial confirmed that surviving ELBW infants randomly assigned to lower SpO_2 target ranges (85% to 89%) had a lower risk of ROP (8.6% vs 17.9%; $p < 0.01$) than those in the higher target group (91% to 95%). However, unexpectedly, a significantly increased mortality was present in the low saturation group (19.9% vs 16.2%; $p < 0.04$).[49] In addition, the BOOST II trial performed in the United Kingdom, Australia, and New Zealand showed similar results, with higher ROP in the babies maintained in the high saturation range and higher mortality in babies kept in the low saturation range.[50] In contrast, the Canadian Oxygen Trial, using a primary outcome that was a composite of death, gross motor disability, cognitive or language delay, severe hearing loss, or bilateral blindness at a corrected age of 18 months, with secondary outcomes of ROP and brain injury, did not find significant differences in death or disability in babies in the lower compared to the higher saturation range.[51] In a meta-analysis that included all the NeOProM studies, with a total of approximately 5000 babies, it was concluded that when targeting SpO_2 in the lower range there was an increased risk of mortality (risk ratio [RR], 1.41 [95% CI, 1.14 to 1.74]) and NEC (RR, 1.25 [95% CI, 1.05 to 1.49]). However, in the lower saturation range there was a significantly decreased risk of ROP (RR, 0.74 [95% CI, 0.59 to 0.92]). The authors of this meta-analysis concluded that SpO_2 targets of 90% to 95% for babies born at <28 weeks' gestation needing supplemental oxygen were recommended until 36 weeks' postmenstrual age.[52]

Although all of these trials had an impeccable design, some concerns especially from a technical perspective have raised doubts about the practical applicability of their conclusions. It is relevant to know that the accuracy of the reading of the pulse oximeters employed was 2.9%. Thus, if the displayed SpO_2 is 88%, true saturation may be in the 85% to 91% range in 68% of observations and in the 82% to 94% range in 95% of observations.[53] In addition, the algorithm used in these trials resulted from the fusion of a high- and a low-range algorithm. The effect of this dual curve was that the SpO_2 values in the region of 87% to 90% (at the junction of the lower and higher algorithm curves) were shifted upward. Readings were therefore factitiously elevated around 2% in the proximity of saturations in the 90% range.[54] Given the relatively small separation in the mean SpO_2 between the high and the low target groups, these technical considerations make interpretation of the data challenging, and the optimal saturation range for extremely preterm infants needing oxygen supplementation remains elusive. It is likely that there is no fixed SpO_2 range or oxygen supply that safely satisfies metabolic demands of all infants born at different gestational ages. Moreover, even for a given gestational age, postnatal age is also a relevant factor to be taken into consideration when establishing oxygen saturation limits. While SpO_2 is relatively easily measured, it is not a direct reflection of tissue oxygen delivery. In addition to oxyhemoglobin saturation, oxygen delivery at the tissue level is affected by oxygen carrying capacity (hemoglobin level) and circulation and may more directly reflect the organism's oxygen sufficiency or excess. Finally, it is important to note that the findings of these trials may be largely related to our limited ability to maintain the SpO_2 within the target ranges during routine care. The exposure to extreme levels of SpO_2 may be more strongly related to the observed outcomes than the target ranges. In these trials the actual SpO_2 levels did not exactly match the target ranges, and the exposure to extremely high or low SpO_2 ranges may have differed between the target ranges. In daily practice, during routine care SpO_2 levels above the target range are frequently tolerated to reduce hypoxemia, but this practice increases the exposure to high SpO_2. Conversely, targeting lower SpO_2 ranges to avoid hyperoxemia can increase exposure to very low SpO_2 levels. Tolerance of high SpO_2 to avert hypoxemia spells or targeting low SpO_2 ranges to avoid hyperoxemia may not be necessary if the maintenance of the intended range of SpO_2 could be improved and exposure to extreme high or low SpO_2 minimized.

Until further evidence is available, keeping preterm babies within a range from 90% to 95% seems a reasonable approach. Minimizing fluctuation in SpO_2 would be desirable, because alternating hypoxia and hyperoxia is known to be a proinflammatory stimulus. To that effect, there is a great deal of interest in improving oxygen saturation targeting by automatic control of FiO_2 (see Chapter 21).

Evolving Oxygen Needs in the First Weeks of Life and New Metabolic Indices

Saugstad et al. suggested that it would be possible to differentiate between two periods with different oxygen limits. Very preterm infants below 32 weeks, postmenstrual age would benefit from lower SpO_2 limits (e.g., 85% to 95%) in a phase of rapid vascular growth and extreme sensitivity to free radical damage owing to an immature antioxidant defense system. During this stage the use of higher oxygen limits would lead to oxidative stress and inflammation in the lung, intestine, or brain, leading to BPD, NEC, or IPVH. However, older neonates (>32 weeks' postmenstrual age) with a more mature antioxidant system and a tendency toward hyperproliferation of the vascular bed of the retina owing to a relative hypoxia of the retinal tissue would benefit from higher SpO_2 ranges (95% to 97%). The latter approach, while based on sound physiologic principles, has not been conclusively established.[55] Hence, in the immediate postnatal period and independent of gestational age, the target saturation during the fetal-to-neonatal transition until postnatal stabilization is completed should be 90%. However, based on the findings of the SUPPORT and BOOST II trials, during the NICU stay, keeping the baby within a range of 90% to 95% seems adequate and safe. However, any attempt to maintain oxygen saturation in a narrow range must be balanced with alarm fatigue, as bedside caretakers must respond to the fluctuations of saturation levels in individual babies. Because there is very likely to be substantial individual variation in the susceptibility to oxidative injury, it would be useful to have at our disposal functional and noninvasive biomarkers, which would allow clinicians to monitor cell aerobic metabolism and evaluate the response to intervention. Traditional biomarkers of hypoxemia such as lactic acid do not significantly correlate with intensity but especially with the duration of hypoxia. Apparently, glycine/branched-chain amino acid or alanine/branched-chain amino acid ratios are far better predictors of duration of hypoxia. In addition, when metabolites from the Krebs cycle such as succinate and propionyl-L-carnitine were also taken into consideration, the correlation with the duration of cell hypoxia was further increased.[56] As of this writing studies are being done on the levels of growth factors, such as insulin-like growth factor and VEGF, and metabolite ratios, which might be used at the bedside in the future to enable the clinician to have reliable information relative to cell oxygenation, which could ensure oxygen sufficiency and avert the initiation of retinal vascular proliferation.[55,56]

Going Home on Oxygen

Chronic lung disease and prolonged oxygen needs after discharge among extremely preterm infants (≤28 weeks' gestation) are a matter of clinical concern. In a 2013 study of 48,877 newborn infants of 23 to 43 week's gestation discharged from the NICUs of 228 hospitals in the United States, rates of BPD varied by gestational age, from 37% in extremely preterm infants to 0.7% in term infants. Of this cohort 1286 infants (2.6%) were discharged on home oxygen, and 722 (56%) of the infants discharged on home oxygen were extremely preterm. Hence, gestational age was by far the most significant risk factor for needing home oxygen; however, other relevant factors were small-for-gestational-age infants, congenital anomalies, need for mechanical ventilation or for FiO_2 >40% in the first 72 hours after birth, and patent ductus arteriosus.[57] The goal of home oxygen therapy is to prevent the effects of chronic hypoxemia, which include pulmonary vasoconstriction and pulmonary vascular remodeling leading to pulmonary hypertension, bronchial constriction leading to airway obstruction, and changes in growth of the ocular vasculature. Improved oxygenation may lead to improved lung growth and repair, better nutritional status, and somatic growth.[58,59] It is relevant to note that although BPD is a predictor of poor developmental outcome, those patients with severe BPD who were discharged home on oxygen did not score worse in neurodevelopmental tests than did patients with BPD that did not need home oxygen supplementation.[60] The decision about sending a baby home with oxygen is not an easy one. Before discharge, the baby has to fulfill a series of requirements or criteria, which are common to most institutions (Box 16-1). As a safety measure oxygen reduction tests can be performed before discharge. The purpose of the oxygen reduction test is to see the nadir of SpO_2 reached in room air after supplemental oxygen has been discontinued. In most units a minimum SpO_2 of >80% should be maintained in air for 30 minutes before discharge, and after discharge clinical signs such as respiratory rate and growth combined with continuous overnight oximetry (or polysomnography) are monitored.

Oxygen Saturation Recommendations

We would suggest that preterm babies should reach an SpO_2 of 90% to 95% in the delivery room at around 5 to 15 minutes after birth depending on gestational age, type of delivery, gender, and response to stabilization maneuvers. Once in the NICU and until the baby reaches 36 weeks' postmenstrual age, the range of SpO_2 should be 90% to 95% according to the latest

---

> **BOX 16-1   Criteria Followed at Our Institution for Decision Making on Sending Preterm Infant Home on Oxygen**
>
> A. Corrected age >34 weeks' gestation
> B. Able to maintain body temperature (axillary 37.0°C) in an open crib
> C. Effective bottle/breast feeding without fatigue or cardiorespiratory compromise
> D. Adequate weight gain in the week before discharge (10 to 15 g/kg/day)
> E. Physiologically mature
> F. Stable cardiorespiratory function with continuous SpO_2 monitoring values within the established range (90% to 95%) in the previous 12 to 24 hours
> G. No apnea of prematurity (no need for caffeine treatment)
> H. No active medical condition needing hospital treatment
> I. Appropriately immunized
> J. Metabolic screening performed
> K. Basic family training (use of the pulse oximeter, basic resuscitation maneuvers) and attachment to an emergency department and outpatient clinic follow-up program
> L. Acceptance by the family

---

publications at the time of writing. If BPD and/or pulmonary hypertension are concomitantly present, a median SpO_2 of 94% should be allowed, meaning that most of the time the baby will be around 95% to 97% saturation. Finally, pulse oximetry should be monitored at home and periodically retrieved for prolonged periods of 8 to 12 hours. During these monitoring periods, the SpO_2 range should be 95% to 97% most of the time. If pulmonary hypertension is under control and the patient is growing, weaning from oxygen should be considered.

REFERENCES

A complete reference list is available at https://expertconsult .inkling.com/.

17

Non-invasive Respiratory Support

Robert Diblasi, RRT-NPS, FAARC, and Sherry E. Courtney, MD, MS

Noninvasive respiratory support refers to support provided to the nasal airway opening of spontaneously breathing infants in the absence of an endotracheal tube. This support consists of continuous positive airway pressure (CPAP), noninvasive intermittent mandatory ventilation (NIMV), also known as noninvasive intermittent positive-pressure ventilation (NIPPV), noninvasive high-frequency ventilation, and noninvasive neurally adjusted ventilatory assist (NIV-NAVA). Although not typically classified as noninvasive respiratory support, humidified high-flow nasal cannula (HHFNC) may provide positive pressure and respiratory assistance as well and is discussed in this chapter. All noninvasive respiratory support devices provide some distending pressure to the lungs, thus increasing transpulmonary pressure during the expiratory phase of breathing. The basic goal of using these devices is to recruit collapsed alveoli and terminal airways, maintain end-expiratory lung volume, preserve gas exchange, and minimize work of breathing.[1] Noninvasive respiratory support also may mitigate lung injury and inflammation by avoiding shear injury (atelectrauma) or repetitive cycling of the lungs at low end-expiratory lung volume. Also, distending pressure helps maintain upper airway patency and reduce obstructive apnea. By avoiding endotracheal intubation, the risks of airway trauma, infection, and airway emergencies may be reduced.

Nasal CPAP (NCPAP) is the most prevalent noninvasive form of respiratory assistance and also the most widely debated. It has been used to support spontaneously breathing infants with lung disease for more than 40 years. Following reports that mechanical ventilation contributes to pulmonary growth arrest and the development of chronic lung disease, there is a renewed interest in using NCPAP as the prevailing method for supporting newborn infants. Animal research has shown that NCPAP is less injurious to the lungs than is mechanical ventilation.[2,3] A report in the presurfactant era[4] suggested that early NCPAP, as an alternative to invasive ventilation, might mitigate lung injury and development of chronic lung disease (CLD) in premature infants,[4] and animal studies supported this view.[2] Three clinical trials suggested that CPAP use was no worse and perhaps better than immediate mechanical ventilation in most infants[5,6] A meta-analysis found decreased death and CLD in infants stabilized and maintained on NCPAP after birth.[7] Despite the successes, little is known about how best to manage patients using NCPAP or other noninvasive strategies. It is also unclear whether some devices used to maintain NCPAP may be better than others in improving outcomes. Additionally, neonates have a high prevalence of NCPAP failure (~35% to 50%).[5,6] Clinicians have devised new intermediary approaches to support neonates that would otherwise fail NCPAP and receive invasive ventilation. These intermediary forms of respiratory support demonstrated increased transpulmonary pressure during inspiration and expiration and will also be reviewed.

BACKGROUND AND HISTORICAL ASPECTS

Many neonatal clinicians believe that noninvasive respiratory support is a relatively recent innovation, but CPAP, though not known by that name at the time, was described for use in newborn infants over a century ago.[8] In his 1914 textbook on diseases of the newborn infant, Professor August Ritter von Reuss describes an apparatus (Fig. 17-1, *A*) that is virtually equivalent to the "bubble CPAP" that is used today (Fig. 17-1, *B*). CPAP helps maintain the functional residual capacity (FRC), thus helping to mitigate the natural physiologic reflex, "grunting," that is frequently exhibited in infants with low lung compliance and low end-expiratory lung volumes (EELVs). Grunting is the dynamic expiratory braking phenomenon resulting from vocal cord adduction and diaphragmatic contraction, which limits airflow during exhalation and maintains transpulmonary pressure and EELV above the critical closing volume of the lungs.[9] Early attempts to replicate the beneficial effects of grunting resulted in the first widely used CPAP systems developed by Gregory et al.[10] In 1971, Gregory et al. were the first to report the successful application of CPAP provided through an endotracheal tube or a head box in a series of spontaneously breathing premature infants with respiratory distress syndrome (RDS) during an era when mortality rates of 60% were common in premature infants receiving invasive mechanical ventilation.

Use of CPAP in neonates during the 1970s was welcomed with enthusiasm as the "missing link" between supplemental oxygen and mechanical ventilation to treat RDS.[11] During this decade a simple, noninvasive approach to providing CPAP was widely used, by application via binasal prongs or oronasal mask.[12,13] Alternative methods of providing CPAP were occasionally described (see subsequent section on delivery of CPAP). During the 1970s, it was commonly believed that air leaks (such as pneumothoraces) were more common with CPAP than with mechanical ventilation. Gastric distension during CPAP was also frequently observed. Hard nasal prongs, nasopharyngeal orotracheal tubes, and oronasal masks often were not tolerated well by neonates. The head chamber (head box) and face chamber, although noninvasive, never gained wide acceptance because of technical difficulties and mechanical disadvantages. The head chamber seals around the infant's neck, thus limiting access to the child's face. It is also difficult to administer in infants weighing less than 1500 g. The devices are very noisy and have been associated with complications such

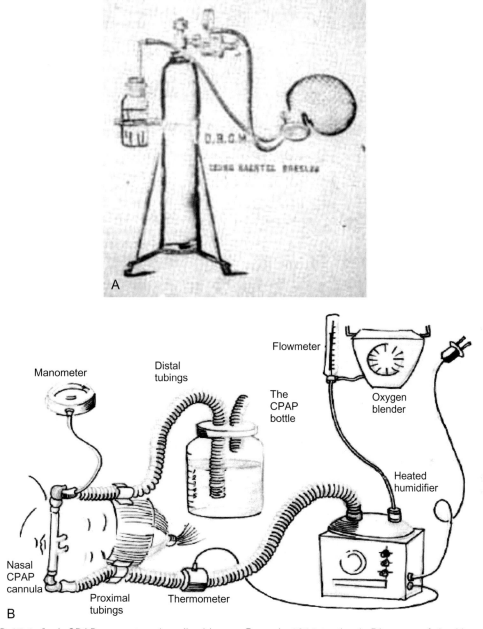

FIG 17-1 A, A CPAP apparatus described in von Reuss's 1914 textbook *Diseases of the Newborn*. Note the tubing that leads from the oxygen tank to the equivalent of a mask-and-bag device. A valve regulates oxygen flow. The distal tubing leaves the mask and is placed in a bottle of water to regulate the pressure. The apparatus is strikingly similar to "bubble CPAP" used in the current era. **B,** A schematic of the bubble CPAP setup. A source of blended gas is administered to the child, in this case via Hudson prongs. The distal tubing is immersed in fluid to a depth of the desired level of CPAP. (**A,** From *Arch Dis Child* 65:68, 1990, used with permission. **B,** From *Pediatrics* 108:759-761, 2001, used with permission.)

as hydrocephalus, nerve palsies, and local neck ulceration from mechanical compression by the neck seal.[14-16] The face chamber was originally described by Alhstrom et al.[17] and consists of the application of CPAP via a mask covering the entire face. The mask is held in place by negative pressure. This system is simple and effective, and there are no reported patient complications or mechanical problems such as loss of pressure during administration. There is reported success in using the

face chamber for treating RDS[17,18] and in weaning infants.[19] The major limitations to both methods are lack of access to the infant's face and the cumbersome method of administration. Other approaches included use of continuous negative pressure applied to the infant's chest wall using a chest wall chamber.[20]

Intermittent mandatory ventilation using an endotracheal tube was first described in the early 1970s. It quickly became the standard of care for supporting the lungs of sick newborn infants and remained so for nearly 3 decades. For these reasons the use of CPAP fell out of favor during this period. Though Kattiwinkel et al.[21] and Caliumi-Pellegrini et al.[22] described the initial experiences using soft short binasal prongs to deliver CPAP in the early 1970s, renewed interest in noninvasive support did not occur until the late 1980s following the report by Avery that infants treated at a hospital using NCPAP seemed to have better outcomes.[4] This ushered in a proliferation of new strategies and more widespread acceptance of NCPAP as a gentle way to maintain airway patency and allow sufficient gas exchange. CPAP and other noninvasive strategies are at the center of some of the mostly intensely focused research in neonatal medicine. Premature infants with RDS represent the most widely studied patient population for all forms of noninvasive support. However, NCPAP is used for other respiratory disorders including transient tachypnea of the newborn,[23] meconium aspiration syndrome,[24,25] primary pulmonary hypertension,[26] pulmonary hemorrhage,[27] patent ductus arteriosus,[28] and consequent pulmonary edema.[29] NCPAP improves lung function following surgical repair of congenital cardiac anomalies[10,30,31] and paralysis of a hemidiaphragm and is also an effective option for infants following surgical repair of diaphragmatic hernias.[32] NCPAP is also effective in managing infants with respiratory insfections, such as congenital pneumonias[33] and respiratory syncytial virus bronchiolitis.[34,35] NCPAP is useful for treating obstructive and central apnea of prematurity and congenital and acquired airway lesions. NCPAP is often used for the management of laryngo-, broncho-, and/or tracheomalacia.[36,37] The positive pressure will distend these large airways and mitigate their tendency to collapse, particularly during expiration. Conceptually, NCPAP should help neonatal pulmonary disorders in which there is excessive lung fluid, including not only transient tachypnea of the newborn and patent ductus arteriosus, but also congestive heart failure, hydrops fetalis, and other causes of pulmonary edema. Data, however, are lacking. NCPAP is contraindicated in patients with upper-airway abnormalities (i.e., cleft palate, choanal atresia, tracheoesophageal fistula), unrepaired diaphragmatic hernia, severe cardiovascular instability, severe apneic episodes, and severe ventilatory impairment (pH <7.25, and $PaCO_2$ >60 mm Hg).

PHYSIOLOGIC EFFECTS OF CPAP

Several short-term studies have evaluated outcomes in infants supported with NCPAP. NCPAP has been shown to reduce tachypnea, increase FRC and PaO_2,[38] decrease intrapulmonary shunting,[39] improve lung compliance,[10] and aid in the stabilization of the highly compliant infant chest wall.[40,41] NCPAP also decreases thoracoabdominal asynchrony[42] and labored breathing index.[43]

Apnea of prematurity (AOP) is a common disorder in premature infants born before 34 weeks' gestation. These infants exhibit various combinations of apnea, bradycardia, and oxygen desaturation. Apnea is classified as obstructive, central, or mixed. Methylxanthines are effective in treating AOP. The sole trial comparing CPAP with methylxanthine therapy was performed more than 25 years ago.[44] In that trial, face mask CPAP at the very low levels of 2 to 3 cm H_2O was compared with theophylline in 32 infants of 25 to 32 weeks' gestation. The investigation found theophylline to be more effective than face mask CPAP with the low setting in reducing (1) prolonged apnea episodes, (2) the need for intubation and ventilation

because of worsening AOP, and (3) the number of bradycardia spells. The Cochrane review regarding CPAP use for AOP concludes that this topic needs additional evaluation.[45] There is widespread use of NCPAP for management of AOP despite the dearth of supportive evidence. Kurtz et al. evaluated the effect of discontinuing CPAP and found that when infants were supported by CPAP they had significantly lower respiratory rates, fewer obstructive apneas, shorter central apneas, and less severe apnea-associated desaturation and spent more time in a state of normal quiet breathing than infants breathing without NCPAP.[46] NCPAP is effective for obstructive apneas because it splints the upper airway open, thereby reducing the risk for pharyngeal or laryngeal obstruction.[47,48]

CLINICAL MANAGEMENT OF PATIENTS ON NASAL CPAP

Clinical management of infants supported by CPAP is based on decades of experience and is often regarded as more of an art than a science. As such, management strategies vary greatly from one institution to another. However, following the publication of several large clinical studies described below, there is more definitive evidence to support clinical management of patients receiving noninvasive support than ever before. Premature infants should be stabilized on NCPAP in the delivery room. Additionally, NCPAP is generally indicated in infants with increased work of breathing (WOB), substernal and suprasternal retractions, grunting, and nasal flaring. The chest radiograph may show poorly expanded and/or increased lung opacification.

Ongoing management for optimal NCPAP levels is based on adequacy of lung inflation without overdistending the lung parenchyma. Determining the optimal level of NCPAP is a technically challenging process, because few objective measurements exist to determine adequacy of lung volume recruitment. Blood gases and chest X-rays can be helpful in determining patient response to NCPAP; however, frequent X-rays and blood gases can also be detrimental to neonatal patients because of repositioning needs, exposure to ionizing radiation, and blood loss. Transcutaneous monitoring of CO_2 and pulse oximetry offer reliable correlates for determining gas exchange in patients supported by NCPAP. In practice, oxygen requirement, which reflects ventilation perfusion matching, is a good proxy of adequacy of lung aeration. The goal is to keep FiO_2 below 0.30 to 0.40 by increasing the NCPAP level stepwise up to 8 cm H_2O, if necessary. Because of the lack of physiologic monitoring, many institutions have embraced respiratory scoring tools, such as the Silverman–Anderson respiratory severity score, to guide clinical management. These scores have been shown to have good reliability between clinicians and can be useful for determining when the patient requires support, ongoing settings adjustments, or weaning[49] during noninvasive support.

Proper airway management is perhaps the single most important aspect for improving outcomes and reducing complications in infants receiving NCPAP. This becomes particularly important because infants are now being supported on NCPAP for long periods of time. Clinicians caring for infants receiving NCPAP must be mindful of selecting the proper prong size. Prongs should fill the entire nares without blanching the tissue. Prongs that are too small will not provide NCPAP pressure because of leakage. They can also increase airway resistance and the imposed WOB and be more easily dislodged. It is essential to secure the prongs well to avoid dislodgment while keeping pressure off the nasal septum.

As previously mentioned, the 1987 publication of Avery et al.[4] surveyed eight neonatal intensive care units (NICUs) to assess the incidence of CLD. The frequency of CLD in that report was lowest at Babies and Children's Hospital, Columbia University, New York, USA. That center reportedly used NCPAP considerably more often than the other seven NICUs. Many clinicians have been influenced by the "Columbia" approach in which bubble CPAP is used early in the course of respiratory distress of both premature and term-gestation infants.

As part of this strategy, clinicians often accept hypercarbia with $PaCO_2$ levels up to 65 mm Hg (8.7 kPa) or even higher, PaO_2 levels as low as or lower than 50 mm Hg (6.7 kPa), and pH values as low as 7.20. This general approach has been used in that institution for more than 30 years.[4] Despite the promulgation and widespread acceptance of this approach, to date there are no published randomized, controlled trials (RCTs) that validate its superiority over any other management strategy or technology. There are no long-term outcome studies comparing neurologic, pulmonary, and other findings among infants treated in this manner with others who are managed differently. Additionally, clinicians should be concerned about the potentially deleterious effects of such high $PaCO_2$ levels, which are beyond the usual limits of "permissive hypercarbia" and can affect cerebral autoregulation and the developing brain (see Chapter 42).[50]

Van Marter and colleagues[51] assessed the differences in outcomes between the Columbia NICU and two NICUs in Boston. Although CLD was less common at Columbia, this review has been criticized because of differences in patient populations, indications for mechanical ventilation, and other treatment strategies, as well as the definition of CLD that was used. Much of the apparent success of the Columbia approach has been attributed to the diligent management of sick neonates by a single senior clinician. A rigorously designed RCT is sorely needed to assess whether bubble CPAP, as opposed to other forms of noninvasive respiratory support, will truly prevent or mitigate CLD. Nevertheless, knowledge of the Columbia experience has contributed to the flurry of research concerning NCPAP since 1990.

METHODS OF GENERATING CONTINUOUS DISTENDING PRESSURE

Following Gregory et al.'s initial publication demonstrating success using CPAP in premature infants,[14] efforts were made to simplify the manner in which continuous distending pressure was generated, as well as the mode of delivery. In the mid-1970s Kattwinkel et al.,[12] as well as Caliumi-Pellegrini and colleagues,[13] described devices in which binasal prongs were used for delivery. Binasal prongs connected to a ventilator for flow and thus pressure delivery were standard for a number of years. In the subsequent section, these and other methods of NCPAP delivery are described.

The pressure delivered via NCPAP can be derived from either a continuous flow or a variable flow source. From the 1970s through the 1980s, only continuous flow was used. Continuous-flow NCPAP consisted of gas flow generated at a source (usually with an infant ventilator) and directed against the resistance of the expiratory limb of the NCPAP circuit. In ventilator-derived NCPAP, variable resistance in a valve is adjusted to provide this resistance to flow.

A second method of continuous-flow NCPAP is bubble or water-seal CPAP (see Fig. 17-1, *B*), the method advocated at the Columbia University NICU.[51,52] With bubble NCPAP, blended gas flows to the infant after being heated and humidified. Typically, binasal prongs, such as the Hudson prongs (Hudson Respiratory Care, Inc., Arlington Heights, Illinois, USA) (Fig. 17-2) or Inca prongs (Ackrad Laboratories, Inc., Cranford, New Jersey, USA), are secured in the infant's nares. The distal end of the expiratory tubing is immersed under either 0.25% acetic acid or sterile water to a specific depth to provide the approximate level of CPAP desired. Clinicians must be cautious when using this method, however, because the level of CPAP may be higher than the submerged depth of the expiratory tubing and is flow dependent with some systems but not all.[53,54] Bench studies of bubble NCPAP[55] have shown that different systems produce inherently different high-frequency pressure profiles. In a neonatal lung/anatomic nasal airway model affixed with a leaky nasal airway interface, detectable high-frequency pressure oscillations were observed in the lung. A new device has been developed that increases the amplitude of pressure oscillations

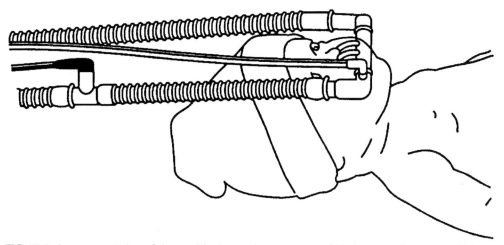

FIG 17-2 A representation of the positioning and appearance of Hudson nasal prongs, which are commonly used for nasal CPAP. (From *Arch Dis Child Fetal Neonatal Ed.* 85:F82-F85, 2001, used with permission.)

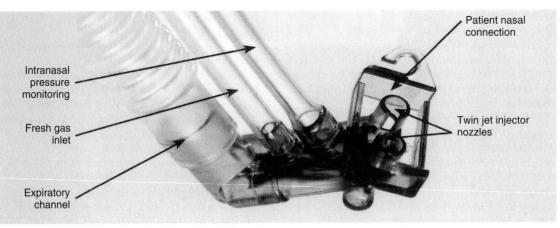

Patient nasal connection

Intranasal pressure monitoring

Fresh gas inlet

Twin jet injector nozzles

Expiratory channel

FIG 17-3 A photograph of the Infant Flow driver pressure generator without the nasal prongs attached. This is a variable-flow CPAP device. Dual injector jets are directed toward the nasal prongs after they are attached. (Courtesy Electro Medical Equipment, Ltd., Brighton, England.)

by altering the configuration by which gas exits into a water column. These pressure oscillations have been shown to deliver volumes that are similar to those generated by high-frequency ventilation. Compared with standard bubble NCPAP, this form of bubble NCPAP has also been shown to substantially reduce WOB in a surfactant-deficient, lung-injured animal model.

Traditionally, bubble NCPAP systems have incorporated pressure generators from ventilator water-seal positive end-expiratory pressure (PEEP) valves or by using homemade systems devised from sterile water bottles. Today, there are three commercially available bubble NCPAP systems. Because of the low cost of maintenance, the simplicity, and no requirement for an electrical power source, these devices are also frequently used to support patients in resource-limited settings (see Chapter 38).[56–59]

Lee and colleagues[60] observed vibrations of infants' chests during bubble CPAP at frequencies similar to those used with high-frequency ventilation. Compared to ventilator-derived CPAP, Lee's group found that bubble CPAP resulted in decreased minute ventilation and respiratory rate. These authors speculated that the observed vibrations enhanced gas exchange. Pillow et al.[61] described similar findings in the lamb model. However, in both of these studies, bubble CPAP was delivered via a nasopharyngeal tube, not nasal prongs. Data obtained using an NCPAP model suggest that these oscillations are quite minimal and unlikely to contribute in a significant way to ventilation.[53] Morley et al.[62] assessed bubble CPAP in a randomized, crossover trial. The bubbles were generated at various rates, from "slow" to "vigorous." These investigators found that bubbling rates had no effect on carbon dioxide, oxygenation, or respiratory rate. The gas-exchange mechanisms of the bubble NCPAP setup must be further explored to elucidate whether there is a to-and-fro oscillatory waveform that truly augments ventilation. One study supporting bubble NCPAP is that of Gupta et al., who evaluated the efficacy and safety of bubble NCPAP compared with the Infant Flow NCPAP system (described below) for the postextubation management of preterm infants with RDS. Extubation failure rate was lower and the duration of support was shorter in infants ventilated <14 days when supported with bubble CPAP following extubation.[63]

A major concern with bubble NCPAP is that these systems may not reliably monitor pressure or provide pressure-relief valves or alarms. This may place infants at greater risk for excessive pressure delivery. As mentioned previously, many noninvasive devices do not provide clinical monitoring of pressure or have alarms. Thus, it is important to provide continuous physiologic monitoring. In a bench model, condensation forming in the expiratory limb of a commercially available bubble NCPAP system resulted in substantially higher NCPAP levels than desired.[64] Whenever possible, stand-alone pressure manometers, alarms, and pressure-relief devices should be used. Also, bedside clinicians must frequently empty the exhalation limb of condensate, provide water traps, or use circuits that incorporate heated wires or are constructed from material that wicks moisture to the environment.

Since 1995, variable-flow NCPAP has come into widespread use. The technique was developed by Moa et al.[65] to reduce the patient's WOB. NCPAP is generated by varying the flow delivered to the infant's nares and a specially constructed nosepiece is employed. These devices use the Bernoulli effect and gas entrainment via dual injector jets directed toward each nasal prong to maintain a constant pressure (Figs. 17-3 to 17-7). With the variable-flow system, when the infant makes a spontaneous expiratory breathing effort, there is a so-called "fluidic flip," which causes the flow of gas going toward the nares to flip around and to leave the generator chamber via the expiratory limb (Fig. 17-7, A and B), thus assisting exhalation. This phenomenon is due to the Coandă effect, which describes the tendency of a fluid or gas to follow a curved surface. A residual gas pressure is provided by the constant gas flow, enabling stable NCPAP delivery at a particular pressure during the entire respiratory cycle.

An extensive description of the physiology of variable-flow CPAP can be found elsewhere.[66–68] Klausner et al.[67] used a simulated breathing apparatus and found the WOB via nasal prongs to be one-fourth that of continuous-flow NCPAP. Pandit et al.[68] assessed WOB in premature infants treated with either continuous-flow or variable-flow NCPAP. They found the WOB to be significantly less with variable-flow NCPAP. Additionally, the variable-flow devices appear to be able to maintain a more uniform pressure level compared to continuous-flow NCPAP.[65,67] This may be the reason for the improved lung recruitment seen with variable-flow NCPAP of this type.[69]

As of this writing two variable-flow NCPAP systems are commercially available. The Infant Flow has been the most extensively evaluated and is marketed by Cardinal Health

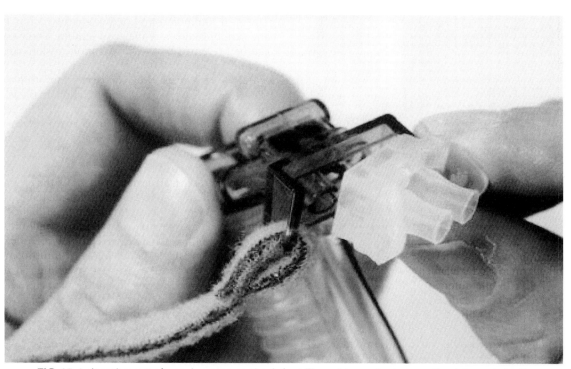

FIG 17-4 Attachment of nasal prongs to the Infant Flow driver prior to insertion into an infant's nares. (Courtesy Electro Medical Equipment, Ltd., Brighton, England.)

(Dublin, Ohio, USA). The Arabella system (Hamilton Medical, Reno, Nevada, USA) has a flow-generating chamber that varies slightly from the Infant Flow system (IFS), although the same principles (Venturi, Bernoulli, and Coandă) apply. These two systems appear to function similarly.[70]

Several investigators have assessed whether differences exist among the various methods of delivering NCPAP. Liptsen et al.[71] compared WOB in bubble vs variable-flow NCPAP in 18 premature infants. These investigators found more labored and asynchronous breathing with bubble NCPAP compared to variable-flow NCPAP. Boumecid and colleagues[32] compared variable-flow NCPAP with ventilator-driven, continuous-flow NCPAP. They described increased tidal volume and improved breathing synchrony with the variable-flow device compared to the ventilator-driven NCPAP. On the other hand, Stefanescu and colleagues found identical rates of extubation failure in preterm infants who had been weaned from mechanical ventilation and randomized to continuous-flow or variable-flow NCPAP.

It is important to note that despite all of the published research showing differences in short-term physiologic outcomes in infants supported with the array of NCPAP devices, there are no definitive data to support or refute using one NCPAP system over another. Moreover, the studies cited above were performed in infants of different gestational ages and weights, which may have had a significant effect on the outcomes reported. Rather than be influenced by these relatively limited studies, it is more important that clinicians familiarize themselves with the equipment they are using and understand the limitations of each device.

NASAL AIRWAY INTERFACES

Multiple nasal devices are available through which continuous-flow NCPAP may be delivered. The devices may be either short (6 to 15 mm) or long (40 to 90 mm). However, long nasal prongs are not recommended because of the high imposed WOB. It is probably more accurate to refer to the former as nasal prongs and to the latter as nasopharyngeal prongs. A single nasopharyngeal prong typically consists of an endotracheal tube that has been cut and shortened and then inserted through one of the nares into the nasopharynx. However, this practice is less common following the advent of binasal short prongs and a Cochrane review suggesting that binasal prongs are more effective.[72]

Nasal prongs commonly used with bubble NCPAP are depicted in Figure 17-8. The nasal prongs used with the Infant Flow driver are depicted in Figs. 17-4 and 17-5. Unfortunately, few comparative data are available to guide clinicians in choosing one type of prong over another. Some prongs, such as those used with the IFS, are specific to the device (Fig. 17-9). Prongs may vary in the type of material, length, configuration, and diameters (both inner and outer). These aspects will affect the resistance to flow in a particular device and, as a result, the pressure entering the device may differ considerably from that entering the child's nares or nasopharynx. DePaoli et al.[73] compared the pressure drop for five different CPAP devices at various rates of gas flow. These authors found great variation among devices in the pressure drop. Although the least amount of drop-off occurred with the IFS, these authors cautioned that their findings do not establish clinical superiority of one mode of NCPAP or nasopharyngeal CPAP (NPCPAP) over any other. DePaoli and colleagues[72] have published a more in-depth appraisal in their Cochrane review characterizing NCPAP devices and pressure sources. As stated above, they concluded that binasal short prongs are more effective than the nasopharyngeal prong for avoiding reintubation. Binasal short prongs remain the most common method of administering NCPAP in neonates. Because infants are generally obligate nose breathers, NCPAP may be facilitated when delivered directly into the nose.

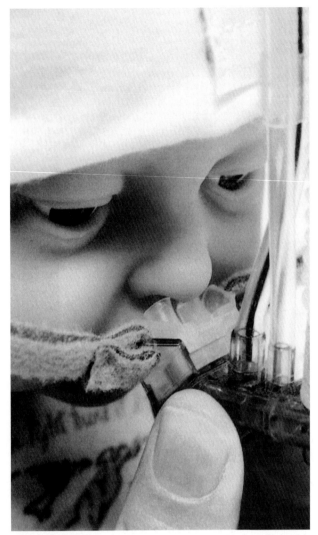

FIG 17-5 Placement of the nasal prongs and Infant Flow driver pressure generator in a mannequin's nares. (Courtesy Electro Medical Equipment, Ltd., Brighton, England.)

The most common complications are obstruction by secretions and skin breakdown at the nasal septum. These complications can be prevented by careful attention to skin care, nasal suctioning, and use of a protective barrier.

Nasal masks are a relatively recent innovation available with the variable-flow systems. A small, soft mask is attached to the pressure generator (Fig. 17-10, *A* and *B*). Such masks are markedly smaller than face masks; hence there is little additional dead space. Nasal masks may be useful when the infant's nares are too small to accept the nasal prongs. Some units also use them in conjunction with nasal prongs, alternating several hours on and off each device to minimize the pressure effects of the prongs on the nares. However, a good seal must be present to prevent pressure loss with the nasal mask. There are no published data concerning the safety and efficacy of nasal masks.

Nasal cannulae (NC) are typically used to provide supplemental oxygen (Fig. 17-11). However, depending on the flow rate, size of the NC, degree of leak, and size of the nares, these devices also provide some distending pressure.[74,75] As no pop-off valve is present on currently available NC, pressure generated is uncontrolled and may be substantial. Some high-flow NC systems do have a pop-off valve. These will be discussed later in this chapter. Cannulae can also be easily dislodged; it is not unusual to pass by a child being treated with NC and to note that the cannulae are not in the nares but on the cheek or in the mouth or elsewhere.

The RAM Nasal Cannula (Neotech, Valencia, California, USA) was originally marketed for use with oxygen therapy but has been shown to be a useful interface for NCPAP and other forms of noninvasive ventilation.[76] It is a short binasal prong designed with a larger bore tubing than standard oxygen or high-flow NC. The resistance and dead space of these prongs are reported to be similar to those of an endotracheal tube, but the dead space consideration is probably less critical, because infants are likely to exhale around the prong, not through the long narrow tubing. One bench study has shown that CO_2 removal is less efficient during simulated NIMV with a RAM cannula compared to binasal short prongs but there

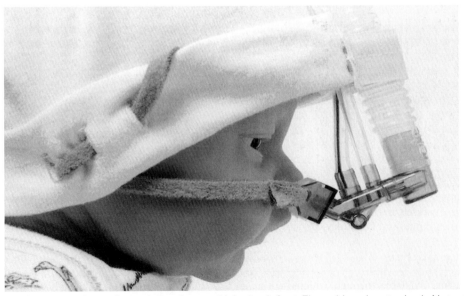

FIG 17-6 Lateral view of a mannequin to which the Infant Flow driver is attached. Note the proper fixation of the device. (Courtesy Electro Medical Equipment, Ltd., Brighton, England.)

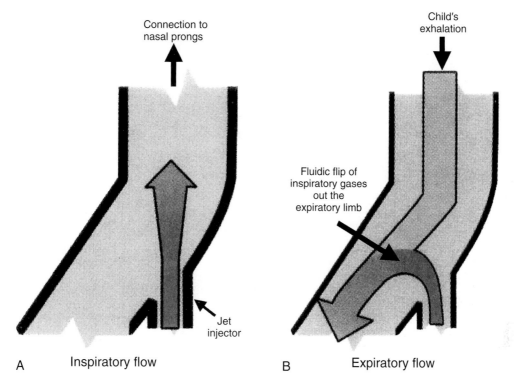

Connection to
nasal prongs

Child's
exhalation

Fluidic flip of
inspiratory gases
out the
expiratory limb

Jet
injector

A   Inspiratory flow   B   Expiratory flow

FIG 17-7 Schematic representations of the "fluid flip" of the variable-flow CPAP device, the Infant Flow driver. **A,** During the child's inspiration, the Bernoulli effect directs gas flow toward each nostril to maintain a constant pressure. **B,** During the child's exhalation, the Coandă effect causes inspiratory flow to "flip" and leave the generator chamber via the expiratory limb. As such, the child does not have to exhale against high inspiratory flow, and work of breathing is decreased compared to continuous-flow CPAP. The residual gas pressure enables stable levels of CPAP to be delivered to the child. (Courtesy Electro Medical Equipment, Ltd., Brighton, England.)

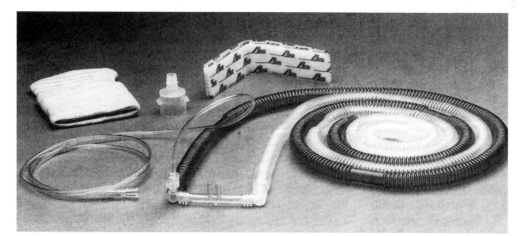

FIG 17-8 The Hudson NCPAP equipment. Note the wide-bore short prongs. Depictions and actual photographs of children being managed with this device are shown in Figs. 17-1, *B*, 17-2, and 17-12. (Courtesy Hudson RCI, Temecula, Calif., USA)

were no differences during NCPAP.[77] Other investigators have shown that even small leaks with the RAM cannula result in large reductions in pressure.[78] However, effective pressures can usually be maintained with small leaks, despite the added tubing length and resistance.[79] This device[80] has gained widespread acceptance to provide NCPAP and NIMV because it is relatively easy to maintain and is fixated similar to an NC.

Anecdotal reports suggest that this nasal airway interface is less injurious to the nasal airway than those that require more complex fixation techniques. However, the long segment of narrow tubing leading from the circuit connector to the prongs creates substantial resistance, such that there is a noticeable drop in pressure from the circuit to the patient interface, especially with the smallest size cannula. It has been observed anecdotally that

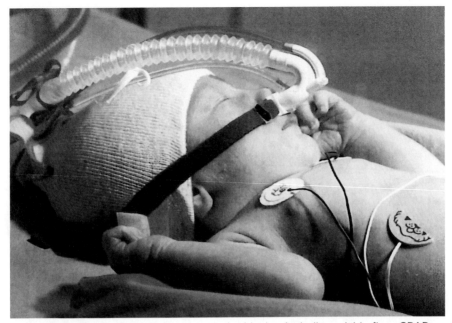

FIG 17-9 Photograph of a baby being managed with the Arabella variable-flow CPAP system. This device has to be fixed properly to optimize function and to prevent injury. (Courtesy Hamilton Medical, Reno, Nev., USA)

when used for NIPPV/NIMV, the ventilator will be cycling and registering substantial peak inflation pressure and therefore not triggering an alarm even when the prongs are completely out of the patient's nose. Consequently bedside staff may be unaware that the infant is not receiving adequate support until oxygen saturation or bradycardia alarms sound. Studies in humans need to assess gas exchange, minute ventilation, and WOB among different nasal airway interfaces.

Infants may lose pressure through their open mouths while undergoing NCPAP or other forms of support. Thus many clinicians actively try to prevent pressure loss by means such as placing a pacifier in the child's mouth or using a strap under the infant's chin to close the mouth (Fig. 17-12). Fortunately, when NCPAP and NPCPAP are applied, there is often enough downward pressure on the palate that it is frequently contiguous to the tongue, providing a natural seal with minimal to no pressure loss through the mouth.

CLINICAL USE OF CPAP: RANDOMIZED, CONTROLLED TRIALS

Several large RCTs have been performed assessing NCPAP for resuscitation or early management in the delivery room and for early management of RDS.

Early CPAP with Rescue Surfactant

Mechanical ventilator-induced lung injury is created by excessive tidal volumes (volutrauma) and/or repetitive cycling of the lungs using insufficient volumes and end-expiratory pressure (atelectrauma), thus propagating the release of inflammatory mediators (biotrauma) in the lungs. Short-term exposure[2,4,51,81-87] to excessive delivered tidal volume during ventilation can exacerbate lung injury and compromise the therapeutic effect of surfactant replacement therapy.[25] Additionally, oxidative stress can occur from excessive FiO_2 administration in the newborn lungs and impair or arrest lung development.

These forms of injury have been implicated as major causes of CLD and other morbidities associated with ventilation of premature lungs (see Chapter 30).

To investigate the use of NCPAP immediately after birth, Morley and colleagues[5] randomized 610 premature infants (25 to 28 weeks' gestation) in the delivery room at 5 minutes of age to NCPAP or to intubation and ventilation in the CPAP or Intubation (COIN) trial. The NCPAP infants were initially treated with either a short single nasal prong or binasal prongs at a pressure of 8 cm H_2O. The primary outcome was the combined endpoint of death or bronchopulmonary dysplasia (BPD), defined as the need for oxygen at 36 weeks' postmenstrual age. Although there was a trend in CPAP babies toward less death/BPD (34% vs 39%), this difference was not statistically significant. There was a 50% decrease in the use of surfactant in CPAP-treated neonates ($p < 0.001$). Although there was a significant decrease in the number of ventilator days in the CPAP group, this difference averaged only 1 day. Of note, the CPAP-treated infants were significantly more likely to develop pneumothoraces (9% vs 3%, $p < 0.001$). Although this is often attributed to the higher initial NCPAP pressure, the more likely explanation is the high threshold for intubation and rescue surfactant (FiO_2 0.60). Many of the pneumothoraces occurred on days 2 to 3 in infants with a high and increasing oxygen requirement, indicative of extensive atelectasis that would result in maldistribution of tidal volume and thus predispose to overdistension and air leak.

In 2010, the National Institute of Child Health and Human Development Neonatal Research Network published the largest trial to date, the SUPPORT trial.[88] In this study 1316 infants were randomized in a factorial design to NCPAP in the delivery room vs intubation and surfactant; participants were also assigned to one of two ranges of oxygen saturation. The primary outcome variable was death or CLD. The early NCPAP and surfactant groups did not differ in the primary outcome, and no increase in pneumothoraces was found. In this trial NCPAP was usually started at 5 cm H_2O, but rescue intubation

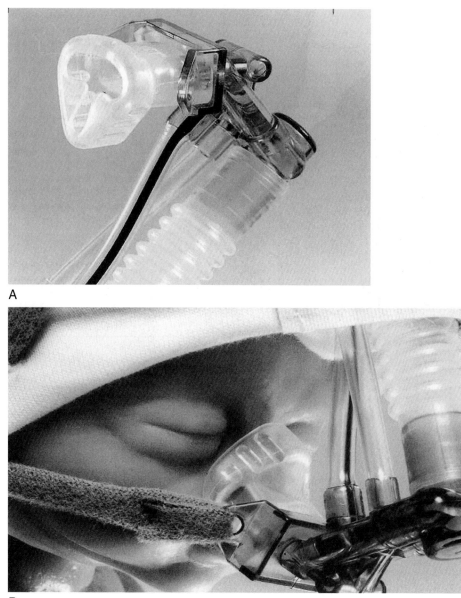

A

B

FIG 17-10 A and B, The nasal mask used with the Infant Flow driver continuous-flow NCPAP system. The mask is attached to the pressure chamber in the same location as nasal prongs. (Courtesy Electro Medical Equipment, Ltd., Brighton, England.)

and surfactant administration occurred at a lower threshold than in the COIN trial. Though two-thirds of the infants in the NCPAP group did ultimately receive surfactant, this group had a shorter duration of mechanical ventilation and less use of postnatal steroids. In post hoc analysis, the infants at 24 and 25 weeks who were randomized to NCPAP had a lower death rate. Importantly, there was no difference in death or neuro-developmental impairment at 18 to 22 months' corrected age[89] and less respiratory morbidity in the NCPAP group.[90]

The Vermont–Oxford Network Study Group studied 648 infants at 27 centers, comparing in a three-arm protocol prophylactic surfactant/mechanical ventilation, prophylactic surfactant/extubation, and bubble NCPAP followed by intubation/surfactant if necessary (the Delivery Room Management or DRM trial). There were no differences in mortality, CLD, or other complications for any of the three groups.

Both intubation and surfactant were needed less in the NCPAP group. This study was stopped early before the planned sample size of 876 infants, because of declining enrollment.[6]

These large studies indicate that, at the very least, early NCPAP is equivalent to early intubation in most cases of newborns of at least 24 weeks' gestation and may be preferable. Additionally, a meta-analysis of prophylactic vs selective surfactant demonstrated less CLD/death when early NCPAP was used, followed by selective surfactant, if needed.[7]

If surfactant is needed, a common approach is the INSURE technique, an acronym whereby infants are *in*tubated, given *sur*factant, and then *ex*tubated to NCPAP. This strategy results in improved short-term outcomes, though long-term outcomes have not been assessed. Importantly, clinicians should be aware that very immature infants or critically ill infants may need continued intubation and ventilator support.

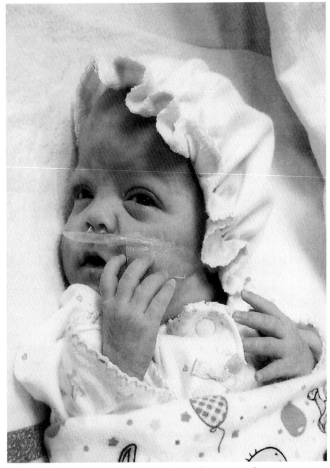

FIG 17-11 Nasal cannulae in place in a growing premature infant. This is a 4-week-old infant of 27 weeks' gestation and birth weight of 960 g. The nasal cannulae are being used in this case to generate NCPAP as therapy for apnea of prematurity.

Until now, surfactant administration has required intubation for drug instillation. However, many other techniques for surfactant administration are now being investigated. Most of these techniques involve the simultaneous application of NCPAP. These alternatives include the use of a small tube passed through the cords, a laryngeal mask, pharyngeal administration, and aerosolized surfactant. None of these techniques has yet been shown to be both equivalent in effect and safer than intubation; however, as of this writing these studies are in their early stages.

Conclusion

Given the randomized trials and Cochrane meta-analyses showing lower rates of CLD/death compared to prophylactic or early surfactant, the American Academy of Pediatrics (AAP) now recommends using NCPAP immediately after birth, with selective surfactant as needed. Intubation solely for the purpose of prophylactic surfactant administration is no longer recommended in the era of early NCPAP; the practice was based on older studies in which the late surfactant group did not receive distending airway pressure, a practice that predictably led to atelectasis and more severe RDS. Additionally, the AAP concludes that there is no evidence for increased adverse outcomes and that, in fact, early NCPAP may lead to a reduction in the duration of mechanical ventilation and use of postnatal steroids.[91]

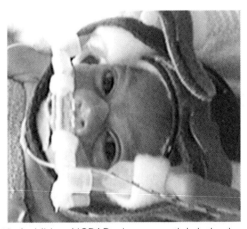

FIG 17-12 A child on NCPAP whose mouth is being kept closed with the use of a strap under the chin. This is done to prevent pressure loss through an open mouth. (From DiBlasi RM. Neonatal noninvasive ventilation techniques: do we really need to intubate? *Respir Care.* 56(9):1273-1294, 2011.)

NONINVASIVE VENTILATION

Noninvasive ventilation (NIV) or NIPPV is a form of support that is typically used for patients failing NCPAP or following extubation from invasive (i.e., intubated) ventilation. Synchronized and nonsynchronized NIMV with a conventional ventilator is the most common form, but some institutions have begun using high-frequency ventilators as well. The concept is attractive: NIV would avoid potential complications of prolonged ventilator support via an endotracheal tube (volutrauma, subglottic stenosis, infections). NIV is not a new concept. It was initially described in the early 1970s when clinicians applied time-cycled pressure-controlled inflations using a ventilator via an oronasal mask. In the mid-1980s, more than half of the level III NICUs in Canada were using this technique.[92] However, this practice was associated with increased risk of neurological injury from the mask fixation.[93-95] In 1985 Garland and colleagues[96] reported an increased risk of gastrointestinal perforation among infants ventilated noninvasively with either nasal prongs or a face mask. Of note, however, subsequent publications concerning NIV have not confirmed higher rates of this complication. Moreover, NIV may have advantages over NCPAP in stabilizing a borderline FRC, reducing dead space, preventing atelectasis, and improving lung mechanics.[97,98] Compared with NCPAP, NIV has been shown in some short-term studies to be associated with larger tidal and minute volumes, reductions in thoracoabdominal asynchrony (chest wall stabilization) and respiratory rates, as well as improved gas exchange and reduction in WOB.[98-103] In general, NIV has been studied to determine its potential usefulness (1) in preventing extubation failure,[104-107] (2) in treating AOP,[107,108] and (3) as a primary mode of treating respiratory disorders.

The most widely used and studied form of NIV is synchronized and nonsynchronized NIMV. The majority of clinical trials in humans have compared outcomes in premature infants between NIMV and NCPAP. Friedlich et al.[105] randomized 41 premature infants, after extubation, to either NPCPAP or nasopharyngeal synchronized mandatory ventilation (NPSIMV). These authors used the Infant Star ventilator (Infrasonics, Inc., San Diego, California, USA) with the StarSync abdominal capsule-triggering device (Graseby capsule, Infrasonics, Inc.) for synchronization. Binasal nasopharyngeal prongs were used in both groups. Treatment failure was defined as one of multiple parameters: (1) pH of 7.25 or less, (2) increased $PaCO_2$, (3) increased FiO_2 requirement, (4) need for an NPSIMV rate greater than 20/min, (5) need for a peak inflation pressure on NPSIMV of 20 cm H_2O or more, (6) need for PEEP on NPSIMV of 8 cm H_2O or more, or (7) severe apnea. They reported significantly fewer extubation "failures" with NPSIMV (1/22, 5%) compared to NPCPAP (7/19, 37%) ($p = 0.016$). Barrington et al.[109] randomized 54 very low birth-weight infants to NCPAP or NPSIMV after extubation. They used binasal Hudson prongs with the Infant Star ventilator as the generating source for both groups, as well as the StarSync triggering device. Extubation failure criteria were similar to those of Friedlich et al. Barrington and colleagues found the NPSIMV group to have a lower incidence of failed extubation (4/27, 15%) compared with the NCPAP group (12/27, 44%) ($p < 0.05$). Khalaf et al.[106] randomized 64 premature infants to either NPSIMV or NCPAP applied after extubation using either the Bear Cub Model BP 2001 (Bear Medical Systems, Inc., Riverside, California, USA) or the Infant Star ventilator with the StarSync triggering device and Argyle nasal prongs (Covidien, Minneapolis, Minnesota, USA). Failure criteria were similar to those of the two previous trials. Treatment failure occurred in 2 of 34 (6%) NPSIMV infants compared to 12 of 30 (40%) NCPAP infants ($p < 0.01$).

Bhandari and colleagues[104] performed an RCT comparing NPSIMV after an initial dose of surfactant followed by mechanical ventilation and then extubation. They found significantly less CLD in the NPSIMV group. This was a small trial with 41 total babies enrolled, so it was not powered to find a difference in CLD. In another small study, Kugelman and colleagues[100] randomized 84 premature infants to NIPPV or to NCPAP. These authors reported a decreased need for mechanical ventilation in the NIPPV group, as well as significantly less BPD. Ramanathan et al. randomized 110 infants to either NIPPV or NCPAP postextubation and found a reduced need for invasive ventilation and a reduction in BPD.[110]

Lampland et al. compared differences in pathophysiologic and pathologic conditions in surfactant-deficient, lung-lavaged piglets supported by invasive SIMV or NPSIMV.[111] Animals supported by NPSIMV had higher arterial blood gas pH, lower $PaCO_2$, and lower respiratory rates. Also, piglets in the invasive SIMV group had higher PaO_2/PAO_2 ratios and more pulmonary interstitial inflammation than did the NPSIMV-treated piglets. The results from this short-term study demonstrate that NPSIMV may be less injurious to the lung and provide better ventilation with less need for support than invasive SIMV.

Results from a large multicenter, international RCT comparing outcomes in premature infants of <1000 g birth weight randomized to either NCPAP or NIV were not able to support any of the above findings.[112] There were no differences in mortality or CLD between the two groups. However, in this trial any form of NCPAP and any form of NIPPV could be utilized. Additionally, the NIV could be used either initially or after extubation (within 28 days). It is thus possible that specific differences due to device or timing of application could have been missed. A Cochrane meta-analysis concluded that NIMV reduces extubation failure and need for reintubation within 48 hours to 1 week more effectively than does NCPAP; however, NIMV has no effect on CLD or mortality.[113]

A major controversy as of this writing surrounding the use of NIMV is whether it would be better to synchronize NIV breaths with the infant's intrinsic efforts. While this is preferred by many clinicians, there are limited technologies to allow this in the face of a large interface leak, especially because the Infant Star ventilator StarSync abdominal capsule-triggering system is no longer available in the United States. Much of the preceding NIMV data have come from trials assessing the efficacy of synchronized NIMV using the StarSync triggering device and Graseby capsule. One study has shown reduced respiratory efforts between synchronized and nonsynchronized NIMV with no differences in tidal volumes, minute ventilation, gas exchange, chest wall distortion, apnea, hypoxemia spells, and abdominal girth.[114]

Bilevel NCPAP or sigh intermittent positive airway pressure (SiPAP) has been marketed as an alternative to constant NCPAP (Viasys, Inc., Conshohocken, Pennsylvania, USA). Using the technology of the Infant Flow driver, these devices can alternate between a lower and a higher CPAP pressure. Synchronization using the Graseby capsule is available in Europe and Canada. In a prospective RCT, Lista et al. compared outcomes in preterm neonates between CPAP and SiPAP as an initial form of support in the acute phase of RDS.[115] Infants supported by SiPAP underwent shorter duration of mechanical ventilation, showed less O_2 dependency, and were discharged sooner. The major flaw in all the comparisons between CPAP and NIPPV/NIV/SiPAP is that they are comparing two different distending pressures; for example, CPAP of 5 cm H_2O is compared with NIPPV of 20/5 at a rate of 25/min. The latter translates to a mean distending pressure of 7 to 8 cm H_2O and it is not clear whether the apparent benefits of these NIV techniques are due to a generation of cyclic tidal volume or simply higher mean airway pressure, i.e., more effective CPAP. A clinical trial is needed that would compare these techniques at an equal mean airway pressure.

Neurally Adjusted Ventilatory Assist

NAVA is a relatively new and unique form of assisted ventilation. It can be used in both intubated and nonintubated patients; here we will concentrate on NIV-NAVA. NAVA controls the ventilator by using the electrical activity of the diaphragm (EAdi). The EAdi signal is obtained by nine miniaturized electrodes embedded on a conventional naso/orogastric tube. When properly positioned in the lower esophagus the EAdi signal represents the spontaneous central respiratory drive (see http://foocus.com/power-point/Chatburn-NAVA-for-Neonates.pdf).

Conveniently, the tube can also be used for feeding. The baseline signal (at end exhalation) represents the tonic activity of the diaphragm, and the peak level represents the inspiratory effort. Signals are recorded in microvolts. The EAdi signal can be used without NAVA support, and as such is a useful tool to assess neural breathing pattern (e.g., neural inspiratory effort, neural respiratory rate, central apnea).

In the NAVA mode, the EAdi signal is used to trigger and cycle-off the ventilator and also determines the amount of pressure delivered to the patient. The level of assistance is proportional to the EAdi signal and NAVA level. The assistance is adjustable and is dependent on a gain factor between EAdi and pressure delivered (so-called "NAVA level," expressed as cm $H_2O/\mu V$). For example, if the NAVA level is 1 cm H_2O and EAdi is 10 μV, the pressure delivered is 10 cm H_2O. Breaths are triggered at 0.5 μV above the baseline EAdi and terminate when the EAdi signal is 70% of the highest value. Thus, the pressure change is equal to the EAdi change times the NAVA level: $\Delta P = \Delta EAdi \times$ NAVA level.

NAVA provides excellent ventilator synchrony as it is based on a neural signal and not affected by circuit leak. Breathing out of synchrony with the ventilator is uncomfortable for the patient and may cause serious side effects, especially in neonates, including increased intracranial pressure and pneumothorax.[116,117]

An EAdi signal will not be present in some situations such as during apnea, overassist, oversedation, or severe brain injury. Thus, use of NIV-NAVA is possible only when the infant has a reasonably stable respiratory drive. NIV-NAVA may not be an option in the extremely low birth-weight infant who is prone to frequent and prolonged apnea or who may not be able to generate an effective EAdi signal. Frequent use of the backup pressure control mode in these cases may not be optimal, as volume-targeted ventilation has been shown to reduce death/CLD, intraventricular hemorrhage, periventricular leukomalacia, pneumothoraces, and hypocarbia compared to pressure-control ventilation.[118]

Nonetheless, NAVA is an intriguing technique, which uses feedback control to optimize synchronization and ventilator support. As of this writing it is available through only one company (Maquet Critical Care, Rastatt, Germany) with their Servo ventilators. Additionally, large randomized trials assessing NAVA have not been done. A randomized crossover trial of 15 infants of <32 weeks compared NIV-NAVA with NIV-pressure support. The authors found better patient–ventilator synchrony with NAVA.[119]

NASAL HIGH-FREQUENCY VENTILATION

In a novel application, van der Hoeven et al.[120] reported the use of nasal high-frequency ventilation (NHFV) in which high-frequency breaths were delivered via a single nasopharyngeal tube in 21 neonates of both preterm and term gestation. NHFV was provided by the Infant Star high-frequency flow interrupter. Six of the 21 neonates had previously received mechanical ventilation, whereas in the other 15 infants, NHFV was used early in the course of their respiratory disease. The authors reported a decline in $PaCO_2$ levels after initiation of NHFV. De La Roque et al.[121] performed a prospective RCT of NCPAP vs NHFV with a Percussionaire IPV-3 ventilator (Percussionaire Corporation, Sagle, Idaho, USA) in 40 term neonates with respiratory distress shortly following cesarean section. Neonates in both groups had similar oxygenation goals, and settings were not changed throughout the study period. Lung disease resolved in all neonates within 10 hours, but neonates supported by NHFV had a shorter duration of respiratory distress and lower oxygen level and duration than did the infants supported by NCPAP.

A bench study has shown that NHFV with a Dräger VN500 ventilator (Lübeck, Germany) may be nearly threefold more efficient for CO_2 clearance than NIMV.[122] Animal studies have shown that short-term application of NHFV may optimize lung recruitment and promote normal alveolarization in preterm lungs better than "gentle" invasive ventilation strategies. A large randomized trial is needed.[123] Carlo has suggested that a potential advantage of NHFV over NIMV is that synchronization is not necessary, because of the relatively high frequencies. However, studies to test this hypothesis in neonates are needed.[124]

Nasal CPAP or Noninvasive Ventilation for Apnea

Management of AOP using NIV has been evaluated in two RCTs.[107,108] Ryan et al.[108] used NIPPV in a crossover study in which 20 premature infants of less than 32 weeks' gestation were being treated for apnea with NCPAP and aminophylline. Infants were randomized either to continue on this regimen or to be treated with NIPPV, using either binasal prongs or nasopharyngeal tubes for a period of 6 hours. The subjects then crossed over to the alternative therapy for an additional 6 hours. There were no differences in the rate of apnea between groups. Lin and colleagues[107] subsequently performed an RCT in which 34 premature infants (gestational age 25 to 32 weeks) were treated with aminophylline and enrolled to be treated with either NCPAP or NIMV. In both groups Hudson nasal prongs were used. In Lin's study, all infants had previously been treated with aminophylline, but were not on any type of positive-pressure support (NCPAP or other support) at the time of enrollment. The infants were treated for a 4-hour period. Those treated with NIPPV had significantly fewer apnea spells ($p=0.02$), as well as a trend toward fewer bradycardia spells ($p=0.09$) compared to neonates managed with NCPAP.

COMPLICATIONS OF NONINVASIVE SUPPORT

Malpositioned Nasal Cannulae

A major difficulty with the use of NC or nasal prongs is keeping them in proper position. One may walk through most NICUs at any given time and note infants with malpositioned or displaced cannulae and prongs. It should be noted that with the variable-flow CPAP systems (the Infant Flow driver, SiPAP, and Arabella devices), meticulous attention must be paid to ensure proper prong fixation. Airway obstruction by secretions, particularly mucus, is a common finding in babies managed with CPAP. Optimal gas humidification, as well as frequent irrigation with saline followed by suctioning, should mitigate airway obstruction. Although nasopharyngeal prongs (single or binasal) may be less likely to be displaced, they are more easily blocked by secretions or can kink and may not be as effective as the shorter prongs.

Inadvertent Positive End-Expiratory Pressure

A number of adverse side effects and complications of NCPAP and nasal ventilation have been described. One is the development of inadvertent PEEP, which can result in air trapping. This is a problem that may occur in ventilated babies, primarily those ventilated via endotracheal tubes. Conceivably, inadvertent PEEP could occur with nasal ventilation. The mechanism is related to fast ventilatory rates and inadequate (too short) expiratory times. Inadvertent PEEP may occur in babies with minimal to no lung disease (such as postoperative patients) or in those with sick lungs. Healthy (i.e., more compliant) lungs have longer time constants. Hence passive exhalation requires a greater amount of time. Clinically, this may appear as hyperexpanded lungs on chest roentgenograms. Air trapping may clinically manifest as hypoxemia and hypercarbia. Clinicians should be suspicious of this entity when oxygenation deteriorates as inspiratory pressure is increased. Air trapping contributes to the development of air leaks. Additionally, air leaks (pneumothorax, pneumomediastinum, and pulmonary interstitial emphysema) may be a direct complication of NCPAP/PEEP.[125-127] The mechanism may be related to overdistension of the more compliant areas of the lung. Pneumothoraces appear to be a problem with babies in whom NCPAP was the primary ventilatory therapy for RDS and appear to be related to uneven distribution of tidal volume when extensive atelectasis is present, as evidenced by a high oxygen requirement. Thus, it is prudent to provide rescue surfactant when oxygen requirement remains >35% to 40% despite provision of adequate CPAP level.[128] We are unaware of any reported increased risk for air leaks when NCPAP is used for postextubation respiratory management or as therapy for AOP. Moreover, there is no apparent increased risk among infants who are nasally ventilated. In any future trials in which CPAP is compared to mechanical ventilation or to other therapies, air leaks remain an important outcome parameter that should be followed and reported.

Carbon Dioxide Retention

Retention of carbon dioxide (CO_2) has been noted with higher levels of NCPAP, particularly at levels at or above $8\,cm\,H_2O$ in patients with compliant lungs. Alveolar overdistension, as well as inadequate expiratory times, may lead to reduced tidal volumes and cause the CO_2 retention. Other manifestations of lung overdistension[129] include increased WOB, impaired systemic venous return, decreased cardiac output, and increased pulmonary vascular resistance. In addition, mechanical ventilation with PEEP may produce a decrease in glomerular filtration rate and a decrease in urine output.[130] Renal effects of NCPAP in preterm infants are notable at higher levels of pressure.[131] These effects on the kidney may be due to decreased cardiac output and thus decreased perfusion to the organs. In addition, inappropriate NCPAP and PEEP are known to increase intracranial pressure.[132] All of these effects are related to inappropriately high levels of CPAP/PEEP, highlighting the need to titrate the level of support to the disease process. Higher CPAP level does not inherently lead to these complications; when lung compliance is poor, CPAP of $8\,cm\,H_2O$ may be needed, but it must be reduced once compliance improves. With the widespread use of screening ultrasonography since 1995, we are unaware of any direct links between NCPAP/PEEP and adverse brain injury in premature or term-gestation neonates.

Decreased Gastrointestinal Blood Flow

Gastrointestinal blood flow may decrease with the application of NCPAP.[133] Additionally, marked bowel distension ("CPAP belly") is frequently recognized in infants treated with this therapy.[134] With NCPAP, administered gas can easily pass into the esophagus. Infants may swallow a considerable volume of gas and present with bulging flanks, increased abdominal girth, and visibly dilated intestinal loops. There may be upward pressure placed on the diaphragm and compromise of the child's respiratory status. Unquestionably, routine placement of an orogastric tube should take place whenever NCPAP is used. The orogastric tube should prevent or alleviate CPAP belly. We are unaware of any direct linkage between NCPAP and necrotizing enterocolitis. Although Garland et al.[96] have reported an increased risk of gastric perforation with nasally ventilated neonates, virtually all more recent investigations of nasal ventilation have not confirmed this association.[113] Moreover, NCPAP alone has not been reported to cause gastric perforation.

Skin Trauma

Nasal prongs may cause trauma to the nose that can be mild (edema or erythema) or severe. Robertson and colleagues[135] have reported a series of cases of severe trauma, including nasal snubbing (Fig. 17-13), flaring of the nostrils (Fig. 17-14),

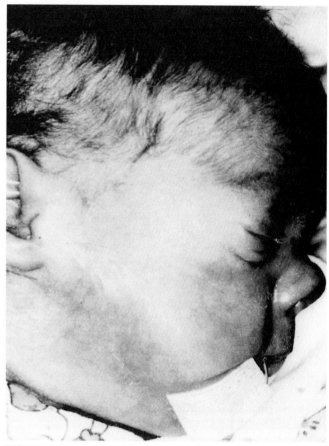

FIG 17-13 Severe nasal "snubbing" noted after prolonged nasal CPAP use in a 3-month-old (24 weeks' gestational age) premature infant. (From Robertson NJ: Nasal deformities resulting from flow driver continuous positive airway pressure. *Arch Dis Child Fetal Neonatal Ed.* 1996 Nov; 75(3): F209–F212, 750-761, used with permission. Courtesy Dr. Nicola Robertson.)

and columella necrosis (Fig. 17-15, *A* and *B*). Nasal deformities may occur with different types of nasal prongs and NCPAP devices.[135,136] Lubrication of the nares with various substances has been used in an attempt to mitigate the contact trauma between the prongs and the internal surfaces of the nose, including antibiotic ointments, steroid ointments and creams, and Ayr gel. We are unaware, however, of any clinical trials assessing such therapy. It is of paramount importance that meticulous attention be paid to appropriate positioning of the nasal prongs, with frequent examinations to assess the possibility of developing injury. With variable-flow devices, some clinicians alternate use of nasal prongs with nasal masks in an attempt to obviate trauma. No trials to date have assessed such management. Good oral hygiene (e.g., with lemon glycerin swabs, saline, or colostrum) should be considered to prevent drying and cracking of the lips.

Last, attempts have been made to use barrier material to protect the nares. One such material is the Cannulaide (Salter Labs, Lake Forest, Illinois, USA). It comes in multiple sizes (Fig. 17-16, *A*) that can be used for varying sizes of preterm infants. Fig. 17-16, *B*, shows a baby with the Cannulaide in place. Other clinicians have used alternative material such as DuoDerm (hydrocolloid gel) or Mepilex (soft silicone) to similarly cushion the nares. There are limited clinical data that assess the effects of any of the aforementioned materials in preventing nasal trauma.

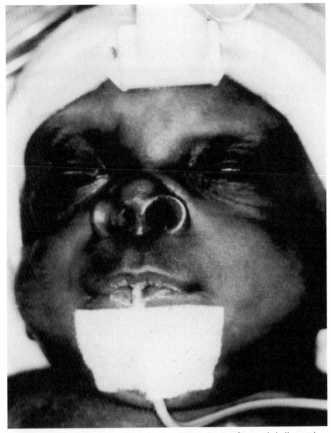

FIG 17-14 A 3-month-old infant with a circumferential distortion noted after prolonged (6 weeks) NCPAP therapy. (From Robertson NJ: Nasal deformities resulting from flow driver continuous positive airway pressure. *Arch Dis Child Fetal Neonatal Ed.* 1996 Nov; 75(3): F209 -F212, 750-761, used with permission. Courtesy Dr. Nicola Robertson.)

Other rare complications have been described in single case reports. Peck et al.[137] described the dislodgement of a single nasal prong that slipped into the child's stomach and ultimately needed endoscopic retrieval. Additionally, a preterm infant developed a pneumatocele approximately 24 hours after NCPAP was instituted.[138] Wong and colleagues[139] described an infant being managed on NCPAP who developed bilateral tension pneumothoraces and extensive vascular air embolism.

CONTRAINDICATIONS TO NASAL CPAP

There are several contraindications to NCPAP.[129,140] These include the following:
- Infants who have progressive respiratory failure and are unable to maintain oxygenation, in general, with $PaCO_2$ levels greater than 60 mm Hg (8 kPa) and/or pH levels of 7.25 or less (although some clinicians allow the pH to be lower than this)
- Certain congenital malformations: congenital diaphragmatic hernia, tracheoesophageal fistula, choanal atresia, cleft palate, gastroschisis
- Infants with severe cardiovascular instability (hypotension, poor ventricular function)
- Neonates with poor or unstable respiratory drive (frequent apnea, bradycardia, and/or oxygenation desaturation) that is not improved by NCPAP

DETERMINING OPTIMAL LEVELS OF NASAL CPAP

What is the best level of NCPAP? We believe it is the level at which oxygenation and ventilation occur in acceptable ranges without evidence of atelectasis or overdistension and with no adverse side effects. Unfortunately, no simple and reliable methods exist to find the most advantageous pressure.[129,132,140] Clearly, each baby's support needs at any given moment cannot be extrapolated to all neonates with similar problems. Some investigators have used esophageal pressures or changes in the inspiratory limbs of pressure–volume curves to guide their efforts to find the elusive pressure level. However, these techniques are not generally available at the bedsides of most clinicians.

In general, to determine whether a particular level of pressure is appropriate, clinicians should assess the infant's clinical condition and the chest radiograph. Oxygen requirement reflects ventilation:perfusion matching and is a good proxy of lung aeration and thus adequacy of distending pressure. Retractions and tachypnea indirectly reflect poor lung compliance; if severe, they suggest the need for a higher level of support. The appearance of the chest radiograph should be assessed for the type of disorder the baby has and the degree of lung expansion. Diseases with atelectasis (volume loss) and increased fluid (e.g., pulmonary edema) should be treated with increasing pressures. Overdistension should be avoided. Most often we start with pressure levels of 5 to 6 cm H_2O and increase as necessary to improve oxygenation. We have used levels as high as 8 to 10 cm H_2O. Occasionally, babies with particularly poor compliance have needed even higher levels. Decreasing oxygen needs suggest improving lung compliance and thus indicate the need to lower CPAP to avoid overexpansion.

Serial chest radiographs will help one assess the degree of lung expansion. If the lungs are overinflated, air trapping may occur and the NCPAP levels should generally be decreased. Additionally, following the child's oxygenation and carbon dioxide levels with appropriate use of arterial or capillary blood gases, as well as oxygen saturation monitoring, will further assist in the assessment of appropriate NCPAP level. As a general rule, we perform blood gas analysis within 30 to 60 minutes after any changes in pressure. If oxygenation worsens or CO_2 levels increase after increases in the pressure, the lungs may be overdistended.

WEANING FROM CPAP

Once an infant is being treated with NCPAP, there are no magic guidelines as to when the child can be weaned off. As we are decreasing the pressures, we assess the baby's oxygen saturation levels, occurrence of apnea and/or bradycardia, and WOB. It is hoped that we have been able to lower the FiO_2 to a relatively low amount. In general, infants who require an FiO_2 greater than 0.40 or are clinically unstable are unlikely to be successfully weaned off NCPAP. Generally, we prefer to decrease pressures down to a relatively low level (~5 cm H_2O) and oxygen to below 25%. Once the NCPAP and oxygen are at this level without increased WOB and the baby does not have substantial apnea, bradycardia, or oxygen desaturation, we attempt to discontinue NCPAP. Infants without oxygen requirement who are breathing comfortably may be trialed off NCPAP with no additional support. There is no evidence to support gradual removal of CPAP for progressively longer periods of time. Infants still

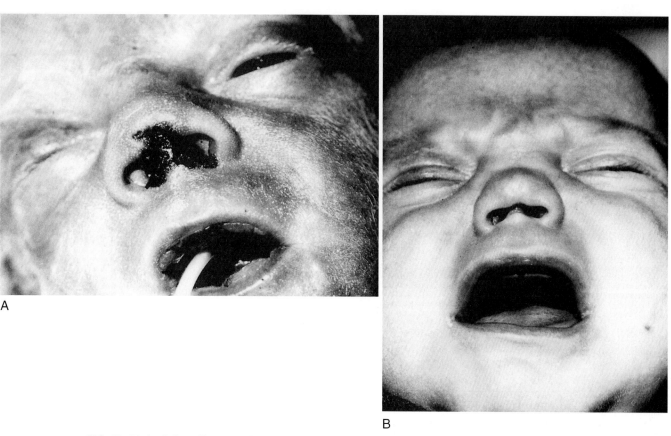

FIG 17-15 **A,** Columella necrosis noted after 3 days of NCPAP. **B,** Progression of the columella necrosis in the same infant to absent columella at 4 months of age. (From Robertson NJ: Nasal deformities resulting from flow driver continuous positive airway pressure. *Arch Dis Child Fetal Neonatal Ed.* 1996 Nov; 75(3): F209 -F212, 750-761, used with permission. Courtesy Dr. Nicola Robertson.)

requiring oxygen or who are still somewhat tachypneic or having mild retractions may require an NC. The baby's subsequent clinical findings and oxygen requirement will guide the clinician as to whether NCPAP needs to be reinstituted. Very preterm infants benefit from continued use of CPAP even in the absence of significant lung disease, because of their excessively compliant chest wall, which lacks the rigidity necessary to oppose the elastic recoil of the lungs and maintain FRC. Some clinicians will routinely keep very low birth-weight infants on NCPAP until 32 to 34 weeks' postmenstrual age to improve lung growth.

HUMIDIFIED HIGH-FLOW NASAL CANNULA

NC are mainly used to deliver supplemental oxygen. Locke et al.[74] demonstrated that NC could deliver significant continuous distending pressure to infants and alter breathing patterns. Because of the uncontrolled pressure, they advised against use of NC for NCPAP. Subsequently, Sreenan et al.[75] compared the use of NC at flows of up to 2.5 L/min with NCPAP generated by a ventilator using Argyle prongs (Covidien, Minneapolis, Minnesota, USA) in premature infants already being treated with NCPAP for AOP. This was a crossover design study in which all infants initially started on NCPAP. After 6 hours, the infants were changed to NC for another 6-hour period. The authors assessed delivered airway pressure by measuring esophageal pressures. Sreenan's group found that comparable continuous distending pressure could be generated by the NC. The amount of flow required to generate

comparable pressures depended upon the infant's weight. There were no differences between the two systems in the frequency and duration of apnea, bradycardia, or desaturation episodes. Typical flow rates that are used for nonhumidified NC are 0.5 to 2 L/min. Because the gases used are nonhumidified, low-flow NC may have a drying effect on nasal secretions that could lead to obstruction or to localized bleeding.

Widespread use of HHFNC (Fig. 17-17) has become common in NICUs since 2005. The premise is that gases at flow rates greater than or equal to 2 L/min are humidified to prevent the adverse effects of dry gas. The higher flow rates are used clinically to provide respiratory support in neonates in lieu of NCPAP or oxygen hoods. Although not specifically approved as devices for generating positive pressure, clinicians generally use HHFNC in the hope that it will be a less invasive form of noninvasive support that will prevent some of the complications of NCPAP (nares injury) and low-flow, nonhumidified NC (thickened secretions, nasal bleeding). The two major commercial devices that are available are produced by Vapotherm, Inc. (Exeter, New Hampshire, USA) and by Fisher & Paykel Healthcare (Auckland, New Zealand).

Two large RCTs have evaluated HHFNC in neonates. Manley et al. randomized 303 infants of less than 32 weeks to either NCPAP (7 cm H$_2$O) or HHFNC (5 to 6 L/min) after extubation. In this noninferiority study, the efficacy of the HHFNC was similar to that of NCPAP, though the result was close to the chosen margin of noninferiority.[141] Yoder et al. studied 432 infants from 28 to 42 weeks and found similar efficacy and

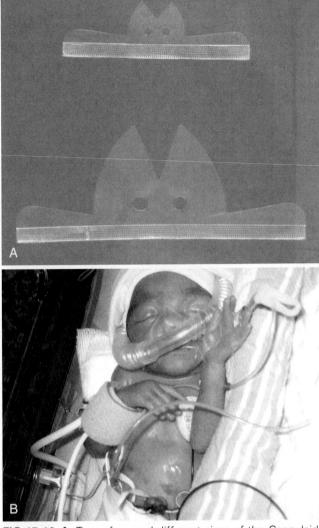

FIG 17-16 **A,** Two of several different sizes of the Cannulaide material that is used to protect the nares during NCPAP therapy. The triangular-shaped upper portions are placed on the external portion of the nose and the NCPAP prongs are inserted through the holes in the lower portion. **B,** A child undergoing therapy with NCPAP with the Cannulaide in place to help protect the delicate tissue of the nose.

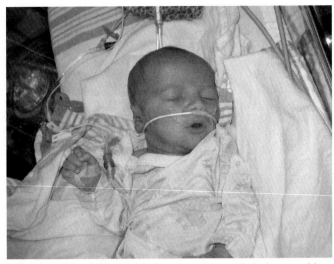

FIG 17-17 Humidified, high-flow nasal cannula being used in a 36-week gestational age infant who had a pneumothorax.

safety of HHFNC compared to NCPAP, using either device postextubation or as initial support.[142]

There are several proposed physiologic mechanisms by which HHFNC is believed to be effective. These include (1) flushing the upper airway dead space of CO_2, allowing for better alveolar gas exchange; (2) providing a flow adequate to support inspiration, thereby reducing inspiratory WOB; (3) improving lung and airway mechanics by eliminating the effects of drying/cooling; (4) reducing or eliminating the metabolic cost of gas conditioning; and (5) providing end distending pressure.[143] Clinicians are unable to continuously measure the pressures generated by HHFNC. Widely variable, extremely high pressures have been noted among infants treated with this therapy.[74,144] The pressure that is generated is unregulated and unpredictable. Thus, it is very important to ensure a large leak when HHFNC is used. This is opposite to the use of NCPAP, in which leak should be minimal to provide the required pressure. The Vapotherm was temporarily removed from the market for approximately 1 year because of the recovery of a bacterium (*Ralstonia* sp.) in infants who were treated with the device. It has since been marketed again with new guidelines on cleaning. There have also been isolated reports of facial burns, a perforated ear drum, and subcutaneous scalp emphysema/pneumocephalus.[145] Woodhead and colleagues[146] found an improved appearance in the nasal mucosa of children treated with HHFNC compared to those managed with nonhumidified NC. Saslow et al.[147] found similar WOB using HHFNC at 3 to 6 L/min compared to NCPAP of 6 cm H_2O. Two groups[144,148] have reported pressure to be dependent on the flow rate that is used, as well as the infant's weight.

Habib et al.[149] observed the effects of pressure generated in a static neonatal lung model using two commercially available HHFNC devices with flow of 0 to 12 L/min and at different leak settings. They demonstrated in a nares model, in which leak was minimized (mouth closed), a systematic increase in simulated tracheal pressures that was proportional to increased flows. In one of the systems (Vapotherm), the measured airway pressures were similar to those reported with NCPAP (~5 to 6 cm H_2O at flows of ~6 to 8 L/min). While this study[149] addressed device performance in a physical model, there are notable safety factors related to the individual devices. Neither of these devices is capable of detecting or limiting pressure at the proximal airway. The Fisher & Paykel HHFNC system (Fisher & Paykel Healthcare, Auckland, New Zealand) has a pressure-relief valve located prior to the humidifier that will limit system pressure (>40 cm H_2O). This provision may reduce the delivered flow to the patient because high circuit pressures are generally required to overcome the resistive properties of the NC. The Vapotherm has a higher pressure threshold than the Fisher & Paykel HHFNC system.

Frizzola and colleagues[150] measured tracheal pressures and gas exchange in 13 lung-injured neonatal piglets supported by NCPAP and HHFNC under high-leak and low-leak conditions. The major finding of this study was that HHFNC tracheal pressures were comparable to NCPAP pressures at the same flow range, and washout of nasopharyngeal dead space was associated with improved ventilation and oxygenation independent of generation of tracheal pressure alone during HHFNC.

A number of short-term studies have evaluated the magnitude of distending pressure in the lung in small groups of infants. Sreenan et al.[75] found that similar end-expiratory pleural pressures could be maintained between a standard oxygen delivery NC (1 to 2.5 L/min) and NCPAP in a group of 40 premature infants with no differences in desaturations, bradycardia, and apnea. However, this pressure is likely to be highly variable because of leak and the relationship between airway and cannula size. Lampland observed similar end-expiratory pleural pressures between HHFNC (2 to 6 L/min) and NCPAP at 6 cm H_2O in premature neonates.[151]

SUMMARY

The use of noninvasive respiratory support such as NCPAP is not a new concept. Apparent benefits were first noted more than 4 decades ago. For a 20-year period, however, treatment with NIV, as well as research concerning the technology, waned. Renewed interest in these therapies came in the late 1980s. With advances in obstetric and neonatal care, survival of increasingly smaller and less mature neonates has become possible. The hope is that NCPAP and other forms of noninvasive respiratory support can lessen iatrogenic injury (particularly CLD) in newborn infants, particularly those of very low birth weight. Though the history of neonatology is replete with widespread enthusiastic acceptance of diverse therapies with a modicum of supportive evidence, recent data about NCPAP are encouraging.

We must continue to carefully evaluate the use of NCPAP and other forms of noninvasive respiratory support so that we may understand the potential benefits and potential disadvantages. The major areas in which these therapies are being used are postextubation management, AOP, and primary treatment of RDS. There are supportive data for NCPAP use at delivery and postextubation. However, NCPAP use for AOP needs more study. There is evidence that early NCPAP use, often even before exogenous surfactant therapy, may reduce the need for mechanical ventilation and reduce the need for surfactant in premature babies with RDS. There is evidence at this time that early NCPAP may reduce the incidence of CLD and mortality. Air leaks may increase with NCPAP use. NCPAP use in the delivery room makes good physiologic sense for infants prone to atelectasis, and recent clinical trials have demonstrated benefit. Data on nasal ventilation are conflicting. Many questions have yet to be answered:

- Does CPAP use increase (or decrease) caloric expenditure?
- What are the long-term pulmonary and neurodevelopmental outcomes among infants that are primarily managed with NCPAP or other types of noninvasive respiratory support?
- What are acceptable ranges of pH, PaO_2, and $PaCO_2$ among infants receiving NIV?
- What forms of noninvasive support are most effective? Safest?
- Should synchronization of nasal ventilation inflations to the infant's breaths be performed, and if so, how? Will NAVA or similar support systems define the future of noninvasive support?

Although noninvasive respiratory support, particularly NCPAP, plays a major role in our management of neonates, there are many additional questions concerning these therapies that have not yet been answered.

REFERENCES

A complete reference list is available at https://expertconsult.inkling.com/.

18

Basic Modes of Synchronized Ventilation

Martin Keszler, MD, FAAP, and Mark C. Mammel, MD

INTRODUCTION

The standard mode of ventilation used in newborn infants prior to the availability of synchronized ventilation was known as *intermittent mandatory ventilation* (IMV). This pressure-controlled, time-cycled mode of ventilation provides a set number of "mandatory" mechanical inflations. The patient continues to breathe spontaneously, using the fresh gas flow available in the ventilator circuit. However, without synchronization of the infant's spontaneous effort, the irregular respiratory pattern of a newborn baby leads to frequent asynchrony between the infant and the ventilator, sometimes resulting in a ventilator inflation that occurs just as the infant is exhaling (Fig. 18-1).[1] High airway pressure, pneumothorax, poor oxygenation, and large fluctuations in intracranial pressures leading to increased risk of intraventricular hemorrhage were the consequences of such asynchrony.[2,3] Heavy sedation or muscle paralysis was often necessary in the past to prevent the baby from "fighting the ventilator."[2-4] These interventions resulted in greater dependence on respiratory support, lack of respiratory muscle training, generalized edema, and inability to assess the infant's neurologic status. The advantages of synchronizing the infant's spontaneous effort with the ventilator cycle, rather than using muscle relaxants, are intuitively obvious and supported by a number of short-term physiologic studies and modestly sized randomized clinical trials demonstrating improved gas exchange and other benefits of synchronized ventilation (Table 18-1).[5-10] Unfortunately, the two largest randomized trials of synchronized ventilation were conducted many years ago using outdated technology (pressure trigger) and had other methodologic issues; both failed to clearly demonstrate benefits of synchronization.[11,12] A Cochrane meta-analysis demonstrated shorter duration of mechanical ventilation with synchronized vs nonsynchronized ventilation but no effect on other important outcomes.[13] The effect of synchronizing the ventilator inflations with the patient's own effort is illustrated in Figure 18-2. This chapter focuses on the commonly used modes of synchronized ventilation. Less widely used modes are discussed in Chapter 21 on Special Ventilation Techniques.

TRIGGER TECHNOLOGY

The availability of effective synchronized ventilation for neonatal applications lagged considerably behind its use in adults because of the technological challenges occasioned by the small size, weak respiratory effort, and short time constants of preterm infants. The ideal triggering device for newborn ventilation must be sensitive enough to be activated by a small preterm infant but must also be relatively immune to auto-triggering. A very rapid response time to match the short inspiratory times and rapid respiratory rates seen in small premature infants is also critically important. An additional challenge is the common presence of a variable leak of gas around uncuffed endotracheal tubes (ETT). The types of triggering devices used in clinical care and their relative advantages are listed in Table 18-2.[14,15] Flow triggering using a flow sensor at the airway opening has proved to be the best method that is currently widely available.[14,15] Either a variable orifice differential pressure transducer (pneumotachometer) or a hot-wire anemometer may be used for flow detection, with the latter being the preferred choice. Flow triggering is much more sensitive than pressure triggering and is capable of detecting a patient effort of as little as 0.2 mL/min.

An attractive new synchronization technology, available as of this writing only on the Maquet Servo ventilators (Maquet, Wayne, N.J.), uses the electrical activity of the diaphragm, detected by transesophageal electromyography, to trigger ventilator inflation. This approach is attractive because it has the shortest trigger delay and is not affected by ETT leakage, thus being particularly suitable for noninvasive synchronized ventilation.[16,17] However, it cannot currently be used independent of the neurally adjusted ventilatory assist mode, which has not yet

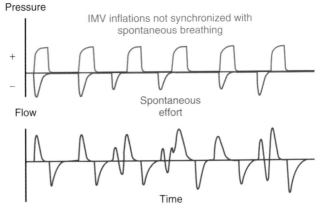

FIG 18-1 Pressure and flow waveforms indicating lack of synchrony between ventilator inflations and patient's spontaneous effort. Positive-pressure inflations are shown in *teal* above the baseline, and the patient's spontaneous effort is shown as negative-pressure deflection in *purple*. Note the consequences of asynchrony with disorganized flow and highly variable tidal volume. *IMV,* Intermittent mandatory ventilation.

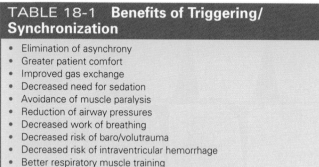

TABLE 18-1 Benefits of Triggering/Synchronization

- Elimination of asynchrony
- Greater patient comfort
- Improved gas exchange
- Decreased need for sedation
- Avoidance of muscle paralysis
- Reduction of airway pressures
- Decreased work of breathing
- Decreased risk of baro/volutrauma
- Decreased risk of intraventricular hemorrhage
- Better respiratory muscle training
- Faster weaning from mechanical ventilation

been adequately evaluated in small preterm infants with immature respiratory control.

While flow triggering is the best widely available method of synchronization, it is not without limitations. The interposition of the flow sensor adds approximately 0.8 mL of dead space to the ventilator circuit, a volume that becomes a larger proportion of the tidal volume as the size of the patient decreases.[18] The second limitation is its susceptibility to auto-triggering in the presence of a leak around the ETT.[19] A substantial leakage flow during the expiratory phase will be erroneously interpreted by the ventilator as an inspiratory effort, potentially resulting in an excessively rapid inflation rate, hypocarbia, or air trapping. Auto-triggering is more of a problem with

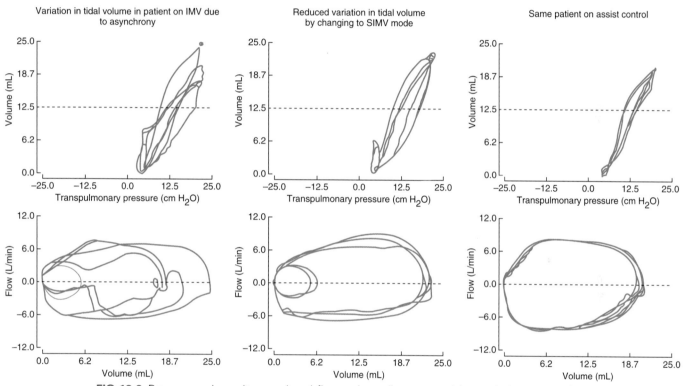

FIG 18-2 Pressure–volume (top row) and flow–volume (bottom row) loops during nonsynchronized intermittent mandatory ventilation (*IMV*), synchronized IMV (*SIMV*), and assist control (*AC*) ventilation in a single patient. Note the large and random variation in the loops with IMV, the more consistent loops but with a large difference between spontaneous breaths and mechanical inflations with SIMV, and the consistent superimposable loops with AC.

TABLE 18-2 Available Trigger Technologies with Their Advantages and Shortcomings

Method/Technology	Advantages	Disadvantages
Airway pressure/pressure transducer	Simple, no added dead space	Lacks sensitivity, causes long trigger delay, high WOB; no tidal volume measurement
Airflow/hot-wire anemometer or pneumotachograph	Good sensitivity, rapid response, provides tidal volume measurement	Added dead space, prone to auto-triggering with ETT leak
Thoracic impedance/ECG leads	No added dead space	Affected by placement, poor electrode adhesion; no tidal volume measurement
Abdominal motion/applanation transducer (Graseby capsule)	Rapid response, no added dead space	Susceptible to artifact with incorrect position; affected by change in patient position; limited availability; no tidal volume measurement
Electrical activity of the diaphragm/transesophageal electromyography	No added dead space, very rapid response, not affected by leak; ideal for NIV	Costly, somewhat invasive; limited availability; no tidal volume measurement

WOB, Work of breathing; *ETT*, endotracheal tube; *NIV*, noninvasive ventilation; *ECG*, electrocardiography.

ventilation modes that support every patient breath and should be suspected when the ventilator rate is >70/min with no evidence of patient inspiratory effort, especially when there is water in the expiratory limb of the ventilator circuit. The simplest way to verify that tachypnea is caused by auto-triggering is to briefly switch the ventilator to continuous positive airway pressure (CPAP) mode. If auto-triggering were occurring, the patient's respiratory rate would immediately be less than the previous rate and usually fall briefly to zero because of the induced respiratory alkalosis. When auto-triggering is recognized, it can be mitigated by making the trigger less sensitive. Unfortunately, the size of the leak can change quite rapidly, requiring constant vigilance and frequent adjustment. Furthermore, when the trigger sensitivity is decreased, increased patient effort is needed to trigger inflation and the trigger delay increases, both of which are highly undesirable (Fig. 18-3). Most devices now allow a fixed amount of leak compensation to mitigate this problem, but a fixed compensation level does not account for the variability of the leak. Specialty neonatal ventilators employ effective leak compensation technology that derives the instantaneous leak flow throughout the ventilator cycle and mathematically subtracts this flow from the raw measurement (Fig. 18-4). This approach eliminates ETT leak-related auto-triggering, but the device may still be affected by water in the expiratory limb of the circuit. The use of heated circuits and modern ventilator circuits with a semipermeable expiratory limb that eliminates water condensation (Evaqua™, Fisher & Paykel, Auckland, New Zealand) has virtually eliminated auto-triggering, allowing trigger sensitivity to remain at the most sensitive value and preserving the rapid response time and minimal work to trigger inflation.

BASIC SYNCHRONIZED MODES

Patient–Ventilator Interactions with Synchronized Ventilation

The key concept in minimizing the need for invasive respiratory support is to avoid heavy sedation and muscle paralysis and to maximally utilize the patient's spontaneous respiratory effort. While allowing the patient to breathe spontaneously during mechanical ventilation has clear advantages as listed above, it leads to considerable challenges for the clinician, who needs to appreciate the complex interaction between the awake, spontaneously breathing infant and the various modes of synchronized ventilation. A key concept in understanding these interactions is an appreciation of the additive nature of the patient inspiratory effort and the positive pressure generated by the ventilator. As illustrated in Figure 18-5, the tidal volume entering the infant's lungs is driven by the transpulmonary pressure, the sum of the negative inspiratory effort of the infant and the positive inflation pressure from the ventilator. Because in a preterm infant, the spontaneous effort is sometimes sporadic and always highly variable, the resulting transpulmonary pressure and tidal volume are typically quite variable. The following paragraphs will attempt to clarify the way an infant's spontaneous respiratory pattern interacts with the common ventilator modes.

Synchronized Intermittent Mandatory Ventilation

Synchronized intermittent mandatory ventilation (SIMV) provides a preset number of inflations, as in standard IMV, but

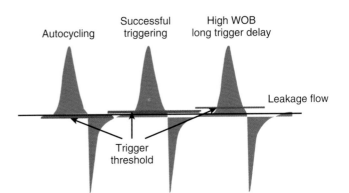

FIG 18-3 Impact of leakage flow on flow triggering. When leakage flow exceeds the trigger threshold, auto-triggering will occur (first ventilator cycle, left). With a trigger sensitivity just above the leakage flow there is rapid response time and no auto-triggering (second cycle, middle). This is the ideal situation, but because leakage flow varies, auto-triggering can recur when the sensitivity is too close to the leakage flow. The danger of auto-triggering can be eliminated by substantially increasing the trigger threshold (making the trigger less sensitive), but this results in increased trigger delay and requires increased effort to trigger the ventilator (third cycle, right). *WOB,* Work of breathing.

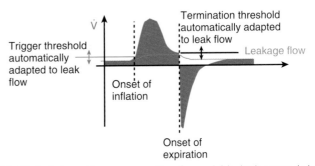

FIG 18-4 Automatic compensation for variable leak around the ETT as implemented on the Dräger Babylog 8000+ and VN 500. The magnitude of leakage flow is derived throughout the ventilator cycle, based on measured pressure and the impedance of the leakage flow, and electronically subtracted from the measured flow. This approach allows the trigger sensitivity to remain at the most sensitive value without danger of auto-triggering (with leaks of up to 70%). The same leak compensation concept is also applied to inflation termination in pressure-support ventilation, which is addressed later in the text. The termination criterion is fixed at 15% of peak flow, and reliable flow cycling will occur even in the face of 70% to 80% leak without premature inflation termination when the leak decreases.

these are synchronized with the infant's spontaneous respiratory effort, if present. SIMV may be pressure or volume controlled, but in neonatal applications it is almost always pressure controlled and time cycled. To prevent mandatory inflations during expiration, there is a brief refractory period so that triggering can occur only within a trigger window. If no spontaneous effort is detected during a trigger window, a mandatory inflation will be given. Spontaneous breaths in excess of the set ventilator rate are not supported. This is not a problem with the relatively rapid set rate typically used in the acute phase of the disease but results in uneven tidal volumes (V_Ts) and high work of breathing during

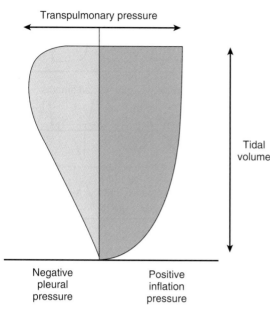

FIG 18-5 With synchronized ventilation, the magnitude of tidal volume on the vertical axis is the result of the combined effort of ventilator and patient. The transpulmonary pressure on the horizontal axis is the sum of the positive inflation pressure from the ventilator (to the right in *blue*) and the negative pressure generated by the patient's inspiratory effort (on the left in *yellow*). Ventilator graphics and calculated compliance and resistance values do not include the patient's spontaneous effort.

weaning in very small infants owing to the high airway resistance of the narrow ETT. As discussed in Chapter 2, resistance to flow is inversely proportional to the fourth power of the radius, making it hard for tiny infants to breathe effectively through the small ETT. The high ETT resistance coupled with the limited muscle strength and mechanical disadvantage of the infant's excessively compliant chest wall results in ineffective spontaneous breathing with a high dead space:V_T ratio. Because anatomic and instrumental dead space is fixed, small breaths that largely rebreathe dead-space gas will contribute minimally to effective alveolar ventilation (alveolar ventilation = minute ventilation − dead space ventilation). To maintain adequate alveolar minute ventilation, a relatively large V_T, typically around 6 mL/kg, is thus required with the limited number of ventilator inflations (Fig. 18-6). From a practical standpoint, the biggest problem with SIMV is that the operator must adjust both rate and pressure (V_T) to facilitate weaning and overall respiratory support.

Assist Control

Assist control (AC) is a conventional mechanical ventilation mode that supports every spontaneous breath (this is the "assist" part) that is sufficient to trigger a ventilator inflation and provides a minimum rate of ventilator inflations in case of apnea (the "control" part). In Europe the mode is sometimes referred to as synchronized intermittent positive-pressure ventilation. AC is a time-cycled mode that can be pressure or volume controlled, but in neonatal applications it is typically pressure controlled. Because every spontaneous breath is supported, AC provides more uniform V_T delivery and lower work of breathing than SIMV (Fig. 18-7). An inspiratory time is set, which may produce an inspiration that is either too long or too short,

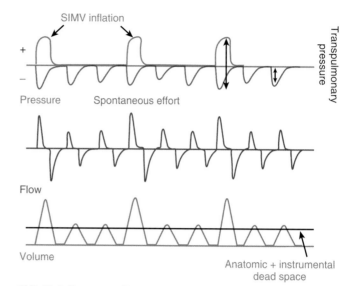

FIG 18-6 Pressure, flow, and volume scalar waveforms during synchronized intermittent mandatory ventilation (*SIMV*). Drawn in *purple* is the spontaneous respiratory effort of the patient, which is not displayed on the ventilator screen, but which contributes to the transpulmonary pressure (*vertical arrow* in top panel) and thus the size of the tidal volume (V_T). Note the large difference in V_T between spontaneous breaths and ventilator inflations. In a small infant with high ETT resistance and weak respiratory effort, the V_T barely exceeds anatomic and instrumental dead space, leading to inefficient rapid shallow breathing.

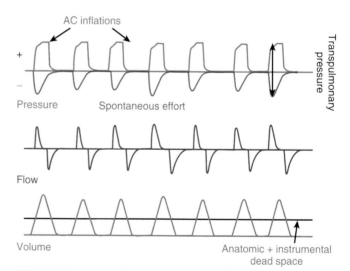

FIG 18-7 Pressure, flow, and volume scalar waveforms during assist control (*AC*). Drawn in *purple* is the spontaneous respiratory effort of the patient, which is not displayed on the ventilator screen. Note the relatively uniform transpulmonary pressure and tidal volume when each patient breath is supported by a ventilator inflation.

a problem that is avoided with the use of flow cycling (see below). The clinician sets a ventilator rate for mandatory "backup" inflations that provide a minimum ventilator rate in case of apnea, and the inflations can be triggered only within the trigger window. The backup rate should be set just below the infant's spontaneous rate, usually 30 to 40 breaths/minute depending on the

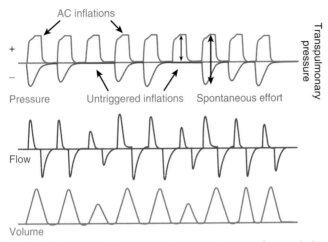

FIG 18-8 Pressure, flow, and volume scalar waveforms during assist control (*AC*) with a backup rate that is too high. Drawn in *purple* is the spontaneous respiratory effort of the patient, which is not displayed on the ventilator screen. Note the occasional untriggered ventilator inflations that result in a smaller transpulmonary pressure when the ventilator cycles before the infant breathes.

baby's size, to allow the infant to trigger the inflations. The goal is to have the infant and the ventilator work together, resulting in lower ventilator pressure. An excessively high backup rate will result in an increased number of untriggered inflations when the ventilator backup rate kicks in before the infant has a chance to breathe (Fig. 18-8).[20] A backup rate that is too low will result in excessive fluctuations in minute ventilation and oxygen saturations during periods of apnea. Because the infant controls the inflation rate, gradual withdrawal of support is accomplished by lowering the peak inflation pressure (V_T) rather than the ventilator rate. In fact, the ventilator rate should never need adjustment once the baby is generating spontaneous respiratory effort. In this fashion, the amount of support provided to each breath is decreased, allowing the infant to gradually take over the work of breathing. This slightly less intuitive weaning strategy and some long-held misconceptions addressed later in this chapter appear to be the reasons for the apparent reluctance of some practitioners to adopt this mode.

Pressure-Support Ventilation

A variety of modes are referred to as pressure-support ventilation (PSV), which greatly complicates communication. As implemented on specialty neonatal ventilators, PSV is a flow-cycled and pressure-controlled continuous spontaneous ventilation mode that supports every spontaneous breath just like AC, with the only difference being flow cycling. Flow cycling means that an inflation is terminated when inspiratory flow declines to a preset threshold, usually 15% of peak flow (Fig. 18-9). Flow cycling eliminates the inspiratory hold (prolonged inflation time [T_I] that keeps the lungs at peak inflation) and thus presumably provides more optimal synchrony. Eliminating the inspiratory hold should limit fluctuations in intrathoracic and intracranial pressure that occur when an infant exhales against the high positive pressure during inspiratory hold. The time needed for the lungs to fill and the flow to decline to the termination threshold is a function of the patient's inspiratory effort and the time constants of the patient's respiratory system. Thus PSV automatically

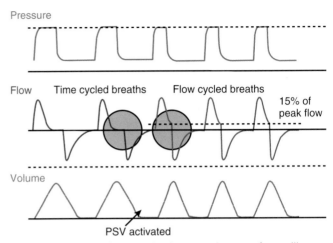

FIG 18-9 Pressure, flow, and volume scalar waveforms illustrating the concept of flow cycling. The left half of the tracing shows time cycling with a fixed inspiratory time that results in a pressure plateau, also known as *inspiratory hold*. The pressure has equilibrated and there is no further inspiratory flow during the latter phase of the cycle. On the right side of the tracing, flow cycling has been activated. The ventilator now cycles into exhalation when flow drops to 15% of peak flow. Flow cycling results in a shorter inflation time (top tracing) and allows the infant to exhale as soon as inspiratory flow is nearly completed. This is a more natural breathing pattern and eliminates active exhalation against the inspiratory hold. *PSV*, Pressure-support ventilation.

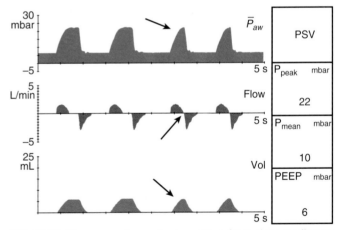

FIG 18-10 Screen capture of a transition from time cycling to flow cycling. The time that flow cycling was activated is indicated by the *black arrows*. Note that the gap between inspiratory and expiratory flow disappears (middle). Also note the shorter inflation time, which results in a drop in mean airway pressure ($\bar{P}_{aw}$) and could lead to atelectasis if positive end-expiratory pressure (*PEEP*) were not adjusted to maintain adequate distending pressure.

adjusts T_I to be appropriate to the changing lung mechanics of the patient. The reader should recognize that changing from basic time-cycled AC to PSV usually results in a shorter T_I and thus lower mean airway pressure and therefore may lead to atelectasis, unless adequate positive end-expiratory pressure (PEEP) is used to maintain mean airway pressure (Fig. 18-10). As with triggering, a substantial leak around the ETT may affect flow cycling.

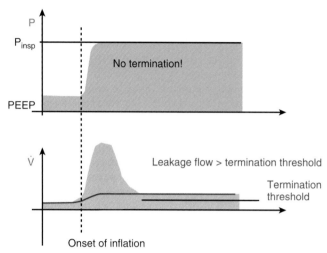

FIG 18-11 Possible consequence of large leak around ETT on flow cycling. When the leakage flow is greater than the termination threshold, flow cycling would not occur. For this reason, manual setting of maximum inflation time is required. Manual adjustment of the termination criteria is necessary on some ventilators; others have an automatic leak adaptation (see Fig. 18-4). *PEEP,* Positive end-expiratory pressure.

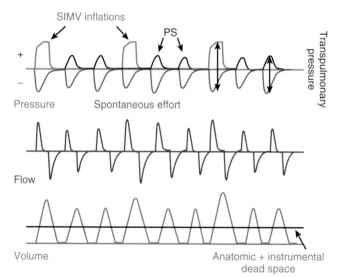

FIG 18-12 Pressure, flow, and volume scalar waveforms during synchronized intermittent mandatory ventilation (*SIMV*) with pressure support (*PS*). Drawn in *purple* is the spontaneous respiratory effort of the patient, which is not displayed on the ventilator screen. Note that the addition of PS to the spontaneous effort now increases the transpulmonary pressure and tidal volume, allowing the tidal volume to reach a more normal value that results in less tachypnea and a more efficient breathing pattern.

When leakage flow is greater than the threshold for inflation termination (known also as termination criteria), flow cycling will not occur (Fig. 18-11). For this reason the user must still set a T_I limit, which should be about 50% longer than the baseline spontaneous inspiratory time, to allow the infant an opportunity to receive a longer T_I when he or she takes a longer, deeper spontaneous breath (i.e., a sigh). Because of the risk of failure to flow cycle due to leak, some devices allow the user to manually set the termination criteria (i.e., the percentage of peak flow that will

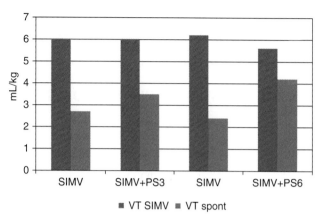

FIG 18-13 The effect of the addition of pressure support (*PS*) during synchronized intermittent mandatory ventilation (*SIMV*) on tidal volume (V_T). The figure was drawn based on data from Osorio et al.[22] Note that in these small infants in the recovery phase of respiratory distress syndrome on SIMV without PS, the spontaneous (spont) V_T was at or below the typical anatomic and instrumental dead space of 3 mL/kg (*blue bar*), whereas the ventilator inflations were about 6 mL/kg (*purple bar*). The addition of 3 cm H_2O of PS increased the spontaneous V_T slightly (second set of bars). Upon return to baseline of SIMV alone the spontaneous V_T again becomes inadequate (third set of bars). The addition of 6 cm H_2O of PS increased the spontaneous V_T to a reasonable physiologic value, allowing the V_T of the ventilator inflations to come down slightly (last set of bars). The PS setting for individual patients should be guided by the V_T that it achieves, with 4 mL/kg being a reasonable goal.

terminate an inflation) up to as much as 25% to 50% of peak flow. The problem once more is that ETT leaks are highly variable, and when the leak decreases, terminating an inflation at 50% or peak flow can result in a rather short T_I and an uncomfortable breathing pattern. Such manual adjustment is obviated by the effective leak compensation known as *leak-adapted pressure support* on the Dräger ventilators, which automatically compensates for leakage flow and maintains effective inflation termination even in the face of very large ETT leak (see Fig. 18-4).

Similar to AC, a backup rate will maintain a minimum inflation rate. In most devices PSV can also be used to support spontaneous breathing between low-rate SIMVs, to overcome the problems associated with inadequate spontaneous respiratory effort and high ETT resistance (Fig. 18-12). Adding PSV to SIMV has been shown to increase minute ventilation and reduce tachypnea,[21] increase the V_T of spontaneous breaths (Fig. 18-13),[22] and lead to more rapid weaning from mechanical ventilation.[23] PSV can also be used as a fully spontaneous mode, which lacks a backup rate and depends instead on an "apnea ventilation" setting that kicks in after a user-preset period of apnea. When used to support spontaneous breaths between SIMV or with CPAP, PSV does not come with a backup mandatory rate, so a reliable spontaneous respiratory effort is required. When used with SIMV, PSV can be thought of as a pressure boost given for each spontaneous breath, lasting only as long as there is inspiratory flow. While this approach is effective, it adds complexity and does not appear to have any advantage over either PSV used alone or AC with appropriate settings, as long as atelectasis is avoided by avoiding heavy sedation and using an adequate level of PEEP.

Withdrawal of support for PSV as a primary mode is accomplished in the same way as for AC. When used in conjunction with SIMV, both the inflation rate and the PSV level should be lowered, again adding a level of unnecessary complexity.

CHOICE OF ASSISTED VENTILATION MODES

With no large randomized trials to provide the necessary evidence base to establish the superiority of one mode or the other, the choice between AC or SIMV, the two most widely used modalities of synchronized ventilation, remains a matter of personal preference or habit. Valid physiologic considerations and short-term studies, however, suggest that modes that support every spontaneous breath are preferable in small preterm infants. Smaller and less variable V_T, less tachypnea, more rapid weaning from mechanical ventilation, and smaller fluctuations in blood pressure with AC, compared to SIMV, have been documented for many years.[8,24,25] Despite indications that SIMV does not provide optimal support in extremely low gestational age newborns with small ETTs, many clinicians continue to use it, especially during weaning from mechanical ventilation,[26] based on the accepted but unsupported dogma that both rate and pressure must be weaned prior to extubation.[8,27] The preference for the lower inflation rate of SIMV appears to be based on the superficially plausible assumption that fewer ventilator inflations are inherently less damaging. However, this belief ignores the fact that the slower ventilator inflation rate is accomplished at the expense of a larger V_T, a variable that is clearly more injurious than a higher ventilator rate, and is also contradicted by available evidence from both animal and human studies.[28,29] Many clinicians also mistakenly believe that assisting every breath prevents respiratory muscle training. This concern reflects a lack of understanding of the complex patient–ventilator interaction during assisted ventilation. As illustrated in Figure 18-5, the V_T with synchronized ventilation is the result of the sum of the negative intrapleural pressure generated by the infant and the positive inflation pressure generated by the ventilator. This transpulmonary pressure, together with the compliance of the respiratory system, determines the resulting V_T. During weaning, as the ventilator inflation pressure is decreased, the infant progressively takes over a greater proportion of the work of breathing with effective training of the respiratory muscles. As weaning progresses, the inflation pressure is decreased to the point at which it only overcomes the added resistance of the ETT and circuit, at which point the infant can be extubated.

GUIDELINES FOR CLINICAL APPLICATION

As discussed previously, specific ventilator settings are a function of the nature and severity of the disease process, the age and size of the patient, and an immediate reassessment of how the patient is responding to the initial settings. A general approach to respiratory support of infants under various conditions is outlined in Chapter 15, and disease-specific ventilation strategies are discussed in greater detail in Chapter 23. Here we will briefly discuss general aspects of how the various synchronized modes may be implemented in the neonatal intensive care unit.

Synchronized Intermittent Mandatory Ventilation

As explained previously, SIMV alone should be avoided in small preterm infants when the inflation rate is <30 but is a reasonable choice when apnea is the primary indication for respiratory support or in larger infants who are able to generate adequate spontaneous V_T. The variables that require user input include PEEP; peak inflation pressure (PIP), when using in pressure-controlled mode, or V_T target, when using in volume-targeted mode; and T_I. Ventilator rate is set indirectly by adjusting expiratory time or directly by setting the rate, depending on the specific ventilator. Care should be taken to choose PIP that results in an appropriate V_T and to adjust it as needed when lung mechanics change. Generally, a volume-targeted mode should be employed (see Chapter 20). Adequacy of the V_T of spontaneous breaths should be assessed, and if these are 3 mL/kg or less and/or the infant remains tachypneic, an increase in ventilator rate, addition of pressure support, or change to AC mode should be seriously considered. Reduction of support is accomplished by reducing inflation pressure and rate. Ventilator rate should not be reduced below 15 inflations/min before extubation.

Assist Control

AC is a mode that allows the patient to control the ventilator rate but provides a minimum number of inflations in case of inadequate or absent respiratory support. The backup rate can be thought of as a safety net that is designed to avoid large fluctuations in minute ventilation in preterm infants with a sporadic respiratory effort. Small preterm infants with respiratory distress syndrome (RDS) have relatively short time constants, and their breathing rate is typically in the 50s and 60s. Thus a backup rate of 40/min is reasonably close to their own rate but not so high that it would interfere with the infant's ability to trigger the ventilator. A backup rate that is too low (e.g., 25 to 30) would result in excessive fluctuations in minute ventilation during periods of apnea that lead to fluctuations in $PaCO_2$ and SpO_2, both of which are undesirable. A slower backup rate of 30 to 35 is appropriate in full-term infants. PIP, PEEP, and T_I are the other variables under user control. As mentioned previously AC can be a pressure-controlled or volume-controlled mode. Pressure-controlled AC may be used with or without volume targeting. When used without volume targeting, the PIP should be carefully chosen to achieve appropriate V_T and adjusted as necessary in response to changing lung mechanics. This need for manual adjustment is obviated by the use of volume targeting, which is preferred. As with all modes of support, adequate gas exchange is not the only indication of adequacy of support. If the infant remains tachypneic after a period of adjustment to the new settings (respiratory rate >70), the reason for the tachypnea should be sought. Autocycling should be ruled out if marked unexplained tachypnea is observed, especially when there is no apparent respiratory effort noted. Any condensed water in the ventilator circuit should be drained, and evidence of a large leak around the ETT should be excluded. If confirmed to be intrinsic to the baby, tachypnea may reflect inadequate V_T, discomfort, or an effort to maintain functional residual capacity when PEEP level is insufficient. If tachypnea persists after optimal patient positioning is ensured and it is verified that the ETT is not pushing on the infant's upper gum (a common cause of discomfort), a trial of higher PEEP should be considered. It should be remembered that AC itself does not cause tachypnea, but because the ventilator rate is driven by the infant's own respiratory rate, AC makes it more obvious to the observer. Moderate tachypnea with a slightly low $PaCO_2$ is sometimes seen in very immature infants with metabolic acidosis. Typically, the pH is not alkalotic and the tachypnea in fact reflects the infant's respiratory compensation for the base deficit that may be the result of perinatal events, low renal threshold for bicarbonate, or intolerance of large amounts of protein in the parenteral nutrition in the first days of life. Changing to SIMV may make the clinician happy by allowing the $PaCO_2$ to rise to what may be seen as a more desirable PCO_2 level, but this will change little else, because it is pH, not $PaCO_2$, that is the primary driver of respiratory effort. Remember, the increase in $PaCO_2$ that may occur comes because SIMV is a less effective support mode and increases the work of breathing required for the baby.

As long as the infant has a reasonably sustained respiratory effort, lowering the backup rate will not affect the overall level of support; weaning from mechanical ventilation is instead achieved primarily by lowering inflation pressure, as well as PEEP and FiO_2.

Pressure-Support Ventilation

When used in conjunction with SIMV, the PSV support is set as x cm H_2O above PEEP (e.g., pressure support [PS] of 8 cm H_2O). There is no backup rate. The choice of the level of support should be guided by the goal of achieving an adequate V_T of about 3.5 to 4 mL/kg for the spontaneous supported breaths. A reasonable starting level may be 6 cm H_2O, titrated upward if needed. The goal is to augment the inadequate respiratory effort of the infant and ensure that spontaneous breathing actually contributes to effective alveolar ventilation. Adequacy of PS can be confirmed by adequacy of spontaneous V_T and resolution of tachypnea. PSV becomes more important as the inflation rate of SIMV is progressively lowered. There is no evidence base on which to base weaning during SIMV + PS, but, keeping in mind the goals of the PS, it seems reasonable to lower the SIMV rate until it is low enough to consider extubation (typically 15/min) and adjust the PS to maintain just adequate V_T during the weaning process. Infants can typically be extubated when they are able to maintain good oxygenation and are generating adequate V_T with a PS of 6 cm H_2O.

When used as a primary mode, the PIP and PEEP are set as with AC (i.e., PIP/PEEP). PSV theoretically results in more optimal synchronization than AC so should probably be the preferred mode in most situations. The exception would be extremely small infants with RDS during the first few days of life, who have such extremely short time constants that the T_I with PSV would be <0.2 s. Such short T_I may contribute to tachypnea and limits the time for intrapulmonary gas distribution. We therefore avoid PSV in infants of <800 g during the first 3 to 4 days of life. It should be kept in mind that the shorter T_I of PSV results in relatively low mean airway pressure and may lead to atelectasis unless adequate PEEP is employed—typically 7 to 8 cm H_2O. If switching from AC to PSV, the simple approach is to make note of the mean airway pressure on AC and then adjust the PEEP to return to the same value after PSV is activated. If an infant remains ventilated beyond a week of life, care must be taken to ensure that the T_I limit is adjusted as needed to allow flow cycling to occur, because airway resistance will be increasing and therefore the time constants are now more prolonged, with the spontaneous T_I now potentially exceeding the set limit.

CONCLUSION

Synchronized mechanical ventilation modes represent a significant advance in respiratory support of newborn infants. Despite a limited evidence base from the published literature, their benefits are generally accepted. While debate continues regarding the specific choice of synchronized modes, there is relatively strong rationale for using modes that support every spontaneous effort in very small infants. Specific details of clinical application should be based on disease-specific strategies and on the advantages and limitations of specific ventilators at the disposal of the clinician. A good understanding of the underlying physiologic principles and the particular aspects of the device in use is critical in providing optimal respiratory support in critically ill newborn infants.

REFERENCES

A complete reference list is available at https://expertconsult .inkling.com/.

19

Principles of Lung-Protective Ventilation

Anton H. van Kaam, MD, PhD

INTRODUCTION

Respiratory failure is a common and serious clinical condition in newborn infants that is associated with an increased risk of neonatal morbidity and mortality.[1-3] Although respiratory failure occurs in both term and preterm infants, it is especially common in the latter group. Despite the fact that many of the very low birth-weight infants can initially be managed on noninvasive respiratory support, such as nasal continuous positive airway pressure, historically almost 70% of them have needed to be supported by invasive mechanical ventilation at some point during their admission.[4] Unfortunately, in its goal to correct gas exchange, mechanical ventilation often results in secondary lung damage, also referred to as ventilator-induced lung injury (VILI).[5] VILI is considered one of the major risk factors for the development of chronic pulmonary morbidity in newborn infants, that is, bronchopulmonary dysplasia (BPD).[6] Studies in both animal models and humans have provided valuable insight into the mechanisms of VILI, and this knowledge has been used to develop so-called lung-protective ventilation strategies, aiming to minimize the risk of (respiratory) morbidity and mortality. This chapter will summarize the basic principles of VILI and the basic concepts of lung-protective ventilation strategies.

NEONATAL RESPIRATORY FAILURE

As noted previously, preterm infants are most at risk of respiratory failure. This is to a large extent explained by the fact that their lungs are both structurally and biochemically immature. This is reflected by surfactant deficiency (neonatal respiratory distress syndrome, i.e., RDS), which results in an increase in elastic recoil forces of the lung due to the higher surface tension at the alveolar/saccular air–liquid interface and a concomitant reduction in lung compliance. In addition, the end-expiratory lung volume (EELV) or functional residual capacity is reduced and unstable, because the excessively high compliance of the chest wall of the preterm infant is unable to counteract the increased recoil forces. A low EELV will lead to a further reduction in lung compliance, an increase in airway resistance, and an increase in work of breathing. Furthermore, collapse of saccules will increase intrapulmonary left-to-right shunting, leading to (severe) hypoxia and to uneven distribution of tidal volume. These physiologic concepts are also applicable to term infants although the immaturity of the respiratory system is much less compared with the preterm infant and the surfactant dysfunction is not caused by surfactant deficiency but surfactant inactivation (meconium aspiration syndrome or pneumonia) or loss of type 2 cell function (e.g., status post asphyxia neonatorum).

Understanding these physiologic concepts is essential when designing and applying so-called lung-protective ventilation strategies.

VENTILATOR-INDUCED LUNG INJURY

Although BPD is considered a multifactorial disease, VILI remains an important determinant in its pathophysiology. Animal studies conducted since 1974 have greatly improved our knowledge about the mechanisms of VILI. These studies have identified the most important risk factors for VILI and its pulmonary and systemic consequences.

Risk Factors for VILI
Volutrauma
In 1974 Webb and Tierney showed that the application of high peak inflation pressures during conventional mechanical ventilation resulted in alveolar and perivascular edema, leading to deteriorating lung mechanics and ultimately death in healthy rats.[7] Additional experiments showed that application of high peak inflation pressures will damage the lung only if the thorax can freely expand and volume can enter the lungs. Preventing this expansion by thoracic strapping (low volume, high pressure) will protect the lung against VILI.[8] These results clearly indicate that the volume entering the lungs (volutrauma) and not the pressure applied to the lungs causes VILI. The importance of volutrauma in the development of VILI has also been confirmed in preterm animal models.[9]

Volutrauma is often thought to be equivalent to high tidal volume ventilation. Although this is true in most cases, it is important to realize that even low tidal volumes can induce volutrauma. First of all and explained in more detail in the next paragraph, low tidal volumes provided at the airway opening can result in regional overdistention if part of the lung is atelectatic. Second, if low tidal volumes are superimposed on a high EELV, the end-inspiratory lung volume can still exceed total lung capacity and result in volutrauma.[10]

Atelectrauma
As previously discussed, neonatal respiratory failure is often accompanied by surfactant deficiency or inhibition, resulting in collapse of small airways and alveoli/saccules (atelectasis). Owing to the heterogeneous nature of lung disease and gravitational effects on the lung, the distribution and behavior of unstable lung units differ at the regional level. Roughly three zones can be identified (Fig. 19-1): (1) alveoli that remain open during the entire ventilatory cycle, (2) alveoli that are recruitable during the inspiration phase but collapse during expiration, and

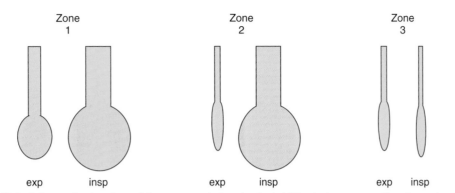

FIG 19-1 Schematic drawing of the zones of alveolar instability during conventional mechanical ventilation. **Zone 1:** alveoli that remain open during the entire ventilatory cycle. **Zone 2:** alveoli that are recruitable during the inspiration phase but collapse during expiration. **Zone 3:** alveoli that remain collapsed during the entire ventilatory cycle. *exp,* Expiration phase; *insp,* inspiration phase.

(3) alveoli that remain collapsed during the entire ventilatory cycle.[11] Alveoli in zone 2 will be subjected to repetitive opening and collapse during conventional (tidal) ventilation. Animal experiments in both adult and preterm models have shown that the repetitive tidal recruitment and collapse are injurious to the lung.[12,13] As alveoli in zone 3 do not participate in tidal ventilation, the tidal volume administered to the lung during conventional ventilation is redistributed to the alveoli in the other two zones. This may increase the risk of regional overdistention (volutrauma) and subsequent VILI.[14]

Oxygen Toxicity

Ventilation with high fractions of inspiratory oxygen concentrations can result in excessive production of oxygen radicals, overwhelming the normal antioxidant-detoxifying capacity of the cell and leading to VILI.[15] Both animal and human studies have indicated that prematurity impairs the ability to increase antioxidant enzymes in response to hyperoxia, making this group of patients extremely vulnerable to oxidative stress often present after preterm birth.[16,17] Low EELV results in high oxygen requirement due to poor ventilation/perfusion matching and intrapulmonary right-to-left shunt, thus contributing to oxidative stress.

Pulmonary and Systemic Consequences of VILI
Structural Injury

Volutrauma can cause direct structural injury to the alveolar–capillary unit. Coexistence of atelectatic and open alveoli may further increase this risk owing to so-called shear forces that exceed transpulmonary pressures.[18] Finally, hyperoxia can have a direct cytotoxic effect on alveolar endothelial and epithelial cells. This loss of structural integrity will increase endothelial and epithelial permeability, leading to pulmonary edema and hemorrhage.[15,19]

Biotrauma

In vitro studies have shown that cyclic stretch of alveolar epithelial cells and alveolar macrophages stimulates the production of proinflammatory cytokines such as tumor necrosis factor α and interleukin-8 (IL-8).[20,21] Ex vivo and in vivo animal studies showed that volutrauma, atelectrauma, and especially the combination of these risk factors result in a significant inflammatory response in the lung.[22-24] Pulmonary inflammation is

further upregulated by hyperoxia, which stimulates neutrophil migration into the alveoli and enhances proinflammatory cytokine response of alveolar macrophages.[19,25,26]

One of the changes induced by the production of proinflammatory mediators like IL-8 is the recruitment of polymorphonuclear (PMN) white blood cells in the lung.[27,28] PMN cells can inflict tissue damage through the release of proteases, the production of reactive oxygen species, and the release of cytokines.[29] The importance of PMN cells in the development of VILI has been shown by Kawano et al., who found little evidence of VILI in rabbits depleted of granulocytes prior to initiation of injurious conventional ventilation.[30]

In addition to upregulation of local inflammation in the lung, there is now also evidence from both experimental and human data that injurious ventilation will also lead to a decompartmentalization of inflammatory mediators into the systemic circulation, possibly leading to multiple organ failure.[22,31-33]

Surfactant Dysfunction

Although surfactant dysfunction is often already present at the start of invasive respiratory support, conventional mechanical ventilation may further compromise its function.

As previously mentioned, VILI is often accompanied by an increased permeability of both the endothelial and the epithelial barriers, promoting an influx of plasma proteins in to the alveolar space.[34,35] It has been shown that these proteins result in a dose-dependent inhibition of surfactant.[36]

Studies investigating the alveolar metabolism of pulmonary surfactant have shown that surfactant exists in different subfractions. The two major subfractions of surfactant obtained from lung lavage material are large aggregates (LA) and small aggregates (SA).[37] LA surfactant is able to lower alveolar surface tension, but SA surfactant is not surface active and is the metabolic product of the LA fraction.[38] Animal experiments have shown that the conversion from LA to SA surfactant is increased when high tidal volumes are applied during ventilation of the injured lung.[39,40] The increased conversion of surfactant has also been documented in newborn and adult patients with acute lung injury.[41,42]

Animal experiments have shown that ventilation can enhance the secretion of endogenous surfactant by the type 2 cells.[43,44] This surfactant can subsequently be squeezed out of the alveolar space into the small airways as a result of compression of the surfactant film when the surface of the alveolus becomes smaller. Ex vivo experiments in rat lungs showed that this movement of surfactant into the airways is directly related to the tidal volume and inversely related to the end-expiratory pressure.[45] Hyperoxia results in both inactivation and decreased synthesis of pulmonary surfactant, resulting in a deterioration of lung mechanics.[46]

Lung Development

Experimental studies in preterm animal models have shown that mechanical ventilation and hyperoxia are able to arrest the normal alveolarization process during lung development.[47-50] This arrest in lung development is considered one of the histologic hallmarks of the "new" BPD and highlights the link between mechanical ventilation, VILI, and the development of BPD.[6]

Susceptibility of Newborn Lungs to VILI

Animal experiments have shown that the magnitude of VILI is highly dependent on the condition of the lung at the start of mechanical ventilation. Exposing the preterm lungs antenatally to intra-amniotic endotoxin before starting mechanical ventilation after birth results in a more pronounced inflammatory response compared to subjecting the lungs to either of these insults alone.[51] The same is true when exposing the lungs to postnatal inflammation by systemic injection of endotoxin.[52] These experiments strongly suggest that the inflammatory status of the lungs is an important mediator in the effect of mechanical ventilation on lung injury. In addition to inflammation, the surfactant status of the lungs also seems to be an important mediator of VILI. Applying high-pressure ventilation to surfactant-deficient lungs results in more VILI compared to similar ventilation given to surfactant-sufficient lungs.[53]

These experimental results suggest that preterm lungs are highly susceptible to VILI, as antenatal inflammation (chorioamnionitis), postnatal inflammation (sepsis, pneumonia), and surfactant deficiency (RDS) are often present in the preterm population and are reasons for starting invasive mechanical ventilation.[54]

Studies in preterm animal models also suggest that just a few injurious inflations administered immediately after birth are sufficient to trigger the cascade of VILI.[9,55]

LUNG-PROTECTIVE VENTILATION: BASIC PRINCIPLES

The basic goal of lung-protective ventilation is to establish an acceptable level of gas exchange while minimizing VILI as much as possible. Based on the experimental data on the pathogenesis of VILI, the cornerstones of a lung-protective ventilation strategy are (1) minimizing end-inspiratory (alveolar) overdistention (volutrauma) and (2) optimizing EELV by reversing atelectasis (recruitment) and stabilizing lung units throughout the ventilatory cycle (avoiding atelectrauma). Applying such a strategy will often improve oxygenation and allow for a reduction in the fraction of inspired oxygen (less oxygen toxicity). A lung-protective ventilation strategy based on these principles is often referred to as an *optimal lung volume strategy* or *open lung ventilation strategy*.[56]

Minimizing Volutrauma

Minimizing volutrauma has mainly been associated with reducing tidal volume during mechanical ventilation. Indeed, animal studies have shown that reducing alveolar overdistention by

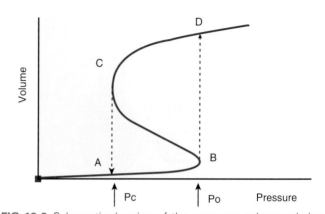

FIG 19-2 Schematic drawing of the pressure–volume relationship of a single alveolus during inspiration and expiration (*solid line*). At the start of the inflation (A) the alveolus is collapsed. At point B, the pressure increase has reached the critical opening pressure (Po), leading to an immediate volume increase (*dashed line*) as the alveolus is recruited (D). As the pressure is slowly decreased there is little volume loss until the critical closing pressure (Pc) is reached at point C. The alveolus immediately collapses to point A. Note that Pc is lower than Po owing to the law of LaPlace.

limiting tidal volumes during mechanical ventilation will attenuate VILI.[8,9,23,55,57] However, it is important to realize that it is equally important to distribute the tidal volume evenly into optimally inflated and adequately recruited lungs; small tidal volumes can still result in (regional) volutrauma if superimposed on a relatively high EELV or administered during heterogeneous lung disease with significant atelectasis.[10,14]

Minimizing Atelectrauma

It is essential to realize that in a diseased lung, the reduction of atelectasis is based on two principles. First, already collapsed alveoli/saccules need to be reopened or recruited by applying sufficient inflation pressure. Second, after recruitment, sufficient (end-expiratory) airway pressure should be applied to stabilize the lung volume and prevent subsequent collapse during expiration. Figure 19-2 shows the pressure–volume (P/V) relationship of an individual alveolus. Staub and colleagues proposed that the behavior of alveoli is quantal in nature.[58] After reaching a critical opening pressure the collapsed alveolus pops open, immediately resulting in a large volume (radius) increase. As follows from the law of LaPlace, which states that the pressure (P) necessary to keep a spherical structure opened is two times the surface tension (γ) divided by the radius (r), the critical closing pressure of the alveolus will be lower than the opening pressure.

The P/V curve of the entire lung, as shown in Figure 19-3, will be the cumulative relationship of all alveoli/saccules of the lung, each with a different severity of lung disease and thus a different opening and closing pressure. The inflation limb of the P/V curve shows the changes in lung volume during incremental airway pressures and usually contains a so-called lower inflection point above which lung volume suddenly increases in a linear fashion. As lung volume approaches total lung capacity (TLC) the inflation limb flattens off. The deflation limb represents the changes in lung volume during decremental airway pressure steps starting at TLC. Again, as explained by the law of LaPlace, lung volume is initially maintained as pressures are lowered but eventually decreases owing to progressive alveolar

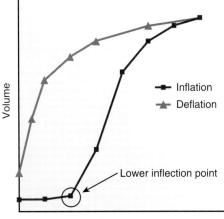

FIG 19-3 Pressure–volume relationship of the lung showing the inflation (*red line*) and the deflation limb (*green line*). Note the clear difference in lung volume between the limbs at identical pressures (*hysteresis*).

collapse as the distending pressure drops below the critical closing pressure. The clear difference in lung volume at identical airway pressures between the inflation and the deflation limb of the P/V relationship is called *lung hysteresis*. Studies in newborn infants have shown that lung hysteresis is present in preterm infants with RDS and term infants with more heterogeneous causes of lung disease.[59-61]

It was initially assumed that lung recruitment occurred primarily around the lower inflection point of the P/V curve. However, observations in adults and newborn infants have indicated that recruitment occurs along the entire inflation limb of the P/V curve.[60,62] Although sometimes stated differently, the *inflation* pressures or volumes, and not positive end-expiratory pressure (PEEP), are responsible for alveolar recruitment during conventional ventilation. PEEP is an expiratory phenomenon, and its main purpose is to stabilize the previously opened alveoli and thereby prevent subsequent collapse during expiration. Failing to recruit the lungs prior to or concomitant with increasing PEEP will not prevent VILI.[13,63] On the other hand, recruiting the lungs but applying insufficient PEEP to prevent subsequent collapse will augment rather than reduce lung injury.[64]

It was also believed that the optimal PEEP levels preventing alveolar collapse should be above the lower inflection point of the P/V curve.[65] However, experimental and human data have shown that the critical closing pressure of the lungs is not related to the lower inflection point.[66,67]

Both mathematical models and animal experiments have shown that adequate recruitment of collapsed alveoli, followed by optimal stabilization with adequate levels of PEEP, will place ventilation on the deflation limb of the P/V curve.[68,69] This position will improve compliance and reduce VILI compared to ventilation on, or close to, the inflation limb of the P/V curve.[63,69]

As most underlying lung diseases causing neonatal respiratory failure are heterogeneous in nature, regional overdistention of relatively healthy lung parts has been a major concern during recruitment. Although this concern seems valid, there is little evidence that recruitment maneuvers actually damage the lungs if accompanied by sufficient PEEP. More importantly, to date most experiments have indicated that derecruitment is more injurious than recruitment.[70,71]

One of the difficulties of practical implementation of lung recruitment is the lack of tools that can assess changes in EELV in ventilated newborn infants at the bedside. Although often used in clinical practice, chest radiography provides only general information on lung aeration at one point in time and does not seem to correlate well with actual lung volumes.[72] This may in part be caused by suboptimal technique in terms of centering of the film and the difficulty in timing exposure at a particular point in the respiratory cycle at rapid respiratory rates. Tracer gas washout techniques can be used to measure changes in EELV, but they do not provide continuous information and are not applicable during high-frequency ventilation.[73] Respiratory inductive plethysmography has been successfully used in newborn infants to measure changes in EELV and to reconstruct the P/V relationship of the lung.[61] However, its application is hampered by signal instability over time, especially in unsedated non-muscle-relaxed infants.[74] Another disadvantage that applies to all of the aforementioned techniques is the inability to differentiate between lung volume changes caused by alveolar *recruitment* (which is the aim of volume optimization) and those caused by alveolar *distention* (of already open alveoli). A more recent imaging technique called *electrical impedance tomography* does provide regional information on changes in lung aeration and has been successfully used in (preterm) infants.[60,74] However, the hardware, software, and patient interface of this technique need to be improved before it can be used in daily clinical practice.

Owing to these limitations of the currently available monitoring tools, most clinicians use oxygenation as an indirect tool to measure changes in lung volume at the bedside. The basic principle is illustrated in Figure 19-4. In a collapsed alveolus, blood flowing through the alveolar–capillary unit will not be able to take up oxygen before returning to the left atrium. This is called *intrapulmonary right-to-left shunting*, which results in hypoxemia. If the alveolus is recruited with sufficient airway pressure, gas exchange will be restored at the alveolar level, resulting in an improvement of the ventilation/perfusion ratio reflected by improved oxygenation. Increasing the airway pressure further will increase the volume of the alveolus (distention) but will not affect the ventilation/perfusion ratio. In the case of overdistention, the capillaries will be compressed, resulting in increased alveolar dead space and hypercarbia. The same concepts also apply when reducing the airway pressure once the alveolus is recruited. This means that oxygenation is able to differentiate between volume changes based on alveolar recruitment and distention.

LUNG-PROTECTIVE VENTILATION: CONVENTIONAL MECHANICAL VENTILATION

Conventional mechanical ventilation is the most frequently used modality in newborn infants.[54] It is a broad term for various modalities that all use the concept of tidal ventilation. In this section we will focus on the various elements of lung protection during conventional mechanical ventilation without going into the specifics of the available conventional ventilation modes. For these details the reader is referred to other chapters in this textbook.

Low Tidal Volume Ventilation

Based on the experimental evidence that higher tidal volumes can lead to VILI, experts have advocated targeting a tidal volume between 4 and 7 mL/kg during conventional mechanical

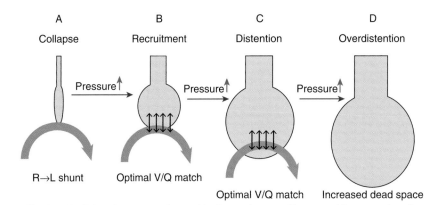

FIG 19-4 Basic principle of oxygenation-guided recruitment illustrated by one alveolar–capillary unit. **A,** Collapsed but perfused alveolus with no uptake of oxygen in the bloodstream. Blood returns to the left atrium in a hypoxic state. This is called *intrapulmonary right-to-left shunting.* **B,** The increased airway pressure exceeds the critical opening pressure of the alveolus, resulting in opening of the alveolus, a (rapid) volume increase, and an uptake of oxygen owing to the optimal ventilation/perfusion match. This process is called *recruitment.* **C,** A further increase in pressure will distend the already open alveolus, resulting in an increase in volume but no change in the optimal ventilation/perfusion match. This process is called *distention.* **D,** A further increase in pressure will result in overdistention of the alveolus, resulting in absent perfusion owing to compression of the alveolar blood vessels. This will result in an increase in (alveolar) dead space and rising Pco_2.

ventilation in (preterm) infants. The evidence to support this recommendation, however, is limited. As of this writing, there are no large randomized controlled trials comparing higher and lower tidal volumes and their impact on clinically relevant outcomes, such as BPD. A small clinical trial comparing a tidal volume of 3 mL/kg with 5 mL/kg in preterm infants with RDS showed an increased inflammatory response in the tracheal aspirates of infants treated with 3 mL/kg.[75] This study seems to suggest that tidal volumes below 4 mL/kg combined with a relatively low PEEP of 3 to 4 cm H_2O may cause lung injury, probably due to alveolar collapse. Other studies have indicated that the optimal tidal volume in terms of gas exchange is probably not a fixed number but instead a dynamic parameter that changes over time.[76]

Tidal Volume Stabilization

Pressure-limited ventilation, the most widely used mode in neonatology, delivers a preset inflation pressure above PEEP during each mechanical inflation. Although the inflation pressure is initially set to target an appropriate tidal volume, the actual delivered tidal volume is dependent on the compliance and resistance of the respiratory system and the patient's own effort. As these variables change, delivered tidal volumes may become too high or too low, thereby increasing the risk of VILI. Applying volume-targeted ventilation will result in a more stable tidal volume and less VILI.[77,78] A systematic review of the (small) randomized controlled trials comparing volume-targeted to pressure-limited ventilation in preterm infants suggests that this approach also translates into a reduced risk of BPD.[79]

Permissive Hypercarbia

In an attempt to reduce tidal volume as much as possible, some clinicians accept higher carbon dioxide levels during mechanical ventilation, a strategy also referred to as *permissive hypercarbia.* Despite the fact that experimental evidence suggests a protective effect on the lungs, studies in ventilated preterm infants did not show a clear benefit in terms of BPD-free survival.[80] Of concern, one of these studies suggested that permissive hypercarbia was associated with worse neurodevelopmental outcome at 2 years' corrected age.[81]

Open Lung Ventilation

As previously mentioned, an open lung ventilation strategy aims to optimize lung volume by recruiting and stabilizing unstable lung units and by ventilating the lungs with low tidal volumes. Animal studies have shown that such an open lung ventilation strategy is feasible during positive-pressure ventilation using relatively high peak inflation pressures and PEEP to, respectively, recruit and stabilize the lung.[82,83] Open lung positive-pressure ventilation (PPV) improves gas exchange and attenuates VILI compared to more conventional ventilation strategies. These beneficial effects are similar during open lung PPV and open lung high-frequency ventilation, suggesting that the open lung ventilation strategy is probably more important than the ventilation mode.

Despite these promising animal data, studies on open lung PPV in human infants are limited. As of this writing, only one study has assessed the short-term benefits of open lung PPV in preterm infants with RDS. This study reported better oxygenation and shorter oxygen dependency.[84]

Several studies explored the short-term effects of various levels of PEEP without a recruitment procedure during conventional mechanical ventilation in preterm infants. Higher levels of PEEP improved functional residual capacity and oxygenation but also resulted in a reduction in lung compliance and higher carbon dioxide levels.[85-87] These findings may reflect failure to achieve lung recruitment before increasing PEEP. Unfortunately, the effects on markers of VILI or the incidence of BPD were not reported. Another study explored the effects of a higher versus a lower PEEP in term infants on extracorporeal membrane oxygenation and showed that lung function was better preserved by using higher PEEP levels, resulting in a more rapid recovery.[88]

LUNG-PROTECTIVE VENTILATION: HIGH-FREQUENCY VENTILATION

In neonatology, high-frequency ventilation (HFV) has been the ventilation mode associated most with lung-protective ventilation. This is probably because HFV, by design, applies very small tidal volumes, thereby reducing the risk of volutrauma. However, animal studies have also shown that HFV will provide lung protection only if combined with an open lung ventilation strategy.[89,90] This means that, in addition to applying the small tidal volumes, collapsed lung units need to be recruited and stabilized with the lowest possible airway pressure. This will place ventilation on the deflation limb of the P/V relationship, taking advantage of the lung hysteresis that is present in both preterm infants with RDS and term infants with more heterogeneous causes of lung disease.[60,61]

Reports on oxygenation-guided lung recruitment during (primary) HFV are limited to preterm infants with RDS. Figure 19-5 shows the basic scheme of this ventilation strategy. Changes in oxygenation are monitored at the bedside using pulse oximetry (SpO$_2$). Assuming that alveolar/saccular collapse resulting in intrapulmonary right-to-left shunt is the main cause of hypoxemia, reversing atelectasis will allow for normal oxygenation with minimal or no supplemental oxygen. For this reason, most clinicians will define an optimally recruited lung as needing an FiO$_2$ less than or equal to 0.25-0.30 to maintain SpO$_2$ within the appropriate target. To minimize the risk of overdistention, the continuous distending pressure (CDP) during HFV is usually set between 6 and 8 cm H$_2$O at the start of the recruitment procedure. The FiO$_2$ is adjusted in such a way that the SpO$_2$ is within the target range. If the FiO$_2$ is >0.30, the lung volume is considered as not being optimal, and the CDP is increased in steps of 2 cm H$_2$O every 2 to 3 minutes. If lung units are recruited, oxygenation will improve, allowing for a stepwise reduction in FiO$_2$ (5% to 10% each step). The CDP is increased stepwise until the FiO$_2$ is <0.30 or oxygenation does not improve during three consecutive pressure steps. At that point, referred to as *opening pressure*, the lung is considered as being optimally recruited. It is essential at this point to reduce the distending pressure because the pressure needed to keep the lungs open will be lower than the opening pressure (law of LaPlace, lung hysteresis). Using a fixed FiO$_2$, the CDP is decreased stepwise (2 cm H$_2$O every 2 to 3 minutes) until SpO$_2$ deteriorates, indicative of alveolar/saccular collapse. The corresponding pressure is called the *closing pressure*. Next, the CDP is increased to the opening pressure for several minutes and then decreased to 2 cm H$_2$O above the *closing pressure*. The corresponding pressure is called the *optimal CDP*.

In addition to oxygenation, changes in (transcutaneous) Pco$_2$ can also assist the clinician in lung recruitment.[91] Pco$_2$ will change depending on the position of ventilation on the inflation and deflation limbs of the P/V relationship. A rise in Pco$_2$ when determining the opening pressure is an indication that the lung is almost fully recruited, as ventilation is moving up the flat part of the inflation limb.

Administering exogenous surfactant will improve both EELV and its stability at lower pressures.[92] This means that following surfactant treatment, the CDP can usually be significantly lowered. A prospective cohort study in preterm infants with RDS subjected to primary HFV provided useful and

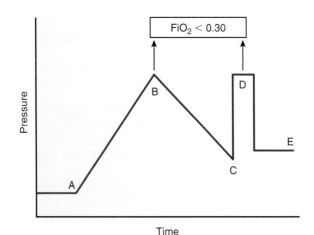

FIG 19-5 Schematic representation using oxygenation to optimize lung volume in preterm infants with RDS. At the start (A) airway pressure is low and FiO$_2$ is high, indicating a high degree of atelectasis and intrapulmonary shunt. Over time, airway pressures are increased stepwise, resulting in alveolar recruitment, a reduction in intrapulmonary shunt, and improvement in oxygenation. The last will allow a stepwise reduction in FiO$_2$, thus preventing hyperoxia. Airway pressures are increased until FiO$_2$ is below 0.30 or oxygenation no longer improves (B). The pressure level at point B is called the *opening pressure*. Airway pressures are reduced stepwise until SpO$_2$ starts to deteriorate, indicating alveolar collapse (C). This pressure level is called the *closing pressure*. After reopening collapsed alveoli with the known opening pressure (D), airway pressure is set 2 cm H$_2$O above the closing pressure to ensure a stabilization of lung volume (E).

practical information on this open lung ventilation strategy during HFV.[93] It showed that the mean opening pressure before surfactant treatment was 20 cm H$_2$O. Optimal recruitment resulting in an FiO$_2$ < 0.30 was feasible in 90% of the infants. It is important to emphasize that the strategy as described uses an individual and dynamic approach. The pressures applied to the lungs are different for each individual patient depending on the severity of lung disease. This is probably the most important reason the incidence of adverse effects of lung recruitment, such as hemodynamic instability and air leaks, is relatively low.

It is also important to acknowledge that oxygenation is an indirect tool for guiding lung recruitment. In case hypoxemia is also caused by extrapulmonary right-to-left shunt owing to persistent pulmonary hypertension or the presence of alveolar debris (pneumonia) impairing normal diffusion in the alveolar–capillary unit, oxygenation is no longer a reliable marker of lung volume. Clinicians should be aware of this drawback.

Although the basic concepts of open lung HFV are also applicable to other causes of respiratory failure, there are some important differences compared to preterm infants with RDS. First, lung disease in older preterm infants or term infants with respiratory failure is much more heterogeneous in nature compared with RDS.[94] Studies have indicated that the time constants of the lungs—that is, the time it takes collapsed lung units to open up or to close after a change in airway pressure—are much longer compared to infants with RDS.[73,95] Furthermore, the heterogeneous nature of lung disease often results in higher optimal pressures and concomitant FiO$_2$ compared to infants with RDS. Finally, lung disease in more mature infants is often accompanied by persistent pulmonary hypertension and, as previously mentioned, this complicates the process of oxygenation-guided lung recruitment during HFV.

The strategy described above is applicable in lung disease accompanied by alveolar/saccular collapse. HFV can also be lung protective during lung disease not characterized by atelectasis, such as lung hypoplasia associated with prolonged premature rupture of membranes and congenital diaphragmatic hernia. However, in these cases it is usually not necessary to apply a recruitment procedure. The optimal lung volume can be maintained with relatively low CDPs. Lung protection is focused on preventing alveolar/saccular overdistention by clearing CO_2 with relatively small tidal volumes.

Most randomized studies of HFV have been done in preterm infants with RDS. The systematic review of all randomized controlled trials comparing HFV to conventional mechanical ventilation shows, at most, a modest reduction in BPD in favor of HFV.[96] However, this effect is weakened by the heterogeneity between trials. Differences in the characteristics of the included patients, supportive therapies, and ventilation strategy used during both HFV and CMV probably account for this heterogeneity. Studies that failed to use or achieve an optimal lung volume strategy did not show any benefit of HFV. Based on the two largest randomized controlled trials, it has been suggested that HFV used with the optimal lung volume strategy might be superior to conventional mechanical ventilation in preterm infants with more severe RDS if consistently used during every ventilation period during hospitalization.[97,98]

As of this writing only one randomized controlled trial has compared HFV to conventional mechanical ventilation in term infants who were candidates for extracorporeal membrane oxygenation, mostly because of meconium aspiration syndrome (MAS).[99] This study showed that high-frequency oscillatory ventilation (HFOV) was an effective mode of ventilation especially when conventional mechanical ventilation failed. However, mortality and significant long-term morbidity did not differ between the groups. This may have been influenced by the relatively advanced age at randomization (40 hours) and the high crossover rate in each treatment arm (>50%). Another randomized controlled trial investigating the use of HFOV and/or inhaled nitric oxide also showed improved oxygenation when switching from conventional ventilation to HFOV in the treatment of MAS.[100] Furthermore, combining inhaled nitric oxide with HFOV was superior compared to combination with conventional mechanical ventilation.

The use of HFV in lung hypoplasia has been reported only in human case reports and case series. Most of these reports described improved survival after adopting HFV in the management of congenital diaphragmatic hernia mostly compared to historical controls.[101,102] Reports that showed no benefit from HFV often used this ventilation mode as a rescue therapy, applying it to those patients who failed (high-pressure) conventional mechanical ventilation, thus subjecting their lungs to volutrauma for a considerable period of time.[103,104] As of this writing, no randomized controlled trial has confirmed this apparently beneficial effect of HFV and its impact on long-term outcome parameters.

LUNG-PROTECTIVE VENTILATION: WEANING AND EXTUBATION

Although a lung-protective ventilation strategy can attenuate lung injury, it can never totally prevent it. For this reason, infants should be weaned from invasive support as soon as possible and transferred back to noninvasive modes of respiratory support. Prolonging mechanical ventilation for more than a few days will already increase the risk of BPD.[3] Furthermore, (protracted) mechanical ventilation has also been associated with an increased risk of adverse neurodevelopmental outcome in preterm infants.[2]

Studies have shown that noninvasive support modes such as continuous positive airway pressure and nasal intermittent PPV will increase the chance of successfully transitioning preterm infants from invasive to noninvasive support.[105,106] This is probably the most important reason protracted ventilation is nowadays less common in preterm infants.

IMPLICATIONS FOR PRACTICE AND RESEARCH

The goal during mechanical ventilation of newborn infants should be to establish adequate gas exchange while minimizing VILI as much as possible. Animal studies suggest that the ventilation strategy is probably more important than the ventilation mode when trying to achieve this goal. Such a lung-protective ventilation strategy should reduce both alveolar/saccular overdistention (volutrauma) and collapse (atelectrauma). When using conventional mechanical ventilation, clinicians should probably aim for a tidal volume between 4 and 7 mL/kg and reduce fluctuations as much as possible by choosing a volume-targeted ventilation mode. In addition, sufficient PEEP should be used to stabilize lung volume at the end of expiration, using oxygenation as an indicator of lung volume. A good alternative for conventional ventilation is HFV. This mode uses very small tidal volumes, thereby reducing the risk of volutrauma. However, HFV will provide optimal lung protection only if combined with an optimal lung volume or open lung ventilation strategy. Again, oxygenation can serve as an indirect monitoring tool for EELV. Finally, patients who require invasive mechanical ventilation should be extubated as soon as possible, limiting the duration of ventilation and the subsequent lung injury as much as possible.

Although invasive mechanical ventilation has been used in newborn infants for almost 50 years, there are still several unresolved issues that need to be addressed in future studies. First, the optimal tidal volume during conventional mechanical ventilation needs to be established in a randomized controlled trial comparing a higher to a lower tidal volume in specific patient populations. Second, the beneficial effects of volume-targeted ventilation reported in a meta-analysis summarizing several small trials need to be confirmed in a large randomized trial. Third, future studies need to confirm the presumed beneficial effect of lung recruitment and stabilization (open lung strategy) during conventional mechanical ventilation. Finally, more direct tools for measuring (changes in) lung volume, such as electrical impedance tomography, are urgently needed. These tools need to be optimized for clinical use and their impact on clinically relevant outcomes tested.

REFERENCES

A complete reference list is available at https://expertconsult.inkling.com/.

20

Tidal Volume-Targeted Ventilation

Martin Keszler, MD, FAAP, and Colin J. Morley, DCH, MD, FRCPCH

As described in Chapter 15, two fundamentally different approaches to positive pressure ventilation are possible. In pressure-controlled (PC) ventilation, the primary control variable governing gas delivery to the lungs is inflation pressure, and the tidal volume delivered to the lungs is the dependent variable that changes as the baby breathes and lung compliance and resistance change. In volume-controlled (VC) ventilation, tidal volume delivery is directly controlled and pressure becomes the dependent variable, changing as necessary to compensate for the baby breathing and to overcome resistive and elastic forces of the lungs (Fig. 20-1).

PC, time-cycled, continuous-flow ventilation has been the standard of care in neonatal ventilation for more than 30 years because early attempts at VC ventilation in small preterm neonates were unsuccessful with the devices available at the time. The perceived advantages of PC ventilation are the ability to directly control the inflation pressure and time and to ventilate despite large leaks around the uncuffed endotracheal tubes used with neonates. A preoccupation with high inflation pressure as the chief culprit in ventilator-induced lung injury and air leak has led to a deeply ingrained "barophobia" that has persisted despite mounting evidence that pressure by itself, without generating excessively large tidal volume, is not the main cause of lung injury.

RATIONALE FOR TIDAL VOLUME-TARGETED VENTILATION

Preclinical studies clearly demonstrate that tidal volume, rather than inflation pressure, is the critical determinant of ventilator-induced lung injury. Dreyfuss and colleagues demonstrated as early as 1988 that severe acute lung injury occurred in animals ventilated with large tidal volume, regardless of whether that volume was generated by a high or low inflation pressure[1] (Fig. 20-2). On the other hand, animals whose chest wall and diaphragmatic excursion were limited by external binding experienced much less lung damage despite being exposed to the same high inflation pressure.[2,3] This work and other similar experiments clearly show that excessive tidal volume, not pressure per se, is chiefly responsible for lung injury. Pressure, without correspondingly high volume, is not by itself injurious to the lungs, although it could be injurious to immature airways.

An equally compelling reason for tidal volume-targeted ventilation (VTV) is the extensive body of evidence documenting that both hypercarbia and hypocarbia are associated with neonatal brain injury.[4-8] Despite increasing awareness of its adverse consequences, inadvertent hyperventilation remains a common problem with pressure-limited ventilation, especially early in the clinical course when the baby starts breathing, lung compliance changes rapidly in response to clearing of lung fluid, surfactant is administered, and lung volume is optimized. Luyt et al. demonstrated that 30% of ventilated infants had at least one blood gas with $PaCO_2 < 25$ torr during the first day of life.[9]

While there are important differences in how volume targeting is achieved with various ventilators, the primary benefit of VTV probably rests in the ability to regulate and maintain an appropriate tidal volume (V_T), regardless of how that goal is achieved. When V_T is the primary control variable, inflation pressure will fall as lung compliance and patient inspiratory effort improve, resulting in real-time weaning of pressure, in contrast to intermittent manual lowering of pressure in response to blood gases. Real-time lowering of pressure avoids excessive V_T and achieves a shorter duration of mechanical ventilation. The inflation pressure will also rise if for some reason the set V_T is not delivered. Two meta-analyses that included a combination of several different modalities of VC and targeted

Volume vs Pressure Ventilation

<u>Volume Control</u>
- Controls the set flow rate
- Cycles when set volume is delivered
- Pressure rises passively

<u>Pressure Control</u>
- Controls the set pressure
- Cycles by time or flow
- Volume depends on compliance

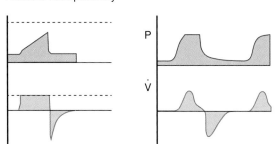

FIG 20-1 Key differences between volume-controlled (VC) and pressure-controlled (PC) ventilation. Volume delivered into the ventilator circuit is the primary control variable in VC. Circuit pressure rises passively and reaches its peak just before exhalation. The device generates whatever pressure is needed to deliver the set volume. Inflation pressure is the primary control variable in PC ventilation. Delivered volume is proportional to inflation pressure and compliance of the respiratory system; therefore the tidal volume will vary with changes in respiratory mechanics.

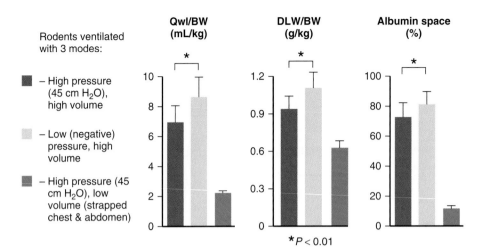

FIG 20-2 Rodents with normal lungs were ventilated with high inflation pressure (45 cm H$_2$O) and no restriction on chest wall movement (*red*), high inflation pressure but with chest wall movement restricted by a tight elastic bandage around chest and abdomen (*blue*), or high negative extrathoracic pressure (*yellow*). Pulmonary edema was assessed by measuring the extravascular lung water content (Qwl/BW). Changes in permeability were assessed by determining the bloodless dry lung weight (DLW/BW) and the distribution space of ^{125}I-labeled albumin (Albumin space). Large tidal volume was associated with high degree of acute lung injury, whether it was generated by high positive inflation pressure or negative pressure. In contrast, despite exposure to the same high inflation pressure, when the tidal volume was limited by restricted thoracic excursion, there was significantly less acute lung injury. (Adapted from Dreyfuss D, Soler P, Basset G, Saumon G. High inflation pressure pulmonary edema. Respective effects of high airway pressure, high tidal volume, and positive end-expiratory pressure. *Am Rev Respir Dis.* 1988;137(5):1159-1164.)

ventilation documented a number of advantages of VC/VTV, compared to pressure-limited ventilation, including significant decrease in the combined outcome of death or bronchopulmonary dysplasia (BPD), lower rate of pneumothorax, less hypocarbia, decreased risk of severe intraventricular hemorrhage/periventricular leukomalacia, and significantly shorter duration of mechanical ventilation (Table 20-1).[10,11] These results are very encouraging, but some limitations should be recognized. Included studies were quite small, used a variety of modalities, and many of the key outcomes reported in the meta-analysis were not prospectively collected or defined. In some of the studies, other variables beyond volume versus pressure targeting also differed. The studies focused on short-term physiologic outcomes, rather than BPD as a primary outcome. Except for one follow-up study based on parental questionnaire, no long-term pulmonary or developmental outcomes have been reported as of this writing.

VOLUME-CONTROLLED VERSUS VOLUME-TARGETED VENTILATION

VC, also known as volume-cycled, ventilators deliver a constant, preset V_T into the ventilator circuit with each inflation. In theory, these ventilators allow the operator to select V_T and respiratory rate and therefore directly control minute ventilation. Pressure rises passively, in inverse proportion to lung compliance, as the V_T is delivered, reaching its peak just before the ventilator cycles off, allowing little time for intrapulmonary gas distribution. The ventilator delivers the set V_T into the circuit, generating whatever pressure is necessary to overcome lung compliance and airway resistance, up to a set safety

TABLE 20-1   Documented Benefits of Volume-Targeted Ventilation

Outcome	No. of Studies	No. of Subjects	RR (95% CI) or Mean Diff (95% CI)
Mortality	11	759	0.73 (0.51-1.05)
BPD at 36 weeks*	9	596	0.61 (0.46-0.82)
Any IVH*	11	759	0.65 (0.42-0.99)
Cystic PVL*	7	531	0.33 (0.15-0.72)
Grade 3-4 IVH*	11	707	0.55 (0.39-0.79)
Pneumothorax*	8	595	0.46 (0.25-0.86)
Any hypocarbia*	2	58	0.56 (0.33-0.96)
Failure of assigned mode*	4	405	0.64 (0.43-0.94)
Duration of supplemental oxygen (days)*	2	133	−1.68 (−2.5 to −0.88)

(Data from Peng W, Zhu H, Shi H, Liu E. Volume-targeted ventilation is more suitable than pressure-limited ventilation for preterm infants: a systematic review and meta-analysis. *Arch Dis Child Fetal Neonatal Ed.* 2014;99(2):F158-165.)
RR, Risk ratio; *BPD*, bronchopulmonary dysplasia; *IVH*, intraventricular hemorrhage; *PVL*, periventricular leukomalacia.
*Indicates a statistically significant benefit of volume-targeted ventilation.

pop-off, typically set at a pressure >40 cm H$_2$O. A maximum inflation time is also set as an additional safety measure. The ventilator cycles into expiration when the preset V_T has been delivered or when the maximum inflation time has elapsed. The latter ensures that with very poor lung compliance, the ventilator does not generate a very prolonged inflation in an attempt to deliver a set V_T that cannot be reached at the pressure pop-off value.

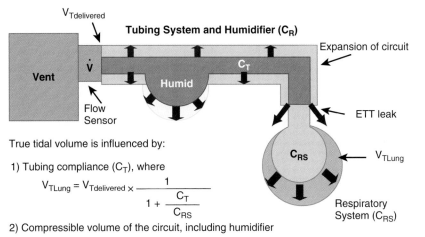

True tidal volume is influenced by:

1) Tubing compliance (C_T), where

$$V_{TLung} = V_{Tdelivered} \times \frac{1}{1 + \dfrac{C_T}{C_{RS}}}$$

2) Compressible volume of the circuit, including humidifier

3) Magnitude of ETT leak

FIG 20-3 Functional limitation of volume-controlled ventilation in newborn infants. Volume-controlled ventilation regulates the volume of gas delivered into the proximal end of the ventilator circuit ($V_{Tdelivered}$). The volume of gas entering the lungs (V_{TLung}) is affected by three factors: (1) tubing compliance (C_T), (2) compressible volume of the circuit and humidifier, and (3) magnitude of the leak around an uncuffed endotracheal tube (ETT). In newborn infants the volume of the lungs is only a fraction of the circuit/humidifier volume and often poorly compliant. Thus the loss of volume to compression of gas in the circuit and to stretching of the compliant circuit is very substantial. Variable leak around ETTs makes compensation very challenging.

The major limitation of any VC ventilator is that what is controlled is *the volume injected into the ventilator circuit and NOT the V_T that enters the patient's lungs*. This limitation is based on the fact that the V_T is measured at the ventilator end of the circuit and does not account for compression of gas in the circuit and humidifier or distention of the compliant circuit.[12] In large patients with cuffed endotracheal tubes (ETTs), this loss is negligible and easily compensated for. But such is not the case in small preterm infants, whose lungs are only a fraction of the total volume of the circuit (Fig. 20-3). Most modern ventilators have provisions to compensate for circuit compliance/gas compression, but this ability breaks down with the ubiquitous and highly variable leak around uncuffed ETTs used in newborn infants. These limitations can be overcome to a degree by using a separate flow sensor at the airway opening to monitor exhaled V_T. This will allow the user to manually adjust the set V_T (also known as V_{del}) to achieve the desired exhaled V_T. Unfortunately, the ETT leak is usually variable, and thus frequent monitoring and adjustment may be necessary. An alternate approach to VC is to rely on clinical assessment of adequacy of chest rise and breath sounds to set the V_{del}, which typically needs to be set at 10 to 12 mL/kg, to achieve effective V_T of 4 to 5 mL/kg, and to make subsequent adjustments based on blood gas measurement. Despite these limitations, VC has been shown to be feasible even in small preterm infants when a flow sensor at the airway opening is used.[13]

NEONATAL TIDAL VOLUME-TARGETED VENTILATION

In contrast to traditional VC ventilation, V_T-targeted ventilation modalities are modifications of pressure-controlled ventilation designed to deliver a target V_T by microprocessor-directed adjustments of inflation pressure or inflation time. Some devices regulate V_T delivery based on flow measurement

during inflation and others during exhalation. Each approach has advantages and disadvantages: leak is greater during inflation and thus exhaled V_T more closely approximates true V_T. Use of exhaled V_T results in regulation of the peak pressure based on the previous ventilator cycle, whereas using inflation volume makes same-cycle control possible, but it is then not possible to compensate for ETT leak in real time. If the inflation volume were 10 mL and the ETT leak 50%, then the baby would be getting a V_T of only 5 mL. When a large ETT leak is present, exhaled V_T may underestimate true volume and inspiratory measurement will overestimate the true V_T that enters the lungs. On balance, the use of exhaled V_T appears to offer the best balance of safety and effectiveness. Newer modalities of VTV have increasingly come to closely resemble volume guarantee ventilation, which focuses on expired V_T, as described below.

VOLUME GUARANTEE

Volume guarantee (VG) is an option available on the Dräger Babylog 8000+, the VN 500 (Dräger Medical, Lübeck, Germany), and the Leoni Plus (Heinen + Löwenstein GmbH, Bad Ems, Germany—not available in the United States). More recently, a version of VG has been implemented on the Avea ventilator (CareFusion, San Diego, CA) and the GE Engström Carestation (GE Healthcare, Chicago, IL). VG may be combined with any of the basic ventilator modes (continuous mandatory ventilation, assist/control [AC], synchronized intermittent mandatory ventilation [SIMV], pressure support ventilation). It is a volume-targeted, time- or flow-cycled, pressure-controlled form of ventilation. The operator chooses a target V_T and a pressure limit up to which the ventilator operating pressure (working pressure) may be adjusted. The microprocessor compares the exhaled V_T of the previous inflation and adjusts the working pressure up or down to target the set V_T (Fig. 20-4).

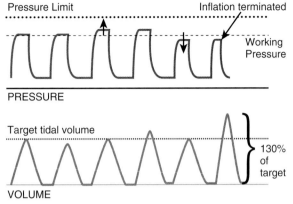

FIG 20-4 Principles of operation of volume guarantee. The device compares the measured tidal volume to the target volume and automatically regulates the PIP (peak inflation pressure, working pressure) within preset limits (as low as end-expiratory pressure to as high as the pressure limit) to achieve the tidal volume that is set by the user. Regulation of PIP is in response to *exhaled* tidal volume to decrease error due to ETT leak. The PIP increase from one cycle to the next is limited to avoid overshoot and undesirable oscillations. If tidal volume exceeds 130% of target, inflation will be terminated at that point (a secondary safety volume-limit function).

The algorithm limits the pressure increment from one inflation to the next to a percentage of the amount needed to reach the target V_T to avoid excessive oscillations, up to a maximum increase of 3 cm H_2O. Consequently, with rapid, large changes in compliance or patient inspiratory effort, several cycles are needed to reach target V_T. If the ventilator is unable to reach the target V_T with the set inflation pressure limit, a "low V_T" alarm will sound, alerting the operator that an assessment is needed. The VG modality, as implemented on the Dräger Babylog 8000+ and VN 500 ventilators, which are designed specifically for newborn infants, employs separate controls for triggered and untriggered inflations. This is an important feature when ventilating spontaneously breathing preterm infants whose respiratory effort is highly variable, because as with all forms of synchronized ventilation, the V_T is determined by a combination of the positive pressure from the ventilator and the negative intrapleural pressure resulting from the spontaneous effort of the infant (Fig. 20-5). Consequently VG leads to a more stable V_T than would be seen in similar modalities that use a single control algorithm (Fig. 20-6). The impact of VG with the dual control algorithm compared to simple PC ventilation is seen in Figure 20-7. A secondary safety feature designed to prevent delivery of excessively large inflations terminates an inflation on the same cycle if the V_T target is exceeded by >30% based on inspiratory volume measurement (corrected for leakage). In an awake, actively breathing infant the variable patient contribution to transpulmonary pressure is always perturbing the equilibrium, causing the V_T to fluctuate around the target V_T. Thus the term volume *guarantee* is arguably a misnomer. However, there is good evidence that a completely constant V_T leads to atelectasis over time; thus a physiologic variability of V_T is actually desirable.[14]

The VG modality, as implemented on a Dräger ventilator, has been studied more thoroughly than other modes of VTV.[15] VG reduces the incidence of hypocarbia and the number of excessively large V_Ts.[16] Specific clinical guidelines for

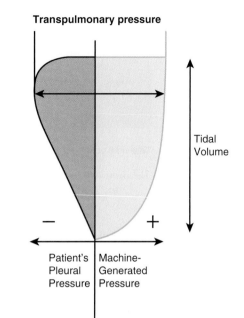

Transpulmonary pressure

FIG 20-5 In an awake, breathing infant the tidal volume that enters the lungs is generated by the transpulmonary pressure, the sum of the negative intrathoracic pressure generated by the infant's spontaneous respiratory effort and the positive inflation pressure generated by the ventilator. Because the respiratory effort of a preterm infant is variable and inconsistent, the infant's contribution to the transpulmonary pressure is variable, thus resulting in a variable tidal volume.

VG have been published and are also provided below and in Table 20-2.[17,18] VG has been shown to be more effective when used with AC than with SIMV, probably because all inflations are subject to volume targeting.[19]

The choice of appropriate V_T (discussed later) depends on infant size, pulmonary diagnosis, and basic synchronization mode. It is critical to appreciate that one size does not fit all when it comes to neonatal V_T settings. The smallest infants require a slightly larger V_T/kg because of the proportionally larger fixed dead space of the flow sensor.[20] Infants with pulmonary conditions that lead to increased alveolar dead space (e.g., meconium aspiration syndrome or BPD) also require relatively larger V_T.[21,22] Depending on the set rate, SIMV requires a larger V_T to deliver the same alveolar minute ventilation, because fewer breaths are supported and volume targeted. As the underlying pulmonary pathology evolves, the V_T target that provides optimal support will also change.

The Babylog 8000+ uses the uncorrected exhaled V_T of the previous inflation to regulate the peak pressure for the current inflation. This measurement begins to progressively underestimate the true V_T with increasing ETT leak, potentially resulting in inadvertent hypocarbia when the ETT leak exceeds about 40%. Progressively larger ETT leak commonly occurs if a preterm infant remains intubated for >2 weeks, because of stretching of the larynx, and may require reintubation with a larger ETT or reversion to PC ventilation, because reliable measurement of V_T is no longer possible with such a large leak. With the VN 500 ventilator, this problem has largely been eliminated, because this ventilator, being specifically designed for newborn infants, employs an effective leak compensation algorithm. We recommend that the leak compensation feature be selected in

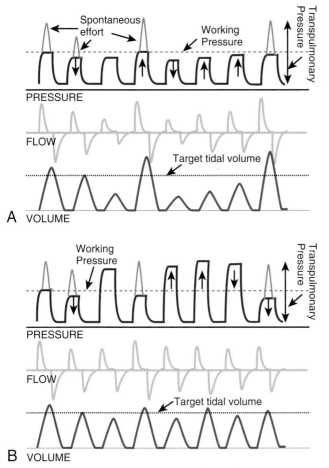

FIG 20-6 **A**, Because the respiratory effort of a preterm infant is variable and inconsistent, the infant's contribution to the transpulmonary pressure is variable, thus resulting in a variable tidal volume. In this graph, the infant's own inspiratory effort is drawn in blue, superimposed on the ventilator pressure. This contribution is not measured or displayed by the ventilator. When an actively breathing infant who was contributing substantially to the transpulmonary pressure fails to take a breath before the next ventilator cycle, there will be a large drop in delivered tidal volume. The ventilator adjusts the working pressure based on the tidal volume of the previous cycle, but the infant again resumes its breathing, resulting in large fluctuations in tidal volume. Because of the limited increment in working pressure from breath to breath, it takes several cycles to reach the target tidal volume when the infant remains apneic. **B**, The VG function as implemented on the Dräger devices has a separate control algorithm to regulate triggered and untriggered inflations. The microprocessor will use the working pressure for the previous cycle of the same type (triggered or untriggered) as a starting point for the adjustment. Consequently, the transpulmonary pressure remains more stable, resulting in more stable tidal volume delivery.

the ventilator default setting to minimize measurement error caused by ETT leakage. The ability to compensate effectively for leaks of up to 75% to 80% is a remarkable technological advance on the VN 500 that makes VG feasible in virtually all infants.

An obvious advantage of VG is that weaning occurs automatically, in real time, and requires fewer blood gas measurements.

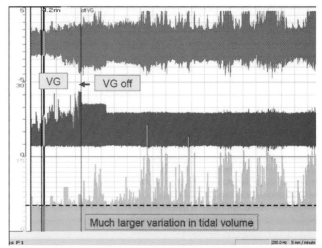

FIG 20-7 The impact of volume guarantee (VG) with dual control algorithm versus PC ventilation. Flow is displayed at the top, pressure in the middle, and tidal volume (V_T) at the bottom. Relatively stable V_T is seen in the first part of the recording while peak inflation pressure (PIP) is highly variable. After VG is turned off, PIP becomes fixed (after it is manually lowered in two steps), while V_T begins to fluctuate from inflation to inflation, because now we see the impact of a fixed PIP on top of a highly variable and sometimes absent spontaneous effort of the baby.

With stable minute ventilation ensured by VG along with noninvasive pulse oximetry monitoring, few invasive blood gas measurements are needed once the appropriate settings are confirmed. This effective closed-loop system is counterintuitive to some practitioners who are accustomed to manual adjustments of ventilator settings. As a consequence, there is sometimes inappropriate lowering of target V_T in an effort to wean the patient off the ventilator. It should be clearly understood that the physiologic V_T required by the patient does not decrease (over time it may actually increase); what goes down is the pressure required to achieve that V_T because of improved compliance of the respiratory system and the infant breathing more effectively. Decreasing the V_T target below the patient's physiologic need will increase the work of breathing[23] and may cause atelectasis and/or delay successful extubation.

SUGGESTED CLINICAL GUIDELINES (SEE ALSO TABLE 20-2)

When starting with VG as the initial mode of support, the V_T target should be chosen carefully, based on the infant's size and pulmonary condition (see Table 20-2). The inflation pressure limit should initially be set between 3 and 5 cm H_2O above the level estimated to be sufficient to achieve that V_T. If the target V_T cannot be reached with this setting, the pressure limit may be increased modestly until the desired V_T is generated. It is important to make sure the ETT is not kinked, malpositioned in the main stem bronchus, or obstructed on the carina, all of which can cause unexpectedly high inflation pressure. Significant volutrauma and/or air leak could result from failure to recognize single-lung intubation. If changing from pressure-limited ventilation in an infant whose $PaCO_2$ is in an appropriate range, it is best to match the average V_T of several

TABLE 20-2   Clinical Guidelines for Volume-Targeted Ventilation

Recommendation	Rationale
Initiation of VTV	
• Implement VTV as soon as feasible	• Compliance and respiratory effort change rapidly soon after birth
• Choose basic mode of synchronized ventilation: PC-AC or PC-PSV is preferred	• These ventilator modes result in more stable V_T and lower work of breathing
• If using SIMV + PSV, be aware that only the SIMV inflations are volume guaranteed	• The PSV pressure is a set value, not subject to VG
• Select backup rate about 10 breaths below spontaneous breathing rate: 30/min for term, 40/min for preterm infants	• Backup rate is a safety net for apnea. If too low, there will be more fluctuation in SpO_2 and minute ventilation; if too high, there will be more untriggered inflations
• Select PEEP appropriate to the infant's diagnosis, current condition, and FiO_2	• Because VG uses lowest possible PIP, adequate PEEP is essential to maintain FRC
• Ensure that flow sensor is calibrated and functioning properly	• Accurate V_T measurement is essential for VTV
• Select target V_T:	• V_T is now the primary control variable
• 4.5 mL/kg for typical preterm infant with RDS	• Typical V_T for average preterm infant
• 5-6 mL/kg if <700 g	• Impact of instrumental DS
• 5-6 mL/kg if MAS, air-trapping	• Increased alveolar DS
• 6 mL/kg if >2 weeks	• Increased anatomic and alveolar DS
• Set PIP limit 3-5 cm H_2O above expected PIP need	• To allow adjustment of working pressure both up and down
• If V_T target not met, ensure ETT is in good position, then increase PIP limit if needed	• ETT obstructed on carina would cause high PIP, ETT in right bronchus would cause high PIP, volutrauma
• Confirm adequacy of support by observing chest rise, auscultating breath sounds, and monitoring SpO_2 and obtaining blood gas	• Recommended V_T targets are population averages; individual patients may need higher or lower V_T
• If converting from PC to VTV, match the V_T generated by PC mode if $PaCO_2$ was satisfactory and increase PIP limit by 3-5 cm H_2O	• Changing primary control variable does not affect relationship of compliance, PIP, and V_T. Allow PIP to float both up and down as needed. Average PIP will be less than or equal to that on PC
Subsequent Adjustment	
• Once range of working PIP is known, set PIP limit 25%-30% above upper end of the range	• Important safety feature to alert provider to changes in support
• Record and present on rounds range of working PIP as well as PIP limit	• PIP limit does not accurately reflect actual level of support
• If indicated, adjust V_T in steps of ~0.5 mL/kg	• This step leads to meaningful change
• Base V_T adjustments on pH, not $PaCO_2$; do not lower V_T target if pH is not alkalotic	• pH, not $PaCO_2$ is the primary control of respiratory drive. Infants compensate for a base deficit by hyperventilating
• Lower PIP limit as needed to keep it 25%-30% above upper end of the range of PIP	• As compliance and respiratory effort improve, working PIP comes down
• Assess patient's respiratory rate, comfort, oxygen requirement, and working pressure, not just blood gas. Increase V_T if necessary to achieve adequate support	• Tachypnea and retractions indicate increased WOB. If V_T is set below patient's physiologic need, the ventilator lowers the PIP and the infant has to work harder to maintain its MV
• Always verify appropriateness of support by clinical assessment, especially if large increase in support appears to be needed	• Machines are fallible. Do not blindly trust any mechanical device
• Use birth weight initially to determine V_T target and remember to adjust for weight gain if the baby remains ventilated	• Short-term changes in weight after birth reflect fluid shifts, but once baby begins to grow, the V_T needs to keep up with current weight
Weaning	
• When pH is low enough to ensure respiratory drive, weaning is automatic; do not lower target V_T to wean, unless patient is alkalotic	• Physiologic V_T need does not decrease, the PIP needed to achieve it does—self-weaning
• Withhold or reduce sedation/analgesia	• Avoid suppressing the respiratory drive
• Do not reduce V_T below 3.5-4 mL/kg	• Setting the V_T below what the infant needs imposes excessive WOB
• Consider raising PEEP to maintain adequate distending pressure as PIP comes down	• Automatic lowering of PIP may lead to atelectasis if PEEP is relatively low
• Avoid using SIMV and do not wean backup rate on PC-AC or PC-PSV	• As PIP comes down, the WOB is gradually shifted from ventilator to infant. The infant controls the ventilator rate
• Observe the graphic display to detect excessive periodic breathing or apnea	• Inconsistent respiratory effort may set up the infant for extubation failure
Extubation	
• Consider extubation if inflation pressure is ≤12-15 cm H_2O with satisfactory blood gas.	• These pressures are low enough to ensure that the infant is able to take over
• Readiness for extubation can be assessed using the SBT	• The SBT has been shown to accurately predict extubation readiness
• Caffeine should always be used prior to extubation of preterm infants ≤32 weeks	• Caffeine reduces extubation failure in preterm infants
• Distending pressure with CPAP, NIPPV, or HHHFNC should always be used for at least 24 hr post extubation	• The use of distending airway pressure after extubation reduces the risk of extubation failure

AC, Assist/control; *CPAP,* continuous positive airway pressure; *DS,* dead space; *ETT,* endotracheal tube; *FRC,* functional residual capacity; *HHHFNC,* high-humidity, high-flow nasal cannula; *MAS,* meconium aspiration syndrome; *MV,* minute ventilation; *NIPV,* nasal intermittent positive pressure ventilation; *PC,* pressure controlled; *PEEP,* positive end-expiratory pressure; *PIP,* peak inflation pressure; *PSV,* pressure support ventilation; *RDS,* respiratory distress syndrome; *SBT,* spontaneous breathing test; *SIMV,* synchronized intermittent mandatory ventilation; *VG,* volume guarantee; *VT,* tidal volume; *VTV,* volume-targeted ventilation; *WOB,* work of breathing.

cycles as measured by the ventilator and increase the pressure limit from 3 to 5 cm H_2O above that used during the PC ventilation, to allow the microprocessor to adjust working pressure up as well as down as needed. It is advisable to keep the pressure 25% to 30% above the upper limit of the range of current working pressure and adjusted periodically as lung compliance and the infant's breathing improves, causing the working pressure to come down. Maintaining this relationship serves as an early warning system and a key safety feature. A persistent "low V_T" alarm indicates that there has been a change in the patient's condition or in the circuit/ETT; this should encourage a prompt evaluation of the reason for a change in respiratory system compliance, ETT position, or patient respiratory effort. Please note that with the Babylog 8000+, when the flow sensor is temporarily removed (such as around the time of surfactant administration or delivery of nebulized medication), if its function is affected by reflux of secretions or surfactant, or it malfunctions for any reason, the working pressure will default to the peak inflation pressure (PIP) limit. If the limit is much higher than the infant requires, dangerously high V_Ts could be reached, and if the situation persists, hypocarbia will develop. Additionally, when the manual inflation function is used, the ventilator will use the PIP limit pressure. Therefore, it is important to keep the PIP limit sufficiently close to the working pressure to avoid volutrauma. Ideally, when the flow sensor is removed for significant periods, such as when nebulizing medications, the PIP should be adjusted to match the average or recent working pressures. To avoid this risk, the newer VN500 defaults to the most recent working pressure when the flow sensor is inoperative. Some clinicians choose to leave the PIP limit at 40 cm H_2O, regardless of the level of working pressure. This simplifies the application of VG and minimizes alarms but defeats important safety features and inactivates the valuable early warning system. The benefits of the interactive closed loop system of VG outweigh the drawbacks. Use of longer alarm delay settings and appropriate pressure limit settings, avoidance of large leak around ETTs, proper ETT positioning, and adequate physical comfort measures or sedation will minimize nuisance alarms. Please see Tables 20-2 and 20-3 for further details and troubleshooting tips.

Subsequent adjustments of V_T should be guided by $PaCO_2$ measurement. Over time, with stretching of the immature upper airway by positive pressure ventilation (acquired tracheomegaly)[24] and the development of BPD, which results in more heterogeneous inflation and air trapping, a modestly higher V_T is required even with permissive hypercarbia.[22] During weaning, pH should be allowed to be low enough to ensure adequate respiratory drive. If sedation is being used, it should be lightened or discontinued. V_T should normally not be weaned below 4 mL/kg to avoid shifting all the work of breathing to the infant. When V_T is set below the infant's physiologic need, the baby will spontaneously generate a V_T above the set value, causing the working pressure to drop all the way to positive end-expiratory pressure (PEEP). This potentially results in excessive work of breathing, with the infant essentially on a prolonged endotracheal continuous positive airway pressure trial, and should be avoided. When the infant is able to maintain good gas exchange with low inflation pressure, extubation should be attempted.

PRESSURE-REGULATED VOLUME CONTROL

The pressure-regulated volume control (PRVC) mode on the SERVO-i ventilator (Maquet, Wayne, N.J.) is a time-cycled,

pressure-controlled assist control mode that uses the V_T of the previous cycle, measured at the ventilator (proximal) end of the circuit, to regulate the inflation pressure needed to achieve the desired V_T. Pressure increment is limited to 3 cm H_2O. Because pressure adjustment is based on the previous breath, regardless of whether it was an assisted breath or an untriggered inflation, variable and/or intermittent patient respiratory effort will cause fluctuations in V_T. The main limitation of the PRVC mode of the SERVO-i ventilator for newborn infants is the overestimation of V_T measured proximally (at the ventilator end of the circuit), rather than at the airway opening. An optional flow sensor at the wye-piece allows for more accurate monitoring of V_T, but the servo regulation of inflation pressure is still based on the proximal flow measurement. Circuit compliance compensation is available to correct for compression of gas in the circuit but is ineffective when there is a leak around the ETT. The reliability of compliance compensation falls with lower infant weight and may result in wide swings of apparent V_T in tiny infants. Therefore, the compliance compensation feature is generally not used in small preterm infants. Because substantial loss of V_T to compression of gas in the circuit occurs, the set V_T must be two to three times larger than the target exhaled V_T at the airway opening.

When initiating PRVC, several methods may be used for setting the target V_T. If a proximal flow sensor is available, it should be used to measure directly the exhaled V_T and adjust the set value (V_{del}) to achieve an exhaled V_T of approximately 5 mL/kg, with the same caveats for matching target V_T to the specific condition as outlined for VG. If the infant is being switched from a pressure-limited mode, a common approach is to set the target volume either (1) to match the volumes (V_{del}) generated by PC ventilation or (2) to generate inflation pressures similar to those being used in PC ventilation. If the infant is being started directly on PRVC without the optional flow sensor, the operator must rely on clinical assessment of chest rise and breath sounds to determine the appropriate V_{del}, keeping in mind that a substantial portion of the V_T will be lost in the circuit. Clinical assessment of the adequacy of support should supplement blood gas analysis. Similar to other VTV modalities, the pressure needed to achieve the target V_T comes down automatically as lung compliance and patient effort improve. The target V_T should not be reduced below 4 mL/kg exhaled volume at the airway opening for the same reasons as described in the previous section on VG. A randomized clinical trial of PRVC on the Servo 300 ventilator compared to pressure-limited SIMV in very low birth-weight infants failed to show any advantage of PRVC.[25]

VOLUME VENTILATION PLUS

Volume ventilation plus (Puritan Bennett 840, Covidien/Medtronic, Minneapolis, Minn.) is a complex mode that combines two different dual-mode volume-targeted inflation types: volume control plus, for delivery of mandatory inflations in AC and SIMV, and volume support, for support of spontaneous breaths in the spontaneous ventilation mode. The ventilator adjusts inflation pressure to target desired V_T. Because V_T is not routinely measured at the ETT, it is functionally similar to the VC and PRVC modes described above. Thus, the selection of volume setting reflects the proximal V_T and must allow for the loss of volume to compression in the ventilator circuit. Proximal flow sensor use is recommended where available with the same targets as above. Again, avoidance of inadvertent main stem bronchus intubation as discussed above is essential. This is a ventilator designed primarily for adult patients and there are no published studies evaluating its clinical performance in small preterm infants.

VOLUME-TARGETED VENTILATION

VTV as implemented on the Hamilton G5 (Hamilton Medical, Reno, Nev.) is a modality that is functionally similar to VG. The device adjusts inflation pressure in response to any deviation of measured V_T from the target value. This is a relatively new modality with no published literature on its safety and effectiveness, but it appears to have functionality similar to that of standard VG, and therefore similar guidelines should be applied to its use.

TARGETED TIDAL VOLUME

Targeted tidal volume (TTV) is a modality on the SLE 4000 and SLE 5000 neonatal ventilators (Specialised Laboratory Equipment Ltd., Croydon, UK). This device is not available in the United States but is widely used outside of North America. The standard TTV is in essence a simple volume limit function. The device increases the rise time of the pressure waveform to improve the chance of effectively limiting V_T to the desired target. To avoid the risk of excessive PIP when the TTV function is turned off, the PIP automatically drops to 5 mbar above the PEEP, and the user must then actively adjust the PIP. Reliance on inspiratory V_T measurement may lead to inadequate V_T delivery with significant leak around the ETT. A recent enhancement referred to as TTV*plus* makes the modality function more like VG by using exhaled V_T measurement and actively modulating inflation pressure to target the desired V_T. A leak compensation feature has also been added.

VOLUME LIMIT

Some older-generation pressure-limited ventilators employ a simple volume limit function that simply terminates inflation when the maximum allowed V_T is delivered. If the inflation pressure is set well above that needed to deliver the limit volume, this strategy will result in very short inflation times and termination of inflation at or near peak flow. This situation exposes the infant's airways to higher than necessary pressure and does not allow inflation to be completed with short intrapulmonary gas dwell time limiting intrapulmonary gas distribution. Additionally, this strategy does not provide a mechanism to ensure adequate V_T delivery should lung compliance deteriorate or patient effort become inadequate. These devices have now been supplanted by more sophisticated algorithms in the newer generation of ventilators but may still be in use in some centers. With these devices, it is important to pay attention to whether the volume limit is being reached on a regular basis and reduce inflation pressure setting to deliver a V_T just below the volume limit.

IMPORTANCE OF OPEN LUNG STRATEGY

The benefits of VTV cannot be fully realized unless we ensure that the V_T is evenly distributed into an "open lung." Although adequate PEEP has long been known to mitigate lung injury, the admonition of Burkhard Lachmann more than 20 years

ago to "Open the lung and keep it open!"[26] has been ignored by many during conventional mechanical ventilation despite a sound physiologic basis and strong experimental evidence in its favor.[27] This is because, as can be seen in Figure 20-8, when partially atelectatic lungs are ventilated, the V_T will preferentially enter the already aerated portion of the lungs, because the pressure required to do so is less than the critical opening pressure of the atelectatic alveoli (LaPlace's law). Thus, ventilating lungs that are partially atelectatic inevitably leads to overexpansion of this relatively healthy portion of the lung with subsequent volutrauma/biotrauma even when the V_T is in the normal range. Additionally, atelectasis leads to exudation of a protein-rich fluid (the hyaline membranes seen by a pathologist) with increased surfactant inactivation and release of inflammatory mediators. Shear forces and uneven stress in areas where atelectasis and overinflation coexist add to the damage. Thus, the open lung concept,[28-30] which ensures that the V_T is distributed evenly throughout the lungs, should be a fundamental component of any lung-protective ventilation strategy (see also Chapter 19).

ALARMS/TROUBLESHOOTING

VTV modes generate alarms not encountered with simple PC ventilation; these become annoying when they are excessive. The alarms are designed to provide feedback as to whether the patient is receiving the desired level of ventilator support. A significant fall in lung compliance, decreased spontaneous respiratory effort, impending accidental extubation, and forced exhalation episodes will all generate "low V_T" alarms. When properly used, this information should improve care in the most vulnerable infants. It is important to evaluate the cause of the alarms and correct any correctable problems. Large leaks result in underestimation of delivered V_T and trigger the low V_T alarm when the device is unable to reach the target V_T at the set PIP limit. With the older Babylog 8000+ and other devices with VG modes that lack effective leak compensation, when the leak exceeds 40% to 50% the VG mode no longer functions reliably owing to an inability to accurately measure V_T. This is much less of a problem with the VN 500 ventilator. The alarms serve an important function and should not be ignored. If the low V_T alarm sounds repeatedly in the absence of excessive leak, increase the pressure limit and investigate the cause. Please see Table 20-3 for troubleshooting advice.

Unnecessary alarms can be avoided by optimizing settings and alarm limits.

Use of longer alarm delay settings, appropriate pressure limit settings, avoidance of large leak around ETTs, and adequate physical comfort measures or sedation will also minimize alarms.

CONCLUSION

There is now strong evidence in support of using V_T as the primary control variable for mechanical ventilation of newborn infants. VTV has been shown to improve a variety of important clinical outcomes, yet its penetration into clinical practice has been surprisingly slow in most parts of the world, Australia, Scandinavia, and Italy being the exceptions. It appears that many clinicians are still unwilling to abandon their comfort zone and embrace the paradigm shift that VTV represents.[31]

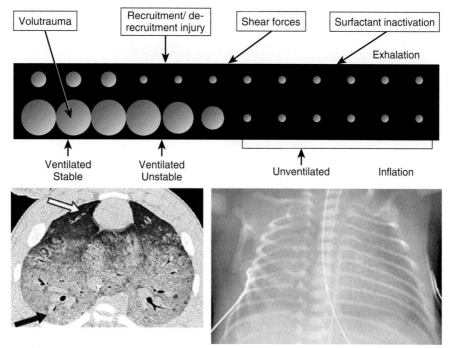

FIG 20-8 The importance of the open lung concept. While anteroposterior chest radiographs make the lungs of an infant with respiratory distress syndrome appear homogeneous (lower right), this is an artifact of a two-dimensional view of a three-dimensional structure. Atelectasis has a gravity-dependent distribution as illustrated on the computer tomography view in the lower left. This situation is diagrammatically represented at the top. Ventilating lungs in the presence of extensive atelectasis results in atelectrauma. Surfactant inactivation in the atelectatic portion, shear forces at the boundary between aerated and unaerated lung, and damage from repeated collapse and opening of unstable alveoli all contribute to lung injury. Perhaps most important, the gas expanding partially atelectatic lungs will preferentially enter the already aerated portion of the lung, which requires less distending pressure than the critical opening pressure of the atelectatic lungs (LaPlace's law). Therefore, even a normal, physiologic tidal volume entering the small proportion of open alveoli will inevitably lead to overexpansion and volutrauma.

TABLE 20-3	Troubleshooting	
Problem	**Possible Cause**	**Suggested Action**

Low V_T alarm—not reaching target Recurrent alarms	• Decreased compliance:
	  • Atelectasis
	  • Pneumothorax/PIE
	  • ETT in RMSB
	  • ETT obstructed on tracheal wall or carina
	  • Abdominal distention
	  • Chest wall edema
	  • Decreased patient effort (oversedation, sepsis)
	  • Baby splinting chest and reducing delivered tidal volume
		• Evaluate breath sounds
		 • Evaluate chest rise
		 • Examine ventilator waveforms
		 • Reposition patient and/or ETT
		 • Assess overall condition
		 • Obtain CXR
		 • Assess patient's level of sedation, activity

	• Increased resistance
	  • Airway secretions
	  • Partial kinking of ETT
	  • Bronchospasm
		• Evaluate breath sounds
		 • Examine ETT, circuit
		 • Listen to patient, examine flow waveform

	• PIP limit too close to WP	• Observe working pressure in relation to PIP limit; the limit needs to be about 5 cm H_2O above upper end of range of working pressure to allow ventilator to increase pressure when baby fails to breathe.
	• Alarm delay is too short	• Increase alarm delay for low V_T; it is not important to know a few inflations fell short of target, but you do want to know if it persists.
	• Large ETT leak	• Check for ETT leak on the ventilator display. Note that when using the VN 500 leak compensation feature the waveforms do not visually indicate the leak, because the ventilator displays the corrected value.
	• Flow sensor malfunction	• Evaluate V_T clinically; recalibrate flow sensor as needed.
	• Forced exhalation episodes	• Recognize these by observing sudden cessation of airflow despite appropriate inflation pressure. These are preceded by a large expiratory flow and the infant is bearing down with a Valsalva maneuver. There is no effective way to abolish these short of muscle relaxation. Setting a higher PIP limit than usual mitigates their effect and achieves faster recovery.

Continued

TABLE 20-3	Troubleshooting—cont'd	
Problem	**Possible Cause**	**Suggested Action**
	• Interrupted exhalation • Some infants intermittently perform expiratory braking and briefly reverse expiratory flow, thus interrupting full exhalation. The ventilator misinterprets this as a new breath and uses the exhaled volume of only the second portion of the exhalation, thus under-estimating the true value of V_T	• Recognize these by a typical brief blip of the expiratory flow above 0 during exhalation. In most infants these are infrequent and benign, but if more regular, may need intervention. Try increasing PEEP to obviate the need for expiratory breaking.
Ventilator is not generating any PIP	• Tubing disconnection • V_T is too low for the infant's physiologic need	• Check for leak, disconnection • Reevaluate V_T setting. If infant consistently generates V_T in excess of the target, the device continues to decrease PIP until it is equal to PEEP.
Ventilator is generating a low PIP, which is not increasing despite low or absent V_T	• Complete ETT obstruction. When the device senses complete ETT or circuit obstruction the PIP drops to about half of the previous value and an alarm sounds. This is a safety feature to avoid a large overshoot of PIP once the obstruction is relieved.	• Check for ETT obstruction or kinked tubing and correct if present. ETT may be obstructed with secretions or viscous surfactant.
Persistently low PaCO$_2$	• Metabolic acidosis • Agitation	• Consider pH, not just PaCO$_2$; the respiratory control center responds to pH and respiratory compensation for a base deficit is normal. • Ensure optimal positioning, comfort. Provide sedation if necessary.
Tachypnea, increased WOB	• V_T set too low • Agitation	• Insufficient support leads to tachypnea and retractions. Reassess appropriateness of V_T setting. • As above

CXR, chest x-ray; *ETT*, Endotracheal tube; *PEEP*, positive end-expiratory pressure; *PIE*, pulmonary interstitial emphysema; *PIP*, peak inflation pressure; *RMSB*, right main-stem bronchus; V_T, tidal volume; *WOB*, work of breathing; *WP*, working pressure.

Availability of equipment is no longer a barrier to acceptance, at least in reasonably well-resourced parts of the world. Some form of VTV is now available on virtually all ventilators used in neonatal intensive care, and the newest devices designed specifically for newborn infants now perform very well even in very small infants. However, it is important to point out that each ventilator functions differently. It is critical that the user become familiar with the specific features and limitations of his or her particular device. The reader is referred to Chapter 25 of this book and to user manuals of their respective devices for further guidance. A ventilator is only a tool in the hands of the clinician, a tool that can be used well, or not. It is probably time to abandon the term *ventilator-induced lung injury* in favor of *physician-induced lung injury*, as it is we who select the ventilator settings!

REFERENCES

A complete reference list is available at https://expertconsult .inkling.com/.

21

Special Techniques of Respiratory Support

Nelson Claure, MSc, PhD, and Eduardo Bancalari, MD

INTRODUCTION

The care of premature infants with respiratory failure has advanced considerably over the past decades, but a substantial proportion of very premature infants survive with some degree of respiratory, visual, and neurodevelopmental impairment. This reality highlights the need for further improvements in the methods and monitoring of respiratory support in this population. There is a wide variety of "standard" modes of respiratory support discussed in other chapters of this book. New strategies and techniques to provide mechanical ventilation and supplemental oxygen to the premature infant have become available as a result of advances in the hardware, software, and sensing technologies that enable a more dynamic control of ventilator functions. The technology is still evolving, and these techniques have not yet come into widespread use for regulatory reasons or because of a paucity of definitive evidence of their benefits. This chapter describes these modalities of respiratory support and discusses the rationale and the evidence for the advantages and possible limitations.

CLOSED-LOOP CONTROL OF INSPIRED OXYGEN

Most premature infants require supplemental oxygen to maintain adequate arterial oxygen levels. However, it is well documented that in routine clinical care, manual adjustment of the fraction of inspired oxygen (FiO_2) commonly fails to keep arterial oxygen saturation (SpO_2) within the prescribed target range. It has been reported that premature infants spend nearly a third of the time with SpO_2 levels above the target range owing to excessive FiO_2.[1,2] The resulting hyperoxemia increases the risk of damage to the eye, brain and other organs, whereas excessive exposure to inspired oxygen increases the risk of oxidant damage to the lungs.[3-8] The same report showed that premature infants spend nearly a fifth of the time with SpO_2 below the target range.[1] This is because hypoxemia episodes are frequently observed in premature infants owing to their respiratory instability. These episodes increase in frequency with postnatal age, especially in infants with chronic lung disease.[9-12] Most of these episodes are spontaneous,[13-15] but some are related to care procedures. The response of the clinical staff can influence the duration and severity of these episodes. However, staff availability to perform this task during standard care is often limited. FiO_2 is increased during the episodes, but the resolution of hypoxemia is not always followed by a prompt return of FiO_2 to baseline, resulting in subsequent hyperoxemia.[16] The occurrence of hypoxemia episodes is in part related to the basal level of SpO_2. Higher SpO_2 levels are often tolerated in infants with frequent hypoxemia episodes in an attempt to prevent their occurrence, but this practice can lead to hyperoxemia.

On the other hand, the use of lower SpO_2 target ranges to avoid hyperoxemia can lead to an increased frequency of episodes of hypoxemia.[17-19]

The impact of staff availability on the maintenance of SpO_2 within target was documented by a decline in the proportion of time with SpO_2 within range as the nurse-to-infant ratio decreased,[20] and this was mainly due to an increased time in hyperoxemia.

Because consistent maintenance of SpO_2 within the prescribed target range is seldom achieved in premature infants receiving supplemental oxygen, exposure to hyperoxemia and hypoxemia is common. Systems for automatic closed-loop control of FiO_2 incorporated into neonatal ventilators have been proposed as a tool to assist caregivers in the maintenance of SpO_2 within the prescribed target range and reduce the exposure to extremes of high and low SpO_2 levels. These systems continuously adjust FiO_2, aiming at keeping SpO_2 within the target range set by the clinician. Figure 21-1 shows representative recordings of SpO_2 and FiO_2 from a premature infant with frequent episodes of hypoxemia during manual and automated FiO_2 control.

Short-term feasibility and efficacy studies have shown that closed-loop FiO_2 control systems are more effective in keeping SpO_2 within the target range than manual control during routine care and equal to or better than a fully dedicated nurse.[21-33] The relative efficacy of automated systems compared to conventional manual adjustment obtained in these clinical studies is shown in Table 21-1. Closed-loop FiO_2 control also produced a consistent reduction in the proportion of time with SpO_2 above the target range compared to manual control.

The proportion of time with SpO_2 below target was not consistently reduced by closed loop compared to manual FiO_2 control. Studies in infants with frequent hypoxemia episodes showed a greater number of mild episodes with SpO_2 slightly below the target range but a consistent reduction in the severe and prolonged episodes of hypoxemia during closed-loop FiO_2 control. This finding illustrates the fact that closed-loop FiO_2 control systems do not prevent hypoxemia episodes but can attenuate their duration and severity.

In these studies, the number of manual changes in FiO_2 was minimal during automatic FiO_2 control. This suggests potential savings in staff workload and the possibility of shifting the staff effort to other areas of clinical care.

SpO_2 alarms are among the most common events in the neonatal intensive care unit. Although not evaluated yet during extended use, systems for automatic FiO_2 control may have an impact on SpO_2 alarm fatigue in the staff. On the other hand, reduced staff attentiveness is a potential unintended consequence of automated FiO_2 control systems. An automatic increase in

FiO_2 during hypoxemia can mask a respiratory deterioration that would otherwise manifest as a persistently lower SpO_2. Hence, it is essential that monitoring of the ventilatory status by the clinical staff remains as usual when these systems are in use and that closed-loop FiO_2 control systems alert the clinician when there is a persistent need for a higher FiO_2.

Neonatal centers have adopted specific target ranges of SpO_2 for premature infants. However, significant discrepancies can exist between the target and the actual range of SpO_2 during routine care. Caution is recommended when setting the range of SpO_2 to be targeted by automatic systems because there may be important clinical implications that become evident when SpO_2 is kept more consistently within such range. This is particularly important because the optimal range of SpO_2 for this population has not been clearly established.

In summary, short-term clinical studies showed that closed-loop FiO_2 control can improve SpO_2 targeting and reduce exposure to hyperoxemia, supplemental oxygen, and episodes of severe

hypoxemia. Whether extended clinical use of this technology can have an impact on long-term visual, respiratory, and neurodevelopmental outcomes in premature infants is still to be determined.

VENTILATION TECHNIQUES

Proportional Assist Ventilation

The underlying lung disease can significantly affect the mechanical properties of the premature infant's respiratory system. Restrictive conditions such as respiratory distress syndrome (RDS) result in a decrease in lung compliance that imposes an elastic load on the infant's respiratory pump, whereas obstructive conditions (increased airway resistance) impose resistive loads. In most cases these higher loads lead to an increased breathing effort to sustain ventilation, resulting in increased work of breathing and increased oxygen consumption and caloric expenditure, as well as distress. When the infant fatigues or the effort is insufficient, the patient develops hypoventilation and respiratory failure.

Proportional assist ventilation (PAV) is a modality in which the pressure generated by the ventilator is increased in proportion to the volume, flow, or both, generated by the infant's inspiratory effort. The gain or proportionality factors by which the positive pressure increases in relation to the measured tidal volume (V_T) or flow are the *elastic gain* (volume proportional, in units of pressure per milliliter of measured volume) or *resistive gain* (flow proportional, in units of pressure per unit of measured flow). The simultaneous increase in ventilator pressure with the infant's spontaneous inspiration augments the patient's own effort and thus can achieve a normal transpulmonary pressure and maintain a normal V_T with less spontaneous inspiratory effort. Generating the same or larger V_T with less inspiratory effort is perceived by the infant as a reduction in the mechanical loads, decreases the work of breathing, and reduces oxygen consumption. The proportional increase in ventilator pressure to the infant's spontaneous effort is illustrated in Figure 21-2.

Studies in infants recovering from RDS showed that PAV produced similar ventilation with lower ventilator and transpulmonary pressures compared to pressure-controlled modalities such as assist/control and intermittent mandatory

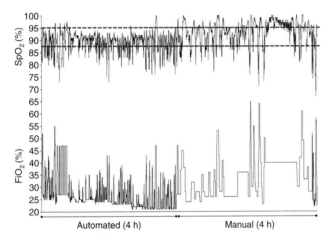

FIG 21-1 The graph shows frequent automated and manual FiO_2 adjustments to keep SpO_2 within the target range (*dotted lines*) in an infant with frequent hypoxemia spells. Automated adjustments reduced periods with SpO_2 above the target range and achieved a consistent reduction of the baseline FiO_2 level over the 4-hour period. (From Ref. 25.)

TABLE 21-1 Maintenance of SpO₂ Target Ranges during Manual and Closed-Loop FiO₂ Control

| | SpO₂ Target Range | % TIME WITHIN TARGET RANGE | |
		Manual FiO₂ Control	Closed-Loop FiO₂ Control
Bhutani, 1992	94%-96%	54	81
Morozoff, 1993	90%-95%	39	50
Claure, 2001	88%-96%	66	75
Urschitz, 2004	87%-96%	82	91
Claure, 2009	88%-95%	42	58
Morozoff, 2009	90%-96%	57	73
Claure, 2011	87%-93%*	39	47
Waitz, 2014	88%-96%	69	76
Hallenberger, 2014	Four centers (90%-95%, 80%-92%, 83%-93%, 85%-94%)	61	72
Zapata, 2014	85%-93%	34	58
Lal, 2015	90%-95%	60	69
Van Kaam, 2015	89%-93%*	54	62
	91%-95%	58	62

*Includes periods with SpO_2 > target range while $FiO_2 = 0.21$.

ventilation.[33-35] The elastic and resistive gains are set to produce the unloading necessary to compensate for the disease-induced respiratory loads. These gains must be individualized to the infant's lung compliance and airway resistance. An elastic gain that exceeds what is needed to compensate for the decrease in lung compliance can result in a runaway increase in pressure. A resistive gain that exceeds what is needed to overcome the increased airway resistance can induce rapid oscillations in pressure. It should be recognized that the underlying assumption of PAV is that the patient's respiratory drive is appropriate and the device is simply overcoming disease-induced mechanical loads. When applied to premature infants with immature respiratory control, there is a potential for this positive feedback system to generate excessive pressures and volumes when an infant is disturbed and briefly generates a large spontaneous inspiratory effort, whereas inadequate support may be provided during periods of hypopnea that are common in preterm infants. Because the system by necessity responds to inspiratory flow and volume, the commonly encountered large leak around the endotracheal tube (ETT) would be interpreted as a large inspiration and given correspondingly a high level of inflation pressure, potentially leading to dangerously large V_T. To minimize the risk of overinflation, the peak pressure and V_T limits must be set appropriately by the clinician.

A clear understanding of the theory behind unloading by PAV is essential because the management of ventilatory support with PAV differs considerably from that of conventional ventilation. Clinicians must understand how to choose the setting of elastic or resistive gains and the possible effects these may have on the infant. When compliance changes, the gain must be adjusted accordingly to maintain the same degree of unloading. This is particularly important as compliance improves, to avoid excessive unloading that could result in large V_T and increase the potential risk for prolonged ventilator dependence due to poor respiratory muscle fitness. Because PAV amplifies only the spontaneous breathing effort, a backup rate of mandatory inflations is required in infants with apnea to prevent hypoventilation.

In summary, published data indicate that PAV is effective in the short term in maintaining comparable ventilation with lower peak ventilator pressure compared to conventional modalities. However, the safety and effectiveness of this approach for long-term support have not been fully established. Further studies are needed to determine if longer term use of this strategy can be advantageous in reducing the need for ventilatory support and improving respiratory outcome. The complexity of this modality and limited availability appear to have limited its penetration into clinical practice. As of this writing, this mode of support is unique to the Stephanie ventilator (F. Stephan GmbH Medizintechnik, Gackenbach, Germany), which is not available in the United States.

NEURALLY ADJUSTED VENTILATORY ASSIST

Neurally adjusted ventilatory assist (NAVA) is a novel modality in which the ventilator pressure is adjusted in proportion to the electrical activity of the diaphragm measured by esophageal electrodes mounted on a modified feeding tube. The ventilator pressure during NAVA is directly proportional to the diaphragmatic activity with a proportionality factor or gain set by the clinician (in units of pressure per microvolt of electrical activity), known as the "NAVA level." When the ventilator pressure is increased simultaneously with and proportionally to the rise in the diaphragm's electrical activity, NAVA can enhance the diaphragm's ability to generate a larger V_T or maintain a similar V_T with less inspiratory effort on the part of the infant. The increase in the ventilator pressure in proportion to the magnitude of the diaphragmatic activity is illustrated in Figure 21-3.

Studies in premature infants have shown that NAVA is effective in synchronizing the positive pressure with the infant's spontaneous inspiration. These studies demonstrated that NAVA maintained similar or better ventilation and gas exchange with lower airway pressures compared to modalities of pressure-controlled ventilation.[36-39] However, the effects of NAVA on breathing effort and ventilatory support were relative to the specific settings of pressure or volume used in the conventional

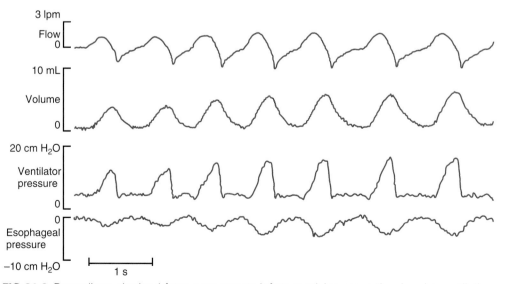

FIG 21-2 Recordings obtained from a premature infant receiving proportional assist ventilation. The increase in positive pressure is proportional to the spontaneous inspiratory effort of the infant measured by esophageal manometry. The increase in inspiratory effort and positive pressure results in a larger tidal volume.

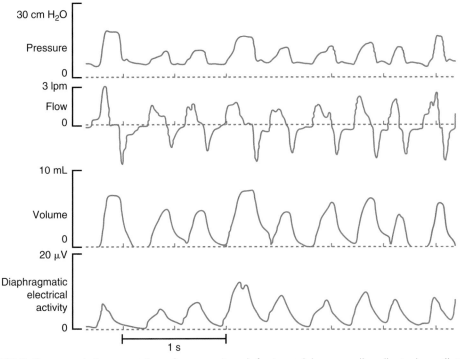

FIG 21-3 Representative recording of a premature infant receiving neurally adjusted ventilatory assist. The increase in the ventilator pressure above positive end-expiratory pressure is proportional to the amplitude of the electrical activity of the diaphragm.

modality used for comparison. NAVA reduced diaphragmatic activity compared to modalities of pressure-controlled ventilation and provided similar V_T with smaller peak pressures.[37,38] In contrast, the activity of the diaphragm was higher during NAVA in comparison to volume-targeted ventilation, but peak airway pressure and V_T were smaller.[39]

Management of the ventilatory support during NAVA differs substantially from conventional modalities. In NAVA the support is adjusted by setting the NAVA gain, but there are no normative or reference values for diaphragmatic activity in preterm infants. Moreover, the electrical activity of the diaphragm cannot be assessed as an absolute value or normalized per body weight, unlike other ventilatory parameters, for example, V_T, to compare among infants or within the same infant over time. Although it is claimed to be safe, there are important aspects regarding the management of NAVA that remain to be explored. Little has been reported on the parameters used to set the NAVA gain and on the possible effects of different NAVA gains in premature infants.[40] Perhaps most important, this technique also assumes a mature respiratory control center, an assumption that is clearly not valid in premature infants, whose respiratory effort is typically irregular and highly variable, with frequent brief pauses interspersed with spurts of vigorous breathing activity. The positive feedback approach that NAVA employs has the potential to amplify this pattern of breathing and could result in the delivery of large V_Ts. Therefore, pressure and volume limits must be set at appropriate levels by the clinician. A backup mechanical support is needed to deal with periods of apnea common in preterm infants.

NAVA is a promising modality of respiratory support, but its impact on short- and long-term respiratory outcomes in premature infants needs to be explored further. As of this writing, this modality is available only on the Maquet Servo ventilator.

Airway Pressure Release Ventilation

Airway pressure release ventilation (APRV) is a modality used primarily in adults with acute respiratory failure as an alternative method to improve oxygenation.[41] APRV is a modality whereby a continuous high positive pressure is applied at the airway with an intermittent release phase. In APRV the higher level positive pressure (P_{high}) is used to maintain lung volume and alveolar recruitment, and the brief release phase is expected to produce some ventilation. However, the bulk of minute ventilation must come from spontaneous respiratory effort of the patient during the application of P_{high}. This alternating pattern of low and high pressure can be thought of as extreme inverse ratio ventilation. It also bears some similarity to the various forms of bilevel continuous positive airway pressure (BiPAP), because of its reliance on spontaneous breathing activity. APRV is usually used as a rescue technique, and unlike BiPAP, the upper pressure level P_{high} is maintained for the majority of the respiratory cycle (T_{high}). The pressure to which the lungs are released is called P_{low}, and the release time is called T_{low}. The technique has primarily been used in adult patients with acute lung injury, in whom there may be some short-term benefits in terms of oxygenation. No clear survival advantage or reduction in complications has been demonstrated. There is insufficient evidence to assess the utility of this technique in newborn infants, with only a handful of case reports available and no controlled trials.

Targeted Minute Ventilation

Standard modes of mechanical ventilation provide a relatively constant level of ventilatory support determined by the peak inflation pressure and ventilator rate. The level of support set by the clinician is adequate in most instances, but in infants who have fluctuations in ventilation due to a weak respiratory pump, immature respiratory drive, or unstable respiratory

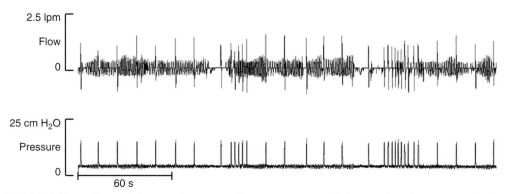

FIG 21-4 Recordings of flow and pressure from a premature infant undergoing targeted minute ventilation. The ventilator rate is automatically reduced during periods of consistent spontaneous breathing (*darker areas* in flow waveform), and it is increased when spontaneous breathing decreases. (From Ref. 42.)

mechanics, the ventilatory support often exceeds the infant's needs, whereas at other times it may be insufficient.

Targeted minute ventilation is based on automatic adjustments to the mandatory rate to maintain minute ventilation above a minimal level. When spontaneous breathing is enough to maintain minute ventilation above the set level, the ventilator rate is automatically reduced or vice versa in the opposite situation. To achieve this goal, the ventilator rate is continually adjusted in inverse proportion to the difference between the measured exhaled minute ventilation and the target level set by the clinician. The ventilator rate is kept between an upper and a lower limit also set by the clinician (Figure 21-4).

The rationale for targeted minute ventilation is that the automatic adjustments to the ventilator rate will maintain a more stable ventilation and gas exchange and reduce the possibility of excessive ventilatory support.

In preterm infants recovering from RDS, targeted minute ventilation achieved a 50% reduction in the synchronized intermittent mandatory ventilation (SIMV) rate without affecting gas exchange compared to conventional SIMV.[42] This study showed that although premature infants can sustain their ventilation for significant periods of time, they frequently have periods when they need much higher ventilator rates. In a subgroup of infants with frequent spontaneous episodes of hypoxemia, targeted minute ventilation attenuated the hypoxemia episodes compared to SIMV. This is in agreement with the findings of a study with an experimental animal model of induced episodes of hypoxemia.[43] In this study, combined adjustments of ventilator rate and peak inflation pressure (PIP) to keep minute ventilation and V_T targets were more effective in reducing hypoxemia than a constant ventilator rate and PIP during conventional SIMV. Simultaneous automatic adjustments of ventilator rate and PIP were even more efficacious in reducing the severity of the hypoxemia episodes. It should be noted that this technique is applicable to the SIMV mode and has been compared only to SIMV. It is not known whether this approach is superior to other modes of synchronized ventilation, such as assist/control and pressure support ventilation as implemented on neonatal ventilators (modes that assist every spontaneous breath), or SIMV with pressure support.

Mandatory Minute Ventilation

Mandatory minute ventilation (MMV) is a ventilatory modality used in the adult that has been adapted for neonates. In MMV

the minute ventilation target is maintained by the product of a constant ventilator rate of volume-targeted mandatory inflations. When minute ventilation exceeds the target level the mandatory inflations stop. MMV is generally used in combination with pressure support to assist every spontaneous breath. In late preterm infants without lung disease, MMV achieved a reduction in the mandatory rate and mean airway pressure compared to SIMV without alterations in gas exchange.[44]

Apnea Backup Ventilation

Apnea backup ventilation is a modality available in most neonatal ventilators. Spontaneous breaths are usually assisted by pressure support, but, in the presence of apnea, the ventilator initiates a preset mandatory rate of mechanical inflations. Although it is available in most neonatal ventilators, its benefits or disadvantages have not been evaluated.

The above modalities can be used only to target a minimum level of minute ventilation or respiratory rate because the ventilator does not prevent increases in spontaneous ventilation or breathing frequency above the target. However, they can inhibit the spontaneous respiratory drive if the set target for ventilation is excessive, resulting in hypocarbia.

Adaptive Backup Ventilation

Adaptive backup ventilation is a modality whereby a mandatory rate is provided during periods of apnea or during episodes of hypoxemia detected by pulse oximetry. In preterm infants recovering from RDS, this modality attenuated the frequency and severity of episodes of hypoxemia compared to the backup mandatory rate for apnea alone.[45]

The results of short-term studies evaluating various modalities of targeted minute ventilation showed that these modalities can better match the mechanical support to the varying ventilatory needs of premature infants. While these findings are promising, the benefits and possible shortcomings of these modalities need to be assessed in longer term clinical trials.

Adaptive Support Ventilation

Adaptive support ventilation (ASV) is an automatic modality of ventilation used in pediatric and adult patients.[46] ASV provides a combination of adjustments to respiratory rate and V_T. For this, the ASV algorithm determines the respiratory rate based on the patient's dead space volume, desired minute ventilation, and respiratory time constant. V_T is calculated by

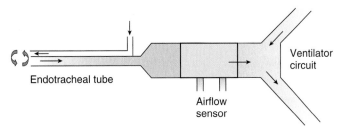

FIG 21-5 Schematic representation of the continuous tracheal gas insufflation concept. A continuous stream of gas is delivered to the distal end of the endotracheal tube (ETT) via capillaries built into the wall of the tube. This produces gas mixing at the distal end, and exhaled gas is washed out through the ETT into the ventilator circuit.

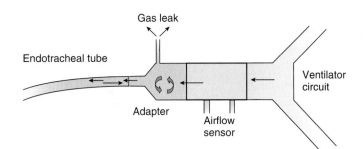

FIG 21-6 Schematic representation of the technique to wash out the instrumental dead space. A continuous gas leakage at the ETT adapter clears the flow sensor of exhaled gases, reducing rebreathing.

dividing minute ventilation by the respiratory rate. The clinician can adjust the target minute ventilation depending on the patient's condition. Thereafter, ASV adjusts the ventilator peak pressure to maintain the target V_T. The set respiratory rate, V_T, and respiratory mechanics are reassessed on a breath-to-breath basis. In periods during which the spontaneous breathing rate decreases, mandatory inflations are provided to maintain the desired rate.

By adapting the respiratory rate depending on the dead space, respiratory mechanics, and consistency of the respiratory drive, ASV aims to maintain adequate minute ventilation and facilitate weaning. ASV represents a novel and sophisticated approach to the management of ventilatory support in pediatric and adult patients, but as of this writing there are no reports on its use in neonates.

Techniques to Reduce Dead Space

Premature infants have a relatively large anatomic dead space.[47] In ventilated premature infants the instrumental dead space, that is, flow sensors and ETTs, is also large in relation to the patient's size.[48,49] The dead space volume (V_D) reduces the efficacy of ventilation, and the reduced CO_2 elimination often results in the need for higher ventilator settings and delayed weaning.

Continuous Tracheal Gas Insufflation

Continuous tracheal gas insufflation (CTGI) is a technique in which a small flow of fresh gas is injected into the distal end of the ETT via small ducts built in the wall of the tube. This supplies fresh gas during inspiration and produces a washout of the ETT during the expiratory phase. Figure 21-5 shows a schematic of the CTGI concept. With CTGI, continuous monitoring of pressure is essential because an obstruction of the main lumen of the ETT can produce a sudden increase in airway pressure.

In premature infants CTGI was shown to be effective in reducing $PaCO_2$ at constant ventilator settings or in keeping $PaCO_2$ unchanged with lower ventilator settings.[50] In a randomized clinical trial, the use of CTGI resulted in faster weaning from mechanical ventilation.[51]

Washout of the Flow Sensor

Continuous washout of the flow sensor is a technique designed to reduce the dead space added by flow sensors used to monitor V_T and synchronize the ventilator with the infant. Although small, flow sensors can increase the V_D/V_T ratio and impair CO_2

elimination in the smaller infants.[48,49] A technique consisting of a small tube inserted into the wall of the ETT adapter was developed to produce a constant outflow of gas and clear the sensor of exhaled CO_2. Figure 21-6 shows a schematic of this technique. Use of this technique in small premature infants reduced $PaCO_2$ and led to a reduction in spontaneous minute ventilation while ventilator settings were kept constant.[52] In another study, $PaCO_2$ and spontaneous ventilation remained unchanged while using this technique during an acute reduction in ventilator rate.[53]

Split-Flow Ventilation

A technique called split-flow ventilation, consisting of a side stream of fresh gas at the ETT adapter, was also shown to be effective in reducing $PaCO_2$ with a lower minute ventilation in premature infants.[54,55]

While appealing on theoretical grounds, the various techniques of dead space reduction have not found their way into clinical practice because they interfere with the ability to accurately measure V_T, adversely affect trigger function and sensitivity, or require specialized equipment, which may not be commercially available. Although the effect of added instrumental dead space is not negligible, it appears to be less of a problem than conventional respiratory physiology suggests. Nassabeh-Montazami et al. demonstrated that small preterm infants are often effectively ventilated with V_T that is near or even below anatomic and instrumental dead space, although this may require higher spontaneous or ventilator respiratory rates.[56] These observations were confirmed by a bench study that demonstrated the ability of V_T below V_D to achieve effective alveolar ventilation, presumably because fresh gas is able to penetrate through dead space gas, rather than pushing it in front of it when a rapid flow of gas passes through narrow ETTs.[57]

SUMMARY

Many of the novel respiratory support techniques discussed in this chapter are promising and address some of the limitations in conventional mechanical ventilation or oxygen administration. Although most of these novel techniques are available or may become available for clinical use in the near future, additional evidence for their safety and benefits in premature infants is necessary before they gain wider clinical application.

REFERENCES

A complete reference list is available at https://expertconsult.inkling.com/.

22

High-Frequency Ventilation

Mark C. Mammel, MD, and Sherry E. Courtney, MD, MS

First described in the 1970s, high-frequency ventilation (HFV) is a form of mechanical ventilation that uses small tidal volumes, sometimes less than anatomic dead space, and very rapid ventilator rates (2 to 20 Hz or 120 to 1200 cycles/min). Potential advantages of this technique over conventional mechanical ventilation (CMV) include the use of lower peak airway pressures, the ability to adequately and independently manage oxygenation and ventilation while using very small tidal volumes, and the preservation of normal lung architecture even when using high mean airway pressures.[1-6] HFV's ability to sufficiently oxygenate and ventilate the fragile preterm lung with peak airway pressures that are lower than those used with CMV, as well as its use for alveolar recruitment and distribution of medications such as inhaled nitric oxide (iNO), makes HFV a crucial constituent of neonatal respiratory therapy. In this chapter, current HFV techniques and technology are described, and their application in the newborn with pulmonary dysfunction is discussed.

Currently, there are three general types of HFV: high-frequency jet ventilation (HFJV), which is produced by ventilators that deliver a high-velocity jet of gas directly into the airway and have passive exhalation; high-frequency oscillatory ventilation (HFOV), which is produced by a device that moves air back and forth at the airway opening and produces limited bulk gas flow; and high-frequency flow interruption (HFFI), which generates pulses of fresh gas and also uses passive exhalation. HFV appears to enhance both the distribution and the diffusion of respiratory gases. Both shift the transition point between convective and diffusive gas transport progressively in a cephalad direction from the acinus into the larger airways. The net effect of this shift is efficient CO_2 elimination relatively independent of mean lung volume.[7]

Conventional pulmonary physiology tells us that the amount of gas available for gas exchange, the alveolar tidal volume (V_A), is the product of the tidal volume (V_T) delivered into the airway minus anatomic dead space (V_D): $V_A = V_T - V_D$. If this relationship is true, V_Ts near anatomic V_D should produce little if any alveolar ventilation. In an attempt to clarify the mechanisms of HFV gas exchange at V_T less than anatomic V_D, Chang[8] demonstrated that multiple modes of gas transport occur, including bulk convection, high-frequency "pendelluft," convective dispersion, Taylor-type dispersion, and molecular diffusion. Whatever the HFV system, the presumed linear relationship between ventilator rate and CO_2 elimination is no longer valid with this mode of ventilation. In fact, during HFOV, CO_2 elimination improves with decreasing ventilator frequency as long as the inspiratory-to-expiratory time ratio (I:E) is held constant. This is because a reduction in frequency produces increased V_T and

minute volume out of proportion to the change, whereas an increased frequency does the opposite. The effects are magnified because minute ventilation is roughly equal to $f \times V_T^2$. The same could be true with HFJV, but with that device the inspiratory time is normally kept at the shortest value, and thus the I:E ratio decreases as frequency goes down and therefore the V_T remains the same.

Although paradoxical at first blush, this inverse relationship reflects the impact of an increasing inspiratory time as frequency is lowered, which results in higher delivered gas volumes. In 1980, Slutsky et al.[9] reported a review of possible gas transport mechanisms during HFV. They suggested that CO_2 elimination during HFV varies according to the product of frequency^a and V_T^b, with b greater than 1 and a less than 1. Since then, many other theoretical and practical reviews have been published, and we know that during HFV carbon dioxide removal is proportional to $f^a \times V_T^b$, where $a < 1$ and $b > 1$. In 2002, Slutsky and Drazen concisely summarized these gas exchange mechanisms (Fig. 22-1).[10] The theoretical mechanisms of gas exchange during HFV are beyond the scope of this clinical chapter. For those interested, there are a number of excellent review articles, as well as a review of physiologic principles in Chapter 2.[11-16]

TYPES OF HIGH-FREQUENCY VENTILATORS

As of this writing, only a small number of HFV devices are approved by the U.S. Food and Drug Administration (FDA) for clinical use. Even though the number of high-frequency ventilators is small, the classification or taxonomy of these ventilators is confusing and at times inconsistent. Froese and Bryan[14] classified HFV into three categories based on the character of exhalation: active, passive, and hybrid. In this chapter we use the more traditional, clinical classification of HFFI, HFJV, and HFOV. Table 22-1 lists all the approved HFV devices in the United States and Canada and their classification. A number of other HFV devices have been studied and are currently being used throughout the world. This chapter focuses primarily on those machines currently approved for clinical use in the United States and Canada.

Determinants of Gas Transport during Mechanical Ventilation

During conventional inflation, the time required for gas to travel from one end of the airway to the other depends on a ventilator's peak inflation pressure (PIP), inspiratory gas flow, and pressure–flow waveforms (compliance of the respiratory system and resistance of the airways). During expiration, the time required for lung emptying depends mainly on lung and chest wall elastic recoil, expiratory resistance, and the ventilator's set positive end-expiratory pressure (PEEP). If inspirations or expirations are long enough, proximal and distal airway pressures equilibrate and gas flow stops. Conditions are static at end inspiration and end expiration. The volume of gas delivered into or out of the lung is determined by the pressure change in the lung and lung compliance ($\Delta V = \Delta P \times CL$). As ventilator rates increase, inspiratory and expiratory times decrease. Eventually, there is inadequate time for proximal and distal airway pressures to equilibrate. Gas flow is continuous. Conditions are no longer static. They are dynamic. The volume of gas delivered into or out of the lung becomes a function of flow rate and time.[17,18]

The key timing factors of gas transport depend upon lung compliance and airway resistance. The product of lung compliance and airway resistance, measured in seconds, is called its *time constant* (see Chapter 2). Time constants describe the time it takes for proximal and terminal airway pressures to equilibrate. After one time constant, there is 63% equilibration; after two, 84.5%; after three, 95%. After five time constants, there is 99% pressure equilibration between the proximal and the terminal airways.[18] When inspiratory time is shortened beyond three time constants, a pressure gradient develops between the proximal and the terminal airways. As inspiratory time becomes shorter, this pressure gradient progressively increases. Because the V_T delivered to the terminal airways is also a function of this gradient, it too becomes a function of inspiratory time. As the pressure gradient between the proximal and the terminal airways increases, the volume of gas delivered into the terminal airways decreases in a predictable way.

Time constants apply equally to inspiration and expiration. Because airway resistance is always greater during expiration,

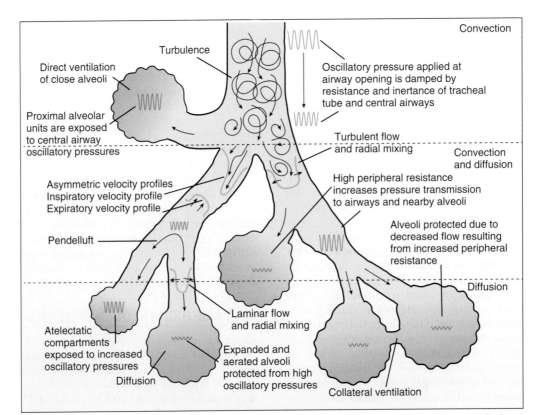

FIG 22-1 Gas transport mechanisms and pressure damping during high-frequency ventilation. Major gas transport mechanisms include convective flow, convection and diffusion, diffusive flow, pendelluft, laminar flow with Taylor dispersion, turbulent flow, cardiogenic mixing, and perialveolar collateral ventilation. (From Slutsky and Drazen. *N Engl J Med*. 2002;347:630.)

TABLE 22-1   Classification and Key Characteristics of High-Frequency Ventilators

Ventilator	HFV Type	CV + HFV	Volume Measurement	Exhalation
SensorMedics 3100A	Diaphragm oscillator	No	No	Active
Dräger V500, VN500	Diaphragm oscillator	Yes	Yes	Active
Fabian HFO	Diaphragm oscillator	Yes	Yes	Active
Leoni Plus	Diaphragm oscillator	Yes	Yes	Active
SLE5000	Reverse jet oscillator	Yes	Yes	Active
VDR-4/Bronchotron	Flow interrupter	Yes	No	Passive
Bunnell Life Pulse	Jet pulse	No	No	Passive

HFV, High-frequency ventilation; *CV*, conventional ventilation.

expiratory time constants are always longer. Experimental evidence suggests that this difference between inspiratory and expiratory resistances increases as ventilator rates increase.[19] Expiratory times less than three time constants do not allow adequate lung emptying and ultimately result in increasing functional residual capacity levels and gas trapping. Because of these factors, inadequate gas delivery during inflation and incomplete lung emptying during expiration limit the effectiveness of gas exchange when using high rates during conventional ventilation (high-frequency positive pressure ventilation, HFPPV).

One can assess for these limiting factors, because today it is relatively easy to estimate respiratory mechanics and the impact of ventilator manipulation at the bedside.[20] Most conventional neonatal ventilators now display measurements of V_T, minute ventilation, airway pressures, and respiratory cycle timing, as well as basic measurements of respiratory mechanics. The simultaneous tracings of proximal airway pressures, gas flows, and volume delivery show whether time constants are violated and create a potential environment for suboptimal gas exchange and/or gas trapping. For example, when gas flow patterns during inflation reach a plateau, proximal and distal airway equilibration has occurred, and prolonging the inspiratory time beyond this point serves only to increase airway pressures. Conversely, decreasing inspiratory time below this point decreases delivered V_T and probably would lead to suboptimal ventilation. Expiratory flow patterns provide similar information regarding lung emptying and gas trapping.

High-Frequency Jet Ventilators

High-frequency jet ventilators deliver short pulses of pressurized gas directly into the upper airway through a narrow-bore cannula or jet injector. High-frequency jet ventilators are capable of maintaining ventilation over wide ranges of patient sizes and lung compliances. These systems have negligible compressible volumes. The only jet device approved for neonatal use in the United States and Canada is the Bunnell jet ventilator; it operates at rates from 240 to 600 cycles/min (4 to 10 Hz), with the most common rates, 240 to 420 cycles/min, being less than those typically used in HFOV. Exhalation during HFJV is a result of passive lung recoil. An open ventilator–patient circuit is essential, and HFJV is used in combination with a CMV to provide PEEP and occasional sigh breaths if needed. V_Ts are difficult to measure but appear to be equal to or slightly greater than anatomic V_D.[21]

In addition to V_Ts delivered through the jet injector, gases surrounding the injector are pulled or entrained into the airway with each jet pulse. The high-flow jet pulse produces a Venturi effect that creates an area of negative pressure at its periphery, entraining ambient gases into the airway. Because of high gas velocities, Venturi effects, and pressure gradients within the delivery system, pressure monitoring is difficult with HFJV. Airway pressures must be measured far enough downstream from the jet injector to minimize Venturi effects. Pressures measured upstream from the jet injector are meaningless unless such effects have been accounted for. Jet ventilation using the Bunnell device is administered via a triple-lumen endotracheal tube adapter. This adapter houses the jet injector port and the pressure monitoring port.

Jet ventilators have been tested extensively in laboratory animals and have been used clinically in adults and neonates for over 30 years.[22-37] The Bunnell Life Pulse jet ventilator (Bunnell, Inc., Salt Lake City, Utah) was designed specifically for infants (Fig. 22-2). Using the triple-lumen endotracheal tube adapter, this device delivers its jet pulse into the endotracheal tube through the adapter's injector port and then servo controls the background pressure, or driving pressure, of the jet pulse to maintain a constant user preset pressure within the endotracheal tube. This device is approved for clinical use in neonates and infants. With HFJV, CO_2 removal can be achieved at lower peak and mean airway pressures than with either HFPPV or HFOV.[3,25,26,36] Although initially primarily used to treat air leak, HFJV is also effective in homogeneous lung disorders such as respiratory distress syndrome (RDS), as a randomized multicenter trial has demonstrated a beneficial pulmonary effect (lower rates of chronic lung disease) with the use of early HFJV over CMV in RDS.[34]

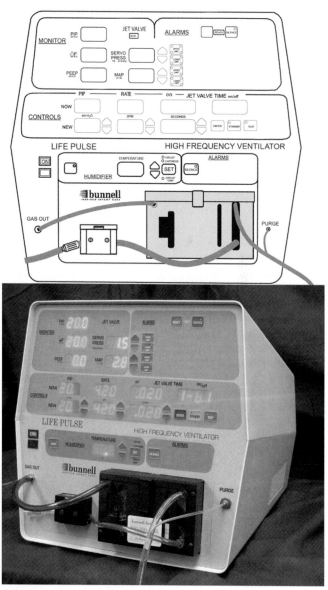

FIG 22-2 The Bunnell Life Pulse jet ventilator. This microprocessor-controlled pressure-limited time-cycled ventilator servo controls delivered airway pressure as measured at the endotracheal tube tip. Frequency range is from 240 to 660 cycles/min. Pressure range is from 8 to 50 cm H_2O. Inspiratory time is adjustable from 0.02 to 0.034 seconds.

HFJV appears to be uniquely effective in nonhomogeneous lung disorders in which CO_2 elimination is the major problem, such as air-leak syndromes (i.e., pulmonary interstitial emphysema [PIE]),[31] or in diseases in which atelectasis and overdistention occur simultaneously. In the former, the long expiratory time and the high-flow jet pulse contribute to the resolution of air leak. In the latter, the ability to provide a low-rate (2 to 6 inflations/min) sigh assists with opening atelectatic areas. It is also safe and effective when used in neonatal transport and can be used with simultaneous delivery of iNO.[37]

In Europe the Monsoon jet ventilator (Acutronic Medical Systems AG, Hirzel, Switzerland) has been used primarily for ear, nose and throat (ENT) surgery and thoracic surgery and has seen limited applications in intensive care for patients with severe respiratory failure and air-leak complications. The device has an integrated humidification and heating system, making it potentially suitable for extended use. It operates at frequencies of 0.2 to 10 Hz, inspiratory time of 20% to 70%, PEEP 10 to 40. No systematic evaluation of safety and effectiveness is available.

High-Frequency Oscillators

High-frequency oscillators (HFOs) are a type of HFV operating at frequencies ranging from 180 to 1200 cycles/min (3 to 20 Hz) to move small volumes of gas in and out of the lungs.[13,38] During HFOV, inspiration and expiration are both active (proximal airway pressures are negative during expiration). In the CareFusion (formerly SensorMedics) 3100A (CareFusion, San Diego, Calif.) a continuous flow of fresh gas flows past the electromagnetically operated piston, generating the oscillations. This bias gas flow is the system's only source of fresh gas. A controlled-leak or low-pass filter allows gas to exit the system (Fig. 22-3).[38] The amplitude of the pressure oscillations within the airway determines the V_Ts that are delivered to the lungs around a constant mean airway pressure. This allows avoidance of high peak airway pressures for ventilation as well as maintenance of lung recruitment by avoidance of low end-expiratory pressures. Though piston pumps or vibrating diaphragms are often used to provide HFOV, newer HFOV devices available in Canada and Europe have a series of Venturi valves that provide effective active expiration and can also measure and control V_T.

As with HFJV, pressure monitoring in HFOV is a problem. During HFOV, airway pressures usually are measured either at the proximal end of the endotracheal tube or within the ventilator itself. Many practitioners question the clinical relevance of such measurements, as they are some distance away from the patient; the relationship of intrapulmonary pressures measured during HFOV to those measured during CMV is difficult to assess accurately. Depending upon the size and resonant frequency of the lung, alveolar pressures can be the same, lower, or even higher than those measured in the trachea.[38-41]

HFOs have been tested extensively in animals and in humans.[1,2,4,38-61] Today the neonatal HFO used in the United States is the CareFusion (formerly SensorMedics) 3100A oscillator (CareFusion, San Diego, Calif.). This ventilator has been approved for clinical use in neonates and does not require a tandem conventional ventilator. This device produces its oscillations via an electromagnetically controlled piston/diaphragm. Frequency (3 to 15 Hz or 180 to 900 cycles/min), percentage inspiratory time, and volume displacement can be adjusted, as well as resistance at the end of the bias flow circuit (Fig. 22-4). Variations in bias flow rate and the patient circuit outflow resistor control mean airway pressures. Ventilation (CO_2 elimination) is proportional to the product of frequency and the square of the V_T ($f \times V_T^2$), and thus a decrease in frequency or increase in V_T by way of an increase in set amplitude should cause increased carbon dioxide removal. The 3100B is a more powerful oscillator that can be used in children and adults. There are many other HFOs that are not currently used in the United States. These include the SLE 5000 (SLE UK Ltd.), the Fabian (Acutronic Medical Systems), the Leoni Plus (Heinen & Lowenstein), the Stephanie and the Sophie (Stephan), the VN500 (Dräger), and the BabyLog 8000+ (Dräger). The Fabian (Fig. 22-5), Leoni Plus (Fig. 22-6), and Dräger devices (Fig. 22-7) are approved for use in Canada. A variety of mechanisms provide HFOV with these ventilators, but they are all true oscillators based on the waveform they generate.

High-Frequency Flow Interrupters

The term *flow interrupter* originally was used to describe a group of ventilators that were neither true oscillators nor true jets. Some had jet-type injectors but delivered their bursts of gas not directly into the airway but into the ventilator circuit some distance back from the trachea and endotracheal tube. For this reason, these machines also were called *setback jets*.

The Infant Star HFV (Nellcor Puritan Bennett, Pleasanton, Calif.), which is no longer in production, was once the most widely used flow interrupter. This ventilator had a set of microprocessor-controlled pneumatic valves that altered inspiratory flow to achieve preset PIPs. Although there was a Venturi system on the exhalation valve to facilitate

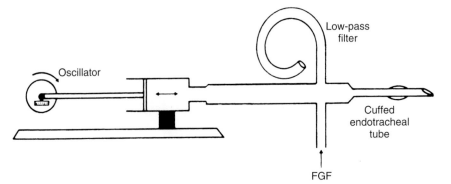

FIG 22-3 High-frequency oscillator. Fresh gases enter the system proximal to the endotracheal tube (FGF). Excess gas and mixed expired gases exit via a low-pass filter. *FGF,* fresh gas flow. (From Thompson WK, et al. *J Appl Physiol.* 1982;52:543.)

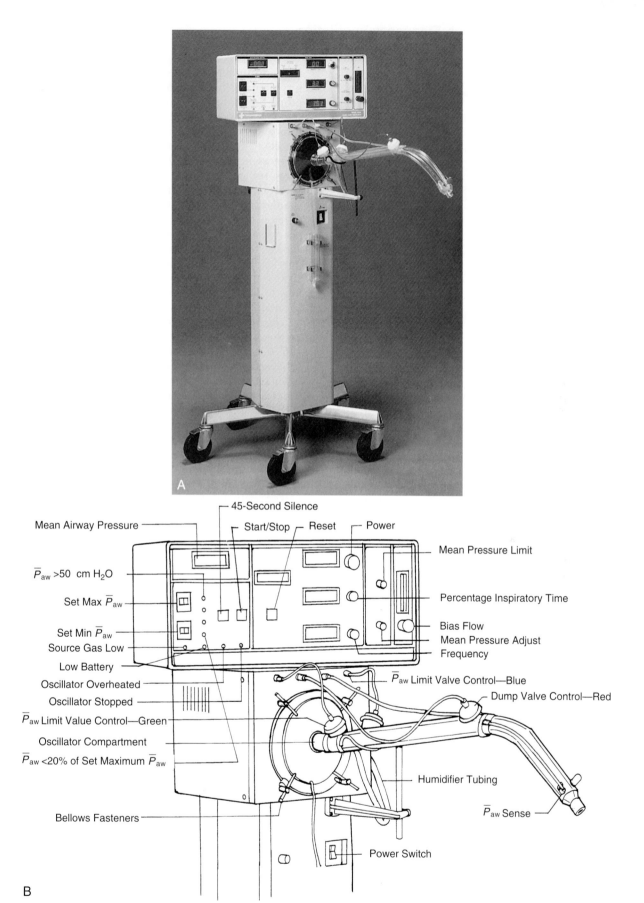

FIG 22-4 A. The SensorMedics 3100A high-frequency oscillator. This electronically controlled and powered ventilator uses a sealed piston with adjustable volume displacement to generate oscillations into the airway. Frequency is adjustable from 180 to 900 cycles/min (3 to 15 Hz). Mean airway pressure can be set between 3 and 45 cm H_2O; oscillatory pressure is adjustable to >90 cm H_2O. Inspiratory time can be set from 30% to 50% of the total cycle. **B.** A schematic representation with labels for key components.

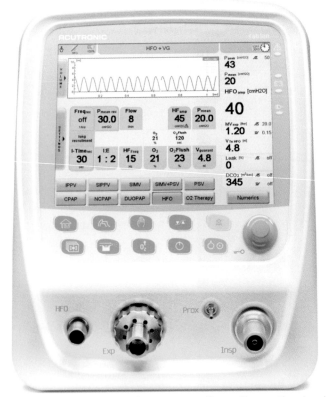

FIG 22-5 The Fabian high-frequency oscillator. Conventional and high-frequency ventilation is available with this device, which is designed for use in patients from 300 g to 30 kg. Frequency is adjustable from 300 to 1200 cycles/min (5 to 20 Hz). Amplitude is set between 5 and 100 cm H_2O, and it uses automatic leak compensation with volume targeting. Mean airway pressure is adjustable between 0 and 40 cm H_2O. Measured and derived respiratory parameters are displayed.

expiration and prevent inadvertent PEEP, exhalation was still largely passive, and air trapping with air leak appeared to be a problem.

Thome and colleagues[62] compared high-frequency flow interrupter (HFFI) ventilation using the Infant Star HFV system to rapid-rate conventional ventilation with several different neonatal ventilators. The outcomes showed no benefit of HFFI ventilation, and babies treated with the Infant Star HFFI had significantly more air leaks. In the "Sy-Fi" study, Craft and colleagues[63] again compared the Infant Star system to CMV in extremely low birth-weight infants and found no difference in air leaks or other pulmonary outcomes with a nonsignificant trend to more air leak with the Infant Star (36% vs 25%).

In recent years, HFFI ventilation has experienced a modest resurgence in the form of several devices from the company of Forrest Bird, the inventor of the first neonatal ventilator, the BabyBird® (Percussionaire Corp., Sagle, Idaho). The Bronchotron® is a pneumatically driven flow interrupter/percussive ventilator increasingly used during transport.[64]

The Bronchotron® is attractive as a transport ventilator because of its light weight, ability to function as both conventional and high-frequency ventilator, and relatively low gas consumption. The ventilator's internal pneumatic timer cycles high-pressure gas flow at a frequency ranging from 3 to 10 Hz.

Rate and amplitude are continuously adjustable. The inspiratory time is determined by the frequency and the mechanical properties of the lungs. The high-frequency gas pulses enter a sliding piston mechanism called a Phasitron® through a Venturi cavity in its central axis. The Phasitron® creates pulses of gas flow by the rapid movement of a spring mechanism that balances inspiratory and expiratory pressures within preset pressures for PEEP or $\overline{P}_{aw}$, acting as both an inspiratory and an expiratory valve. In the inspiratory phase, the pulse of gas is augmented by entrained gas proportional to the pressure difference before and after the Venturi. During expiration, the piston springs back, opening an exhalation port, and gas is allowed to exit the patient through an adjustable resistor that provides PEEP and regulates mean airway pressure. The mean airway pressure, frequency, and flow (which adjusts the gas flow to the Phasitron® and controls the pulse amplitude) are continuously adjustable.

The main limitation of the device is the lack of real values for the ventilator variables—all dials are marked with values of 1 to 10, but these numbers do not readily translate to values to which a clinician can relate. Adjustments must be made based solely on clinical observation of chest movement and patient response. Frequency is displayed as cycles/min (not Hz), and mean airway pressure can be measured intermittently by flipping a toggle switch and changing the phasic pressure display to an integrated mean. The phasic pressure displayed by the rapidly oscillating needle of a mechanical gauge is difficult to read. The other major concern is a lack of alarms or other safety features.

The safety and efficacy of the Bronchotron® are not well documented; the device was "grandfathered" by the FDA, meaning that it was approved based on its "substantial equivalence" to a device in existence prior to the effective date of the law (1979). In a preclinical study in saline-lavaged newborn piglets the Bronchotron® and the 3100A oscillator achieved similar gas exchange when the devices were adjusted to deliver identical V_T at the same mean airway pressure and frequency, but a higher pressure amplitude was needed with the Bronchotron®.

The VDR-4® (Percussionaire Corp., Sagle, Idaho) is a time-cycled, pressure-controlled, pneumatically driven high-frequency percussive ventilator similar to the Bronchotron® but more complex and designed for hospital use. The device delivers gas from a pressurized source through a pneumatic timing cartridge system. The source gas is interrupted to produce a pulsatile flow, which enters the breathing circuit via the Phasitron® as with its sister device. Warmed, humidified gas is entrained to augment V_T. V_T delivery is determined by flow velocity, inspiratory duration, and supplementary gas entrainment. The VDR-4® is composed of two subsystems: conventional and high frequency. The conventional component can deliver up to 70 inflations per minute with independent control of inflation time and pressure. The high-frequency component can deliver frequencies from 0.5 to 30 Hz, amplitudes from 0 to 100 cm H_2O, and inspiratory to expiratory time ratio from 1:1 to 1:5. A variety of conventional and high-frequency combinations can be used. Like the Bronchotron®, the VDR was approved by the FDA without requiring proof of safety and efficacy. The literature regarding the safety and efficacy of this device is limited to a few small studies in adult and pediatric patients and a single case series of six newborn infants.[65] There is also some interest in using this device to deliver HFV vial the nasal route.[66]

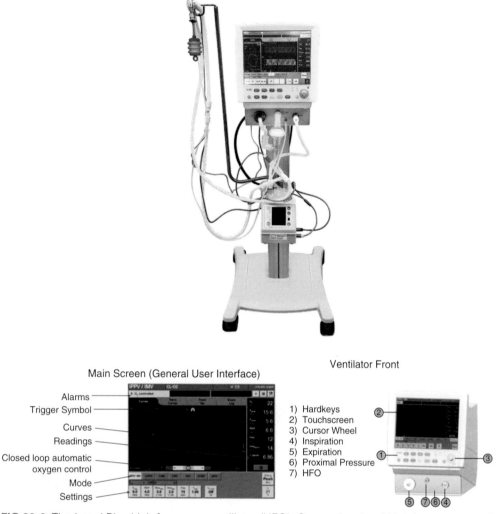

Main Screen (General User Interface)

Ventilator Front

Alarms
Trigger Symbol
Curves
Readings
Closed loop automatic
oxygen control
Mode
Settings

1) Hardkeys
2) Touchscreen
3) Cursor Wheel
4) Inspiration
5) Expiration
6) Proximal Pressure
7) HFO

FIG 22-6 The Leoni Plus high-frequency oscillator (HFO). Conventional and high-frequency ventilation is available with this device, which is designed for use in patients up to 30 kg. Frequency is adjustable from 300 to 1200 cycles/min (5 to 20 Hz). Amplitude is set between 0 and 80 cm H_2O, and it uses automatic leak compensation with tidal volume measurement and targeting. Mean airway pressure is adjustable between 0 and 30 cm H_2O. Measured and derived respiratory parameters are displayed.

Because all conventional pressure-preset neonatal ventilators will generate rates up to 150 inflations/min, theoretically all of them can be used to produce rapid-rate conventional ventilation, sometimes referred to as HFPPV. Use of a conventional ventilator at these rates is now mostly of historical interest. The term *HFPPV* most often refers to mechanical ventilators operating at rates between 60 and 150 inflations/min (1 to 2.5 Hz). Sjostrand[67] pioneered this technique in Sweden using specially designed ventilators with extremely low compressible volumes. He and his colleagues studied more than 2000 adults and children during surgery and 32 neonates with RDS.[68] He concluded that in most clinical situations, HFPPV provided adequate respiratory support. In 1980, Bland et al.[69] reported improved outcomes in 24 infants with RDS using conventional volume-preset infant ventilators operating at rates ranging from 60 to 110 inflations/min. In 1991, a multicenter randomized trial compared HFPPV using rates of 60 inflations/min to CMV using rates up to 40 inflations/min. The infants treated with HFPPV had fewer

pulmonary air leaks.[70] Few people today would consider a rate of 60 inflations/min in the neonate as HFV.

Though CMVs can operate at rates up to 150 inflations/min, few of these machines were designed with such frequencies in mind. In vitro and in vivo studies of conventional pressure-preset infant ventilators show that all have maximum operating frequencies beyond which their performance deteriorates and inadvertent PEEP becomes a problem.[71-75]

The first such in vitro study measured delivered tidal and minute volumes as ventilator rates increased progressively from 20 to 150 inflations/min.[71] All the machines tested had maximal effective rates beyond which minute ventilation decreased exponentially. For the compliance and resistance values studied, these maximum effective rates ranged from 75 to 100 inflations/min (Fig. 22-8, *A*). A subsequent animal study showed remarkably similar results. This study also noted that as CMV rates increased and minute ventilation decreased, functional residual capacities progressively increased.[72] Hird et al.[75] studied human neonates and

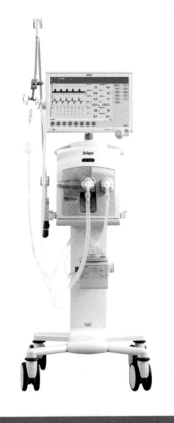

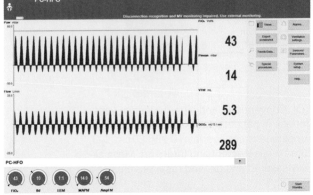

FIG 22-7 The Dräger VN500 neonatal ventilator. This ventilator provides both conventional and high-frequency ventilation using the same platform. Frequency is adjustable from 0 to 1200 breaths/min (0 to 20 Hz). Mean airway pressure ranges from 5 to 50 cm H$_2$O. Amplitude is adjustable from 5 to 90 cm H$_2$O. Tidal volumes are displayed, and a volume guarantee option is available with a range of tidal volume from 0.2 to 40 mL. Pressures, respiratory cycle timing, tidal and minute volumes, and basic respiratory system mechanics are measured or calculated during ventilation and displayed. Sigh inflations are available at a rate ranging from 1 to 30 and pressure of 6 to 80 cm H$_2$O.

confirmed such gas trapping at higher rates as well, in particular in paralyzed infants. Fontan et al.[73] studied rabbits and saw predictably reduced compliance and V$_T$ values at higher rates.

When in vitro studies of ventilator performance were repeated using currently available neonatal ventilators, performance was more consistent as rates increased, but marked intradevice variability was demonstrated at similar pressures

(Fig. 22-8, *B*).[17] These studies all suggest that CMVs cycling at the upper limits of their frequency range to produce HFPPV require higher, not lower, airway pressures to maintain adequate gas exchange. Thus, some other form of HFV is much more commonly employed today, but as of this writing, in the United States, this requires changing to a different device. In Europe and Canada, ventilators that switch from conventional ventilation (CV) to HFOV are easily available.

CLINICAL APPLICATIONS OF HIGH-FREQUENCY VENTILATION

Elective versus Rescue High-Frequency Ventilation

HFV has been studied in animal models for over 30 years. The majority of animal data supports the superiority of HFV over CMV, in terms of both short-term physiology and pressure exposure and in lung pathology over days to weeks. Animal studies suggest that HFV works at lower proximal airway pressures than CMV, reduces ventilator-induced lung injury and lung inflammatory markers, improves gas exchange in the face of air-leak syndromes, is synergistic with surfactant, and decreases oxygen exposure. Unfortunately, these findings have not been consistently reproduced in the human studies of HFV versus CMV, when looking at HFV either as an initial, elective mode of ventilation or as a rescue mode of ventilation when CMV has failed to provide adequate gas exchange.

As of this writing there have been 16 randomized controlled trials (RCTs) of elective use of HFV versus CMV for the treatment of neonates with respiratory insufficiency, primarily in babies with RDS of prematurity.[30,33,34,48,54-63,70,76] The studies include HFV in the forms of HFPPV, HFFI, HFJV, and HFOV. The majority of the studies (11 of 16) were unable to demonstrate any significant difference in pulmonary outcomes between babies treated with HFV versus CMV. The remainder of the studies demonstrated a small yet significant reduction in bronchopulmonary dysplasia (BPD) in the HFV-treated groups.[34,50,55,57,59] In 2009, the Cochrane database provided a review and meta-analysis of clinical trials of elective HFOV versus CMV in preterm infants with acute pulmonary dysfunction.[77] The review demonstrated no evidence of effect on mortality and no clear advantage to the preferential use of elective HFO over CMV as the initial ventilation strategy in premature babies with respiratory distress. An individual patient data meta-analysis confirmed these results.[78]

An "optimal lung volume" strategy with HFOV, piston oscillators, lack of lung-protective strategies in the CMV groups, early use of HFO (less than 6 hours), I:E of 1:2, and extubation to continuous positive airway pressure rather than a trial of CV were associated with the trials that demonstrated a reduction in chronic lung disease in the HFO groups. The Cochrane database also reviewed the elective use of HFJV versus CMV and from the three studies reviewed concluded that there may be a decreased risk of BPD in the elective HFJV groups.[79] However, the authors raised questions about these apparent positive findings because of significant heterogeneity among the studies and the fact that one study showed increased adverse neurologic outcomes in the HFJV group. This finding appears to be related to the significant hypocarbia seen in the HFJV group and was also apparent in a subgroup analysis of the larger multicenter trial.[34] The fact that two studies of HFV using the same device in a virtually identical population obtained very different results highlights the importance of using an appropriate ventilation strategy. Overall, grouped analysis of all randomized, controlled

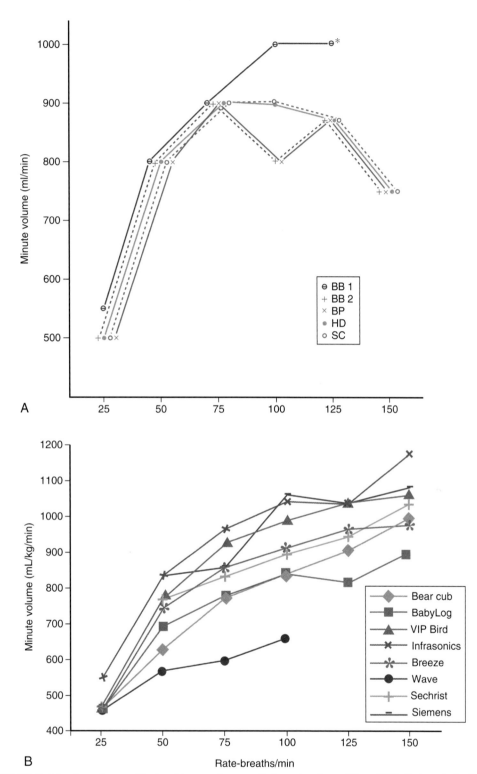

FIG 22-8 Minute volume effects of increasing ventilator rates from 25 to 150 inflations/min (horizontal axis). **A,** Ventilators examined: BB1, BabyBird 1; BB2, BabyBird 2; BP, Bourns BP200; HD, Healthdyne; SC, Sechrist. Ventilator settings: peak inspiratory pressure 25 cm H$_2$O; positive end-expiratory pressure 5 cm H$_2$O; inspiration to expiration ratio (I:E) = 1:2 (beyond 75 inflations/ min, BB1 minute volumes were measured at 1:1 I:E); flow 10 L/min. *(From Boros, et al. Pediatrics. 1984;74:487.)* **B,** Ventilators examined: Bourns Bear Cub, Dräger BabyLog 3000, VIP Bird, Infrasonics Infant Star, Newport Breeze, Newport Wave, Sechrist 100 V, and Siemens 300. Studies were performed using a lung simulator at fixed compliance and resistance values, peak pressures of 25 cm H$_2$O, end-expiratory pressure of 5 cm H$_2$O, and I:E of 1:2. *(From Mammel and Bing. Clinics in Chest Medicine. 1996;17:603.)*

studies to date would not support the selective use of early and elective HFV over CMV in premature babies with respiratory insufficiency. This is very likely due to the improved methods of CV in use today, including volume-targeted ventilation.

One of the early HFV versus CMV RCTs, the HIFI study, raised concerns, as the HFOV-treated group demonstrated increased incidence of intraventricular hemorrhage (IVH) and/or periventricular leukomalacia (PVL).[48] More alarming, the neurodevelopmental outcomes at 16 to 24 months postterm age were significantly worse in the HFO-treated group.[80] Two subsequent large, multicenter, randomized trials by Courtney et al.[57] and Johnson et al.[56] demonstrated no difference in the rates of IVH or PVL between the HFOV- and the CMV-treated groups nor did the individual patient meta-analysis by Cool et al.[78] Studies by Truffert et al.[81] and Marlow et al.[82] have now provided long-term neurodevelopmental follow-up at 2 years of age from their initial RCTs of HFOV versus CMV in preterm babies with RDS. Both studies concluded that elective use of HFOV does not portend any worsening of the long-term neurologic status. Truffert and colleagues state that early use of HFOV may in fact be associated with a better neuromotor outcome at 2 years of age. Zivanovic et al. found superior lung function at 11 to 14 years of age in the infants from the Johnson et al. trial.[83] Although valuable, more follow-up data are necessary before widespread generalizations can be made regarding predicted long-term outcomes.

So, if elective use of HFV has not demonstrated any clear advantage over CMV for RDS, what about the use of rescue HFV when CMV appears to be failing to provide adequate gas exchange? To date, there are four RCTs in premature and term infants assessing HFV as a rescue technique after failing CMV.[31,35,84,85] The data set is limited and includes two studies using HFJV and two studies using HFOV. In a first trial treating premature infants, the HIFO trial demonstrated improved gas exchange and lower rate of new air leak with HFOV. There was no effect on existing air leak and no difference in overall pulmonary outcomes and a marginally increased rate of severe IVH.[84] Keszler's trial, which specifically enrolled infants with PIE, showed improvement of PIE in the HFJV group versus those who remained on CMV.[31] In the two trials treating older preterm babies (more than 34 weeks), there was notable improvement in gas exchange and treatment success in the HFV groups; however, there was no significant difference in the incidence of BPD or death between those rescued with HFV and those who remained on CMV.[35,85] A meta-analysis of rescue HFV versus CMV in the Cochrane database demonstrates that there is no long-term benefit conferred on the patient by using rescue HFOV or HFJV over continued CMV.[86-88] Whether lumping results from HFV studies using different modes of HFV in different populations together is appropriate is a debatable point. The HFJV study did, in fact, demonstrate improved survival attributable to HFJV when the effect of crossover was taken into account.[31] Of note, most of these HFV rescue trials were performed when the administration of exogenous surfactant and maternal antenatal steroids were not routine standard of care. More importantly, there have been no long-term neurodevelopmental or pulmonary outcome follow-up data published from these rescue trials. Therefore, use of rescue HFV over continued CMV is not necessarily the better option; as always, each clinical situation will require careful consideration of the treatment possibilities from each mode of therapy.

Some circumstances may respond to the use of HFV more than others. Persistent pulmonary hypertension requiring nitric oxide therapy, with or without meconium aspiration or other lung disease, often responds best when HFOV is used for support.[89] Similarly, postsurgical support for infants with gastroschisis, omphalocele, necrotizing enterocolitis, and other similar problems may benefit from HFV therapy in the face of lung disease and increased intra-abdominal pressures. Finally, potentially viable infants with pulmonary hypoplasia from different causes often require prolonged ventilator support, with the ongoing risk of acute pulmonary air-leak syndromes. HFV for these babies may help provide the bridge needed for growth and clinical assessment.

Lung Protective Strategies with HFV: Limiting Pressure While Optimizing Volume

Much progress has been made in the treatment of neonatal respiratory failure over the past few decades. In particular, antenatal steroids and exogenous surfactant replacement have decreased neonatal mortality and morbidity in premature infants.[90-93] However, lung injury and pulmonary morbidities secondary to mechanical ventilation remain an ongoing problem in the care of premature infants. Of most concern, chronic lung disease in the form of BPD, defined as a persistent oxygen need at 36 weeks, postmenstrual age, develops in 40% of 22- to 29-week infants who survive to 36 weeks, with increasing frequency and severity as gestational age decreases.[94] Clearly, dilemmas remain regarding optimization of both timing and mode of mechanical ventilation to decrease neonatal pulmonary morbidities. HFV has been explored aggressively as a potential ventilation strategy that would avoid the large V_{TS} (volutrauma) and repetitive shear stress of the expansion and collapse with each CMV inflation (atelectrauma) that contributes to the development of BPD.

Although the body of literature comparing HFV and CMV is sizeable, it is difficult to compare one study to another because there is significant variation in ventilation strategies. In particular, when meta-analyses are performed, the heterogeneity among RCTs becomes obvious. The meta-analysis performed by Bollen and colleagues[95] demonstrated that variation in ventilation strategies in both the HFV and the CMV groups most likely explains the observed differences in outcomes compared with other variables. These findings lead to key questions: Would the outcomes of these studies be different if all had employed similar ventilation strategies, and what would be the most appropriate HFV and CMV ventilation strategies? The search for the optimal lung-protective strategy is ongoing.

Animal models have shown that low V_T and increased PEEP during CMV will lessen ventilator-induced lung injury (VILI).[96-99] With both HFV and CV, animal studies have demonstrated that recruiting the lung to ensure open and stable alveoli can attenuate VILI.[100-103] Reducing V_T to avoid VILI will prevent the most important cause of VILI, volutrauma. Modestly increasing PCO_2 (45 to 55 torr) to further decrease volutrauma and barotrauma has been termed *permissive hypercarbia*. The approach of recruiting and stabilizing the open alveoli has been termed *optimal lung volume* or *open lung* strategy. Taken together, these two concepts have been termed *lung-protective ventilation*. However, there is much debate as to how to actually employ lung-protective ventilation strategies at an infant's bedside, because there are no strict criteria or guidelines and some of the guiding data are from adult literature.[104,105] Nonetheless, most studies and reviews refer to an "open lung" strategy when there is a predefined FiO_2 target of 0.25 to 0.30 being used as a surrogate for optimal lung recruitment.[106,107] To that end, V_{TS} of less than 7 mL/kg with high ventilator rates and

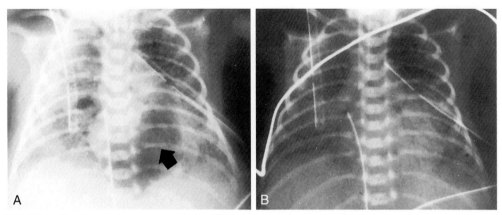

FIG 22-9 Chest roentgenogram of a 1300-g infant with severe hyaline membrane disease (**A**) before and (**B**) 4 hours following high-frequency jet ventilation (HFJV). Pulmonary interstitial emphysema and air trapped within the pulmonary ligament (*arrow*) were markedly decreased following HFJV. (From Pokora T, et al. *Pediatrics*. 1983;72:27.)

"permissive hypercarbia" on laboratory evaluation are generally considered to be "lung protective" with the goal to limit lung volume and alveolar overdistention (see Chapters 13 and 15).

HFV would appear to be ideal for a lung-protective strategy because it delivers very small V_Ts at low airway pressures while maintaining lung recruitment around a constant mean airway pressure. However, randomized clinical trials as of this writing do not consistently demonstrate benefits of HFV over CMV in terms of long-term morbidities and mortality.[1,77-82,85-87] These findings, or lack thereof, have been ascribed to the inconsistent, and at times poorly defined, ventilation strategies in the HFV and/or CMV arm.[108,109] Although we have many ventilator tools, there are few neonatal studies to guide us down one "best path" for optimum treatment. However, two meta-analyses, as well as a Cochrane database review, have concluded that volume-targeted CV decreases BPD, hypocarbia, pneumothorax, PVL, and grade 3/4 IVH.[110-112] Still, ventilation strategies vary greatly from neonatal intensive care unit (NICU) to NICU across North America and the world. As pointed out by van Kaam and Rimensberger, there is much left to learn, including whether recruitment maneuvers and higher levels of PEEP could further optimize low V_T CMV and whether the use of HFV over CMV can demonstrate decreased morbidity and mortality if the same lung-protective strategy is used in both groups.[109] It is becoming increasingly apparent that lung recruitment is necessary for lung protection and that PEEP should be used as needed in different disease states to stabilize lung volume. Whether HFV will be shown to be generally superior to CV when similar strategies are used remains to be seen. However, it appears that lung volume recruitment may be easier to accomplish with HFV, at least psychologically, because there seems to be less resistance to using higher mean airway pressure with HFOV than to increasing PEEP with CV.

APPLICATIONS OF HIGH-FREQUENCY VENTILATION IN SPECIFIC DISEASES

Respiratory Distress Syndrome

RDS continues to be the primary form of respiratory failure requiring treatment with mechanical ventilation in neonates. Treatment of acute RDS is based on principles of lung volume

recruitment and optimization and is described in detail below under "Clinical Guidelines."

Air-Leak Syndromes

Today HFV is generally accepted as a safe and effective treatment for severe pulmonary air leaks. This application was one of the original clinical uses of HFV, sometimes with dramatic results (Fig. 22-9).[24,25,44] There are very few RCTs evaluating the management of air-leak syndromes with HFV versus CMV. A British trial compared the incidences of pulmonary air leaks in 346 neonates treated with either HFPPV or CMV. Twenty-six percent of the infants treated with CMV developed air leaks compared to 19% of those who received HFPPV.[70] Mortalities, durations of ventilation, and incidences of chronic lung disease (CLD) and IVH were similar. Keszler et al.[31] compared HFPPV and HFJV in 144 infants with severe PIE. Sixty-one percent of those treated with HFJV improved, compared to only 37% treated with HFPPV. Forty-five percent of those who did not respond to HFPPV and were transferred to HFJV improved, whereas only 9% of the infants who did not respond to HFJV and were transferred to HFPPV improved. In addition, HFJV appeared to ventilate patients using lower proximal airway pressures. In another multicenter HFOV RDS trial (the HIFO study), the effect of HFOV on the treatment of air leak was examined.[84] Air leaks, either PIE or pneumothorax, were present in 26 (30%) of 86 patients randomized to HFOV and in 22 (24%) of 90 patients randomized to CMV. Although a low-pressure strategy might be presumed in a study of this type, HFOV patients still required higher airway pressures for gas exchange. Air leaks occurred in 42% of HFOV patients who entered the study without air leak, compared to 63% of CMV patients ($p < 0.05$). Although HFOV patients who entered the study with air leaks tended to do better than their counterparts treated with CMV, the differences were not significant.

Of all the forms of HFV considered thus far, HFJV has been the most successful with respect to the incidence and treatment of air-leak syndromes. All things considered, most forms of HFV appear to lessen the incidence of ventilator-associated pulmonary air leaks, whereas the data for the benefit for preexisting pulmonary air leaks are more convincing for HFJV. The question remains, why do pulmonary air leaks improve during HFV? One theory is that HFV produces smaller pressure fluxes within the distal airways. Pressures in the upper airway equilibrate and gas is delivered distally at a more constant distending pressure. Pressure differentials between airway and intrapleural space lessen. There is less stretching of the injured tissue. Less gas escapes during peak inflation and there are greater opportunities for self-repair. HFJV may be particularly good for air leaks because of the short inspiratory time (0.02 seconds), with relatively long expiratory time, and the extremely high accelerating inspiratory flow. An air leak will persist when gas is delivered at a pressure that opens the injured tissue, creating a low-resistance path for flow. The leak will continue during an inspiration for as long as the pressure exceeds that needed to stent the leak open. During CV or HFOV, because of both the inspiratory time and the characteristics of gas flow, a leak may persist, whereas during HFJV, it may rapidly close.

The low occurrence rates of bronchopleural and tracheoesophageal fistulas in neonates preclude the ability to perform adequate randomized clinical trials of management with HFV versus CMV. However, a few studies have formally evaluated the amount of air leak through these types of fistulas using HFV versus CMV. In the management of infants with bronchopleural fistula, Gonzales and colleagues[113] showed a decrease in chest tube air leak when using HFJV versus CMV. Goldberg et al.[114] and Donn et al.[115] report similar experiences in managing infants with tracheoesophageal fistulas with HFJV. Furthermore, case reports, such as that by Bloom et al.,[116] and animal studies, such as that by Orlando et al.,[117] relay findings of an observed benefit to the use of HFV in the ventilatory stabilization of patients with tracheoesophageal or bronchopleural fistula. Although these findings are positive, the lack of RCTs makes it difficult to provide an evidence-based recommendation for the use of HFV over CMV in the treatment of bronchopleural or tracheoesophageal fistulas. As such an evidence base may never exist, the evidence available does support a trial of these therapies in these difficult conditions when more conventional approaches are failing.

Pulmonary Hypoplasia, Persistent Pulmonary Hypertension, and Inhaled Nitric Oxide

Infants with various forms of pulmonary hypoplasia may derive at least some short-term benefit from HFV. Some of these infants have associated, equally lethal, abnormalities. In such situations, HFV may provide a brief respite for diagnostic studies to identify potential survivors or confirm diagnoses for family members. In infants with congenital diaphragmatic hernia (CDH), HFV may be a useful "bridge" therapy to cannulation for extracorporeal membrane oxygenation (ECMO), although iNO has not been shown to significantly change outcomes.[118,119] In the hypoplastic lung, because the number of gas-exchanging units is small, it is only logical to assume that ventilation at rapid rates using low V_Ts would be most effective. Because of the variety of conditions associated with pulmonary hypoplasia and their relative rarity, controlled studies are difficult to design or perform, and clear evidence-based guidelines simply are not available.

Infants with pulmonary hypoplasia associated with CDH may derive some benefit from HFV. To date there are no published controlled studies, only clinical anecdotes. There are many early case reports of infants with pulmonary hypoplasia associated with CDH treated with HFV. Most of the patients improved initially but had poor long-term outcomes if the hypoplasia was severe. In most of the patients, arterial blood gas measurements improved at lower proximal airway pressures; however, few patients survived. These reports predated ECMO.

Carter et al.[120] studied 50 infants referred for ECMO who were first treated with HFOV. Forty-six percent improved and did not

require ECMO. Four infants had pulmonary hypoplasia associated with CDH. None responded positively to HFOV. All required ECMO. Baumgart et al.[121] reviewed results of 73 neonatal ECMO candidates who first were treated with HFJV. Nine infants had pulmonary hypoplasia associated with CDH; only three survived. deLemos et al.[122] reviewed the outcomes of 122 neonatal ECMO candidates first treated with HFO. Fifty-three percent did not require ECMO; however, only 5 of 20 patients who had pulmonary hypoplasia associated with CDH responded positively to HFOV and did not require ECMO. A smaller series of 12 infants, described by Stoddard and colleagues,[123] showed much better outcomes with HFO. Eleven of the 12 babies with CDH did not require ECMO and ultimately survived. Migliazza and colleagues[124] retrospectively reviewed 111 babies with CDH treated with early HFOV for both preoperative stabilization and postoperative care. They saw a 69.4% survival overall, compared to a predicted 69% survival based on the CDH Study Group formula. A 2007 review summarizing "best-evidence practice strategies" discussed HFOV; they found no consistent approach and no new evidence supporting HFOV over conventional approaches to respiratory support.[125]

The sole RCT evaluating the presumed benefits of HFOV in infants with CDH failed to recruit a sufficient number of subjects and was abandoned when an interim analysis showed no hint of benefit of HFOV as applied in that trial. Forty-one patients (45%) randomized to conventional mechanical ventilation died/had BPD compared with 43 patients (54%) in the high-frequency oscillation group. Patients initially ventilated by conventional mechanical ventilation were ventilated for fewer days (P = 0.03), less often needed extracorporeal membrane oxygenation support (P = 0.007), inhaled nitric oxide (P = 0.045), sildenafil (P = 0.004), had a shorter duration of vasoactive drugs (P = 0.02), and less often failed treatment (P = 0.01) as compared with infants initially ventilated by high-frequency oscillation.[125a]

Despite some reports of success, overall, HFV has not been very successful in the treatment of severe pulmonary hypoplasia associated with CDH, at least as an independent treatment. As with other forms of pulmonary hypoplasia, however, HFV often can stabilize critically ill patients until their ultimate prognosis becomes clear. Another common use of HFV is in conjunction with iNO as a treatment for severe respiratory failure secondary to persistent pulmonary hypertension. Detailed discussion regarding the current evidence to support this combined therapy in preterm and term neonates can be found in Chapter 14.

CLINICAL GUIDELINES

Most clinical guidelines are, by their nature, arbitrary; they reflect the experiences, biases, and, at times, idiosyncrasies of their authors. Many clinicians do not consider HFV first-line therapy in the neonatal population; however, many quickly move to it when problems develop during CMV.[126] Some practitioners use HFV early in the course of uncomplicated RDS. Likewise, some wean to extubation from HFV. Others choose a return to CMV prior to extubation. Because of these many clinical variations and the lack of data from which to generalize, the following guidelines must be tempered by experience and modified as new information becomes available. What follows is a description of HFV use in a variety of situations, using two different HFV strategies: (1) limiting pressure exposure, which is used in air leaks, CDH, and most other rescue situations, and (2) optimizing lung volume, which is used in RDS or other conditions in which diffuse atelectasis is a major issue.

Limiting Pressure Exposure
High-Frequency Jet Ventilators

The only high-frequency jet ventilator currently in general use for neonates is the Bunnell Life Pulse.

HFJV settings will depend on the clinical condition. For air leak, the lowest possible rate should be used, which will provide the longest expiratory time. A rate of 240 is often effective in larger infants, 320 to 360 in small preterm infants. Inspiratory time should be left at 0.02 unless a very large infant is being treated, in which case a longer inspiratory time may be needed to generate the required PIP. As is true with both conventional and oscillatory ventilation, mean airway pressure supports end-expiratory lung volume. During HFJV, this is mainly controlled by using PEEP adjustment. Sufficient PEEP is essential for maintenance of lung volume; use of too low a PEEP is a common mistake with HFJV. For air-leak syndromes, a conventional sigh breath should not be used. For other conditions a rate of 420 is usually preferred for preterm infants. A slower rate of 280 to 360 is appropriate for large infants, particularly if there is increased airway resistance, which increases the time needed for passive exhalation. PIP should be sufficient for CO_2 elimination. A transcutaneous monitor to continuously assess CO_2 levels is very important for HFJV and HFOV, as overventilation may occur rapidly, with decreased cerebral blood flow and an increased risk of brain injury and pulmonary air leak.

For nonhomogeneous lung disease with atelectasis and overdistention, a CMV "sigh" rate of 2 to 6 inflations/min may help open atelectatic areas. A common error with HFJV is to use a CV rate instead of appropriate PEEP to increase mean airway pressure. Generally speaking, if addition of a sigh breath improves oxygen saturation, this suggests that end-expiratory lung volume, which is supported by mean airway pressure, is too low. During HFOV with the Dräger BabyLog in an animal model, sigh breaths were useful during lung recruitment but not after recruitment was complete.[127] The PIP of the CMV rate should approximate a pressure that would provide a normal V_T of 4 to 6 mL/kg.

Whether or not the sigh breaths interrupt the cycling of the high-frequency jet ventilator is not as important as the V_T delivered. Once HFJV settings are established, mean airway pressures should be adjusted as necessary to maintain a balance between the lowest possible pressure and the oxygen exposure.

After HFJV is initiated, some patience is required. During HFJV, airway pressures equilibrate more slowly than during CMV. One must allow adequate time for the system's servomechanisms to adjust the HFJV driving pressure to achieve the targeted pressures. Patients usually stabilize within 15 to 30 minutes. Continuous CO_2 monitoring is important during this time. After this initial equilibration period, interval arterial blood gases are measured. Usually CO_2 elimination improves, and it may do so at lower mean airway pressures. Oxygen requirements may transiently increase. Because this strategy is designed to minimize pressure exposure, increases in FiO_2 may be necessary to eliminate air leaks. Because the effectiveness of HFJV depends on the ability of the jet of gas to stream down the center of the airway unimpeded, it is important to ensure that the head is in midline and the tip of the endotracheal tube is at least 1 cm above the carina. If the head is turned to the side, the jet stream will hit the wall of the trachea, rendering it less effective and possibly contributing to mucosal injury. If the tube is too close to the carina, the flow of gas may be preferentially directed to one or the other main stem bronchus. Most commonly, HFJV is a rescue therapy; relatively short-term exposure to HFJV (generally a few days) often will result in substantial clinical improvement. As patients improve,

HFJV PIP can be decreased in decrements of 1 to 2 cm H_2O while acceptable pH and $PaCO_2$ values are maintained. One should also aim to decrease FiO_2 levels as arterial oxygen saturation values allow. Be sure that adequate PEEP is maintained, even in the presence of air leak. Even with a low-pressure strategy, lung end-expiratory volumes must be supported adequately. When HFJV PIP values are below 18 to 20 cm H_2O and FiO_2 values fall below 0.4, consider extubation to noninvasive ventilation.

If the patient is returned to CMV prior to extubation, set the jet ventilator to standby mode. Set the CMV rate to 60 inflations/min (an arbitrary number) and wean based on patient–ventilator interaction. Adjust CMV PIP levels to deliver V_Ts of 4 to 6 mL/kg by using a volume-targeted CMV mode. Adjust FiO_2 levels as necessary to maintain arterial oxygen saturation values in the desired range. If, after returning to CMV, the patient's general condition worsens or FiO_2 or $PaCO_2$ levels increase significantly, return to HFJV for at least another 24 hours.

High-Frequency Oscillatory Ventilators

In the United States, the most commonly used neonatal high-frequency oscillatory ventilator is the SensorMedics 3100A. With this device, in contrast to HFJV, use of an endotracheal tube adapter is not necessary. Initial HFOV frequency for a premature infant is commonly set between 10 and 15 Hz. Generally, there is seldom a need to change the frequency; however, if the frequency is altered, it is important to be mindful of the effect of frequency on effective V_T discussed earlier in this chapter. This ventilator's "power" control sets the amplitude of its airway pressure oscillations ($\ddot{A}\Delta$), the prime determinant of CO_2 removal. Increasing airway pressure amplitude increases chest wall movement and decreases $PaCO_2$ values, sometimes dramatically. Use of a transcutaneous monitor will provide important data on minute-to-minute gas exchange. Decreasing airway pressure amplitude decreases chest wall movement and increases $PaCO_2$ values. Initially, the amplitude control is set at a level that adequately produces chest wall vibration or "jiggling" of the chest and abdomen; at times it can be as high as 35 to 40 cm H_2O when HFOV is used in rescue mode. Some physicians simply use a visual assessment as to adequacy of the chest wall movement to set the initial amplitude value, and others use an amplitude value of approximately double the mean airway pressure as a starting point and adjust as necessary for adequate chest wall movement. After assessment of the initial $PaCO_2$ value on HFOV, the amplitude is then adjusted up or down as necessary to produce the desired $PaCO_2$ levels. If a transcutaneous monitor is not available, assessment of $PaCO_2$ values every 15 minutes will be needed until the patient is stabilized within the goal range. Continued vigilance is essential, because changes in lung compliance may occur quite rapidly and result in large swings in $PaCO_2$ because of the geometric relationship of V_T and CO_2 removal.

Outside the United States, several HFOV devices have the ability to monitor V_T and display a calculated value for CO_2 removal, termed *DCO2*. Tracking this number allows the clinician to detect changes in ventilation and respond quickly, similar to what tracking transcutaneous CO_2 allows. Even more attractive is the ability of some of these devices to maintain a target V_T by means of a volume guarantee (VG) mode, analogous to conventional VG. With HFOV + VG, once an appropriate V_T is identified, that V_T can be maintained despite changes in lung mechanics by automatic adjustment of pressure amplitude, analogous to adjustment in PIP with CMV. When the VG mode is used with HFOV, changes in frequency will not produce the usual changes in minute ventilation, because the V_T will be unaffected by the frequency change. As of this writing, there is limited information about the effectiveness of this refinement, but it promises to reduce the risk of hypocarbia during HFOV.

During HFOV (as well as HFJV), mean airway pressure is the main determinant of lung volume. Small changes in $\overline{P}_{aw}$ can produce large changes in lung volume, either overdistention or atelectasis. The airway pressures are measured within the oscillator circuit, not in the endotracheal tube or proximal airway. These pressures may or may not reflect the actual pressures within the patients' airways. Though mean airway pressure is relatively consistent, oscillation pressures are rapidly damped across the endotracheal tube and further within the airways (Fig. 22-10). $\overline{P}_{aw}$ should exceed that used during CMV by approximately 2 to 3 cm H_2O when using a 33% inspiratory time (1:2 I:E ratio). Owing to the flow characteristics of the 1:2 I:E ratio, this will provide a $\overline{P}_{aw}$ approximately equal to what was given on CMV. This gradient does not exist when a 1:1 ratio is used, as is common with some devices used outside the United States. In theory, the longer expiratory time of the 1:2 I:E ratio means that the expiratory flow and thus pressure during the active exhalation is lower than during the inspiratory phase, making airway collapse less likely to occur. Mean airway pressure can then be adjusted depending on chest radiographs and oxygenation. Once the patient stabilizes or starts to improve, airway pressures should be decreased, as long as FiO_2 is below 0.30 and $PaCO_2$ values are normal. The ÄΔ should be lowered if $PaCO_2$ levels are below target. During HFOV weaning, if FiO_2 increases, consider a 1-to 2-cm H_2O increase in $\overline{P}_{aw}$ to stabilize lung volume. Some advocate intermittent lung volume recruitment maneuvers when FiO_2 increases to reestablish adequate end-expiratory lung volume. If things do not improve or worsen, a chest radiograph may be needed. When the FiO_2 is below 0.3 to 0.4, the chest radiograph is significantly improved,

and the $\overline{P}_{aw}$ is 7 to 9 cm H_2O, infants can be extubated to noninvasive ventilation. In some situations or for heavily sedated infants, return to CMV may be needed.

Optimizing Lung Volume

The strategy of optimizing lung volume is critical. As was described previously in this chapter, adequate recruitment of lung volume is the key to protection and preservation of lung architecture as well as to potentiation of endogenous and exogenous surfactant.[100,128-131] Because lung volumes are difficult to assess at the bedside, other surrogates must be employed. Respiratory inductive plethysmography (RIP) has been studied in animals and in neonates to define the inspiratory and expiratory pressure–volume (P-V) relationship.[132,133] A study in lambs reported direct estimation of lung volume change during HFV using RIP.[133] Similarly, electrical impedance tomography (EIT), which measures differences in electrical impedance from changes in lung tissue conductivity, may become a useful clinical adjunct for assessment of lung volume changes during mechanical ventilation.[134-136] Although more precise and informative than SaO_2 measurements, RIP and EIT remain research tools at this time. Therefore, SaO_2 (combined with FiO_2) and chest radiographic findings are used most commonly as surrogates for changes in lung volume.[107,132]

Optimizing lung volume maximizes the advantages of lung hysteresis by defining the P-V relationship of the lung during treatment. In the laboratory, this is done by inflating the lung to near-maximum volume, then deflating the lung to closing volume. The lung is reinflated to a point above closing volume but below maximum volume. This technique allows ventilation to move from the inspiratory limb of the P-V curve to the expiratory limb, allowing effective ventilation and oxygenation at lower pressures. The delineation of an individual patient's P-V relationship is still difficult but has been done successfully in neonates (Fig. 22-11). De Jaegere and colleagues have eloquently described this technique.[107] Some specific techniques for optimization of lung volume during HFJV and HFOV are discussed below. However, a general schematic applicable to all techniques of ventilation is shown in Figure 22-12.

With a sustained inflation (SI), the lung may be maximally inflated at a high $\overline{P}_{aw}$ for 15 to 30 seconds, which also moves ventilation onto the expiratory limb of the P-V relationship. This then allows maximal preservation of lung volume at lower pressures, with the potential for the greatest protection from VILI. The lung changes rapidly during the course of illness; theoretically, providing ventilation on the descending limb of the P-V relationship offers potential protection from these rapid changes. Figure 22-13 schematically demonstrates this potential advantage as well as potential pitfalls using basic physiologic principles.

High-Frequency Jet Ventilators

HFJV is initiated as previously described. So-called optimal PEEP is used to recruit lung volume and decrease oxygen requirements. In fact, this is merely the appropriate application of $\overline{P}_{aw}$ to recruit and maintain lung volume. In surfactant deficiency syndromes, surfactant can be administered either immediately after intubation during CMV or during HFJV. At this time, there is no convincing evidence that surfactant administration is either more efficient or safer during any form of HFV, although adequate volume recruitment prior to

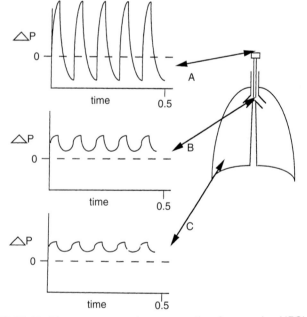

FIG 22-10 Airway pressure drop across the airway using HFOV. (The graph was adapted from unpublished observations using the SensorMedics 3100A.) **Curve A,** Pressure measured at the proximal endotracheal tube. **Curve B,** Pressure measured at the carina. **Curve C,** Pressure measured in the distal airways.

instillation clearly improves surfactant distribution and function.[131] Mean airway pressure levels are increased in increments of 1 to 2 cm H_2O until arterial oxygen levels no longer increase. When initial recruitment is complete, PIP levels must be adjusted based on transcutaneous CO_2 monitoring or very frequent blood gases to avoid hypocarbia. When oxygen saturation levels are satisfactory, $\overline{P}_{aw}$ (PEEP) may be weaned by 1 to 2 cm H_2O to prevent overdistention and to shift the P-V relationship to the expiratory portion of the curve. Then FiO_2 rather than PEEP should be decreased to prevent atelectasis. When FiO_2 falls below 0.30 to 0.40, further decreases in $\overline{P}_{aw}$ may be made. A technique of stepwise pressure increases, using SaO_2 as a volume surrogate, with a decrease in PEEP after recruitment, is effective during HFJV as it is during HFOV. A study in preterm lambs showed decreased final pressure

requirements, improved compliance, and reduced inflammatory markers using this technique.[137]

HFJV removes CO_2 very efficiently, possibly more so than HFOV. If hypocarbia and alkalosis develop, decrease the PIP. It is important to understand that lowering PIP while PEEP remains unchanged will lead to a drop in $\overline{P}_{aw}$. To avoid an unintended drop in $\overline{P}_{aw}$, PEEP needs to be increased sufficiently to offset the drop in PIP, thus avoiding loss of lung recruitment. If FiO_2 increases and a chest radiograph shows atelectasis, PEEP should be increased for higher $\overline{P}_{aw}$ and increased end-expiratory lung volume. If FiO_2 remains stable, sufficient lung volume recruitment has been achieved. When $\overline{P}_{aw}$ falls to 8 to 10 cm H_2O, PIP levels to less than 20 cm H_2O, and FiO_2 to 0.30-0.40, an attempt to return to CMV or extubation to noninvasive ventilation may be made in the fashion previously described.

High-Frequency Oscillatory Ventilators

The ventilator frequency and amplitude are set as previously described; $\overline{P}_{aw}$ initially is set 2 to 3 cm H_2O higher than that used during CMV when a 1:2 I:E ratio is used. Recruitment of lung volume may be accomplished by $\overline{P}_{aw}$ increases and decreases as previously described or by increasing $\overline{P}_{aw}$ by 5 to 10 cm H_2O above baseline for 10 to 30 seconds as an SI maneuver. HFOV is continued during the SI. While data from controlled trials remain limited, the best evidence as of this writing would favor the technique shown in Figure 22-12. Using either technique, mean airway pressure should be reduced after improvement in oxygenation is seen. Failure to do so would result in overdistention of the lungs, which become more compliant once recruited and secondarily adversely affect venous return and cardiac output. As noted earlier, this will maximize the effects of lung hysteresis.

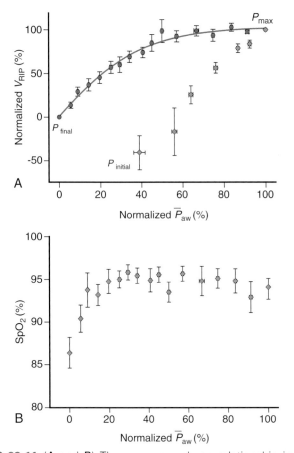

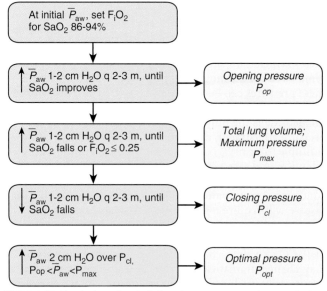

FIG 22-11 (A and B) The pressure–volume relationship in 12 infants with respiratory failure during treatment with high-frequency oscillatory ventilation. Diamonds show the inflation limb, circles the deflation limb of the curve. Inflation curves were established in individual patients by increasing $\overline{P}_{aw}$ from the baseline clinical value by 2 cm H_2O every 10 minutes until no further increase in SaO_2 was seen or SaO_2 decreased; deflation curves were established by decreasing $\overline{P}_{aw}$ from the maximum value by 2 cm H_2O until baseline pressures were reached, then decreases were continued by 1 cm H_2O until SaO_2 fell to 85% for more than 5 minutes or a $\overline{P}_{aw}$ of 5 cm H_2O was reached. Volume changes were estimated using respiratory impedance plethysmography. (From Tingay DG, et al. *Am J Respir Crit Care Med.* 2006;173:414.)

FIG 22-12 Technique for defining the pressure–volume relationship of the lungs during treatment. Using systematic stepwise increases and decreases in $\overline{P}_{aw}$, the clinician can find the opening pressure, maximum pressure (total lung volume), and closing pressure of each individual patient and target the optimal pressure for ventilation. (Adapted from De Jaegere, et al. *Am J Respir Crit Care Med.* 2006;174:639.)

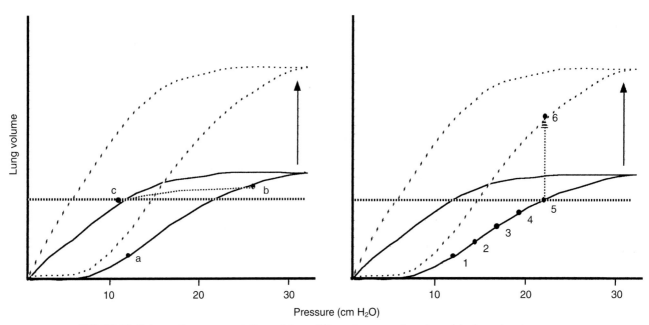

FIG 22-13 Schematic representation of two different approaches to achieving alveolar expansion, and the theoretical effect of a sudden improvement in lung compliance. The horizontal dashed line indicates the desired mean lung volume. The solid curve is a pressure–volume (P-V) relationship of a surfactant-deficient lung prior to the development of structural injury. The dashed line shows the P-V curve of the lung after some recovery has occurred. On the left, a brief sustained inflation from opening pressure (point a) to pressure point b inflates the lung to the desired volume. Pressure is then decreased to point c, moving to the deflation limb of the curve. In the improved lung, volume at point c is still maintained within the desired range at low pressure. On the right, progressive increases in mean airway pressure occur on the inflation limb (points 1 to 5). Target volume is achieved, but at higher pressure. If the lung then improves, rapid overdistention could occur when pressure is maintained, but volume increases (point 6). (Adapted from Froese AB. Neonatal and pediatric ventilation: physiological and clinical perspectives. In: Marini JJ, Slutsky AS, eds. *Physiological Basis of Ventilatory Support*. New York: Marcel Dekker, Inc.; 1998, p. 1346.)

If stepwise pressure increases are used, reduction in $\overline{P}_{aw}$ in increments of 1 to 2 cm H_2O is made every 1 to 2 minutes. Oxygenation should be well maintained as long as $\overline{P}_{aw}$ remains above the lung's closing pressure. Because neither of these pressures can be accurately predicted and lung volume changes can be only estimated, careful clinical observation at the bedside is the only solution. After lung recruitment and pressure adjustment, decrease FiO$_2$ to less than 0.3 and then continue to wean $\overline{P}_{aw}$. Amplitude is adjusted upward for CO$_2$ retention and vice versa for hypocarbia. Optimal rate (Hz) depends on the size of the patient and the underlying lung condition. Larger patients or patients with obstructive lung disease will require a lower frequency, and smaller patients or those with restrictive disease will do better on a higher frequency. As noted previously, one way to produce changes in PaCO$_2$ involves changing frequency. However, since V$_T$ may change dramatically and the magnitude of the change is not easily predicted, it is more appropriate to change the amplitude or power setting. Increasing oxygen requirements despite appropriate volume recruitment maneuvers suggest impaired cardiac output, fixed intrapulmonary shunting, air-leak syndrome, or other problems not amenable to lung volume recruitment. When mean airway pressures fall between 7 and 9 cm H_2O, consider extubation to noninvasive ventilation or, if necessary, returning to CMV in the fashion previously described.

PROBLEMS, COMPLICATIONS, AND QUESTIONS WITHOUT ANSWERS

Will HFV become the preferred means of support for neonates with respiratory failure? As of this writing, there is inadequate information to make this leap. There are a number of practical problems associated with the clinical use of any HFV. Although approved for general use, the role of HFV remains undefined in many respects. Each HFV system is different. Generalizations and recommendations developed for one system may or may not apply to the next.[138-142] There are few standards; however, HFV, whether in the form of HFPPV, HFFI, HFOV, or HFJV, is used in virtually all NICUs today. Many different HFV systems are in use around the world; there is a lack of adequate direct comparisons between various forms of HFV. HFJV and HFOV can be extremely effective in many different clinical situations, but all systems have their complications and their limitations. Perhaps most importantly, the results of studies not only reflect the characteristics of the devices but are greatly affected by the strategies and skill with which they are used, making interpretation of clinical trials complicated.

In the absence of a good technique for monitoring lung volumes at the bedside, can HFV produce lung overdistention by quietly trapping gas? We know HFV may produce higher end-expiratory volumes at lower proximal airway pressures. Increased end-expiratory lung volumes may also result in increased end-expiratory alveolar pressures. Under such circumstances, $\overline{P}_{aw}$ exceeds mean proximal airway pressures. Such silent distending pressure is commonly referred to as *inadvertent PEEP* (see Chapter 2). Because this pressure cannot be easily measured, the extent to which it produces problems is a conundrum. In some circumstances, it probably causes substantial difficulty with ventilation.

Does HFV produce lung underdistention? Under normal circumstances, small monotonous V_Ts delivered at relatively constant pressures result in progressive atelectasis. Early HFOV primate studies document that this does occur, but the problem is almost always due to inadequate $\overline{P}_{aw}$ with resulting low end-expiratory lung volumes. To combat this problem, many clinicians periodically vary V_Ts using either manual or mechanical sigh breaths or periodic SI maneuvers. These techniques recruit alveoli and prevent atelectasis. Is this a better technique than simply increasing $\overline{P}_{aw}$? What is the best way to vary V_T during HFV? Newer machines available in Europe and Canada provide volume targeting, which is not well studied in HFV but offers real promise.[141,142] Is SI better than gradual increases and then decreases in $\overline{P}_{aw}$? A 2009 study investigated four techniques for lung volume recruitment: stepwise increases in $\overline{P}_{aw}$, using a 20-second SI, using six 1-second repeated SIs, and setting a single higher $\overline{P}_{aw}$ without change.[143] The stepwise increases in $\overline{P}_{aw}$, followed by a reduction in pressure after the maneuver was completed, produced the greatest increase in thoracic gas volume, the best redistribution of aeration, and the greatest change in SaO_2. A bedside technique for rapid accurate assessment of changes in lung volume is needed to assist the clinician no matter the technique.

High-frequency techniques have been associated with rare complications. A number of early reports linked tracheal inflammation and tracheal obstructions to various forms of HFV.[24,25,144-156] These complications were serious and at times fatal. They occurred in both adults and neonates. Initially these lesions were believed to result from inadequate humidification of respiratory gases. This no longer appears to be the entire answer. Ophoven et al.[144] compared the tracheal histopathology seen in animals after CMV and HFJV using different humidification systems. Although humidity was important, regardless of the humidification system used, HFJV always produced more inflammation and damage in the proximal trachea than did CMV. The histologic injury patterns observed in these animals were virtually identical to those seen in human patients exposed to HFJV. Similar animal studies compared the tracheobronchial histopathology seen after HFPPV, HFJV, and CMV.[147,150-154] HFJV and HFPPV produced nearly identical tracheal lesions. This unique tracheal injury now is referred to as *necrotizing tracheobronchitis* (NTB) (Fig. 22-14). This problem has been extensively studied in the laboratory. It now appears that NTB is associated with a number of factors and occurs during all forms of HFV. Ventilator rates and ventilatory strategies, airway humidification, FiO_2 levels, the severity of the underlying illness, duration of ventilation, alterations in epithelial permeability, and infections all seem to play roles.[36,147-157] While true NTB is uncommon today, possibly because of different

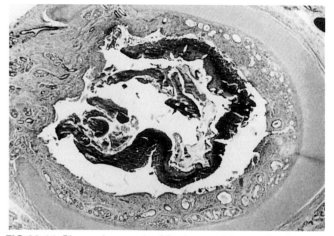

FIG 22-14 Photomicrograph of fatal necrotizing tracheobronchitis. This section was obtained from the trachea just above the carina. The entire mucosal surface has become necrotic and completely obstructs the tracheal lumen. (From Boros SJ, et al. *J Pediatr.* 1986;109:95.)

humidification systems, improved equipment and different use patterns such as optimal lung volume and surfactant therapy, it may still occur.[154] Airway obstruction from inspissated secretions, a precursor to NTB, should be suspected any time the combination of acute hypercarbia associated with decreased chest wall movement is observed during HFV; reintubation often solves the problem. Emergent bronchoscopy may be required if reintubation is unsuccessful.

A review from the presurfactant era suggested that between 2% and 4% of HFV-treated patients have either clinical or microscopic evidence of NTB.[148] No data are available to assess the impact of surfactant administration on the incidence of NTB. Although it also occurs during CMV, NTB continues to be more likely during HFV. Acute hypercarbia, respiratory acidosis, and a sudden decrease in chest wall movement during HFV signal possible NTB. Aggressive airway suctioning, use of airway bronchoscopy, and reintubation can be potentially life saving. Far more often, especially with HFJV, the problem is simply related to endotracheal tube malposition (too close to the carina, angled relative to the trachea) or to accumulated secretions that need to be suctioned.

The most serious potential side effect of HFV is concern that an increase in long-term neurologic injury may occur, resulting from an increase in early PVL or severe IVH. This concerning finding, originally reported in the HIFI trial, was also seen in a study of HFJV reported by Wiswell et al.[33,48] These injuries seem to be linked to the strategy of ventilation used in these studies. Neither of these studies delineated a standardized technique for lung volume recruitment, and hypocarbia during treatment was common. As noted previously in this chapter, meta-analyses of randomized trials of HFV have concluded that, in studies using an "optimal lung volume" strategy, there is no evidence of increased neurologic injury.

SUMMARY

HFV is an exciting and useful form of mechanical ventilation. In some circumstances it can produce gas exchange at lower airway pressures than during CMV, and it allows safer application of high mean airway pressures when necessary for oxygenation. This technique is superior to CMV in airway leak syndromes and may be a useful rescue technique and/or bridge to ECMO. It has clear usefulness as a rescue or temporizing measure in pulmonary hypoplasia, persistent pulmonary hypertension, and other forms of neonatal respiratory failure unresponsive to CMV. In neonatal RDS, HFV, perhaps in association with surfactant therapy, may yet play a major role in improving long-term pulmonary outcomes. Today HFV is no longer a treatment in search of a disease, but neither is it the panacea for all forms of neonatal respiratory failure that many initially hoped it would be. HFV is now a standard form of neonatal therapy for a wide variety of respiratory conditions, despite inadequate information about its efficacy. Newer models of HFV may provide even better therapy for neonatal respiratory diseases. While it is unlikely that new multicenter RCTs will be performed, research continues on ways to better use these techniques.

REFERENCES

A complete reference list is available at https://expertconsult .inkling.com/.

23

Mechanical Ventilation: Disease-Specific Strategies

Bradley A. Yoder, MD

When noninvasive respiratory support is insufficient to achieve adequate gas exchange, insertion of an endotracheal tube and mechanical ventilator support may be necessary. Once it is determined that mechanical ventilation is needed, a variety of factors should be considered in choosing the mode of support. One factor is the type of mechanical ventilator to use: specifically either one of the "conventional approaches" or high-frequency ventilation. There are a number of conventional and high-frequency devices from which to choose; most are covered in greater detail in other chapters and will not be specifically addressed here. A second factor to be considered is the mode of ventilator support to be applied. Specifically, for conventional mechanical ventilation several different support modes may be selected on each device; again these are covered in more detail elsewhere in this book. A third factor to consider is the presumed benefits related to targeted gas exchange values and decreased work of breathing versus the relative risk of ventilator-induced lung injury (VILI). Perhaps most important, one needs to consider the underlying pathophysiology and its potential evolution over time. Finally, even from the time of initiating mechanical ventilator support, it is essential that the clinician has an active approach or plan for weaning and extubation (see also Chapter 24).

This chapter will discuss our approach to ventilator management in several of the most common neonatal respiratory disorders. It should be understood that there are a variety of devices and approaches other than those described here that one could employ resulting in safe, effective respiratory support of the ill neonate. Therefore, we will emphasize the key pathophysiologic features of each of the disorders and how the pathophysiology relates to the specific approach to mechanical ventilation. We firmly believe that the single most important factor associated with safe and successful ventilator management of the neonate is the person operating the device, not the device itself. A thorough understanding of the device, the mode applied, and the pathophysiology being managed, as well as a consistent, attentive approach to the specific infant being cared for, is essential to any success in managing respiratory problems in critically ill neonates.

RESPIRATORY DISTRESS SYNDROME

It is indeed ironic that over 40 years after the introduction of continuous positive airway pressure (CPAP) as the first effective therapy for neonatal respiratory distress syndrome (RDS), and despite the marked technological advances that have been made during that time span, there has been a renewed emphasis on the application of noninvasive

approaches, such as nasal CPAP, for respiratory support of neonatal lung disease.[1] Despite the increasing success with noninvasive respiratory support, many neonates still require mechanical ventilator support for RDS, particularly those at the lowest gestational ages, and these are the ones that will be addressed here.

Key Pathophysiologic Features (Table 23-1)
Surfactant
A comprehensive overview of surfactant and its role in neonatal RDS is beyond the scope of this presentation. The reader is referred to Chapter 31 of this book and other publications for additional information.[2-5] Quantitative, qualitative, and metabolic disturbances in surfactant play key roles in the pathophysiology of neonatal RDS. The net effect is decreased compliance of distal airspaces that can lead to atelectasis, ventilation:perfusion mismatch, and intrapulmonary shunt.[2,5] Surfactant proteins play a critical role not only in the function of surfactant but also in the lung's response to infection. The indications for and approach to surfactant replacement therapy for neonatal RDS continue to be an area of very active investigation and will not be addressed in this chapter.[6-8]

Lung Liquid
Normal lung growth is regulated, in part, via fluid secreted into the potential airspace across the alveolar epithelial cells. Lung liquid secretion is generated via upregulated Cl^- channels that actively transport Cl^- into the lung lumen, with Na^+ and H_2O following via an osmotic gradient.[9] During fetal life the epithelial Na^+ channel that promotes Na^+ and fluid absorption from the airspace in postnatal life is downregulated. Delayed upregulation of all three subunits of the epithelial Na^+ channel has been found in preterm infants with RDS, persisting in some to at least 1 month of age.[10] Additional factors that may contribute to persistent fetal lung liquid formation and delayed reabsorption of airspace fluid following preterm delivery include variable expression and activity of aquaporin channel proteins and persistent function of the secretory Cl^- channels.[11]

Developmental Lung Biology
Development of the mammalian lung is a complex, highly orchestrated process that is subject to interruption from numerous insults, particularly premature birth. The progressive stages of lung development are well described and include embryonic, pseudoglandular, canalicular, saccular, and alveolar stages.[12] Vasculogenesis and angiogenesis, processes critical to lung growth and differentiation, are tightly connected throughout

TABLE 23-1 Pathophysiology of Respiratory Distress Syndrome of Prematurity

Factor	Effect	Possible Intervention
Surfactant	Reduced quantity	Antenatal steroid therapy
	Impaired metabolism	Surfactant replacement
	Reduced surfactant proteins	Surfactant-specific proteins
	Disrupted function–proteins	Additional surfactant therapy
Lung liquid	Reduced clearance	Antenatal steroid therapy
	Sustained production	Postnatal steroid therapy
Mechanical	Reduced airspace compliance	Surfactant therapy
	High chest wall compliance	Positive end-expiratory pressure
	Increased airway compliance	Low inspiratory tidal volumes
Development	Canalicular–saccular stage	Antenatal steroid therapy
	Thickened mesenchyme	Maternal stress
	Immature capillary development	Effect of subclinical chorioamnionitis (?)
Inflammation	Altered surfactant metabolism	Antenatal steroid therapy
	Disrupted membrane integrity	Prevention/treatment of chorioamnionitis
	Interrupted lung development	Postnatal steroids and other antiinflammatories

TABLE 23-2 Indications for Trial of Noninvasive Respiratory Support

Indication	Comment
Consider noninvasive respiratory support initially for:	• All infants of ≥26 weeks gestation
After 10 minutes of resuscitation if:	• Indication for intubation has resolved but requires FiO_2 0.3-0.5 to maintain targeted SpO_2
After surfactant administration if:	• FiO_2 <0.4 and decreasing while maintaining targeted SpO_2 • No marked retractions • No suspected airway obstruction • >5 minutes since surfactant delivered
While on mechanical ventilation if:	• On high-frequency oscillation (see Table 23-4) • On conventional ventilation (see Table 23-4)
Other	• Consider early/preextubation caffeine for infants of <32 weeks' gestation • Wean/discontinue sedation/narcotics prior to extubation

FiO_2, Fraction of inspired oxygen; *SpO_2*, oxygen saturation.

TABLE 23-3 Possible Indications for Intubation and Mechanical Ventilation in Neonates

Indication	Comment
Infant of <26 weeks' gestation	Consider for prophylactic surfactant therapy (NB: recent evidence no longer supports this)
Absent/poor respiratory effort	Inadequate/sporadic effort, poor air entry
Apnea/bradycardia	Refractory; recurrent; requiring PPV
Hypoxemia	FiO_2 > 0.4-0.6 to maintain targeted PaO_2/SpO_2
Hypercarbia	$PaCO_2$ > 60-65 mm Hg with pH < 7.20
Severe distress	Marked retractions on noninvasive support
Suspected airway obstruction	Severe micrognathia, oropharyngeal mass, other
Cardiovascular collapse	Heart rate <60 or shock; CPR
Congenital malformations	Diaphragmatic hernia, choanal atresia, other

PPV, Positive pressure ventilation; *FiO_2*, fraction of inspired oxygen; *PaO_2*, partial pressure arterial oxygen; *SpO_2*, oxygen saturation; *$PaCO_2$*, partial pressure arterial carbon dioxide; *CPR*, cardiopulmonary resuscitation.

lung development. Postnatal viability first becomes possible for the human fetus during the latter phase of the canalicular stage, which occurs between 20 and 28 weeks' gestation, or approximately 50% to 70% gestation. During this stage, rudimentary air sacs begin to form off the terminal airways, simple interstitial capillaries begin to organize around these potential airspaces, and type I and type II epithelial cells begin to differentiate, with type II cells beginning to produce surfactant.[12] It must always be remembered that preterm birth, with subsequent exposure to increased ambient oxygen, unplanned gaseous inflation of the distal airspace, microbial colonization associated with prolonged tracheal intubation, and disturbances in nutrition, initiates a dramatic change in lung growth and development. The effects on lung growth and function, particularly at gestations of <30 weeks, may be lifelong, even for infants not diagnosed with bronchopulmonary dysplasia.[13,14] It is in the context of this immature stage of lung development, and the potential for adverse effects, that the following discussion on ventilatory support for neonatal RDS should be considered.

Relevant Principles of Ventilation

In our neonatal intensive care unit (NICU) we most commonly use high-frequency oscillatory ventilation (HFOV) as the initial mode of support for those infants that require mechanical ventilation for neonatal RDS, at any gestational age. It is important to emphasize that there is no clear evidence that HFOV provides increased benefit (nor risk) compared to more conventional approaches to mechanical ventilation (i.e., volume targeted, surfactant treated) in terms of short-term outcomes such as initial gas exchange and subsequent diagnosis of bronchopulmonary dysplasia (BPD) prior to initial discharge.[15] Our approach to conventional ventilation, which is primarily volume targeted in nature, will also be discussed. Regardless

of the mode of ventilation employed, the primary objective in the management of neonatal RDS is to minimize the initial use and/or duration of exposure to any form of invasive mechanical ventilation through aggressive application of early noninvasive modes of respiratory support (Tables 23-2 and 23-3), as well as the application of written guidelines to promote weaning and extubation from mechanical ventilation when applied (Table 23-4). The key to management includes recognition of the predominant pulmonary pathophysiology, which for RDS is typically a diffuse "alveolar" disease, coupled with the potential to disrupt immature lung development through pathways leading to or associated with VILI.[16-18] The management of the very preterm infant is additionally confounded by the underlying inflammatory milieu that is often present in association with clinical/subclinical chorioamnionitis and impaired intrauterine growth.[19-21] The key to all lung-protective ventilation strategies in infants with diffuse alveolar disease (i.e., diffuse microatelectasis) is the recruitment and maintenance of optimal lung

TABLE 23-4   Guidelines for Recommending Extubation Based on Current Infant Weight, Mode of Ventilatory Support, and Ventilator Settings, Assuming Stable Airway and Minimal Apnea

	WEIGHT (G)			
	<1000	**1000-2000**	**2000-3000**	**>3000**
High-Frequency Ventilation				
$\bar{P}_{aw}$	8	9-10	10-12	12
ΔP/amp	16	18	20	22
FiO$_2$		<0.40		
PC-SIMV and PSV				
PIP	<16	16-20		20
PEEP	<6	<7		<8
PS		<6-8		
FiO$_2$		<0.40		
Rate		16-20 bpm		
SIMV + VG and PSV				
PIP	<16	16-20		20
PEEP	<6	<7		<8
V$_T$		4-5 mL/kg		
PS		<6-8		
FiO$_2$		<0.40		
Rate		16-20 bpm		

FiO$_2$, Fraction of inspired oxygen; *$\bar{P}_{aw}$,* mean airway pressure; *ΔP/amp,* change in pressure (amplitude); *PIP,* peak inspiratory pressure; *PEEP,* positive end-expiratory pressure; *PS,* pressure support; *PC-SIMV,* pressure control–synchronized intermittent mandatory ventilation; *PSV,* pressure support ventilation; *V$_T$,* tidal volume; *VG,* volume guarantee.

inflation and avoidance of excessive tissue stretch. In our NICU, we are more comfortable achieving these goals with HFOV, although similar strategies can be achieved with conventional ventilation.

High-Frequency Ventilation

With HFOV the key is to achieve initial airspace recruitment and then to maintain optimal lung inflation and gas exchange at the lowest acceptable mean airway pressure ($\bar{P}_{aw}$) (Tables 23-5 and 23-6). The process for achieving this goal includes (1) an initial stepwise escalation in $\bar{P}_{aw}$ to recruit atelectatic airspaces indicated by the ability to significantly reduce FiO$_2$ (commonly referred to as the "opening pressure" for the lung); (2) a subsequent stepwise reduction in $\bar{P}_{aw}$ to a point at which FiO$_2$ needs to be again escalated to maintain targeted SpO$_2$ (commonly referred to as the "closing pressure" for the lung); and (3) increasing the $\bar{P}_{aw}$ back above the closing pressure (typically by 2 to 3 cm H$_2$O in surfactant-treated infants) to maintain an end-expiratory lung volume that allows effective gas exchange while minimizing pressure/volume effects on the cardiovascular system, thus "optimizing" oxygen delivery at the tissue/cellular level. A number of studies have described this approach using such measurements as SpO$_2$, respiratory inductance plethysmography, high-resolution computed tomography (CT) scan, and forced oscillatory technique.[22-25] Other than SpO$_2$, these tools are not currently available in most practice settings. We typically provide early surfactant replacement therapy to all preterm infants intubated for RDS

and then begin the process of optimizing lung inflation. We do not usually reduce $\bar{P}_{aw}$ to closing pressure but more commonly will incrementally reduce the $\bar{P}_{aw}$ by 1 to 2 cm H$_2$O once FiO$_2$ has been reduced to <0.25 (Table 23-7). Although radiographic lung volumes may not be ideal for assessing optimal lung inflation, when combined with clinical observations such as heart rate and blood pressure, as well as the temporal changes in FiO$_2$ and SpO$_2$, one can usually maintain adequate lung inflation and gas exchange while minimizing the risks of either overinflation or atelectasis.

Ventilation, or the removal of CO$_2$ during HFOV, is dependent on tidal volume (V$_T$) and rate. As described elsewhere in this book, V$_T$ has a relatively greater effect on minute ventilation than rate. Factors affecting V$_T$ during HFOV include lung compliance and resistance, inspiratory time, and the amplitude or power of the oscillatory breath. It is critical to remember that changes in frequency during HFOV can markedly affect V$_T$ (increased as frequency decreases and decreased as frequency increases). Dynamic changes in lung volume and compliance that accompany increased lung inflation can significantly affect not only oxygenation but also ventilation through effects on V$_T$.[24] As dramatic shifts can occur in Pco$_2$ during HFOV, we recommend either frequent blood gas assessment or transcutaneous Pco$_2$ monitoring during the initial implementation of HFOV, particularly in the most immature infants. As shown in Table 23-7, adjustments in amplitude are more commonly made in response to measured Pco$_2$ than are changes in frequency. We practice a mild permissive hypercarbia approach at all gestational and postnatal ages.[26-28] More pronounced hypercarbia has not been shown to be of benefit in a randomized trial.[29]

Conventional Ventilation

Our approach to conventional ventilator support for neonatal RDS is almost always a volume-targeted, synchronized intermittent mandatory ventilation (SIMV) mode, unless a large (>50%) air leak occurs around the endotracheal tube, in which case we will use a pressure-controlled mode.[30] The same guiding principles should be used in initiating and adjusting support as noted above. Typical initial ventilator settings for SIMV are shown in Tables 23-5 and 23-6. We prefer to initiate support with slightly higher positive end-expiratory pressure (PEEP) values, in the 6- to -8 cm H$_2$O range, in an effort to improve recruitment. Subsequent reductions in PEEP are based on FiO$_2$, SpO$_2$, and chest radiographs. V$_T$s are usually set at around 5 mL/kg; clinical assessment of chest movement as well as analysis of ventilator-derived lung mechanics is performed to ensure V$_T$ is adequate. If a pressure-controlled mode is required, usually due to excessive air leak around the endotracheal tube, we attempt to limit the peak pressure via clinical assessment as well as frequent monitoring of delivered V$_T$ (again targeting volumes of 4 to 6 mL/kg). We employ early caffeine therapy in infants of <32 weeks' gestation and attempt to minimize sedation to encourage spontaneous respiratory efforts. Pressure support is commonly employed to minimize work of breathing, yet encourage diaphragmatic activity, while intubated (Table 23-6).[31] The preference for SIMV is subjective, not evidence based; many other centers use assist/control or pressure support ventilation as the primary mode with equal success.

Extubation

An aggressive approach to weaning and extubation is encouraged. This includes (1) written guidelines for weaning from

TABLE 23-5   Suggested Initial Approach to Mechanical Ventilation by Condition and Ventilatory Mode

Respiratory Disorder	Conventional Ventilation (Volume-Targeted, SIMV+PS, or A/C)	High-Frequency Ventilation
RDS	Surfactant therapy Volume target (V_T) 4-6 mL/kg Rate 30-60 bpm I-time 0.30-0.35 seconds PEEP 5-8 cm H_2O PS to achieve ~¾ set V_T	Surfactant therapy Oscillator: Frequency 8-10 Hz; $\bar{P}_{aw}$ 10-16; ΔP ~2× $\bar{P}_{aw}$—adjust to vibrate chest/abd Jet: Rate 360-420; PEEP as needed to optimize lung inflation (typically 7-10); minimal or no backup rate
MAS	Surfactant therapy; ±iNO V_T 5-6 mL/kg Consider rate ≤30 I-time 0.35-0.50 seconds PEEP 4-7 cm H_2O; set/adjust Based on lung inflation PS to achieve ~¾ set V_T	Surfactant therapy; ±iNO Oscillator: Frequency 6-8 Hz w/ΔP to vibrate chest/abd; $\bar{P}_{aw}$ as needed for ~9 rib lung inflations Jet: Rate 240-360; may need increased I-time; minimal or no backup rate; PEEP as needed Flow interrupter: Rate 240-360; convective rate 6-12; convective I-time ≥1 second; PEEP as needed
Lung hypoplasia/diaphragmatic hernia	V_T 4-5 mL/kg; PIP <26 cm H_2O Rate 40-60 bpm I-time 0.25-0.40 seconds PEEP 4-6 cm H_2O Surfactant only for RDS features	Oscillator: Frequency 8-10 Hz; $\bar{P}_{aw}$ @ 10-13 depending on weight; ΔP ~2× $\bar{P}_{aw}$—adjust to vibrate chest/abd; I:E 33% Jet: Rate 360-420; PEEP 5-8 cm H_2O as needed to optimize lung inflation; minimal/no backup rate
BPD, early/mild–moderate form BPD, chronic–severe form	Volume-targeted: V_T 5-8 mL/kg; rate 20-40 bpm I-time 0.35-0.45 seconds PEEP 5-8 cm H_2O PS to achieve ~¾ set V_T V_T: May need 6-10 mL/kg (or higher) owing to increased dead space I-time 0.50-0.70 seconds; longer to overcome airway resistance Rate 20-30 bpm; slower to allow adequate lung emptying PEEP: Quite variable; may need 8-12 cm H_2O to "stent" airway open	Oscillator: Similar to MAS Jet: Similar to MAS except consider minimal backup rate to optimize lung recruitment HFV not commonly applied for managing chronic–severe BPD; anecdotal reports suggest HFJV used with the "MAS approach" may be more effective than HFOV
PPHN	iNO as indicated Avoid lung hyperinflation, correct atelectasis Adjunct therapies	iNO as indicated Optimize lung inflation, avoid both over- and underinflation Adjunct therapies

ABD, abdomen; *A/C*, Assist/control; *BPD*, bronchopulmonary dysplasia; *HFJV*, high-frequency jet ventilation; *HFOV*, high-frequency oscillatory ventilation; *HFV*, high-frequency ventilation; *I:E*, inspiratory to expiratory ratio; *iNO*, inhaled nitric oxide; *MAS*, meconium aspiration syndrome; $\bar{P}_{aw}$, mean airway pressure; *PEEP*, positive end-expiratory pressure; *PPHN*, persistent pulmonary hypertension of the newborn; *PS*, pressure support; *PIP*, peak inflation pressure; ΔP, change in pressure (amplitude); *RDS*, respiratory distress syndrome; *SIMV*, synchronized intermittent mandatory ventilation; V_T, tidal volume.

TABLE 23-6   Initial Recommended Settings for Mechanical Ventilator Support of Infants with Respiratory Distress Syndrome by Current Weight and Ventilatory Support Mode

	WEIGHT (G)		
Mode	<1000	1000-2500	>2500
HFOV	**Initial Settings**		
Rate	10 Hz	10 Hz	8-10 Hz
$\bar{P}_{aw}$ (cm H_2O)	10-12	10-14	12-16
ΔP	2× $\bar{P}_{aw}$	2× $\bar{P}_{aw}$	2× $\bar{P}_{aw}$
SIMV	**Initial Settings**		
Rate	30-60	30-40	20-40
V_T (mL/kg)	~5	~5	~5
PEEP (cm H_2O)	5-8	5-8	6-9
I-time (s)	Start at 0.3-0.4, adjust PRN based on graphics		
PS (cm H_2O)	Start at 8-12, adjust to ~⅔ PIP for V_T		

HFOV, High-frequency oscillatory ventilation; $\bar{P}_{aw}$, mean airway pressure; ΔP, change in pressure (amplitude); *SIMV*, synchronized intermittent mandatory ventilation; V_T, tidal volume; *PEEP*, positive end-expiratory pressure; *PRN*, as needed; *PS*, pressure support; *PIP*, peak inspiratory pressure.

TABLE 23-7   Recommended Adjustments for High-Frequency Oscillatory Ventilation by Ventilator Parameter Based on Oxygen Requirements and Ventilation

Parameter	Adjustment
Rate	Typically no change in frequency except: ↓ if ΔP > 2-3 × $\bar{P}_{aw}$ ↑ if ΔP < $\bar{P}_{aw}$
$\bar{P}_{aw}$ (cm H_2O)	Increase/decrease as follows based on FiO_2: ↑ by 2-3 if FiO_2 >50% ↑ by 1-2 if FiO_2 25%-50% No change or ↓ by 1 if FiO_2 <25% ↓ by 2-3 after surfactant therapy
ΔP	Increase/decrease based on Pco_2 or $TcPco_2$: ↑ 5-10 if Pco_2 >65 mm Hg ↑ 2-5 if Pco_2 55-65 mm Hg ↓ 2-5 if Pco_2 35-45 mm Hg ↓ 5-10 if Pco_2 <35 mm Hg

ΔP, Change in pressure (amplitude); $\bar{P}_{aw}$, mean airway pressure; *FiO_2*, fraction of inspired oxygen; *Pco_2*, partial pressure of carbon dioxide (capillary or arterial); *TcPco_2*, partial pressure of transcutaneous carbon dioxide.

TABLE 23-8 Recommended Adjustments for Volume-Targeted Synchronized Intermittent Mandatory Ventilation by Ventilator Parameter Based on Oxygen Requirements and Ventilation

Parameter	Adjustment
Rate	Wean rate as tolerated for Pco_2 <50
	Minimum SIMV rate 15-20
V_T (mL/kg)	Wean as indicated for Pco_2 <50
	Do not wean off V_T <4 mL/kg
PEEP (cm H_2O)	Wean as indicated when FiO_2 <0.25
	Follow lung inflation by CXR
	Typically do not wean off <5 cm H_2O
I-time (s)	Typically do not adjust
PS (cm H_2O)	Wean as indicated based on PIP for V_T
	Change to tube compensation if <5 cm H_2O

V_T, Tidal volume; Pco_2, partial pressure of carbon dioxide (capillary or arterial); *PEEP*, positive end-expiratory pressure; *CXR*, chest radiograph; *PS*, pressure support; *PIP*, peak inspiratory pressure; *SIMV*, synchronized intermittent mandatory ventilation.

all modes of mechanical ventilation (Table 23-8); (2) encouragement of active weaning by respiratory therapists as well as physicians and nurse practitioners; (3) written extubation criteria from both conventional ventilation and HFOV; (4) a policy that mandates daily assessment during clinical rounds of whether the infant meets extubation criteria; and (5) promotion of all approaches to noninvasive respiratory support. With this approach we have demonstrated a quality improvement process by which almost 90% of infants who meet criteria can be extubated within 24 hours of doing so, with an overall reduction in ventilator days by 40% and a median duration of mechanical ventilation of <1 day for infants of >27 weeks' gestation.

Evidence-Based Recommendations

The best evidence base for management of RDS includes initial management with noninvasive modes of respiratory support and, for those infants requiring intubation, surfactant replacement therapy.[6,32] There is also good evidence to support the use of a volume-targeted rather than pressure-limited approach to conventional mechanical ventilation.[30] Although there is evidence to support the use of a "lung-protective" approach to mechanical ventilation in adults with RDS,[33] such trials do not exist (and probably would not be undertaken) for neonatal RDS.[17,18] Although we preferentially employ HFOV in the management of neonatal RDS, there is no convincing evidence from randomized controlled trials (RCTs) in the era of surfactant availability and advanced conventional techniques that HFOV using an "open-lung" approach results in improved outcomes compared to lung-protective, volume-targeted approaches via conventional mechanical ventilators.[15]

Gaps in Knowledge

Despite over 50 years of experience with mechanical ventilation in the support of neonates with RDS, there remain important gaps in our knowledge. One of the most important needs is the extension of pulmonary follow-up studies beyond the first few years of life. There is now compelling evidence, primarily from pre-surfactant survivors, that altered lung growth and function may persist into early adulthood, with the potential

to result in significant functional issues as the lung undergoes normal age-related declines in physiologic function.[34] Some studies have suggested that the use of much later functional assessments, rather than the short-term definitions of BPD, supports the early, sustained use of HFOV over more conventional modes of ventilation.[35-37] Nonetheless, at this time there is no clear evidence to that effect, and, when properly employed, one approach cannot be clearly advocated over the other. Additional studies are also needed to evaluate the potential benefits or harms of newer approaches to mechanical ventilator support for neonatal RDS, such as neurally adjusted ventilator assist,[38] and the use of different approaches to early noninvasive support, including high-amplitude bubble CPAP and high-frequency nasal ventilation.[39,40]

MECONIUM ASPIRATION SYNDROME

Although meconium-stained amniotic fluid is a relatively common occurrence, particularly as gestation increases beyond 40 weeks, true meconium aspiration syndrome, or MAS, is relatively infrequent and appears to be decreasing in frequency over the past few decades.[41-44] Despite its relatively low incidence, approximately 50% of infants diagnosed with MAS may require ventilator support.[45-47]

Key Pathophysiologic Features

MAS has a complex, multifactorial pathophysiology that is primarily inflammatory, with a variable obstructive component.[41,42,48,49,50] Key features include altered surfactant metabolism/function, obstruction of the airways, and increased pulmonary vascular resistance and/or reactivity (Fig. 23-1). These components lead to disordered surfactant metabolism and function, epithelial and endothelial membrane injury, and partial or complete obstruction of large and small airways, superimposed on an altered pulmonary vascular bed related to both inflammation and prenatal/postnatal hypoxia–ischemia. Perhaps more than any other neonatal disorder, the clinical features of MAS may be quite variable from one infant to the next and can change fairly rapidly during the course of caring for a single infant. As such, the ventilatory approach must be individualized and frequently assessed based on the predominant pathophysiology at the time. Clinical examination, radiographic features, and echocardiography may all play a role in determining the variable dominant pathophysiologic processes. This section will focus on the ventilatory approach to MAS; other adjunctive therapies may also be indicated, including surfactant replacement, antibiotics, vasodilator use, and antiinflammatory treatments, but will not be discussed in detail.

Surfactant Dysfunction

Disturbances in surfactant metabolism and function lead to decreased compliance of distal airspaces leading to atelectasis and intrapulmonary shunt.[49,51-53] From the perspective of ventilator management, the primary goal is attempting to establish an optimal functional residual volume through recruitment and maintenance of poorly inflated airspaces while attempting to minimize overinflation of unaffected regions of the lung and those areas where airway obstruction predisposes to air trapping. Beyond the use of surfactant replacement therapy in an effort to improve lung compliance, lung inflation is optimized through judicious application of PEEP and/or $\overline{P}_{aw}$.

**Meconium aspiration syndrome
pathophysiology**

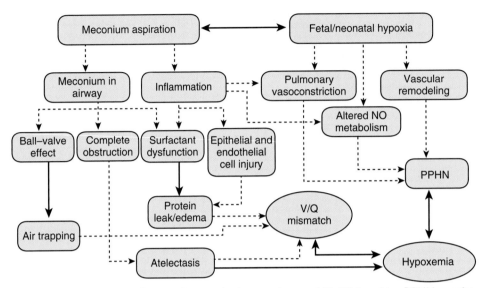

FIG 23-1 Pathophysiology of meconium aspiration syndrome. *NO*, Nitric oxide; *PPHN*, persistent pulmonary hypertension of newborn; *V/Q*, ventilation-perfusion.

Airway Resistance

Severe MAS is often accompanied by elevated airway resistance due to obstruction from inhaled/aspirated meconium.[42,54] In animal models of MAS, there is an early acute phase of near-complete obstruction of the large airways, followed by movement of the meconium into smaller more distal airways.[48,55] Given that the prenatal conditions that typically predispose to MAS are extant well before delivery, the vast majority of neonates with significant MAS have already moved the bulk of any inhaled meconium into the distal airways/airspaces.[41] Typically, aspiration of meconium results in overall increased lung resistance. Given the small diameter of more distal airways, the potential exists for partial or complete obstruction, or a "ball–valve" effect (Fig. 23-2). The former prevents gas from getting into the distal gas-exchange space, leading to atelectasis; the latter allows some gas into the distal airspace but impedes gas from escaping during the exhalation phase, leading to air trapping and overinflation. Saccular overinflation not only directly impairs gas exchange but can also further aggravate oxygenation through compressive effects on the pulmonary microvasculature. It is this combination of disturbed airway mechanics coupled with surfactant dysfunction creating a nonhomogeneous lung disease that makes severe MAS so difficult to manage.

Pulmonary Hypertension

Unlike most other neonatal lung disorders, pulmonary hypertension is a common and significant problem in infants with severe MAS.[56-58] Fetal hypoxemia and inflammation are thought to be primary contributors to underlying pulmonary hypertension.[48,49,58-60] Abnormalities in nitric oxide metabolism contribute to the underlying dysfunction in pulmonary vasomotor tone.[58,61,62] As noted previously, air trapping and compression of the pulmonary vascular bed can also contribute to pulmonary hypertension. Adjunctive therapy with inhaled nitric oxide (NO) and other pulmonary vasodilators, as well as inotropic support of the systemic vascular system, may be required for management of the pulmonary hypertension.

Relevant Principles of Ventilation

Although we most commonly use HFOV, other approaches to high-frequency ventilation (HFV) and/or volume-targeted conventional ventilation can be used in the initial management of MAS (Tables 23-5 and 23-9). The key to management includes recognition of the predominant underlying pulmonary pathophysiology. While the majority of infants with MAS do not require ventilator support, those infants that do are usually quite ill and often have a mixed pattern of both over- and underinflated lung segments, as well as severe persistent pulmonary hypertension of the newborn (PPHN).

High-Frequency Ventilation

With HFOV the key to success is to use a lower rate, typically 6 to 8 Hz, and to set the initial $\overline{P}_{aw}$ based on the overall pattern of lung inflation. For infants with significant air trapping we start at 6 Hz with a $\overline{P}_{aw}$ similar to that on conventional ventilation. Amplitude, or ΔP, is then adjusted to generate vibration of the chest to midabdomen. This approach provides a slightly greater oscillatory V_T and longer expiratory phase, both of which lead to improved ventilation. For those infants with MAS who have relatively poor lung inflation, the $\overline{P}_{aw}$ is typically started at 3 to 5 cm H_2O above that on conventional ventilation. Subsequent adjustments in $\overline{P}_{aw}$ are made based on FiO_2 response and radiographic assessment of lung inflation. In most babies with MAS we typically adjust amplitude, not frequency, to further affect ventilation. If high-frequency jet ventilation (HFJV) is employed, it is important to use a lower rate (in the range of 240 to 360 cycles per minute) as exhalation is passive and air trapping is a significant risk if the rate is too high. On occasion it may be helpful to minimally increase the inspiratory time (I-time) (from 0.02 to 0.03 seconds) to gain increased V_T with high-frequency pulses. When employing HFJV, a backup rate

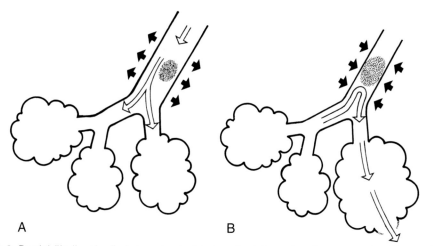

FIG 23-2 Partial "ball–valve" air trapping behind particulate matter (i.e., meconium) in an airway, which leads to alveolar overexpansion and rupture. **(A)** Tidal gas passes beyond the meconium on inspiration when the airway dilates, but **(B)** cannot exit on expiration when airways constrict. (From Goldsmith JP. Continuous positive airway pressure and conventional mechanical ventilation in the treatment of meconium aspiration syndrome. *J Perinatol.* 2008;28(suppl 3):S49-S55; used with permission.)

TABLE 23-9 Suggested Initial Approach to Ventilator Support of Meconium Aspiration Syndrome by Ventilatory Mode and Suspected Underlying Pathophysiology

Ventilatory Approach	Airway Obstruction w/Gas Trapping	Alveolar Disease w/Low Lung Volumes	Pulmonary Hypertension
Pathophysiology	↑ Resistance ↑ Time constant ↑ Lung volumes	↓ Surfactant function ↓ Compliance ↑ V/Q mismatch	↓ NOS Hypoxemia Acidosis
Conventional (SIMV)			
Pressure-controlled	PIP to move chest; lower I-time ≤30; PEEP 4-6 cm H$_2$O; PS ~⅔ set PIP	Surfactant therapy; monitor lung volume; higher PEEP as needed to maintain EELV	iNO; SpO$_2$ 92%-98%; consider other vasodilator therapy; optimize sedation
Volume-targeted	V$_T$ 5-6 mL/kg; limit rate to ≤30; PEEP 4-6 cm H$_2$O; PS to achieve ~¾ set V$_T$	Same as above	Same as above
High Frequency			
Oscillatory	Hz 6-8 ΔP vibrate chest/abd	$\bar{P}_{aw}$ as needed for 9 rib lung expansion	Same as above
Jet	HF rate 240-360 May need ↑ I-time Minimal/no backup rate	PEEP as needed for 9 rib lung expansion; backup rate 2-5	Same as above
Flow interrupter	HF rate 240-360 Convective rate 6-10	PEEP as above Set convective I-time close to 1 second	Same as above

NOS, Nitric oxide synthase; *V/Q,* ventilation-perfusion; *SIMV,* synchronized intermittent mandatory ventilation; *PIP,* peak inspiratory pressure; *PEEP,* positive end-expiratory pressure; *PS,* pressure support; *V$_T$,* tidal volume; *EELV,* end-expiratory lung volume; *iNO,* inhaled nitric oxide; *SpO$_2$,* oxygen saturation; *ΔP,* change in pressure (amplitude); $\bar{P}_{aw}$, mean airway pressure; *HF,* high frequency.

may be helpful if some element of lung recruitment is indicated, using V$_T$ inflations rather than large increases in PEEP. However, backup conventional sighs should be set at a relatively low frequency, typically two to five breaths per minute (bpm) (see Tables 23-5 and 23-9). On occasion we also use the Bird VDR-4 for high-frequency flow interruption. Though not as "user friendly" as other neonatal ventilators, this device can be quite effective to aid in the removal of airway secretions for infants with large amounts of airway meconium. It is important to again remember that exhalation is passive, and

thus lower rates (240 to 360) should be used to minimize risk of air trapping. Typically we use convective inflations between 5 and 10 bpm and set the I-time for convective inflations close to 1 second (see Tables 23-5 and 23-9).

Conventional Ventilation

We almost always use a volume-targeted, SIMV-based approach to conventional ventilator support (see Tables 23-5 and 23-9). The same guiding principles should be used in initiating and adjusting support as noted above. When air trapping is the predominant pathologic problem, it is more often caused by dynamic PEEP due to insufficient expiratory time. Set PEEP should be limited (typically ≤6 cm H_2O) and the ventilator rate should be kept relatively low (typically ≤30 bpm), with shorter I-times to ensure adequate expiratory time to minimize gas trapping. However, because both inspiratory and expiratory time constants are prolonged, the inspiratory times must be adequate to achieve complete V_T delivery. For infants in whom the predominant pathology is alveolar disease with low lung volumes due to surfactant inactivation, PEEP should initially be set at higher levels (6 to 8 cm H_2O) and adjusted as needed to achieve an acceptable end-expiratory lung volume. We also commonly use pressure support to assist spontaneous breaths with a goal of support between two-thirds and three-quarters the set pressure/V_T of the SIMV inflations. Because the pathophysiology of MAS includes increased alveolar dead space, these infants require slightly larger V_T/kg than similar infants with more homogeneous lung disease.[63]

Irrespective of the ventilatory approach used, frequent clinical, radiographic, and laboratory assessments are indicated to optimize gas exchange and minimize VILI. This monitoring is even more important following surfactant therapy and during the initial 12 to 24 hours of support as the predominant pathophysiology can and does change quickly.

Evidence-Based Recommendations

There is a very limited "evidence" base to support the multiple management schemes employed for MAS. Although numerous trials have been conducted comparing different modes of conventional ventilation, or conventional to high-frequency ventilation, in term and preterm neonates with respiratory failure, no randomized trials have specifically compared different approaches to mechanical ventilation in a population of babies limited to a diagnosis of MAS. Therefore, the use of SIMV rather than assist/control (A/C) is a matter of practice style preference, not specifically evidence based, although it could be argued that there may be greater potential for air trapping with A/C. There is increasing evidence from RCTs involving mechanically ventilated infants diagnosed with MAS related to the potential benefit of surfactant therapy (including bolus and lavage approaches)[64-66] as well as early corticosteroid therapy (including systemic and inhaled approaches).[67,68] There is evidence that HFV may improve the effectiveness of inhaled NO by promoting optimal lung inflation.[69]

Gaps in Knowledge

Although the evidence related to the benefits of surfactant therapy is compelling, additional studies are needed to better define the optimal at-risk population, timing, and dose of this therapy. Trials of corticosteroid therapy are relatively few and small; additional trials are needed to further clarify the overall benefit to risk effect of this intervention. The complete lack of RCTs comparing different approaches to ventilatory support in babies diagnosed with MAS (such as pressure-controlled versus volume-targeted, SIMV versus A/C, conventional ventilation versus HFV, or HFOV versus HFJV) leaves a large gap in our knowledge about optimal ventilator management of this group of patients. Given the overall decreasing incidence of MAS and the relatively limited number of babies diagnosed with MAS who require mechanical ventilation, such studies may never be carried out, but at a minimum will require a multicenter approach.

TABLE 23-10	**Published "Protocols" for Management of Neonates with Congenital Diaphragmatic Hernia**[70-74]	
Ventilator Mode	**Conventional**	**High-Frequency Oscillation**
Peak pressure/ΔP	<25-26 cm H_2O	30-50
PEEP	2-5 cm H_2O	N/A
$\bar{P}_{aw}$	<12 cm H_2O	13-17 cm H_2O
Rate	40-60 bpm	10 Hz
I-time/I:E	0.30 s	1:1
PaCO$_2$	45-65 mm Hg	45-65 mm Hg
PaO$_2$ Preductal	60-80 mm Hg	60-80 mm Hg
Postductal	>30 mm Hg	>30 mm Hg
SpO$_2$ Preductal	85%-95%	85%-95%
Postductal	>70%	>70%
Chest radiograph	~8 ribs contralateral lung	~8 ribs contralateral lung

ΔP, Change in pressure (amplitude); *PEEP*, positive end-expiratory pressure; $\bar{P}_{aw}$, mean airway pressure; *I:E*, inspiratory to expiratory ratio; *PaCO$_2$*, partial pressure arterial carbon dioxide; *PaO$_2$*, partial pressure arterial oxygen; *SpO$_2$*, oxygen saturation.

CONGENITAL DIAPHRAGMATIC HERNIA AND LUNG HYPOPLASIA DISORDERS

Congenital diaphragmatic hernia (CDH) has remained one of the most challenging and frustrating major birth defects to manage. Since 1995, a number of treatment strategies have evolved, but there have been no large RCTs targeted specifically to the postnatal management of neonates with CDH. Despite this fact, a general consensus related to a few specific management concepts has emerged (Table 23-10).[70,71] First, the existence of a specific set of guidelines targeting early neonatal care of CDH infants is associated with improved center-specific survival.[70-73] Second, despite the absence of a clear evidence base, there is general agreement that immediate surgical repair of the diaphragmatic defect is not only unnecessary but probably detrimental.[74-77] However, specific indications for optimal timing of repair remain unclear.[78,79] Third, adoption of a gentle approach to ventilator support has been associated with reported improvements in morbidity and mortality.[80-82] However, it is unclear what the best ventilation mode is to provide gentle support. It was hoped that information from a large RCT comparing initial ventilator support with high-frequency oscillation to volume-targeted conventional ventilation would help provide answers to this question.[74] However, that study was terminated early for slow enrollment and failed to identify a significant difference in CDH outcome related to the initial ventilator mode.

Key Pathophysiologic Features
Lung Hypoplasia
The most obvious pathophysiologic problem for the infant with CDH is impaired lung growth, primarily due to the space-occupying effect of abdominal viscera in the thoracic cavity. It is probable that not only the volume of abdominal organ herniation, but also how early in gestation herniation occurs, compromises lung liquid formation, and developmental defects in lung morphogenesis also contribute to the severity of lung hypoplasia.[83,84] This is evidenced by the association of decreased survival as diaphragmatic defect size increases[85] and improved survival with fetal tracheal occlusion for severe lung hypoplasia based

on very low lung-to-head ratios.[86] In addition to decreased lung size, there also appear to be altered lung development and disturbances in surfactant metabolism of both the ipsilateral and the contralateral lung with CDH,[87-91] though not all investigators agree on the adverse effects of CDH on surfactant stores or metabolism.[92] The specific mechanisms for development of the diaphragmatic defect remain unclear and are beyond the scope of this chapter. The use of animal models has contributed greatly to the understanding of possible molecular and genetic factors that may be associated with CDH, and the reader is referred to other reviews for more information.[93-95]

Pulmonary Vascular Bed

Given that angiogenesis and vasculogenesis of the pulmonary circulation and capillary network are closely linked, impaired vascular development accompanies the altered lung growth found in CDH.[96] A variety of pulmonary vascular abnormalities have been described in animal models and neonates with CDH, including impaired growth and development of pulmonary arteries and arterioles as well as increased arteriolar medial muscle thickness,[97,98] altered expression of angiogenic factors including vascular endothelial growth factor,[99-101] decreased endothelial NO synthase expression,[102,103] impaired response to NO metabolites,[104] increased expression and activity of phosphodiesterase 5,[105] and increased expression/levels of endothelin-1 and endothelin receptor A.[106,107] The effect of decreased vascular growth and impaired endothelial cell function is an impaired pulmonary vascular response at birth to inflation and oxygen. Additionally, the postnatal response to inhaled NO (iNO) also appears to be impaired.[108,109] PPHN continues to be a major contributor to the continuing relatively high mortality rate among infants with CDH, with limited improvement since 1995 despite a variety of new therapeutic approaches.[110-113]

Cardiac Development

Often overlooked in the pathophysiology of CDH is the contribution related to impaired growth and function of the left ventricle (LV).[114-116] The severity of the LV hypoplasia correlates with the severity of the diaphragmatic defect/hernia and appears to be more significant in left-sided compared to right-sided defects.[117] Some investigators have suggested that significant LV dysfunction related to the hypoplasia contributes to postnatal PPHN through increased pulmonary venous congestion and have recommended against early iNO use to minimize this problem.[118] Despite the apparent impact of left-sided CDH on LV growth and function, and suggested treatment with a variety of vasoactive therapies, no controlled trials have been performed to determine the optimal approach for management of this problem.[110,112,119-121]

Relevant Principles of Ventilation

Since 2005 there has been a general acceptance of using a "lung-sparing" or "gentle" approach to mechanical ventilation of neonates with CDH.[70-72,81,82] Most developed protocols initially employ conventional ventilation, with recommended ventilator settings as shown in Table 23-10. In our NICU we use HFOV as the initial mode of support for all infants with CDH (Table 23-11), an approach that has evolved since 1995.[122] Differences in our initial support parameters for HFOV compared to those established for the VICI Trial[74] include (1) we initiate HFOV with a lower $\bar{P}_{aw}$, usually 12 cm H_2O, and limit initial maximum $\bar{P}_{aw}$ to <16 cm H_2O; (2) we often start at a

---

TABLE 23-11 Recommended Initial Ventilator Settings for Neonates with Congenital Diaphragmatic Hernia

	HFOV	HFJV	SIMV-A/C
ΔP/PIP	24-28	20-25 cm H_2O	V_T 4-5 mL/kg
Max PIP		30 cm H_2O	≤25 cm H_2O
$\bar{P}_{aw}$/PEEP	11-13 cm H_2O	11-13/6-8 cm H_2O	4-6 cm H_2O
Max $\bar{P}_{aw}$	≤16 cm H_2O	≤16 cm H_2O	
Frequency	8-10 Hz	360-420 bpm	40-60 bpm
I:E/I-time	1:2	0.02 seconds	0.3 seconds
FiO₂	Goal <0.50	Goal <0.50	Goal <0.50
SpO₂ Preductal			
First hour	>80%	>80%	>80%
Goal	92%-98%	92%-98%	92%-98%
"Tolerated"	>90%	>90%	>90%
PaCO₂			
Goal	45-55 mm Hg	45-55 mm Hg	45-55 mm Hg
"Tolerated"	<65 mm Hg	<65 mm Hg	<65 mm Hg
Chest X-ray	9-10 rib inflation contralateral lung	9-10 rib inflation contralateral lung	9-10 rib inflation contralateral lung

HFOV, High-frequency oscillatory ventilation; *HFJV,* high-frequency jet ventilation; *SIMV,* synchronized intermittent mandatory ventilation; *A/C,* assist/control; ΔP, change in pressure (amplitude); V_T, tidal volume; *PIP,* peak inspiratory pressure; $\bar{P}_{aw}$, mean airway pressure; *PEEP,* positive end-expiratory pressure; *I:E,* inspiratory to expiratory ratio; *FiO₂,* fraction of inspired oxygen; *SpO₂,* oxygen saturation; *PaCO₂,* partial pressure arterial carbon dioxide.

BOX 23-1 Recommended Respiratory Support Parameters for Consideration of Operative Repair of Congenital Diaphragmatic Hernia

Infant "stable" for at least 24 hours as follows:
- FiO₂ <0.50 with SpO₂ ≥92%
- $\bar{P}_{aw}$ <16 cm H_2O and ΔP <30
- PaCO₂ <55 mm Hg
- PA pressures ≤2/3 systemic (TR jet <3.0 m/s)

Note: If calculated oxygenation index is consistently <7.0 for >24 hours and persistent pulmonary hypertension of the newborn is stable, survival following operative repair is >98%.

FiO₂, Fraction of inspired oxygen; *SpO₂,* oxygen saturation; $\bar{P}_{aw}$, mean airway pressure; ΔP, change in pressure (amplitude); *PaCO₂,* partial pressure of arterial carbon dioxide; *PA,* pulmonary artery; *TR,* tricuspid regurgitation; *OI,* oxygenation index; *PPHN,* persistent pulmonary hypertension of newborn.

---

lower frequency, typically at 8 Hz; (3) we use an I:E ratio of 1:2 rather than 1:1; and (4) we attempt to maintain contralateral lung inflation at 9 or 10 ribs rather than 8. It is important to emphasize that there is no clear evidence that HFOV provides increased benefit (or risk) compared to HFJV or conventional mechanical ventilation, nor is there evidence to support a specific approach to HFOV, such as the one presented here, compared to that recommended in the VICI Trial. More recently others have published observational or retrospective studies describing their approaches to the initial use of HFOV in the management of neonatal CDH.[76,123-125] We typically continue support with HFOV until after repair of the diaphragm, which is most often performed in the NICU (Box 23-1).

For infants with minimal evidence of respiratory compromise we may change to conventional ventilation using a volume-targeted approach (Table 23-11), and these more stable infants more often go to the operating room for repair. Though the use of HFJV has been reported by other investigators, most often it has been used as a rescue therapy in lieu of HFOV, and the parameters employed have not been well described.[126,127] There is clinical evidence to suggest that HFJV may be the optimal approach for ventilation of babies with CDH with an ability to ventilate using small V_T and lower $\bar{P}_{aw}$ while minimizing adverse cardiovascular effects.[128] Initial settings we employ for the application of HFJV to infants with CDH are shown in Table 23-11.

Irrespective of the ventilatory approach used for managing CDH, several key concepts must be kept in mind. First, the lung is small, with a functional residual capacity that may be considerably less than normal.[129] Given the effects that both atelectasis and hyperinflation have on pulmonary microvasculature and vascular resistance, careful attention must be paid to optimizing lung inflation.[130] In that regard, the $\bar{P}_{aw}$ needed to achieve optimal lung inflation may be less than that required for a normal-sized lung, even with the reported surfactant abnormalities. Second, it is considerably more difficult to determine optimal $\bar{P}_{aw}$ and lung inflation under conditions of lung hypoplasia with minimal to no surfactant dysfunction than for infants with diffuse alveolar disease. Attempting to employ the stepwise increase in $\bar{P}_{aw}$ as suggested under the RDS section is not recommended in babies with CDH as it is too easy to provide a higher $\bar{P}_{aw}$ than is necessary without any identifiable improvement in oxygenation, particularly with the underlying issue of pulmonary hypertension. An alternate, but unproven, approach is to start at a lower $\bar{P}_{aw}$ and gradually adjust upward based on radiographic lung inflation. Third, though the minute ventilation necessary to achieve eucarbia should be the same as for infants with normal lungs, use of a V_T on the higher end of normal (i.e., 6 mL/kg) may have greater risk for initiating lung injury secondary to inadvertent volutrauma in hypoplastic lungs.[131] The fact that studies by Landolfo and Sharma[129,132] report relatively normal to high V_T to achieve effective ventilation should not be taken to indicate that $V_T > 5$ mL/kg ought to be employed in babies with CDH. It is unclear, however, whether higher rates (i.e., 60 bpm) and lower V_T (4 mL/kg) or higher V_T (6 mL/kg) at lower rates has any difference in short- or long-term outcomes for CDH. However, given the decreased complement of alveoli in this condition, physiologic V_T of 5 mL/kg would probably result in volutrauma, as this volume is directed into a fraction of the normal number of terminal airspace units; this reality provides a sound physiologic rationale for the use of HFV in infants with CDH.[132] In this context it is also important to note that those infants with the greatest degree of lung hypoplasia have increased dead space-to-V_T ratios, suggesting that more of the applied V_T is lost as ineffective dead space ventilation.[133] Last, oxygenation is dependent as much on the impaired pulmonary vascular bed as it is on relative lung volumes. Adjustments in ventilator support must be made with the recognition that altered oxygenation could be due to increased pulmonary vascular resistance related to factors other than changes in ventilator support.

Pulmonary Hypertension

The management of pulmonary hypertension in lung hypoplasia disorders remains controversial.[110,112,113] There are no large RCTs demonstrating short- or long-term benefit for many of

TABLE 23-12   Potential Vasodilator Therapies Considered for Management of Pulmonary Hypertension in Infants with Congenital Diaphragmatic Hernia

Therapy	Mechanism	Comments
Lung "specific"		*No proven benefit by RCTs*
Inhaled NO[138]	↑ cGMP production	Commonly used
Sildenafil[130]	PDE5 inhibitor; ↓ cGMP breakdown	Often used later in course
Inhaled PGI2[140]	↑ cAMP production	Highly alkaline
"Nonspecific"		*No proven benefit by RCTs*
Milrinone[141]	PDE3 inhibitor; ↓ cAMP breakdown	Vasodilator, inotrope, lusitrope
Intravenous PGI2[140]	↑ cAMP production	Systemic effect; hypotension
Bosentan[142]	Blocks endothelin receptors	Potential hepatotoxicity
Norepinephrine[143]	2× activation; ? ↑ NO production	↑ SVR:PVR ratio
Vasopressin[144]	? ↑ NO production	↑ SVR:PVR ratio
Intravenous PGE1[123]	Inhibits cyclooxygenase	PDA "off-loads" RV
Cinaciguat[145]	↑ cGMP; activates soluble guanylate cyclase	No use in neonates to date

NO, nitric oxide; *PGI2*, prostaglandin I2 (prostacyclin); *cGMP*, cyclic guanosine monophosphate; *cAMP*, cyclic adenosine monophosphate; *RCT*, randomized controlled trial; *PDE*, phosphodiesterase; *SVR:PVR*, systemic-to-pulmonary vascular resistance; *PDA*, patent ductus arteriosus; *RV*, right ventricle; *PGE1*, prostaglandin E1.

the approaches that have been used, including iNO[108,110-113] (Table 23-12).[119,134-141] The reader is referred to Chapters 32 and 33 of this book and to review articles for a more thorough discussion of therapeutic approaches to PPHN.[58,111,118,134] As previously noted, a critical component of PPHN management in all neonatal lung conditions includes optimization of lung inflation.[25,122,128,130,142] Currently, there is no proven clinical approach to such lung optimization for infants with lung hypoplasia/CDH. The combination of clinical examination, monitoring indices of gas exchange, and serial chest radiographs is most commonly used.

Evidence-Based Recommendations

There is almost no evidence base for clinical management of CDH.[70,71,112,143] The few randomized trials that have been performed, such as for "delayed operative repair,"[75] include only small numbers of infants and were done prior to the current era in which gentle ventilation is almost uniformly employed. Though a wide range of therapies are employed for management of PPHN, none of these approaches has been systematically studied in babies with CDH, and as of this writing the most recent reports suggest that anecdotal use has not been associated with improved outcomes in large study populations.[110,112,113]

Gaps in Knowledge

Nearly all approaches to ventilatory and cardiovascular support of newborns with CDH require systematic investigation. There is a uniform consensus that gentle ventilation improves outcomes, though the optimal approach and device remain unclear. Identifying better clinical tools to determine optimal lung inflation,

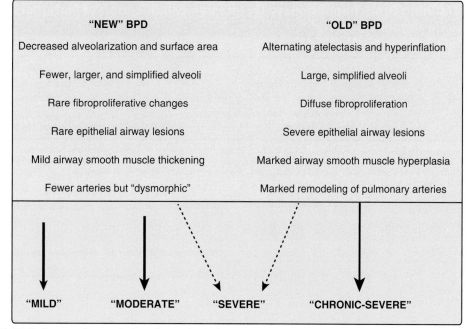

FIG 23-3 Contrasting pathology for and relative association with definitions of bronchopulmonary dysplasia (BPD): "old" (pre-surfactant era) versus "new" (post-surfactant era).

such as the forced oscillatory technique,[25] should be investigated in babies with CDH. Another area of interest is the optimal preductal/postductal saturation to target; many centers still target a higher SpO$_2$, whereas others suggest that a lower preductal SpO$_2$ may be reasonable. Finally, in addition to postnatal studies, investigations of maternal–fetal interventions to improve lung growth and/or vascular development should be continued or developed. A number of investigations related to fetal tracheal occlusion are ongoing.[144] Animal investigations suggest that pharmacologic approaches may also be an option to improve fetal lung and vascular development in CDH.[145-147]

BRONCHOPULMONARY DYSPLASIA*

BPD is the most common morbidity affecting surviving preterm infants, described in various studies at rates of over 40% for infants of <29 weeks' gestation.[148-151] Efforts have been made to differentiate the "old" form of BPD, first described clinically by Northway and colleagues in 1967,[152] from a "new" form of BPD suggested from human and animal studies in the 1990s[153-155] (Fig. 23-3). The epidemiology of BPD has clearly changed over time, with the vast majority of infants diagnosed with BPD now at <29 weeks and <1000 g birth weight, and most probably being of the new BPD variant with underlying impaired alveolarization.[148-151] Nonetheless, though much less common, preterm infants with an underlying pathophysiology consistent with old BPD continue to survive with severe chronic respiratory failure.[151,156] Any effort to discuss the ventilatory approach to BPD must take into consideration the wide range of clinical variability and diagnostic criteria used to make this

diagnosis[155,157,158] (Table 23-13). Infants diagnosed with mild BPD may require supplemental oxygen for only the first few weeks of life, whereas infants with severe–chronic BPD continue to require positive pressure support beyond 36 to 40 weeks of postmenstrual age. These represent distinctly different ends of the BPD spectrum. Additionally, in the context of BPD care it is important to differentiate approaches aimed at prevention of BPD from the management of established severe–chronic lung disease. This section will focus on the latter group of patients, requiring ongoing ventilator support beyond the initial weeks of life and extending into the first year or beyond. Approaches designed to prevent or ameliorate BPD are discussed elsewhere in this chapter as well as in other chapters throughout this book. Also not specifically addressed in this chapter is the important concept that management of the infant with severe BPD is best served through a multidisciplinary approach to care including primary/specialized nursing and respiratory therapy support, neonatal nutritionists, and occupational/physical therapists. Additionally, other pediatric subspecialty providers may need to be members of the care team for infants with severe BPD, including pulmonology, cardiology, radiology, and otolaryngology, as well as pediatric surgery.

Key Pathophysiologic Features

Infants with established chronic lung disease are very different from premature newborns with RDS and those with mild BPD, requiring an individualized approach based on the underlying pathophysiology of the lung (Table 23-14). Other important factors to consider in their overall management include nutritional approaches,[159] assessment for pulmonary hypertension,[160] and the possible influence of gastroesophageal reflux and aspiration on injury to the airway and lung parenchyma.[161,162]

Lung Pathology

Abnormalities are well described for both the airways and the gas exchange areas of the lungs (Table 23-14). The most notable

---

*Editor's Note: The reader is referred to Chapter 35 for a detailed discussion of the management of BPD. Although the management recommendations in both chapters are in general agreement on key principles, there is some variation in the specific recommendations, reflecting the paucity of high-quality evidence in this population.

TABLE 23-13   Defining Bronchopulmonary Dysplasia—Modification of National Institutes of Health Consensus Conference Criteria[206]

Gestational Age–Birth	<32 weeks	≥32 weeks
Assessment age	36 weeks' PMA, or D/C to home	>28 but <56 days' postnatal age, or D/C to home
"Mild"	In room air at 36 weeks, or D/C to home	In room air by 56 days' age, or D/C to home
"Moderate"	FiO₂ >21% but <30% at 36 weeks' PMA, or D/C to home	FiO₂ >21% but <30% at 56 days' age, or D/C to home
"Severe"*	FiO₂ >30% ± NIV# at 36 weeks' PMA, or D/C to home	FiO₂ >30% ± NIV# at 56 days' age, or D/C to home
"Severe–chronic"*	Need for ventilator support at 36 weeks' PMA	Need for ventilator support at 56 days' age

*The NIH Consensus Conference definition describes only "severe bronchopulmonary dysplasia"; in this table those babies continuing to require mechanical ventilator support are differentiated from those with increased FiO₂ need and/or other higher level noninvasive support (NIV#, positive pressure support including nasal ventilation, nasal, continuous positive airway pressure, or high-flow NC > 2 Lpm). *PMA*, Postmenstrual age; *D/C*, discharge; *FiO₂*, fraction of inspired oxygen; *NC*, nasal cannula.

TABLE 23-14   Pathophysiology of the Lung in Bronchopulmonary Dysplasia

Respiratory Site	Issues
Upper Airways	
Glottis	Arytenoid inflammation/edema
Trachea	Subglottic stenosis; malacia
	Infection
Bronchus	Granuloma/stenosis
	Stenosis
	Malacia
Small/lower airways	Hyperplasia of epithelium and mucous glands
	Bronchoconstriction/increased secretions
	Associated vasculature
	Smooth muscle hypertrophy
	Increased reactivity/tonic constriction
Distal airspace	Alveolization
	Decreased gas exchange surface area
	Hypoxemia
	Capillary/vascular growth
	Impaired growth
	Increased vascular resistance
	Risk for pulmonary hypertension
	Heterogeneous lungs (focal atelectasis/hyperinflation)
	Increased ventilation/perfusion shunt

TABLE 23-15   Abnormalities of Lung Function among Infants with Bronchopulmonary Dysplasia

Parameter	Abnormality
Lung Volume	
Overall lung volume	Decreased[166-168]
Functional residual volume	Decreased[169-173]
Compliance	Reduced[170-172]
Gas exchange	Impaired diffusion[164,166-168]
Airway Function	
Expiratory flow velocity	Decreased[168-172]
Resistance	Increased[170-172]

features include interrupted alveolarization with reduced number and increased size of the remaining saccular–alveolar structures, thickened mesenchymal/septal tissues, disrupted growth and development of the pulmonary microvasculature, and varying degrees of fibrosis.[153-155,163,164] More severe changes in airway pathology, similar to that reported in pre-surfactant era old BPD, can be seen in infants requiring prolonged ventilatory support, though this appears to be relatively uncommon among infants with new BPD.[153-155,163] Additionally, infants with more severe forms of BPD may often have impaired cartilaginous development of the large and small airways, leading to tracheo/bronchomalacia.[165]

Lung Mechanics and Function

Decreased lung volumes and alveolar surface area resulting from the interrupted alveolarization and accompanying reduced lung microvasculature lead to impaired gas exchange[164,166-168] (Table 23-15). Most studies report decreased lung compliance in infants with BPD, though this may not be sustained into later life.[169-171] Among infants with more severe forms of BPD,

heterogeneous lung disease with regions of atelectasis and air trapping can also impair oxygenation owing to increased ventilation/perfusion mismatch and intrapulmonary shunts.[158] Increased resistance related to airway injury can contribute to the air trapping noted above affecting ventilation.[169-173] Failure to adjust V_T owing to increased physiologic dead space also may impair gas exchange.[174]

Relevant General Principles of Mechanical Ventilation

Even among infants with less severe forms of BPD there is increased anatomic and functional dead space. Thus, mild increases in delivered V_T may be necessary to achieve reasonable ventilation goals (PCO_2 values in the range of 45 to 55 mm Hg for arterial samples and 50 to 65 mm Hg for capillary samples).[174] In the developing stages of BPD, beyond 7 to 14 days of age but prior to several weeks of age, the optimal approach to ventilator support is fairly similar to that recommended for the management of RDS (Table 23-5). The exception may be the above-mentioned need for some increase in V_T (Table 23-16). With more chronic, severe forms of BPD, the severity of airway disease and more heterogeneous saccular–alveolar disease significantly changes the approach to ventilatory support (Table 23-16). With chronic–severe BPD even higher V_T may be needed, sometimes as high as 10 to 12 mL/kg. There are several potential reasons for this: (1) similar to infants with milder forms of BPD, there is interrupted/impaired alveolarization with reduced gas exchange surface area; (2) nonheterogeneous lung disease is accompanied by increasing nonfunctional lung volume due to increased areas of atelectasis coupled with areas of overinflation (increased alveolar dead space) and (3) dilatation of the large airways due

TABLE 23-16 **Suggested Approaches to Mechanical Ventilation for Infants Diagnosed with Bronchopulmonary Dysplasia (BPD) Based on Relative Severity of BPD**

Mild/Moderate BPD	Chronic–Severe BPD
Tidal volume (V_T) 5-8 mL/kg	V_T: May need 6-10 mL/kg due to increased dead space
I-time 0.35-0.45 seconds	I-time: 0.4-0.6 seconds; longer to overcome inspiratory airway resistance (?)
PEEP to "optimize" lung inflation	Rate: 20-30 bpm, to allow adequate lung emptying during exhalation
Pressure support ~¾ V_T	PEEP: Quite variable; often 8-10 needed to "stent" airway open
Rate 20-40 based on infant effort	SpO_2 goals: 92%-98%
SpO_2 goals: 88%-98% based on GA	Target $PaCO_2$: 50-60 torr
Target $PaCO_2$: 45-60 torr	

PEEP, Positive end-expiratory pressure; *SpO₂*, oxygen saturation; *GA*, gestational age; *PaCO₂*, partial pressure of arterial carbon dioxide.

to exposure to cyclic stretch from positive pressure ventilation (acquired tracheomegaly);[175] and (4) there may be loss of V_T related to expansion of floppy large airways and/or to back-pressure leakage around the endotracheal tube related to high airway resistance. Increased airway resistance should be managed via longer inspiratory times to allow for more complete distribution of V_T. Additionally, modification of the slope of gas delivery from a square-wave form to a more bell-shaped form may also improve the flow of gas through these airways. Owing to the local and/or regional abnormalities in airway resistance and airspace compliance, a longer expiratory time is also needed for the multicompartmental BPD lung to effectively empty during the exhalation phase. Thus the combination of higher V_T, longer inspiratory times, and low rates (allowing for increased exhalation time) is indicated for infants who remain ventilator dependent with more chronic–severe forms of BPD. Finally, both tracheal and bronchomalacia can develop in infants with chronic–severe BPD.[165,176] For infants with these lesions, increased PEEP levels are required to prevent closure of the larger airways prior to complete exhalation of the inspired V_T.[177,178] At times we have used PEEP as high as 14 cm H_2O to prevent airway collapse, improve expiratory airway mechanics, and reduce trapped gas lung volumes. However, the application of high PEEP must be used cautiously because of the potential to further aggravate areas of localized/regional lung overinflation. At times additional diagnostic studies may prove useful in helping to define both the severity of heterogeneous lung disease and the presence/location of significant airway lesions, including endoscopy[165,176] and dynamic high-resolution spiral CT scans.[179,180] Other evaluations that may be considered for infants with chronic–severe BPD include pulmonary function testing, an echocardiogram or cardiac catheterization to evaluate for pulmonary hypertension, and testing for gastroesophageal reflux and aspiration. In select cases we have obtained a lung biopsy to evaluate for other processes that may contribute to severe chronic lung disease of infancy.[181]

The importance of airway dysfunction in the nonventilated as well as the mechanically ventilated infant with BPD is highlighted by studies evaluating the functional and mechanical effect of helium–oxygen mixtures. The low viscosity of the helium–oxygen allows for increased laminar flow and decreased turbulent flow through obstructed airways. In the study by Migliori and colleagues, helium–oxygen was associated with decreased peak inflation pressures, increased minute ventilation, and a 50% reduction in work of breathing; additionally, improved gas exchange (partial pressure of transcutaneous

oxygen ($TcPo_2$) and $TcPco_2$) was noted during both intubated and noninvasive support.[182] In a more recent study, relatively brief exposures (1 hour) to a helium–oxygen mixture again were accompanied by improvements in peak expiratory flow, dynamic compliance, exhaled V_T, and minute ventilation of 25% to 37%, with an associated 50% reduction in FiO_2 needs.[183] When the helium–oxygen mixture was discontinued, lung mechanics and FiO_2 needs returned to baseline values.

Tracheostomy

Some infants with chronic–severe BPD may require tracheostomy. The reported rate of tracheostomy in populations of very preterm infants at high risk for BPD is around 3% to 5%.[156,184] The optimal time to move toward tracheostomy is unclear at this time in terms of postnatal age and/or duration of mechanical ventilation. Data from retrospective studies of large neonatal data sets suggest that most infants have been ventilator dependent for more than 2 to 3 months before tracheostomy is considered.[184,185] In our practice we tend to delay tracheostomy unless we have evidence for earlier development of trachea/bronchomalacia, but there appear to be developmental and other benefits to earlier tracheostomy. In one of these studies tracheostomy after 120 days was associated with worse neurodevelopmental outcome,[184] but this was an observational study with many potential confounders. A prospective randomized trial would be required to determine the optimal time and conditions for this serious procedure. Nonetheless, clinical practice appears to already be shifting in favor of earlier tracheostomy placement.

Pulmonary Hypertension

Pulmonary hypertension is a relatively common problem among infants with more severe forms of BPD, with rates ranging from 20% to 50% depending on the population and approach to evaluation.[160,186,187] Mechanisms for pulmonary hypertension in this population include reduced vascular bed associated with impaired alveolarization, increased vascular smooth muscle proliferation and reactivity, and pulmonary vascular effects of localized areas of atelectasis or hyperinflation.[188] Diagnosis of pulmonary hypertension in babies with BPD requires a deliberate investigative approach. Echocardiography is the mainstay for diagnosis, but occasionally cardiac catheterization is needed for both diagnosis and evaluation of response to various therapies. Management of BPD-associated pulmonary hypertension includes adequate oxygenation (we recommend SpO_2 values >92%; but not hyperoxemia),[189,190] adjustment of support to prevent significant respiratory acidosis, avoidance of lung overinflation, and occasional use of adjunctive therapies. A number of potential pulmonary vasodilators are available and in use, including iNO,[191] sildenafil,[189,192] inhaled or intravenous prostacyclin, and bosentan.[193] It is important to note, however, that no RCTs have been performed as of this writing to establish the efficacy and safety of these therapies in the treatment of infants with BPD.[190] General management of infants with severe BPD is further discussed in Chapter 35.

Evidence-Based Recommendations

There is almost no high-quality evidence base supporting a specific approach to mechanical ventilation for infants with significant BPD. The approaches described here are based on clinical experience linked to known/suspected underlying pathophysiology. The best approach for BPD is preventing it,[194,195] but that has proved a difficult task to accomplish.[196-198]

Gaps in Knowledge

Given the fairly broad pathophysiologic spectrum and the relatively limited number of infants with chronic–severe BPD, even large specialized centers will have difficulty in performing randomized studies targeting specific ventilatory approaches to the care of this population of infants. Multicenter approaches, such as the Neonatal Research Network, the Children's Hospital Neonatal Database collaborative,[156] and the BPD Collaborative,[199] may be able to provide large enough patient populations to perform such studies.

Though comparative effectiveness studies of treatments for severe BPD are urgently needed, research also needs to focus on interventions aimed at the prevention of BPD. Although much effort and money have been expended in the pursuit of a single "magic bullet" for the prevention of BPD, given the multifactorial pathophysiology of BPD, studies designed around "systems" approaches to preventing BPD—that is, "best demonstrated practices"[200,201]—and/or combination therapy approaches[202,203] are more likely to prove useful.

Finally, trials must be sufficiently funded to evaluate not just relatively short-term outcomes such as BPD at 36 or 40 weeks' gestation, or even at 2 to 5 years of age, but well beyond those time points. Current long-term studies, primarily of infants born prior to the uniform availability of surfactant, suggest that even preterm infants not diagnosed with BPD have reduced lung growth and impaired lung function relative to infants born at term.[14,34,204] Given the fact that lung function normally begins to decline around the end of the third decade of life, minimizing the interruption of alveolarization associated with very preterm birth, and exacerbated through processes leading to BPD should be a top research priority.[37,205]

SUMMARY

A variety of respiratory disorders may be encountered in the neonatal period, the most common of which have been discussed in this chapter. A firm understanding of the underlying pathophysiology, and how it may change over time, is necessary to optimally apply any approach to mechanical ventilation. A variety of ventilatory modes are available, and there is limited evidence to strongly support one mode or approach over another for most of these conditions. Given the limited evidence base for much of the care we provide, there is much to be gained through controlled interventional trials within collaborative networks. It is critical to recognize that the lungs of all newborns are not developmentally complete (not just the most premature) and may be more susceptible to VILI. Protocols for weaning and extubation are strongly recommended. The most important factor associated with safe and successful ventilator management of the sick neonate is the person operating the ventilator rather than the ventilator itself.

REFERENCES

A complete reference list is available at https://expertconsult .inkling.com/.

24

Weaning from Mechanical Ventilation

Guilherme Sant'Anna, MD, PhD, FRCPC, and Martin Keszler, MD, FAAP

BACKGROUND

Although it is a life-saving intervention, mechanical ventilation is associated with many complications (Box 24-1), making timely and safe weaning an important imperative. However, the process of discontinuing mechanical ventilation in newborn infants with significant pulmonary morbidity and those who are extremely premature remains a major challenge, made more complex by the variety of modes of respiratory support currently in use. There is no consensus about the most appropriate way to wean babies from mechanical ventilation, and their management remains largely subjective, depending on institutional practices and individuals' training or preferences. Unfortunately, many important gaps in knowledge remain in the science of weaning from mechanical ventilation and assessment of extubation readiness in neonates, which results in significant variations in periextubation practices worldwide.[1] In this chapter we provide a comprehensive review of this subject and some evidence-based recommendations to guide clinical practice for weaning from mechanical ventilation, assessment of extubation readiness, and postextubation management.

WEANING FROM VENTILATORY SUPPORT

Weaning from mechanical ventilation is the process of decreasing the amount of ventilatory support, with the patient gradually assuming a greater proportion of the overall work of ventilation. As mentioned in Chapter 15, weaning and extubation at the earliest possible time are among the a priori goals of mechanical respiratory support. In addition to the obvious goal of reducing ventilator-induced lung injury, early weaning will reduce the risk of nosocomial sepsis, reduce patient discomfort and need for sedation, minimize the development of oral aversion with subsequent feeding difficulties, and facilitate parental bonding and developmentally appropriate care. Therefore, as soon as the patient's condition stabilizes and the underlying respiratory disorder that led to the initiation of ventilation begins to improve, weaning should be initiated. This approach differs from that employed in the past (and persisting in some centers) when patients were heavily sedated or even paralyzed during the acute phase of the illness and weaning from mechanical ventilation did not begin until some arbitrary weaning criteria were met.[2,3] In the early days of mechanical ventilation of newborn infants, there was a widespread practice of keeping infants on mechanical ventilation until they reached the arbitrary weight of 1 kg. This practice, long ago abandoned, was based on the assumption that small preterm infants would

expend too much energy to breathe and were unlikely to remain extubated. This concept was in large part related to the practice of extubating preterm infants to an oxygen hood rather than to continuous positive airway pressure (CPAP). Today we know that with appropriate noninvasive support many extremely low birth-weight infants are able to be extubated within a few days of birth and thrive. Those who remain ventilator dependent beyond the first week of life have a much higher risk of bronchopulmonary dysplasia (BPD). A retrospective study of infants of ≤1000 g and ≤28 weeks demonstrated a seventeenfold increase in the risk of any BPD in infants ventilated for >7 days, compared to those extubated on days 1 to 3, with a 62% incidence of moderate or severe BPD in the babies extubated for the first time beyond 7 days of age.[4]

Many different modes of invasive respiratory support are used in neonates, and the specific mechanics of weaning from mechanical ventilation are to a large extent a function of the mode of support in use. The basic types of mechanical ventilation are (1) pressure-controlled ventilation, (2) volume-controlled or volume-targeted ventilation, and (3) high-frequency ventilation (HFV). The basic process of weaning for the various pressure-controlled synchronized modes is described in Chapter 18, and the basic steps for pressure-controlled ventilation and HFV are summarized in Box 24-2. A detailed discussion of weaning using volume-targeted ventilation is available in Chapter 20. Available data support the preferential use of (1) any mode of synchronized ventilation over unsynchronized intermittent mandatory ventilation (IMV),[5] (2) modes that support each spontaneous breath over synchronized IMV (SIMV),[2,6,7] and (3) volume-targeted over pressure-controlled ventilation.[8,9] Some important concepts that should be kept in mind to facilitate weaning include the following: (1) Weaning too slowly may be more dangerous than weaning too fast, as it may result in excessive lung injury and hypocarbia. (2) Weaning should be attempted throughout the day, not just during rounds. (3) When gas exchange is satisfactory and the work of breathing is not excessive, weaning should be attempted. (4) Volume-targeted ventilation effectively addresses concepts 1 to 3 by lowering inflation pressure in real time in response to improving lung mechanics and patient effort. Ventilatory settings at which to consider extubation readiness in infants 2 weeks of age or younger are provided in Box 24-3. These reflect general consensus and are based on values used as extubation criteria in many randomized controlled trials (RCTs). However, they are not based on prospectively obtained trial data.

BOX 24-1   Complications of Mechanical Ventilation in Newborns

Ventilator-Induced Lung Injury (Volutrauma)
Atelectasis
Overdistention
Bronchopulmonary dysplasia

Air-Leak Syndromes
Pulmonary interstitial emphysema
Pneumothorax
Pneumomediastinum
Pneumopericardium

Airway Trauma
Vocal cord injury
Subglottic stenosis
Subglottic cysts
Granulomas
Tracheobronchomalacia
Palatal deformities
Nasal septal defects

Endotracheal Tube Complications
Obstruction
Displacement
Accidental extubation

Infection
Ventilator-associated pneumonia
Late-onset sepsis

Cardiovascular
Decreased cardiac output

Neurologic
Hypocarbia (cerebral vasoconstriction)
Neurodevelopmental impairment

BOX 24-2   Basic Weaning Strategies with Pressure-Controlled Modes and High-Frequency Ventilation

Desired Result	Action: SIMV	Action: AC or PSV	Action: HFV
↑ Pco$_2$	⇓ PIP, rate	⇓ PIP	⇓ Amplitude
↓ Po$_2$	⇓ FiO$_2$, PEEP	⇓ FiO$_2$, PEEP	⇓ FiO$_2$, MAP

SIMV, Synchronized intermittent mandatory ventilation; *AC,* assist control; *PSV,* pressure-support ventilation; *HFV,* high-frequency ventilation; *PIP,* peak inflation pressure; *FiO$_2$,* fractional inspired oxygen concentration; *PEEP,* positive end-expiratory pressure; *MAP,* mean airway pressure.

WEANING FROM PRESSURE-LIMITED VENTILATION

With SIMV, weaning is accomplished by reducing both peak inflation pressure (PIP) and the ventilator rate. The rate should not be reduced much until PIP has been reduced to relatively low values (<20 cm H$_2$O) that indicate improved lung compliance. Lowering the set rate while the lungs are still quite stiff is likely to impose a high work of breathing and result in rapid shallow spontaneous breathing requiring an excessively large tidal volume

BOX 24-3   Ventilatory Settings at Which Extubation Should Be Considered in Infants ≤2 Weeks of Age.

Conventional Ventilation (AC, SIMV, PSV)
- SIMV: PIP ≤16 cm H$_2$O, PEEP ≤6 cm H$_2$O, rate ≤20, FiO$_2$ ≤0.30
- AC/PSV, BW <1000 g: MAP ≤7 cm H$_2$O and FiO$_2$ ≤0.30
- AC/PSV, BW >1000 g: MAP ≤8 cm H$_2$O and FiO$_2$ ≤0.30

Volume Ventilation
- Tidal volume ≤4.0 mL/kg (5 mL/kg if <700 g or >2 weeks of age) and FiO$_2$ ≤0.30

High-Frequency Oscillatory Ventilation
- BW <1000 g: MAP ≤8 cm H$_2$O and FiO$_2$ ≤0.30
- BW >1000 g: MAP ≤9 cm H$_2$O and FiO$_2$ ≤0.30

High-Frequency Jet Ventilation
- BW <1000 g: PIP ≤14 cm H$_2$O, MAP ≤7 cm H$_2$O, and FiO$_2$ ≤0.30
- BW >1000 g: PIP ≤16 cm H$_2$O, MAP ≤8 cm H$_2$O, and FiO$_2$ ≤0.30

Older infants may be able to be extubated from higher pressures or tidal volumes.

AC, Assist control; *SIMV,* synchronized intermittent mandatory ventilation; *PSV,* pressure-support ventilation; *PIP,* peak inflation pressure; *PEEP,* positive end-expiratory pressure; *FiO$_2$,* fractional inspired oxygen concentration; *BW,* birth weight; *MAP,* mean airway pressure.

(V_T) for the low-rate SIMV inflations to maintain adequate alveolar minute ventilation. In small preterm infants, it is advisable to add pressure support (PS) when SIMV rate is reduced below 30/minute. The combination of SIMV + PS resulted in more rapid weaning from mechanical respiratory support than SIMV alone in extremely low birth-weight (ELBW) infants[7] and significantly lower work of breathing.[10] If SIMV is used without PS, the rate should not be reduced below 15 inflations/minute. There are no studies to inform the best method of weaning from SIMV + PS. It seems reasonable to reduce the SIMV rate gradually to 10 while also reducing the PIP as necessary to avoid excessive V_T and maintain PS at a level sufficient to achieve acceptable V_T for the spontaneous breaths, typically 4-5 ml/kg.

With assist control and PS ventilation as a stand-alone mode, the infant controls the ventilator rate; therefore, lowering the set rate, which acts as a backup only in the case of apnea, has no real impact on reducing ventilator support. Weaning is accomplished by lowering the PIP and gradually transferring the work of breathing to the infant. For a brief period of several hours just prior to extubation, it may be reasonable to reduce the backup rate to 20 inflations/minute to better recognize any inconsistent respiratory effort that may have been masked by a higher backup rate.

WEANING FROM HIGH-FREQUENCY VENTILATION

Many clinicians are more comfortable changing from HFV to conventional modes prior to extubation, but extubation directly from both jet and oscillatory ventilation is not only possible, it may even be desirable. Clark et al. reported that infants who remained on high-frequency oscillatory ventilation (HFOV) until extubation had a lower incidence of BPD than those ventilated conventionally, but infants who were changed to SIMV after 72 hours of HFOV did not seem to benefit equally.[11] Similarly, the large HFOV trial by Courtney et al., which required infants to remain on HFOV for 14 days or until extubation, reported a lower rate of BPD and shorter duration of ventilation, compared with conventional ventilation,[12] whereas a similar study published in the same issue of the *New England Journal of Medicine*, which allowed early crossover from HFOV to conventional ventilation, showed no such benefits.[13] The way HFOV support is reduced is based on empiric data and experience, with few experimental data to guide the clinician. In general, both pressure amplitude and mean airway pressure are reduced progressively as tolerated, the former to reduce minute ventilation, the latter to avoid overexpansion as lung compliance and oxygenation improve. There is no consensus regarding "extubatable" settings during HFV, but in general, extubation is considered when mean airway pressure is around 8 cm H_2O with FiO_2 less than 0.30. Frequency is not reduced as a means of reducing support. With most HFOV devices, delivered V_T increases as frequency decreases, so that reducing ventilator frequency has the opposite effect compared to that on conventional ventilation. Some clinicians increase the HFOV frequency as an indirect means of reducing V_T, but this approach of making ventilation more inefficient seems counterintuitive and not specifically supported by evidence.

Weaning from high-frequency jet ventilation more closely parallels conventional ventilation, with stepwise reduction in peak and mean pressures. The primary means of reducing support is reduction in pressure amplitude, which is the difference between PIP and positive end-expiratory pressure (PEEP). With both jet and oscillatory ventilation, when support is reduced enough to allow mild respiratory acidosis, spontaneous breathing will be observed as the infant begins to take over more of the respiratory effort. When there is good spontaneous effort and the settings are judged to be sufficiently low, extubation should be attempted. There are no studies of extubation readiness for infants on HFV.

GENERAL STRATEGIES TO FACILITATE WEANING

Permissive Hypercarbia

Permissive hypercarbia is a ventilatory strategy that accepts higher than normal $PaCO_2$ levels (between 45 and 65 mm Hg), as long as the pH is ≥7.20, while using lower rates and/or V_Ts. This strategy may reduce injury to the developing lung through a variety of mechanisms, which include more efficient CO_2 removal, better ventilation–perfusion matching, stabilization of or increase in respiratory drive facilitating weaning, and improvement in cardiac output. Permissive hypercarbia appears to be an effective strategy to allow continued use of noninvasive support and avoidance of mechanical ventilation. This approach, though widely practiced, has not actually been directly evaluated as an isolated intervention in randomized trials. Nonetheless, it is generally accepted as appropriate and was an important part of several large trials comparing delivery room management.[14,15] It remains unclear if permissive hypercarbia is effective in facilitating weaning. Mariani et al. showed shorter duration of mechanical ventilation with a trend to less BPD in a single-center randomized pilot trial comparing target $PaCO_2$ of 35 to 45 mm Hg to 45 to 55 mm Hg for the first 96 hours of life.[16] A subsequent multicenter trial targeting an even higher level of hypercarbia failed to replicate these findings, possibly because unlike in the pilot study, a clear separation in between the two arms could not be achieved.[17] Furthermore,

the trial was stopped early after enrollment of 220 infants because of increased complications associated with the other intervention involved in this 2 × 2 factorial design trial. There was a nonsignificant trend to less BPD at 36 weeks (63% vs 68%), and fewer infants required mechanical ventilation at 36 weeks' postmenstrual age.

The largest trial that incorporated permissive hypercarbia as part of a strategy to avoid mechanical ventilation and hasten extubation before and during the first 14 days of mechanical ventilation was the Surfactant, Positive Pressure, and Oxygenation Randomized Trial (SUPPORT).[14] The study compared a strategy of routine intubation and surfactant administration in the control arm to primary use of noninvasive support in the delivery room and permissive hypercarbia. The target PCO_2 was >65 mm Hg with a pH >7.20 in the group assigned to noninvasive support and <50 mm Hg and a pH >7.30 in the routine intubation group. There was no difference in the primary outcome of BPD/death (47.8% vs 51.0%), but subgroup and secondary analysis showed decreased mortality in infants with gestational age (GA) between 24 and 25 weeks (23.9% vs 32.1%, $p = 0.03$), lower rates of mechanical ventilation and surfactant supplementation, shorter duration of mechanical ventilation, and less use of postnatal corticosteroids for BPD.[14] However, a secondary analysis of data from SUPPORT reported increased risk of adverse outcomes, such as severe intraventricular hemorrhage, and death, with both high $PaCO_2$ and fluctuating $PaCO_2$.[18] A single-center trial focusing solely on permissive hypercarbia enrolled 65 infants of between 23 and 28 weeks' gestation who received mechanical ventilation within 6 hours of birth. Infants were randomized to a $PaCO_2$ target of either 55 to 65 or 35 to 45 mm Hg for the first week of life. The trial was stopped early after enrolling about one-third of the projected sample size. BPD or death occurred in 64% of the infants in the hypercarbia group and 59% of control infants ($p = NS$). A concerning finding was that permissive hypercarbia was associated with trends toward higher mortality and higher incidence of neurodevelopmental impairment with a significantly increased combined outcome of mental impairment or death ($p < 0.05$). The authors concluded that permissive hypercarbia, as performed in that study, did not improve clinical outcome and may actually be associated with a worse neurodevelopmental outcome.

As of this writing, the most recent randomized trial was the Permissive Hypercapnia in Extremely Low Birthweight Infants (PHELBI) trial, which compared permissive hypercarbia and more traditional PCO_2 targets. The high-target group aimed at $PaCO_2$ values of 55 to 65 mm Hg on postnatal days 1 to 3, 60 to 70 mm Hg on days 4 to 6, and 65 to 75 mm Hg on days 7 to 14; the control group target was PCO_2 40 to 50 mm Hg on days 1 to 3, 45 to 55 mm Hg on days 4 to 6, and 50 to 60 mm Hg on days 7 to 14. The trial was stopped after interim analysis when it became evident that the probability of showing a benefit of the intervention became vanishingly small. Ultimately, 359 infants of 400- to 1000-g birth weight were analyzed. The rate of the combined outcome of BPD or death in the permissive hypercarbia group versus control (36% vs 30%; $p = 0.18$), death (14% vs 11%; $p = 0.32$), and grade III to IV intraventricular hemorrhage (15% vs 12%; $p = 0.30$) showed nonsignificant trends favoring the control group.[19] As with the previous randomized trials, the $PaCO_2$ in the hypercarbia group, although higher than in the control group, was generally below the target range, despite significantly lower ventilator settings. This highlights the practical limitation of targeting a significant respiratory acidosis in infants who are not heavily sedated or paralyzed—the baby's own respiratory drive will cause increased spontaneous respiratory effort, which may lower the $PaCO_2$ below the target range but also cause tachypnea, retractions, and agitation, necessitating either heavy sedation, which is associated with substantial adverse effects,[20] or an increase in respiratory support. The above studies, taken together with observational studies that suggested that $PaCO_2$ values >60 to 65 mm Hg during the first few days of life were associated with increased risk of severe intraventricular hemorrhage (IVH), especially when rapid changes occur,[21–23] indicate that marked permissive hypercarbia is not beneficial and may in fact be harmful. Mild degrees of permissive hypercarbia similar to the control arm of the PHELBI trial[19] are based on sound physiologic principles and are generally accepted as safe and effective in reducing the need for mechanical ventilation.

Permissive Hypoxemia

Less aggressive oxygenation targets became incorporated into neonatal care without the benefit of large randomized trials in an effort to reduce oxidative stress and adverse effects on the lungs and other organs. Early observational studies suggested that lower oxygen saturation targets were associated with less retinopathy of prematurity, less chronic lung disease, and faster weaning from mechanical ventilation.[24–27] The safety of this permissive hypoxemia approach was called into question by a series of studies attempting to define the optimal target saturation as measured by pulse oximetry (SpO_2). Five trials with similar designs including a prespecified composite outcome of death/disability at 18 to 24 months' corrected GA were conducted to compare two different ranges of oxygen saturation (high, 91% to 95%, and low, 85% to 89%). Two systematic analyses of these trials have been published. An increased relative risk for mortality and necrotizing enterocolitis and a reduced risk for severe retinopathy of prematurity was noted in the low, compared to the high, oxygen saturation target group.[28] There were no differences regarding BPD (physiologic definition), brain injury, or patent ductus arteriosus between the groups. Another systematic review found no difference in the prespecified composite outcome of death/disability (risk ratio [RR], 1.02; 95% CI, 0.92 to 1.14) or mortality before 24 months (RR, 1.13; 95% CI, 0.97 to 1.33).[29] A significant increase in hospital mortality was found in the restricted oxygen group (RR, 1.18; 95% CI, 1.03 to 1.36). However, even though many questions remain unanswered, it has been suggested that SpO_2 targets should be raised between 90% and 95% in infants with GA <28 weeks until 36 weeks' postmenstrual age.[28] Permissive hypoxemia therefore does not appear to be a useful strategy to accelerate weaning from mechanical ventilation.

WEANING PROTOCOLS

The availability of a variety of ventilators and ventilatory modes and the diverse backgrounds and training of neonatal practitioners contribute to highly variable approaches to mechanical ventilation practices with significant intra- and intercenter differences in outcome.[30] Such variability can be harmful. The use of ventilation protocols driven by health care providers is an effective way of decreasing unnecessary variations in practice.[31,32] Indeed, in adults the use of ventilation protocols has been demonstrated to improve weaning from mechanical

ventilation, with no complications and decreasing costs.[33,34] Several studies involving patients in the pediatric intensive care setting similarly indicated benefits of protocol-driven weaning.[35–37] In neonates, especially in the preterm population, the highest level of evidence is lacking and weaning practices remain very physician-dependent, but some evidence in favor of weaning protocols in newborn infants is available. In a retrospective study, Hermeto et al. demonstrated a significant improvement in short-term respiratory outcomes in preterm infants after a respiratory therapy-driven protocol was implemented.[38] Despite the lack of solid evidence, a Canadian survey showed that almost 40% of the neonatal intensive care units (NICUs) have already adopted the use of protocols for mechanical ventilation.[39] A 2002 paper suggested that experienced NICU nurses are more effective at weaning infants from mechanical ventilation than physicians in training, adding another potential avenue to facilitate weaning.[40]

ADJUNCTIVE THERAPIES

Adjunctive therapies are interventions designed to help preterm infants maintain adequate gas exchange and respiratory effort during the weaning and postextubation periods. Some of these therapies have been investigated by large RCTs, whereas for others there is still a glaring lack of evidence to support or refute their use. A more complete discussion of pharmacologic therapies can be found in Chapter 34.

Caffeine

When given to infants receiving mechanical ventilation, caffeine was associated with faster weaning, within 2 to 7 days after initiation of the treatment.[10,44] Caffeine also improved important outcomes such as extubation failure, number of days on invasive and noninvasive ventilation, and neurodevelopment at 18 to 22 months of age. The most appropriate dose is still not well defined[41] but caffeine is commonly administered at 10 mg/kg/day of caffeine citrate once a day given 24 hours after a loading dose of 20 mg/kg. Higher doses have been shown to be beneficial in single-center studies.[42,43] The most appropriate age at which caffeine should be initiated has also not been established.[44] Caffeine is usually started soon after birth, but some centers prefer to initiate caffeine only around the time of extubation, either prophylactically or in infants with significant episodes of apnea after extubation. Furthermore, additional evidence is needed to better define when to safely discontinue caffeine for extremely preterm infants and possible long-term side effects.[45]

Diuretics

High fluid intake and low weight loss during the first 10 days of life is associated with an increased risk of death or BPD in preterm infants.[46] A meta-analysis on this subject concluded that restricted water intake reduces the risk of patent ductus arteriosus (PDA) and necrotizing enterocolitis with trends toward reduced risks of BPD, intracranial hemorrhage, and death.[47] These findings naturally led clinicians to consider therapies to address fluid overload as a means of improving lung function and reducing the need for respiratory support. However, diuretics have been shown to be ineffective in the treatment of the acute phase of respiratory distress syndrome, even though it is clearly associated with fluid retention.[48] Furosemide is the most commonly used diuretic in the newborn period.

Furosemide decreases interstitial lung water and improves lung mechanics in the short term, and thus it is commonly used in infants who are difficult to wean from mechanical ventilation, especially when there is evidence of fluid overload. However, it is important to recognize the lack of objective evidence for its effectiveness in the long term. It is also important to note that furosemide stimulates the renal synthesis of prostaglandin E2,[49] a potent dilator of the ductus arteriosus, and therefore should be used with caution within the first days of life.[50]

Closure of Patent Ductus Arteriosus

Left-to-right shunting of blood through a widely patent ductus arteriosus can cause pulmonary edema and decreased lung compliance. PDA is associated with increased mortality and morbidity and BPD, and difficult weaning from mechanical ventilation in preterm infants is commonly attributed to a "hemodynamically significant PDA." Treatment (pharmacologic and/or surgical) was routinely instituted to facilitate weaning. However, aggressive PDA treatment is a practice that has been questioned based on analyses of individual RCTs and meta-analyses.[51,52] Pharmacologic ductal closure is effective in reducing the need for ductal ligation, but no long-term benefits of PDA treatment were documented. Both medical and surgical PDA closure have significant associated risks, and spontaneous PDA closure commonly occurs, supporting a more conservative approach.[53] Thus, the role of treatment of PDA in facilitating weaning from mechanical ventilation remains unclear.

Avoidance of Routine Sedation

In preterm infants, a systematic review has evaluated the routine use of opioids in neonates receiving mechanical ventilation and found insufficient evidence to recommend it.[54] Indeed, the use of morphine in this population has been reported as potentially harmful.[20] In a multicenter randomized trial the use of additional analgesia with morphine was associated independently with increased rates of IVH and air leaks and longer duration of mechanical ventilation, nasal CPAP, and oxygen therapy.[20,55] In an observational study the use of morphine given for preemptive analgesia or without ongoing, patient-specific measures of pain was associated with prolonged hospitalization.[56] In this study, the implementation of a nursing-driven comfort protocol significantly reduced this type of morphine use. Morphine administration to ventilated preterm infants has also been associated with subtle neurobehavioral differences during childhood.[57] Therefore, routine use of morphine analgesia/sedation cannot be recommended as it clearly impairs weaning from respiratory support.

Nutritional Support

Adequate nutritional support is critical to any patient receiving intensive care. Nutrition and lung growth and development are interdependent, with the former playing a critical role in the prevention and management of BPD.[58,59] Most preterm infants with moderate or severe BPD experience growth failure predominantly due to suboptimal nutritional intake, which in turn can worsen BPD by further compromising lung repair and growth.[59] Indeed, high rates of extrauterine growth restriction have been described in critically ill preterm infants.[60,61] Therefore, adequate nutritional management of these infants should start immediately after birth to enhance ventilation weaning and lung repair and growth and ultimately minimize respiratory morbidity.

Chest Physiotherapy

Chest physiotherapy, such as percussion and vibration followed by suction, in infants receiving mechanical ventilation was assessed in a systematic review updated in 2009. A total of three trials involving 106 infants were included, and analysis identified insufficient evidence to adequately assess the efficacy and/or adverse effects of this therapy.[62]

Systemic Corticosteroids

The updated Cochrane meta-analysis concluded that the use of early postnatal systemic corticosteroids (<8 days of age) at various doses facilitates weaning and decreases the risk of BPD in preterm infants but also increases the risk of short-term complications and long-term neurologic sequelae.[63] Later use (beyond 7 days of age) also reduced BPD at 36 weeks, facilitated earlier weaning, and reduced mortality at 28 days and at 36 weeks. There was a trend toward a higher rate of cerebral palsy (CP), but this was offset by lower mortality.[64] Following the initial reports of steroid association with increased rates of CP the use of corticosteroids dropped sharply, with a subsequent increase in the rates of BPD.[65] In 2005, a meta-regression analysis of several RCTs demonstrated that the risk of death or CP varies with the a priori level of risk for BPD, with a negative relationship between these variables in the control group.[66] An update of this analysis showed that the results were unchanged by the addition of more studies, but a slightly narrower confidence interval with a slightly greater statistical significance was observed.[67] Based on this evidence, clinicians should use prediction equations or their own local data to identify the highest risk infants who are likely to have a net benefit from postnatal corticosteroid treatment with respect to survival free of CP. Most of the concerns about neurologic sequelae focus on dexamethasone. As of this writing, whether hydrocortisone administered between 14 and 28 days of age is effective in facilitating weaning and reducing the risk of BPD is being investigated in a large randomized trial conducted by the National Institute of Child Health and Human Development (NICHD) Neonatal Research Network.

Inhaled Corticosteroids

Inhaled steroids have long been used in the management of preterm infants on mechanical ventilation. Published surveys from 2014 and 2015 indicate a relatively high and variable use of inhaled steroids,[68,69] despite the lack of evidence to support the routine use of inhaled steroids in infants receiving mechanical ventilation.[70] A large multicenter trial in Europe (NEUROSIS) has finished patient enrollment, but final results have not been published as of this writing.[71] While the apparent lack of efficacy of inhaled steroids may be a function of ineffective delivery systems, the use of inhaled steroids to facilitate weaning cannot be recommended, unless data from the European trial provide convincing evidence to the contrary.

ASSESSMENT OF EXTUBATION READINESS

With no clear evidence to guide extubation practice, the decision to extubate is most often based on the clinical judgment of the responsible physician, based largely on personal training and experience and taking into account the evolution of blood gases, oxygen needs, and ventilator settings. Predictably, this leads to substantial variation in practice and frequent failure of extubation. Reported success of extubation ranges from 60% to 73% in

ELBW infants.[72,73] Higher success rates (80% to 86%) have been reported in some series that included larger preterm infants.[74,75] Infants who fail and require reintubation are exposed to significant risks and discomfort and may experience deterioration of their respiratory status due to atelectasis. Hypoxemia and/or hypercarbia prior to reintubation may expose them to additional risks. Reintubation itself causes discomfort, may be traumatic, and is often accompanied by bradycardia, hypercarbia, and alterations in cerebral blood flow and oxygenation.[76,77] It is, however, also worth noting that a relatively large number of infants experience inadvertent extubation and remain extubated subsequently.[78] Those infants may have been exposed to mechanical ventilation (MV) and the associated ventilator-induced lung injury for longer than necessary. Protracted MV is clearly not benign; in preterm baboons 5 days of elective MV resulted in a greater degree of brain injury compared to only 1 day of ventilation.[79] Based on data from the NICHD Neonatal Research Network, Walsh et al. showed that each week of additional MV was associated with a significant increase in the likelihood of neurodevelopmental impairment.[80] Additionally, the endotracheal tube acts as a foreign body, quickly becoming colonized and acting as a portal of entry for pathogens, increasing the risk of ventilator-associated pneumonia and late-onset sepsis.[81] Clearly, both premature extubation and unnecessarily prolonged MV are undesirable.

Unfortunately, there is a striking paucity of high-quality data to guide the clinician regarding optimal ways to wean from respiratory support as well as judging an infant's readiness for extubation. Many attempts at developing tools to predict extubation readiness have been evaluated, but typically these were small, single-center studies. Box 24-4 lists various potential predictors of extubation readiness, which are reviewed below.

Lung Mechanics and Minute Ventilation

Measurements of lung and respiratory system compliance and resistance, V_T, functional residual capacity, and lung volume have been investigated but did not consistently improve the ability to determine successful extubation.[74,82–85] Furthermore, most of these studies were performed long ago and may no longer apply to current clinical practice. More recently, the application of a *pressure–time index* assessing respiratory muscle (diaphragm) strength was able to predict successful extubation with high sensitivity and specificity, indicating a decreased diaphragmatic efficiency in neonates who fail extubation.[75] However, this promising tool was evaluated only in a small single-center study that enrolled relatively large infants of up to 36 weeks of gestation. Whether the results of this study are applicable to the smallest and most immature infants who are at the greatest risk of failure remains to be determined.

The use of the minute ventilation test as measured by a ventilator pulmonary function monitor showed mixed results. A randomized controlled but unblinded trial reported faster extubation but a higher extubation failure rate with the use of a minute ventilation test compared to clinical decision making alone.[86] In another study, the percentage of time an ELBW infant could breathe with spontaneous expiratory minute ventilation above a predetermined threshold during a 2-hour challenge of endotracheal tube CPAP was shown to predict readiness for extubation with high sensitivity and specificity.[73] This small study used a 2-hour challenge, but infants were extubated from very low ventilatory settings, making it likely that a number of infants could have been successfully extubated much earlier. Such a long period of endotracheal CPAP imposed substantial stress on the infant and could not be recommended.

Clinical Assessment: Spontaneous Breathing Trials

Spontaneous breathing trials (SBTs), also known as trials of endotracheal (ET) CPAP, have long been used to assess extubation readiness in a variety of populations, but the number of studies in newborn infants is quite small. Several early trials done more than 20 years ago used ET CPAP trials ranging from 6 to 24 hours; a meta-analysis of those studies concluded that preterm infants should be extubated directly from low ventilatory settings without a trial of ET CPAP.[87] The basic principle of an SBT as used today is to test the patient's capacity to sustain adequate ventilation and oxygenation during a brief loading challenge before removal of the endotracheal tube. In neonates, this challenge is usually done by leaving the patient to breathe through the endotracheal tube with PEEP but no other support for 3 to 10 minutes. In a prospective observational study, a 3-minute SBT was shown to identify suitability for extubation in very low birth-weight infants with high accuracy.[88] With the implementation of this prediction tool as part of clinical practice, infants were extubated earlier and from higher ventilatory settings but with similar rates of extubation failure.[89] This reinforces the idea that the adoption of a standardized approach to assess extubation readiness may be of great value in expediting weaning by streamlining practice.

Several aspects of SBT, such as the optimal level of PEEP to be used, duration of the test, and definition of SBT pass or failure, remain uncertain. In the meantime, units that have already adopted the routine utilization of such a test should closely follow the impact of its implementation on important short- and long-term outcomes.[89]

Analysis of the Dynamics of Physiologic Signals Prior to Extubation

Several physiologic variables exhibit rhythms that are essential to life. These rhythms fluctuate irregularly over time and are characterized by a highly elaborate, apparently random output that arises from nonlinear biological mechanisms interacting with the fluctuating environment.[90] The application of physiologic variability measurements as markers of well-being has a long tradition in medicine. Extremely regular dynamics are often associated with disease, including periodic breathing, certain abnormal heart rhythms, cyclical blood diseases, and epilepsy. Analysis of biological signal variability has also been used

BOX 24-5 Key Elements of Postextubation Management

Respiratory Support
- Continuous positive airway pressure
- Nasal intermittent positive-pressure ventilation
- Heated humidified high-flow nasal cannula

Adjunctive Therapies
- Caffeine
- Racemic epinephrine
- Chronic diuretics
- Chest physiotherapy
- Inhaled and/or systemic steroids

in the prediction of clinical outcomes.[91] In adults, variations in cardiac and respiratory rhythms have been demonstrated as good predictors of ventilation weaning and extubation readiness.[92–95] In preterm infants, investigations of the dynamics of physiologic signals are limited to a few studies, most of them using heart rate characteristics as predictors of sepsis or physiologic signals to develop a score able to predict later critical illness.[96-99] In preterm infants with birth weight of ≤1250 g undergoing their first extubation attempt, the power spectrum analysis of heart rate variability, used in combination with a successful SBT, improved the accuracy of the SBT alone to predict extubation failure.[100] In another group of preterm infants, analysis of respiratory variability calculated during a 3-minute SBT showed a good predictive ability to differentiate the outcome of extubation success and failure.[101] Using this same cohort and applying support vector machine methodology, an analysis of cardiorespiratory variability was conducted. Results demonstrated an ability to identify 80% of the preterm infants who went on to fail their first extubation attempt.[102] Currently, in a large multicenter prospective observational study we are as of this writing collecting cardiorespiratory signals prior to extubation, with the objective to develop an automated prediction tool for extubation readiness in this preterm population.

In summary, no single approach applied prior to disconnection from MV has been convincingly demonstrated to decrease the incidence of extubation failure in the extremely preterm population. Thus, the need to improve a clinician's ability to correctly predict extubation readiness in these infants warrants further investigation.

POSTEXTUBATION MANAGEMENT

Some form of distending airway pressure should always be employed for at least 24 hours after extubation. For the more immature infants this period should be extended for much longer. The use of CPAP following extubation of preterm infants has been shown to reduce extubation failure compared to headbox or oxygen hood.[103] The rationale for the use of distending pressure is the excessively compliant rib cage of the ELBW infant, which is unable to maintain adequate functional residual capacity. The preterm infant normally uses grunting as a means to generate an internal distending pressure, but after being intubated for some time, the infant's vocal cords are edematous, preventing effective grunting.

The most commonly used types are CPAP, nasal intermittent positive-pressure ventilation, and heated humidified high-flow nasal cannula therapy (Box 24-5). Details about these therapies

are provided in Chapter 17 of this book. In addition, several adjunctive therapies may be useful during the postextubation period (see Box 24-5).

Adjunctive Therapies
Caffeine
As previously discussed, caffeine became a common therapy in the management of preterm infants with respiratory problems following the positive results of RCTs.[104,105] A Cochrane meta-analysis documented a relative risk of failed extubation of 0.48 for infants exposed to methylxanthines before extubation.[106] Thus in preterm infants at risk of apnea of prematurity, caffeine should virtually always be administered prior to extubation, if it has not been initiated previously. The optimal dose to achieve successful extubation may be higher than the standard dose used for apnea. An RCT by Steer et al. demonstrated a significant reduction in extubation failure for infants receiving 20 mg/kg/day dosing, compared to controls (15.0% vs 29.8%; RR, 0.51; 95% CI, 0.31 to 0.85; number needed to treat [NNT], 7).[43] A significant difference in duration of MV was seen in infants of <28 weeks' GA receiving the high dose of caffeine (14.4 ± 11.1 days vs 22.1 ± 17.1 days; $p = 0.01$).

Nebulized Racemic Epinephrine and Dexamethasone
Nebulized racemic epinephrine is commonly used to treat acute airway edema for postextubation stridor in newborn infants. Although anecdotal experience and short-term studies support its use,[107] a Cochrane meta-analysis last updated in 2010 failed to identify any randomized studies that evaluated important clinical outcomes.[108] There is a similar paucity of clear evidence in support of nebulized dexamethasone, but it is in common use for this indication based largely on anecdotal experience.

Postnatal Corticosteroids for the Prevention and Treatment of Postextubation Stridor
Two studies examined the use of systemic steroids for the prevention of postextubation stridor in newborn infants. A meta-analysis revealed that the results were heterogeneous, with no overall statistically significant reduction in postextubation stridor (RR, 0.42; 95% CI, 0.07 to 2.32).[109] A study that selected high-risk neonates treated with multiple doses of steroids around the time of extubation showed a significant reduction in stridor.[110] Neither study had sufficient statistical power to evaluate the need for reintubation, an outcome that deserves evaluation in further investigations. Despite the equivocal data, the use of a short burst of low-dose corticosteroids has become quite widespread, largely based on favorable anecdotal experience. Because corticosteroids have important side effects, it is prudent to reserve such therapy for infants who have been intubated for prolonged periods, who have a history of traumatic or multiple endotracheal intubations, or who previously failed extubation owing to subglottic edema.

Chest Physiotherapy
Four small RCTs have evaluated the effects of active respiratory physiotherapy, chest wall percussion and vibration followed by oropharyngeal suctioning, during the periextubation period. A systematic review of these trials showed a lack of clear evidence to support the use of this therapy.[111] However, frequent chest physiotherapy performed every 1 to 2 hours was associated with a reduction in the need for reintubation within the first 24 hours post extubation. There was no decrease in the

BOX 24-6   Risk Factors for Extubation Failure in Neonates

General
- Sedation (narcotics or benzodiazepines)
- Multiple endotracheal intubations
- Difficult or traumatic intubation
- Neurologic or neuromuscular disorder
- Genetic disorders
- Airway abnormalities
- Positive fluid balance
- Acidosis prior to extubation (pH <7.20)
- Hemodynamic instability
- Sepsis and necrotizing enterocolitis

Preterm Infants
- Low gestational age (<26 weeks)
- Low postmenstrual age
- Extremely low birth weight (<1000 g)
- Low current weight
- Male gender
- Intraventricular hemorrhage (grade III and/or IV)
- Hemodynamically unstable patent ductus arteriosus
- Lack of caffeine administration preextubation
- Extubation from high ventilatory settings (FiO₂ and rates)
- Inadequate provision of noninvasive respiratory support after extubation

incidence of postextubation lobar collapse and insufficient information to adequately assess important short- and longer term outcomes, including adverse effects. Caution is required when interpreting any possible positive effects of this therapy because the studies are old and enrolled a small number of larger, more mature infants, and results were not consistent across the trials.

EXTUBATION FAILURE

In clinical trials, extubation failure has been defined either by using specific clinical criteria or by the perceived need for reintubation. The time frame in various RCTs has commonly ranged from 24 to 72 hours but occasionally is up to 1 week after extubation.[112] However, the increased use of aggressive noninvasive respiratory support during the postextubation period has further complicated the interpretation of the time frame for failure, because it may simply delay failure. Therefore, the time interval to define successful extubation should probably be longer than 72 hours, perhaps 1 week for infants with a birth weight of <1000 g.[112] Lack of a consensus on extubation failure definition makes it difficult to determine acceptable failure rates for different GAs and to better understand the risks associated with failure. The major risk factors for extubation failure in neonates are presented in Box 24-6.

In the care of the critically ill patient, the need for reintubation is frequent, challenging, and independently associated with increased morbidity and mortality in adult patients.[113] Of course, a central question is whether extubation failure is simply a marker for the underlying severity of the disease or directly contributes to a poor prognosis. From the adult and pediatric literature, there is some evidence that extubation failure, reintubation, or prolongation of MV adversely affects survival independent of the underlying illness severity.[113–117] In extremely preterm infants, especially infants born at <26 weeks and birth weight <750 g, rates of extubation failure are very high. Concerns of neonatologists dealing with extubation and subsequent reintubation are related not only to the inability to accurately predict extubation readiness but also the challenges confronted in attempting to safely reestablish the airway, which may directly affect important clinical outcomes in this fragile population. Three single-center studies provide some insight into this problem in preterm infants. Chawla et al. demonstrated extubation failure to be an independent risk factor associated with higher morbidity rates,[118] and Kaczmarek et al. reported on significantly higher rates of retinopathy of prematurity in infants who failed extubation compared to successfully extubated infants.[100] In contrast, the largest of the three studies reported that infants who were extubated early but subsequently reintubated because of extubation failure did not have higher rates of BPD or death than babies who were first extubated at a later time and did not need reintubation.[4] The data are somewhat difficult to interpret because the rate of reintubation in this observational study ranged from 70% to 81% and did not differ among infants first extubated on days 1 to 3, days 4 to 7, or beyond 1 week.[4] Larger, well-designed multicenter studies are needed to better clarify this issue. In the meantime, we must continue to strive to extubate infants as early as possible, while attempting to optimize the chance of success. Despite those efforts, extremely preterm infants will frequently require reintubation. Therefore, both interventions need to be carefully planned and performed under well-controlled conditions by the most experienced personnel.

SUMMARY

Weaning from invasive ventilation and subsequent extubation continue to be challenging problems in urgent need of further study. Available evidence indicates that early extubation is desirable, but our ability to predict the level of support at which this can be accomplished safely remains limited, especially in very preterm infants. There is strong evidence that volume-targeted ventilation accelerates weaning from MV. There is also strong support for the use of caffeine and distending airway pressure following extubation. Evidence for other adjuncts to weaning and extubation is less well established. Improved tools for predicting successful extubation in this vulnerable population are currently being explored with the goal of reducing extubation failure and need for subsequent reintubation.

REFERENCES

A complete reference list is available at https://expertconsult.inkling.com/.

25

Description of Available Devices

Robert L. Chatburn, MHHS, RRT-NPS, FAARC, and Waldemar A. Carlo, MD

INTRODUCTION TO VENTILATORS

A ventilator is defined as an automatic machine designed to provide all or part of the work required to generate enough ventilation to satisfy the body's respiratory needs. Devices like resuscitation bags or a T-piece resuscitator are used to assist breathing but are not automatic and are not considered mechanical ventilators.

There was a time (the late 1970s) when textbooks[1,2] describing ventilators emphasized individual mechanical components and pneumatic schematics of mechanical ventilators. Today, ventilators are incredibly complex mechanical devices controlled by multiple microprocessors running sophisticated software. Figure 25-1 shows a simplified pneumatic schematic diagram of a current-generation intensive care ventilator.

To keep this chapter practical, we restrict our description of ventilator design to a simplified discussion about general principles. From an engineering systems point of view, a ventilator can be viewed as having three main design characteristics: power inputs, power conversion and control, and power outputs. Beyond that, we need to understand some of the common design features of both the operator–ventilator interface (i.e., the control panels and displays) and the ventilator–patient interface (i.e., the tubing and adjunctive equipment that connects the ventilator to the patient).

Power Inputs

Work is force acting through a distance. For example, if you are asked to walk up a flight of steps, you do work in moving the mass of your body a certain distance above the earth. If you are asked to run up the steps, you may be disappointed to know that you are doing the same amount of work because it does not feel the same. What you are feeling is related to power, the rate of doing work. Similarly, it takes a certain amount of work as you inhale a breath. The larger the breaths and the faster you breathe, the more work you do per minute and the more power your body expends. Thus, power is a useful concept in understanding how ventilators are designed and operated.

Modern ventilators are powered by either electricity or compressed gas (early iron lung ventilators could actually be manually powered). Power is defined as the rate of doing work and is usually expressed in units of watts. Electrical power is calculated as the product of voltage and current required to operate the ventilator (watts = volts × amperes).[3] Electricity, either from wall outlets (e.g., 110 to 220 V A/C, at 50/60 Hz) or from batteries (e.g., 10 to 30 V DC), is used to run compressors or blowers of various types. Batteries are used for transport or emergency power.

Alternatively, the power to expand the lungs is supplied by compressed gas. Pneumatic power in watts is equivalent to a flow of 1 L/s moving in response to a pressure gradient of 1 kPa.[3] Compressed gas is usually supplied to ventilators from tanks or from wall outlets in the hospital (in the United States, hospitals supply about 50 psi from wall outlets). Some ventilators use compressed gas to power both lung inflation and the control circuitry, making them practical for transport and emergency use. Typically, ventilators are powered by separate sources of compressed air and compressed oxygen. This permits the control of oxygen concentrations between 21% (O_2 concentration in room air) and 100%. Although wall outlets supply air and oxygen at 50 psi, most ventilators have internal regulators to reduce this pressure to a lower level (e.g., 20 psi) to allow for safe operation in the case of fluctuating supply pressure. Compressed gas has all moisture removed. Otherwise, there could be condensed liquid in the tubing system, which could ruin ventilator pneumatic systems. Therefore, the gas delivered to the patient must be warmed and humidified to avoid drying out the lung tissue. A description of heating and humidification devices is beyond the scope of this chapter but is well described in current textbooks.[4]

Power Conversion and Control

Input power must be converted (e.g., from electrical to pneumatic) to get the desired outputs of pressure, volume, and flow. Electrical power is converted to pneumatic power with either a compressor or a blower. A compressor generates a relatively low flow of gas at ambient pressure to a storage container at a higher level of pressure (e.g., 20 to 50 psi). Compressors are used to create stores of compressed air in hospitals. Smaller versions are also built into intensive care ventilators (avoiding the need for connection to the hospital supply). In contrast, a blower (also called a turbine) is smaller, consumes less electrical power, and generates relatively larger flows of gas directly to the ventilator output with a relatively moderate increase of pressure (e.g., 2 psi). Blowers are typically built into home care and transport ventilators, and more powerful versions are starting to appear in intensive care unit (ICU) ventilators.

Flow Control Valves

Once pneumatic power is produced, it must be controlled to achieve the desired output of flow to the patient. Flow is manipulated in various ways to achieve predetermined patterns of patient–ventilator interaction called "modes of ventilation" (see Chapter 15). Inexpensive microprocessors became available in the 1980s and led to the development of digital flow control

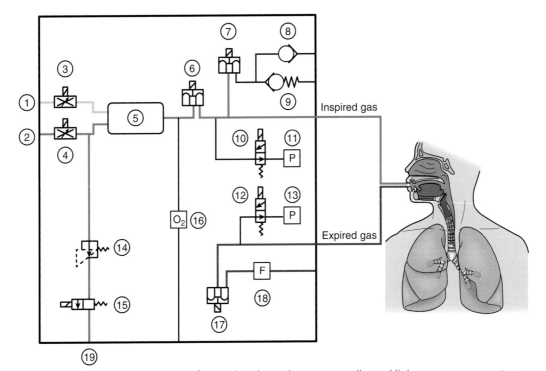

FIG 25-1 Simplified schematic of a modern intensive care ventilator. High-pressure gas enters the ventilator through the gas inlet connections for oxygen and air (1, 2). Mixing takes place in a reservoir (5) and is controlled by two valves (3, 4). Inflation flow from the reservoir is controlled by a separate proportional valve (6). On the inspiratory circuit there is a safety valve (7) and two non-return valves (8, 9). In normal operation the safety valve is closed so that inflation flow is supplied to the patient's lungs. When the safety valve is open, spontaneous inspiration of atmospheric air is possible through the emergency breathing valve (8). The emergency expiratory valve (9) provides a second channel for expiration when the expiratory valve (17) is blocked. Also on the inspiratory circuit are an inflation pressure (P) sensor (11) and a pressure sensor calibration valve (10). The exhalation circuit consists of the expiratory valve (17), expiratory pressure sensor (13) with its calibration valve (12), and an expiratory flow (F) sensor (18). The expiratory valve is a proportional valve and is used to adjust the pressure in the patient circuit. It has an expiratory flow sensor. Conversion of mass flow to volume (barometric temperature and pressure saturated) requires knowledge of ambient pressure, measured by another pressure sensor (not shown). Pressure in the patient circuit is measured by two independent pressure sensors (11, 13). Oxygen flow to the nebulizer port (19) is controlled by a pressure regulator (14) and a solenoid valve (15). (Reproduced with permission Mandu Press Ltd.)

valves. Digital control allows a great deal of flexibility in shaping the ventilator's output pressure, volume, and flow.[5] Such valves are used in the current generation of intensive care ventilators used for neonates.

The output control valve works in coordination with another valve, called the expiratory valve or "exhalation manifold." When inflation is triggered, the output control valve opens, the expiratory valve closes, and the only path left for gas is into the patient. When inflation is cycled off, the output valve closes, flow from the ventilator ceases, and the exhalation valve opens, allowing the patient to exhale to the atmosphere. An additional function of the exhalation valve is to adjust the instantaneous expiratory flow path resistance to control the level of positive end-expiratory pressure (PEEP). There is a complex interaction between the output flow control valve and the exhalation valve enabling many different pressures, volume, and flow waveforms to be generated.

Control Subsystems

The output flow valve and the exhalation valve behavior are coordinated by the ventilator's control system.[6] Most ventilators use electronic control circuits with microprocessors and complex software algorithms to manage monitoring (e.g., from pressure and flow sensors) and control functions. The differences among modes of ventilation (and the ventilators themselves) are due to the control system software as much as to the hardware. Software determines how the ventilator interacts with the patient, i.e., the modes available.[7]

Power Outputs

As we have seen, the ventilator takes input power (e.g., electricity) and converts it to flow. Then it generates output as the power that supports the work of breathing for the patient. This output power is a function of the ventilator settings, such as frequency and preset inflation pressure, as are often used in the ventilation of infants.[8]

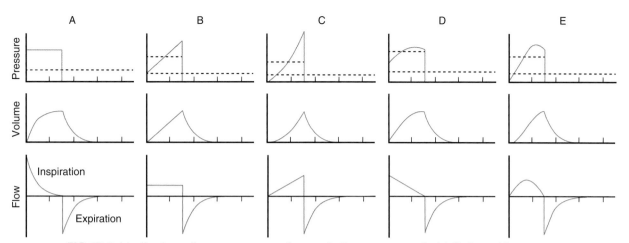

FIG 25-2 Idealized ventilator output waveforms. **A,** Pressure-controlled inflation with a rectangular pressure waveform. **B,** Volume-controlled inflation with a rectangular flow waveform. **C,** Volume-controlled inflation with an ascending-ramp flow waveform. **D,** Volume-controlled inflation with a descending-ramp flow waveform. **E,** Volume-controlled inflation with a sinusoidal flow waveform. The short dashed lines represent mean inflation pressure, and the long dashed lines represent mean pressure for the complete respiratory cycle (i.e., mean airway pressure). Note that mean inflation pressure is the same as the pressure limit in A. These waveforms were created as follows: (1) defining the control waveform using a mathematical equation (e.g., an ascending-ramp flow waveform is specified as flow = constant × time), (2) specifying the tidal volume for flow- and volume-control waveforms, (3) specifying the resistance and compliance, (4) substituting the preceding information into the equation of motion for the respiratory system, and (5) using a computer to solve the equation for the unknown variables and plotting the results against time. (Reproduced with permission from Mandu Press Ltd.)

The clinically relevant outputs of a mechanical ventilator are the pressure, volume, and flow waveforms it generates in supporting the patient's work (or more accurately, power) of breathing along with the measured or calculated data it generates and displays to the operator. A "waveform" is simply a graphic representation of a variable as a function of time. Most modern ICU ventilators have graphic displays that plot the variables of interest (pressure, volume, or flow) on the vertical axis with time on the horizontal axis. The best way to understand this subject is to start with idealized waveforms, meaning the waveforms that would exist in an ideal world with perfect machines and no interferences from leaks or patient breathing efforts. These waveforms can be easily generated for educational purposes by using graphs of mathematical models using a spreadsheet program like Excel. Understanding idealized waveforms, one can more easily interpret real-world waveforms displayed on ventilators.

Idealized Pressure, Volume, and Flow Waveforms

Typical waveforms available on modern ventilators are illustrated in Figure 25-2. These waveforms are defined by mathematical equations that characterize the ventilator's control system. They do not show the minor deviations, or "noise," caused by extraneous factors such as vibration, flow turbulence, or the patient's spontaneous breathing efforts. Remember that most ventilators have manual or automatic scaling of the horizontal and vertical axes, and this can dramatically affect the appearance of waveforms. Interpretation of ventilator waveforms requires an in-depth understanding of a number of underlying concepts (see UNDERSTANDING MODES OF VENTILATION below).

Ventilator Alarm Systems

Ventilators used for neonates in the hospital environment have a wide range of alarms. The most important alarms cover events that are life-threatening, like loss of input power or microprocessor malfunction.[9] Other alarms cover events that can lead to life-threatening situations if not corrected quickly. These include things like high or low airway pressure, tidal volume, and minute ventilation or unusual ventilator settings such as an *I:E* ratio greater than 1:1. The ventilator may also provide alarms for external monitors such as pulse oximeters and capnometers.

Operator–Ventilator Interface: Displays

The operator interface allows the operator to adjust settings and to monitor the status of the ventilator and patient. Interface designs vary widely, ranging from just a few hardware knobs and gauges to digital touch screen "virtual displays" and hybrids that have hardware knobs and buttons combined with digital displays. Obviously, the more complex the ventilator the more complex the operator interface (e.g., a simple transport ventilator compared to an ICU ventilator). Yet among the complex ventilators there is still a wide range of "user friendliness" of interface design, and there is a need for standardization.[10]

As far as monitored patient data are concerned, there are four basic ways to present the information: as numbers or text, as waveforms, as trend lines, and in the form of abstract graphic symbols.

Alphanumeric Values

Data represented in numeric form include both settings and measured values such as fraction of inspired oxygen (FiO_2),

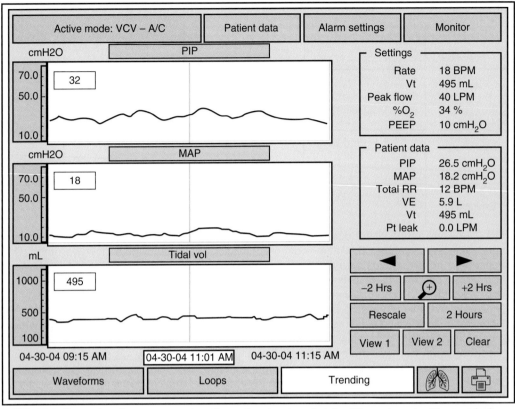

FIG 25-3 Example of an operator interface showing trend data. (Reproduced with permission from Cleveland Clinic.)

peak, plateau, mean and baseline airway pressures, inhaled/exhaled tidal volume, minute ventilation, and frequency. A wide range of calculated parameters may also be displayed, including resistance, compliance, time constant, percentage leak, I:E ratio, and peak inspiratory/expiratory flow, to name just a few. Alarms and alerts are commonly displayed as text messages. Some ventilators also present brief instructions to the operator about settings and alarms, and there may even be excerpts from the operator's manual. See the sections below describing specific ventilators to see examples of the operator's interface.

Trends

Aside from the current values of ventilator settings and measured values, we are often interested in how parameters related to mechanical support change over time. Therefore, many ventilators provide trend graphs of just about any parameter they measure or calculate. These graphs show how the monitored parameters change over variable periods of time (Fig. 25-3). Significant events or gradual changes in patient condition can be easily identified. In addition, ventilators often provide an alarm log. This is usually a text-based list documenting such things as the date, time, alarm type, urgency level, and events associated with alarms including when activated and when canceled. Such a log could be invaluable in the event of a ventilator failure leading to a legal investigation.

Waveforms and Loops

Most ventilators display graphical depictions of pressure, volume, and flow waveforms (see Chapter 12). These waveforms are quite useful for adjusting ventilator settings or evaluating respiratory system mechanics.[11,12] They are essential for assessing sources of patient–ventilator asynchrony such as missed triggers, flow asynchrony, and delayed/premature cycling and making appropriate corrections.[13] Sometimes it is more useful to plot one variable against another as an *x–y* or "loop" display. Pressure–volume loop displays are useful for identifying optimum PEEP levels (to avoid atelectrauma) and optimum tidal volume (to avoid volutrauma).[14] Ideally, loop displays for such usage should be made with patients who are paralyzed or heavily sedated (to avoid errors due to patient effort effects) and with very slow inflations (i.e., quasi-static curve), but that is rarely possible in newborn infants. Caution must be exercised because ventilators display loops under any ventilating circumstances, and hence the display may be meaningless when the patient is actively breathing. An example of a composite display showing numeric values, waveforms, and loops is shown in Figure 25-4.

Patient–Ventilator Interface: Circuits

The ventilator output is connected to the patient input (i.e., the airway opening) by means of the *patient circuit*. There are three basic configurations (Fig. 25-5). Home care and transport ventilators often use only one tube, called a single limb circuit, with a pneumatically controlled exhalation valve (Fig. 25-5, top) rather than having the exhalation valve built into the ventilator. The exhalation valve is controlled by a pressure signal from the ventilator, conveyed through small-bore tubing. This signal determines the timing of flow into and out of the patient for mandatory inflations and also may control the PEEP level.

Intensive care ventilators usually have the exhalation valve built into the ventilator and are connected to the patient with a double-limb circuit (Fig. 25-5, middle).

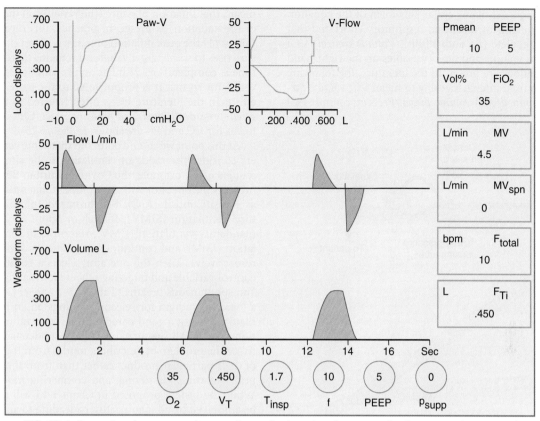

FIG 25-4 Example of a composite ventilator display showing numeric data, waveforms, and loops. (Reproduced with permission from Cleveland Clinic.)

Noninvasive ventilation may use a mask instead of an artificial airway. Ventilators designed specifically for mask ventilation often have single limb circuits that are used without an exhalation valve (Fig. 25-5, bottom). In this case, the circuit or the mask has a carefully sized opening or port. The port provides a known leak. The relationship between circuit pressure and flow through the leak is programmed into the ventilator's microcontroller. Thus, the ventilator can estimate the flow and hence the volume delivered to the patient by measuring the pressure in the circuit, calculating the leak flow, and deducting that from the total flow delivered by the blower.

Some intensive care ventilators measure flow at the airway opening using a small, usually disposable sensor. There are two basic types of flow sensors used with ventilators (Fig. 25-6). One is called a *pneumotachometer*. It has a flow-resistive element such as a screen or plastic flap in the flow path. The pressure on both sides of the resistor is conducted to pressure sensors in the ventilator through small-diameter stiff tubing. The difference between the two pressures is proportional to flow. The second type of flow sensor is called a *hot-wire anemometer*. Very thin wires are placed in the flow path and heated. Gas flow passing over the wires carries away the heat. Therefore, the amount of energy required to maintain a stable temperature in the wires is proportional to flow.

UNDERSTANDING MODES OF VENTILATION

A detailed description of the classification of ventilation modes can be found in Chapter 15. Here, we briefly define some basic terms related to mechanical ventilation in general, with specific applications to neonatal ventilation highlighted along the way. The classification of modes is based on 10 basic technological concepts (maxims) that underlie all modes of ventilation. These concepts are each fairly simple and intuitively obvious. But taken together, they result in a classification system applicable to any mode on any ventilator.[15,7]

Defining a Breath/Inflation

A breath/inflation is defined as one cycle of positive flow (inspiration) and negative flow (expiration) defined in terms of the flow–time curve (Fig. 25-7). A breath is a spontaneous breath. An inflation (followed by exhalation) is a ventilator-generated "breath." For the purpose of the proposed classification, a "spontaneous breath" (inflation) is one for which inflation is started (triggered) and stopped (cycled) by the patient. A mandatory inflation is one for which inflation is either started or stopped (or both) by the ventilator independent of the patient.

Assistance with Volume or Pressure Control

A ventilator assists breathing using either "pressure control" or "volume control" based on the equation of motion for the respiratory system:

$$P(t) = EV(t) + R\dot{V}(t) \qquad (25\text{-}1)$$

This equation relates pressure (P), volume (V), and flow ($\dot{V}$) as continuous functions of time (t) with the parameters of elastance (E) and resistance (R). If any one of the functions (P, V, or $\dot{V}$) is predetermined, the other two are derived. The term *control variable* refers to the function that is controlled (predetermined or preset) during a ventilator cycle. This form of the equation assumes that the patient makes no inspiratory effort and that expiration is complete (no auto-PEEP). *Volume control (VC)* means that *both* volume and flow (variables on the right-hand side of the equation) are preset. In the literature, the following terms are often used interchangeably to mean VC: *volume targeted, volume limited,* and *volume preset. Pressure control (PC)*

means that inflation pressure (the variable on the left-hand side of the equation) is preset. In practice, this means one of two things: (1) the peak inflation pressure is preset (i.e., airway pressure rises to some target value and remains there until inflation time is complete) or (2) inflation pressure is controlled by the ventilator so that it is proportional to the patient's inspiratory effort. In the literature PC is often referred to as *pressure targeted, pressure-limited,* and *pressure preset.* Characteristic waveforms for VC and PC are shown in Figure 25-8.

At this point we should point out that some ventilator designers consider the mode of ventilation to be simply the breath sequence. For example, the Covidien Puritan Bennett (PB) 840 presents the operator with the option of first setting the "mode" as Assist/Control (A/C), Synchronized Intermittent Mandatory Ventilation (SIMV), Bilevel, or Spont (being continuous mandatory ventilation (CMV), intermittent mandatory ventilation (IMV), and continuous spontaneous ventilation (CSV), respectively). Then the operator selects a combination of the control variable and targeting scheme for mandatory inflations and spontaneous breaths (Tables 25-1 and 25-2). While this is a logical paradigm for selecting settings on an individual ventilator, it is not a good paradigm for a general mode classification system. All manufacturers have (understandably) tended to see the problem of describing modes from the narrow vision of their particular product rather than from the larger issue of understanding, classifying, and comparing modes in general. While the system proposed in Chapter 15 will probably never be embraced by all manufacturers, leading to an industry-wide set of standards for ventilator design, we can still hope that they at least describe modes the same way in their operator manuals. And even if that never happens, end users are now free to apply this knowledge on their own to understand and use the available technology.

To make this chapter practical for the user, we provide only a brief description of the unique features of each device and the available modes. We provide the list of available modes and their classification in the accompanying tables. For a general discussion of mode classification and definitions of the modes, please see Chapter 15.

UNIVERSAL INTENSIVE CARE VENTILATORS USED FOR NEONATAL VENTILATION

Up until the 1980s, there was an unequivocal need to have separate adult and infant ventilators, mainly because of technological

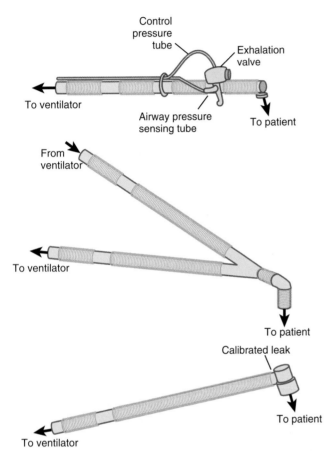

FIG 25-5 Three basic types of patient circuits. **Top,** Single-limb circuit with exhalation valve often used on home care or transport ventilators. **Middle,** Double-limb circuit usually used on intensive care ventilators. **Bottom,** Single-limb circuit without exhalation valve used on noninvasive ventilators. (Reproduced with permission from Cleveland Clinic.)

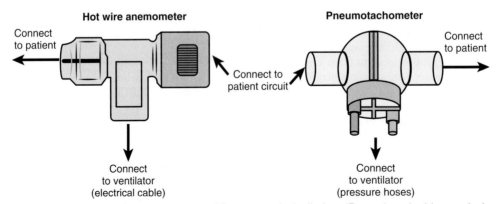

FIG 25-6 Examples of flow sensors used for neonatal ventilation. (Reproduced with permission from Cleveland Clinic.)

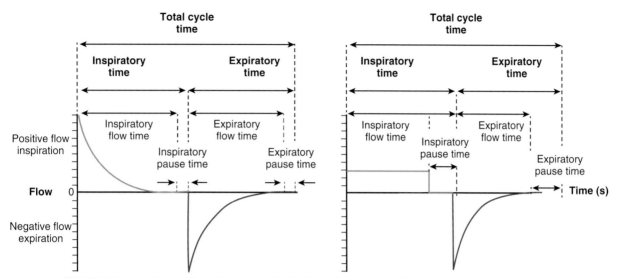

FIG 25-7 A breath is defined in terms of the flow–time curve. The curve for pressure control (with constant pressure) is shown on the left and for volume control (with constant flow) on the right. Important timing parameters related to ventilator settings are labeled. (Reproduced with permission from Mandu Press Ltd.)

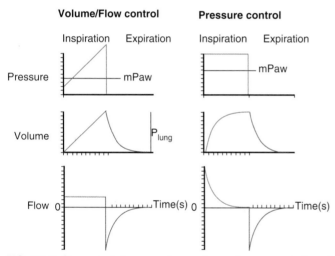

FIG 25-8 Characteristic waveforms for volume control and pressure control. Note that mean airway pressure (*mPaw*) is less for volume control than for pressure control given the same tidal volume and inspiratory time. (Reproduced with permission from Mandu Press Ltd.)

limitations related to delivering small volumes to children and newborns. Today, most of the high-end ICU ventilators used in the United States are able to ventilate the whole range of patients from premature infants (weighing a few hundred grams) up to obese adults (over 400 kg). This is an amazing technological feat but by necessity involves certain compromises. Because the adult market is much larger than the neonatal and pediatric market, these devices are primarily adult ventilators that extend their reach into neonatal-size patients but do not address some of the unique aspects of neonatal physiology, allow for precise tidal volume measurement at the airway opening or ventilation in the presence of large leaks due to the use of uncuffed endotracheal tubes. Thus some of these devices may not be optimal for the smallest preterm infants. The most common "universal" ventilators are described below (in alphabetical order).

Note that the tables showing the modes for each ventilator pair the arbitrary names created by the manufacturers with the standardized ventilator mode taxonomy described in Chapter 15.

Modes commonly referred to as *volume targeted* in the pediatric literature include both modes classified as VC and those that are classified as PC with adaptive targeting of tidal volume (either of which may have any of the three breath sequences).

CareFusion AVEA

Description
The CareFusion AVEA ventilator (Fig. 25-9) is designed for intensive care ventilation of adult, pediatric, and neonatal patients.

Operator Interface
The AVEA's operator interface has a touch screen, buttons, and a control knob. Settings are entered by touching a virtual button on the screen to select the desired setting, turning the knob to select the setting value, and then pressing the ACCEPT button to finalize the setting. The real buttons provide various features related to menu navigation, alarm silencing, suctioning, temporary 100% oxygen delivery, manual breath trigger, inspiratory hold, and expiratory hold.

Modes
Modes are selected by pressing the virtual button with the desired mode name. There are 10 basic mode names (Table 25-3). All modes can be flow or pressure triggered. In addition, there are "advanced settings" that can be used to modify the main modes (Table 25-4). Some of these advanced settings actually change the mode, resulting in many more modes by classification (Table 25-5).

The advanced settings increase both flexibility and confusion. For example, the mode named Volume Control A/C is classified as VC continuous mandatory ventilation with set-point targeting (VC-CMVs). However, adding the "Vsync" and "Flow Cycle" advanced settings to this mode turns it into PC

TABLE 25-1 Targeting Schemes Commonly Used for Neonatal Ventilation

Name	Abbreviation	Description	Advantage	Disadvantage	Example Mode Name	Ventilator	Manufacturer
Set-point	s	Operator sets all parameters of pressure waveform (pressure control modes) or volume and flow waveforms (volume control modes)	Simplicity	Changing patient conditions may make settings inappropriate	Pressure Control A/C	Babylog VN500	Dräger
Servo	r	Output of the ventilator (pressure/volume/flow) automatically follows a varying input. Currently implemented as inspiratory pressure proportional to inspiratory effort.	Proportion of total work of breathing supported by the ventilator is constant regardless of inspiratory effort	Requires estimates of artificial airways and/or respiratory system mechanical properties	Proportional Assist Ventilation Plus	PB 840	Covidien
Adaptive	a	Ventilator automatically sets target(s) between breaths in response to varying patient conditions	Can maintain stable tidal volume delivery with pressure control for changing lung mechanics or patient inspiratory effort	Automatic adjustment may be inappropriate if algorithm assumptions are violated or they do not match physiology	Pressure-regulated Volume Control	SERVO-i	Maquet

(Used with permission of Mandu Press Ltd.)

TABLE 25-2 Mode Setting Options for the Covidien PB 840 Ventilator*

Mode	BREATH CATEGORY	
	Mandatory	Spontaneous
A/C	VC	NA
	PC	
	VC+	
SIMV	VC	PS
		TC
	PC	PS
		VS
		PA
		TC
	VC+	PS
		TC
Bilevel	PC	PS
		TC
Spont	NA	PS
		VS
		PA
		TC

*The word "mode" in this case refers to the breath sequence (continuous mandatory ventilation, intermittent mandatory ventilation, and continuous spontaneous ventilation), which are given names (assist/control, synchronized intermittent mandatory ventilation, and spontaneous, respectively).

A/C, assist/control; *NA*, not applicable; *PA*, proportional assist; *PC*, power control; *PS*, pressure support; *SIMV*, synchronized intermittent mandatory ventilation; *TC*, tube compensation; *VC*, volume control; *VC+*, volume control plus; *VS*, volume support.

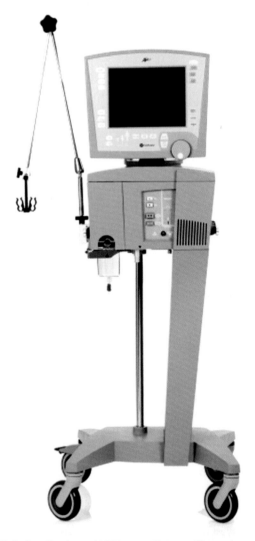

FIG 25-9 CareFusion AVEA ventilator. (Reproduced with permission from CareFusion).

TABLE 25-3   The 10 Basic Mode Names for CareFusion AVEA

Setting	VOL/AC	VOL SIMV	PRES A/C	PRES SIMV	PRVC A/C	PRVC SIMV	CPAP/PSV	APRV/ BIPHASIC	TCPL A/C	TCPL SIMV
Frequency	x	x	x	x	x	x			x	x
Volume	x	x			x	x				
Peak flow	x	x							x	x
Inspiratory pressure			x	x				x	x	x
Inspiratory time			x	x	x	x		x	x	x

TABLE 25-4   Advanced Modes for the CareFusion AVEA

Advanced Setting	Action
Volume limit	For pressure control modes, sets a volume cycle threshold. Note that volume cycling of a pressure support breath changes it from spontaneous to mandatory.
Machine volume	For pressure control modes, allows a volume target and flow and activates dual targeting. The operator sets the target volume and the ventilator calculates the target flow as the volume divided by the set inspiratory time. If flow decays to this flow target and the volume has not been delivered, then inspiration switches to volume control with constant flow until the volume has been delivered. Inspiratory time remains constant. Machine volume overrides flow cycle setting if activated.
Flow cycle	For pressure control modes, changes the cycle criterion from time to flow and sets the threshold for inspiratory flow termination as a percentage of peak flow.
Demand flow	For volume control modes, sets a ventilator-determined pressure target and activates dual targeting. If inspiratory pressure decreases 2 cm H_2O (because of patient inspiratory effort), volume control switches to pressure control. If the set volume is delivered and flow is equal to the set flow, inspiration is volume cycled. Otherwise, inspiration is flow cycled at 25% of peak flow.
Vsync	Switches the mode from volume control to pressure control with adaptive targeting. Inspiratory pressure is automatically adjusted to maintain an average tidal volume equal to the set volume.

TABLE 25-5   All Modes Available on the CareFusion AVEA

Mode Name	MODE CLASSIFICATION				
	Control Variable	Breath Sequence	Primary Breath Targeting Scheme	Secondary Breath Targeting Scheme	Tag
Volume A/C	Volume	CMV	Set point	N/A	VC-CMVs
Volume SIMV	Volume	IMV	Set point	Set point	VC-IMVs,s
Volume SIMV with artificial airway compensation	Volume	IMV	Set point	Set point/servo	VC-IMVs,sr
Volume A/C with demand flow	Volume	IMV	Dual	Dual	VC-IMVd,d
Volume SIMV with demand flow	Volume	IMV	Dual	Set point	VC-IMVd,s
Volume SIMV with demand flow and artificial airway compensation	Pressure	IMV	Dual	Set point/servo	VC-IMVd,sr
Pressure A/C	Pressure	CMV	Set point	N/A	PC-CMVs
Time-cycled pressure-limited A/C	Pressure	CMV	Set point	N/A	PC-CMVs
Pressure A/C with machine volume	Pressure	CMV	Dual	N/A	PC-CMVd
Pressure A/C with volume guarantee	Pressure	CMV	Adaptive	N/A	PC-CMVa
Time-cycled pressure-limited A/C with volume guarantee	Pressure	CMV	Adaptive	N/A	PC-CMVa
Volume A/C with Vsync	Pressure	CMV	Adaptive	N/A	PC-CMVa
Regulated volume control A/C	Pressure	CMV	Adaptive	N/A	PC-CMVa
Pressure A/C with flow cycle	Pressure	IMV	Set point	Set point	PC-IMVs,s
Pressure A/C with flow cycle and artificial airway compensation	Pressure	IMV	Set point	Set point/servo	PC-IMVs,sr
Pressure SIMV	Pressure	IMV	Set point	Set point	PC-IMVs,s
Pressure SIMV with artificial airway compensation	Pressure	IMV	Set point	Set point/servo	PC-IMVs,sr
CPAP/pressure support ventilation with volume limit	Pressure	IMV	Set point	Set point	PC-IMVs,s
CPAP/pressure support ventilation with volume limit and artificial airway compensation	Pressure	IMV	Set point	Set point/servo	PC-IMVs,sr
Infant nasal IMV	Pressure	IMV	Set point	Set point	PC-IMVs,s
Infant nasal IMV with artificial airway compensation	Pressure	IMV	Set point	Set point/servo	PC-IMVs,sr
Airway pressure release ventilation/biphasic	Pressure	IMV	Set point	Set point	PC-IMVs,s

Continued

TABLE 25-5   All Modes Available on the CareFusion AVEA—cont'd

Mode Name	Control Variable	Breath Sequence	Primary Breath Targeting Scheme	Secondary Breath Targeting Scheme	Tag
			MODE CLASSIFICATION		
Time-cycled pressure-limited A/C with flow cycle	Pressure	IMV	Set point	Set point	PC-IMVs,s
Time-cycled pressure-limited SIMV with artificial airway compensation	Pressure	IMV	Set point	Set point/servo	PC-IMVs,sr
Time-cycled pressure-limited SIMV	Pressure	IMV	Dual	Set point	PC-IMVs,s
Pressure SIMV with volume guarantee	Pressure	IMV	Adaptive	Set point	PC-IMVa,s
Pressure SIMV with volume guarantee and artificial airway compensation	Pressure	IMV	Adaptive	Set point/servo	PC-IMVa,sr
Time-cycled pressure-limited A/C with flow cycle and volume guarantee	Pressure	IMV	Adaptive	Set point	PC-IMVa,s
Time-cycled pressure-limited SIMV with volume guarantee	Pressure	IMV	Adaptive	Set point	PC-IMVa,s
Time-cycled pressure-limited SIMV with volume guarantee and artificial airway compensation	Pressure	IMV	Adaptive	Set point/servo	PC-IMVa,sr
Volume A/C with Vsync and flow cycle	Pressure	IMV	Adaptive	Set point	PC-IMVa,s
Volume SIMV with Vsync	Pressure	IMV	Adaptive	Set point	PC-IMVa,s
Volume SIMV with Vsync and artificial airway compensation	Pressure	IMV	Adaptive	Set point/servo	PC-IMVa,sr
Pressure-regulated volume control A/C with flow cycle	Pressure	IMV	Adaptive	Adaptive	PC-IMVa,s
Pressure-regulated volume control SIMV with flow cycle	Pressure	IMV	Adaptive	Set point	PC-IMVa,a
Pressure-regulated volume control SIMV	Pressure	IMV	Adaptive	Set point	PC-IMVa,s
Pressure-regulated volume control SIMV with artificial airway compensation	Pressure	IMV	Adaptive	Set point/servo	PC-IMVas,s
Time-cycled pressure-limited A/C with flow cycle, volume guarantee, and artificial airway compensation	Pressure	IMV	Adaptive/servo	Set point/servo	PC-IMVar,sr
Volume A/C with Vsync, flow cycle, and artificial airway compensation	Pressure	IMV	Adaptive/servo	Set point/servo	PC-IMVar,sr
Pressure-regulated volume control A/C with flow cycle and artificial airway compensation	Pressure	IMV	Adaptive/servo	Set point/servo	PC-IMVas,as
Pressure-regulated volume control SIMV with flow cycle and artificial airway compensation	Pressure	IMV	Adaptive/servo	Set point/servo	PC-IMVar,sr
Time-cycled pressure-limited A/C with flow cycle and artificial airway compensation	Pressure	IMV	Set point/servo	Set point/servo	PC-IMVsr,sr
CPAP/pressure support ventilation	Pressure	CSV	Set point	N/A	PC-CSVs
CPAP/pressure support ventilation and artificial airway compensation	Pressure	CSV	Set point/servo	N/A	PC-CSVsr

(Used with permission of Mandu Press Ltd.)

a, adaptive; *A/C*, assist/control; *ar*, adaptive and servo; *as*, adaptive and set point; *CMV*, continuous mandatory ventilation; *CSV*, continuous spontaneous ventilation; *d*, dual; *IMV*, intermittent mandatory ventilation; *N/A*, not applicable; *PC*, pressure control; *r*, servo; *s*, set point; *SIMV*, synchronized intermittent mandatory ventilation; *sr*, set point and servo; *VC*, volume control.

intermittent mandatory ventilation with adaptive and set-point targeting (PC-IMVa,s), a completely different mode.

Leak compensation is used to compensate for baseline leaks, which may occur at the patient–mask interface or around the patient's endotracheal tube. It provides only baseline leak compensation and is not active during breath delivery. Machine volume uses inspiratory tidal volume as its target and thus would overestimate actual tidal volume in the presence of a large leak around an uncuffed endotracheal tube.

Airway Pressure Release Ventilation/Biphasic. Airway pressure is maintained at a relatively high level for most of the respiratory cycle with intermittent release to a lower value. This is in essence extreme inverse ratio ventilation with a very long inspiratory time and brief exhalation. Spontaneous breaths are permitted both between and during mandatory inflations

and account for the bulk of minute ventilation; therefore adequate respiratory effort is needed. (Please see Chapter 21 for a functional description of airway pressure release ventilation (APRV).)

Artificial Airway Compensation. When Artificial Airway Compensation is turned on, the ventilator calculates the pressure at the airway opening required to deliver the set inflation pressure to the distal (carina) end of the endotracheal tube, as if the pressure drop across the artificial airway did not exist. This calculation takes into account flow, gas composition (heliox or nitrogen/oxygen), FiO$_2$, tube diameter, tube length, and pharyngeal curvature based on patient size (neonatal, pediatric, adult). This compensation occurs only during inflation. Artificial airway compensation is active in all pressure support (spontaneous) and flow-cycled PC inflations (spontaneous or mandatory depending on machine or patient triggering).

CPAP/Pressure Support. All spontaneous breaths are pressure supported if the pressure support level is set above zero.

CPAP/Pressure Support with Volume Limit. All spontaneous breaths are pressure supported: When a patient-triggered inflation exceeds the set volume limit, inflation is terminated.

Infant Nasal CPAP. This is available for the neonatal patient size setting only. This mode is designed to work with standard two-limbed neonatal patient circuits and nasal prongs.

Infant Nasal IMV. This mode is available for the neonatal patient size setting only. It is designed to work with standard two-limbed neonatal patient circuits and nasal prongs.

Mandatory inflations are delivered at a set rate. Spontaneous breaths are allowed but receive no support.

Pressure A/C. All inspiratory efforts trigger a pressure-controlled inflation (provided the ventilator detects the effort). A preset frequency of mandatory inflations provides a backup rate in case of apnea.

Pressure A/C with Flow Cycle. Activation of flow cycle makes every inflation patient cycled. A backup rate will trigger the ventilator at the preset rate in case of apnea. Flow-cycled A/C is equivalent to pressure support on many devices.

Pressure A/C with Machine Volume. All inspiratory efforts trigger a pressure-controlled inflation. In this mode the ventilator switches from PC to VC if inflation flow decays to a machine-determined threshold before the preset tidal volume is reached. Inflation continues at a constant flow for preset inspiratory time until the set *inspiratory* tidal volume is delivered. Thus this mode will not function well in the presence of a large endotracheal tube leak.

Pressure A/C with Volume Guarantee. This mode is available for the neonatal patient size setting only.

All inspiratory efforts trigger a time-cycled, pressure-controlled inflation and are volume targeted, based on the *exhaled* tidal volume measured at the airway opening. An upper pressure limit and average tidal volume target is set by the user, and the device will adjust the delivered inflation pressure to maintain the set target tidal volume. A backup rate will trigger the ventilator at the preset rate in case of apnea.

Pressure-Regulated Volume Control A/C (Not Available for Neonatal Ventilation). Pressure-regulated volume control (PRVC) delivers pressure-controlled inflations that support every breath for which the pressure level is automatically modulated to achieve a preset *inspiratory* volume. Initially, a decelerating-flow, volume-controlled test inflation to the set tidal volume is delivered to the patient. The ventilator then sets the target pressure based on the peak inflation pressure of the test inflation for the subsequent pressure-controlled inflations. The inflation pressure is then adjusted automatically by the ventilator to maintain the target volume. The maximum step change between two consecutive inflations is $3 \, cm \, H_2O$. The maximum tidal volume delivered in a single inflation is determined by the volume limit setting.

Pressure-Regulated Volume Control A/C with Flow Cycle (Not Available for Neonatal Ventilation). This mode is as above, but flow cycled.

Pressure-Regulated Volume Control SIMV with Flow Cycle (Not Available for Neonatal Ventilation). This mode is as above, but only a preset number of mandatory breaths is delivered in synchrony with inspiratory efforts (if present). Spontaneous breaths are possible between mandatory breaths. Machine-triggered inflations occur at the set rate if no respiratory effort is detected.

Pressure-Regulated Volume Control SIMV (Not Available for Neonatal Ventilation). This mode is as above, but with time, not flow, cycling.

Pressure SIMV. This mode is pressure-controlled SIMV.

Pressure SIMV with Volume Guarantee (Available for Neonatal Patient Size Setting Only). The volume guarantee is the same as with A/C. Mandatory inflations are delivered at a preset rate and synchronized with inspiratory effort (if present).

Time-Cycled Pressure-Limited A/C (Available for Neonatal Patient Size Setting Only). Every inspiratory effort triggers a time-cycled pressure-limited inflation. Pressure-limited modes are flow controlled with a pressure limit, as opposed to pressure-controlled modes that are directly pressure controlled. The practical implication of this distinction is that it is possible that the pressure limit may not be reached if inspiratory flow is low and the inspiratory time is long. On the other hand, peak inspiratory flow may be set higher than what may occur with a pressure controlled inflation, perhaps improving patient-ventilator synchrony. A backup rate will cycle the ventilator at the preset rate in case of apnea.

Time-Cycled Pressure-Limited A/C with Flow Cycle. Every inspiratory effort triggers a flow-cycled pressure-limited inflation. This mode is equivalent to pressure support on other devices.

Time-Cycled Pressure-Limited A/C with Flow Cycle and Volume Guarantee. This mode is as above, but with volume guarantee.

Time-Cycled Pressure-Limited A/C with Volume Guarantee (Available for Neonatal Patient Size Setting Only). This mode is as above, but time, not flow, cycled.

Time-Cycled Pressure-Limited SIMV (Available for Neonatal Patient Size Setting Only). Pressure-limited, time-cycled mandatory inflations are delivered at a preset rate and synchronized with inspiratory efforts (if present). Spontaneous breaths are possible between mandatory inflations.

Time-Cycled Pressure-Limited SIMV with Volume Guarantee (Available for Neonatal Patient Size Setting Only). This mode is as above, but with volume guarantee.

Volume A/C. Every inspiratory effort triggers a volume-controlled inflation. A set tidal volume is delivered using a constant flow over a specified amount of time during each mandatory inflation. The amount of pressure required to deliver the tidal volume will vary according to the compliance and resistance of the respiratory system. Tidal volume measurement is based on volume entering the ventilator circuit. Endotracheal tube leak will cause a problem.

Volume SIMV. Volume controlled mandatory inflations are delivered at a preset rate and synchronized with inspiratory efforts (if present). Spontaneous breaths are possible between mandatory inflations. Machine-triggered inflations occur at the set rate if no respiratory effort is detected. A set amount of volume is delivered using a constant flow over a specified amount of time during each mandatory inflation. The amount of pressure required to deliver the tidal volume will vary according to the compliance and resistance of the respiratory system.

Covidien PB 840

The Puritan Bennett 840 ventilator (Fig. 25-10) is designed for invasive and noninvasive ventilation of adult, pediatric, and neonatal patients. It is electrically controlled and pneumatically powered (requires external compressor).

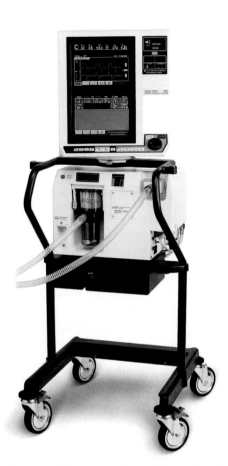

FIG 25-10 Covidien PB 840 ventilator. (Reproduced with permission from Covidien.)

Operator Interface

The operator interface uses a touch screen, buttons, and a control knob. Settings are entered by touching a virtual button on the screen to select the desired setting, turning the knob to select the setting value, and then pressing the ACCEPT button to finalize the setting. The physical buttons control menu navigation, alarm silencing, temporary increase in oxygen concentration, manual inflation trigger, inspiratory hold, and expiratory hold.

Modes

Modes on the PB 840 are set by selecting the breath sequence and the control variables separately. The operator interface uses the term *mode* to refer to what we have described in Chapter 15 as the breath sequence (i.e., CMV, IMV, CSV). Menu selections include A/C (Assist/Control), SIMV (Synchronized Intermittent Mandatory Ventilation), Spont (Spontaneous), CPAP (Continuous Positive Airway Pressure), and BILEVEL. Mandatory inflation types available are PC, VC, and VC+ (VC Plus). Spontaneous breath types available are PS (Pressure Support), TC (Tube Compensation), VS (Volume Support), PA (Proportional Assist), and NONE. An Apnea mode is available with default settings based on the patient ideal body weight (entered during the setup routine), circuit type, and mandatory inflation type. These settings can be changed.

The modes available on the PB 840 are shown in Table 25-6.

Assist/Control Pressure Control. Every inspiratory effort triggers a pressure-controlled, time-cycled inflation. A preset rate of backup apnea ventilation is available in case of apnea.

Assist/Control Volume Ventilation Plus. Every inspiratory effort triggers a pressure-controlled, time-cycled inflation with adaptive pressure adjustment. Tidal volume measurement is at the ventilator end of the circuit using inspiratory tidal volume. The manufacturer's specifications indicate that with a set value of 5 mL, 95% of the time, the actual delivered tidal volume was between 2.3 and 3.9 mL on a test lung. Endotracheal tube leaks lead to further underestimation of tidal volume. An optional proximal

TABLE 25-6   Modes Available on the Covidien PB 840

Mode Name	MODE CLASSIFICATION				
	Control Variable	Breath Sequence	Primary Breath Targeting Scheme	Secondary Breath Targeting Scheme	Tag
A/C volume control	Volume	CMV	Set point	N/A	VC-CMVs
SIMV volume control with pressure support	Volume	IMV	Set point	Set point	VC-IMVs,s
SIMV volume control with tube compensation	Volume	IMV	Set point	Servo	VC-IMVs,r
A/C pressure control	Pressure	CMV	Set point	N/A	PC-CMVs
A/C volume control plus	Pressure	CMV	Adaptive	N/A	PC-CMVa
SIMV pressure control with pressure support	Pressure	IMV	Set point	Set point	PC-IMVs,s
SIMV pressure control with tube compensation	Pressure	IMV	Set point	Set point	PC-IMVs,r
Bilevel with pressure support	Pressure	IMV	Set point	Set point	PC-IMVs,s
Bilevel with tube compensation	Pressure	IMV	Set point	Servo	PC-IMVs,r
SIMV volume control plus with pressure support	Pressure	IMV	Adaptive	Set point	PC-IMVa,s
SIMV volume control plus with tube compensation	Pressure	IMV	Adaptive	Servo	PC-IMVa,r
Spont pressure support	Pressure	CSV	Set point	N/A	PC-CSVs
Spont tube compensation	Pressure	CSV	Servo	N/A	PC-CSVr
Spont proportional assist	Pressure	CSV	Servo	N/A	PC-CSVr
Spont volume support	Pressure	CSV	Adaptive	N/A	PC-CSVa

(Reproduced with permission of Mandu Press Ltd.)

a, adaptive; *CMV,* continuous mandatory ventilation; *CSV,* continuous spontaneous ventilation; *IMV,* intermittent mandatory ventilation; *N/A,* not applicable; *PC,* pressure control; *r,* servo; *s,* set point; *VC,* volume control.

sensor is available to monitor actual tidal volume. A preset rate of backup apnea ventilation is available in case of apnea.

Assist/Control Volume Control. Every inspiratory effort triggers a volume-controlled inflation. A set amount of volume is delivered using a constant flow over a specified amount of time during each mandatory inflation. The amount of pressure required to deliver the tidal volume will vary according to the compliance and resistance of the respiratory system. A preset rate of backup apnea ventilation is available in case of apnea. Tidal volume measurement is at the ventilator end of the circuit using inspiratory tidal volume.

Bilevel (with Pressure Support). This is a form of low-rate pressure controlled IMV that allows spontaneous breathing throughout the ventilatory cycle. Inspiratory pressure and PEEP are called $PEEP_H$ and $PEEP_L$ respectively. The bulk of minute ventilation depends on the spontaneous respiratory effort.

Bilevel (with Tube Compensation). This mode is as above. Spontaneous breaths occur throughout the entire cycle. Tube compensation reduces the work of breathing.

SIMV Pressure Control (with Pressure Support). A set number of spontaneous breaths trigger a pressure-controlled inflation. Machine-triggered inflations occur at the set rate if no respiratory effort is detected. Spontaneous breaths in excess of the set rate are supported with a user set pressure above PEEP.

SIMV Pressure Control (with Tube Compensation). Pressure controlled mandatory inflations are delivered at a preset rate and synchronized with inspiratory efforts (if present). Spontaneous breaths are possible between mandatory inflations and may be assisted with pressure support. Spontaneous breaths in excess of the set rate have reduced work of breathing with tube compensation that adjusts inspiratory pressure in proportion to inspiratory flow throughout inspiration to overcome endotracheal tube resistance.

SIMV Volume Control with Pressure Support. Volume controlled mandatory inflations are delivered at a preset rate and synchronized with inspiratory efforts (if present). Spontaneous breaths are possible between mandatory inflations and may be assisted with pressure support. VC is based on tidal volume measurement at the ventilator end of the circuit using inspiratory tidal volume.

SIMV Volume Ventilation Plus (with Pressure Support). Every inspiratory effort (if detected) triggers a mandatory pressure controlled breath with adaptive targeting to automatically adjust inflation pressure to achieve the preset average tidal volume. Machine-triggered inflations occur at the set rate if no respiratory effort is detected. Tidal volume measurement is at the ventilator end of the circuit using inspiratory tidal volume, which leads to underestimation of delivered tidal volume. Endotracheal tube leaks lead to further underestimation of tidal volume. An optional proximal sensor is available to monitor actual tidal volume. Spontaneous breaths in excess of the set rate may be assisted with a user-set pressure above PEEP.

SIMV Volume Control Plus (with Tube Compensation). This mode is as above, but with tube compensation rather than pressure support.

Spont Pressure Support. This mode is spontaneous ventilation on CPAP with all spontaneous breaths supported by a set pressure above PEEP.

Spont Volume Support. This is the same as pressure support but with adaptive targeting such that inflation pressure is automatically adjusted to achieve the preset average tidal volume, based on inspiratory tidal volume measurement at the ventilator end of the patient circuit.

Neonatal Ventilation

A NeoMode option determines values for allowable settings based on patient circuit type and ideal body weight (range for neonates is 0.3 to 7.0 kg or 0.66 to 15 lb).

Dräger Evita XL

The Dräger Evita XL ventilator (Fig. 25-11) is designed for invasive and noninvasive ventilation of adult, pediatric, and neonatal patients. It is electrically controlled and pneumatically powered (requires an external compressor). This is an older model that is still widely used, but is now becoming supplanted by the Evita V500 and Babylog VN500.

Operator Interface

The operator interface uses a touch screen, buttons, and a control knob. Settings are entered by touching a virtual button on the screen to select the desired setting, turning the rotary knob to select the setting value, and then pressing the knob to finalize the setting. Other virtual buttons provide various features related to menu navigation, alarm silencing, temporary 100% oxygen delivery, manual breath trigger, inspiratory hold, and expiratory hold.

Modes

Modes are selected by mode name (e.g., CMV, SIMV, etc.), using tabs on the touch screen. Relevant ventilator setting screens are displayed according to the mode tab. The settings are also grouped by tab, giving access to basic settings (e.g., tidal volume for VC modes and inspiratory pressure for PC modes) and additional settings. Some additional settings are simple, like trigger sensitivity or automatic tube compensation. Others are more complex, such as AutoFlow. Activating AutoFlow changes the mode from VC with set-point targeting to PC with adaptive targeting, a completely different mode. All modes can be flow or pressure triggered. Table 25-7 shows the modes available on the Dräger Evita XL.

Airway Pressure Release Ventilation. Airway pressure is maintained at a high level for most of the respiratory cycle

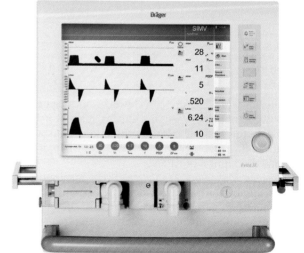

FIG 25-11 Dräger Evita XL ventilator. (Reproduced with permission from Dräger.)

TABLE 25-7   Modes Available on the Dräger Evita XL

Mode Name	MODE CLASSIFICATION				
	Control Variable	Breath Sequence	Primary Breath Targeting Scheme	Secondary Breath Targeting Scheme	Tag
Continuous mandatory ventilation	Volume	CMV	Set point	N/A	VC-CMVs
Continuous mandatory ventilation with pressure-limited ventilation	Volume	CMV	Dual	N/A	VC-CMVd
SIMV	Volume	IMV	Set point	Set point	VC-IMVs,s
SIMV with automatic tube compensation	Volume	IMV	Set point	Set point/servo	VC-IMVs,sr
SIMV with pressure-limited ventilation	Volume	IMV	Dual	Set point	VC-IMVd,s
SIMV with pressure-limited ventilation and automatic tube compensation	Volume	IMV	Dual	Set point/servo	VC-IMVd,s
Mandatory minute volume ventilation	Volume	IMV	Adaptive	Set point	VC-IMVa,s
Mandatory minute volume ventilation with automatic tube compensation	Volume	IMV	Adaptive	Set point/servo	VC-IMVa,sr
Mandatory minute volume with pressure limited ventilation	Volume	IMV	Dual/adaptive	Set point	VC-IMVda,s
Mandatory minute volume with pressure limited ventilation and automatic tube compensation	Volume	IMV	Dual/adaptive	Set point/servo	VC-IMVda,sr
Pressure controlled ventilation plus assisted	Pressure	CMV	Set point	N/A	PC-CMVs
Continuous mandatory ventilation with AutoFlow	Pressure	CMV	Adaptive	N/A	PC-CMVa
Continuous mandatory ventilation with AutoFlow and tube compensation	Pressure	CMV	Adaptive/servo	N/A	PC-CMVas
Pressure controlled ventilation plus/pressure support	Pressure	IMV	Set point	Set point	PC-IMVs,s
Pressure controlled ventilation plus/pressure support and tube compensation	Pressure	IMV	Set point/servo	Set point/servo	PC-IMVsr,sr
Airway pressure release ventilation	Pressure	IMV	Set point	Set point	PC-IMVs,s
Airway pressure release ventilation with tube compensation	Pressure	IMV	Set point/servo	Set point/servo	PC-IMVsr,sr
Mandatory minute volume with AutoFlow	Pressure	IMV	Adaptive	Set point	PC-IMVa,s
Mandatory minute volume with AutoFlow and tube compensation	Pressure	IMV	Adaptive/servo	Set point/servo	PC-IMVar,sr
Synchronized intermittent mandatory ventilation with AutoFlow	Pressure	IMV	Adaptive	Set point	PC-IMVa,s
Synchronized intermittent mandatory ventilation with AutoFlow and tube compensation	Pressure	IMV	Adaptive/servo	Set point/servo	PC-IMVar,sr
Continuous positive airway pressure/pressure support	Pressure	CSV	Set point	N/A	PC-CSVs
Continuous positive airway pressure/pressure support with tube compensation	Pressure	CSV	Set point/servo	N/A	PC-CSVsr
SmartCare	Pressure	CSV	Intelligent	N/A	PC-CSVi

(Reproduced with permission of Mandu Press Ltd.)

a, adaptive; *ar*, adaptive and servo; *as*, adaptive and set point; *CMV*, continuous mandatory ventilation; *CSV*, continuous spontaneous ventilation; *d*, dual; *IMV*, intermittent mandatory ventilation; *N/A*, not applicable; *PC*, pressure control; *VC*, volume control *s*, set point; *d*, dual; *sr*, setpoint and servo; *a*, adaptive; *da*, dual and adaptive; *as*, adaptive and set point; *ar*, adaptive and servo; *i*, intelligent.

with intermittent release to a lower value. Spontaneous breaths occur both between and during mandatory breaths and provide the bulk of minute ventilation. Thus a reliable respiratory effort is needed. (Please see Chapter 21 for functional description of APRV.)

Continuous Mandatory Ventilation. Every inspiratory effort triggers a volume controlled mandatory inflation synchronized with inspiratory effort (if present). Machine triggered mandatory inflations are delivered at the preset frequency.

Continuous Mandatory Ventilation with AutoFlow. Every inspiratory effort (if detected) triggers a mandatory pressure controlled inflation with adaptive targeting to automatically adjust inflation pressure to achieve the preset average tidal volume. Machine triggered mandatory inflations are delivered at the preset frequency.

Continuous Positive Airway Pressure/Pressure Support. This mode is spontaneous breathing on CPAP with each breath receiving a set amount of pressure support above CPAP. Reliable respiratory drive is necessary.

Pressure-Controlled Ventilation Plus Assist. This is called Assist/Control on the newer V500 model. Every inspiratory effort triggers a time-cycled, pressure-controlled inflation. A backup rate ensures a minimum machine-triggered rate.

Pressure-Controlled Ventilation Plus/Pressure Support. Pressure controlled mandatory inflations are delivered at a preset rate and synchronized with inspiratory efforts (if detected). Spontaneous breaths are possible between mandatory inflations. Spontaneous breaths are permitted both between and during mandatory inflations and may be pressure supported.

Synchronized Intermittent Mandatory Ventilation. Pressure controlled mandatory inflations are delivered at a preset rate and synchronized with inspiratory efforts (if present). Spontaneous breaths are possible between mandatory inflations and may be assisted with pressure support, if that option is selected.

Synchronized Intermittent Mandatory Ventilation with AutoFlow. This mode is as above, but with adaptive pressure targeting to achieve the set tidal volume.

Neonatal Ventilation

The Evita XL may be used for ventilation of premature infants with the NeoFlow option. This option offers flow measurement at the wye-piece, which provides precise volume monitoring independent of compliance of the patient circuit in addition to accurate triggering. The automatic compensation for leaks allows for direct adjustment of tidal volume down to 3 mL.

Dräger Evita Infinity V500

The Dräger Evita Infinity V500 ventilator (Fig. 25-12) is designed for invasive and noninvasive ventilation of adult and pediatric patients. With additional software and optional flow measurement at the wye-piece it can also ventilate neonatal patients. It is electrically controlled and pneumatically powered (requires external compressor). A specialty neonatal version of this ventilator, the VN500, is discussed in the next section.

Operator Interface

The operator interface has a touch screen, buttons, and a control knob. Settings are entered by touching a virtual button on the screen to select the desired setting, turning the rotary knob to select the setting value, and then pressing the knob to finalize the setting. Other buttons provide various features related to menu navigation and alarm silencing. The Smart Pulmonary View allows for real-time visualization of pulmonary function data (compliance and resistance).

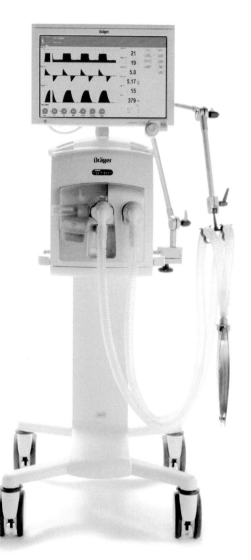

FIG 25-12 Dräger Evita Infinity V500 ventilator. (Reproduced with permission from Dräger.)

		MODE CLASSIFICATION			
Mode Name	Control Variable	Breath Sequence	Primary Breath Targeting Scheme	Secondary Breath Targeting Scheme	Tag
Volume control continuous mandatory ventilation	Volume	CMV	Set point	N/A	VC-CMVs
Volume control assist control	Volume	CMV	Set point	N/A	VC-CMVs
Volume control assist control with pressure-limited ventilation	Volume	CMV	Dual	N/A	VC-CMVd
Volume control synchronized intermittent mandatory ventilation	Volume	IMV	Set point	Set point	VC-IMVs,s
Volume control synchronized intermittent mandatory ventilation with automatic tube compensation	Volume	IMV	Set point	Set point/servo	VC-IMVs,sr
Volume control synchronized intermittent mandatory ventilation with pressure-limited ventilation	Volume	IMV	Dual	Set point	VC-IMVd,s
Volume control synchronized intermittent mandatory ventilation with pressure-limited ventilation and automatic tube compensation	Volume	IMV	Dual	Set point/servo	VC-IMVd,sr
Volume control mandatory minute volume ventilation	Volume	IMV	Adaptive	Set point	VC-IMVa,s
Volume control mandatory minute volume ventilation with automatic tube compensation	Volume	IMV	Adaptive	Set point/servo	VC-IMVa,sr

TABLE 25-8 Modes Available on the Dräger Evita Infinity 500 Ventilator

Continued

TABLE 25-8 Modes Available on the Dräger Evita Infinity 500 Ventilator—cont'd

Mode Name	Control Variable	Breath Sequence	Primary Breath Targeting Scheme	Secondary Breath Targeting Scheme	Tag
Volume control mandatory minute volume with AutoFlow/volume guarantee	Volume	IMV	Adaptive	Set point	VC-IMVda,s
Volume control mandatory minute volume with AutoFlow/volume guarantee and automatic tube compensation	Volume	IMV	Adaptive/servo	Set point/servo	VC-IMVdar,sr
Volume control mandatory minute volume with pressure-limited ventilation	Volume	IMV	Dual/adaptive	Set point	VC-IMVda,s
Volume control mandatory minute volume with pressure-limited ventilation and automatic tube compensation	Volume	IMV	Dual/adaptive	Set point/servo	VC-IMVda,sr
Pressure control assist control	Pressure	CMV	Set point	N/A	PC-CMVs
Pressure control assist control with automatic tube compensation	Pressure	CMV	Set point/servo	N/A	PC-CMVsr
Volume control continuous mandatory ventilation with AutoFlow/volume guarantee	Pressure	CMV	Adaptive	N/A	PC-CMVa
Volume control continuous mandatory ventilation with AutoFlow/volume guarantee and automatic tube compensation	Pressure	CMV	Adaptive/servo	N/A	PC-CMVar
Volume control assist control with AutoFlow/volume guarantee	Pressure	CMV	Adaptive	N/A	PC-CMVa
Volume control assist control with AutoFlow/volume guarantee and automatic tube compensation	Pressure	CMV	Adaptive/servo	N/A	PC-CMVar
Pressure control continuous mandatory ventilation	Pressure	IMV	Set point	N/A	PC-IMVs
Pressure control continuous mandatory ventilation with automatic tube compensation	Pressure	IMV	Set point/servo	N/A	PC-IMVsr,sr
Pressure control synchronized intermittent mandatory ventilation	Pressure	IMV	Set point	Set point	PC-IMVs,s
Pressure control synchronized intermittent mandatory ventilation with automatic tube compensation	Pressure	IMV	Set point/servo	Set point/servo	PC-IMVsr,sr
Pressure control biphasic positive airway pressure	Pressure	IMV	Set point	Set point	PC-IMVs,s
Pressure control biphasic positive airway pressure with automatic tube compensation	Pressure	IMV	Set point/servo	Set point/servo	PC-IMVsr,sr
Pressure control airway pressure release ventilation	Pressure	IMV	Set point	Set point	PC-IMVs,s
Pressure control airway pressure release ventilation with automatic tube compensation	Pressure	IMV	Set point/servo	Set point/servo	PC-IMVsr,sr
Pressure control pressure support ventilation	Pressure	IMV	Set point	Set point	PC-IMVs,s
Pressure control pressure support ventilation with automatic tube compensation	Pressure	IMV	Set point/servo	Set point/servo	PC-IMVsr,sr
Volume control synchronized intermittent mandatory ventilation with AutoFlow	Pressure	IMV	Adaptive	Set point	PC-IMVa,s
Volume control synchronized intermittent mandatory ventilation with AutoFlow and automatic tube compensation	Pressure	IMV	Adaptive/servo	Set point/servo	PC-IMVar,sr
Spontaneous continuous positive airway pressure/pressure support	Pressure	CSV	Set point	N/A	PC-CSVs
Spontaneous continuous positive airway pressure/pressure support with automatic tube compensation	Pressure	CSV	Set point/servo	N/A	PC-CSVsr
Spontaneous continuous positive airway pressure/variable pressure support	Pressure	CSV	Bio-variable	N/A	PC-CSVb
Spontaneous continuous positive airway pressure/variable pressure support with automatic tube compensation	Pressure	CSV	Bio-variable/servo	N/A	PC-CSVbr
Spontaneous continuous positive airway pressure/volume support	Pressure	CSV	Adaptive	N/A	PC-CSVa
Spontaneous continuous positive airway pressure/volume support with automatic tube compensation	Pressure	CSV	Adaptive/servo	N/A	PC-CSVar
Spontaneous proportional pressure support	Pressure	CSV	Servo	N/A	PC-CSVr
SmartCare	Pressure	CSV	Intelligent	N/A	PC-CSVi

(Reproduced with permission of Mandu Press Ltd.)

a, adaptive; *ar,* adaptive and servo; *CMV,* continuous mandatory ventilation; *CSV,* continuous spontaneous ventilation; *d,* dual; *IMV,* intermittent mandatory ventilation; *N/A,* not applicable; *PC,* pressure control; *VC,* volume control ; *s,* set point; *d,* dual; *b,* bio-variable; *a,* adaptive; *i,* intelligent; *sr,* set point and servo; *da,* dual and adaptive; *dar,* dual, adaptive, and set point; *ar,* adaptive and servo; *sr,* set point and servo; *br,* bio-variable and servo.

Modes

Modes are selected by the mode name (e.g., VC-AC, VC-SIMV, etc.), using tabs on the touch screen. Relevant ventilator setting screens are displayed according to the mode tab. The settings are also grouped by tab, giving access to basic settings (e.g., tidal volume for VC modes and inflation pressure for PC modes) and additional settings. Some additional settings are simple, like trigger sensitivity or automatic tube compensation. Others are more complex, such as AutoFlow. Activating AutoFlow changes the mode from VC with set-point targeting to PC with adaptive targeting, a completely different mode. All modes can be flow or pressure triggered. Table 25-8 shows the modes available on the Dräger Evita Infinity V500.

Pressure Control Airway Pressure Release Ventilation. This is a form of pressure controlled IMV that allows spontaneous breathing throughout the ventilatory cycle. Airway pressure is maintained at a relatively high level (P_{high}) for most of the respiratory cycle with intermittent release to a lower value (P_{low}). (Please see Chapter 21 for functional description of APRV.)

Patient triggering of mandatory inflations is possible using the AutoRelease feature. This triggers inspiration once a pre-set expiratory flow threshold is reached. When AutoRelease is turned on, the switch from P_{high} to P_{low} is synchronized with the patient's breathing. Spontaneous breaths occur both between and during mandatory breaths and provide the bulk of minute ventilation. Thus a reliable respiratory effort is needed.

Pressure Control Assist Control. Every inspiratory effort triggers a time-cycled, pressure-controlled inflation. A backup rate of apnea ventilation ensures a minimum machine-triggered rate.

Pressure Control Biphasic Positive Airway Pressure. The device cycles between two levels of airway pressure with spontaneous breathing throughout the cycle. It can be considered a form of Pressure Control SIMV, except that cycling of mandatory cycles is synchronized with the end of a superimposed spontaneous breath (if present).

Pressure Control Continuous Mandatory Ventilation. The ventilator generates mandatory pressure-limited inflations at a set machine-triggered rate. Spontaneous breaths are permitted both during and between mandatory breaths, so this is a form of IMV not CMV.

Pressure Control Pressure Support. Every inspiratory effort triggers a pressure-controlled, flow-cycled inflation. A backup rate of apnea ventilation ensures a minimum machine-triggered rate.

Pressure Control Synchronized Intermittent Mandatory Ventilation. Pressure controlled mandatory inflations are delivered at a preset rate and synchronized with inspiratory efforts (if present). Spontaneous breaths are possible between mandatory inflations and may be assisted with pressure support if that option is selected.

Spontaneous Continuous Positive Airway Pressure/Pressure Support. This mode is spontaneous breathing on CPAP, with each breath receiving a set amount of pressure support above CPAP. Reliable respiratory drive is necessary.

Spontaneous Continuous Positive Airway Pressure/Volume Support. This is the same as pressure support but with adaptive targeting such that inflation pressure is automatically adjusted to achieve the preset average tidal volume. Reliable respiratory drive is necessary.

Volume Control Continuous Mandatory Ventilation with AutoFlow. The ventilator generates mandatory volume-targeted, time-cycled inflations at a set machine-triggered rate. Spontaneous breaths are possible, but not synchronized.

Volume Control Assist Control with AutoFlow. Every inspiratory effort triggers a time-cycled inflation, which is volume-targeted. This results in a decelerating flow pattern and is really a form of PC with adaptive targeting of pressure to achieve a target tidal volume with the minimum pressure necessary. A pressure limit that determines the upper limit of adaptive pressure range is set by the user. A backup rate ensures a minimum machine-triggered rate.

Volume Control Synchronized Intermittent Mandatory Ventilation with AutoFlow. This mode is as above, but only a set number of spontaneous breaths trigger a mandatory inflation. Machine-triggered inflations occur at the set rate if no respiratory effort is detected. Spontaneous breaths in excess of the set rate are permitted but receive no support.

Neonatal Ventilation

The neonatal mode offers flow measurement at the wye-piece, which provides precise volume monitoring independent of compliance of the patient circuit in addition to accurate triggering. The measured values for minute ventilation and tidal volume are not corrected for leakage and are therefore lower than the actual minute and tidal volumes applied to the patient if a leakage occurs. When leakage compensation is activated, the measured volume and flow values as well as the curves for flow and volume are displayed with leakage correction. The Dräger Evita Infinity V500 compensates for leakages up to 100% of the set tidal volume. Exhaled tidal volume is used for volume targeting.

Maquet SERVO-i

The SERVO-i ventilator (Fig. 25-13) is intended for invasive and noninvasive ventilation of adults, children, and infants with respiratory failure or respiratory insufficiency in hospitals or health care facilities and for in-hospital transport.

Operator Interface

The operator interface uses a touch screen, buttons, and knobs. The touch screen is used to select control variables, and the main control knob allows adjustment of settings (by turning) and confirmation of settings (by pressing). The supplemental control knobs provide quick setting adjustments of oxygen percentage, tidal volume, inflation pressure, and PEEP. The buttons provide for manual inflation trigger, temporary 100% oxygen breaths, inspiratory hold, and expiratory hold. Other buttons are related to alarms, system information, and navigation.

Modes

Mode names are selected by pressing buttons on the touch screen. Once a mode name is chosen, the screen changes to show the available settings options. All modes can be flow or pressure triggered.

Automode is a term to describe the automatic transition between controlled ventilation and supported ventilation, depending on the adequacy of respiratory effort. It is a form of IMV in which mandatory inflations are suppressed if the spontaneous breath rate is higher than the preset mandatory rate. This is similar to assist/control and pressure support modes

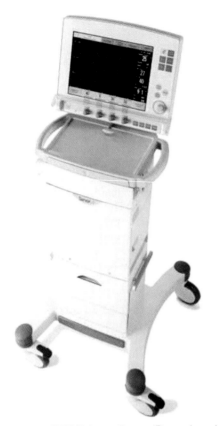

FIG 25-13 Maquet SERVO-i ventilator. (Reproduced with permission from Maquet.)

as implemented on neonatal ventilators in which a backup rate automatically takes over when spontaneous breathing is absent.

The modes available on the SERVO-i are shown in Table 25-9.

Automode (Pressure Control to Pressure Support). Mandatory pressure controlled inflations are delivered at a preset rate. Patient-triggered inflations are delivered with pressure support.

Automode (Pressure-Regulated Volume Control to Volume Support). Mandatory inflations are delivered at a preset rate with adaptive targeting to achieve a preset average tidal volume. Patient-triggered inflations are delivered with pressure support also using adaptive targeting.

Automode (Volume Control to Volume Support). Mandatory inflations are delivered at a preset rate with volume control. Patient-triggered inflations are delivered with pressure support using adaptive targeting to achieve the preset average tidal volume.

BiVent. This is essentially bilevel CPAP with spontaneous breathing throughout, which provides the bulk of minute ventilation; thus it requires intact respiratory drive.

Neurally Adjusted Ventilatory Assist. Neurally adjusted ventilatory assist (NAVA) uses the electrical activity of the diaphragm (EAdi) to trigger and cycle inflation and delivers pressure in proportion to patient inspiratory effort. Triggering by EAdi ensures complete synchronization, irrespective of circuit leaks; thus it is ideal for noninvasive support. However, NAVA is a positive feedback mechanism that assumes mature respiratory control. Pressure and volume are variable and controlled by the patient's inspiratory effort. A gain (the NAVA level) is applied to the electrical signal from the diaphragm to translate that signal to an inflation pressure.

Note: If the EAdi signal is lost, the ventilator switches to Pressure Support. It returns to NAVA if the signal is regained. Mandatory inflations occur only when the EAdi signal is absent or the patient is apneic.

Pressure Control. Mandatory pressure-controlled breaths are machine triggered at a preset frequency or patient triggered and machine cycled. Spontaneous breaths are not allowed.

Pressure-Regulated Volume Control. PRVC delivers pressure-controlled inflations that support every breath, in which the pressure level is automatically modulated to achieve a preset

TABLE 25-9   Modes Available on the Maquet SERVO-i

Mode Name	MODE CLASSIFICATION				
	Control Variable	Breath Sequence	Primary Breath Targeting Scheme	Secondary Breath Targeting Scheme	Tag
Volume control	Volume	IMV	Dual	Dual	VC-IMVd,d
SIMV (volume control)	Volume	IMV	Dual	Dual	VC-IMVd,s
Automode (volume control to volume)	Volume	IMV	Dual	Adaptive	VC-IMVd,a
Pressure control	Pressure	CMV	Set point	N/A	PC-CMVs
Pressure-regulated volume control	Pressure	CMV	Adaptive	N/A	PC-CMVa
SIMV (pressure control)	Pressure	IMV	Set point	Set point	PC-IMVs,s
BiVent	Pressure	IMV	Set point	Set point	PC-IMVs,s
Automode (pressure control to pressure support)	Pressure	IMV	Set point	Set point	PC-IMVs,s
SIMV pressure-regulated volume control	Pressure	IMV	Adaptive	Set point	PC-IMVa,s
Automode (pressure-regulated volume control to volume support)	Pressure	IMV	Adaptive	Adaptive	PC-IMVa,a
Spontaneous/CPAP	Pressure	CSV	Set point	N/A	PC-CSVs
Pressure support	Pressure	CSV	Set point	N/A	PC-CSVs
Neurally adjusted ventilatory assist	Pressure	CSV	Servo	N/A	PC-CSVr
Volume support	Pressure	CSV	Adaptive	N/A	PC-CSVa

(Reproduced with permission of Mandu Press Ltd).
a, adaptive; *CMV*, continuous mandatory ventilation; *CSV*, continuous spontaneous ventilation; *d*, dual; *IMV*, intermittent mandatory ventilation; *N/A*, not applicable; *PC*, pressure control; *r*, servo; *s*, set point; *VC*, volume control.

exhaled volume measured at the ventilator end of the circuit. The ventilator delivers a test volume-controlled inflation and initiates ventilation with pressure-controlled inflations at the pressure derived from the test inflation. The inflation pressure is then adjusted automatically based on the exhaled tidal volume of the previous inflation to maintain the target volume. The maximum step change between two consecutive inflations is 3 cm H_2O. Its classification is PC-CMVa.

SIMV Pressure-Regulated Volume Control. This mode is as above, but only a set number of spontaneous breaths are supported. Machine-triggered inflations occur at the set rate if no respiratory effort is detected. Spontaneous breaths are allowed but receive no support.

Pressure Support. Every inspiratory effort triggers a pressure-controlled, flow-cycled inflation. A backup rate of apnea ventilation ensures a minimum machine-triggered rate.

SIMV Pressure Control. Mandatory pressure controlled inflations are delivered at a preset rate. Spontaneous breaths are permitted between mandatory inflations but receive no support.

SIMV (Volume Control). Mandatory volume control breaths are delivered at a preset rate. Spontaneous breaths are permitted between mandatory inflations but receive no support. This mode uses dual targeting (see the explanation of dual targeting in Chapter 15). Therefore, if the patient's inspiratory effort is large enough (airway pressure drop 3 cm H_2O), inflation will switch from VC to PC with flow cycling.

Spontaneous/CPAP. This is spontaneous breathing on a set level of CPAP. Minute ventilation is fully supplied by patient effort.

Volume Control. Every inspiratory effort triggers a volume controlled inflation. Machine triggered breaths are delivered at a preset rate. This mode uses dual targeting (see the explanation of dual targeting in Chapter 15). Therefore, if the patient's inspiratory effort is large enough (airway pressure drop 3 cm H_2O), inflation will switch from VC to PC with flow cycling.

Volume Support. All spontaneous breaths trigger flow-cycled inflations with a variable amount of pressure support to target average inspiratory tidal volume at the target level. Apnea ventilation can be provided to ensure a minimum level of support.

Neonatal Ventilation

An optional neonatal flow sensor is available with an airway adapter dead space of less than 0.75 mL and weight of 4 g. This allows flow readings as close to the patient as possible to provide accurate tidal volume measurement. Volume targeting, however, still uses volume measured at the ventilator end of the patient circuit, not airway opening.

GE Healthcare Engström Carestation

The Engström Carestation (Fig. 25-14) is designed to be used with adult patients down to infants with a body weight of 5 kg or greater. If the neonatal option is installed on the ventilator, patients weighing down to 0.5 kg may be ventilated with the Engström.

Operator Interface

The operator interface has a touch screen, buttons, and a control knob. Settings are entered by touching a virtual button on the screen to select the desired setting, turning the rotary knob to select the setting value, and then pressing the knob to finalize the setting. Other buttons provide various features related

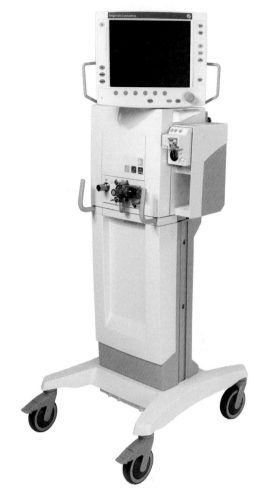

FIG 25-14 GE Healthcare Engström Carestation ventilator. (Reproduced with permission from GE Healthcare.)

to menu navigation, temporary increased oxygen delivery, and alarm silencing.

Modes

Modes on the Engström Carestation are selected by mode name (e.g., VCV, PCV, SIMV-VC) using a menu. Specific mode settings are selected using other menus and can be flow or pressure triggered. Available modes are shown in Table 25-10.

Airway Resistance Compensation. Airway resistance compensation adjusts the target delivery pressure to compensate for the resistance caused by the endotracheal tube or tracheostomy tube used. The compensation is applied to the inspiratory phase of all pressure-controlled, CPAP, and pressure-supported breaths.

Bilevel Airway Pressure Ventilation. Pressure controlled mandatory inflations are delivered at a preset rate. Inspiratory pressure and PEEP are called P_{high} and P_{low} respectively; this mode is commonly referred to as bi-level CPAP. The patient can breathe spontaneously while at either of the pressure levels. Spontaneous breaths provide most of the minute ventilation.

Bilevel Airway Pressure Ventilation–Volume Guaranteed. This mode is as above, but the P_{high} level is automatically adjusted to achieve a set inspired tidal volume when the ventilator goes from P_{low} to P_{high}.

Constant Positive Airway Pressure/Pressure Support. This mode requires reliable respiratory drive, allowing the patient to

TABLE 25-10　Modes Available on the GE Healthcare Engström Carestation

Mode Name	MODE CLASSIFICATION				
	Control Variable	Breath Sequence	Primary Breath Targeting Scheme	Secondary Breath Targeting Scheme	Tag
Volume controlled ventilation	Volume	CMV	Set point	N/A	VC-CMVs
Volume controlled ventilation with pressure limit	Volume	CMV	Dual	N/A	VC-CMVd
Synchronized intermittent mandatory ventilation–volume controlled	Volume	IMV	Set point	Set point	VC-IMVs,s
Synchronized intermittent mandatory ventilation–volume controlled with airway resistance compensation	Volume	IMV	Set point	Set point/servo	VC-IMVs,sr
Synchronized intermittent mandatory ventilation–volume controlled with pressure limit	Volume	IMV	Dual	Set point	VC-IMVd,s
Synchronized intermittent mandatory ventilation–volume controlled with pressure limit and airway resistance compensation	Pressure	IMV	Dual	Set point/servo	VC-IMVd,sr
Pressure controlled ventilation	Pressure	CMV	Set point	N/A	PC-CMVs
Pressure controlled ventilation with airway resistance compensation	Pressure	CMV	Set point/servo	N/A	PC-CMVsr
Pressure controlled ventilation–volume guaranteed	Pressure	CMV	Adaptive	N/A	PC-CMVa
Pressure controlled ventilation–volume guaranteed with airway resistance compensation	Pressure	CMV	Adaptive/servo	N/A	PC-CMVar
Synchronized intermittent mandatory ventilation–pressure controlled	Pressure	IMV	Set point	Set point	PC-IMVs,s
Synchronized intermittent mandatory ventilation–pressure controlled with airway resistance compensation	Pressure	IMV	Set point/servo	Set point/servo	PC-IMVsr,sr
Bilevel airway pressure ventilation	Pressure	IMV	Set point	Set point	PC-IMVs,s
Bilevel airway pressure ventilation with airway resistance compensation	Pressure	IMV	Set point/servo	Set point/servo	PC-IMVsr,sr
Bilevel airway pressure ventilation–volume guaranteed	Pressure	IMV	Adaptive	Set point	PC-IMVa,s
Bilevel airway pressure ventilation–volume guaranteed with airway resistance compensation	Pressure	IMV	Adaptive/servo	Set point/servo	PC-IMVar,sr
Synchronized intermittent mandatory ventilation–pressure controlled volume guaranteed	Pressure	IMV	Adaptive	Set point	PC-IMVa,s
Synchronized intermittent mandatory ventilation–pressure controlled volume guaranteed with airway resistance compensation	Pressure	IMV	Adaptive/servo	Set point/servo	PC-IMVar,sr
Constant positive airway pressure/pressure support	Pressure	CSV	Set point	N/A	PC-CSVs
Constant positive airway pressure/pressure support with airway resistance compensation	Pressure	CSV	Set point/servo	N/A	PC-CSVsr
Volume guarantee pressure support	Pressure	CSV	Adaptive	N/A	PC-CSVa
Volume guarantee pressure support with airway resistance compensation	Pressure	CSV	Adaptive/servo	N/A	PC-CSVar

(Reproduced with permission of Mandu Press Ltd.)

a, adaptive; *ar,* adaptive and servo; *CMV,* continuous mandatory ventilation; *CSV,* continuous spontaneous ventilation; *IMV,* intermittent mandatory ventilation; *N/A,* not applicable; *PC,* pressure control; *VC,* volume control; *s,* set point; *d,* dual; *r,* servo; *a,* adaptive; *sr,* set point and servo; *ar,* adaptive and servo.

breathe on CPAP. The ventilator provides a set pressure level above the CPAP level to support each spontaneous breath. The patient determines his or her own rate, tidal volume, and inspiratory timing.

Pressure Controlled Ventilation. A set pressure level is delivered during each mandatory inflation, which can be machine or patient triggered. The pressure is delivered using a decelerating flow, and the inflation is held for a set amount of time. The amount of volume provided will vary according to the compliance of the respiratory system. May be used in SIMV or A/C mode.

Pressure Controlled Ventilation–Volume Guarantee. Every inspiratory effort triggers a pressure controlled mandatory inflation using adaptive targeting to achieve a preset average tidal volume. Machine triggered breaths are delivered at a preset rate.

Synchronized Intermittent Mandatory Ventilation–Pressure Controlled. Mandatory pressure controlled inflations are delivered at a preset rate and synchronized with inspiratory efforts (if present). Spontaneous breaths are allowed between mandatory inflations but receive no support.

Synchronized Intermittent Mandatory Ventilation–Pressure Controlled Volume Guaranteed. Mandatory pressure controlled inflations are delivered at a preset rate using adaptive targeting to achieve a preset average tidal volume. Spontaneous breaths are allowed between mandatory inflations but receive no support.

Synchronized Intermittent Mandatory Ventilation–Volume Controlled. Every inspiratory effort triggers a mandatory volume controlled inflation. Spontaneous breaths are allowed between mandatory inflations but receive no support. Machine-triggered inflations occur at the set rate if no respiratory effort is detected.

Synchronized Intermittent Mandatory Ventilation–Volume Controlled with Pressure Limit. This mode is as above, but uses dual targeting. Inflation begins at the set inflation flow and switches to PC when inflation pressure meets the inflation pressure target (P_{limit} setting).

Volume Controlled Ventilation. Mandatory volume-controlled inflations are machine triggered at a preset frequency or patient triggered and machine cycled. A set amount of volume is delivered using a constant flow over a specified amount of time during each mandatory inflation. The amount of pressure required to deliver the tidal volume will vary according to the compliance and resistance of the respiratory system.

Volume Controlled Ventilation with Pressure Limit. This mode uses dual targeting. Inflation begins at the set inflation flow and switches to PC when inflation pressure meets the inflation pressure target (P_{limit} setting). Mandatory inflations may be machine triggered at a preset frequency or patient triggered and machine cycled when the set tidal volume is delivered or maximum inflation time reached.

Neonatal Ventilation

The neonatal option on the Engström Carestation provides ventilation for intubated neonatal patients weighing down to 500 g. This is accomplished by using a proximal flow sensor at the patient wye-piece, which connects to the ventilator with a cable. This sensor allows the ventilator to deliver flows as low as 0.2 L/min and as high as 30 L/min.

SPECIALIZED NEONATAL VENTILATORS

Specialized neonatal ventilators are more common outside the United States, and there are many brands to choose from. Within the United States, there is currently only one specialized ICU infant ventilator available, the Dräger VN500 Babylog, and one specialized noninvasive ventilator, the CareFusion Infant Flow SiPAP device.

Dräger Babylog VN500

The Dräger I VN500 is the only specialty neonatal ventilator available in the United States. It differs from the universal ventilators in a number of features specifically designed to address the unique characteristics of the neonatal patient described in Chapter 15. The VN500 shares the basic layout, controls, and hardware components with its adult counterpart, the V500, but its software provides excellent leak compensation to allow for ventilation with uncuffed endotracheal tubes with precise flow sensing and triggering as well as leak-adapted breath termination in the face of endotracheal tube leaks as large as 80%. There is a dual control algorithm for triggered and untriggered inflations in the volume-targeted mode of VG to allow more stable tidal volume in very preterm infants with immature respiratory control and intermittent respiratory effort. The Dräger Babylog VN500 (Fig. 25-15) is intended for the ventilation of neonatal patients from 0.4 kg (0.88 lb) up to 10 kg (22 lb) and pediatric patients from 5 kg (11 lb) up to 20 kg (44 lb) body weight. It is

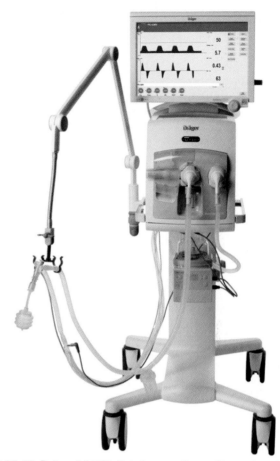

FIG 25-15 Dräger VN500 Babylog ventilator. (Reproduced with permission from Dräger.)

electrically controlled and pneumatically powered (requires an external compressor).

Operator Interface

The operator interface is similar to that of the Dräger Infinity V500 and uses a touch screen, buttons, and a control knob. Settings are entered by touching a virtual button on the screen to select the desired setting, turning the rotary knob to select the setting value, and then pressing the knob to finalize the setting. Other buttons provide various features related to menu navigation and alarm silencing.

Modes

Modes are selected by mode name (e.g., Pressure Control A/C, Pressure Control Pressure Support, etc.), using tabs on the touch screen. The settings screens are also tabbed, giving access to basic settings and additional settings. The additional settings include trigger sensitivity, automatic tube compensation, and volume guarantee. There are no VC modes available on the Babylog VN500. Table 25-11 shows the modes available on the Babylog VN500.

Pressure Control Assist Control. Every inspiratory effort triggers a pressure-controlled inflation. A set pressure level is generated using a decelerating flow and the inflation is held for a set amount of time (is time-cycled). The amount of volume provided will vary according to the compliance of the respiratory system. A set rate provides mandatory inflations in case of apnea.

TABLE 25-11   Modes Available on the Dräger Babylog VN500

Mode Name	Control Variable	Breath Sequence	Primary Breath Targeting Scheme	Secondary Breath Targeting Scheme	Tag
			MODE CLASSIFICATION		
Pressure control A/C	Pressure	CMV	Set point	N/A	PC-CMVs
Pressure control A/C with automatic tube compensation	Pressure	CMV	Set point/servo	N/A	PC-CMVsr
Pressure control A/C with volume guarantee	Pressure	CMV	Adaptive	N/A	PC-CMVa
Pressure control A/C with volume guarantee and automatic tube compensation	Pressure	CMV	Adaptive/servo	N/A	PC-CMVar
Pressure control continuous mandatory ventilation	Pressure	IMV	Set point	Set point	PC-IMVs,s
Pressure control continuous mandatory ventilation with automatic tube compensation	Pressure	IMV	Set point/servo	Set point/servo	PC-IMVsr,sr
Pressure control SIMV	Pressure	IMV	Set point	Set point	PC-IMVs,s
Pressure control SIMV with automatic tube compensation	Pressure	IMV	Set point/servo	Set point/servo	PC-IMVsr,sr
Pressure control pressure support ventilation	Pressure	IMV	Set point	Set point	PC-IMVs,s
Pressure control pressure support ventilation with automatic tube compensation	Pressure	IMV	Set point/servo	Set point/servo	PC-IMVsr,sr
Pressure control airway pressure release ventilation	Pressure	IMV	Set point	Set point	PC-IMVs,s
Pressure control airway pressure release ventilation with automatic tube compensation	Pressure	IMV	Set point/servo	Set point/servo	PC-IMVsr,sr
Pressure control mandatory minute volume ventilation with volume guarantee	Pressure	IMV	Adaptive	Set point	PC-IMVa,s
Pressure control continuous mandatory ventilation with volume guarantee	Pressure	IMV	Adaptive	Set point	PC-IMVa,s
Pressure control continuous mandatory ventilation with volume guarantee and automatic tube compensation	Pressure	IMV	Adaptive/servo	Set point/servo	PC-IMVar,sr
Pressure control SIMV with volume guarantee	Pressure	IMV	Adaptive	Set point	PC-IMVa,s
Pressure control SIMV with volume guarantee and automatic tube compensation	Pressure	IMV	Adaptive/servo	Set point/servo	PC-IMVas,sr
Pressure control pressure support ventilation with volume guarantee	Pressure	IMV	Adaptive	Set point	PC-IMVa,s
Pressure control pressure support ventilation with volume guarantee and automatic tube compensation	Pressure	IMV	Adaptive/servo	Set point/servo	PC-IMVar,sr
Spontaneous CPAP/pressure support	Pressure	CSV	Set point	N/A	PC-CSVs
Spontaneous CPAP/pressure support with automatic tube compensation	Pressure	CSV	Set point/servo	N/A	PC-CSVsr
Spontaneous proportional pressure support	Pressure	CSV	Servo	N/A	PC-CSVr
Spontaneous proportional pressure support with automatic tube compensation	Pressure	CSV	Servo	N/A	PC-CSVr
Spontaneous CPAP/volume support	Pressure	CSV	Adaptive	N/A	PC-CSVa
Spontaneous CPAP/volume support with automatic tube compensation	Pressure	CSV	Adaptive/servo	N/A	PC-CSVar

(Used with permission of Mandu Press Ltd.)
a, adaptive; *ar*, adaptive and servo; *CMV*, continuous mandatory ventilation; *CSV*, continuous spontaneous ventilation; *IMV*, intermittent mandatory ventilation; *N/A*, not applicable; *PC*, pressure control; *r*, servo; *s*, set point; *sr*, set point and servo.

Pressure Control Assist Control with Volume Guarantee. This mode is as above, but with volume guarantee. The operator selects the upper limit of pressure adjustment and target tidal volume. Volume guarantee automatically adjusts inflation pressure based on exhaled tidal volume of the previous breath, measured at the airway opening to target the set tidal volume. Effective dynamic leak compensation allows accurate tidal volume measurement even with moderately large endotracheal tube leak.

Pressure Control Airway Pressure Release Ventilation. Airway pressure is maintained at a relatively high level for most of the respiratory cycle with intermittent release to a lower value.

Patient triggering of mandatory inflations is possible using the AutoRelease feature. This triggers exhalation once a preset expiratory flow threshold is reached. When AutoRelease is turned on, the switch from P_{high} to P_{low} is synchronized with the patient's breathing. Spontaneous breaths provide the bulk of minute ventilation—thus adequate respiratory effort is required.

Pressure Control Continuous Mandatory Ventilation. Mandatory inflations occur at a set rate and are machine triggered and time-cycled. Spontaneous breaths are permitted both between and during mandatory inflations.

Pressure Control Continuous Mandatory Ventilation with Volume Guarantee. This mode is as above, but with volume guarantee.

Pressure Control Mandatory Minute Volume Ventilation with Volume Guarantee. A set number of inspiratory efforts trigger pressure-controlled, time-cycled inflations with volume guarantee. Mandatory inflations are suppressed if minute ventilation from spontaneous breaths is above the preset minute ventilation target (i.e., product of tidal volume and frequency). Spontaneous breaths in excess of the set rate are not volume guaranteed.

Pressure Control Pressure Support Ventilation. Every inspiratory effort triggers a pressure-controlled, flow-cycled inflation. A backup rate provides a minimum rate of machine-triggered, flow-cycled inflations in case of apnea.

Pressure Control Pressure Support Ventilation with Volume Guarantee. This mode is as above, but with volume guarantee.

Pressure Control Synchronized Intermittent Mandatory Ventilation. Pressure controlled mandatory inflations are delivered at a preset rate and synchronized with patient effort, if any. Spontaneous breaths are allowed between mandatory inflations but receive no support. Machine-triggered inflations occur at the set rate if no respiratory effort is detected.

Pressure Control Synchronized Intermittent Mandatory Ventilation with Volume Guarantee. This mode is as above, but with volume guarantee. Spontaneous breaths are not volume guaranteed.

Spontaneous Continuous Positive Airway Pressure/Pressure Support. Spontaneous breathing with pressure support of every spontaneous breath to a fixed level above CPAP. Unlike Pressure Control Pressure Support, there is no set backup rate; instead, apnea ventilation kicks in after a period of apnea.

Spontaneous Continuous Positive Airway Pressure/Volume Support. This mode is as above, but with adaptive targeting to achieve a preset average tidal volume. This is not really a neonatal mode, but may be used in pediatric patients.

Spontaneous Proportional Pressure Support. Every inspiratory effort triggers a pressure controlled inflation with servo targeting that makes inflation pressure proportional to inspiratory effort. This mode assumes mature respiratory control and thus is probably not ideal for preterm infants.

High-Frequency Oscillatory Ventilation (with Volume Guarantee). Outside the United States, the VN500 ventilator has a high-frequency oscillatory ventilation (HFOV) option that has the ability to measure tidal volume and maintain a set tidal volume by means of a volume guarantee option. As of this writing, the HFOV option is not available in the United States.

CareFusion Infant Flow SiPAP

The CareFusion Infant Flow SiPAP (Fig. 25-16) is designed for noninvasive ventilation of infants using either nasal prongs (Fig. 25-17) or a nasal mask (Fig. 25-18). The Infant Flow SiPAP is available in a Plus or a Comprehensive configuration. The Plus configuration provides NCPAP (nasal CPAP) and time-triggered BiPhasic modes with and without breath rate monitoring. CareFusion defines "BiPhasic" as time-triggered, time-cycled pressure assists at two separate pressure levels (i.e., bilevel CPAP). Using the ventilator mode taxonomy described in this book, the name BiPhasic is classified as PC intermittent mandatory ventilation, though for the purpose of the Food and Drug Administration SiPAP

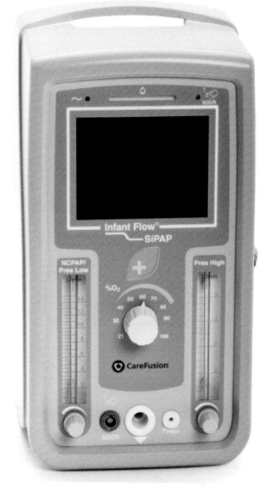

FIG 25-16 CareFusion Infant Flow SiPAP noninvasive ventilator. (Reproduced with permission from CareFusion.)

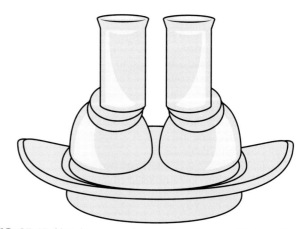

FIG 25-17 Nasal prongs for noninvasive ventilation. (Reproduced with permission from Cleveland Clinic.)

is not a ventilator. The Comprehensive configuration offers these features plus a patient-triggered BiPhasic mode with apnea backup inflations.

Operator Interface

The operator interface consists of an LCD touch screen display with a key pad. There are separate flowmeter controls for

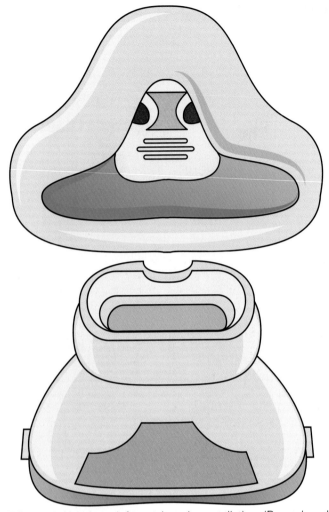

FIG 25-18 Nasal mask for noninvasive ventilation. (Reproduced with permission from Cleveland Clinic.)

TABLE 25-12   Modes on the CareFusion Infant Flow SiPAP

Mode Name	Control Variable	Breath Sequence	Primary Breath Targeting Scheme	Secondary Breath Targeting Scheme	Tag
BiPhasic	Pressure	IMV	Set point	Set point	PC-IMVs,s
Nasal CPAP	Pressure	IMV	Set point	N/A	PC-CSVs

(Used with permission of Mandu Press Ltd.)
CSV, continuous spontaneous ventilation; *IMV,* intermittent mandatory ventilation; *N/A,* not applicable; *PC,* pressure control; *s,* set point.

adjustment of NCPAP and inflation pressure above CPAP and an oxygen blender control. LEDs along the top of the front panel indicate power on, connection to wall AC, active alarms, and transducer interface connection to the driver.

Modes

Modes on the Infant Flow SiPAP are selected by name—that is, CPAP, BiPhasic, and BiPhasic *tr* (triggered). The available modes are shown in Table 25-12.

BiPhasic. The device cycles between two levels of CPAP (e.g., 6 and 9 cm H_2O) at an operator-selected rate, with spontaneous breathing occurring throughout and accounting for the bulk of minute ventilation.

BiPhasic tr. This mode is as above, but with patient triggering. This mode as of this writing is not available in the United States. It requires the use of an abdominal sensor for the trigger signal.

CPAP. The device can also be used to provide standard CPAP.

SUMMARY

A wide variety of devices is available for invasive and noninvasive respiratory support of newborn infants. Most ventilators used in neonatal ICUs offer a plethora of modes, some of which have not been adequately evaluated in newborn infants. It is incumbent on the users to learn the advantages and limitations of the devices used in their neonatal ICU and to become familiar with the ventilation modes commonly used in newborn infants. The key to success is to understand that ventilators are merely tools in our hands that need to be used with care and attention to the particular disease pathophysiology with a clear idea of the goals of mechanical ventilation. In general, one should optimize the settings on whatever mode is in use and avoid frequent changes between modes, without a clear rationale for why such change is being made. The ventilator descriptions in this chapter are meant to provide an overview of their functionality and available options. The reader is referred to the user's manual for each device for further details.

REFERENCES

A complete reference list is available at http://expertconsult .inkling.com/

Delivery Room Stabilization, and Respiratory Support

Louise S. Owen, MBChB, MRCPCH, FRACP, MD, Gary M. Weiner, MD, FAAP, and Peter G. Davis, MBBS, MD, FRACP

INTRODUCTION

Rapid and complex physiologic changes occur around the time of birth. The keys to a successful transition are the clearance of lung fluid and the establishment of a functional residual capacity (FRC). These changes are accompanied by an increase in pulmonary blood flow and the onset of regular respiration. Most infants achieve the transition unaided, but approximately 10% need help to establish spontaneous breathing in the first minutes of life.[1] Positive-pressure ventilation is required by approximately 1% of newborn infants[2] and chest compressions and/or drug therapy in fewer than 2 in 1000[3] live births. Successful aeration of the lungs may reduce the need for more extensive resuscitation. Therefore, ensuring that clinicians acquire and maintain the basic skills necessary to deliver effective respiratory support is vital.

Intrapartum-related neonatal death and neonatal encephalopathy impose a substantial burden worldwide, particularly in resource-limited settings.[4] In response to this problem, since 2005 the evidence base available to guide clinicians has grown considerably. The International Liaison Committee on Resuscitation (ILCOR) has evaluated and synthesized the available evidence and produced four iterations of guidelines, most recently, as of this writing, in 2015.[5] From these guidelines each national resuscitation council (the Neonatal Resuscitation Program Steering Committee in the United States) formulates recommendations suitable for application in its own country.

This chapter outlines the important developments in the assessment and management of babies in the first minutes of life.

PHYSIOLOGY OF TRANSITION, ASPHYXIA, AND RESUSCITATION

Physiology of Normal Transition

At birth, the first spontaneous breath generates a large negative pressure, up to $-100\,\mathrm{cm\,H_2O}$,[6] inflating the lungs and driving lung fluid distally into the interstitial tissues.[7] Studies of the initiation of respiration in well term infants from more than 50 years ago,[6] and more recently data from preterm infants,[8] demonstrate that the first breaths have a short, deep inspiration, followed by a prolonged phase of chest muscle contraction with a closed[6] (braking), or partially closed (crying), glottis,[8] and then finally a small-volume, short expiration. These breaths push back the air–liquid interface; more volume is inspired than expired and the FRC is established.[9]

As the lungs are aerated, pulmonary vascular resistance falls, and flow through the ductus arteriosus changes from right-to-left to left-to-right. Pulmonary blood flow rises, increasing first the cardiac output and then the heart rate and blood pressure.[10,11]

Within three breaths carbon dioxide (CO_2) starts to be exhaled, increasing to levels of ~50 mm Hg (~67 kPa) after 1 minute.[12] Observational studies of newborn term and preterm infants not requiring resuscitation show that the heart rate is typically <100 beats per minute (bpm) at 1 minute of age and rises quickly to >160 bpm by 3 minutes.[13]

Before the umbilical cord is cut, the left ventricular preload is dependent on umbilical blood flow. When the cord is cut, preload and cardiac output fall. As the lungs aerate, pulmonary vascular resistance falls and pulmonary venous return provides most of the ventricular preload. Therefore, delaying cord clamping until after lung aeration may stabilize preload and cardiac output and reduce potential swings in arterial pressures and blood flows, leading to a more stable circulatory transition.[10,14]

Physiology of Asphyxia

Many pre- and peripartum events can reduce the supply of oxygenated blood to the fetus, resulting in varying degrees of fetal hypoxia–ischemia. Classic studies of acute total hypoxia–ischemia (asphyxia) in animal models[15] have guided our understanding of neonatal asphyxia. The physiologic changes and their response to resuscitation are shown in Figure 26-1.

At the onset of hypoxia, breathing movements become deep and rapid. As the level of consciousness falls, respiratory efforts stop. This is the period of primary apnea, during which heart rate falls to ~100 bpm and blood pressure transiently rises before falling. Prior to lung aeration, left ventricular preload comes from umbilical blood flow; early clamping of the umbilical cord in infants who have not aerated their lungs, and who therefore do not have any pulmonary venous return, may exacerbate hypoxia by reducing preload and cardiac output.[10]

As cardiac output falls, there is an increase in noncerebral vascular resistance, redirecting remaining cardiac output to the brain to maintain cerebral blood flow and maximize cerebral oxygen delivery. Spinal reflexes, no longer inhibited by higher (conscious) brain activity, trigger the classic diving reflex: respiratory efforts recommence as slow, deep, effortful gasps. This period lasts for several minutes while heart rate, blood pressure, and oxygen levels fall, and carbon dioxide, lactate, and acidosis increase. Hypoxia and acidosis increase vasoconstriction of the pulmonary vasculature, resulting in reduced pulmonary blood flow, lower left atrial pressure, increased right-to-left shunting, and exacerbation of hypoxia. Animal studies show that eventually all respiratory efforts cease (terminal or secondary apnea), the myocardium fails, cardiac output and blood pressure drop,[16] and without intervention the animal dies. In human infants, this sequence may last up to 20 minutes after the onset of hypoxia.[17]

However, animal models have focused on acute *total* asphyxia, whereas asphyxia in newborn infants may be intermittent, subacute, or chronic. The varying types of asphyxia make it difficult to translate the knowledge gained from animal models to the different pathophysiologies seen in newborn infants.

Physiology of Resuscitation

The primary aims of resuscitation are to sustain life and prevent brain injury. In the newborn setting the focus is on lung aeration, to reduce pulmonary vascular resistance and increase pulmonary blood flow, and to move oxygenated blood to the coronary arteries to reperfuse the myocardium and increase cardiac output. Newborn resuscitation guidelines focus primarily on good ventilatory support to achieve these goals. Even partial lung aeration will significantly increase pulmonary blood flow.[18]

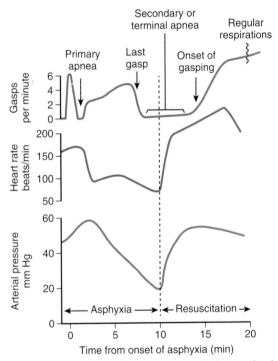

FIG 26-1 Changes in physiologic factors during asphyxia and resuscitation in newborn rhesus monkeys. (Adapted from Adamsons Jr K, Behrman R, Dawes G, et al. The treatment of acidosis with alkali and glucose during asphyxia in foetal rhesus monkeys. *J Physiol.* 1963;169:679; Dawes GS. *Foetal and Neonatal Physiology.* Chicago: Year Book Medical Publishers; 1968.)

Infants at the stage of primary apnea may go on to make a successful transition through gasping reflexes; however, at birth it is not possible to be sure of the duration of compromise, or whether the presenting apnea is primary or terminal. The earlier in the asphyxial process that resuscitation is started, the more likely it is to be successful. Animal studies demonstrate that resuscitative efforts are more likely to be successful during primary apnea, and the longer the delay in initiating resuscitation after the last gasp, the longer the time to the first gasp after resuscitation begins. For every 1-minute delay, the time to first gasp extends by ~2 minutes, and the time to onset of spontaneous respiration extends by ~4 minutes.[15] The decision whether to intervene at birth is complicated by the fact that healthy babies may not take their first breath for more than 30 seconds,[6] and if decisions to intervene are made too early, unnecessary interventions may be applied. However, if decisions are delayed, there may be further cardiorespiratory compromise. In considering whether to intervene, it is helpful to remember that an infant who has good tone is unlikely to be severely hypoxic, and the key sign of an infant's condition in the minutes after birth, and response during stabilization, is the heart rate.

ANTICIPATION AND PREPARATION FOR RESUSCITATION

The need for respiratory support and other interventions immediately after birth is a relatively frequent emergency. Approximately 5% to 10% of term and late preterm newborns will receive some assistance to establish spontaneous respirations, and the probability increases significantly in the presence of known risk factors.[19,20] Similar to other emergencies, the best outcome is achieved when there is a skilled, organized, and efficient response from a highly effective team. Ensuring such a response requires comprehensive training, deliberate practice, and careful preparation.

Training

All health providers working with newborns should complete a standardized neonatal resuscitation training course. Examples include the Neonatal Resuscitation Program, developed by the American Academy of Pediatrics and the American Heart Association, and the Newborn Life Support course organized by the U.K. Resuscitation Council. Using adult education principles, these programs focus on the cognitive, technical, and teamwork skills required to resuscitate a newborn in the hospital. Other courses teach similar skills for births occurring outside the typical delivery room setting. By simulating both common and unusual neonatal emergencies, providers can identify weaknesses in their skills and develop proficiency. Although a participant's knowledge and skills improve after a resuscitation course, both have been demonstrated to decay rapidly over time.[21,22] Without deliberate practice, providers are unlikely to acquire and maintain competence with infrequently used technical skills such as tracheal intubation and emergency vascular access. Even basic assisted ventilation skills have been shown to decay within months of course completion.[22] The ideal frequency of retraining has not been established; however, several studies have shown that low-intensity/high-frequency practice, as short as 6 minutes every month, may improve skill retention.[23,24]

Teamwork

A complex neonatal resuscitation requires health providers to precisely execute multiple assessments and interventions within minutes of birth. Although the individual team members may have mastered the skills to resuscitate a newborn, they will not be able to use their skills optimally unless they work together as a team. Poor teamwork and communication are the most common causes of potentially preventable deaths in the delivery room.[25] Simply assembling a team of expert health providers does not ensure that they will work well together. Without practice, even a group of highly skilled neonatal providers are likely to work inefficiently in the high-intensity setting of an unexpected resuscitation. High-fidelity simulation and multidisciplinary teamwork training have been shown to improve teamwork skills and the outcome of resuscitation.[26-28]

A common analogy is to compare the resuscitation team with a race car pit crew. Pit crews practice their teamwork in advance and use highly scripted protocols that distribute the work load to ensure that the correct task is performed efficiently by the correct team member. Similarly, high-performance resuscitation teams precisely execute structured protocols that allow them to recognize important patterns, share information efficiently, and trigger the appropriate response. Each team member's roles and responsibilities are well defined before the resuscitation begins. The team is directed by an identified leader who gives clear direction, delegates responsibilities, and maintains awareness of the entire clinical situation without becoming distracted by individual procedures.

Anticipation

Before every birth, the neonatal health providers should review the pregnancy history with the obstetric care team to determine which personnel should be present at the time of birth. Using a comprehensive list of risk factors, Aziz[29,30] demonstrated that approximately 80% of newborns who require resuscitation can be identified before birth (Table 26-1) and that the risk can be stratified into categories that correlate with the need for positive-pressure ventilation. When the neonatal team was called to attend a birth, 22% of newborns received positive-pressure ventilation. When the pregnancy was considered high risk, 47% of newborns received positive-pressure ventilation. In a logistic regression model, an increased risk of requiring positive-pressure ventilation was associated with maternal hypertension, oligohydramnios, maternal infection, preterm multiple pregnancy, opiates received during labor, meconium-stained fluid, breech presentation, abnormal fetal heart rate patterns, delivery at 34 to 35 weeks' gestation, emergency cesarean birth, and

shoulder dystocia. However, the individual risk factors had limited discriminatory power and identified many births for which no intervention was needed. To avoid missing a newborn who required resuscitation, the neonatal team attended approximately two-thirds of all births. Moreover, the absence of risk factors did not exclude the possibility that the newborn would require assistance. Among births with no identified risk factor, 7% of newborns received positive-pressure ventilation. This highlights the importance of having adequate personnel available to immediately resuscitate the newborn at every birth.

Preparation

After evaluating the perinatal risk factors, the necessary personnel should be assembled. The numbers and qualifications of the health providers will vary depending upon the specific circumstances. Every birth should be attended by at least one qualified health provider whose only job is to manage the newborn.[31] At a minimum, this person must be proficient at newborn assessment, the initial steps of newborn care, and positive-pressure ventilation. A rapid and reliable method of calling for additional help is imperative. If important risk factors are identified, at least two qualified providers should be present at the time of birth. Regardless of the setting, every hospital that delivers newborns should have a qualified resuscitation team proficient in all resuscitation skills immediately available if a complex resuscitation is required. The full team should be present at the time of birth if the need for a complex resuscitation is anticipated. If the newborn has cardiorespiratory collapse, multiple procedures will need to be completed without delay. In smaller hospitals the team may comprise personnel from different disciplines, including anesthesiology for airway management and emergency medicine or pediatrics for vascular access.

Once the appropriate personnel are assembled, if there is time before delivery a preresuscitation briefing or "Time Out" should be performed, to discuss the maternal history, review the clinical situation, identify a team leader, plan the response and the possible contingencies, delegate roles and responsibilities, and prepare the necessary equipment (Tables 26-2 and 26-3). The equipment necessary to initiate positive-pressure ventilation should be checked and ready for immediate use at every birth. All equipment necessary to perform a complex resuscitation should be readily available if needed and should be checked and ready for immediate use if a complex resuscitation is anticipated. Using a standardized prebirth checklist helps to ensure adequate preparation, allows rapid identification of missing equipment, improves communication and teamwork, supports quality assurance data collection, and facilitates postresuscitation debriefing.[32,33]

TABLE 26-1 Risk Factors for Neonatal Resuscitation

Antepartum Risk Factors	Intrapartum Risk Factors
Preterm birth at less than 36 weeks' gestational age	Abnormal fetal heart rate pattern (category II or III)
Intrauterine growth restriction	Prolapsed cord
Polyhydramnios	Placenta previa
Oligohydramnios	Placental abruption
Maternal diabetes	Meconium-stained fluid
Maternal hypertension	Shoulder dystocia
Major fetal anomaly or hydrops	Breech or transverse presentation
Maternal infection	Vacuum or forceps birth
Chorioamnionitis	Emergency cesarean birth
	Opiates received in labor
	General anesthesia

(Data from Aziz K. Ante-and intra-partum factors that predict increased need for neonatal resuscitation. *Resuscitation*. 2008;79:444-452.)

TABLE 26-2 The Preresuscitation "Time Out"

Introduce team members
Review maternal history and risk factors
Identify team leader
Review anticipated clinical scenarios
Describe the planned response and contingencies
Delegate roles and responsibilities
Prepare supplies and equipment
Are special consultants or equipment needed?
"If any team member identifies concerns or safety issues, alert the team leader immediately."

TABLE 26-3 Neonatal Resuscitation Supplies and Equipment

NEONATAL RESUSCITATION SUPPLIES AND EQUIPMENT

Basic Supplies
Radiant warmer with servo-control sensor
Warm towels/blankets
Clock with second hand
Stethoscope
Pulse oximeter, sensor, and sensor cover
Electronic cardiac monitor and leads
Gloves and gowns

Suction Equipment
Bulb syringe
Mechanical suction
Suction catheters (5-6 F, 8-12 F)
8-F feeding tube and 20-mL syringe
Meconium aspirator

Positive-Pressure Ventilation Equipment
Resuscitation bag or T-piece and mask
Compressed air and oxygen
Oxygen blender and flowmeter tubing

Intubation Equipment
Laryngoscope (sizes 0 and 1)
Tracheal tubes (ID 2.5, 3.0, 3.5)
Stylet
Measuring tape
Tape or securing device
Scissors
CO_2 detector
Laryngeal mask or other supraglottic device

Medications
Epinephrine 1:10,000 (0.1 mg/mL)
Normal saline (50- to 250-mL bag)
Syringes (1, 3, 20, to 60 mL)

Umbilical Vessel Catheterization Kit
Sterile gloves
Antiseptic solution
Umbilical tie
Small clamp (hemostat)
Forceps
Scalpel
Umbilical catheters (single lumen), 3.5F or 5F
Three-way stopcock
Syringes (3-5 mL)
Intraosseous needle (18 gauge or 15 mm)

For Very Preterm
Food-grade plastic wrap or bag
Exothermic mattress

For Thoracentesis and Paracentesis
Antiseptic solution
18- or 20-gauge percutaneous catheter-over-needle device
Three-way stopcock
Syringe (20- to 60-mL)

TABLE 26-4 The Apgar Score

Sign	SCORE		
	0	1	2
Heart rate	Absent	Slow (<100 bpm)	>100 bpm
Respirations	Absent	Slow, irregular	Good, crying
Muscle tone	Limp	Some flexion	Active motion
Reflex irritability	No response	Grimace	Cough, sneeze, cry
Color	Blue or pale	Pink body, blue extremities	Completely pink

effectiveness of resuscitation. However, both methods of clinical measurement have been shown to be inconsistent and systematically underestimate heart rate by approximately 15 to 20 bpm relative to measurement by electrocardiogram.[37] Assessment of respiration is also difficult. Although no studies have evaluated spontaneously breathing infants, assessment of chest rise in those being ventilated indicates that observers differ substantially in their perceptions of chest rise and there is considerable disparity between clinical assessment and objective tidal volume measurements.[38] Not surprisingly, studies of the precision and accuracy of the Apgar score have shown that experienced observers differ considerably in their assessments.[39] Hence, clinicians need to be aware of the limitations of clinical signs obtained in the delivery room.

Pulse Oximetry and Electrocardiography

Pulse oximetry has been used for decades to safely administer oxygen to infants in the intensive care unit. Advances in technology have enabled reliable readings of both oxygen saturation and heart rate to be obtained within the first 90 seconds of life.[40] Continuous display, particularly of heart rate, means that resuscitation can be continued without interruption for intermittent auscultation. The sensor should be attached to the right hand or wrist to measure preductal saturations. Normal ranges of saturation measurements[41] and heart rate[13] have been defined by monitoring healthy term infants not requiring any interventions after delivery. Electrocardiography provides an alternative method of measuring heart rate in the delivery room and is now the recommended method of obtaining an accurate number immediately after birth.[5] Katheria et al. have shown that it provides data more quickly than the pulse oximeter.[42] Both methods require further evaluation to determine whether their use improves outcomes for at-risk infants.

CLINICAL ASSESSMENT, APGAR SCORE, SATURATION, AND HEART RATE MONITORING

Initial assessment of the newborn baby must be rapid and accurate to identify babies who need resuscitation and to evaluate the effectiveness of interventions.

Clinical Evaluation

The Apgar score was first published in 1953 and represents an important landmark in the care of newly born infants. It marked the author's reaction to the scant attention paid to newborns in the delivery room at that time: "nine months observation of the mother surely warrants one minute's observation of the baby."[34] For many decades the score (Table 26-4) and its five components have been used "as a basis for discussion and comparison of the results of obstetric practices, types of maternal pain relief and the effects of resuscitation."[35] Conventionally, scores are assigned at 1 and 5 minutes of life, although it has been acknowledged that assessment and intervention may be required before 1 minute. The precision and accuracy of the component signs have been evaluated. Observers have been found to disagree about the presence or absence of cyanosis, and the correlation between color and oxygen saturation is poor.[36] Assessment of color no longer forms part of the ILCOR guidelines for resuscitation.[5] Heart rate determined by auscultation of the chest or palpation of the cord has long been considered critical in monitoring the need for and

INTERVENTION BASICS: WARMTH, POSITION, SUCTION, STIMULATION

The basic steps of newborn care include ensuring adequate warmth, positioning the baby's head and neck so that the airway is open, clearing the airway of secretions if necessary, and providing gentle stimulation.

Warmth

Newborns lose heat and rapidly become hypothermic without adequate attention to thermal regulation. Hypothermia after birth is associated with increased mortality and morbidity including respiratory distress, late-onset sepsis, metabolic acidosis, and hypoglycemia. The delivery room should be appropriately warm and free from draughts. Immediately after birth, a vigorous term newborn may be placed on the mother's chest or abdomen and covered with a warm, dry blanket. Warmth will be maintained by drying the newborn's skin and maintaining direct skin-to-skin contact with the mother. A nonvigorous newborn should be placed on a warm, dry blanket under a prewarmed radiant heat source, the skin dried, and the wet linen removed. The baby should remain uncovered to allow visualization and effective radiant warming. Newly born infants without evidence of hypoxic injury should have their temperature maintained between 36.5 and 37.5°C. If the baby remains under the radiant warmer for more than a few minutes, a servo-controlled temperature sensor should be used to adjust the radiant warmer's output and avoid overheating.

Very preterm newborns will require additional interventions to prevent hypothermia, which are discussed later in this chapter.

Position

The infant should be placed supine with the head and neck in a neutral or slightly extended position. This has been called the "sniffing" position (Fig. 26-2). This position opens the baby's airway, aligns the posterior pharynx and trachea, and allows unrestricted air movement. Excessive flexion or extension of the baby's neck may cause airway obstruction. If the baby has a prominent occiput, it may be helpful to place a small towel or blanket roll under the baby's shoulders to lift the shoulders and straighten the neck.

Suction

If the newborn is vigorous after birth, a soft cloth or towel may be used to gently wipe the baby's face, mouth, and nose. Among vigorous newborns, there is no benefit to routine oropharyngeal, nasopharyngeal, or gastric suction, and this practice may interfere with pulmonary transition and the initiation of feeding.[43-45] Gentle oral and nasal suction should be reserved for babies who are having difficulty breathing, who have secretions obstructing their airway, or who require positive-pressure ventilation. Prolonged, vigorous, or deep pharyngeal suction should be avoided because it may cause bradycardia and traumatize tissues.

Meconium-Stained Amniotic Fluid

The approach to babies born through meconium-stained amniotic fluid has evolved over recent years. Large, multicenter, randomized trials have shown no benefit from routine intrapartum oropharyngeal suction or from tracheal suction of the vigorous newborn.[46,47] Previous treatment guidelines from ILCOR recommended selective tracheal intubation and suction for nonvigorous newborns in an attempt to prevent meconium aspiration syndrome.[5] These recommendations were based on nonrandomized observational studies completed in the 1970s.[48,49] A 2015 small randomized controlled trial among nonvigorous infants born through meconium-stained fluid found that tracheal suction did not reduce the incidence of meconium aspiration syndrome or other adverse outcomes.[50] At present, there is no high-quality evidence to support a recommendation for routine intubation and tracheal suction of nonvigorous newborns born through meconium-stained fluid. Given the potential complications associated with tracheal intubation, additional evidence from randomized controlled trials is needed to inform this practice. The 2010 ILCOR statement recommends against routinely performing endotracheal suction of babies born through meconium-stained amniotic fluid.[5]

Stimulation

The process of positioning and drying the newborn often provides sufficient stimulation to initiate spontaneous respirations. If the newborn is not breathing, brief additional stimulation by rubbing the newborn's back, trunk, or extremities may be

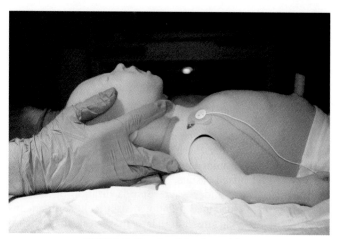

FIG 26-2 The "sniffing" position.

helpful. If the baby does not rapidly initiate spontaneous respirations, positive-pressure ventilation is indicated. Continuing to stimulate an apneic newborn is not helpful and delays appropriate interventions.

OXYGEN

Oxygen is perhaps the most widely used drug in neonatology, but until recently remained poorly evaluated. An appreciation of its life-sustaining properties is now balanced by an understanding of its potential toxicity, even from a relatively short period of resuscitation. A substantial body of evidence from animal models is now supplemented by findings from human trials, which indicate that the use of 100% oxygen increases mortality rates compared with the use of air.[51] However, uncertainty remains regarding the effects on long-term neurodevelopment.[52] International guidelines for the resuscitation of term infants now recommend commencing resuscitation with air. Kattwinkel suggested using pulse oximetry in the delivery room to titrate oxygen therapy to achieve normoxia.[53] The establishment of a normal range for term babies provides targets for clinicians, but the optimal increments and timing of changes remains uncertain. It is vital that operators continue to ensure adequate ventilation throughout the resuscitation and are not distracted by making frequent adjustments to oxygen concentrations. Although no compelling evidence exists, current ILCOR guidelines recommend the use of 100% oxygen whenever cardiac compressions are provided. The use of oxygen in the preterm infant may have a different risk/benefit profile, and recommendations are detailed in a subsequent section of this chapter.

VENTILATION

Any newborn infant who does not initiate regular respiration, or who fails to respond to initial measures of drying, wrapping, and gentle stimulation, should be given positive-pressure support. This is typically first applied noninvasively using a face mask or nasal prong(s) and a pressure-generating device. If the infant is making inadequate respiratory effort, continuous positive airway pressure (CPAP) may be sufficient to aid lung inflation, to establish FRC, and to regularize breathing.[54] An infant who has no respiratory effort, or is bradycardic (heart rate <100 bpm), or remains hypoxic despite CPAP support, should be given positive-pressure inflations, ideally with positive end-expiratory pressure (PEEP).[55] The aim of positive-pressure ventilation is to provide effective ventilation and gas exchange, without causing lung injury, which can occur within a few large-volume positive-pressure inflations (volutrauma).[56-58] Actions to prevent lung injury include avoiding large tidal volumes and facilitating formation and maintenance of FRC.

Observation of the first breaths in well infants suggests that prolonged (sustained) initial inflations may be advantageous;[6,8] this idea is supported by studies of sustained inflation in preterm animal models, which show rapid lung inflation without overexpansion, immediate development of appropriate FRC, and uniformly aerated lungs[59] without serious side effects.[60] Randomized trials of sustained inflations at birth in preterm infants have produced mixed results,[61-64] and as of this writing further large trials are under way.[65] Standardization of pressure and duration for sustained inflations is difficult; spontaneous breathing, glottic closure,[66] and face mask leak make delivered tidal volumes variable.[67] Sustained inflations have been included in some resuscitation guidelines, whereas others state insufficient evidence to recommend their implementation.[5]

The ideal target volumes for ventilation of term and preterm infants after birth have not been established; animal studies demonstrate that initial high tidal volumes are detrimental.[68] Aiming for volumes <8 mL/kg seems reasonable,[69] but tidal volumes are difficult to measure with standard delivery room equipment and are consequently rarely targeted or measured at birth. Clinicians rely on setting peak pressure and clinical signs as a proxy for "appropriate" volume delivery. Guidelines suggest peak pressures should begin in the range of 20 to 30 cm H_2O,[5] and these have been shown to produce adequate tidal volumes.[70] Infants without any respiratory effort may require higher pressures initially, which should be reduced as the lungs aerate and become more compliant.[71] The actual delivered volume will vary owing to many factors: spontaneous breathing effort, lung compliance, laryngeal closure, face mask leak, obstruction at the mouth and nose, and the resuscitation device used. The result is that delivered tidal volumes vary widely and can be much higher than those generated during spontaneous breathing.[72] A rising heart rate is a good sign that effective ventilation is being delivered[5] and is preferable to using achievement of peak pressure or assessing chest rise, neither of which is reliable.[38,73]

Although use of PEEP in the delivery room is not strongly supported by clinical evidence, it is a well-established technique with convincing animal data to support its use in establishing FRC, whether or not a sustained inflation is given.[55,59,74] A "standard" level of PEEP may not suit all infants, and published guidelines do not recommend specific levels. The reported typically used level of PEEP in the delivery room is 5 cm H_2O.[75] Infants who have not fully established FRC are likely to have higher oxygen requirements and may benefit from higher PEEP.[76]

Ventilation rates of 40 to 60 per minute are recommended (unless chest compressions are being given concurrently) and match the typical respiratory rates of healthy newborns. The duration of each inflation is operator dependent and may, following the initial inflations, be best timed to coincide with and to reflect spontaneous inspiratory times of newborn infants,[77] at about 0.3 seconds. Set gas flow will vary with the pressure device being used. T-piece ventilation is susceptible to fluctuations in PEEP and tidal volume with flow changes, and the manufacturer's recommendations regarding flow should be followed.[78,79]

If, during mask ventilation, chest wall movement is poor or absent and heart rate does not improve, corrective steps need to be taken. These include repositioning of the head to ensure neutral position and reapplication of the mask to reduce leak and

nasal obstruction. Other measures to consider include increasing the applied peak pressure, opening the mouth, suctioning secretions, holding the mask on the face with two hands, and using an oropharyngeal airway.[31]

Once heart rate exceeds 100 bpm and spontaneous breathing is established, positive-pressure ventilation can be stopped; CPAP should be continued in premature infants. Positive-pressure ventilation must continue if spontaneous respiration is inadequate or if the heart rate remains less than 100 bpm. Endotracheal intubation should be considered for infants who do not develop adequate respiratory effort or who remain bradycardic and/or hypoxic despite adequate mask ventilation. Options for the management of preterm infants who require ongoing respiratory support include intubation and surfactant administration in the delivery room or initial CPAP support with rescue intubation and surfactant treatment only if required.[5,80]

PRESSURE SOURCES

In resource-limited settings there may be no device available to generate positive-pressure support. Mouth-to-mouth resuscitation can be used, but it carries the risk of infection. Mouth-to-mask[81] or mouth-to-tube[82] ventilation may be viable options and carry somewhat lower risks of infection.[83]

Worldwide, many devices are available for generating positive pressure in the delivery room (Fig. 26-3). The choice of device may be made based on cost; availability of a gas supply; desire to deliver sustained inflations, PEEP, and CPAP; or personal preference (Table 26-5).

Self-inflating bags (SIBs) reexpand after compression. They are the only devices that can be used without a gas supply and may be the most useful for those with limited resources. Several types and sizes of SIBs exist; the smallest size, ~240 mL, is for newborns. The peak pressure delivered by an SIB depends on how hard and fast the bag is squeezed. Although SIBs usually incorporate a valve to limit the maximum delivered pressure, it can be inadvertently or manually overridden to deliver higher pressures. Pressures >100 cm H_2O have been reported, resulting in excessive tidal volumes.[84] It is difficult to give consistent peak pressures with an SIB,[85] even when using a manometer. If a PEEP valve is attached, some PEEP can be generated, but again this is inconsistent[86] and lower with slower inflation rates.[86,87] SIBs cannot deliver CPAP or sustained inflations[88] and therefore may not be the optimal device for stabilizing preterm infants. SIBs entrain room air during reexpansion but can still deliver up to 70% inspired oxygen when used without a reservoir bag.[89]

A flow-inflating bag (FIB) needs a continuous gas supply to inflate the bag. Like the SIB, delivered pressure and volume depend on how hard the bag is squeezed. A pressure-limiting valve can be attached, and a manometer is recommended to increase the consistency of peak pressure delivery.[90,91] PEEP can be generated by controlling the rate of gas flow from the back of the bag, although this requires experience; many operators find the FIB more difficult to use than the SIB.[92] Experienced FIB users can deliver sustained inflations with an FIB, but the delivered pressure fluctuates.[88] It is very difficult to deliver reliable CPAP using an FIB.

A T-piece device is flow-controlled and pressure-limited; it also requires a continuous gas supply to operate. Gas flow through a ported expiratory valve is used to generate PEEP. Peak pressure is achieved by occluding the port in the expiratory valve with a

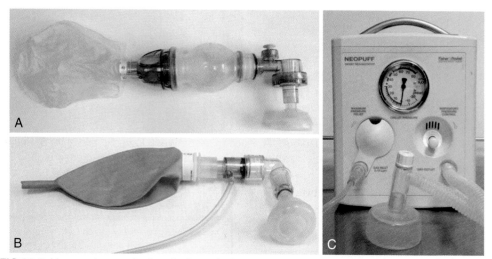

FIG 26-3 Neonatal resuscitation devices. **A,** A 240-mL self-inflating bag with an oxygen reservoir attached (Laerdal Medical, Stavanger, Norway). **B,** A flow-inflating bag or anesthetic bag (Parker Healthcare Pty, Mitcham, Australia). **C,** A T-piece pressure-limited device (Neopuff Infant Resuscitator; Fisher & Paykel, New Zealand).

TABLE 26-5 Comparison of Attributes across the Range of Positive-Pressure-Generating Devices

Device	Self-Inflating bag	Flow-Inflating bag	T-Piece	Ventilator
Can function without gas supply	✓	–	–	-
Achieves accurate, consistent peak pressure	–	–	✓	✓
Measures delivered peak pressure	–	–	✓	✓
Potential to deliver sustained inflation	–	Possible with experience	✓	-
Delivers PEEP	Possible with PEEP valve	Possible with PEEP valve	✓	✓
Delivers CPAP	–	–	✓	✓
Delivered pressures are independent of gas flow	✓	✓	–	✓
Measures delivered tidal volume	–	–	–	Possible with some ventilators

CPAP, continuous positive airway pressure; *PEEP,* positive end-expiratory pressure.

finger. Inflation time depends on how long the port is occluded. T-pieces are easy to use and are preferred by both experienced and inexperienced operators.[91] T-pieces deliver more accurate and consistent peak and PEEP pressures than other devices, resulting in more stable tidal volume delivery,[93] including with new operators.[94] However, operators are less responsive to changing lung compliance than when using other devices.[95] The T-piece effectively delivers CPAP while the port is open,[93] and occlusion of the port efficiently delivers sustained inflations of any duration or pressure.[88] Therefore, T-pieces may be the optimal device for providing respiratory support for preterm infants at birth.[91] However, no clinical trials have demonstrated superiority of one resuscitation device over another.[96] If either a T-piece device or an FIB is used, there must be a backup SIB for use in the event of failure of the compressed gas source.

Finally, infants can also be stabilized using a ventilator. Ventilators can provide accurate delivery of peak and PEEP pressures, sustained inflations, CPAP, synchronization, and tidal volume measurement.[97]

INTERFACES

Positive-pressure ventilation is most often delivered via a face mask. Although the principles of face mask ventilation are simple, good technique is essential. To achieve reasonable stable tidal volumes, a good seal must be achieved between the mask and the face. Without a good seal, there will be substantial leak around the mask, and inadequate ventilation will ensue. Masks are available in a number of sizes and shapes. The most commonly used masks are round and have cushioned rims. Choosing the correct mask size is important. The mask should extend from the chin tip but not encroach upon the eyes. For a single operator, the two-point top hold provides the most stable application. The mask should be rolled rather than directly placed onto the face. A finger positioned on the baby's chin tip may be used to align the lower edge of the mask, which can then be rolled gently upward (Fig. 26-4).[98] An alternative interface is a cut-down endotracheal tube placed 3 to 4 cm inside the nose. A randomized trial

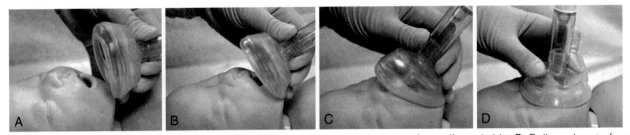

FIG 26-4 Application of face mask and recommended hold. **A**, Place mask between lower lip and chin; **B**, Roll mask onto face; **C**, Ensure top of mask is over bridge of nose; **D**, Apply downward pressure to flat part of mask to ensure good contact with face.

of 300 infants showed no difference in efficacy between this interface and a face mask.[99]

ENDOTRACHEAL INTUBATION

Indications for intubation after birth vary depending on gestational age, respiratory effort, response to noninvasive ventilation, and the skill and experience of the resuscitator. International resuscitation guidelines suggest intubation be considered at several stages[5]: if the heart rate is <100 bpm after 30 seconds of effective positive-pressure ventilation, if the infant continues to be apneic despite adequate mask ventilation, if mask ventilation is prolonged or ineffective, or if there are congenital anomalies affecting transition, such as diaphragmatic hernia. Infants without a detectable heartbeat should be intubated and ventilated as soon as possible; the endotracheal route of adrenaline administration may be needed prior to intravenous access being established. Neonatal intubation is a difficult skill to acquire and maintain. Fewer infants are now intubated and skills are declining. Junior trainees are successful in less than half of intubation attempts;[100] they take longer to perform intubations, frequently longer than the recommended 30 seconds, with consequent clinical deterioration in the infant.[100]

INTUBATION EQUIPMENT AND PROCEDURE

Equipment for endotracheal intubation should be readily available wherever infants may be born. The required items are outlined in Table 26-6. The infant should be placed supine in a neutral position, avoiding both flexion and hyperextension of the neck, which make the glottis hard to visualize.

The tip of the laryngoscope should be advanced over the tongue, either to the vallecula or over the top of the epiglottis and elevated (not rotated) to reveal the vocal cords (Fig. 26-5). The laryngoscope should remain midline and support the tongue toward the left of the mouth, leaving sufficient space to see the larynx while passing the endotracheal tube (ETT). If the laryngoscope is advanced too far, the larynx will not be visible. Gentle external cricoid pressure may help to bring the anterior larynx into view.

Initially, the ETT should be inserted to the level of the vocal cord marker. At this depth, the tube is expected to be above the carina; however, the marker position varies by manufacturer and should not be used as the primary method of determining the insertion distance. Previous recommendations suggested an insertion depth, measured from the ETT tip to the infant's upper lip, estimated by adding 6.0 cm to the infant's weight (kg). This formula tends to overestimate the insertion depth and may inadvertently insert the

TABLE 26-6 Recommended Equipment and Supplies for Endotracheal Intubation

Positive-pressure delivery device (self-inflating bag/flow-inflating bag with manometer and positive end-expiratory pressure valve if possible, or T-piece device)
Air/oxygen supply with flowmeter and blender
Neonatal cushioned round face masks in range of sizes
Pulse oximeter (attached to right hand/wrist)
Laryngoscope(s) with straight blades, Miller sizes 00, 0, and 1
Uncuffed, uniform-diameter, radio-opaque, endotracheal tubes, with a standard curve, depth marked, in sizes 2.5-, 3.0-, 3.5-, and 4.0-mm internal diameter
Stylet (optional)
Magill forceps (for nasal intubation)
Neonatal stethoscope
Colorimetric carbon dioxide detector
Suction equipment and suction catheters (5-, 6-, 8-, and 10-F size)
Equipment to secure the endotracheal tube in place (adhesive tape/ ties/hat)

tube into the infant's right main stem bronchus, especially in extremely low birth-weight infants. Two more recent methods of estimating the insertion depth have been validated in term and preterm newborns. Updated estimates based on the baby's weight or gestational age have been shown to accurately predict the insertion depth (Table 26-7).[101] Another method measures the distance (cm) between the newborn's nasal septum and ear tragus (nasal–tragus length or NTL). The tube is inserted the distance of NTL +1 cm with the appropriate centimeter mark located at the infant's upper lip.[102] The ultimate goal is to place to ETT in the midtrachea and align the tip of the ETT between the first and the second thoracic vertebrae.

A stylet can be used for ETT insertion; however, there is no evidence that this improves the rate of successful intubation.[103] The stylet must not protrude beyond the tip of the ETT, as this could result in tracheal damage. It is also easy to inadvertently dislodge a correctly placed ETT when removing a stylet. Magill forceps are often required to advance the ETT through the vocal cords during nasal intubation.

The placement of the ETT must always be verified; the best clinical indicator is a rapid increase in heart rate. Correct placement can be assessed by observing the tube passing through the vocal cords, auscultating air entry in both axillae, observing condensation inside the ETT during expiration, and observing chest rise during positive pressure inflations. However, these signs can be misleading, and the use of an end-tidal CO_2 detector on the ETT connector is recommended.[5] The depth of ETT tube insertion should be assessed with chest radiography.

Properly Positioned in Vallecula

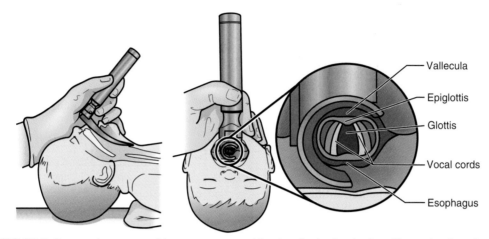

FIG 26-5 Proper placement of laryngoscope and landmarks for intubation. (From the American Heart Association/American Academy of Pediatrics. *Textbook of Neonatal Resuscitation.* Dallas: American Heart Association; 2006:5-13.)

TABLE 26-7 **Guidelines for Endotracheal Tube Size**

Weight (g)	Gestation (weeks)	Endotracheal Tube Size i.d. (mm)	Insertion Depth "Tip-to-Lip" Oral Endotracheal Tube (cm)
500-600	23-24	2.5	5.5
700-800	25-26	2.5	6.0
900-1000	27-29	2.5/3.0	6.5
1100-1400	30-32	3.0	7.0
1500-1800	33-34	3.0	7.5
1900-2400	35-37	3.0/3.5	8.0
2500-3100	38-40	3.5	8.5
3200-4200	41-43	3.5/4.0	9.0

i.d., internal diameter.
(Data from Kempley ST, Moreiras JW, Petrone FL. Endotracheal tube length for neonatal intubation. *Resuscitation.* 2008;77(3):369-373.)

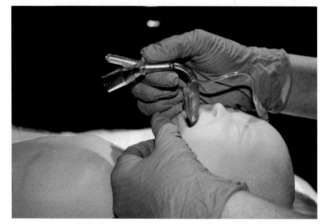

FIG 26-6 A laryngeal mask airway.

LARYNGEAL MASK AIRWAY

Supraglottic devices, such as a laryngeal mask, are effective alternatives to face mask and ETT ventilation. Several designs are available, but most include a small elliptical mask with an inflatable rim attached to an airway tube (Fig. 26-6). The device is inserted into the baby's mouth and advanced along the palate into the posterior pharynx, and the mask is positioned over the laryngeal inlet. After insertion, the rim around the mask is inflated and forms a seal over the glottis. A resuscitation bag or a T-piece is attached to a connector on the airway tube for positive-pressure ventilation. Supraglottic devices do not require the operator to visualize the vocal cords and do not require an instrument for insertion. Their major limitation is the lack of small sizes, meaning that it is usually not possible to use a laryngeal mask airway in an infant smaller than 1500 g, or about 31 weeks of gestational age.

Clinical trials and case series among term and late preterm newborns have shown that laryngeal masks compare favorably with both face mask ventilation and tracheal intubation during neonatal resuscitation.[104,105] The time required for mask insertion is short, the first-attempt success rate is high, and operators require relatively little training to acquire the insertion skill. In comparison to face mask ventilation, one quasi-randomized trial showed that the laryngeal mask decreased the need for subsequent tracheal intubation.[106]

The most commonly reported use during neonatal resuscitation has been as a rescue airway when both face mask ventilation and tracheal intubation were unsuccessful. This includes support of newborns with a wide variety of orofacial anomalies that prevent resuscitators from achieving an effective seal with a face mask or that obstruct the upper airway. Because the operator does not need to visualize the vocal cords during mask insertion, the device may be inserted successfully when an oral obstruction prevents laryngoscopy.[107] Published examples include newborns with a small mandible or large tongue complicating a wide variety of congenital syndromes.[108] In addition, the laryngeal mask has been used to secure the airway during helicopter and ambulance transport when laryngoscopy for intubation is not feasible.[109,110] A supraglottic device may provide a life-saving airway during an unanticipated emergency. These devices should be readily available in every birth setting, and all neonatal resuscitators should become proficient in their use.

MONITORING

As noted previously, effective ventilation is the key to successful resuscitation. This means delivering a tidal volume that is sufficient to achieve adequate gas exchange, but not so much as to cause lung damage. As few as six large inflations can cause severe lung injury in a preterm lamb model of resuscitation.[56] Leak around the face mask and obstruction to gas flow may lead to reduced tidal volumes, which may result in an unsuccessful resuscitation. Clinical assessment of lung inflation based on chest rise during ventilation is imprecise and inaccurate.[38] For many years clinicians have used ventilators in the intensive care unit that measure and display flow and volume of gas entering and leaving the lung. Stand-alone respiratory function monitors are available to perform similar functions in the delivery room. A recording of effective face mask ventilation is shown in Figure 26-7. This technology enables clinicians to detect ineffective ventilation due to excessive mask leak (Fig. 26-8) or airway obstruction (Fig. 26-9) and then adjust the mask position or inspiratory pressure to obtain optimal tidal volumes (Fig. 26-10). A small pilot randomized trial demonstrated the feasibility of this approach and showed that operators responded to the information provided by the monitor and reduced mask leak and excessive tidal volumes.[111] Respiratory monitoring is not yet widely available and larger trials are required before this technique is widely adopted. Nevertheless, this technology has potential for improving training in mask ventilation as well as providing valuable information during resuscitation of high-risk infants.

A simple alternative to respiratory function monitoring is provided by colorimetric carbon dioxide detectors. Leone and colleagues describe the use of these devices to demonstrate airway patency during mask ventilation.[112] Blank et al. demonstrated further proof of concept by showing that color change preceded improvement in heart rate and oxygen saturations.[113] This technique has considerable potential, particularly in resource-limited settings.

CHEST COMPRESSIONS

Fewer than 1 per 1000 term and late preterm newborns receive chest compressions in the delivery room.[3,20] Most newborns requiring resuscitation have primary respiratory failure and require only effective positive-pressure ventilation to recover. If gas exchange is impaired over a prolonged period of time, progressive hypoxemia and acidosis may deplete myocardial energy stores and depress myocardial function to the point that assisted ventilation alone will not be sufficient. In this setting, chest compressions may be required to augment circulation and allow the myocardium to recover. Compressions increase coronary artery blood flow by increasing the diastolic pressure gradient between the ascending aorta and the coronary sinus.[114]

Chest compressions should be started if the newborn's heart rate remains less than 60 bpm after at least 30 seconds of effective

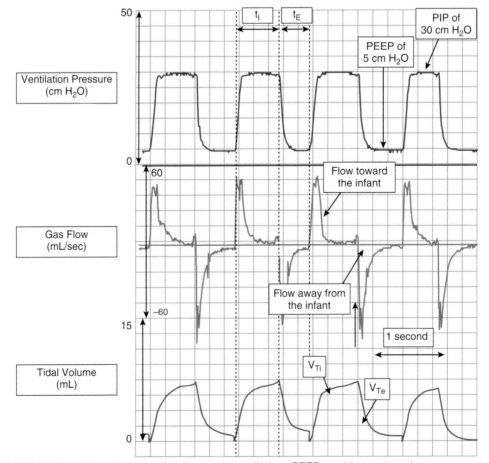

FIG 26-7 Recording showing effective mask ventilation. *PEEP,* positive end-expiratory pressure; *PIP,* peak inflation pressure.

positive-pressure ventilation that aerates the newborn's lungs.[5] Effective positive-pressure ventilation must be achieved before starting chest compressions. In most cases, ventilation should be provided through a properly inserted ETT before initiating compressions.

Current guidelines recommend compressing the chest using two thumbs centered on the middle of the sternum, over the lower third of the chest, with the hands and fingers encircling the chest (Fig. 26-11).[5] In comparison to the previously recommended two-finger method, the two-thumb method improves the quality and consistency of compressions and decreases compressor fatigue.[115] Compressions should be given with sufficient force to depress the sternum approximately one-third of the depth of the chest. Computed tomography studies of a small series of hospitalized infants resuscitated with arterial pressure catheters in place suggest that this depth provides adequate cardiac output while limiting the risk of injury from compressions.[116-118] Once an ETT is secured, the individual providing ventilations may move to the side of the bed and allow the compressor to stand at the head of the bed. This position allows the compressor to continue two-thumb compressions while permitting access to the baby's umbilicus for another team member to insert a catheter for medication administration.

There is ongoing controversy regarding the recommended ratio of compressions and ventilations during neonatal resuscitation. During adult cardiopulmonary resuscitation (CPR), high rates of uninterrupted compressions with infrequent pauses for ventilation are recommended to maintain coronary artery perfusion pressure. Once a secure airway is established, adult and pediatric CPR is performed with continuous chest compressions and asynchronous ventilations. Unlike adult cardiac arrests, most neonatal cardiac arrests are preceded by respiratory failure. At the time of arrest, blood in the neonate's left ventricle has a low oxygen tension and high carbon dioxide tension. It is, therefore, important to provide effective ventilation during neonatal compressions to ensure that blood reaching the coronary arteries is sufficiently oxygenated. The recommended compression method synchronizes compressions with ventilations. Three rapid compressions are administered followed by a short pause to interpose one ventilation, yielding a total of

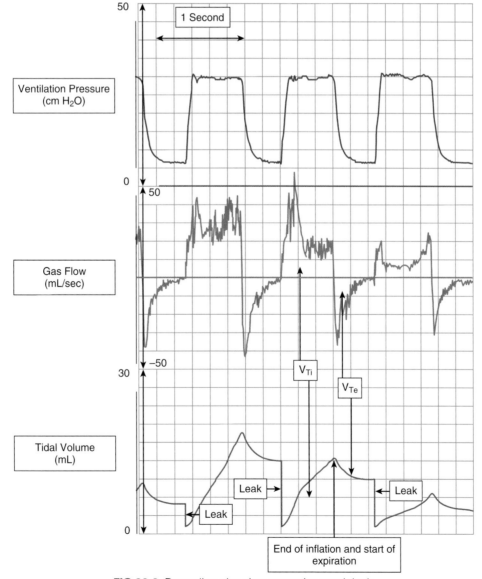

FIG 26-8 Recording showing excessive mask leak.

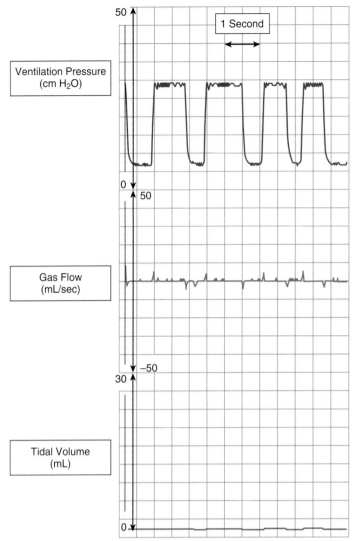

FIG 26-9 Recording showing airway obstruction.

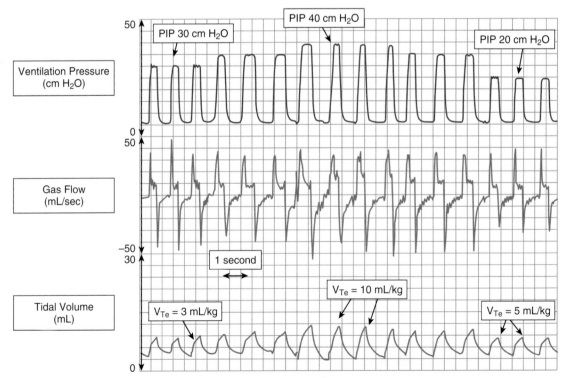

FIG 26-10 Adjustment of peak inflation pressure (PIP) to attain effective tidal volume.

90 compressions and 30 ventilations each minute.[5] Manikin models indicate that this 3:1 ratio results in better compression depth and ventilation dynamics than the 15:2 ratio recommended for adults and older children.[119,120] Small studies evaluating sustained inflations during compressions and continuous compressions with asynchronous ventilations have been completed in animal models; however, there are as of this writing no human studies.[121,122] Although the ideal oxygen concentration for ventilation during chest compressions is not known, current guidelines recommend ventilating with 100% oxygen until the heart rate exceeds 60 bpm and a reliable pulse oximetry reading can be obtained.[5]

Chest compressions should be continued until the baby's heart rate increases above 60 bpm. In an effort to avoid frequent interruptions, the heart rate should be checked after 60 seconds of compressions.[5] Physical examination methods of determining the baby's heart rate are inaccurate, and a pulse oximeter may not achieve a reliable signal during cardiovascular collapse. An electrocardiogram provides a more accurate and continuous measure of the newborn's heart rate[33,123] and is the current recommendation of the most recent ILCOR guidelines.[5] Other methods of monitoring the return of effective circulation during compressions have been investigated. During asystole, blood is not flowing to the lungs and carbon dioxide is not exhaled. Once circulation is restored, carbon dioxide is carried to the lungs and exhaled. A study performed in a piglet model showed that detecting the return of exhaled carbon dioxide (>14 mm Hg) by continuous capnography during compressions correlated with the return of an audible heart rate greater than 60 bpm.[124] There are no studies in human newborns evaluating this method as of this writing.

EPINEPHRINE

Medications are also rarely needed during neonatal resuscitation.[125] However, if the myocardium is so compromised by hypoxia and ischemia that it does not recover function with effective ventilation, chest compressions are indicated and there is a high likelihood that epinephrine will also be required. Epinephrine is a catecholamine that constricts vascular smooth muscle by stimulating α-adrenergic receptors. The resulting increase in systemic vascular resistance increases coronary artery perfusion pressure and enhances the efficacy of chest compressions. In addition, epinephrine increases the rate and strength of cardiac contractions.

Epinephrine is indicated if the newborn's heart rate remains less than 60 bpm after 30 seconds of ventilation that inflates the lungs followed by an additional 60 seconds of effective ventilation coordinated with chest compressions.[5] In most cases, ventilation will have been provided through a properly placed ETT. The recommended dose is 0.1 to 0.3 mL/kg of the 1:10,000 concentration (0.1 mg/mL) administered rapidly into the central venous circulation (Table 26-8).[5] If an adequate response is not achieved, the dose may be repeated every 3 to 5 minutes.

Medications rapidly reach the central venous circulation after administration into an umbilical venous catheter or an intraosseous needle inserted into the proximal tibia.[126] Although experienced neonatal providers commonly use the umbilical vein for emergency access, a simulation study using a neonatal model found that umbilical venous catheter insertion took longer than intraosseous needle placement.[127] Intraosseous needles are commonly used by prehospital providers and in pediatric emergency departments. They should be readily available with standard neonatal resuscitation supplies, and neonatal health providers should be trained in how to insert them. Peripheral veins are not recommended for emergency medication administration during resuscitation because cannulation is unlikely to be successful in the setting of cardiovascular collapse, and drug delivery to the central circulation is likely to be impaired. Delays in epinephrine administration can be prevented by anticipation, preparation, and training. If risk factors for severe neonatal depression are identified, such as persistent fetal bradycardia, the epinephrine and the equipment for emergency vascular access should be prepared before the baby is born.

While vascular access is being secured, some clinicians may choose to administer one dose of epinephrine via the ETT. Although endotracheal administration is an option, animal and human studies indicate that drug absorption is unreliable and endotracheal epinephrine is less effective.[128] Among newborns who did not respond to an initial dose of endotracheal epinephrine, most (77%) had return of spontaneous circulation after receiving an intravenous dose.[125] If endotracheal epinephrine is administered, a higher dose (0.5 to 1 mL/kg) is recommended.[5] This dose should not be administered intravenously and the syringe containing the higher dose should be clearly labeled "Endotracheal use only." If the baby's heart rate does not increase after one dose of endotracheal epinephrine, subsequent doses should be administered using the intravenous or intraosseous route.

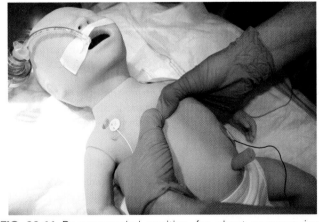

FIG 26-11 Recommended position for chest compressions with two thumbs centered on the middle of the sternum, over the lower third of the chest, with the hands and fingers encircling the chest.

TABLE 26-8 **Neonatal Resuscitation: Emergency Medications**
Epinephrine (1:10,000 = 0.1 mg/mL)
• UVC or IO needle: 0.1-0.3 mL/kg
• ETT (*less effective*): 0.5-1 mL/kg
• Infuse rapidly
• Repeat every 3-5 min
Normal Saline (0.9 NaCl)
• UVC or IO needle: 10 mL/kg
• Infuse over 5-10 min
• May repeat 10 mL/kg if inadequate response

ETT, endotracheal tube; *IO*, intraosseous; *UVC*, umbilical venous catheter.

VOLUME EXPANSION

Newborns may develop hypovolemic shock secondary to acute blood loss from a fetal–maternal hemorrhage, bleeding vasa previa, placental laceration, or umbilical cord prolapse or disruption. Signs of hypovolemic shock include pallor, weak pulses, poor perfusion, decreased capillary refill, and persistent bradycardia. The source of acute blood loss is not always apparent. Volume expansion is indicated if the baby does not respond to epinephrine and has clinical signs of hypovolemic shock, or risk factors that suggest the possibility of unrecognized blood loss. Routine volume expansion should not be considered in the absence of hypovolemia because of evidence that it worsens pulmonary edema without improving blood pressure or acidemia.[129]

Normal saline is a readily available isotonic crystalloid solution, and it is the most commonly recommended volume expander. The initial dose of normal saline for hypovolemic shock is 10 mL/kg infused over 5 to 10 minutes (see Table 26-8).[5] If the baby does not improve, an additional 10 mL/kg may be infused. In unusual circumstances, additional volume expansion may be considered; however, caution should be used to avoid infusing excessive volume and increasing demands on the newborn's heart. Although 5% albumin may lead to a short-term increase in blood pressure compared to volume expansion with crystalloid solution, it is not recommended for use during resuscitation because of the additional cost, unavailability for immediate use, theoretical risk of infection, and lack of demonstrated clinical benefit.[129] Emergency, non-cross-matched, type O, Rhesus-negative packed red blood cells should be rapidly available from the hospital blood bank and considered for the acute replacement of a large volume of blood loss.

SPECIAL CASES

Preterm Neonates

Preterm infants, particularly those born at less than 32 weeks' gestation, should be delivered in settings with adequate physical resources and trained personnel available. Maintenance of normal body temperature is vital. Preterm infants are especially prone to hypothermia because of their large surface area-to-mass ratio and thin epidermis. Plastic bags and wraps are shown to be effective in maintaining temperature[130] and are now accepted as the standard of care for infants of less than 28 weeks' gestational age. ILCOR recommends that infants be placed in plastic bags or wraps without drying and managed under a radiant warmer.[5] Temperatures need to be regularly measured and hyperthermia avoided, as it is associated with increased risk of adverse outcomes. Maintenance of delivery room temperatures of at least 26°C (~79°F) is also recommended. If respiratory support is required, it may be beneficial to use warmed and humidified gases, to limit evaporative heat loss.[131]

Recommendations regarding the optimal method of respiratory support have changed in recent years. Whereas some preterm infants are in poor condition at birth and require immediate resuscitation, the majority cries and breathes spontaneously[132] and requires help with stabilization rather than immediate intubation. Following a series of multicenter randomized trials[133-135] the American Academy of Pediatrics has issued a statement indicating that CPAP is an appropriate alternative to immediate intubation and ventilation.[136] If intubation is required, surfactant should be administered and the ETT removed as soon as possible. If intermittent positive pressure is required during the first minutes of life, PEEP is likely to be beneficial in facilitating rapid aeration of the lungs and should be used if available.[5] The ideal concentration of oxygen to begin resuscitation and the optimal targets of oxygen saturation remain to be determined for preterm infants. Investigators have noted that in preterm infants, commencing resuscitation with air leads to saturations that fall below the recommended range.[137,138] For infants of less than 33 weeks' gestation, it seems reasonable to begin resuscitation with 30% oxygen and adjust the concentration to maintain saturations within the range seen in full-term infants.

Congenital Diaphragmatic Hernia

Congenital diaphragmatic hernia (CDH) is a defect of the diaphragm, most commonly on the left side, which allows the abdominal viscera to herniate into the fetal chest. Compression from the herniated contents disturbs development of the lungs and pulmonary vasculature, causing varying degrees of pulmonary hypoplasia and pulmonary hypertension. Despite advances in care, most newborns with CDH develop severe respiratory failure shortly after birth and the mortality risk remains high.

Whenever possible, the birth should occur at an experienced high-risk center with a coordinated team capable of offering advanced resuscitation, cardiorespiratory care, and neonatal surgery. Birth outside of an experienced high-risk center has been associated with a higher risk of mortality.[139,140]

Before the birth, the resuscitation team should prepare a comprehensive management plan; the use of a standardized protocol has been shown to decrease CDH mortality.[141] Positive-pressure ventilation with a face mask should be avoided to prevent gaseous distention of the herniated abdominal contents and increased lung compression. Most experts recommend intubating immediately after birth and initiating ventilation with low peak pressures.[142] A nasogastric tube should be inserted promptly and placed on continuous suction to decompress the abdominal contents. An umbilical arterial catheter or radial arterial line should be placed for continuous blood pressure monitoring and blood gas sampling. An umbilical venous catheter is helpful for fluid and medication administration; however, the catheter may not advance properly if the liver is herniated into the chest. Volume expansion and inotropic support may be required to maintain normal blood pressure and minimize right-to-left shunting associated with pulmonary hypertension. Functional echocardiography may be helpful to optimize blood pressure support.

The goal of delivery room management is to achieve an acceptable preductal oxygen saturation without causing lung injury from high ventilating pressure, excessive tidal volume, and oxygen toxicity. The CDH EURO Consortium recommends maintaining preductal oxygen saturation between 88% and 95%, postductal saturation above 70%, and arterial P_{CO_2} between 45 and 60 mm Hg.[142] During the first 2 hours of life, the consortium suggests that lower preductal saturation may be acceptable if the baby is gradually improving and organ perfusion is maintained.

Fetal Hydrops

Fetal hydrops usually presents as subcutaneous edema with abdominal ascites and pleural or pericardial effusions. The most common associated diagnoses are congenital heart problems, abnormalities in heart rate, twin-to-twin transfusion, congenital anomalies, chromosomal abnormalities, congenital viral infections, and congenital anemia.[143]

The delivery room resuscitation team should anticipate complex problems, including restricted ventilation from pleural effusions and ascites, pulmonary hypoplasia, pulmonary edema, surfactant deficiency, pulmonary hypertension, severe anemia, intravascular volume depletion, and myocardial dysfunction.[144] An experienced team with proficiency in endotracheal intubation, emergency vascular access, thoracentesis, and paracentesis should be present in the delivery room. Multiple procedures may be required in a short period of time, and specific roles should be delegated in advance. The equipment to perform these procedures should be prepared before birth and ready for immediate use. Ultrasonography performed just before birth is helpful to identify the location of fluid collections and plan interventions. If there is a large pleural effusion or significant ascites, the obstetric provider may remove fluid before delivery.

After birth, respiratory distress should be expected. The resuscitation team should be prepared to promptly intubate the trachea and provide positive-pressure ventilation. Tracheal intubation may be difficult if there is soft tissue edema or a neck mass. If the abdomen is distended and interfering with ventilation, paracentesis should be performed. Only enough fluid to permit diaphragmatic excursion and effective ventilation should be removed. If pleural effusions interfere with ventilation, thoracentesis may be required in the delivery room. If the baby is born preterm, surfactant administration may be helpful. Once the airway has been secured and ventilation has been established, umbilical arterial and venous catheters are needed to monitor arterial blood pressure, obtain blood samples, and infuse fluids. Despite marked edema, the newborn may have intravascular volume depletion, and careful volume expansion with normal saline or packed red blood cells may be needed. Hypoglycemia, metabolic acidosis, and hypothermia are common problems and should be anticipated. If severe anemia is present, an isovolemic partial volume exchange transfusion with type O, Rh-negative packed red blood cells cross-matched against the mother may be required to avoid volume overload.

ETHICS

Deciding Whether to Commence Resuscitation

Noninitiation of resuscitation at birth can be ethically acceptable under certain circumstances. Families with fetuses known to be affected by anencephaly, confirmed trisomy 13 or 18, or severe brain, cardiac, lung, or renal malformations may opt not to offer support at birth. For infants at very low gestational age, the decision of whether to initiate intensive care is complex. Initiation of resuscitation in the delivery room does not mandate continued provision of intensive care. Later withdrawal of intensive care support may allow time to elicit more clinical information and to counsel the family. Parents should be informed that a decision made before birth to initiate resuscitation may need to be altered, depending upon the infant's response to resuscitation and his or her subsequent progress. Redirection of care toward palliation is considered ethically equivalent to noninitiation of support.

International guidelines have provided some consistency in the development of gestational age–based guidelines regarding resuscitation.[145] Initiation of resuscitation is nearly always indicated where there is a high survival rate and acceptable morbidity. Typically this includes babies with gestational age of 25 weeks or more. No published guidelines advise initiation of resuscitation for infants born before 22 weeks' gestation. Between these two time points there is a gray zone, in which the wishes of the parents, the experience and beliefs of

the clinicians, and local policy and guidelines will influence whether resuscitation is offered, advised, or given.[146] In Japan it is standard practice to offer resuscitation to infants born at 22 weeks' gestation, whereas in Switzerland resuscitation is not recommended to those <24 weeks' gestation.[147] Guidance from the Nuffield Council on Bioethics in the United Kingdom recommends that threatened delivery below 25 weeks warrants discussion with parents, with resuscitation normally advised between 24 and 25 weeks; parents' wishes should take precedence at 23 to 24 weeks, with a recommendation not to resuscitate at 22 to 23 weeks unless parents insist following counseling.[148] In contrast, the American Academy of Pediatrics guidance[149] avoids reliance on gestational age alone to guide decision making, instead making less directive recommendations, which take estimated weight, sex, receipt of antenatal steroids, and multiple versus singleton pregnancy into consideration. If there is uncertainty surrounding the gestational age, a therapeutic trial may be an option. However it should be noted that clinicians are very poor at predicting which infants will do well in the long term on the basis of their appearance at birth.[150]

The gestational age recommendations are based on the poor outcomes associated with extreme preterm birth, but determining outcome for extremely low gestational age infants is challenging. It is a self-fulfilling prophecy that if resuscitation is not offered at certain gestations, then survival will be very low. Therefore true survival, if all infants were offered intensive support, is very hard to measure. In Japan, where initiation of support at 22 weeks is common, 37% of 22-week infants are reported to survive to hospital discharge.[151] In contrast, in the British EPICURE study from 2006, in which resuscitation at 22 weeks was not recommended, only 2% of 22-week infants survived to discharge.[152] Overall survival below 25 weeks has increased since 2005, but rates of serious morbidity have either remained static or increased,[152] meaning that the number of preterm survivors with or at risk of later health problems has increased. For infants born at 22 to 25 weeks overall mortality is still ≥50%; rates of surviving minimally or unimpaired are <20% for those born below 25 weeks' gestation, but <5% for those born at 22 and 23 weeks' gestation.[153] Poor neurodevelopmental outcome is often cited as a reason for noninitiation of resuscitation, as is poor long-term quality of life. However, quality of life is subjective; physical or intellectual impairment does not necessarily equate to poor quality of life.[146] Teenage children born extremely preterm rate their life quality similarly to that of term-born teenagers.[154]

Deciding Whether to Stop Resuscitation

It is reasonable to want to avoid prolonged resuscitation where the outcome is likely to be death or survival with severe disability. Therefore, clinicians have sought to determine how much intervention, and for how long, is most appropriate. Data from the late 1990s showed that two-thirds of term infants who received epinephrine in the delivery room (DR) survived and two-thirds of survivors had no neurologic deficit at 1 year.[155] However, survival was only 30% in the subgroup of infants <29 weeks' gestation, and although almost 80% of preterm survivors were normal at 1 year, overall 78% of the group either died or had neurodevelopmental disability. These data brought into question the appropriateness of epinephrine use in the preterm population in the DR. More recent data from a review of outcomes of infants of <1500 g in the Vermont Oxford Network showed that of the 6% who received chest compressions and/or epinephrine (CPR/Epi) in the DR, 63% survived (compared with 88% of those who did not receive CPR/Epi),[156] and more than half survived without evidence of severe intraventricular hemorrhage. For the subgroup <1000 g, survival was 54% (75% in controls).[156] Other follow-up data report that for infants of <32 weeks' gestation, or <1000 g who received CPR/Epi in the DR, the risk of adverse neurologic outcome was two to three times higher than those who did not.[157,158]

A report in 1991 showed that within a cohort of infants with an Apgar score of 0 at 1 minute (n = 93), almost two-thirds initially responded to resuscitation and one-third ultimately survived to discharge. Followed-up survivors (23/33) had normal development in 61% of cases. However, in the subgroup who still had an Apgar of 0 at 10 minutes of life (n = 58), 98% died and the single survivor had poor neurologic outcome. These results led to the recommendation that resuscitation should be stopped if there is no return of spontaneous circulation at 10 minutes of life.[159] These findings were demonstrated again in a more recent (2007) cohort of infants with Apgar of 0 at 10 minutes, showing that 94% died or had severe neurodevelopmental disability.[160] However, two larger studies, in the era of hypothermia use for neuroprotection, reported a lower rate of death or severe neurodevelopmental disability, 73% to 76%,[161,162] inferring that almost a quarter survived without major neurodevelopmental sequelae. These data may influence recommendations for resuscitation duration in the future, but currently the ILCOR guidelines conclude that discontinuation of resuscitation may be justified after "10 minutes of continuous and adequate resuscitative efforts of an infant with no heartbeat and no respiratory effort."[163]

POSTRESUSCITATION CARE

Examination/Monitoring

Infants who required resuscitation after birth have an increased risk of medical problems involving multiple organ systems. These complications may be anticipated and promptly addressed by careful assessment and appropriate monitoring. Even newborns who required only brief (<1 minute) positive-pressure ventilation after birth have a higher risk of short-term respiratory and neurologic complications and should have postresuscitation monitoring.[19] The nature and duration of monitoring are dependent upon the newborn's condition and identifiable risk factors.

A thorough examination should be performed to identify anomalies that may have contributed to cardiorespiratory compromise after birth and any evidence of trauma from the birth or resuscitation procedures. The newborn should be evaluated for signs of ongoing respiratory distress such as retractions, nasal flaring, or grunting. The chest should be auscultated to assess the presence of bilateral breath sounds. If cyanosis is apparent when the baby is quiet and resolves with crying, ensure that both nares are patent. The abdomen should be examined for evidence of trauma, distention, masses, or unusual flattening ("scaphoid"). If the baby required prolonged resuscitation, a standardized neurologic examination including alertness, pupillary response, sucking, tone, and reflexes should be completed to rule out encephalopathy.

Vital signs should be monitored frequently during postresuscitation care. Term and late-preterm babies who received positive-pressure ventilation have an increased risk of pneumothoraces (2% to 5%) and ongoing respiratory distress requiring assisted ventilation (5% to 16%).[19] Delayed transition increases the risk of persistent pulmonary hypertension, and caregivers should be attentive to signs of worsening hypoxemia. Chest radiography and arterial blood gases may be indicated to inform treatment decisions. Hypotension may occur due to hypovolemia, peripheral vasodilation, myocardial dysfunction, or sepsis. Routine volume expansion without evidence of hypovolemia, however, is not recommended and may contribute to worsening respiratory distress.[129] Babies who required significant resuscitation may require pharmacologic agents to support their blood pressure. Hypotension, hypoxia, and acidosis can decrease renal blood flow and cause renal failure associated with acute tubular necrosis. Babies who required significant resuscitation should have their urine output, body weight, and serum electrolyte levels checked frequently. Perinatal stress increases glucose consumption and may causes hypoglycemia. Milk feeds may be delayed because of clinical instability, and intravenous fluids may be required to maintain the blood glucose in the normal range. Blood glucose levels should be checked at regular intervals until milk feeds are established and the infant is able to maintain a normal glucose level. Newborns with hypotension, hypoxemia, and acidosis may develop apnea and seizures associated with hypoxic–ischemic encephalopathy.

Therapeutic Hypothermia for Hypoxic–Ischemic Encephalopathy

Death and long-term neurodevelopmental sequelae are the most important consequences of peripartum hypoxia. Neuronal death following a severe insult occurs in two phases.[164] Immediate primary neuronal death due to primary energy failure is followed by a latent period of at least 6 hours. A secondary, delayed neuronal death phase ensues, during which a substantial proportion of cell loss occurs. The 6-hour "therapeutic window" allows amelioration of injury through brain cooling by rescuing cells from apoptotic death and reducing cerebral metabolic rate. The Cochrane review on this topic found 11 randomized trials, which recruited 1505 term and late-preterm infants with evidence of peripartum asphyxia. Infants typically had Apgar scores of 5 or less at 10 minutes, required ventilation at 10 minutes, or had cord or arterial pH <7.1 within 1 hour of birth and had evidence of encephalopathy.[165] Infants treated with either whole-body or selective head cooling were compared with standard treatment. Cooling reduced the risk of death or neurodevelopmental disability to 18 months of age (relative risk 0.75 (0.68 to 0.83); number needed to treat 7 (5 to 10)). Both whole-body and selective head cooling are effective, and both moderately and severely encephalopathic patients appear to benefit from cooling. The benefits of cooling outweighed the short-term adverse effects of sinus bradycardia and thrombocytopenia. Therapeutic cooling should be undertaken according to protocols similar to those used in the randomized trials and in settings with sufficient resources in terms of both staff and equipment. Infants who undergo therapeutic hypothermia should be followed up throughout childhood to identify and support those with neurodevelopmental impairment.

REFERENCES

A complete reference list is available at https://expertconsult.inkling.com/.

27

Respiratory Care of the Newborn

Robert DiBlasi, RRT-NPS, FAARC, and John T. Gallagher, MPH, RRT-NPS, FAARC

Respiratory care encompasses a set of practices, usually implemented by a multidisciplinary team (physician, respiratory therapist, nurse), to ensure the optimal delivery of respiratory support to newborn infants with respiratory distress or other problems. These practices include resuscitation, artificial airway management, invasive and noninvasive monitoring of gas exchange, airway clearance, and aerosolized drug administration. A thorough understanding of these techniques will help clinicians provide optimal invasive and noninvasive respiratory support to sick neonates and simultaneously avoid iatrogenic injury such as skin breakdown, airway injury and inflammation, infection, ventilator-induced lung injury, and other complications. Unfortunately many of these interventions have not been rigorously studied, and the recommendations and suggestions in this chapter are often based on low-quality evidence and experience.

TECHNIQUES TO PROVIDE POSITIVE-PRESSURE VENTILATION

Manual Ventilation

Positive-pressure ventilation can be provided through a face mask or through an endotracheal tube either with a mechanical ventilator or with one of the three commonly used manual resuscitators: the self-inflating bag, the flow-inflating ("anesthesia") bag,[1] and the T-piece resuscitator.[2] Each possesses inherent features that distinguish one from the other. The clearest differences are found in their ability to control ventilating pressures, their reliance upon a gas source, and their potential to deliver free-flow oxygen, continuous positive airway pressure (CPAP), positive end-expiratory pressure (PEEP), and sustained inflations.

Both flow-inflating and self-inflating bags come in a wide variety of configurations, but all configurations share some basic attributes, including an oxygen inlet, patient outlet, flow-control valve, and pressure manometer attachment site. The self-inflating bag, as the name implies, reinflates after squeezing and does not require the flow of oxygen to reinflate. However, this bag with an oxygen source can deliver only about 40% oxygen because as the bag reinflates, room air is drawn into the bag and mixes with 100% oxygen from the oxygen source. A reservoir will not allow room air to come into the bag; therefore, the self-inflating bag attached to an oxygen source with a reservoir is able to deliver 90% to 100% oxygen to the baby.

Two other important characteristics of most self-inflating bags are a pressure-relief ("pop-off") valve, which is set at 30 to 40 cm H_2O, and a nonrebreathing valve, which is built into the

bag and prevents the reliable delivery of free-flow oxygen.[3] To deliver free-flow oxygen, the operator needs to disconnect the oxygen tubing from the bag and hold the oxygen tubing close to the nose of the baby. In contrast, the flow-inflating bag is an excellent source of free-flow oxygen, especially with the use of the appropriate-sized mask attached to the bag. Finally, both of these bags require a pressure manometer to provide safe and effective ventilation to the newborn.[3] Table 27-1 compares the two ventilation bags (or manual resuscitators).

The self-inflating bag is the only resuscitator that can operate with or without a gas source, making it ideal for transport. Because of its design, however, it cannot deliver free-flow oxygen or "blow-by oxygen." Some devices incorporate a reservoir hose coming from the back that can be used for this purpose. Improvements in sensitive valve mechanisms now allow spontaneous breathing and CPAP without having to squeeze the bag and at a relatively low work of breathing. Sustained inflations are not reliably given across all available models of self-inflating bags.[4] PEEP can be delivered with a self-inflating bag but only with an adjunctive PEEP valve affixed to the exhalation port on the resuscitator. The self-inflating bag does not reliably control ventilating pressures and volumes even when the device is equipped with a manometer and pressure-relief valve.[5]

A flow-inflating bag, as the name suggests, requires flow from a pressurized gas source to operate. Its design allows for free-flow oxygen delivery as well as CPAP during spontaneous breathing and PEEP during positive-pressure ventilation. Inspiratory pressure, PEEP, and/or CPAP is very difficult to maintain with these systems because the clinician must coordinate a mask seal and regulate egress of flow using the thumb valve while observing chest rise and pressure readings on a manometer. One study showed more excessive PEEP (defined as >10 cm H_2O for >10 seconds) with the flow-inflating bag than with the self-inflating bag.[6] Flow-inflating bags have traditionally been believed to be superior to self-inflating bags because they allow the clinician to feel changes in lung compliance better than with a self-inflating bag.[7-9] Repeated laboratory scenarios have found that the flow-inflating bag produced more variable tidal volume and PEEP than the self-inflating bag.[10] Studies have also shown that this sense of "feeling compliance changes" with a flow-inflating bag is less reliable than with a self-inflating bag.[11] In fact, experienced physicians were unable to detect when an endotracheal tube was occluded in a lung model 75% of the time. Additionally, experienced respiratory therapists specializing in neonatology were shown not to distinguish changes in compliance better with a flow-inflating bag than with a self-inflating bag.[10]

TABLE 27-1	Neonatal Manual Resuscitators	
	Self-Inflating Bag	**Non-Self-Inflating Bag**
Types	Laerdal, Hope II, PMR 2, and a host of disposable equivalents	"Anesthesia bag" with spring-loaded or variable-orifice bleed port
Operator	Requires education on bag characteristics	Requires both experience and knowledge of bag characteristics for adjustment of flow and bleed
Oxygen–air source positive FiO_2 delivery	Operates with room air	Requires compressed gas
	Efficacy of O_2 delivery dependent on correct use of closed reservoir system and closure of pop-off valve (use of open reservoir or pop-off valve reduces FiO_2)	Delivers FiO_2 of gas source unambiguously
	Many brands deliver room air on spontaneous breaths (in-house verification of brand performance is recommended)	Oxygen delivery same on spontaneous breaths as it is on mandatory breaths
Pressure delivery	Having excessive trust in pop-off feature is unwise; occlusion of pop-off valve and use of manometer allow performance equal to that of non-self-inflating bags	With manometer attached, any pressure can be easily given
Comments	Relatively complex mechanism with possibility of failure, particularly when reusable units are reassembled	Simple, reliable mechanism dependent on gas supply
	If pop-off pressure is adequate, allows removal of bulky manometer for transport	Manometer is bulky

Most manual ventilation devices used during resuscitation have been shown to result in variability in delivered volumes and pressures. Displayed tidal volume permits better detection of compliance changes than monitored or preset pressures.[12] Future devices are needed to display volume to avoid hypo/hyperventilation and lung injury in neonates.

The T-piece resuscitator is the newest and most sophisticated of the manual resuscitator designs. Similar to the flow-inflating bag, it requires a pressurized gas source to operate and can be used to administer free-flow oxygen and CPAP to a spontaneously breathing patient. Its greatest advantage lies in its ability to regulate ventilating pressures.[13]

Face Masks for Ventilation

In cases in which the baby requires manual ventilation prior to endotracheal intubation, a ventilation bag with a manometer and the appropriate-sized mask should be used. The mask should be clear and have a soft, form-fitting cushion that extends around the circumference. The alternative is the rigid but anatomically shaped Rendell-Baker/Soucek mask, which may have less dead space but has been demonstrated to be more difficult to use, often resulting in ineffective ventilation.[14]

Endotracheal Intubation

Endotracheal intubation is commonly required during neonatal resuscitation at birth or postnatally in an infant with apnea or severe respiratory failure. Certain anatomic lesions may cause obstruction at the level of the nasopharynx, larynx, and upper trachea and may necessitate endotracheal intubation of affected neonates during initial resuscitation.[15] Beginning at the nasal level, these lesions include bilateral or severe unilateral choanal atresia or stenosis, pharyngeal hypotonia, and micrognathia, such as may be seen in the Robin sequence (which may include cleft palate and glossoptosis). At the level of the larynx, obstructive problems may include laryngomalacia (or laryngotracheomalacia), laryngeal web, bilateral vocal cord paralysis, and congenital subglottic obstruction. In addition, critical airway obstruction may be secondary to other lesions that may compress the airway and impair normal respiration. These may include cystic hygroma, goiter, or hemangioma. Many of these

lesions, particularly those causing significant fixed obstruction at the level of the larynx or below, may render endotracheal intubation extremely difficult and may require emergency tracheostomy (see Chapter 25).

Infants in the neonatal intensive care unit may require endotracheal intubation and positive-pressure ventilation because of respiratory failure related to a variety of causes. Two common scenarios that merit particular consideration include preterm infants with worsening respiratory distress syndrome and infants with postextubation respiratory failure.

A variety of competing factors will influence the decision to intubate an infant who has worsening respiratory distress syndrome (RDS). The symptoms of untreated RDS will tend to worsen during the first 48 to 72 hours of life, until the infant begins to make significant amounts of endogenous surfactant. Therefore, an infant with moderately severe respiratory insufficiency and distress during the first 24 hours of life may merit intubation and ventilation in anticipation of worsening disease, whereas an infant with comparable disease severity at 3 or 4 days of life may avoid intubation in anticipation of spontaneous improvement.

Although the optimal timing of surfactant administration for treatment of RDS is controversial, the available data suggest that early treatment and multiple doses are more effective, and this observation may thus lead to earlier intubation. On the other hand, positive-pressure ventilation delivered through an endotracheal tube is well known to cause lung injury, particularly if large tidal volumes are used. Some centers that make extensive use of nasal CPAP to avoid intubation and mechanical ventilation have reported fewer apneic events, less need for (re)intubation, and low rates of chronic lung disease.[16] However, these finding were not duplicated in randomized controlled trials.[17,18] Different practitioners will weigh these competing factors differently, and the indications for intubation of an infant with RDS will vary depending on the clinical circumstances and local practices.

Postextubation respiratory failure is a common occurrence in preterm infants, occurring in as many as one-third of infants. Causes of respiratory failure in these infants include central or obstructive apnea, respiratory insufficiency leading to progressive atelectasis, and early chronic lung disease. While premature infants represent a large percentage of the patient population treated in the neonatal intensive care unit (NICU), term or postterm babies can become critically ill and develop life-threatening respiratory failure. This can result from congenital diaphragmatic hernia, primary pulmonary hypertension, meconium aspiration, sepsis, and pneumonia. Early application of nasal CPAP directly following extubation has been shown to result in lower incidence of respiratory failure, need for mechanical ventilation, and risk of developing bronchopulmonary dysplasia (BPD) in preterm neonates than extubation to no respiratory support, but CPAP may fail in 25% to 40% of infants.[19-21] Some evidence suggests that intermediary forms of noninvasive ventilation (NIV) or noninvasive intermittent mandatory ventilation may be more effective in preventing postextubation respiratory failure.[22] Other techniques to avoid reintubation include the use of methylxanthines. Indications for reintubation include progressive respiratory acidosis, increased work of breathing, grunting, stridor, significant oxygen requirement, or severe apnea.

It is not uncommon to have significant respiratory failure following extubation due to upper airway edema or subglottic stenosis, especially if the patient received prolonged ventilator support or multiple intubations or had traumatic intubation. Patients who develop respiratory failure following extubation often present with stridor, grunting, nasal flaring, and prolonged exhalation. These infants are at significant risk for severe clinical deterioration and cardiopulmonary arrest. Often, infants with a known risk of failed extubation attempts will be given intravenous steroids to reduce inflammation prior to extubation. Many clinicians will monitor the endotracheal tube leak displayed on the ventilator to determine the degree of airway edema present. However, this practice may not accurately reflect whether the neonatal patient will develop distress following extubation. Also, cuffed endotracheal tubes have been introduced into the NICU arena. Attempts should be made to reduce the cuff volume and prevent excessive pressure on the tracheal mucosae but only if the patient is able to be ventilated appropriately. In the event that there is airway compromise from edema following extubation, inhaled aerosolized racemic epinephrine can be delivered to reduce swelling, but there are no data to support or refute this practice.[23] Nonetheless, many NICUs will have supplies ready at the bedside of high-risk neonates in the event that they develop stridor and respiratory distress. Additionally, clinicians should also have reintubation supplies ready at the bedside in case the patient develops severe respiratory failure. If the baby is unable to maintain adequate ventilation despite interventions, then reintubation and suctioning should be accomplished. There are multiple reasons for extubation failure; Box 27-1 provides a comprehensive list. Extubation failure should prompt a search for a cause that can be corrected before the next extubation attempt.

Routes of Intubation

Intubation can be performed orally or nasally. The choice of route depends on the circumstances and the preference of the clinician. Both oral and nasal endotracheal intubation have their unique complications and share a few as well.[24-26] Oral intubation is easier, faster, and less traumatic to perform, and it may be preferable in an emergency. Available data have failed to demonstrate statistically significant differences between oral and nasal intubation with respect to tracheal injury, frequency

---

BOX 27-1 Major Causes of Extubation Failure

I. Pulmonary
  A. Primary disease not resolved
  B. Postextubation atelectasis
  C. Pulmonary insufficiency of prematurity
  D. Bronchopulmonary dysplasia
  E. Eventration or paralysis of diaphragm
II. Upper Airway
  A. Edema and/or excess tracheal secretions
  B. Subglottic stenosis
  C. Laryngotracheomalacia
  D. Congenital vascular ring
  E. Necrotizing tracheobronchitis
III. Cardiovascular
  A. Patent ductus arteriosus
  B. Fluid overload
  C. Congenital heart disease with increased pulmonary flow
IV. Central Nervous System
  A. Apnea (extreme immaturity)
  B. Intraventricular hemorrhage
  C. Hypoxic ischemic brain damage/seizures
  D. Drugs (phenobarbital)
V. Miscellaneous
  A. Unrecognized diagnosis (e.g., nerve palsy, myasthenia gravis)
  B. Sepsis
  C. Metabolic abnormality

---

of tube retaping, or tube replacement.[27] However, a higher incidence of postextubation atelectasis has been noted in nasally intubated patients, especially in preterm infants with birth weight less than 1500 g; atelectasis was associated with a marked reduction in nasal airflow through the previously intubated nares and stenosis of the nasal vestibule.[28,29] Midface hypoplasia has been reported to be associated with long-term intubation for BPD.[30]

On the other hand, proponents of nasal intubation believe that fixation of the tube to the infant's face is easier and more stable because it minimizes the chance for accidental dislodgment and decreases tube movement, which can result in subglottic stenosis. Prolonged oral intubation can result in palatal grooving[31] and defective dentition.[32] Furthermore, there is evidence that acquired subglottic stenosis is increased in patients who were orally intubated and whose birth weight was less than 1500 g. The same study and one other offer evidence that the nasotracheal tube is easier to stabilize than an oral tube and that extubation occurs less frequently than in oral intubation.[26,33] Acquired subglottic stenosis secondary to oral intubation may be a sequela of tracheal mucosal damage from the endotracheal tube itself or from repeated intubations. Most significantly, severe damage can occur from the up-and-down movement of the endotracheal tube.[27] Even with perfect fixation of the tube, up-and-down movement of 7 to 14 mm has been reported owing to the varying degrees of flexion of the neck. The caretaker team can minimize palatal grooving and defective dentition by rotating the fixation site from side to side during periodic retaping. Devices are available commercially that serve as palate protectors for prolonged intubation of very low birthweight infants (Gesco Pla-nate, MedChem Products, Woburn, Massachusetts, USA). Continuing attention to the quality of fixation, together with stabilization of the infant's head position, minimizes tube shifting and accidental extubation with the oral approach. However, both the oral and the nasal techniques will continue to have a place in the care of the ventilated neonate. Problems associated with oral and nasal endotracheal tube use are summarized in Box 27-2.

Equipment

The equipment needed for intubation is listed in Box 27-3, and the guidelines for choosing the correct tube size and suction catheters are listed in Tables 27-2 and 27-3.[1]

The use of tubes of appropriate size minimizes trauma, airway resistance, and excessive leak around the tube. A standard kit containing all of the equipment, as listed in Box 27-3, can be prepared and stocked, but it must be checked regularly to ensure that all of the necessities are present. The infant should be placed under a radiant warmer for endotracheal intubation.

A laryngoscope with a Miller No. 0 or No. 1 blade should be used to visualize the vallecula, epiglottis, and glottis. The No. 0 blade is used for almost all newborns. The No. 1 blade is used for infants who are several months of age or newborns whose birth weight is greater than 4 to 5 kg.[1,34] A Miller No. 00 blade has been touted for use in extremely low birth-weight infants because its smaller blade is more easily accommodated in the mouths of micropreemies. However, because the light source is set back farther from the blade tip, some clinicians believe the visualization is not as good as with the No. 0 blade.

Types of Tubes

The endotracheal tube should be made of a nontoxic, thermolabile, nonkinking material that molds to the airway. The tube should meet the standards of the American Society for Testing and Materials F1242-89 and be radiopaque or have a radiopaque line. Cuffed endotracheal tubes are not routinely used in neonates because the bulk of the cuff may prevent the practitioner from inserting a tube with as large a diameter as would otherwise be possible. There is always a serious concern that the inflated cuff may damage the very sensitive airway mucosa of the small baby. If sealing the space around the tube becomes a priority, cuffed tubes are now available (Sheridan, Teleflex, Morrisville, North Carolina, USA).

The type of endotracheal tube used most commonly is the Murphy endotracheal tube (Fig. 27-1). The Murphy tube is preferred for long-term ventilation. Most often, Murphy tubes have centimeter markers to show the overall depth of the tube, as well as vocal cord guide markers near the tip. These markers, under laryngoscopic visualization, show the clinician the depth within the trachea. Standard default markers should be used with caution because of the range of anatomic variation. In one review of the length of the black area at the tip of endotracheal tubes produced by four major manufacturers, the marker length varied by 10 mm in 2.5-mm internal-diameter tubes.[35]

BOX 27-2 Problems in Newborn Infants with Oral and Nasal Endotracheal Tubes

Common Problems

- Postextubation atelectasis—more common with nasal endotracheal tubes
- Pneumonia/sepsis
- Accidental extubation
- Intubation of main stem bronchus
- Occlusion of tube from thickened secretions
- Tracheal erosion
- Pharyngeal, esophageal, tracheal perforation
- Subglottic stenosis

Problems Unique to Nasal Endotracheal Tubes

- Nasal septal erosion
- Stricture of the nasal vestibule

Problems Unique to Oral Endotracheal Tubes

- Palatal grooving
- Interference with subsequent primary dentition

Data from Spitzer AR, Fox WW. The use of oral versus nasal endotracheal tubes in newborn infants. *J Calif Perinatol Assoc* 4:32, 1984.

BOX 27-3 Equipment Needed for Intubation

- Laryngoscope with premature (Miller No. 0) and infant (Miller No. 1) blades; Miller No. 00 optional for extremely premature infant
- Batteries and extra bulbs
- Endotracheal tubes, sizes 2.5, 3.0, 3.5, and 4.0 mm i.d.
- Stylet
- Suction apparatus (wall)
- Suction catheters: 5.0, 6.0, 8.0, and 10.0 F
- Meconium aspirator
- Oral airway
- Stethoscope
- Non-self-inflating bag (0.5 L), manometer, and tubing; self-inflating bag with reservoir, manometer optional for self-inflating bag
- Newborn and premature mask
- Source of compressed air/O_2 with capability for blending
- Humidification and warming apparatus for air/O_2
- Tape: ½-inch pink (Hy-Tape)
- Scissors
- Magill neonatal forceps
- Elastoplast (elastic bandages)
- Cardiorespiratory monitor
- Carbon dioxide monitor or detector
- Pulse oximeter (SpO$_2$)

TABLE 27-2 Selecting the Appropriate-Sized Endotracheal Tube

Tube Size (Inside Diameter in mm)	Weight (g)	Gestational Age (week)
2.5	<1000	<28
3.0	1000-2000	28-34
3.5	2000-3000	34-38
3.5-4.0	>3000	>38

From Kattwinkel J, ed. *Neonatal Resuscitation Textbook*. 5th ed. Elk Grove Village, Ill., American Academy of Pediatrics and the American Heart Association, 2006. Used with permission of the American Academy of Pediatrics.

TABLE 27-3 Selecting the Appropriate-Sized Suction Catheter

Endotracheal Tube Size (mm)	Catheter Size (French)
2.5	5 or 6
3.0	6 or 8
3.5	8
4.0	8 or 10

From Kattwinkel J, ed. *Neonatal Resuscitation Textbook*. 5th ed. Elk Grove Village, Ill., American Academy of Pediatrics and the American Heart Association, 2006. Used with permission of the American Academy of Pediatrics.

A Murphy tube has a tip bevel that allows smooth passage through the nares and a side hole whose purpose is to allow ventilation even if the tip is partially obstructed or is placed in the right main stem bronchus. Some clinicians avoid using side-hole ("Murphy eye") tubes for prolonged ventilation because of anecdotal evidence that these tubes can abrade the trachea and cause scarring. Exclusive use of these endotracheal tubes in one institution was associated with an increased incidence of subglottic stenosis that ended when use of the tubes was discontinued. It can be adequately maintained in the correct position if the lip marker is placed on the tube at the lip level and it is fixed to the face. After proper placement is determined, the marker can be used as a reference to ensure that the tube's position remains constant. The Murphy tube is pliable (and becomes even less firm when it is allowed to remain under a radiant warmer while preparations are made for resuscitation). Many clinicians prefer to use an obturator or stylet to facilitate insertion. The stylet should not extend beyond the distal tip of the tube to avoid tracheal damage from the insertion process.

The vicious cycle of asphyxia is frequently in progress in the critically ill neonate who requires emergent tracheal intubation. The process of intubation in such an infant can exacerbate the difficulties that he or she is already experiencing. Intubation is associated with severe bradycardia, hypoxia, and elevation of arterial blood pressure and intracranial pressure.[36]

Depth of Tube Insertion

In addition to direct visualization of the tube as it passes through the glottis, there are a number of suggested "rules of thumb" for initial estimation of proper depth of tracheal tube placement. These rules use the centimeter markings on the side

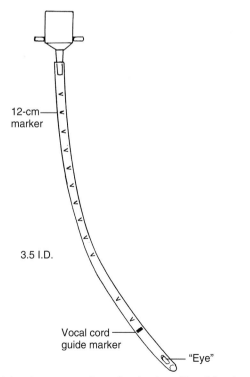

FIG 27-1 Murphy-type endotracheal tube. The Murphy type is straight and relatively soft, with markings to show depth of insertion in the airway and in the trachea. An "eye" is present at the tip.

of a standard Murphy tube to gauge the depth of placement. The most common rule uses birth weight and a simple formula, the rule of 7-8-9. An endotracheal tube is advanced 7 cm to the lip for a 1-kg infant, 8 cm for a 2-kg infant, and 9 cm for a 3-kg infant. The rule of 7-8-9 is not appropriate for infants with hypoplastic mandibles (e.g., those with Pierre Robin syndrome) or short necks (e.g., those with Turner syndrome).[37] While the 7-8-9 rule appears to be an accurate clinical method for endotracheal tube placement in neonates weighing more than 750 g, when applied to infants weighing <750 g, caution is warranted. This may lead to an overestimated depth of insertion and potentially result in clinically significant consequences.[38] Nasotracheal tube insertion is generally governed by adding 1 cm to the 7-8-9 rule.

Determination of Placement

Placement of the endotracheal tube after intubation is determined first clinically and then by chest radiograph. Clinical determination includes the following:
- Improvement or maintenance of heart rate in the normal range
- Good color, pulses, and perfusion after the intubation
- Good bilateral chest wall movement with each breath
- Equal breath sounds heard over both lung fields
- Breath sounds heard much louder over the lung fields than are heard over the stomach
- Presence of inspiratory and expiratory tidal volume measurements
- No gastric distention with ventilation
- Presence of vapor in the tube during exhalation
- Direct visualization by laryngoscope of the tube passing between the vocal cords
- Presence of exhaled CO_2 as determined by a CO_2 detector and/or an end-tidal CO_2 monitor or capnography[39]
- Tip-to-lip measurement: Add 6 to the newborn's weight in kilograms (rule of 7-8-9)

The chest radiograph should be performed to demonstrate that the tube is in the mid trachea. Tube position can change during the X-ray procedure if the infant's neck is in a flexed or extended position. Endotracheal tube (ETT) position can be confirmed on X-ray by following both of the main stem bronchi back to the carina and cephalad to the tip of the tube.[1] Occasionally a lateral radiograph is necessary to confirm placement in the trachea. Only one study has been conducted to compare differences in outcomes related to radiographic placement of the ETT.[40] They concluded that the ETT tip should be kept at the level of the first or second thoracic vertebrae in extremely premature babies to reduce the incidence of nonuniform lung aeration and adverse pulmonary outcomes.

Tube Fixation

Secure fixation of the ETT is important, not only to prevent accidental extubation but also to minimize tube movement during ventilation and other interventions such as suctioning, chest physiotherapy (CPT), surfactant administration, and positioning the patient. An insecure fixation of the tube is one of the most common reasons accidental extubation can occur. Accidental extubation and repeated intubations have been demonstrated to be associated with the development of subglottic stenosis, as well as increased mortality.[24,25] The likelihood of accidental extubation also has been associated with younger gestational age, higher level of consciousness, higher

Labels on figure:
- 12-cm marker
- 3.5 I.D.
- Vocal cord guide marker
- "Eye"

volume of secretions, and slippage of the tube.[25] It also is clear that there is no consensus as to which tube fixation method is most effective. The technique shown in Figure 27-2 represents a modification of the method originally described by Gregory.[41] Another approach that was initially described by Cussel et al.[42] is to secure an umbilical clamp with a drilled hole in the center with tape to the face. Several modifications have been described using this technique. Compared with standard taping to the upper lip, methods using a modified umbilical clamp have been shown to substantially reduce unplanned or accidental extubation in neonatal patients (Fig. 27-3 and Table 27-4).[43]

Other studies have compared standard taping to approved commercially available fixation devices, and the ETT location was shown to be directly attributable to the type of fixation being used.[44] Another important development is that tincture of benzoin is no longer used, especially in extremely low birth-weight infants (micropreemies). Also, some of these techniques can be used to secure nasotracheal tubes (Fig. 27-4) without the use of tincture of benzoin. Several devices for fixation of neonatal ETTs and adhesive materials are available from various manufacturers. (See also discussion in Chapter 7.)

Acquisition and Maintenance of Intubation Skills

Intubation of the trachea is a complex psychomotor skill taught to a variety of health care professionals. Although ventilation can be accomplished successfully using a bag and mask, there are many instances in which neonatal tracheal intubation is required. The challenge is maintaining a high skill level for a procedure that may be performed only sporadically by individual providers.

Depending on the clinical setting, intubation skill may be required of attending physicians, residents, nurses, respiratory therapists, and paramedics. Institutional or departmental policies may require or expect that certain individuals be proficient at intubation yet may be unable to provide opportunities to maintain proficiency. The challenge is that, without regular practice, individual intubation skill level decreases over time,[45] and the complications from an unskilled intubation may be severe.[46,47]

Initial training in intubation often occurs in a clinical skills lab using plastic manikins made specifically for the purpose of intubation. This is typically the first exposure to the skill of intubation for medical students as well as for other disciplines. Courses such as the Neonatal Resuscitation Program and the Pediatric Advanced Life Support course include intubation education, practice, and testing on a manikin. The fact that students are "tested" on their ability to intubate a plastic manikin airway model may lead some to think that they are now "proficient." It is important to emphasize that such courses provide only limited exposure to the intubation skill and that the ability to intubate a plastic manikin does not immediately translate to the bedside. However, improvements in the manikin, especially the anatomy and "feel" of the airway, have made this simulation experience more readily transferable to actual clinical situations.

Studies have shown that, over time, cognitive knowledge remains but the actual hands-on skill level declines[48] and that ongoing review and proctored skills practice are needed to maintain a level of proficiency.[49] A 10-year study of neonatal intubations performed by pediatric residents at one institution showed that median success rates varied from 33% for PL 1 residents to 40% for PL 2 and PL 3 residents. Success rates for residents with greater than 20 intubation attempts

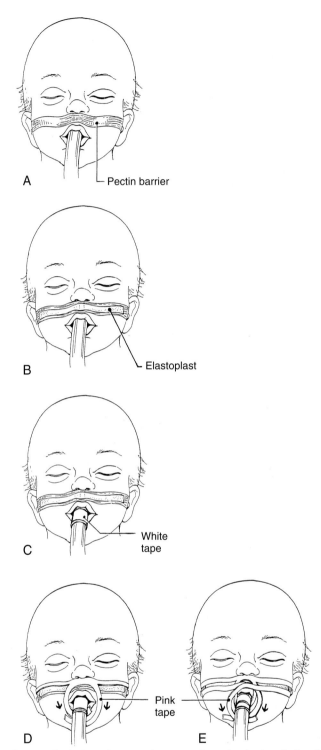

FIG 27-2 Technique for securing an endotracheal tube. **A,** Pectin barrier is applied to the infant's face from ear to ear and over the upper lip. **B,** A ¼-inch-wide elastic bandage (Elastoplast) is applied over the pectin barrier. **C,** A short strip of cloth tape or elastic bandage is wrapped around the tracheal tube to mark its point of passage at the mouth. The centimeter marking under the tape should be charted. **D,** Pink tape cut in the shape of an H is applied over the elastic bandage, with its ends extending beyond the bandage. The lower arms of the H are then wrapped around the tube. **E,** Single, ¼-inch strips of pink tape are secured over the lower part of the elastic bandage and wrapped around the tube. As an alternative to using an H-shaped piece of tape, the entire taping procedure can be done with a series of single strips of tape.

was 49%, whereas those residents with fewer than 20 attempts had a 37% success rate.[50] These same pediatric residents may go on to take positions in which they are expected to and need to have intubation proficiency, yet the study showed that they did not have the opportunity during their training to achieve a high level of success at the procedure. Another study found that, although pediatric residents stated that they felt confident with neonatal intubation skills, objective findings showed that they did not meet the study-specified definition of technical competence.[51]

Neonatal and pediatric transport teams typically use a combination of registered nurses, respiratory therapists, paramedics, and physicians, and there are many teams that run primarily as nurse–therapist or nurse–paramedic. Because team members are expected to perform advanced level skills, team training generally includes skills such as intubation, umbilical line, and needle aspiration/chest tube insertion. In addition to a didactic and skills practice orientation, transport team members should attend regular update and competency sessions. Experts recommend that team members perform a minimum number of transports to maintain skills and, if the number of transports is low, there be other mechanisms to simulate transport team function.[52]

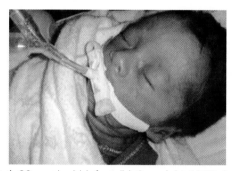

FIG 27-3 A 32-week-old infant (birth weight 1840 g) with cord clamp in place. (From Loughead JL, Brennan RA, DeJuilio P, Camposeo V, Wengert J, Cooke D. Reducing accidental extubation in neonates. *Jt Comm J Qual Patient Saf*. 2008 March; 34(3):164-170, 125.)

TABLE 27-4 **Using a Modified Umbilical Clamp**
1. Umbilical cord clamps are converted into ETT stabilizers by drilling holes through their center such that when closed they will snugly accommodate ETTs of 2.5-, 3.0-, 3.5-, 4.0-, and 4.5-mm inside diameters.
2. The clamps are opened, cleaned, individually packaged, and marked with size.
3. With the infant orally intubated, the clamp is secured around the ETT just above the lip with the ETT fitting within the predrilled hole. The clamp fits snugly but does not narrow the internal diameter of the ETT.
4. Skin barrier is applied to the infant's clean buccal surfaces bilaterally.
5. Adhesive tape is applied over the skin barrier and the tube is secured using the Y-tape method. The base portion of the Y tape is secured to the face, and the top arms are wrapped one around the ETT and one around the clamp. The second Y tape is applied in a mirror fashion to the other cheek.
6. Appropriate placement of the clamp allows the child to fully close lips and mouth.
7. NICU RNs and RCPs are accountable for assessing ETT placement and stability with every vitals check, position change, and suction and as needed. Repositioning and/or retaping of the ETT occurs as needed and is performed with two caregivers to minimize accidental dislodgment during the procedure. During retaping, the clamp and ETT remain in place and only the tape and skin barrier are replaced. Tape reinforcement is discouraged.

ETT, endotracheal tube; *NICU*, neonatal intensive care unit; *RNs*, registered nurses; *RCPs*, respiratory care practitioners.
Data from Loughead JL, Brennan RA, DeJuilio P, Camposeo V, Wengert J, Cooke D. Reducing accidental extubation in neonates. *Jt Comm J Qual Patient Saf* 34(3): 164-170, 125, 2008.

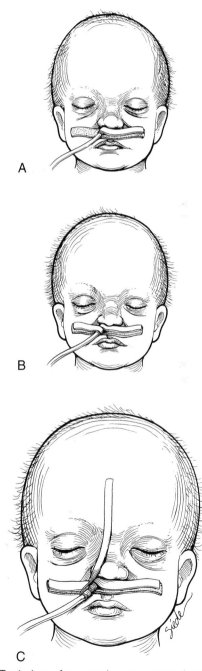

FIG 27-4 Technique for securing a nasotracheal tube. **A,** A ¼-inch strip of elastic bandage is applied over the upper lip, and a ¼-inch strip of Hy-Tape (*pink*) is applied from the right side of the face and around the tube. **B,** A second piece of tape is applied from the left side of the face and around the tube. **C,** A third piece of tape is applied down the bridge of the nose and around the tube.

Since 1990 there have been many changes related to the indications for intubation of the neonate. Historically, all newly born infants with meconium staining of the amniotic fluid require intubation and suctioning. The latest Neonatal Resuscitation Program (NRP) recommendations call for intubating only those infants with meconium staining who are not vigorous. Newer oxygen delivery methods, such as high-flow nasal cannula and nasal CPAP, allow more infants to be cared for without the need for intubation. Ready availability of high-risk perinatal units and NICUs ensures that more critically ill neonates are born at a center with high-level skills. All of these advances are good for the neonate, but they have unfortunately resulted in a decreased number of intubations available for pediatric residents and other practitioners, necessitating alternate methods to ensure that competence in airway management is maintained.

Health care educators need to be creative in providing the initial intubation education and also in monitoring and facilitating the continuing education of those individuals expected to respond to a neonatal emergency. A blended learning approach can integrate online learning with supervised manikin practice. Although expensive, animal intubations (usually cats) can provide an excellent practice model but must be done adhering to the NIH Office of Animal Care and Use guidelines. The airline industry has long been using simulators for initial training and for continuing education and competency evaluation. The simulator manikin setup is expensive but provides an excellent learning model that functions in real time. Patient simulations are generally enjoyed by students (generic and professional) and are perceived by the students to be of benefit.[53,54] The newest neonatal simulator manikins, although expensive, provide an excellent resource for this training.

Looking to the future, educators should consider the use of virtual reality simulation. Virtual reality simulators are available to teach trauma assessment and skills and also diagnostic bronchoscopy. In one study the virtual reality bronchoscopy simulator was used to train new students in doing a diagnostic bronchoscopy. With minimal time practicing on the simulator, the new students were able to attain a level of proficiency similar to that of more experienced bronchoscopists.[55] Virtual reality simulation can be used for initial education and practice and at regular intervals to reinforce skills.

Laryngeal Mask Airway

The laryngeal mask airway (LMA) has been available for a number of years as an alternative to endotracheal intubation in babies, infants, children, and adults.[1] It is mentioned but not recommended for routine use in the new NRP textbook,[1] and a variety of papers discuss its use in various clinical scenarios, including the following:

- In neonatal resuscitation of term and larger preterm infants (size 1 LMA)
- In the difficult airway, such as in the Robin sequence, and other situations when micrognathia is profound
- As an aid to endotracheal intubation
- As an aid in flexible endoscopy
- In surgical cases in place of endotracheal intubation[56-59]

The success rate of insertion of the LMA has been reported to be greater than 90% in a number of descriptive studies of small series of infants and children[60] (see Chapter 4 for further discussion of LMA use).

NONINVASIVE VENTILATION AND CONTINUOUS POSITIVE AIRWAY PRESSURE

Avoiding ventilator-induced lung injury is a common goal of neonatal intensive care and has led to considerable interest in less invasive means of providing effective respiratory support. Neonates who might require respiratory support short of intubation and mechanical ventilation include those with apnea of prematurity, mild to moderate RDS, and atelectasis caused by respiratory insufficiency, as well as recently extubated infants at risk for postextubation respiratory failure. Nasal CPAP has traditionally been a widely used support modality in these infants. It has the advantage of being well studied and is known to improve pulmonary mechanics and to stabilize the upper airway.[61] The use of CPAP and noninvasive ventilation is discussed in more detail in Chapter 17.

HEATED HUMIDIFIED HIGH-FLOW NASAL CANNULA

Humidified high-flow nasal cannula (HHFNC) devices have come into widespread use in NICUs. These devices differ from traditional nasal cannula therapy in that the gas flow to the patient is warmed and humidified up to the point of patient contact, allowing the use of higher gas flows without causing nasal drying, mucosal trauma, and patient cooling. Gas flow rates used in neonatal HHFNC therapy may range between 2 and 8 L/min. The higher gas flows that can be attained with HHFNC have led many to view this therapy as a viable alternative to nasal CPAP that is less bulky and easier to maintain.

The level and consistency of CPAP that can be attained with HHFNC have been examined in several small case series reports, with variable results.[62-65] There is general agreement that HHFNC can produce a clinically significant level of CPAP, particularly at higher flow rates. However, several variables appear to play an important role in determining the level of CPAP attained, including patient size,[62] cannula diameter,[66] and whether the mouth is open or closed.[62] In some instances, particularly when the nasal cannula completely occludes the nares, dangerously high levels of CPAP may be produced.[66] It should be noted that, unlike nasal CPAP devices, HHFNC devices at this time do not incorporate a safety pop-off valve in their design, raising the possibility that very high pressures could be transmitted to the lungs. Until better safety and efficacy data are available, HHFNC should be used with caution and not be viewed as a substitute for nasal CPAP devices.

MONITORING DURING RESPIRATORY SUPPORT

Monitoring during Noninvasive Respiratory Support

Infants are supported with noninvasive respiratory support using nasal CPAP (NCPAP) or NIV to prevent intubation or following weaning and extubation from invasive support. Such patients may require more attention at the bedside than a patient who is being ventilated invasively. Patients receiving this form of support do not have accurate or reliable mechanics or tidal volume measurements. Also, many of these devices are limited by a lack of alarms. As such, ongoing assessment, gas exchange, and evaluation of work of breathing are vital to the management and success of this form of support. Patients receiving noninvasive approaches can be instrumented with physiologic monitoring to include SpO_2, transcutaneous CO_2, heart rate, and blood pressure. Routine blood gases are not frequently obtained and are reserved for situations in which the patient has developed clinical deterioration and for correlating values with noninvasive monitoring. Chest X-rays are a poor surrogate for determining lung volumes during noninvasive support. Unfortunately, there are no approved devices for monitoring inspiratory and end-expiratory lung volumes. Novel technology using electrical impedance tomography may prove to be useful once it has been developed for newborns. Because of the lack of physiologic monitoring, many institutions have embraced respiratory scoring tools (i.e., Silverman–Anderson Respiratory Severity Score) to guide clinical management. These scores have been shown to have good interrater reliability among clinicians and can be useful for determining when the patient requires support or ongoing settings adjustments and for weaning.

Airway management is a time-consuming endeavor but perhaps the single most important aspect for improving outcomes and reducing complications in infants receiving noninvasive support. This detailed approach is more art than science, and the increased use of noninvasive support since 2005 has provided new experience that is summarized in some excellent resources.[67,68] Many neonates are being supported for weeks and sometimes months with this support. Briefly, clinicians caring for infants receiving CPAP should select prongs of the optimal size and ensure that the prongs are not displaced. Prongs that are too small increase the resistance to gas flow and work of breathing and are associated with excessive leaks. An optimally sized prong fills the entire opening without blanching the external nostril. The infant's nostrils should be suctioned periodically, and the nasal airway evaluated for skin breakdown. There are many approaches that are used to prevent nasal breakdown, including (1) alternating between nasal prongs and mask, (2) nasal barrier devices, and (3) nasal airway interfaces/fixation that are less likely to cause sustained pressure on the nasal airway.

As mentioned previously, many noninvasive devices do not provide clinical monitoring of pressure or alarms. Disconnection of the patient from the device (e.g., dislodged prongs) may not result in an alarm to indicate low pressure. Two such devices, bubble NCPAP and HHFNC, do not have integrated alarms as a standard system component. Thus, it is important to provide continuous physiologic monitoring. In a bench model, condensation forming in the expiratory limb of a commercially available bubble NCPAP system resulted in substantially higher CPAP levels than desired.[69] Whenever possible, stand-alone pressure manometers, alarms, and pressure-relief devices should be used. Also, bedside clinicians must provide measures to frequently empty the exhalation limb of condensate, provide water traps, or use circuits that incorporate heated wires or are constructed from material that wicks moisture to the environment.

Monitoring during Conventional and High-Frequency Ventilation

Electrocardiography, blood pressure, and serial arterial and/or capillary blood gases have been the traditional mainstays of bedside monitoring of the newborn, and they still have an important role. In general, the emphasis on noninvasive monitoring has resulted in the development and availability of new technologies that allow close monitoring without invasive procedures. The following is a list of those instruments:

- Transcutaneous monitoring of Po_2 and Pco_2
- Pulse oximetry to provide continuous measurement of hemoglobin saturation with O_2
- End-tidal CO_2 monitoring

See Chapters 7 and 17 for a more in-depth discussion of these noninvasive monitoring techniques.

Nearly all of the neonatal mechanical ventilators that are currently available provide airway graphics monitoring. A complete understanding of airway graphics can be vital for determining response to different therapies (i.e., surfactant and bronchodilators), clinical improvement and deterioration, equipment malfunction, and appropriate setting changes. In the NICU, there is also the additional difficulty of dealing with ETTs that are uncuffed, leading to large positional leaks around the ETT, which can lead to autocycling and missed trigger attempts by the patient. Assessing airway graphics can be useful, in cases such as these, for providing improved patient comfort. Airway graphics and tidal volume monitoring are best accomplished using a proximal flow sensor in neonates. Tidal volume monitoring and targeting have steadily become a widely accepted practice in most NICUs. Seminal animal studies have shown that ventilation for 15 minutes with a volume of 15 mL/kg has been shown to cause lung injury and as few as three overdistending breaths at birth have been shown to compromise the therapeutic effect of subsequent surfactant replacement.[70-72] Conversely, small or inadequate volumes can also cause lung injury.[73,74] Tidal volume is also an important measurement in volume-targeted ventilation. Compared with pressure ventilation, volume-targeted ventilation has been shown to reduce pneumothorax, days of ventilation, hypocarbia, periventricular leukomalacia or grade 3-4 intraventricular hemorrhage, and combined outcome of death/BPD. Monitoring expiratory volumes at the level of the ventilator valves may overestimate tidal volume delivery and reduce the accuracy of airway graphics, despite attempts to adjust for circuit tubing compliance with the ventilator.[75] Proximal flow sensors are prone to accumulating secretions, malfunctioning, creating torque on the ETT, and adding mechanical dead space. The benefit of a flow sensor outweighs all of these risks. Flow sensors may not accurately predict the delivered volumes when tube leaks are present but measured expiratory volume is usually more accurate than inspiratory tidal volumes for predicting the delivered volume in these cases. Appropriate bedside maintenance of flow sensors, calibration, and standardized cleaning procedures are important clinical quality measures.

For infants on high-frequency ventilation (HFV), pulmonary care involves new technology and keen observation.[76,77] These critically ill babies require a definite team approach, including an experienced respiratory therapist and nurse, and the traditional tools, including cardiorespiratory monitoring, intermittent arterial blood gases (from an arterial line), and "wiggle" assessment. A sample of a protocol used in the infant special care unit at one institution includes the following:

Assessments every hour:
- Vital signs from monitors, including heart rate, arterial blood pressure, body temperature
- Vibration (or wiggle) assessment (scale +1 to +3)
- Capillary refill
- Comfort level
  Assessments every 4 hours—"hands-on assessment":
- Auscultation of breath sounds on oscillator
- Palpation of pulses
- Nasogastric tube placement can be assessed without having to take the baby off of the ventilator

Assessments every 8 hours—ventilator is turned off but the patient remains on the circuit or backup rate (high-frequency jet ventilation):

- Heart rate, position of point of maximum intensity of heart, presence or absence of a heart murmur
- Bowel sounds
  Other assessments:
- Arterial blood gases after initiation of HFV: hourly for 6 hours, every 2 hours for 6 hours, and every 4 hours and as needed thereafter
- Tidal volumes (when available)
- Chest radiograph schedule: just prior to being placed on HFV, within 1 hour of initiation of HFV, every 12 hours twice, and then daily and as needed
  - Continuous monitoring of oxygen saturation using the pulse oximeter

HUMIDIFICATION AND WARMING DURING RESPIRATORY SUPPORT

The ETT bypasses the normal humidifying, filtering, and warming systems of the upper airway; therefore, heat and humidity must be provided to prevent hypothermia, inspissation of airway secretions, and necrosis of airway mucosa. Filtration of dry gases before humidification also is needed because of the contamination sometimes found in medical gas lines.

Assuming all other forms of infant warming are provided, ventilation with nonhumidified gases is a major reason for development of hypothermia[78] in neonates. Inadequate humidification of the respiratory tract may reduce mucociliary clearance and predispose infants to airway obstruction by secretions, thereby increasing the risk of gas trapping and air leak.[79] Also, dry gases have been associated with severe lung injury in animal models.[80] Higher inspired gas temperatures are associated with a lower incidence of pneumothorax and a decreased severity of chronic lung disease in ventilated very low birth-weight infants compared to lower temperatures.[79]

The use of heat–moisture exchangers, or artificial noses, in neonates should be discouraged because they have been shown to increase ventilation requirements, increase CO_2 levels, lower body temperature, and increase artificial airway blockage. They are particularly ineffective in the presence of large ETT leaks. In most cases, heat–moisture exchangers are reserved for short-term use, such as neonatal transport. A heated water humidifier is necessary to ensure that inspired gases are delivered at or near body temperature (37°C) and that they achieve near-total saturation with water vapor. In the past, nebulizers were used in some applications, particularly with oxygen administration with a hood after extubation. Use of this system has been discarded because of impairment in oxygenation and the possibility of water intoxication caused by excess delivery of particulate water droplets and because of the presence of excessive noise.

A modern servo-controlled heated humidifier, with high- and low-temperature alarms and heated wires that prevent accumulation of condensation, should provide adequate humidification with proper operation. O'Hagan et al.[81,82] observed wide variation in the delivery of relative humidity, even when the temperature was maintained above 34.7°C; this variation resulted in failure to meet the American National Standards Institute guidelines for humidifier performance.[83] This may account for the findings of O'Hagan et al.,[82] who observed a significant increase in morbidity when temperatures below 36.5°C were maintained at the airway. These studies have led to the recommendation that relative humidity, as well as temperature, be monitored continuously. Miyao et al.[84] suggest that even maintenance of the Institute's standards (70% humidity at 37°C) may be inadequate, particularly if heated wire circuits are used. Use of circuits with heated wires was adopted primarily because of the frequency with which condensation needed to be drained and because of infection control considerations. The heated wire circuits were intended to enable the clinician to heat the gas inside the circuit to a temperature above that at which it left the humidifier, ensuring adequate absolute humidity without condensation in the circuit. This feature, which results in delivery of a hot gas with a lower relative humidity, may have caused the problems noted earlier.[84]

The increased temperature of a gas shifts the isothermal boundary (the point at which the gas completes equilibrium to body temperature and humidity levels) to a point closer to the airway opening. At first glance, this seems beneficial because less mucosa is exposed to the humidity deficit of the gas. However, because the effect of a given humidity deficit is concentrated on a smaller area of the mucosa, there is the potential for a greater degree of damage. Moreover, use of higher airway temperatures means that, even with lower humidity, there is relatively less opportunity for humidified air from within the lung to recondense some of its humidity upon exhalation. The result is an increase in the humidity deficit (the difference in total water content of inspired gas and the water content it achieves within the lung). The potential for adverse effects with use of the heated wire circuit is exacerbated by inadequate monitoring of humidity levels. If the wire is so hot that the circuit is dry, it is not known whether the relative humidity is 70% (the nominally acceptable American National Standards Institute value) or less.[82]

Traditionally, probes for monitoring inspired gas have been placed as close as possible to the patient connection so that the effect of the trip down the inspiratory line on the inspired gas can be monitored. Unfortunately, in some neonatal circumstances, the probe is continuously in the presence of a heated field and may register the effect of this heat by radiation and/or convection, totally apart from the effect of the inspired gas. If this temperature is sensed by a servo controller, the humidifier and the heated wires may automatically heat less because the temperature is actually being controlled by another heat source (Fig. 27-5). An extension adapter, which is provided by most manufacturers, allows the probe to be placed outside of the heating field, thus remedying this problem. This extension does not need to incorporate heated wires because the gas temperature is maintained by the heated field on entry.

The use of inline water traps is recommended for decreasing the resistance to flow caused by condensate and for ensuring stability of oxygen concentrations. Novel materials have been used in the latest generation of infant ventilator circuits to minimize mobile condensate in the expiratory limb by allowing water vapor to diffuse through the tubing wall. In theory, these circuits may minimize alarms, excessive pressure and volume delivery to the infant, and work of breathing.

Ventilator-acquired pneumonia (VAP) and other respiratory infections can arise and are prevalent in neonates because of prolonged mechanical ventilation, frequent reintubation, low gestational age, and low birth weight.[85] VAP has been associated with higher mortality rates than in those unaffected by this disease. There is concern that the frequency at which

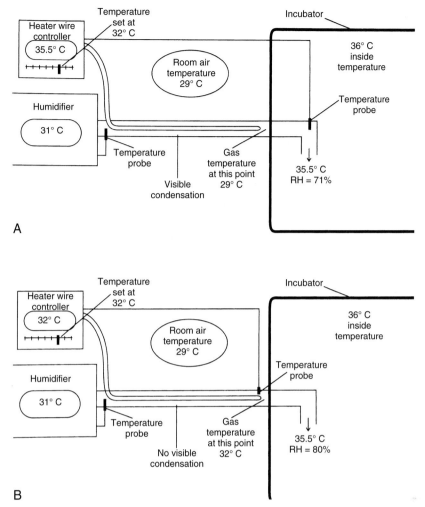

FIG 27-5 A, Temperature probe located inside a heated field tends to indicate a heat representative of the heated field rather than of the inspiratory gas before entry into the field. The humidifier does not provide the heat that is being detected by the wire controller. The heat source is particularly difficult to assess because most heated wire circuits operate with humidifiers that do not provide a display of the temperature of the gas immediately after it leaves the humidifier. **B,** Proper placement of the probe. If the probe is only slightly outside a radiant warmer field, it may need to be shielded, particularly if phototherapy is in use. *RH,* relative humidity. (From Chatburn RL. Principles and practice of neonatal and pediatric mechanical ventilation. *Respir Care*. 1991;36:560.)

ventilator circuits and humidifiers are changed may affect the rate of VAP.[86] However, one study showed that there were no differences in VAP between a 7-day circuit change and a 14-day change.[85] Some sources suggest changing the patient circuit only when visibly soiled to avoid opening the circuit. Other attempts at reducing VAP include changing manual resuscitators once per week, changing equipment on stand-by every 12 hours, elevating the head of the bed, and draining circuit fluid frequently.

AIRWAY CLEARANCE TECHNIQUES

Patients who have an ETT are predisposed to damage to the airway lining, weak or ineffective cough, and improper humidification of the airways. This can result in accumulated secretions in the airways and consequent gas trapping, air leak, and poor gas exchange. Based on two extensive literature reviews, "successful suctioning of an intubated patient improves air exchange and breath sounds, decreases the peak inspiratory pressure, decreases airway resistance, increases compliance, increases tidal volume delivery, improves arterial blood gas values, improves oxygen saturation, and removes secretions."[87,88]

There are significant risks to endotracheal suctioning, including atelectasis and loss of lung volume due to high negative suction pressures,[89-92] hypoxemia,[93-95] cardiovascular instability,[96,97] and changes in cerebrovascular volume.

One study showed that ETT suctioning significantly increases intracranial pressure in preterm infants on assisted ventilation in the first month of life. These changes appear to be independent of changes observed in oxygenation and ventilation.[98,99] ETT suctioning has been found to be a risk factor for VAP in ventilated infants.[100]

Use of a closed "inline" suctioning system has been promoted to decrease respiratory contamination and pulmonary infections. Inline suction systems use a suction catheter integrated into the patient circuit using a specialized adapter, and the catheter is protected with a transparent sleeve. Closed suction is perceived by nursing staff to be easier, less time consuming, and better tolerated by patients. The suction depth is determined by the length of the tube, the adapter, and the preferred suction depth using colored markings that can be visualized in a small window. Deep suctioning should be avoided, and attempts should be made to remove secretions from within the tube and slightly beyond (~0.5 cm). Visual bedside charts, like the one used at the authors' center (Fig. 27-6), can be useful for guiding proper suction depths using inline or closed suction devices.

Disadvantages of these systems include increased expense and potential increase in system air leaks. Also, the catheter or portion of the catheter can be left in the airway accidentally, causing airway obstruction.

Closed suction obviates the physiological disadvantage of ventilator disconnection. In one study, a total of 39% of infants in the supported with closed suction devices group and 44% of infants in the disconnected from the ventilator to use and open airway suction technique group had significant differences in airways colonized with gram-negative bacilli. Also, closed suction is perceived by nursing staff to be easier, less time consuming, and better tolerated by small premature infants requiring mechanical ventilation for a week or longer.

Depending on the severity of lung disease, ETT suction may cause transient loss of lung volumes throughout the lung. It has been suggested that the lowest possible suction pressure that adequately removes secretions from the tube should be used. Suction pressures of 50 to 100 cm H_2O have been shown to be safe and effective in neonates, and suction time should not exceed 10 to 15 seconds.[88] The number of catheter passes should be minimized to <3 to avoid irritation to the airway mucosa.[101]

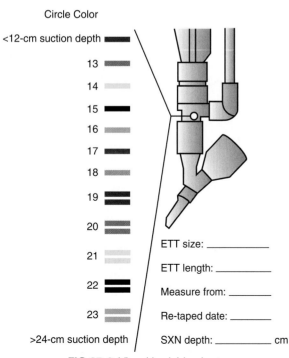

Circle Color

<12-cm suction depth

13
14
15
16
17
18
19
20
21
22
23

>24-cm suction depth

ETT size: _____

ETT length: _____

Measure from: _____

Re-taped date: _____

SXN depth: _____ cm

FIG 27-6 Visual bedside chart.

The patient should also be allowed to recover between each catheter pass.

One study investigated whether closed endotracheal suctioning reduces the frequency of hypoxemia and bradycardia in extremely low birth-weight neonates compared to open suctioning. There were no differences in heart rate between the two treatment strategies. The magnitude and frequency of hypoxemic events were lower with the closed suction than with the open suction technique.[102] Despite significant derecruitment with ETT suction, there was rapid recovery resulting in an increase in end-expiratory lung volume immediately after suction. The lung volume remained increased for the next 2 hours, suggesting that the benefit of suction persists much longer than many of the previous studies have described.[103]

ETT suction causes transient loss of lung volume. Catheter size exerts a greater influence than suction method, with closed suction protecting against derecruitment only when a small catheter is used, especially in the nondependent lung.[104]

Routine endotracheal suctioning with an open system has increasingly become less desirable not only for infection control purposes but also because intermittent manual ventilation is needed. As mentioned previously, this practice is typically associated with variable tidal volume ventilation. Removing a patient from the ventilator and initiating hyperinflation and hyperoxygenation with 100% FiO_2 may produce oxygen free radicals and may be associated with the development of retinopathy of prematurity and lung injury. Preoxygenation has been shown to result in less hypoxemia and faster return to baseline oxygenation prior to suction than no preoxygenation.[105] The latest guidelines suggest that the FiO_2 is adjusted to 10% to 20% above the current FiO_2 on the ventilator. Many ventilators have a suction key that can be configured to deliver a preset FiO_2 for oxygenation prior to suctioning. Manual ventilation with excessive tidal volumes can also initiate lung injury in the developing lung. Also, removing the patient from the ventilator can cause clinical destabilization and introduce bacteria into the circuit, placing infants at greater risk for developing ventilator-acquired infections. The use of manual resuscitation and sigh breaths should be avoided whenever necessary in neonates.

Suctioning should be performed by experienced personnel because complications from the trauma of this procedure may lead to hypoxemia,[106-108] cardiovascular compromise, barotrauma, and intraventricular hemorrhage. The frequency of ETT suctioning of infants ventilated in the NICU has been widely debated. One study showed that a low-frequency suctioning regimen (every 8 hours plus as needed) and a higher frequency suctioning regimen (every 4 hours plus as needed) were associated with similar frequencies of nosocomial bloodstream infections, VAP, bacterial airway colonization, frequency of reintubation, need for postural drainage, severity of BPD, neonatal mortality, duration of mechanical ventilation, and duration of hospitalization.[109]

The interval should be individualized and documented at the bedside; an example of a suctioning regimen is illustrated in Figure 27-7. Following are a few suggestions on how to optimize benefits and prevent complications (Table 27-5).

Many clinicians will use bulb suction during deliveries or to suction the upper airway prior to endotracheal suctioning. There is evidence that suggests that most bulb suction devices will not provide pressures <100 mm Hg. Excessive pressure may be damaging to the sensitive oral mucosa of the infant's upper airway.

The once routine practice of instilling normal saline prior to endotracheal suctioning is now discouraged. With the present focus on VAP, studies that have shown a marked increase in the number of bacteria present in the lower airway after normal saline administration versus no normal saline have forced nurses and respiratory therapists to reevaluate suction procedures (see Chapter 24).[110]

An American Association of Respiratory Care guideline has provided excellent information for suctioning and may be useful to optimize benefits and prevent complications during suctioning of a ventilated patient:[87]

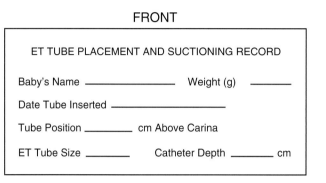

FRONT

ET TUBE PLACEMENT AND SUCTIONING RECORD

Baby's Name _____   Weight (g) _____

Date Tube Inserted _____

Tube Position _____ cm Above Carina

ET Tube Size _____   Catheter Depth _____ cm

BACK

INTERTECH / OHIO

TUBE SIZE	CUT (cm)	CATHETER DEPTH (cm)
2.5	11	14.5
3.0	13	17.0
3.5	13	17.0
4.0	14	18.0

FIG 27-7 Bedside "suction card" with values to be reverified after every chest radiograph has been obtained. Values are based on tube position relative to the carina. Suction depth must be reduced if the tip is not 2 cm above the carina. The table on the back of the card allows compensation for the extra length of the endotracheal tube's 15-mm adapter.

(1) Endotracheal suctioning should be performed only when secretions are present and not routinely.

(2) Preoxygenation should be considered if the patient has a clinically important reduction in oxygen saturation with suctioning.

(3) Performing suctioning without disconnecting the patient from the ventilator is suggested.

(4) Use of shallow suction is suggested instead of deep suction, based on evidence from infant and pediatric studies.

(5) Routine use of normal saline instillation prior to endotracheal suction should not be performed.

(6) Endotracheal suctioning without disconnection (closed system) is suggested for neonates.

(7) It is suggested that a suction catheter that occludes less than 70% of the lumen of the ETT is used.

(8) The duration of the suctioning event is limited to less than 15 seconds.

Other guidelines that may be useful include (1) providing the proper equipment; (2) awareness of FiO_2 settings and ventilator parameters; (3) performing noninvasive monitoring of oxygenation before, during, and after suctioning; (4) having the proper suction catheter size; and (5) using normal saline for irrigation, 0.1 to 0.5 mL/kg ONLY if secretions are deemed to be thick and tenacious upon assessment (see Tables 27-1 and 27-2 and Figs. 27-7 and 27-8).

Many hospitals have embraced practices to prevent VAP (called "bundles") such as (1) strict hand hygiene, (2) limited circuit breaks, (3) inline suction, (4) palate protectors, (5) circuit changes for new equipment, (6) weaning protocols, (7) taping and confirmation of tube placement, and (8) scheduled oral care. These strategies have been shown to reduce VAP rates, need for reintubations, and length of hospital stay[111] as well as having substantial cost savings.[112]

Chest Physiotherapy

CPT is a common but controversial airway clearance technique for infants in the NICU. Generally, appropriate indications for CPT include (1) evidence of retained pulmonary secretions, (2) weak or ineffective cough, (3) focal lung opacity on chest X-ray consistent with mucous plugging and/or atelectasis, and (4) intrapulmonary shunt requiring oxygen. CPT involving

TABLE 27-5	**Endotracheal Suctioning in Newborn Infants**		
	Hodge	**Hagedorn et al.**	**Fletcher and MacDonald**
Irrigation solution	Saline, but not routinely	Saline	Saline
Amount for irrigation	0.1-0.2 mL/kg	0.25-0.5 mL	Not specified
Catheter size	0.5-0.66 of tube diameter	Not specified	0.5 of tube diameter
Depth of insertion	Length of tube only	Length of tube only	1 cm beyond tip of tube
Hyperinflation	PIP 10%-20% above baseline	Match PIP	PIP or PIP plus up to 10 cm H_2O
Hyperventilation	Equal to total respiratory rate	Equal to ventilatory rate	Rate 40-60 breaths/min with long inspiratory time
Oxygen enhancement	10%-20% above baseline	If clinically indicated	10% above baseline
Suction pressure	50-80 cm H_2O	80-100 mm Hg	"Lowest possible"
Duration	Not specified	5-10 s	15-20 s disconnect time
Intermittent vs continuous	Not addressed	Continuous on withdrawal	Not addressed
Head turn	No	No	Turn head for selective bronchial suction

PIP, peak inspiratory pressure.
Data from Hodge D. Endotracheal suctioning and the infant: A nursing care protocol to decrease complications. *Neonat Network* 9:7, 1991; Hagedorn MI, Gardner SL, Abman SH: Respiratory diseases. In: Merenstein GB, Gardner SL, eds. *Handbook of Neonatal Intensive Care.* St. Louis, CV Mosby, 1989, 381; Fletcher MA, MacDonald MG. *Atlas of Procedures in Neonatology.* 2nd ed. Philadelphia, JB Lippincott, 1993, 292.

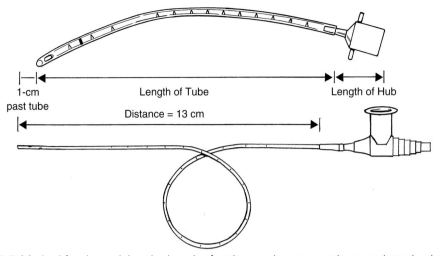

FIG 27-8 Method for determining the length of catheter advancement in an endotracheal tube. Knowledge of the placement of the tube and of the length of the tube can be applied to the use of a calibrated suction catheter for providing consistent catheter advancement to a level 1 cm above the carina.

postural drainage in concert with percussion or vibration has been shown to be beneficial in removing secretions and preventing atelectasis in recently extubated neonates.[113] It also has been shown to result in removal of more secretions from intubated neonates.[114] Furthermore, oxygenation has been shown to be enhanced after completion of CPT.[113] The benefit of this procedure may lie in the periodic redistribution of the gravity-dependent regions of the lung from positioning, rather than in the physical removal of secretions.

Two systematic reviews found no evidence from randomized controlled trials to support the use of CPT to improve oxygenation, reduce length of time on the ventilator, reduce stay in the ICU, resolve atelectasis/consolidation, and/or improve respiratory mechanics versus usual care.[115,116]

CPT was traditionally thought to assist in clearance of secretions in infants with bronchiolitis but according to a Cochrane meta-analysis, CPT did not improve the severity of the disease or the respiratory parameters or reduce the length of hospital stay or oxygen requirements in hospitalized infants with acute bronchiolitis not on mechanical ventilation.[117] It is unclear at this time whether there is a benefit in infants with other respiratory infections receiving mechanical ventilation.[118] Another review found that routine use of CPT in ventilated neonates does not improve outcomes and may induce hypoxemia and increase oxygen requirements.[119] Two separate studies compared short-term outcomes between neonates supported with CPT and those without CPT after extubation and found no differences in radiologic evidence of atelectasis.[120] While the benefit of such techniques remains in question, CPT does not go entirely without some risk to the patient. CPT has also been found to be poorly tolerated, with side effects such as esophageal reflux, tachypnea, tachycardia, hypoxemia, rib fracture, and severe central nervous system complications, especially in newborns.[121,122]

CPT use should be individualized in each baby because, as noted earlier, the use of these techniques has been associated with a variety of negative effects, especially in infants born weighing less than 1000 g. This group of extremely low birth-weight infants frequently is on a minimal stimulation plan of care for the first 3 to 5 days of extrauterine life, thus minimizing any pulmonary care interventions.[123] The paucity of airway secretions in this group of infants during this time has led some clinicians to suction only on an "as needed" basis or not at all.

Positioning of the Patient

Postural drainage involves the use of different positions in which the different main stem bronchi are positioned vertically so that drainage from the smaller bronchi moves into the larger bronchi (Figs. 27-9 to 27-16). The approach has been combined with CPT in the past. The two forces at work during this procedure are gravity and airflow. Any area of the bronchial tree that is to be drained (with the exception of the medial basal segment) must be uppermost.[124] These positions may not be practical for implementation in critically ill babies who have chest tubes or ETTs, who have undergone surgery, or who are at great risk for intraventricular hemorrhage. Optimally, the infant should be monitored during CPT; potential monitors include transcutaneous O_2 or CO_2 or pulse oximeter. Significant oxygen desaturation during the procedure should cause the caretaker to pause and initiate measures necessary to correct hypoxemia.

Percussion and Vibration

Two types of hand pressure can be applied to the neonatal chest to expedite adequate drainage: percussion and vibration. Percussion (chest physiotherapy) in the neonate can be performed with small plastic cups with padded rims or with soft circular masks with their adapters plugged so that the air pockets are maintained. The chest is percussed over the area to be drained for 1 to 2 minutes. Percussion may be reserved for infants who weigh more than 1500 g and are older than 2 weeks of age because of the potential risk for intraventricular hemorrhage.

The traditional view of vibration is that it is effective only during exhalation because it causes secretions to move from the periphery of the lungs with the outflow of air. This technique requires careful observation of chest movements. For vibration,

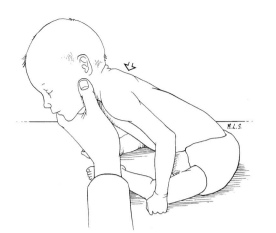

FIG 27-9 Drainage of the posterior segments of the upper lobe. The infant is leaned over at a 30-degree angle from the sitting position. The clinician claps and vibrates over the upper back on both sides.

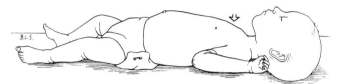

FIG 27-10 Drainage of the anterior segments of the upper lobe. While the infant is lying flat on his or her back, the clinician claps and vibrates between the nipples and the clavicle on both sides.

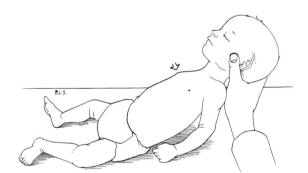

FIG 27-11 Drainage of the apical segment of the upper lobe. The infant is leaned backward about 30 degrees from the sitting position, and the clinician claps or vibrates above the clavicle on both sides.

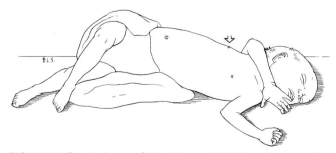

FIG 27-12 For drainage of the right middle lobe, the caregiver elevates the hips to about 5 inches above the head. He or she rolls the infant backward one-quarter turn and then claps and vibrates over the right nipple. For drainage of the lingular segments of the left upper lobe, the caregiver places the infant in the same position but with the left side lifted upward; he or she then claps and vibrates over the left nipple.

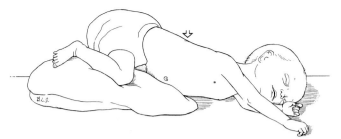

FIG 27-13 Drainage of the lateral basal segments of the lower lobes. The caregiver places the infant on the left side with the hips elevated to a level about 8 inches above that of the head. The caregiver rolls the infant forward one-quarter turn and then claps or vibrates over the lower ribs. Note that the position shown is for draining the right side. For draining the left side, the same procedure is followed, except that the infant is placed on his or her right side.

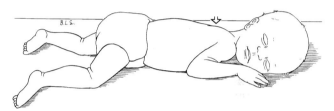

FIG 27-14 Drainage of the superior segments of the lower lobe. The clinician places the infant flat on the stomach and then claps or vibrates at top of the scapula on the back side of the spine.

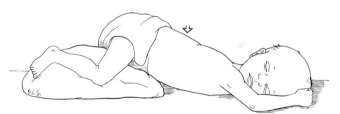

FIG 27-15 Drainage of the posterior basal segments of the lower lobe. The clinician places the infant on the stomach with the hips at a level 8 inches above that of the head. He or she then claps and vibrates over the lower ribs close to the spine on both sides.

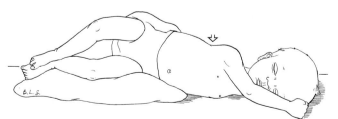

FIG 27-16 Drainage of the anterior basal segment of the lower lobes. The caregiver places the infant on the left side with the hips at a level about 8 inches above that of the head. He or she then claps and vibrates just beneath the axilla. Note that for drainage of the opposite anterior basal segment, the infant is turned on the right side.

the wrist is extended and the arm muscles are contracted in a manner similar to that used for isometric exercises. The result can be described as a controlled quiver. The placement of fingers flat against chest walls of infants suffices. A light touch with rapidly vibrating fingers has been considered effective in mobilizing secretions in neonates.[123] Because few practitioners feel comfortable with this manual technique, vibrations can be done with a small hand vibrator or a commercially available pulmonary vibrator. It is unclear whether gentle vibrations produced by these devices are transmitted to the lungs. Nonetheless, clinicians prefer them simply because they "soothe" the patient.

Vibration is tolerated by a greater number of patients than is percussion. The duration of vibration therapy is subject to the infant's tolerance and can be monitored on the basis of the parameters discussed previously.[123]

ADMINISTRATION OF MEDICATIONS INTO THE RESPIRATORY TRACT

Surfactant Treatment

Surfactant treatment of established RDS has been shown to decrease the incidence of air-leak complications and death.[124]

Intratracheal surfactant replacement therapy, administered via the ETT, has been an essential component of the prevention and treatment of RDS in premature infants since the early 1990s (also see Chapter 22). Multiple trials have compared prophylactic surfactant administration, usually given within the first 10 minutes of life in the delivery room, with later rescue treatment of established RDS in infants at substantial risk for the development of RDS. A meta-analysis of these trials demonstrated that prophylactic surfactant administration leads to significant reductions in the risk of air-leak complications and death.[125] More recent trials have further demonstrated that prophylactic surfactant administration reduces the incidence of RDS and length of time on mechanical ventilation compared to rescue treatment.[126] These benefits are most pronounced in those infants born at less than 30 weeks of gestation who have not been exposed to antenatal steroids.[127,128] Current recommendations from the American Academy of Pediatrics (AAP) Committee on the Fetus and Newborn suggest that prophylactic surfactant be considered for those premature infants at highest risk for RDS.[129] However, the use of prophylactic surfactant is quite variable in neonatal units across the country.[130] One reason for this variation in practice is widespread interest in early application of NCPAP, rather than prophylactic intubation and surfactant treatment, for the prevention and early treatment of RDS (see Chapter 8). Early NCPAP may have the potential to reduce the incidence of BPD without an increase in other morbidities.[16] However, a 2008 randomized, controlled trial demonstrated that early NCPAP, compared with early intubation, did not significantly reduce the rate of death or BPD.[17]

Surfactant Administration

This section addresses the technical aspects of surfactant administration, including dosage forms, amounts, and administration techniques. Other aspects of surfactant treatment are discussed in Chapter 22.

The surfactant pool size in lungs of healthy, full-term neonates is about 100 mg/kg.[131] Infants with RDS have a surfactant pool size that is approximately 10% of that seen in the healthy, full-term lung.[132] Surfactant doses for prevention or treatment of RDS are aimed at achieving a surfactant pool size comparable to that in the full-term lung while also allowing for some uneven distribution of exogenous surfactant and surfactant inactivation by protein exudates. Thus surfactant doses in the range of 50 to 200 mg/kg have been used in various clinical studies.[133] Currently available commercial surfactant preparations contain varying amounts of phospholipids, but the recommended dosage amounts give 100 to 200 mg/kg phospholipids per dose (Table 27-6). All currently available surfactant preparations are obtained by extraction from animal lungs and are available in a liquid form for intratracheal instillation, although a new, completely synthetic surfactant (lucinactant) has been tested in humans. Compared in clinical trials, lucinactant was found to have rates of mortality and morbidity similar to those of beractant and poractant alfa.[134] Differences in recommended dosage volume may lead the clinician to favor a particular surfactant preparation in certain clinical situations.

Surfactant replacement therapy should be performed only by clinicians who are proficient at administering surfactant and capable of handling adverse events. Recommended modes of surfactant administration are based on those used in research protocols, but there are limited human data comparing techniques of surfactant administration. Surfactant is generally administered through a small-bore catheter inserted into the ETT, although the Infasurf package insert suggests instillation through a side-port adapter.[135] Animal data suggest that administering surfactant by bolus or rapid intratracheal infusion results in more even distribution of surfactant than giving the surfactant by very slow continuous intratracheal infusion.[136] Surfactant doses are typically divided into two or four aliquots. In animal studies, distribution of intratracheally instilled surfactant has been largely determined by gravity and unaffected by the position of the chest.[137] As such, leaving the chest in a horizontal position may result in even distribution of surfactant to the lungs. Placing the infant in a reverse Trendelenburg position should be avoided to avoid increased intracranial pressures.

Tracheal suctioning should be avoided immediately following surfactant administration and as long as 6 hours if ventilation can be adequately maintained. Safe and effective administration and monitoring by the respiratory therapist or nurse at the bedside are critical to the success of surfactant administration in infants. Careful patient assessment and continuous monitoring of work of breathing, FiO_2, compliance, pulmonary airway

TABLE 27-6	Surfactant Preparations Data from Package Inserts			
		Phospholipid Content, mg/mL	RECOMMENDED DOSE (ML/KG)	
Surfactant	Source		Initial	Repeat
Infasurf	Calf lung	35	3	3
Survanta	Cow lung	25	4	4
Curosurf	Pork lung	80	2.5	1.25

graphics and tidal volumes with a proximal flow sensor, chest radiograph, and SpO$_2$ are useful for clinicians when responding to deterioration or improvement in the patient's condition.[138] These tools may provide important information for stopping therapy, weaning, and/or escalation of mechanical respiratory support and assessing the need for subsequent dosing.

Very limited data suggest that delivery of surfactant by nebulization might result in improved distribution of surfactant,[139] but this approach requires further study in humans. It was discovered that surfactant delivery could be accomplished sooner by nebulization in an LMA group, with efficacy equal to that of direct instillation with an ETT. While far from conclusive this method holds hope for areas in which ETT intubation skills are lacking.[140] Also, new research focused on minimizing invasive ventilation by injection of surfactant through the nasopharynx during delivery[141] or by using a thin catheter[142] may show promise in the future.

Optimization of Aerosol Drug Delivery

The common practice of administering aerosolized medications before bronchopulmonary hygiene and suctioning is based on custom more than scientifically verified practice. The pharmacology of drug action is discussed in Chapter 21.

Although delivery of aerosolized medication has a number of advantages over systemic dosing, recent information has helped in the design of a few reliable aerosol delivery systems (Boxes 27-4 and 27-5 and Table 27-7).[143] The basic fundamental characteristics of factors that influence neonatal aerosol delivery and deposition are listed in Box 27-4. These factors can be divided into two groups: host-related factors and aerosol system–related factors.[143] Box 27-5 lists the characteristics of "the ideal aerosol delivery system." Table 27-7 compares the advantages and disadvantages of the three most frequently used aerosol delivery systems: the pressurized metered-dose inhaler (pMDI) and the jet and ultrasonic nebulizers.[143] However, even with the progress being made in the design of aerosolized medication delivery systems, the clinician may need to test a variety of delivery devices and decide which system is most efficacious for each individual patient. The same may have to be done with the type and dose of aerosol medication[144,145] to establish a bronchodilator dose, that is, measuring a patient's response to a specific drug and dose using bedside pulmonary function methods detailed in Chapter 18 rather than using predetermined dose tables. Apart from bronchodilators, novel inhaled drugs are being delivered via the aerosolization pathway, including hypertonic saline, surfactant, pulmonary vasodilators, and antibiotics. It is important to understand the variables unique to the aerosol route that can affect the drug delivery device. The small internal diameter and high resistance of the neonatal ETT and humidity impair aerosol delivery in the intubated patient compared with the nonintubated patient. In studies with animals, humans, and bench models, from 0.19% to 2.14% of the total drug amount in the nebulizer cup was administered to the lung or lung model when conventional jet nebulizers were used[144,145] compared with 10% of the total dose that was shown to be deposited in the lungs of nonintubated patients.[146] There are several different approaches for delivering inhaled drugs to patients. A review of aerosol practices in infants reviews the safety and efficacy of these disparate practices.[147] Briefly, spontaneously breathing patients who receive blow-by, face mask, and infant hood treatments should receive the treatments using a nebulizer that uses a gas source to direct the aerosol to the infant's airway opening or a pMDI with a valved holding chamber. Vibrating mesh nebulizers should be used for drug delivery during HHFNC, CPAP, NIV, and invasive mechanical ventilation.

The greatest challenge with drug delivery in infants is getting the patient to tolerate a mask treatment. The mask should have low dead space and should be tightly fitted to the face. A crying infant receives substantially lower drug deposited in the lungs (<1%) and more on the face than one who is resting or sleeping (~5%).[148-150] Blow-by aerosol[151] therapy is accomplished using a gas-powered jet nebulizer placed within a reasonable distance from the patient, and the aerosol plume is directed toward the oral or nasal airway opening with an aerosol mask or T-piece. While this practice may result in less crying or distress, it has been shown to result in negligible drug delivery in patients and anatomically accurate lung/airway models (~0.3%).[150,152] Drug delivery using a jet nebulizer attached to a hood may be as effective as a face mask treatment and better tolerated by the patient.[153,154]

With currently available methods, the placement and operation of a nebulizer are important for maximizing drug delivery to the lung. The nebulizer should be placed in the inspiratory limb and proximal to the patient wye-piece (not directly between the ventilator Y and the ETT) during invasive infant ventilation. If using a gas-powered jet nebulizer with a time-cycled pressure-limited ventilator with a fixed flow, the operational flow used with the nebulizer should be adjusted from a blended gas source, and the ventilator flow should be reduced

---

BOX 27-4 Overview of Factors That Influence Neonatal Aerosol Delivery and Deposition

Host-Related Factors
- Anatomic (nasal breathing, size of oropharynx, airways, lung development)
- Physiologic (breathing pattern, inspiratory flow rate, tidal volume, pulmonary mechanics)
- Pathophysiologic (inflammation, mucus, atelectasis, fibrosis)

Aerosol System–Related Factors
- Characteristics of the medication (particle size, shape, density, output)
- Generator (pressurized metered-dose inhaler [pMDI] or nebulizer)
- Delivery devices–patient interfaces (face mask or endotracheal tube)
- Conditions (ventilatory, environmental)
- Provider technique (optimum use of pMDI with spacer)

Data from Cole C. The use of aerosolized medicines in neonates. *Neonat Respir Dis* 10:4, 2000.

BOX 27-5 The Ideal Aerosol Delivery System

- High efficiency in aerosol delivery
- Predictable and reproducible (in same patient and different patients)
- Easy to use and maintain
- Efficient to administer
- Convenient
- Cost-effective
- Environmentally safe

Data from Cole C. The use of aerosolized medicines in neonates. *Neonat Respir Dis* 10:4, 2000.

TABLE 27-7	**Advantages and Disadvantages of Aerosol Generators in Neonates**	
Aerosol Generator	**Advantages**	**Disadvantages**
Pressurized metered-dose inhaler (pMDI)	• More consistent aerosol particle size and output • Less time consuming • Less preparation time • Less contamination • Less expensive than single-use nebulizers • Some hydrofluoroalkane formulations have more optimal aerosol particle size	• Technique problems • Lack of pure medications • Not all medications available in pMDI • New hydrofluoroalkane formulations need clinical studies
Jet nebulizer	• Tidal breathing • Passive cooperation • Can be used for long periods to deliver high doses • Wide range of medications	• Expensive and inconvenient • Inefficient and highly variable aerosol output • Numerous environmental factors affect aerosol particle size and output • Poor aerosolization of suspensions and viscous solutions • Preparation time • Time consuming to administer • Contamination potential • Requires compressed gas
Ultrasonic nebulizer	• Potentially more efficient than jet nebulizer and pMDI • Tidal breathing • Passive cooperation • Can be used for long periods to deliver high doses	• Expensive and inconvenient • Requires power source • Contamination potential • Limited medications available for use • Preparation time • Time consuming to administer

Data from Cole C. The use of aerosolized medicines in neonates. *Neonat Respir Dis* 10:4, 2000.

transiently to maintain pressure and volume delivery to the patient.[155] On the other hand, for more sophisticated microprocessor-controlled ventilators, a gas-powered jet nebulizer may cause the ventilator to alarm and/or affect the patient's ability to flow trigger-assisted ventilator inflations. A vibrating mesh nebulizer does not add flow to the ventilator system. This may improve triggering and reduce excessive pressure and volume delivery to the patient. Bench and animal studies have shown that the vibrating mesh nebulizer is capable of providing between 10.74% and 12.6% of the drug placed in the nebulizer during neonatal ventilation.[156] While it appears that vibrating mesh nebulizers represent a potentially safer and more efficient drug delivery system than jet nebulizers during ventilation, the cost of this drug delivery system may not be feasible for many institutions. Reports have also shown that drug delivery is more efficient with a vibrating mesh nebulizer during neonatal high-frequency compared to conventional ventilation.

Most infant ventilators now require proximal flow sensors to be placed at the airway under normal operation. Medication condensate from a nebulizer treatment can accumulate within these sensitive flow sensors, affecting patient triggering, quality of airway graphics, tidal volume accuracy, ventilator operation, and drug delivery. As such, the proximal flow sensor is typically removed for a short-term nebulizer treatment. While humidity has been shown to reduce aerosol delivery, a humidifier should not be disabled during a nebulizer treatment.

There is renewed interest in providing aerosolized drugs to patients supported by noninvasive support. Several studies have evaluated aerosol drug delivery during HFNC in neonatal lung models, but this practice cannot be suggested at this time.[157-160] A 2014 study compared bronchodilator drug delivery using a vibrating mesh nebulizer between HFNC, sigh intermittent mandatory ventilation (SiPAP), and bubble CPAP.[161] Drug delivery to a lung model was quite low (<1.5%) with all

testing conditions. Overall, SiPAP provided lower drug mass than HFNC and bubble CPAP, probably because of drug loss in the nasal pressure generator. There were also no differences between different nebulizer circuit positions for HFNC and SiPAP but during bubble CPAP, nebulizer placement at the humidifier provided greater drug delivery than when placed proximal to the patient nasal airway interface.

Improvements in nebulizer efficiency and safety as well as a better understanding of how nebulizers can be integrated in the array of delivery options for infants will be useful for future drug preparations and research. Owing to the improved efficiency of nebulizers and the small particle size, many investigators are intensely focused on ways to deliver aerosolized surfactant. Preclinical studies in mechanically ventilated preterm animals have shown improved outcomes and are likely to be used more frequently in the NICU in the future.[162]

CLINICIAN-BASED VENTILATOR AND WEANING PROTOCOLS

High variability in medical practice may have contributed, in part, to higher health care costs and poor adherence to evidence-based interventions. Evidence-based protocol strategies have been developed to reduce the lack of concordance in an attempt to improve clinical outcomes. Where evidence is lacking, expert opinion has been used to guide the development of management guidelines or protocols and reduce unnecessary variations in practice. In the respiratory care setting, non-physician-driven protocols have been shown to result in improvement in cost and allocation of appropriate resources to patients when respiratory therapy protocol–based care was used in adults.[163-168] The message is less clear in neonates receiving mechanical ventilation, and this is probably because of the array of lung diseases treated in the NICU.

Only one study has evaluated the impact of the implementation of a ventilation protocol driven by registered respiratory therapists on respiratory outcomes of premature infants. This included strict guidelines for outcomes, which were assessed at 1 and 2 years following implementation of the protocol and compared with historic controls. Following implementation of the protocol, there were significant and sustained reductions in time of first extubation attempt, duration of mechanical ventilation, and rate of extubation failure.

A protocol that used early extubation to NCPAP after 24 hours of ventilation has been shown in animals to result in less apnea and need for more intubations compared to those supported with invasive ventilation for 5 days.[169] However, outside of animal studies, mechanical ventilator weaning protocols are scant in the medical literature. The one study that has compared outcomes in infants between a weaning protocol and no intervention failed to show any differences.[170] As such, weaning practices vary widely from one institution to the next.

According to a survey among U.S. NICUs weaning decisions are frequently physician dependent and not evidence based, with only 36% of respondents having a guideline (31%) or written protocol (5%) for ventilator weaning.[171] Reasons for this lack of definitive data may include that fact that there is no single reliable physiologic parameter or pulmonary function test in neonates that determines readiness for extubation. Further, many neonates have leaky ETTs, making tidal volume and minute ventilation difficult to measure. The optimal time for extubation is determined by a variety of parameters, including mean airway pressure, oxygen requirement, ventilatory requirements (see Chapters 9 and 10 on modes of ventilation), estimation of negative inspiratory force, static compliance, and, most importantly, the appearance of the baby. Gillespie et al.[172] have suggested placing the infant on endotracheal CPAP for 10 minutes while monitoring the spontaneous minute ventilation. The ability of the infant to spontaneously generate at least 50% of the minute ventilation that was seen during assisted ventilation predicted readiness for extubation and shortened the time to successful extubation. The clinician may also use intermittent bagging of the infant to get a sense of the compliance of the lung. The baby's primary problem and the clinical course and duration of assisted ventilation can provide helpful information regarding the appropriate timing for extubation. Some experts believe that a transition period from assist mode, pressure support, and/or extubation to CPAP is an excellent way to facilitate extubation, Sometimes a methylxanthine is used during the weaning process because its effects include "reminding the newborn to breathe" and increasing the efficiency of the diaphragm, especially in very low birth-weight infants.[173,174] If the infant has been on assisted ventilation for several days and there is concern about edema and inflammation in the upper airway, one or two doses of dexamethasone, given 24 to 48 hours prior to extubation, may be helpful.

All caretakers involved in the management of these babies need to be aware of the safety issues with regard to the transmission of pathogenic organisms by bodily fluids and closely follow the Occupational Safety and Health Administration standards outlined in Appendix 30.

RESUSCITATION AND STABILIZATION AT DELIVERY

The NRP is a training program for providers of newborn resuscitation created by the AAP and the American Heart Association to provide a comprehensive stepwise algorithm for the assessment and resuscitation of the newborn infant at delivery.[1] A core feature of this algorithm is the provision of adequate respiratory support and establishing effective ventilation using a variety of resuscitation devices, while repeatedly assessing the patient's response to the support provided and adjusting the technique of respiratory support.

Furthermore, endotracheal intubation may be considered at several points during a resuscitation; however, the timing of intubation may be influenced by the skill and experience of the provider as well as the clinical circumstances. Potential indications for endotracheal intubation during delivery room resuscitation include (1) tracheal suctioning of meconium (this is no longer recommended by the NRP), (2) need for prolonged positive-pressure ventilation, (3) administration of prophylactic surfactant, (4) presence of obstructive upper airway lesions requiring an artificial airway, and (5) cases in which air distention of the gastrointestinal (GI) tract is undesirable, such as with congenital diaphragmatic hernia.

Positive-pressure ventilation should be initiated during neonatal resuscitation when the infant is bradycardic (heart rate less than 100) or apneic despite stimulation or when there is persistent hypoxemia despite supplemental oxygen administration.[1] Under these circumstances, positive-pressure ventilation should be initially provided with a resuscitation bag and mask or T-piece resuscitator. Ultimately, intubation for positive-pressure ventilation should be considered if bag and mask ventilation is ineffective or if the need for prolonged positive-pressure ventilation is anticipated.

One of the most recent advances in manual ventilation of the newborn has been the introduction of the sustained lung inflation.[175] The process involves using one of the resuscitation devices previously discussed to administer a single high pressure to the infant's lungs in an effort to better establish the functional residual capacity. The pressure is sustained for a designated amount of time and then reduced to a standard CPAP level to assist spontaneous breathing. This maneuver remains controversial, but emerging evidence suggests that such a maneuver may decrease the need for mechanical ventilation in the first few days of life.[176,177]

Infants born with congenital diaphragmatic hernia frequently require positive-pressure ventilation at delivery because of respiratory distress with cyanosis. Provision of positive-pressure ventilation with bag and mask will drive large amounts of air into the upper GI tract, causing distention of a bowel that has herniated into the chest. Such bowel distention will cause further lung compression and compromise respiratory function. For this reason, infants with diaphragmatic hernia should be promptly intubated in the delivery room if resuscitation is required.[1] Some clinicians also advise that these infants should be paralyzed with a muscle relaxant to prevent spontaneous breathing from causing bowel distention. An orogastric tube should also be placed to evacuate any air that does enter the stomach. The diagnosis of diaphragmatic hernia is often confirmed by antenatal ultrasound studies and should be suspected in any infant with a scaphoid abdomen, unilaterally diminished breath sounds, and persistent respiratory distress.

REFERENCES

A complete reference list is available at https://expertconsult .inkling.com/.

28

Nursing Care

Debbie Fraser, MN, RNC-NIC

Neonates needing respiratory support require close monitoring to detect subtle changes that can signal either the need for weaning or a deterioration requiring additional intervention. An interdisciplinary team with expertise in managing small and sick infants should provide care to these infants. It is important that all care providers including nurses have a good understanding of developmental physiology, pathophysiology, pharmacotherapeutics, and the needs of the newborn and family.

As we learn more about the morbidities experienced by very low birth-weight infants and other newborns requiring respiratory assistance, it has become clear that technology alone will not result in further improvements in outcome unless accompanied by exquisite attention to the neonate's environment and the small details that result in an optimal outcome. Because nurses spend the most concentrated period of time at the bedside, they are likely to be the most familiar with the neonate and most likely to detect changes in the patient's condition.

ASSESSMENT OF THE NEONATE

Newborns should be assessed at the time of admission to the neonatal intensive care unit (NICU) and also at regular intervals each day. An evaluation is made of each body system and is documented in the medical record at least once per shift and according to unit policy. Prior to assessing the infant, it is important to review the history including that of the family, mother, labor and delivery, and problems and interventions since birth (Table 28-1). Expected findings will vary according to the infant's gestational and chronologic age.

Assessment should begin with a period of observation prior to disturbing the infant. This is followed by auscultation and palpation. General observation encompasses the infant's color, tone, and activity levels. The presence of cyanosis of the lips or mucous membranes should be noted. All infants should be centrally pink; acrocyanosis is common especially in the first hours and days after birth. Term infants are normally flexed and cycle through periods of sleep and activity. Premature infants are more likely to have decreased tone and activity levels; therefore, it is important to observe each infant for subtle changes over time.

In appropriately grown term infants the chest circumference is approximately 2 cm less than the occipital–frontal head circumference, or between 30 and 36 cm in diameter.[1] A small or bell-shaped chest may be seen in infants with pulmonary hypoplasia or neuromuscular abnormalities, whereas a barrel chest with an increase in the anteroposterior diameter is seen in conditions associated with air trapping such as meconium aspiration, advanced chronic lung disease, or transient tachypnea of the newborn.

The chest should be examined for symmetry, shape, and movement. Particular attention is given to work of breathing, use of accessory muscles, and chest wall movement. Normal respiratory rate is 30 to 60 breaths per minute with relaxed diaphragmatic movements. Tachypnea is one of the most common manifestations of respiratory disease, especially diseases with decreased compliance such as respiratory distress syndrome (RDS). Infants are preferential nose breathers but will often breathe through their mouth in the presence of nasal obstruction. In infants receiving mechanical ventilation, excessive chest wall excursion may be seen when ventilator pressures exceed what is required for adequate gas exchange.[2] Diminished chest wall movement may signal a loss of lung volume related to atelectasis or obstruction of the airway. Asymmetrical chest movement may indicate the presence of a pneumothorax.

Auscultation of breath sounds should be done over both the anterior and the posterior surfaces of the chest comparing one side to the other. Breath sounds are diminished in the presence of air leaks, atelectasis, or fluid in the pleural space. Infants with RDS may have faint breath sounds with a sandpaper-like quality in the latter part of inspiration. Sounds may be accentuated in the presence of consolidation such as occurs with pneumonia. Fine crackles are a normal finding in the first few hours after birth as fetal lung fluid is cleared. Beyond that period, crackles may be heard in infants with RDS or bronchopulmonary dysplasia (BPD). More prominent crackles reflect fluid in the alveoli and airways. Wheezes are not common in neonates but may be heard in infants with BPD. Stridor occurs as a result of upper airway obstruction and is most commonly heard after extubation. Both wheezes and rubs are more commonly heard in ventilated infants as a result of narrowing of the airway in the presence of an endotracheal tube. Infants receiving high-frequency ventilation will have altered breath sounds that range from jackhammer in nature (jet ventilation) to more high-pitched and vibratory. Higher-pitched or musical sounds are heard in the presence of secretions. Auscultation of the chest includes an assessment of heart sounds listening for any irregularities, extra beats, or murmurs.

Palpation of the chest is performed to assess for the presence of masses, edema, or subcutaneous emphysema. It is also a useful technique to assess air entry in infants receiving high-frequency ventilation. Using the palm of the hand, compare one side of the chest to the other. Differences in the strength of the vibrations between one side of the chest and the other may indicate an air leak, secretions, or a displaced endotracheal tube. Chest examination findings are summarized in Table 28-2.

TABLE 28-1 Elements of a Neonatal History

Family History

Genetic conditions

Maternal and paternal occupations

Siblings—ages, health status

Socioeconomic status, living conditions

Environmental risks/exposures

Maternal History

Age, previous pregnancies including complications in those pregnancies

Blood type, Rh status, Group B *Streptococcus* status, serology results, HIV and hepatitis B status

Results of prenatal screening tests including glucose tolerance testing

Preexisting medical conditions

Complications of pregnancy

Exposure to teratogens, tobacco, alcohol, and drugs

Prenatal steroids

Labor and Delivery

Onset of labor (premature, spontaneous or induced)

Complications during labor—maternal fever, bleeding, fetal heart tracing

Time of membrane rupture, amniotic fluid quantity and quality

Medications during labor (pain medications, magnesium sulfate, other)

Type of delivery (spontaneous vaginal, operative)

Apgar scores and resuscitation required

PAIN ASSESSMENT

Pain is often referred to by some clinicians as the "fifth vital sign," and the importance of its assessment cannot be overemphasized. It is well recognized that neonates in the NICU experience numerous painful treatments and procedures on a daily basis.[3,4] There are a number of pain assessment tools that have been validated for use in the neonatal population.[5,6] However, there are a number of gaps and shortcomings in current practice in regard to the selection of, use of, and response to pain assessment tools.[6,7] Each NICU should use a validated assessment tool that is appropriate for its patient population. Staff should be educated on the use of the tool, and protocols should be in place to provide guidance regarding the appropriate response to elevated pain scores. Regular audits should be undertaken to ensure compliance with pain assessment and management protocols.

RESPIRATORY CARE

Providing care to an infant in the NICU is best accomplished through the efforts of a multidisciplinary team. When the infant is receiving respiratory support, additional monitoring of both the patient and the equipment is essential. Special concerns while caring for infants requiring assisted ventilation include maintaining targeted oxygen saturation parameters, providing nasal continuous positive airway pressure (CPAP) or non-invasive ventilation, maintaining a secure and patent airway, management of the infant on high-frequency ventilators and inhaled nitric oxide, preventing ventilator-acquired pneumonia, and detecting and intervening in cases of sudden respiratory deterioration.

TABLE 28-2 Examination of Newborn Chest

EXAMINATION OF THE NEWBORN CHEST		
	Normal Findings	**Abnormal Findings**
Inspect	Oval chest shape, narrow at top and flares at bottom with narrow anteroposterior diameter	Bulging of chest
	Prominent xiphoid process	Concavity of chest
	Flexible chest wall, mild retractions with crying	Increased anteroposterior diameter (barrel chest)
	Symmetric chest movement in synchrony with abdomen during respirations	Depressed sternum (pectus excavatum/funnel chest)
		Protuberant sternum (pectus carinatum/pigeon breast)
	Breath rates 30-40/min in term infants and 40-60/min in preterm infants	Asymmetric chest wall movement, flail chest
		Asynchronous respirations/paradoxical breathing ("seesaw")
	Nipples well formed and prominent, symmetrically positioned; may have milk secretion	Retractions
		Tachypnea
	Pink color; harlequin color change	Supernumerary nipples
		Erythema and tenderness of breasts
Palpate	Clavicles and ribs intact	Widely spaced nipples
	Breast nodule 3-10 mm	Central cyanosis, jaundice, pallor, mottling
	PMI left of lower sternum	Precordial impulse visible beyond first hours of life in term infant
Auscultate	Equal bronchovesicular breath sounds	Lump over clavicle
	Lusty cry	Crepitus
	No murmur or soft murmur	Lack of breast tissue
		Shifts in PMI
		Fremitus
		Crackles, rhonchi, wheeze, stridor, rubs, bowel sounds in chest
		Grunting
		Cough
		Weak, whining, or high-pitched cry
		Hoarseness, stridor
		Harsh murmur (grade 2-3) in first hours of life

PMI, point of maximal intensity. Data from Koszarek K, Ricouard D. Nursing assessment and care of the neonate in acute respiratory distress. In: Fraser D, ed. *Acute Respiratory Care of the Neonate.* 3rd ed. Petaluma, Calif., NICU INK Books, 2012:65-108.

Oxygen Saturation Monitoring

It is important that neonates receiving respiratory support have their oxygen status monitored on a continuous basis. The optimal oxygen saturation targets in premature infants have not been definitively determined and are usually set by unit protocol. Reducing the targeted oxygen saturation ranges in premature infants to between 85% and 93% substantially decreased rates of grades III and IV retinopathy of prematurity.[8] The SUPPORT Trial[9] found a small but statistically significant increase in early deaths in the group of infants in the lower oxygen saturation range. This has prompted some experts to recommend keeping oxygen saturations above 90% in the early neonatal period until more definitive data are available.[10] Similarly the BOOST-II trial, which enrolled 2108 infants born at less than 28 weeks' gestation before enrollment was stopped, demonstrated a significant increase in the combined outcomes of death and disability at 2 years of age in neonates randomized to an oxygen saturation target range of 85% to 89% compared to those in the target range of 91% to 95% (BOOST-II Australia and United Kingdom Collaborative Groups, 2016). The authors of a meta-analysis of the SUPPORT, the COT (Canadian Oxygen Trial), and the three BOOST-II studies concluded that an oxygen saturation target range of 90% to 95% should be used until further data become available.[11]

Target saturation levels are also dependent on the infant's underlying condition and the goals of care. In infants with persistent pulmonary hypertension, it may be desirable to maintain a higher oxygen saturation level, whereas in those infants with cyanotic congenital heart disease, a target saturation as low as 75% may be acceptable.[12]

Maintaining tight control of oxygen levels presents a significant challenge for clinicians. Among the challenges is the significant lability displayed by ventilated premature infants related to their disease conditions, responses to environmental stimuli, and need for ongoing interventions such as suctioning and other invasive procedures. Education and awareness regarding the need for narrow oxygen target ranges is also a challenge. A multicenter audit found that nurses were compliant with pulse oximetry alarm limits around 70% of the time.[13] Another multicenter study reported that, although lower alarm limits were set correctly 91% of the time, higher alarm limits were set correctly only 23% of the time, with 76% of the limits set too high and 24% of the limits set at 100%. In 2013, The Joint Commission issued a sentinel alert statement related to medical device alarm safety that highlighted the potential danger of alarm fatigue, a problem familiar to those responding to repeated oxygen saturation alarms.[14]

A number of successful quality improvement projects designed to address oxygen targeting and alarm fatigue have been reported. One of the early reports came from Chow and colleagues,[15] who developed an oxygen targeting policy followed by an extensive staff education and audit process. The authors describe an initial resistance to change among staff, difficulties in consistency in implementation on different shifts, and the need for initial training, followed by retraining. Since Chow and colleagues reported on the results of their initiative, many NICUs have undertaken similar quality improvement projects to remind staff of the need to carefully monitor oxygen saturation and maintain much tighter control of parameters, avoiding hyperoxia in infants at high risk of retinopathy of prematurity (Fig. 28-1). Carefully evaluating the number and types of procedures that a ventilated neonate receives is also necessary

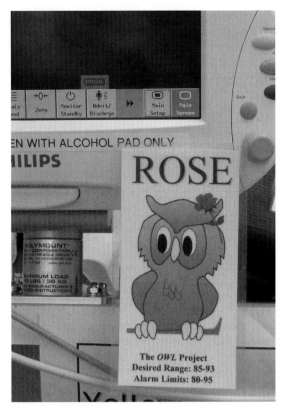

FIG 28-1 Pulse oximetry sign.

to reduce episodes of hypoxia and resulting hyperoxia when increased FiO_2 is administered.

Positioning and Containment

Premature and seriously ill neonates undergo a significant number of hands-on assessments or procedures in a 24-hour period. A descriptive study showed that infants averaged eight painful procedures per day during the first 2 weeks of NICU stay;[16] the authors encouraged neonatal units to question the need for each and every potentially harmful invasive procedure.

Procedures often result in significant and prolonged reductions in oxygenation.[17-19] The extent of hypoxemia and overall distress can be dramatically reduced when personnel modify their caregiving according to the infant's responses. Careful observations of oxygenation and behavioral reactions in infants receiving CPAP or mechanical ventilation with appropriate, individualized interventions can reduce the amount of stress the infant experiences. Many NICUs are moving to provide cue-based care, that is, providing routine care to the infant only during times when the infant is awake.

Supporting the infant's body position can also reduce the stressful effects of procedures and other interventions. Swaddling, rolls, and the use of other containment techniques have been shown to improve physiologic and behavioral organization during weighing, suctioning, and heel sticks and provide comfort from pain.[20] Placing an infant on assisted ventilation in the prone position increases oxygenation, improves sleep, and reduces stress compared to the supine position,[20,21a] possibly by increasing lung volumes and residual capacities.[21b] The Cochrane review of 12 trials (285 infants) comparing various positions for ventilated infants found that prone positioning slightly improved oxygenation, but that there was no evidence of sustained improvement for infants who were positioned prone. One study found lower bacterial colonization in infants who were cared for in an alternating lateral position compared to those neonates cared for in a supine posture.[22]

Infant positioning is also a risk factor for the development of intraventricular hemorrhage. In an evidence-based review of the literature on midline head positioning, Malusky and Donze[23] identified 11 articles that met the inclusion criteria for the review. Despite some differences in the study populations and methods of evaluation, several studies found changes in cerebral blood flow with position changes.[24] Three studies found a significant decrease in intracranial pressure when infants were positioned with their heads in midline.[24-26] The authors of this review concluded that there was support for maintaining infants <32 weeks in a midline (neutral) head position with the head of the bed elevated 30 degrees for the first 72 hours of life.

Nasal Continuous Positive Airway Pressure

One of the key strategies in preventing barotrauma and chronic lung disease is avoiding endotracheal tube-mediated mechanical ventilation. As a result of this shift away from intubation, the use of noninvasive ventilation strategies including nasal CPAP (NCPAP) has increased dramatically. Caring for an infant receiving CPAP is challenging. A major factor contributing to success or failure with NCPAP lies in the comfort level and knowledge of the team providing the care.[27] One study reported significant improvements with the success of early NCPAP over a 4-year period, indicating a substantial learning curve for all professionals involved, including nurses, respiratory therapists, and physicians; extensive and ongoing education included information on how and why CPAP works and on complications and troubleshooting.[28]

Assessment of infants on NCPAP also includes overall evaluation of respiratory status including retractions and respiratory effort, breath sounds, oxygenation, and P_{CO_2} levels. Although there may be retractions and P_{CO_2} levels in the range of 45 to 65 torr, if the infant generally appears comfortable, he or she can be maintained on NCPAP. Signs of distress include P_{CO_2} greater than 65, FiO_2 requirement greater than 60% consistently, and increased retractions, tachypnea, and apnea. These signs may be indications that the infant is failing NCPAP and that noninvasive ventilation or intubation plus assisted ventilation is needed. Assessment of an infant on CPAP includes careful assessment of the cheeks, philtrum, and nasal structures for any evidence of redness, erythema, or injury.[29]

Complications from NCPAP include airway or prong blockage by secretions, and injury to the skin and nasal septum, abdominal distension, feeding intolerance, and a slight increase in the risk of pneumothorax and necrotizing enterocolitis.[30,31] Careful auscultation of breath sounds is needed, as well as attention to the pressure limits on the CPAP delivery device. Excessive abdominal distension is addressed by gastric decompression with an orogastric tube, although this complication may often hinder the advancing of enteral feedings and lead to numerous abdominal X-rays. One study documented that gastric emptying actually occurred earlier in infants receiving NCPAP.[32]

Maintenance of continuous flow and appropriate CPAP pressures is affected by the infant's position and overall comfort. The prongs or mask interface need to be properly positioned, and the infant's mouth needs to be closed to ensure the maintenance of appropriate CPAP levels. To reduce the risk of the infant developing atelectasis, avoid removing the mask or

prongs for routine care in the first 24 to 48 hours and minimize the disruption of CPAP as much as possible until the infant is ready for weaning.[29]

One of the biggest challenges encountered while caring for the infant on NCPAP is protecting the nasal septum and surrounding structures from injury. Nasal injury is more common in more premature infants and in those infants requiring CPAP for long periods of time. Types of nasal injury include nasal snubbing, flaring or widening of the nares, and necrosis of the columella nasi.[33,34] The nasal septum is fragile, and the interfaces between the infant's nose and the CPAP system, either prongs or mask, may cause pressure on facial structures. There are limited data about the effect of using CPAP masks in premature infants, although many NICUs have adopted the use of masks alternating with nasal prongs in an effort to reduce nasal trauma. Diligence in ensuring the appropriate positioning of prongs relative to the nose and frequent repositioning is necessary. The CPAP hat should fit snugly and should rest just above the infant's eyebrows. Prongs should be the correct size to fit snugly in the nares without excessive pressure on the septum and should be positioned to avoid blanching of the skin around the nose. Straps should be snug but not to the point of creating indentations on the cheeks.

Despite meticulous care practices, tissue injury may occur on the philtrum of the lip or the nasal septum (Fig. 28-2).[35] Hydrocolloid "shields" have been shown to offer some protection against injury[31] but do not prevent all injuries because pressure is often the problem, rather than friction. Once the skin barrier has been injured, use of these products may promote further breakdown.[36] Application of an antimicrobial ointment such as mupirocin may be beneficial to reduce the risk of infection through this portal of entry.

Administration of oxygen under pressure through nasal prongs can be excessively irritating to nasal mucosa, resulting in increased production of secretions, especially in the first few hours after initiation.[37] The use of warmed, humidified gas is imperative. Although there is currently no empirical evidence for exactly how best to care for the airway of infants on NCPAP,[38] suctioning of the nares to maintain patency is required. Suctioning should be based on assessment of the patient and not routinely scheduled.[29,37] Frequent suctioning causes trauma to the nares and nasopharynx and may increase the risk of infection through skin breakdown. Other hazards of suctioning include bradycardia or cardiac dysrhythmias. Using techniques such as round-tipped plastic suction devices can minimize trauma from mucosal bleeding and swelling. Saline or sterile water drops instilled prior to suctioning may be helpful in loosening secretion and lubricating the catheter.[39]

Repositioning is essential for a number of reasons, including neurodevelopmental outcomes, and is recommended every 4 to 6 hours.[25] Prone positioning may also be beneficial in infants receiving NCPAP because lying prone seems to aid in keeping the infant's mouth in a closed position, decreases abdominal distension, and also keeps the infant calmer. Offering a pacifier and providing containment using swaddling or nesting techniques can be beneficial in both promoting comfort and improving respiratory support. The use of a chin strap may prevent air leaks and loss of CPAP pressure.[40]

Mechanical Ventilation

There are a wide variety of neonatal ventilators in the market, each with a unique set of properties and settings. Everyone

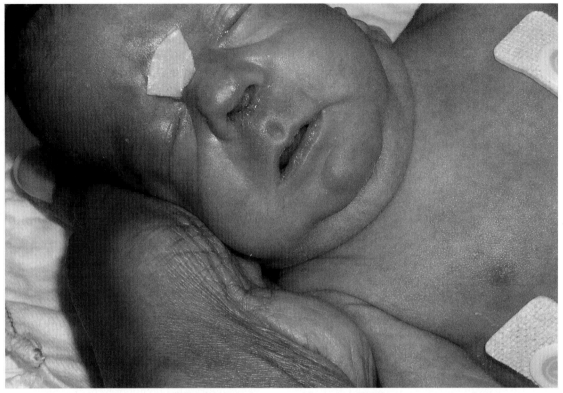

FIG 28-2 Damage caused by nasal CPAP.

providing care to the infant on mechanical ventilation should have an understanding of the machine itself and the interface between the machine and the baby. Careful assessment of the infant's breathing pattern, chest movement, respiratory rate, and oxygenation should be undertaken each shift and each time ventilator parameters are adjusted. This information is then documented in the patient record along with any diagnostic tests (X-rays or blood gases) that are performed. There are some issues unique to mechanical ventilation that should be considered in the care of the infant. These include airway security, endotracheal tube (ETT) movement and position, suctioning of the ETT, and prevention of ventilator-acquired pneumonia.

Airway Security

Accidental dislodgment of the ETT can result in serious complications including acute hypoxia, bradycardia, and potential damage to the trachea or larynx. Factors associated with accidental extubation include agitation, ETT suctioning, weighing, turning the patient's head, loose tape, short ETTs, and retaping the ETT.[41] The incidence of accidental extubations reported in the literature is variable[42] but approximates three to six events per 100 ventilator days, although this rate has been decreased to as low as <1 by neonatal units through quality improvement projects.[43]

Many different techniques have been described to secure ETTs, ranging from adhesives with bonding agents or pectin barriers to using metal or plastic bows to prevent slipping of the ETT.[42] Some commercially available products for securing neonatal ETTs have incorporated similar ideas in their products. Because the common link in all these methods is the use of adhesives, an in-depth review of adhesive application and removal in the neonate is in the section on skin care below.

Endotracheal Tube Movement and Malposition

The position of the ETT may be altered with inadequate fixation of the tube, changes in patient position, and flexion and extension of the head. Because the trachea of a term newborn is quite short (mean 57 mm) and even shorter in premature infants, small movements of the ETT can result in displacement, causing the tube to move into the right main stem bronchus with flexion or into the neck with extension (Fig. 28-3).[44,45] In addition to potentially altering ventilation and blood gas parameters and causing tracheal damage, ETT movement can result in misinterpretation of the ETT position on X-rays. The infant's head should be carefully positioned when obtaining X-rays and placed in a "neutral" position to avoid extension or flexion. The ETT should be positioned with the bevel opening to the same side the head is facing to avoid having the bevel abut against the tracheal wall with head movement or position changes (Fig. 28-4).[46]

Each NICU should develop a standard practice that is consistently used to avoid confusion during intubations and ETT retaping. A card specifying the depth at which the ETT is inserted should be posted at each bedside, with the centimeter marking that is at the patient's lip displayed. Adhesion of the ETT taping should be inspected often and the ETT retaped whenever necessary to prevent accidental dislodgment. Regular monitoring of unplanned extubations can be incorporated into quality improvement audits.[43]

Suctioning

The presence of an ETT causes irritation to tissue and increased secretions. It is necessary to clear this artificial airway periodically to maintain ventilation for the infant. ETT suctioning has been associated with a number of complications in infants including hypoxemia, bradycardia, atelectasis, airway trauma, and pneumothorax.[17] Systemic adverse effects are also of

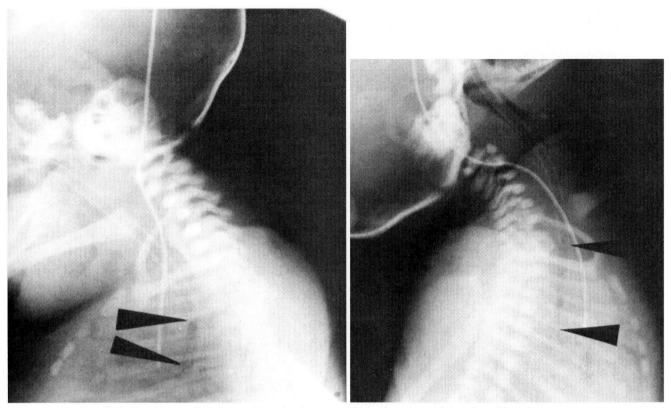

FIG 28-3 X-rays showing endotracheal tube position changes with head position changes.

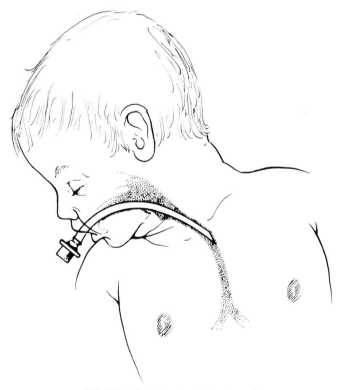

FIG 28-4 Endotracheal tube bevel.

concern, including increased blood pressure, changes in intracranial pressure, and an increased risk of infection.[17] Neonates should be suctioned only when it is assessed to be needed, that is, when breath sounds are moist or congested, when secretions are visible, when there is a change in the infant's respiratory rate and pattern, or when the infant is bradycardic, hypoxic, or agitated with no known cause.[12,47] During high-frequency oscillatory or jet ventilation, it is not always obvious when suctioning is needed, and some nurseries implement routine suctioning every 4 to 8 hours for patients on high-frequency ventilation (HFV).

To reduce trauma to the tracheal mucosa, the suction catheter should be inserted to a premeasured depth that includes the ETT and the adaptor.[2] Normal saline has been used for many years to lubricate the ETT; however, there is concern that saline interferes with the innate immune properties in the airway mucosa.[48] Other studies report potential adverse effects of saline instillation on oxygenation[49] and a potential to exaggerate complications of suctioning such as changes in intracranial pressure, trauma to the airway mucosa, and bradycardia.[47] In addition, there is concern that saline instillation does not lead to increased secretion recovery and may be a risk factor in ventilator-associated pneumonia by way of moving the biofilm that occurs in the ETT further into the distal airway. Given the potential for adverse effects and a lack of evidence supporting the benefit of routine nasal saline instillation, this practice is not recommended.[47,50]

Suctioning techniques have also been examined in an attempt to determine the least harmful method of suctioning. Cone and colleagues[17] compared routine suctioning with a two-person procedure. They found that the use of four hands for suctioning resulted in an increase in oxygen saturation during the observation period compared to presuctioning levels and that infants displayed more stress and defensive behaviors after routine one-person suctioning compared to four-handed suctioning.

Closed suctioning (CS) systems that are placed inline with the ETT and ventilator circuit are now used in many nurseries (Fig. 28-5). The research comparing open and closed

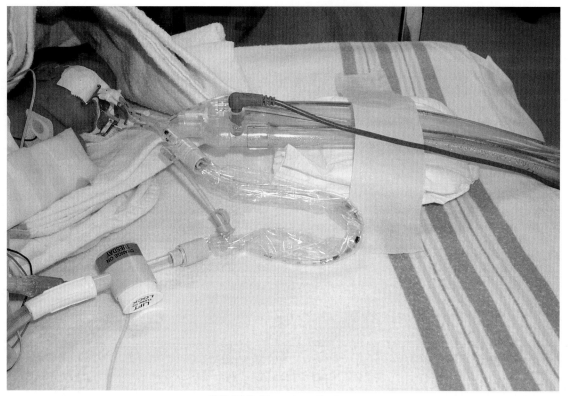

FIG 28-5 Closed suctioning.

suctioning practices has not been definitive in determining which system is more advantageous. A Cochrane review evaluated four studies using a crossover design that included 252 infants and found a reduction in the number and severity of hypoxic events and a decrease in the number and severity of bradycardia with CS. The authors concluded, however, that the evidence was not strong enough to recommend CS as the only acceptable method for suctioning ventilated neonates.[51] Other potential advantages to CS include ease of use, with only one person needed, and reduced loss of lung volumes during suctioning.[47] One study of CS in intubated adults reported that loss of lung volume during CS was reduced compared to open-system suctioning but that end-expiratory lung volumes recovered more slowly in patients suctioned with a closed system vs those suctioned with an open system. This suggests that closed systems may not be totally protective of lung volumes.[52]

Ventilator-Associated Pneumonia

Preventing nosocomial infection in the NICU and in other hospitalized patients, including ventilator-associated pneumonia (VAP) and catheter-related bloodstream infections, is now mandated by The Joint Commission (formerly the Joint Commission on Accreditation of Healthcare Organizations). The assumption is that these complications are preventable by measures undertaken by care providers in the NICU. Many controversies remain regarding the diagnosis of VAP in neonates, and little evidence exists about how to best prevent VAP in the NICU. One of the most pressing challenges is diagnosing VAP. While the Centers for Disease Control and Prevention has developed diagnostic criteria for infants <1 year of age, there is a lack of objective criteria specific to VAP in neonates, and obtaining a lung specimen, the gold standard for adult diagnosis, is impractical in neonates.[53a]

Risk factors for the development of VAP include prematurity, days of mechanical ventilation, ETT suctioning, the need for reintubation, antibiotic exposure, and use of sedation, feeding, or parenteral nutrition with days of mechanical ventilation being the most significant risk.[53b] Although the presence of a bloodstream infection is identified as a risk for VAP, it appears that most infections are attributed to exogenous sources such as the hands of health care workers, biofilm on the ETT, and contamination from the ventilator circuit.[54]

A number of VAP-prevention guidelines have been developed for adults[55,56] and, in many cases, have been extrapolated for use in the neonatal population. Some of the empirically based VAP prevention strategies for neonates on assisted ventilation include the following: (1) avoiding the use of mechanical ventilation and extubating infants as soon as possible, (2) avoiding repeated intubations, (3) maintaining separate ETT suctioning tubing and oral suctioning tubing, (4) changing the ventilator circuit only when visibly contaminated, (5) avoiding saline instillation with ETT suctioning, (6) suctioning the ETT only when needed, (7) keeping the head of the bed elevated 30 degrees, (8) performing mouth care every 4 hours, and (9) performing appropriate hand hygiene. Although these interventions have not yet been rigorously studied, many NICUs are attempting to reduce their VAP rate by bundling similar interventions in the hope of potential benefit.[54,57,58] VAP is also discussed in more detail in Chapter 30.

High-Frequency Ventilation

Nursing care for the infant on HFV, either via oscillator or via jet ventilators, requires a unique set of knowledge and skills.[59,60] Assessment of the infant receiving HFV is frequent and extensive, differing from routine nursery assessment related to the absence of tidal breathing. Auscultation is aimed at detecting changes in the pitch of breath sounds, with high-pitched sounds suggestive of secretions. It is not possible to auscultate the apical pulse or to detect the presence of a heart murmur while the infant is on HFV. Observing and palpating for chest vibration and other parameters of ventilation adequacy are employed. In many cases, the infant's condition while undergoing HFV can change very rapidly because of both the infant's underlying pulmonary pathology and the device in use. It is possible to interrupt or pause the ventilator briefly during the assessment process to auscultate spontaneous breath sounds and listen for heart murmurs; however, this can also destabilize the infant. Coordination among multidisciplinary team members is recommended for these assessment periods, so that the time during which the patient is removed from HFV is kept to a minimum.

CS should be used to prevent disconnecting the infant from ventilation during suctioning. Many NICUs use in-bed scales, weigh infants infrequently, or simply do not weigh patients receiving HFV to prevent destabilizing the respiratory system or accidental extubation. Depending on which high-frequency ventilator is used, positioning and turning infants on HFV may require two persons, one to rotate the infant while another caregiver briefly disconnects the ventilator circuit while the ventilator itself remains in a fixed location. The infant should be positioned to maintain the head in alignment with the body rather than turned to the side. This prevents obstruction of the flow of gases and disruption in ventilation.

Inhaled Nitric Oxide

The use of inhaled nitric oxide (iNO) is now commonplace for newborns receiving assisted ventilation. Originally approved for the treatment of pulmonary hypertension, iNO is now also used to treat premature infants with BPD.[61] Care of the newborn receiving iNO includes careful monitoring of the gas administration and preventing any interruption of iNO administration during hand ventilation, turning, moving, or suctioning; CS systems are recommended. Monitoring of methemoglobin levels, suggested in studies of full-term infants treated with iNO for pulmonary hypertension (especially those on higher concentrations), was not found to be necessary in premature infants treated with iNO for BPD.[62] However, a National Institutes of Health Consensus Statement found no advantage to the use of iNO in infants of <34 weeks' gestation.[63] Gradual weaning from iNO is necessary even in patients who are "nonresponders" because of the downregulation of the patient's endogenous nitric oxide production during treatment with iNO and the potential for destabilizing patients with marginal oxygenation and reserves.

Sudden Deterioration

A sudden deterioration can occur as a result of a multitude of factors in the ventilated neonatal patient. The cause of acute deterioration is not always apparent and two clinicians are often necessary at the bedside. After the baby is disconnected from the mechanical device, hand ventilation with a resuscitation bag connected to a manometer is initiated immediately. The FiO_2 is increased until oxygen saturation reaches the infant's target range. Breath sounds are immediately auscultated; if equal bilaterally, the tube is likely to be in proper position and free from obstruction. If the breath sounds are distant, or if air entry is detected in the gastric areas accompanied by distension, or an audible cry is heard, the ETT may have slipped into the esophagus. An end-tidal CO_2 monitor or detection device will show an absence of CO_2 during expiration. The ETT should be immediately removed and bag and mask ventilation provided until

it is determined whether reintubation is necessary. If replaced, the ETT should be securely taped at the same level as the previous tube, and an X-ray obtained to confirm appropriate ETT position.

If the breath sounds are louder on the right side, the ETT may have slipped into the right main tem bronchus. A chest X-ray can confirm this diagnosis or perhaps identify an air leak in the left lung. If the ETT extends into the right bronchus, the left lung or the upper lobe of the right lung may appear to have atelectasis on X-ray. The appropriate adjustment to the ETT position is determined by measuring the tube position from the X-ray and then repositioning and taping the ETT securely.

If the ETT is plugged with secretions, breath sounds may be diminished bilaterally, with decreased rise of the chest wall during hand ventilation. Initially, the ETT is suctioned to attempt to remove the secretions. If this measure is unsuccessful, the ETT is removed and bag and mask ventilation initiated until the ETT is replaced.

A large pneumothorax typically presents with cyanosis, bradycardia, decreased blood pressure, narrowing pulse pressure, and diminution of the QRS complex on the ECG. The point of maximal impulse of the heart may be shifted away from the side with the air leak, and breath sounds may be diminished or absent on the affected side. The diagnosis of a pneumothorax can be confirmed with transillumination of the chest with a high-density fiber-optic light source or with a chest X-ray. When the infant is significantly compromised it may be necessary to decompress the chest with needle aspiration before the diagnosis is confirmed radiographically. Once the air is evacuated and the patient stabilized, a chest tube is inserted and attached to a drainage system to assist in air removal.

GENERAL CARE OF THE NEONATE

Infants requiring care in the NICU, especially those ill enough to need respiratory support, require expert assessment and ongoing care. Respiratory diseases, with the potential for episodes of hypoxemia, predispose infants to complications such as retinopathy of prematurity, necrotizing enterocolitis, infection, and chronic lung disease. Optimizing the infant's environment to reduce the likelihood of complications is an important part of caring for these infants. Issues requiring special consideration include temperature management, nutrition, skin care, pain management, and developmental care.

Thermal Instability

Both hyperthermia and hypothermia place neonates at risk of complications. Hyperthermia is more likely to be iatrogenic as a result of exogenous sources of heat such as too many layers of clothing or blankets, an elevated incubator temperature, or excessive radiant heat. Hyperthermia increases the neonate's metabolic rate leading to tachycardia, tachypnea, increased oxygen consumption, increased insensible water loss, and poor weight gain.[64]

Because of the large surface area-to-body weight ratio and an inability to generate heat through shivering, all newborn infants are more susceptible to hypothermia compared to older infants. The risk of hypothermia is accentuated in premature infants who have limited subcutaneous tissue, reduced brown fat stores, and decreased tone and muscle activity. Evaporative heat losses are higher in very low birth-weight (VLBW) infants as a result of the thin epidermal skin layer.

Hypothermia has been shown to increase the risk of morbidity and mortality especially in VLBW infants. In a study of 5277 infants with birth weights between 401 and 1499 g, admission temperature was inversely related to mortality with a 28% increase in mortality for each 1°C decrease.[65] A more recent study of 1764 infants born between 22 and 33 weeks' gestation demonstrated a 1.64-fold increase in early neonatal death in infants with admission temperatures of <36°C.[66] Cold stress results in increased oxygen consumption and an increased risk of worsening respiratory distress, hypoxemia, hypoglycemia, and metabolic acidosis.[64] Longer term hypothermia slows postnatal growth, as calories are used for heat production rather than weight gain.

Careful temperature monitoring should be undertaken for all neonates, especially those at increased risk of hypothermia. Provision of a neutral thermal environment is critical in minimizing oxygen consumption and caloric expenditure. Additional thermal support is provided through the use of double-walled incubators or servo-controlled radiant warmers. Increased humidity is recommended for VLBW infants as a means of reducing transepidermal evaporative heat loss. Polyethylene bags or wraps are recommended for VLBW infants immediately after birth in the delivery room to reduce both evaporative and convective heat losses[67]

Nutrition

The contribution of postnatal growth failure to long-term neurodevelopmental outcomes in premature infants has been clearly recognized.[68-70] In addition, poor growth after birth in low birth-weight infants has been noted to be a risk factor for retinopathy of prematurity[71] and has been implicated in the development of adult-onset conditions such as diabetes and cardiovascular disease.[72-74] The increased work of breathing common to infants with respiratory disease results in increased caloric consumption and may prevent adequate oral intake of nutrients. Adequate growth has been identified as an important strategy in mitigating the risk of BPD.[75-77]

Attaining adequate growth rates in premature infants is challenging for a number of reasons. Most fat and energy stores are accrued in the third trimester, leaving preterm infants with limited caloric reserves at birth. At the same time these infants often experience a delay in achieving adequate intake of nutrients and may have periods of relative undernutrition related to feeding intolerance or fluid restrictions. Concurrently premature and sick infants require increased calories for tissue repair, generation of heat, and work of breathing. Early optimal nutrition for VLBW infants is a key pillar in preventing postnatal growth restriction and the related complications. Strategies to optimize nutrition include early parenteral nutrition with adequate protein and lipid intake, ensuring adequate protein intake with parenteral nutrition until oral feeding reaches adequate levels, minimal enteral feedings introduced on day 1 of life, advancement of feeds at a rate of 20 mL/kg/day, use of maternal or donor breast milk, and the appropriate fortification of calories and nutrients beginning when oral feeds reach 60 to 100 mL/kg/day.[78-80] Growth rates should be monitored carefully and individual adjustments made when anticipated growth rates are not achieved.

Skin Care

In premature infants the uppermost layer of the epidermis of the skin, the stratum corneum, is histologically thinner, and fibrils that connect the top two layers of the skin, the epidermis and the dermis, are fewer and more widely spaced compared with term infants.[81] Thus premature infants are more vulnerable to skin injury and stripping of the epidermis. Risk factors for skin injury include gestational age less than 32 weeks, edema, and adhesives applied to the skin to secure tubes, lines, and monitoring equipment. Although pressure sores are very rare in neonates, they may occasionally be seen on the ears or occiput of critically ill neonates on HFV or extracorporeal membrane oxygenation unless frequent repositioning and use of gel pillows or mattresses is employed.

Assessment of preterm infants should include frequent inspection of the skin for color, perfusion, turgor, edema, pressure points, and evidence of injury. A breech in skin integrity is a risk factor for sepsis, and attention should be given to preventing damage to the skin. Acutely ill infants should have their skin cleansed when it is soiled, with full baths reserved for more stable infants. To avoid drying out the skin, pH-neutral soaps should be used sparingly. Any product applied to the skin should be evaluated to determine if it contains dyes, perfumes, or drying agents and should be assessed for potential absorption of any chemically active ingredients. Emollients are not routinely used in some NICUs because of concern for infection[82] but may be needed when the infant's skin is dry and cracking. Again, care should be taken to select agents that have been tested in the neonatal population.

The use of products for skin antisepsis prior to invasive procedures such as intravenous starts, line placement, or heel sticks is an important part of preventing infection. Most products capable of killing bacteria are potentially harmful to the fragile skin of premature infants. Alcohol products are drying, whereas products containing iodine may be absorbed, leading to systemic problems. Topical antiseptic products should be approved for use in neonates and should be removed from the skin after the procedure using sterile water.[12]

Adhesive Application and Removal

The traumatic effects of adhesive removal have been documented on premature infants and include reduced barrier function, increased transepidermal water loss, erythema, and skin stripping.[83,84] Solvents are not recommended for adhesive removal in newborns because these contain hydrocarbon derivatives or petroleum distillates that have potential toxicity when absorbed. Skin irritation and injury have been reported related to the use of a solvent in a premature infant.[84] Pectin-based skin barriers such as HolliHesive and DuoDerm are used between skin and adhesive and mold well to curved surfaces while maintaining adherence in moist areas. Although studies initially described less visible trauma to skin from pectin barriers,[81] a study using direct measurements of skin barrier function found that pectin barriers caused a degree of trauma similar to that of plastic tape.[83] Despite this finding, pectin barriers and similar hydrocolloid adhesive products continue to be used in the NICU because they mold well to curved surfaces and adhere even with moisture.

The use of bonding agents, such as tincture of benzoin or Mastisol, increases the adherence of adhesives and may result in skin stripping and damage because they cause the adhesive to adhere more tenaciously to the epidermis than the fragile bond between epidermis and dermis, especially in the premature infant. An alcohol-free plastic polymer skin protectant, Cavilon (3M, St. Paul, MN), has been shown to reduce measurable damage from adhesives in adults[85] and reduce visible disruption in newborns.[86] It is approved for use in infants greater than 30 days of age.[87] The effect of repeated applications of barrier films on adherence or their effectiveness in moist environments has not been studied as of this writing.

Preventing trauma from adhesives can be accomplished by minimizing use of tape when possible, dabbing cotton on tape to reduce adherence, and using hydrogel adhesives for electrodes. However, hydrogel adhesives are not adequate when attaching life-support devices such as ETTs. Delaying tape removal may be helpful, because many adhesives attach less well to skin when in place for over 24 hours. Remove adhesives slowly and carefully, using water-soaked cotton balls and pulling the adhesive parallel to the skin surface, folding the adhesive onto itself.[83] Removal also can be facilitated using emollients or mineral oil if reapplication of adhesives at the site is not necessary.

Pressure Ulcers and Skin Breakdown

Although the incidence of ischemic injury related to pressure ulcers is low in NICU patients compared to adults, infants at risk for this complication include those on HFV and extracorporeal membrane oxygenation because they are more difficult to turn or move. In addition, they are generally critically ill and may be hypotensive, which can lead to peripheral tissue hypoperfusion. They may also be edematous because of leaking capillaries and may need excessive fluid or blood products to maintain blood pressure. Paralyzing medications such as pancuronium and vecuronium, or high levels of sedation, create poor tone and decreased movement,[88] which also increases the risk of skin breakdown.

Sites for pressure ulcers in newborns on assisted ventilation include the occiput of the head and the ears, because of the heavy weight of the infant's head compared to the body. In addition, the circuit connected to the ETT is often secured to avoid displacing the tube, and thus the infant cannot turn or move the head without assistance.[89]

Prevention of pressure ulcers to the head and ears involves using surfaces that alleviate pressure points. These include water mattresses or pillows, air[90] and gel mattresses, pillows, and wedges that equalize the pressure around the head and ears. Turning the infant a minimum of every 4 hours is necessary, along with careful inspection of skin surfaces. Even when turning side to side is not feasible, lifting the head, shoulders, and hips and supporting these areas with pressure-reducing surfaces is helpful. Once a pressure ulcer occurs, wound care is necessary using moist healing techniques and principles.[88,91,92]

Managing Pain

There are a variety of interventions that have been shown to reduce pain and agitation in NICU patients. It is important that strategies be put in place to prevent and manage infant pain and agitation. Exposure to painful procedures in otherwise healthy term infants has been shown to result in short-term hyperanalgesia.[93] Repeated exposure to stress and pain in the neonatal period has been shown to have long-term detrimental effects including a reduction in brain white matter, decreased growth in the parietal and temporal lobes, and impaired brain organization.[94,95] Additional studies have shown that repeated early pain exposures in premature infants result in poorer cognitive and motor function at 8 and 18 months' corrected age and altered cortical brain-wave patterns in the resting brain at school age.[96,97]

TABLE 28-3 Strategies to Minimize Stress and Overstimulation

- Swaddle or provide boundaries to promote flex position.
- Place prone with arms and knees flexed or side-lying with hands in midline.
- Move the infant slowly during position changes and contain limbs to avoid startle response.
- Avoid hyperextending neck or arms.
- Coordinate care activities to reduce handling and sleep disruptions.
- Provide care during times when the infant is awake rather than according to a fixed schedule.
- Prior to handling, bring the infant to a quiet alert stage by talking in a soft voice and touching the infant gently.
- Reduce environmental noise in the unit.
- Implement periods of "quiet time" on each shift with lights dim and noise minimized.
- Cover the incubator to reduce exposure to bright lights.
- If medically stable, dress and bundle the infant.

Data from Koszarek K, Ricouard D. Nursing assessment and care of the neonate in acute respiratory distress. In: Fraser D, ed. *Acute Respiratory Care of the Neonate*. 3rd ed. Petaluma, Calif., NICU INK Books, 2012:65-108.

The first and most important strategy should be to decrease the number of stressful procedures (Table 28-3). Skin-to-skin care,[98] facilitated tucking,[99,100] and swaddling[101] have been shown to reduce agitation and pain responses to acute painful procedures and may be useful as adjunctive strategies for the management of ongoing pain.[102]

Oral sucrose has been shown to reduce crying when offered to newborns during painful procedures such as heel-stick blood sampling. Dipping a pacifier in sucrose was also shown to significantly reduce pain responses in premature infants.[101] However, there is controversy regarding the efficacy and long-term effects of repeated doses of sucrose.[103]

Routine administration of opiates and sedatives for ventilated infants remains controversial.[102] Use of opiates for ventilated infants during routine caregiving procedures has been reported to improve oxygenation and blood pressure stability[104] and is the most effective treatment of moderate to severe pain.[6] However, opioids may interfere with the infant's own respiratory effort and prolong weaning from assisted ventilation.[6,105] In a large randomized trial, there were no benefits seen with the continuous administration of morphine to ventilated preterm infants.[106] A systematic review of 13 studies involving more than 1500 infants found that there was insufficient evidence to recommend routine use of opioids in neonates receiving mechanical ventilation because pain scores did not decrease with treatment and morphine did not reduce adverse effects (death, intraventricular hemorrhage, and periventricular leukomalacia).[107]

In addition, the safety profile for morphine in preterm infants has not been established. A secondary analysis of infants in the NEOPAIN trial found that head circumference and body weight at 5 to 7 years of age were smaller/lower in premature infants treated with morphine compared to infants receiving a placebo.[108]

Narcotic abstinence syndrome (NAS) is a risk when higher doses of opioids are administered over a prolonged period of time. In a study of 19 neonates receiving fentanyl for at least 24 hours, symptoms of withdrawal were seen in 53%. Higher doses and longer duration of administration increased the likelihood of withdrawal.[109] Signs of NAS including irritability, tachypnea, jitteriness, increased tone, vomiting, diarrhea, sneezing, hiccoughs, and skin abrasions may be seen when narcotics are weaned rapidly.[110]

Abrupt discontinuation of opioids should be avoided and these infants weaned in a slow and planned manner. Monitoring for signs of abstinence should also be part of the weaning plan.

Medications are best used judiciously, taking into account the stage of illness, therapeutic goals, and individual infant characteristics. Other causes of agitation should be considered, including inadequate ventilation. In many cases, patient comfort is often the best indicator of the appropriateness of selected ventilator support modes, perhaps more useful than blood gases. The infant's response to all interventions should be assessed and documented. Clear communication among health care team members is critical to ensure that pain is appropriately managed and the potential side effects of pain medication limited.

Developmental Care

The NICU environment is known to be bright, noisy, and over-stimulating to premature or sick infants who may not have the capacity to cope. The seminal work of Heidelise Als[111] provided the basis for our understanding of newborn adaptation as an integration of physiologic and behavioral systems. An inability to cope with environmental stimuli causes dysfunctional autonomic, state, and motor responses. The ability to cope with stimuli such as light, noise, touch, and pain is inversely proportional to gestation age, with very preterm infants lacking the self-regulatory mechanisms to promote stability. A number of studies have examined various interventions aimed at modifying the NICU environment to support optimal preterm infant development. Attempts at systematically reviewing developmental care interventions have been hampered by a lack of consistency among interventions. Studies examining individual interventions have shown benefit; however, evaluation of a broader group of interventions such as the Newborn Individualized Developmental Care and Assessment Program have failed to demonstrate long-term benefits.[112] Despite lack of clear long-term benefits of a formalized developmental care program, there is a large body of literature that shows the detrimental effects of stress, including excessive noise and handling.[113-115] A comprehensive plan of care for VLBW infants should include strategies to promote uninterrupted sleep, reduce stressful procedures, and promote self-regulation through supportive positioning, encouraging nonnutritive sucking, and hand-to-mouth behaviors. Parents should be taught to recognize both approach and avoidance signals displayed by their infant and should be encouraged to modify their interactions according to the infant's developmental stage.

Skin-to-Skin Holding

Skin-to-skin or kangaroo care confers significant benefits for both newborns and their parents. Short-term benefits include stabilizing heart rate, oxygen saturation, and breathing patterns;[116] improved sleep–wake cycles;[116,117] increased growth rate;[118] decreased response to pain;[98,119] improved breast-feeding duration; and greater maternal attachment.[116] Longer-term benefits of kangaroo care have not been well established but the short-term benefits may have a positive effect on neurodevelopmental outcomes by affecting brain development at critical periods. Kangaroo care in the NICU has been identified as significant in reducing parental stress and facilitating parent–infant bonding.[120-122]

Kangaroo care can be done with ventilated infants (Fig. 28-6) and is an important part of family-centered care. A prospective study of 53 premature infants with a mean weight of 1253 g (range 631 to 1700 g), including 5 ventilated infants, found that

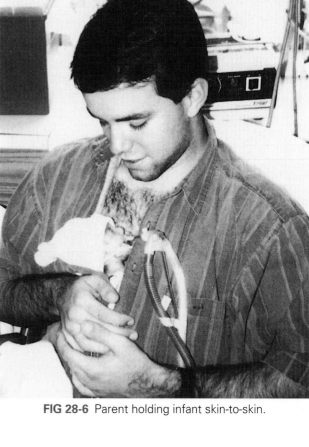

FIG 28-6 Parent holding infant skin-to-skin.

the infants remained clinically stable with more efficient gas exchange, with no risk of hypothermia even for infants weighing less than 1000 g.[123] Practical issues during skin-to-skin holding include transfer techniques from bed/incubator to parent, selecting chairs that support parent and infant comfortably, and monitoring during holding. Transfer techniques include carefully moving the baby to the seated parent or having the parent stand while the infant is placed on is or her chest; then the parent carefully lowers himself or herself with the infant onto the chair. Other nurseries have invested in special lounge or reclining chairs that can be raised to the level of the infant's incubator, which then provide a comfortable way for the parent to relax during holding for prolonged periods. Continuous monitoring of heart rate, oxygenation, and skin temperature is necessary to determine each individual infant's tolerance during holding. Careful monitoring of all physiologic parameters is necessary during skin-to-skin holding to assess each infant's response to this valuable experience and to determine when nursing intervention is needed.

The knowledge level and comfort with skin-to-skin care among nurses and other health care providers has been identified as a barrier to the implementation of skin-to-skin holding.[121,124] Education programs to enhance knowledge and comfort should be undertaken to increase the utilization of skin-to-skin holding for infants receiving respiratory support.

CARE OF THE FAMILY

Providing support for the family is the responsibility of all members of the health care team and that family should be viewed as an integral part of the team. Most NICUs have adopted a family-centered care (FCC) approach to neonatal care that recognizes the importance of integrating family members in care decisions. FCC is based on principles of participation and partnership that come from empowering family members to be involved in their infant's care.[125] Providing open access to the unit for parents, having parents participate in infant caregiving, and maintaining open communication are basic principles of FCC.[126]

Having an infant that requires NICU care is an extremely stressful event for parents and extended family members. It is important to recognize the impact of having a newborn in an intensive care setting and to recognize the social and cultural influence that may shape the parents' approach to coping and communication. True FCC is built on a trusting relationship between parents and health care team members. That trusting relationship begins with open and honest communication.

Fostering parental partnership should begin when a high-risk pregnancy is identified. Providing information and an opportunity to meet members of the team helps to increase family members' awareness and comfort level before they are faced with the overwhelming situation of having their baby admitted to the NICU. Parents should receive an orientation to the unit and should be provided with written (and sometimes audiovisual) material that they can refer to. Material should include an overview of visiting policies, an introduction to members of the health care team, and contact information. This written material is the ideal place to reinforce important roles the parents can play such as providing breast milk, participating in skin-to-skin holding, and helping to provide care for their infant. In many units parents are given the opportunity to participate in rounds at their infant's bedside and/or to meet with the team on a regular basis to discuss their infant's care. Where available, parent or peer-support groups are valuable, especially for families who do not have extended family nearby.[127]

Each family presents with unique strengths and weaknesses and has a varying capacity for coping in a crisis situation. Understand the family dynamics and coping strategies will assist care providers in meeting the family "where it is at" and working together to build capacity for providing care for the family's infant.

SUMMARY

In conclusion, the daily care of newborns who are receiving respiratory support involves knowledge that extends beyond pulmonary anatomy, physiology, and technology. Care of these infants requires advanced knowledge of multiple organ systems, precision in caregiving, and creative problem solving. Also critical to successful outcomes is attention to developmental care and FCC during this vulnerable period for infants and their families.

REFERENCES

A complete reference list is available at https://expertconsult.inkling.com/.

29

Nutritional Support

Laura D. Brown, MD, Edward F. Bell, MD, and William W. Hay, Jr., MD

Optimal nutritional support is fundamental for the survival, good health, growth, and development of newborn infants who require intensive care, particularly those who require assisted ventilation. Most of these infants suffer disorders that place them at risk for poor nutrition as a result of increased metabolic rate, limited gastrointestinal function, and limited capacity for metabolic processing of ingested nutrients. Hypoxia, circulatory insufficiency, fluid and electrolyte imbalance, acid–base disorders, and deficiencies in anabolic hormones also complicate the ability to sustain optimal growth. Furthermore, physiologically unstable preterm or "sick" infants often face limitations in the tolerance and processing of enterally and parenterally delivered nutrients. As a result of such poor nutrition, impaired somatic growth is common in these infants, which directly and adversely restricts lung growth and recovery from lung injuries,[1] as well as brain growth, which produces abnormal neurodevelopmental outcomes.[2-5]

The most widely accepted standard for developing nutritional goals for preterm infants is the intrauterine growth rate of a fetus of corresponding postmenstrual age.[6,7] Intrauterine growth rates, body composition, and energy expenditure are all used to define the nutritional requirements of the healthy, growing preterm infant. For term infants, the growth and nutrient intake of healthy breast-fed infants are used as references. Surprisingly, much less attention has been paid to how the physiology of illness affects growth, metabolism, and nutrient requirements.[8] For example, the goals of nutritional support for infants who require assisted ventilation are to prevent catabolism and exhaustion of endogenous energy resources, to achieve growth in lean body mass, and to promote healing, growth, and maturation of the lungs, brain, and other vital organs. These nutritional goals must be met without impairing respiratory gas exchange or tissue oxygen delivery. Thus, the nutritional support for infants with respiratory distress syndrome (RDS), chronic lung disease (CLD), and bronchopulmonary dysplasia (BPD) requires special consideration.

NUTRITIONAL REQUIREMENTS

Water Requirement

Water is a key element in nutritional management, because energy, protein, and other nutrients cannot be delivered without water, and optimal water intake is important for all infants who require assisted ventilation.[9] Water is required for growth and is produced in small amounts as a by-product of cellular metabolism. Water comprises a large fraction of body weight in preterm and term infants,[10] declining after birth with improvement in renal function[11] triggered, at least in part, by atrial

natriuretic peptide.[12] Body water balance and thus weight may not decrease, however, and in fact often increase with aggressive fluid intake from intravenous (IV) solutions (both dextrose only and total parenteral nutrition (TPN) solutions). Normal infants with good kidney and lung function generally tolerate high rates of IV fluid. In contrast, physiologically unstable infants, such as preterm infants with RDS requiring supplemental oxygen and ventilators, often have poor renal function in the first days after birth. Excessive water intake with limited renal function leads to fluid accumulation in the lung, which worsens lung function and increases the need for potentially injurious oxygen and ventilator support. Knowledge of the factors that affect water balance is essential in estimating water requirements, especially for preterm and critically ill infants who require assisted ventilation, because excessive water balance, particularly with increased salt intake, can compromise lung function. Pulmonary edema due to fluid overload can contribute to decreased pulmonary compliance and increased airway resistance.[1] A Cochrane review showed that restricted water intake significantly reduced the risk of patent ductus arteriosus and tended to reduce the risk of BPD.[13]

Insensible Water Loss

Smaller, less mature infants lose more water by evaporation because of greater surface area–to–body weight ratios, thinner and more permeable skin, dry ambient air, higher respiratory rates, and increased humidity gradient between the upper respiratory airway and the gas mixture they breathe. Antenatal corticosteroids given to promote fetal maturation reduce the insensible water loss (IWL) of very preterm infants during the first few days of life, presumably by enhancing epidermal barrier function.[14] Several devices also have been shown to decrease IWL. Transparent thermal blankets can reduce IWL by preterm infants in incubators.[15] Polyethylene occlusive skin wrapping also reduces the IWL of infants under radiant warmers, including during resuscitation in the delivery room.[16] In recent years, IWL has been much reduced with improved humidification of incubators,[17] ventilators, and respiratory gas circuits that allow spontaneous breathing by the infant, such as continuous positive airway pressure (CPAP) or heated high-flow nasal cannula.[18]

Renal Water Excretion

The amount of water required for urine production depends on the renal solute load and the renal concentrating ability. The term newborn infant can produce urine as dilute as 50 mOsm per liter and can concentrate to a maximum osmolality only slightly above plasma. The preterm infant's kidney is limited to a narrower range of concentrating ability, producing a higher renal sodium excretion rate.[19]

The renal solute load comes from two sources: *exogenous*, primarily electrolytes and metabolic products of nutrients, and *endogenous*, products of catabolism or changes in body composition.[20] In practice, the amount of solute excreted by the kidney is larger than the exogenous or potential solute load, because many of these infants are in a catabolic state; in such cases, the exogenous solute intake is usually low, so that the actual solute excretion is still generally less than what the sick or physiologically unstable infant's kidneys can excrete (about 35 mOsm/kg/day). In contrast, growing infants deposit some of the exogenous solute in the body (approximately 1 mOsm per gram of weight gain) so that the actual solute load is less than the potential. An infant receiving preterm formula with a potential renal solute load of 24 mOsm/100 kcal at 125 kcal/kg/day (30 mOsm/kg/day) and gaining 15 g/kg/day of weight would excrete about 15 mOsm/kg/day. Avoiding excess solute load is desirable, particularly to avoid accumulation of salts and water in the lung that could lead to increased oxygen and ventilator requirements. It is unusual, though, with modern TPN solutions, enteral nutrient mixtures, and enteral supplements, to exceed renal solute excretion capacity, even in very preterm infants.

The critically ill infant who requires assisted ventilation may have special problems with renal handling of water. Hypoxia or hypotension during the course of the illness may compromise the kidney function by causing tubular or cortical injury. During the anuric or oliguric phase of acute tubular necrosis (ATN), the renal water excretion is markedly reduced, and its allowance in the maintenance water calculation should be reduced accordingly. In the diuretic phase of ATN, water excretion through the kidney is markedly increased.

The renal function of infants with RDS is similar to that of infants of the same gestational age without respiratory disease so long as normal blood gas and acid–base status can be maintained. However, in a large case series, RDS was an independent predictor of renal impairment, presumably due to associated hypoxia and acidosis that may have reduced renal perfusion.[21] Most preterm infants, including those with RDS, have an increase in urine volume on the second or third day of life,[22,23] which is accompanied by a rise in plasma atrial natriuretic peptide[24] and contraction of the extracellular water compartment.[12] These changes are often temporally associated with improvement in respiratory function. There is no evidence, however, that renal function is affected by specific methods of assisted ventilation, such as conventional ventilation or high-frequency oscillation.[25] Furthermore, there is no evidence to support routine administration of diuretic therapy to promote diuresis in preterm infants with RDS.[26]

Energy Requirement

Healthy preterm infants gain weight at rates similar to the fetus of corresponding postmenstrual age (15 to 18 g/kg/day). An average intake of 110 to 130 kcal/kg/day from preterm infant formula or human milk is generally sufficient to support normal growth and metabolism of very low birth-weight preterm infants, provided protein intake is adequate.[27] This broad range of energy intake is designed to accommodate the needs of rapidly growing, extremely low birth-weight infants, who may need higher energy delivery for growth, as well as larger, more mature preterm infants who may require less. Moreover, infants receiving high energy intakes develop excess body fat without accelerating their gain in fat-free mass.[28-30] The energy from the diet that is not lost in the stool or urine (about 10% of intake) is either expended for metabolism or stored in the body for growth. Energy is expended during rest (about 50 kcal/kg/day for preterm infants) and also for activity, thermoregulation, postprandial or synthetic energy expenditure, and growth (Table 29-1).[7,27,31-34] Calorie needs vary depending on whether the infant is enterally or parenterally fed. The energy expended during growth in human infants has been estimated to be 5.5 kcal/g of new tissue deposited for protein and 1.6 kcal/g for fat.[35] Estimates of the overall energy cost of growth range from about 2.9 to 6.0 kcal/g.[36] The energy cost of physical activity in healthy, preterm infants accounts for only about 3% of the total daily energy expenditure.[37]

Energy demands, oxygen consumption, and resting energy expenditure are 15% to 25% higher in infants with respiratory disease such as apnea, RDS, and BPD and those on mechanical ventilation,[38] an important factor to consider when providing nutrition to this vulnerable population. Energy expenditure is increased during therapy with caffeine for apnea of prematurity.[39] Preterm infants with RDS have increased oxygen consumption in the first 1 to 2 days of life, and oxygen consumption is directly correlated with the amount of ventilator support the infant requires.[40,41]

Energy expenditure is increased with more severe RDS requiring higher levels of ventilatory support and oxygen administration, which together are associated with higher risk of BPD.[42-44] Spontaneously breathing infants with BPD also have increased rates of energy expenditure,[45-48] in conjunction with lower energy intake and poor weight gain.[49] Increased oxygen consumption is not entirely due to increased work of breathing, however, as strategies implemented to improve pulmonary function do not necessarily decrease oxygen consumption.[50] Low energy intake (<100 kcal/kg/day) also increases the risk of severe retinopathy of prematurity (ROP) in extremely preterm infants.[51]

Protein Requirement

The provision of parenteral or enteral protein soon after birth is essential to prevent negative nitrogen balance and promote protein accretion. Preterm infants have lower lean mass and higher body fat by postmenstrual age 40 weeks compared to

TABLE 29-1 Energy, Protein, and Nutrient Requirements for Preterm Infants

Nutrient	ADVISABLE INTAKE (PER KG/DAY)	
	<1000-g Infant	1000- to 1500-g Infant
Energy (kcal)	110-130	110
Protein (g)	3.5-4.5	3.5-4.0
Sodium (mmol)	3.6	3.0
Potassium (mmol)	2.5	2.2
Chloride (mmol)	3.2	2.6
Calcium (mg)	150-220	120-200
Phosphorus (mg)	60-140	60-140
Magnesium (mg)	8-15	8-15
Iron (mg)	3.0-4.0	2.0-3.0
Zinc (mg)	1.0-3.0	1.0-3.0
Copper (mg)	0.2	0.2

normally growing fetuses at term.[52] Specifically, infants with BPD have decreased lean body mass, indicating that current levels of protein intake might be inadequate.[53,54] Thus, providing an optimal balance of protein and energy is critically important to maximize lean tissue and organ growth.[28] The protein requirement of the healthy term infant in the first month of life is approximately 2.0 g/kg/day. Estimates of the protein requirement of preterm infants are higher than for term infants and range between 3.5 and 4.5 g/kg/day depending on gestational age (see Table 29-1).[32,55,56] These estimates are supported by experimental studies of protein turnover, nitrogen balance, tissue accretion, and growth.

Preterm infants, including those who require assisted ventilation, benefit from IV amino acids starting as soon after birth as possible.[57-59] In a retrospective analysis of a large multicenter database, early initiation of IV amino acids was associated with better growth, as assessed by gain in weight, length, and head circumference from birth to 36 weeks' postmenstrual age.[60] Although this study did not evaluate lung growth specifically, linear and head growth measurements are better indicators of lean tissue growth (including the lung) than weight measurements alone. Furthermore, the severity of BPD is reduced among infants who receive more nutrition during the first 3 weeks after birth.[61] In adults, branched-chain amino acids such as leucine in IV nutrient solutions can modulate respiratory distress, decreasing Pco_2 and stimulating the ventilatory response to hypercarbia, corresponding to an enhanced ventilatory sensitivity.[62] In preterm infants of ~30 weeks' gestation, providing higher concentrations of branched-chain amino acids in parenteral nutrition results in increased dynamic lung compliance, decreased pulmonary resistance, and fewer episodes of apnea,[63] findings also observed in neonatal piglet studies.[64] Finally, infants given a nutrient-enriched formula through 3 months of age demonstrate greater linear growth and lean and bone mass growth when fed higher intakes of protein, calcium, phosphorus, and zinc than are provided in standard formulas.[53]

Lipid Requirement

Lipids are important as a source of energy for metabolism and growth. For preterm infants, a reasonable range of fat intake is 4.4 to 6.0 g of fat per 100 kcal (40% to 55% of energy intake).[32] Only two fatty acids are known to be essential (cannot be synthesized in the body) for humans: α-linolenic acid, an ω3 fatty acid, and linoleic acid, an ω6 fatty acid. Milk and most formulas contain adequate amounts of these two essential fatty acids, linoleic acid and α-linolenic acid, from which the essential long-chain polyunsaturated fatty acids (LC-PUFAs), such as arachidonic acid (AA) and docosahexaenoic acid (DHA), respectively, are derived. These LC-PUFAs play particularly important biological roles in development as immune modulators and components of membrane phospholipids and are essential for normal development of the central nervous system.[65,66] Preterm infants have insufficient capacity for de novo synthesis of LC-PUFAs, requiring that these substrates are received from the diet. For infants fed intravenously, the requirement for LC-PUFAs can be met by providing 0.5 to 1.0 g/kg/day intake in the form of IV lipid emulsion.[31]

Lipid emulsions are a key component of parenteral feeding regimens for infants who require assisted ventilation, providing an important source of energy. Early introduction of soybean oil–based emulsions in preterm infants was shown to have detrimental effects on pulmonary gas exchange and hemodynamics,[67,68] though a meta-analysis of this practice did not show beneficial or adverse effects on growth, death, or CLD.[69]

ω3 LC-PUFAs such as DHA and AA are found in human milk. There is no evidence from clinical trials that adding LC-PUFAs to commercial term infant formulas confers benefits.[70] However, based on theoretical benefits that they could improve visual acuity,[71] neurodevelopmental outcomes,[72] and lung development,[1,73] and evidence from studies that show no harm,[65] they are commonly added to commercial infant formulas.

Decreased DHA and AA levels in preterm infants are associated with an increased risk of BPD.[74] Preterm infants born to mothers randomized to high-dose supplements to augment DHA in their breast milk showed a reduced incidence of BPD compared to standard-dose supplements.[75] It might be that LC-PUFA requirements for extremely low birth-weight infants are much higher than what is seen in term breast milk; thus, higher supplemental doses of DHA might be of greater benefit and require further investigation.[66]

Carbohydrate Requirement

Approximately half of an infant's energy needs are normally provided by carbohydrate metabolism. Moreover, glucose is the primary energy source for brain metabolism. In the preterm infant, glucose is largely derived from exogenous carbohydrate sources once glycogenolysis has exhausted stored hepatic glucose. Gluconeogenesis develops soon after birth and is not easily suppressed by increases in plasma glucose or insulin concentrations, thus contributing to a common problem of hyperglycemia in preterm infants.[76,77] Maintenance of normal plasma glucose concentrations is fundamental, as the vital organs (brain and heart) take up glucose according to plasma concentration and not IV infusion rates or rates of hepatic glucose production. When plasma glucose concentrations decline, the newborn brain may use ketone bodies as additional energy sources, but these are usually limited in very preterm and small-for-gestational-age infants with intrauterine growth restriction (IUGR) who have low body stores of fat.[78]

Preterm and stressed infants are at risk for developing hyperglycemia, especially those with respiratory distress, mechanical ventilation, and restricted cardiac output and circulation. Such infants often are intermittently hypoxic, which adds to increased glucagon, adrenaline, and glucocorticoid secretion. These stress-reactive hormones reduce insulin secretion and insulin action and promote glucose production from both glycogenolysis (acutely) and gluconeogenesis (over a sustained period). They also contribute to protein breakdown. Hyperglycemia leads to increased cellular allostatic load, in which excess carbon cannot be fully oxidized, producing increased amounts of reactive oxygen species that cause cellular breakdown (Table 29-2).[79]

Other complications of hyperglycemia frequently develop in neonates when maximal glucose oxidative capacity (>12 mg/kg/min) is exceeded, including increased energy expenditure (glucose-to-fat synthesis is energy expensive), increased oxygen consumption (and hypoxia), increased carbon dioxide production,[48,80] increased fat deposition in excess of lean mass, and increased fatty infiltration of heart and liver.[81,82] Such problems may underlie the increased morbidity and mortality in infants with severe and/or persistent hyperglycemia.[83]

TABLE 29-2 Toxicity from Hyperglycemia and Excess Allostatic Load

Excess Glucose, Cortisol, and Mitochondrial Allostatic Load (Acute as well as Chronic)

Increased cortisol and catecholamine levels

Hyperglycemia

Increased insulin*

Increased cell glucose uptake

Increased Mitochondrial Allostatic Load

Mitochondrial fragmentation

Increased reactive oxygen species production

Accumulation of mitochondrial DNA damage

Decreased energy-producing capacity

Increased susceptibility to cell death

Cellular Dysfunction

Oxidative stress

Molecular damage

Telomere shortening

Cell loss, apoptosis

Energy deficiency

Systemic Inflammation

Increased circulating proinflammatory cytokines

*Also antiinflammatory, by suppressing proinflammatory transcription factors (nuclear factor B, activator protein-1, and early growth response-1).

Mechanisms for enteral carbohydrate digestion and absorption mature in a defined sequence in the human fetus. Sucrase, maltase, and isomaltase are usually fully active by 24 to 28 weeks' gestation, but lactase lags behind the others and is not fully active until term.[84] For this reason, most preterm formulas contain lower lactose content than that in human milk. However, there is evidence that intestinal lactase activity increases to adequate functional levels within a few days after the initiation of enteral feedings, even in infants born as early as 28 weeks' gestation.[85,86] Furthermore, despite the late gestational rise in lactase activity, both term and preterm infants seem to tolerate the carbohydrates in human milk and commercial formulas quite well. Activity of pancreatic amylase remains low until after term.[84] Salivary amylase activity is present even in very preterm infants.[87]

Other carbohydrates such as mannose and inositol, as well as oligosaccharides (prebiotics), play an important role in nutrition and organ development for the preterm infant. Mannose is an essential carbohydrate for protein glycosylation and normal neural development.[88] Mannose is a component of oligosaccharides, which contribute to the establishment of nonpathogenic intestinal flora, and play a major role in intestinal health for both term and preterm infants.[89] Inositol is particularly important for lung development, as it is integral in the formation of surfactant phospholipid production. Inositol is present in high concentrations in human milk and can be synthesized by newborn infants of gestational age 33 weeks or more.[90] There is evidence that lower inositol concentrations are associated with more severe RDS[91] and that inositol supplementation may reduce the incidence of RDS.[92] Benefits of routinely supplementing preterm infant nutrition with inositol are being investigated.[93]

Mineral Requirements

The requirements of sodium, potassium, and chloride are all between 2 and 4 mmol/kg/day (see Table 29-1).[7] The requirement of sodium may be even higher for preterm infants, particularly in the first week of life because of urinary sodium losses. Urinary excretion of electrolytes depends on intake. Typical urinary concentrations of sodium are 20 to 40 mmol/L and of potassium 10 to 30 mmol/L.[9] When the infant is receiving diuretic therapy, urinary sodium concentrations can reach 70 mmol/L or higher, and these large losses must be considered when electrolyte needs are assessed. This is particularly important as insufficient sodium intake impairs longitudinal growth and weight gain.[94]

The recommended intakes of calcium and phosphorus depend on the route of administration. If given enterally, absorption rates might be limiting. The fraction of calcium absorbed depends on the type of milk or formula and the infant's gestational and postnatal age. If given parenterally, the limits of mineral solubility become a significant factor. Adequate enteral intake of calcium for term infants in the first 6 months of life is about 70 mg/kg/day. The calcium requirement for preterm infants is much higher, 150 to 220 mg/kg/day, because of more active bone formation and remodeling (see Table 29-1).[33,95] Adequate enteral intake of phosphorus for term infants is ~30 mg/kg/day but is higher for preterm infants (60 to 140 mg/kg/day) to ensure adequate bone mineralization. Fortification of human milk is necessary to ensure adequate intakes of calcium and phosphorus to preterm infants who are fed human milk by bottle or tube, particularly with mature mother's milk and donor milk.[96] Recommended IV intakes of calcium and phosphorus are lower than enteral requirements, ranging from 65 to 100 mg/kg/day for calcium and 50 to 80 mg/kg/day for phosphorus.[33] The risk factors in preterm infants for calcium and phosphorus deficiency and subsequent rickets are gestational age less than 27 weeks or birth weight less than 1000 g, long-term parenteral nutrition (>4 to 5 weeks), severe BPD requiring diuretics and fluid restriction, long-term steroid treatment, a history of necrotizing enterocolitis (NEC), and intolerance to enteral formula or human milk.[95]

Adequate intake of magnesium for enterally fed term and preterm infants is about 10 mg/kg/day (see Table 29-1). Intravenous intake of 7 to 10 mg/kg/day is recommended for infants receiving TPN for prolonged periods.[33]

Iron intake should be 2 to 4 mg/kg/day for both term and preterm infants who are enterally fed[34] but increased to 6 mg/kg/day for preterm infants with anemia of prematurity who are receiving recombinant erythropoietin.[31,97] Up to three-fourths of preterm infants will develop iron deficiency anemia in their first half-year of life if they do not receive enough iron from supplements or formula.[98] One study found improved neurocognitive outcomes when iron supplements were started at 2 weeks vs 8 weeks after birth,[99] and a recent meta-analysis found improved mental performance and psychomotor development when iron supplements were started soon after birth.[100] The American Academy of Pediatrics guidelines recommend that 2 to 4 mg/kg/day of iron should be provided to growing preterm infants beginning at 2 weeks of age.[31] Risk of iron overload and toxicity (e.g., possible increased risk of ROP, increased risk of infection, and impaired growth) from unnecessary iron supplementation following red blood cell transfusions also must be considered[101]; commonly, iron supplementation is delayed for 2 weeks after a transfusion. Each red blood cell transfusion in preterm infants typically adds 8 mg/kg iron, and hepatic iron stores as well as serum ferritin concentrations are highly correlated to the number of blood transfusions received.[102,103] Formula-fed infants

TABLE 29-3   Vitamin and Mineral Requirements for Preterm Infants

	Advisable Intake (per day)
Vitamin A	400-3330 IU/kg
Vitamin D	400-1000 IU
Vitamin E	3.3-16.4 IU/kg
Vitamin K	4.4-28 µg/kg
Vitamin C	20-55 mg/kg
Thiamin (B1)	140-300 µg/kg
Riboflavin (B2)	200-400 µg/kg
Niacin (B3)	1.0-5.5 mg/kg
Pyridoxine (B6)	50-300 µg/kg
Biotin	1.7-16.5 µg/kg
Pantothenic acid	0.5-2.1 mg
Folic acid	35-100 µg
Cobalamin (B12)	0.1-0.8 µg/kg

should receive iron-fortified formula, beginning with the first formula feedings,[104,105] to help counter anemia of prematurity and to ensure adequate iron supply to the growing brain, as iron is preferentially taken up by red blood cells.[34] Because individual infants vary considerably in their hematocrit at birth, delayed cord blood clamping, transfusions, blood sampling, and erythropoietin treatment, it is helpful to monitor their iron status and need for iron supplementation by following serum ferritin concentrations.[102] Research to define the benefits and risks of iron supplementation and fortification of milk and formula in preterm infants is sorely lacking.[34]

The advisable enteral intakes of zinc and copper are 1 to 3 and 0.1 to 0.2 mg/kg/day, respectively. Zinc has been shown to improve growth specifically in extremely low birth-weight preterm infants with CLD receiving human milk.[106] Other minerals such as selenium, manganese, iodine, chromium, and molybdenum are also required in trace amounts (Table 29-3).[107]

Vitamin Requirements

Vitamin A is essential for growth and differentiation of epithelial tissues, including those in the lung. Preterm infants have low stores of vitamin A at birth, and preterm infants with lung disease have lower plasma vitamin A levels than those without lung disease.[108] Thus, vitamin A deficiency may contribute to the development of BPD. A large randomized clinical trial showed a reduction in the risk of death or BPD (defined as a requirement for supplemental oxygen at 36 weeks' postmenstrual age) with vitamin A supplementation, 5000 IU given intramuscularly three times a week for 4 weeks.[109] A systematic review of eight clinical trials of vitamin A supplementation to preterm infants confirmed the beneficial effect of vitamin A in reducing the risk of death or oxygen requirement at 1 month of age by 7% (relative risk 0.93, 95% confidence interval 0.88 to 0.99). Neurodevelopmental assessment of surviving infants showed no differences between groups at 18 to 22 months' corrected age.[109] The number needed to treat was 20 to allow survival of one more infant without BPD. In the review, other morbidities and mortality were not significantly reduced by vitamin A supplementation. Despite its efficacy, vitamin A supplementation has not become standard practice,[110] in part because of the need for repeated intramuscular injections, as absorption from the gastrointestinal tract does not appear to be sufficient.

Vitamin D is essential for bone health. As with other fat-soluble vitamins, the body stores of vitamin D are low at birth, especially in preterm infants.[111] Infants who require assisted ventilation have no exposure to ultraviolet light in the hospital and limited exposure after discharge and thus have minimal cutaneous synthesis of vitamin D. The recommended enteral intake of vitamin D is 200 to 400 IU per day regardless of body weight.[95,112] This dose is probably sufficient to maintain adequate (>50 nmol/L) serum concentrations of vitamin D and to prevent vitamin D-deficiency–associated rickets.[33] Higher doses (800 to 1000 IU per day) have been recommended for vitamin D–deficient newborns[113] (see Table 29-3). The major circulating metabolite of vitamin D after its 25-hydroxylation in the liver is 25-hydroxyvitamin D. Levels may be monitored in infants at risk for developing rickets, including those infants with extreme prematurity, short bowel syndrome, cholestasis, and long-term exposure to diuretics and/or steroids.

Vitamin E is a major natural antioxidant in the body. It protects lipid-containing cell membranes against oxidative injury and is thought to play a role in preventing neonatal oxygen toxicity. The recommended enteral vitamin E intake, 3.3 to 16.4 IU/kg/day, is sufficient to compensate for variation in vitamin E absorption and distribution and in the intake of other nutrients known to influence vitamin E requirement, such as iron and LC-PUFAs.[107] The amount of vitamin E required to prevent lipid peroxidation in vulnerable tissues depends on the PUFA content of the tissues and diet.[114] Thus, it also is advisable to keep the dietary ratio of vitamin E to PUFAs at or above the level of 0.6 mg of D-α-tocopherol (0.9 IU) per gram of PUFAs.[114] Recommended IV doses of vitamin E are 2.8 IU/kg/day as α-tocopheryl acetate.[115] Though studies have shown efficacy of vitamin E supplementation in reducing the risk of ROP and intraventricular hemorrhage, excessive intake of vitamin E has the potential for severe toxicity including risk of sepsis.[116] Consequently, routine administration of high-dose vitamin E supplements is not recommended, even though a single enteral dose of vitamin E at birth may help correct the relative vitamin E deficiency that has been found in some very preterm infants in the first days of life.[117]

Vitamin K is essential to prevent hemorrhagic disease of the newborn in the first weeks of life.[118,119] A single dose of intramuscular vitamin K (1.0 mg) is effective in the prevention of classic hemorrhagic disease of the newborn.[120] Subsequent supplementation with vitamin K is necessary to prevent deficiency, especially for critically ill infants, who often receive broad-spectrum antibiotics (reducing vitamin K synthesis by gut bacteria) and may have other abnormalities of hemostasis or hepatic function.

Infants with fat malabsorption due to cholestatic liver disease or short bowel syndrome are at risk for developing fat-soluble vitamin deficiency. Thus, additional fat-soluble vitamin supplementation may be necessary in these patients. Additional nutrients, such as water-soluble vitamins and other trace substances, are required for recovery and healthy growth of preterm infants (see Table 29-3).

PARENTERAL NUTRITION

Parenteral nutritional support is essential for providing a continuous supply of both macro- and micronutrients to the preterm infant starting immediately after birth and as enteral feedings are being advanced, particularly in those infants who cannot tolerate enteral feedings.

Intravenous Access

Indwelling short polyvinyl chloride catheters provide safe and convenient access to the peripheral venous circulation. Hand and arm sites are preferred, but scalp veins are sometimes necessary. The most common significant complication of peripheral IV infusions is tissue necrosis at the site of extravasation.[121] The infusion site must be carefully observed to detect extravasation as soon as possible. Infusions with glucose concentrations greater than 12.5 g/dL should be avoided in peripheral veins.

Central vein catheters, usually Silastic, are used for longer term IV delivery of nutrients to newborn infants. Umbilical vein catheters are placed immediately after birth into most preterm and sick term infants who require iv nutrition and other treatments. The *percutaneously inserted central catheter* is the preferred technique for long-term central venous access. With good care, the risk of infectious complications is very low, but removing such lines as soon as possible is essential to reduce rates of line sepsis and other complications such as thrombosis or extravasation of infused fluid into the pleural or pericardial space.[122] The *surgically placed central vein catheter* is typically used for infants who have required gastrointestinal surgery for gut malformation (especially gastroschisis) or NEC and for whom extensively prolonged parenteral nutrition is anticipated.

Composition of Total Parenteral Nutrition

Preterm infants who are ill enough to require assisted ventilation should receive IV nutrition as soon as possible after birth. The initial infusion should consist of 10% dextrose in water to prevent hypoglycemia, though occasionally this concentration of dextrose will induce hyperglycemia in the extremely low birth-weight infant. It is now abundantly clear that providing IV amino acids to sick preterm infants as soon as possible after birth can improve protein balance and can increase protein accretion.[123] Most neonatal intensive care units now use a "starter" TPN solution that provides at least 2 g/kg/day of amino acids in addition to 10% dextrose. A relative restriction of water intake during the first day or two of life allows for a physiologic state of negative water and sodium balance that accompanies the mobilization of extracellular water.[9] A standard starting rate for IV fluids is 80 mL/kg/day, with titration of the infusion rate based on environmental humidity (more for infants under open warmers, less for infants in high-humidity incubators), use of humidified air–oxygen mixes in ventilator or CPAP circuits, and when the onset of diuresis and natriuresis develops.[23]

Sodium is added by day 3 to deliver 2.5 to 3.6 mmol/kg/day, provided the serum sodium concentration is not elevated. Initially withholding sodium from preterm infants who have RDS in the first 24 to 48 hours of life helps reduce water accumulation in the lung.[124] The sodium is usually given as sodium chloride or sodium acetate, depending on the degree of metabolic acidosis.[125] Potassium chloride or acetate also is added to the infusate on day 2 or 3 to give 2.0 to 2.5 mmol/kg/day, provided the serum potassium concentration is normal and adequate urine flow is established. By the end of the first week of life, maintenance delivery of sodium and potassium should be achieved (see Table 29-1).

Intravenous calcium and phosphorus supplementation should be started in high-risk infants as soon as possible after birth, if the serum calcium level is low, and certainly if the infant is showing signs of hypocalcemia (tremulousness, seizures, apnea, or cardiac arrhythmia). The usual dosing range of parenteral calcium in the form of calcium gluconate is 0.6 to 2.5 mmol/kg/day (25 to 100 mg/kg/day of elemental calcium), and the dose is titrated based on either the total serum calcium level (with consideration for albumin binding) or the ionized calcium level (with consideration for cardiac output and neurologic status).[33,126] Phosphorus is given as sodium phosphate with a dosing range of 0.75 to 2.5 mmol/kg/day (18 to 80 mg/kg/day of phosphate). The Ca/P ratio should be kept at 1:1 on a molar basis and 1.3:1 on a mg/mg basis to maximize accretion of both minerals. Caution should be used if calcium is infused into a peripheral IV catheter, as tissue necrosis and sloughing can occur. Some intensive care units avoid peripheral calcium administration entirely except in emergencies (hypocalcemic seizures, shock). Magnesium supplementation ranges from 0.12 to 0.4 mmol/kg/day (3 to 10 mg/kg/day).

Full IV amino acid nutrition, including carbohydrate, protein, minerals, and vitamins, should be started as soon as possible after birth, preferably within the first 24 hours, and should be continued at this rate if a delay in advancement to full enteral feedings is anticipated. Lipid emulsions should normally be given as a part of any infant's parenteral nutrition regimen.[127] The IV lipid product in the United States is derived from soybean oil; while it does contain the essential fatty acids, linoleic acid and α-linolenic acid, it lacks their downstream products, AA, eicosapentaenoic acid (EPA), and DHA. This product also contains relatively large amounts of phytosterols, which appear to induce hepatic inflammation and lead to cholestasis and parenteral nutrition-associated liver disease (PNALD).[128] Lipid emulsions must be started within the first few days of life at a minimum dose of 0.5 to 1.0 g/kg/day to avoid essential fatty acid deficiency in infants who cannot be fed enterally. The maximum infusion rate should not exceed 2 to 3 g/kg/day, and the infusion is usually administered over 20 or more hours each day. Hypertriglyceridemia and/or hyperglycemia can result from parenteral lipid administration. Plasma triglyceride levels can be monitored periodically, especially in extremely low birth-weight infants, to assess lipid tolerance. Additionally, IV lipid intake may be associated with decreased binding affinity of bilirubin for plasma protein and increased free bilirubin concentration in very preterm infants.[129]

Newer generation lipid emulsions that contain mainly ω3 LC-PUFAs, such as EPA and DHA, or a mixed emulsion of both ω3 and ω6 LC-PUFAs but with a preponderance of ω3 LC-PUFAs, are available outside of the United States, as of this writing. Evidence from research and practice in other countries demonstrates that the dose and composition of ω3 fatty acids in lipid emulsions may play important roles in reducing development and progression of PNALD.[130-134]

ENTERAL NUTRITION

Most preterm infants, even those who require assisted ventilation, can and should be fed enterally by gavage tube, starting as soon as possible after birth, using the mother's own colostrum and subsequent maternal or donor human milk and/or formula. Most early feeding regimens follow a gut-priming approach, starting with small amounts (<24 mL/kg/day) and advancing as tolerated over several days toward full enteral feeding.

Advantages of Enteral Nutrition

Enteral feeding provides nutrients to support growth and metabolism but also, even in very small amounts, promotes intestinal development and function.[135] Feeding stimulates secretion of gut hormones and regulatory peptides,[136] motility,[137] and intestinal growth.[138] These effects are most prominent with feeding of maternal milk,[138] which also contributes to gut health by facilitating and augmenting the innate gut immune system[139] and establishing a more normal gut microbiome, which is increasingly being recognized as essential for both short- and long-term health.[140-142] Enteral feeding, even in small amounts, helps to prevent the cholestasis that often develops with TPN.[143]

Enteral feedings are contraindicated in those infants with active NEC or hemodynamic instability (marked hypotension). Caution must be exercised when considering enteral feeding of infants with poor intestinal motility or ileus, such as those who are postoperative, on extracorporeal membrane oxygenation, or heavily sedated with narcotics. Use of paralytics, per se, is not an absolute contraindication to enteral feeding because nondepolarizing neuromuscular blocking agents block transmission at the neuromuscular junction in skeletal muscle[144] but not in smooth muscle. In general, trophic feedings, particularly of mother's milk, should be considered for all infants, with feeding advancement dependent on individualized feeding tolerance and signs of intestinal motility.

Methods of Gavage Feeding

Gavage feedings are indicated in infants who are unable to be fed by nipple or in infants requiring tracheal intubation, noninvasive ventilation, or higher levels of CPAP. Either oral or nasal feeding tubes can be used. Nasal tubes are easier to secure. Nasal feeding tubes partially obstruct the infant's airway and may not be feasible for those infants requiring CPAP, but they offer no disadvantage for infants who are intubated.

Intermittent ("bolus") gavage feeding at 2- or 3-hour intervals is the most commonly used method for enteral feeding. Intermittent "slow" infusion (e.g., 3 hours of volume given over 1 to 2 hours) has been shown to improve gastric emptying and duodenal motility compared to rapid bolus delivery.[145]

An alternative method of intragastric feeding is to infuse the milk or formula continuously through an indwelling nasogastric or orogastric tube at a constant rate controlled by an infusion pump. This method offers the theoretical advantages of allowing greater volumes to be absorbed without taxing the limited gastric capacity of smaller preterm infants and of avoiding the volume-related abdominal distention and restricted movement of the diaphragm that may occur in some infants with respiratory failure. Unpredictable nutrient delivery, however, is a significant problem with continuous feeding, because human milk fat separates from the nonfat milk and is left in the tubing or syringe.[146,147] This problem can be averted by positioning the infusion pump so that the opening of the syringe is pointed upward, ensuring that the fat is still delivered even if it separates, and by minimizing the length of the extension tubing. Analysis of clinical trials did not find consistent differences in the effectiveness of continuous versus intermittent bolus intragastric feeding, with the exception of a single small study that showed earlier discharge of patients with a birth-weight of less than 1000 g when fed by the continuous method.[148]

Transpyloric feeding, done by placing the tube directly into the duodenum or jejunum, has been used successfully to feed critically ill infants. Transpyloric feeding is technically more difficult, requires X-ray or ultrasound confirmation of tube placement, and generally offers no advantage over intragastric feeding; moreover, some evidence of harm exists with transpyloric feeding, including gastrointestinal (GI) disturbances and mortality.[149] This technique, therefore, is not recommended as a primary feeding method for ventilated infants and should be restricted to short-term use in those infants who cannot tolerate gastric feedings because of excessive gastroesophageal reflux.

Nonnutritive sucking of a pacifier during gavage feedings has been tested as a way of compensating for the lack of oral stimulation in tube-fed infants. A systematic review based on published studies showed shorter hospital stay and a trend toward more rapid weight gain with nonnutritive sucking.[150] When an infant no longer requires mechanical ventilation or CPAP, has achieved stable cardiorespiratory status, and has demonstrated adequate sucking and swallowing of secretions, nipple feedings may be introduced. The transition to oral feedings typically requires more time for infants who required assisted ventilation and those who were most preterm at birth.[151]

Minimal Enteral Feedings and Enteral Feeding Advancement

Accumulating evidence strongly supports early initiation of low-volume enteral feedings ("minimal enteral feeding" or "trophic feeds"), preferably with maternal colostrum. Minimal enteral feedings represent the administration of small feeds (<24 mL/kg/day) over a short but defined period of time to promote GI development, motility, and function in the preterm infant and can improve growth and time to reach full enteral feeding.[152-155] Minimal enteral feeding has not been shown to increase the risk of NEC.[156] The duration that minimal enteral feeds are provided depends on several factors, including degree of prematurity, presence of intestinal underperfusion in utero (such as in the IUGR infant), degree of perinatal hypoxic–ischemic injury, or need for medications after birth that might reduce intestinal perfusion (inotropic support, indomethacin).

Enteral feeding advancement is usually by 15 to 30 mL/kg/day, though no advantage has been demonstrated in terms of protection from NEC by slower (15 to 20 mL/kg/day) vs faster (30 to 35 mL/kg/day) feeding advancement in very low birth-weight infants.[157] If the enteral feeding advancement spans several days, this method must be combined with IV nutritional support. Gastric residual volumes are checked commonly, but their value in assessing feeding tolerance is widely debated, and there is little consensus about the meaning of any one volume. If significant gastric residuals are found repeatedly and are increasing, especially in the context of other signs of enteral feeding intolerance such as abdominal distention, the infant should be carefully evaluated for signs of systemic infection, NEC, and intestinal obstruction. Full enteral feedings (approximately 120 mL/kg/day, depending on caloric density) usually can be achieved over 7 to 10 days.

Composition of Enteral Nutrition
Human Milk

Few medical interventions offer as much advantage to preterm and critically ill infants as human milk feeding. Human milk stimulates the development of beneficial GI flora, provides antimicrobial factors that protect against infections, and provides hormones and growth factors to stimulate organ growth and health.[158-161] The most compelling early benefit of human milk is its dose-related protective effect against NEC in preterm infants.[162-165] The most important long-term benefit is the favorable impact of human milk feeding on neurodevelopmental outcome.[166-169] The American Academy of Pediatrics states that human milk is the recommended basis of nutrition for the preterm infant.[170] Thus, it is important for hospitals that care for sick and preterm infants to provide good lactation support services. These services should include parent education and information, electric breast pumps, convenient pumping and storage facilities, and the services of trained lactation specialists. Mothers of infants who require intensive care including assisted ventilation should be strongly encouraged to provide their milk for their infants. There is increasing evidence that an exclusive human milk diet (human milk fortified with human milk protein–based fortifier) confers additional protection against NEC compared to bovine-based milk protein.[171,172]

Universally, however, it has been observed through carefully controlled, randomized trials, that the preterm infant will not grow at the normal rate of fetal growth if fed human milk alone. Multicomponent fortification of human milk is required for preterm infants to meet their increased daily requirements of energy, protein, vitamins, and minerals.[96]

Donor Human Milk

Donor human milk is a pasteurized product from accredited milk banks. It is used when maternal milk is insufficient or unavailable, because of the multitude of benefits associated with the use of human milk in preterm infants as described above.[173] Donor milk is pasteurized to prevent the transmission of infection, but this also negates most of the antiinfective properties of milk. Nevertheless, infection rates and NEC rates are lower with donor milk than with formulas, indicating that the processing of donor milk does not result in increased infections.[174] There are differences in composition between maternal and donor milk as well, especially in protein content, but also energy, lactose, and DHA content; these differences are particularly noted between human milk donated by women later in lactation after having delivered term infants compared with milk expressed by mothers delivering preterm infants.[175] Thus, close attention must be paid to appropriate fortification of donor human milk to meet the nutritional requirements for optimal growth of preterm infants.

Formulas

Cow's milk–derived formulas have been modeled after the composition of human milk to provide biologically available protein mixtures with appropriate protein/energy ratios for normal growth. Preterm formulas are designed to meet the additional protein, energy, and micronutrient requirements of the preterm infant. New generations of "high-protein" preterm formulas are now available that contain even higher protein contents to achieve the recommended protein delivery of 3.6 to 4.5 g/kg/day for extremely low birth-weight preterm infants.[55] Cow's milk–based protein-hydrolyzed formulas and human milk fortifiers are now available and may reduce GI inflammation; this is an area of ongoing research.

TABLE 29-4 **Considerations for the Preterm Infant with Respiratory Insufficiency**
Poor nutrition is associated with abnormal lung development
Careful restriction of fluid and sodium intake during the first postnatal days may reduce the risk of BPD
Excessive fluid volumes increase pulmonary edema and contribute to lung injury
RDS and BPD increase the infant's metabolic needs for energy and protein
Steroid therapy and chronic disease have negative effects on protein balance
Diuretic therapy can waste electrolytes (Na, K) and calcium
Early nutritional support and feeding guidelines are associated with the prevention of BPD
Excessive carbohydrates (>12.5 mg/kg/min) will increase carbon dioxide production disproportionate to oxygen consumption
Lipids (ω3 LC-PUFAs) are a good alternative source of concentrated energy
Adequate provision of amino acids prevents catabolism of respiratory and diaphragmatic muscle protein
Intramuscular vitamin A supplementation during the first month of life is associated with a reduction in death/BPD

BPD, bronchopulmonary dysplasia; *LC-PUFAs*, long-chain polyunsaturated fatty acids; *RDS*, respiratory distress syndrome.

SPECIAL NUTRITIONAL CONSIDERATIONS FOR INFANTS WITH BRONCHOPULMONARY DYSPLASIA

BPD is the most common pulmonary morbidity seen in very low birth-weight preterm infants, with an incidence approaching 50% among infants born before 29 weeks' gestation.[176] Preterm infants who develop BPD are at risk of postnatal growth failure.[177] Although there have been no randomized, controlled trials on the effects of early nutrition on the risk of developing BPD,[178] there is evidence that improvement in nutritional status can provide beneficial effects for lung growth and healing. Analysis from a large database demonstrated that infants who received more nutritional support during the first 3 weeks of life (and who were less critically ill, defined as having required mechanical ventilation for <7 days) were less likely to develop moderate to severe BPD.[61] However, severity of illness and early nutritional practices were both independently associated with morbidity, including BPD.[179] In a retrospective analysis, infants with BPD who received more protein in the first 20 days of life grew with greater velocity and had better head circumference growth.[180] In a prospective, nonrandomized study, preterm infants with BPD fed individually tailored fortified breast milk and/or preterm formula (with 130 kcal/kg/day energy intake and 3.2 g/kg/day protein intake) vs standard fortification showed greater weight gain velocity and less postnatal growth restriction.[181]

Nutritional factors that are important to consider for infants who require assisted ventilation and/or who have developed BPD are summarized in Table 29-4. In summary, it is critically important to provide adequate nutrition to all infants requiring assisted ventilation, thereby allowing each infant the best possible chance for recovery of lung function and normal growth and development.

REFERENCES

A complete reference list is available at https://experconsult .inkling.com.

30

Complications of Respiratory Support

Tara M. Randis, MD, MS, Jennifer Duchon, MDCM, MPH, and Richard Alan Polin, BA, MD

INTRODUCTION

Neonates requiring intensive care represent a particularly vulnerable population because of their frequent need for intubation (as part of resuscitation), prolonged mechanical ventilation, and susceptibility to hospital-acquired infections. Hospital-acquired infections in neonates increase costs, prolong hospitalization, and are major causes of morbidity and mortality.[1-4] In pediatric intensive care patients and adults, ventilator-associated pneumonia (VAP) is the second most commonly occurring health care–associated infection. However, the rate of VAP in infants and neonates, especially those with underlying pulmonary disorders, is not as clear. The diagnosis of VAP is problematic because it occurs in ventilated infants who are likely to have other reasons for respiratory decompensation (e.g., atelectasis or heart failure secondary to a patent ductus arteriosus). Moreover, procedures commonly used to diagnose VAP in adults (e.g., bronchoscopy, lung biopsy, protected brush specimen, and bronchoalveolar lavage) are rarely used in the neonatal population.

The current definition used by the National Healthcare Safety Network (NHSN) of the Centers for Disease Control and Prevention (CDC) for the diagnosis of VAP in infants (this definition is not specific for neonates but is applied to them) requires new and persistent radiographic infiltrates and worsening gas exchange in infants who are ventilated for at least 48 hours and who exhibit at least three of the following criteria: temperature instability with no other recognized cause, leukopenia, change in the characteristics of respiratory secretions, respiratory distress, and bradycardia or tachycardia.[5] The strictness of this definition makes it likely that the diagnosis of VAP is underreported in the United States. The 2013 data from the NHSN report an incidence of 1.0 to 1.1/1000 ventilator days for infants weighing <1000 g in level III neonatal intensive care units (NICUs).[6] Rates of VAP/1000 ventilator days in the International Nosocomial Infection Control Consortium are eightfold higher.[7]

In 2011, the CDC convened a working group consisting of critical care organizations, infection control groups, and epidemiology organizations to address the lack of precision in the diagnosis of VAP.[8] As a result, a new term was developed, ventilator-associated event, or VAE. Within the VAE surveillance algorithm, three definition tiers were recognized. A ventilator-associated condition is defined by worsening oxygenation in a patient ventilated for at least 2 days (etiology not specified). The second tier is termed IVAC (infection-related ventilator-associated complication). Patients with an IVAC exhibit hypoxemia accompanied by general and objective evidence of inflammation/infection. To meet this definition antibiotics must be administered for at least 4 days. The third tier is possible or

probable VAP, which requires additional laboratory evidence of white blood cells on Gram stain and/or positive cultures. The new definition is meant to improve epidemiologic surveillance, but it is clearly not easily adaptable to the NICU setting.

This chapter reviews the epidemiology, pathogenesis, diagnosis, prevention strategies, and treatment of VAP in the newborn infant.

EPIDEMIOLOGY

The most recent surveillance data as of this writing suggest that the incidence of VAP may be decreasing. Patrick et al. examined the incidence of health care–associated infections among critically ill children in 173 U.S. hospitals from 2007 to 2012 and noted the rate of VAP had decreased from 1.6 to 0.6/1000 ventilator days.[9] An NHSN report indicates a pooled mean incidence rate varying from 0.3 to 1.6/1000 ventilator days (Table 30-1) in U.S. level II/II NICUs.[6] This represents a greater than 50% decrease from that reported in 2004.[10] Cernada et al. note that regional economic development has a major influence on the incidence of VAP. Reported rates in developed countries range from 2.7 to 10.9/1000 ventilator days, whereas those in developing nations are as high as 37.2/1000 ventilator days. Variability in the diagnostic criteria used also contributes to the wide range of reported incidence rates in the literature.

Critically ill neonates are at high risk for hospital-acquired infections. Extrinsic factors such as inconsistent hand hygiene practices and overcrowding in NICUs contribute to the high incidence of health care–associated infections.[11,12] Increased susceptibility of the neonatal host is multifactorial in nature and includes immaturity of the immune system (particularly infants weighing less than 1500 g) and the need for invasive monitoring, central catheters, prolonged intravenous alimentation, and mechanical ventilation. In a large prospective surveillance study, Van der Zwet et al. identified low birth weight (odds ratio (OR) 1.37; confidence interval (CI) 1.01, 1.85) and mechanical ventilation (OR 9.69; CI 4.60, 20.4) as risk factors for hospital-acquired pneumonia.[13] Hentschel et al. observed a difference in the hospital-acquired pneumonia rates between intubated infants and those receiving nasal continuous positive airway pressure (NCPAP) (12.8 vs 1.8/1000 ventilator or NCPAP days).[14]

A number of studies have examined specific risk factors for VAP among critically ill neonates. Yuan et al. conducted a retrospective cohort study in 259 patients who were ventilated more than 48 hours.[15] By logistic regression analysis, the following variables independently predicted VAP: reintubation (OR 5.3; CI 2.0, 14.0), duration of mechanical ventilation (OR 4.8; CI 2.2, 10.4), treatment with opiates (OR 3.8; CI 1.8, 8.5), and frequency of

TABLE 30-1   Pooled Means and Percentiles of the Distribution of Ventilator-Associated Pneumonia Rates for Level II/III NICUs in 2013

Birth-Weight Category (g)	No. of Locations[†]	No. of VAPs	Ventilator Days	Pooled Mean	10%	25%	50% (median)	75%	90%
			PEDIATRIC VENTILATOR-ASSOCIATED PNEUMONIA RATE*				PERCENTILE		
≤750	118 (86)	53	33,351	1.6	0	0	0	1.6	7.7
751-1000	133 (80)	25	17,568	1.4	0	0	0	0	4.1
1001-1500	150 (58)	12	10,163	1.2	0	0	0	0	6.7
1501-2500	156 (43)	2	8910	0.2	0	0	0	0	0
>2500	154 (48)	4	11,616	0.3	0	0	0	0	0

*(No. of pediatric VAP/No. of ventilator days) × 100.
[†]The number in parentheses is the number of locations meeting minimum requirements for percentile distributions (i.e., ≥50 device days for rate distributions, ≥50 patient days for device utilization ratios) if less than the total number of locations. If this number is <20, percentile distributions were not calculated.
VAP, ventilator-associated pneumonia.
Data from National Healthcare Safety Network.[79]

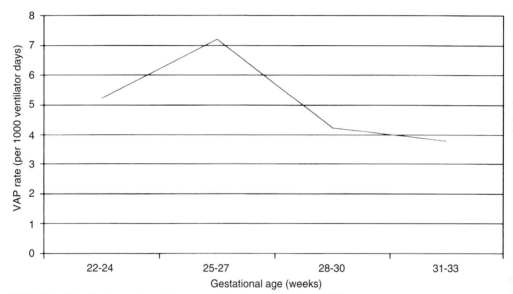

FIG 30-1 Distribution of ventilator-associated pneumonia (*VAP*) rates per 1000 ventilator days among neonates with gestational ages of 22 to 33 weeks. (From Apisarnthanarak A, Holamann-Pazgal G, Hamvas A, et al. *Pediatrics.* 112:1283-1289, 2003.)

endotracheal suctioning (OR 3.5; CI 1.6, 7.4). Low gestational age and/or birth weight have also been identified as risk factors for VAP.[13,16,17] Data from the CDC's NHSN (2006-2008) at 304 participating hospitals revealed a VAP rate of 2.36/1000 ventilator days among neonates weighing less than 750 g and 0.72/1000 ventilator days in those >2500 g.[18] A prospective cohort study by Apisarnthanarak et al. reported a VAP incidence of 6.5/1000 ventilator days in infants less than 28 weeks' gestational age, compared with 4/1000 ventilator days in those of ≥28 weeks' gestation (Fig. 30-1).[16] The same authors found that after adjustment for the duration of endotracheal intubation, a preceding bloodstream infection (with an unrelated organism) was an independent risk factor for VAP (OR 3.5; CI 1.2, 12.3). This finding may reflect a subpopulation of infants with compromised immune function. Interestingly, the occurrence of VAP in this study was strongly associated with an increased likelihood of mortality (OR 3.0; CI 1.2, 12.3). A 2014 meta-analysis published by Tan et al. identified the following risk factors for the development of VAP: length of stay in NICU (OR 23.45), reintubation (OR 9.18), enteral feeding (OR 5.59), mechanical ventilation (OR 4.04), transfusion (OR 3.32), low birth weight (OR 3.16), prematurity (OR 2.66), parenteral nutrition (OR 2.30), bronchopulmonary dysplasia (OR

2.21), and tracheal intubation (OR 1.12).[19] Additional risk factors for VAP have been described in the pediatric ICU literature (presence of a genetic syndrome, bronchoscopy, and the use of steroids, antibiotics, and histamine-type 2 receptor blockers).[20-23] However, their association with VAP in the neonatal population remains unclear.

PATHOGENESIS

VAP occurs when bacterial, fungal, or viral pathogens gain entrance to the normally sterile lower respiratory tract. Only rarely does the organism gain entry to the lung through hematogenous dissemination or by bacterial translocation from the gastrointestinal tract.[24,25] Pathogens responsible for VAP originate from exogenous sources (hands of health care workers, ventilator circuit, biofilm of endotracheal tube) or endogenous sources (colonized oropharyngeal, tracheal, and gastric secretions) (Fig. 30-2).[26] The organism gains entry to the respiratory tract by colonizing the endotracheal tube and the upper airway, by tracheal suctioning, or by direct aspiration of gastrointestinal contents. Cuffed endotracheal tubes are not generally used in the NICU. This practice provides

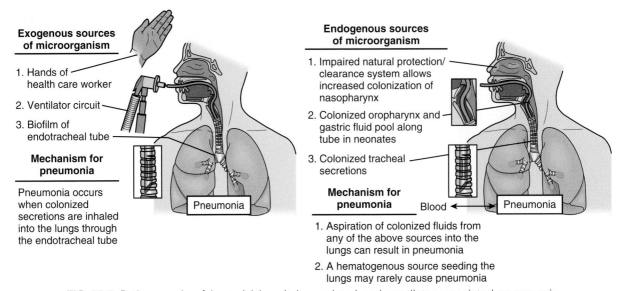

FIG 30-2 Pathogenesis of bacterial hospital-associated and ventilator-associated pneumonia. (Data from Garland JS. *Neoreviews.* 15:e225-e235, 2014.)

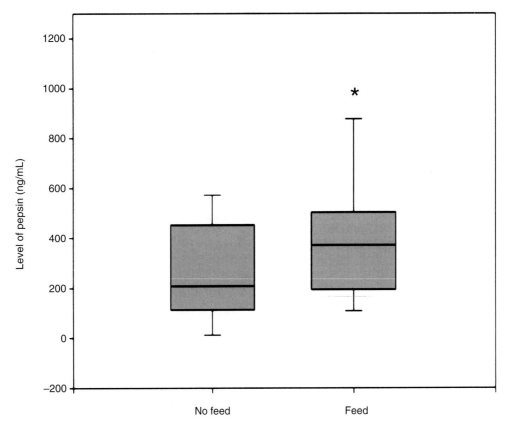

*P = 0.02

FIG 30-3 The levels of pepsin when infants were unfed and during the feed. Median concentration of pepsin was significantly lower in the unfed state compared with the concentration during feeding. (From Farhath S, Aghai ZH, Nakhla T, et al. *J Pediatr Gastroenterol Nutr.* 43:336-341, 2006.)

easier access for microorganisms to the lower respiratory tract of neonates. Furthermore, microscopic aspiration may be more common than previously appreciated.[27,28] Farharth et al. quantified pepsin, a marker of gastric contents, in tracheal aspirate samples from 45 ventilated newborn infants.[27] Pepsin was detected in 92.8% of tracheal aspirate samples. The mean concentration of pepsin was significantly lower when the infants were unfed (Fig. 30-3). Methylxanthines increased tracheal aspirate pepsin levels,[27] and infants who developed bronchopulmonary dysplasia (BPD), or developed BPD or died before 36 weeks' gestation, had significantly higher levels (Fig. 30-4).[28] Pepsin levels were also higher in infants who developed severe BPD versus those with moderate BPD (Fig. 30-5).

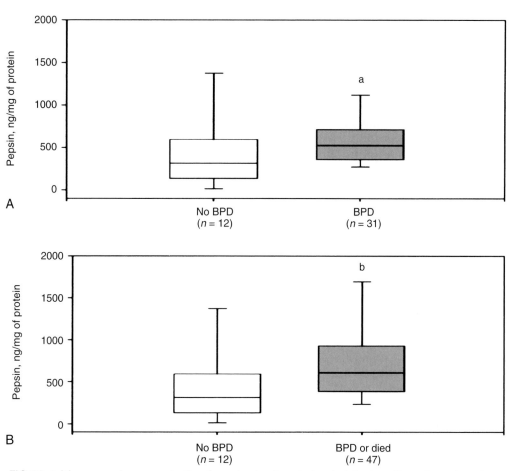

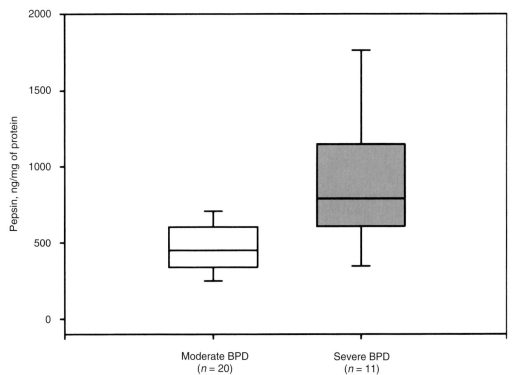

FIG 30-4 Mean pepsin concentration from tracheal aspirates in infants with no bronchopulmonary dysplasia (*BPD*) and from infants with BPD, or with BPD or who died before 36 weeks' gestation. (From Farhath S, Zhaoping H, Nakhla T, et al. *Pediatrics*. 121:e253-e259, 2008.)

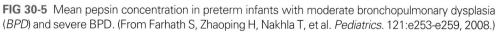

FIG 30-5 Mean pepsin concentration in preterm infants with moderate bronchopulmonary dysplasia (*BPD*) and severe BPD. (From Farhath S, Zhaoping H, Nakhla T, et al. *Pediatrics*. 121:e253-e259, 2008.)

MICROBIOLOGY

In NHSN surveys of adult and pediatric hospitals, *Staphylococcus aureus* and gram-negative organisms, primarily *Pseudomonas* and *Klebsiella* species, have remained the predominant pathogens over time.[18] Apisarnthanarak et al.[16] recovered gram-negative microorganisms from the respiratory secretions in 94% of VAP episodes. *Staphylococcus aureus* was recovered in about one-quarter of infants with VAP, and multiple organisms were recovered from the airway in 58% of episodes. Yuan et al.[15] recovered gram-negative bacteria in the majority of infants with VAP. Table 30-2 shows the predominant pathogens, stratified by birth weight, associated with VAP among NICU patients from the CDC's NHSN surveillance system from 2006 through 2008. Historically most health care–associated pneumonia is felt to be polymicrobial in nature. However, this may be reflective of sampling techniques, which are typically noninvasive and nonspecific in neonates, such as endotracheal tube suctioning. Cernada et al.[29] found that when targeted techniques for sample collection such as bronchoalveolar lavage are performed, polymicrobial VAP represented merely 16.7% of episodes.

DIAGNOSIS

The diagnosis of VAP is problematic.[30] As noted above, the NHSN and CDC definitions are of value for epidemiologic studies, but of limited help for identifying infants with VAP.[31] Complicating this issue is that most infants with suspected VAP have underlying lung disease that predisposes them to atelectasis and episodes of clinical deterioration. Additionally, it is not uncommon for general radiologists to report the presence of an infiltrate on a chest radiograph in an otherwise asymptomatic infant.[32]

In adults with fever, pulmonary infiltrates, and clinical criteria for VAP, only 42% had a definitive diagnosis of pneumonia and 66% had a noninfectious etiology.[33,34] Moreover, postmortem examinations demonstrated that only 35% of patients with a new or progressive infiltrate had histopathologic evidence of a pneumonic process.[35,36] In ventilated adults, invasive techniques have been used to quantify the bacterial load as a way to distinguish infection from colonization. The airway of the newborn infant is colonized soon after intubation with a variety of potential pathogens, and a specimen taken from the endotracheal tube will not differentiate colonization from infection. Therefore, cultures of tracheal aspirates have low sensitivity, specificity,

and positive predictive accuracy for the diagnosis of VAP.[37] In a national survey from the United Kingdom regarding the diagnosis and management of VAP, only 57.8% obtained an endotracheal aspirate before starting empirical antibiotics.[38] The American Thoracic Society and Infectious Diseases Society of America guidelines[39] suggest using, in adult patients, a threshold of 10^3 for quantitative culture from a protected specimen brush sample, 10^4 for quantitative culture of bronchoalveolar lavage (BAL) fluid, and 10^5 or 10^6 for quantitative culture of tracheal aspirates. A meta-analysis of 23 studies in adult patients of quantitative BAL cultures and 18 studies of protected specimen brush cultures suggested the diagnostic value of these methods.[24,40] However, a Cochrane review published in 2008 found no evidence that the use of quantitative cultures (vs qualitative cultures) reduced either mortality or time spent in the ICU.[41] Furthermore, the use of quantitative cultures has been criticized because it may delay initiation of antibiotic therapy and there is the possibility of a false negative test secondary to preexisting use of antibiotics.[42] Most recently, some pediatric intensive care units have begun to use a modified pulmonary infection score, mCPIS (using temperature, leukocyte count, chest radiography, pulmonary secretions, PaO_2/FiO_2 (mm Hg), and cultures of nonbronchoscopic BAL), in the diagnosis of VAP. In a 2014 study[43] of children who met the CDC criteria for VAP, a score of ≥6 had a sensitivity of 94%, a specificity of 50%, a positive predictive accuracy of 64%, and a negative predictive accuracy of 90%. Therefore, the score was best at identifying children who were unlikely to have VAP, but not nearly as good at identifying patients with VAP. There are no studies using the mCPIS in neonates.

A few studies in neonates have evaluated the value of nonbronchoscopic BAL in neonates. In this technique, a suction catheter is placed into the endotracheal tube until resistance is met and then a small amount of sterile saline is placed and then suctioned back. Köskal et al.[44] obtained BAL specimens from 145 intubated newborn infants and did quantitative counts and smears for white blood cells on the BAL fluid. Using CDC criteria for VAP, 44 infants (30%) were diagnosed as infected and 90% of those infants ($n = 40$) had positive BAL cultures. The percentage of neutrophils containing intracellular bacteria was significantly higher in infants with VAP (vs colonized, asymptomatic infants), as was the presence of leukocytes in BAL fluid (84% vs 26%). Quantitative cultures (greater than 10^5 cfu/mL) also distinguished infants with VAP from colonized asymptomatic infants. The sensitivity and specificity of intracellular bacteria and quantitative cultures were 94% and 90% respectively.

	BIRTH WEIGHT, N (%)					
Pathogen	≤750 g	751-1000 g	1001-1500 g	1501-2500 g	>2500 g	Overall
Pseudomonas species	78 (19)	29 (12)	12 (12.1)	7 (17.9)	8 (17.0)	134 (16.1)
Staphylococcus aureus	50 (12)	43 (18)	18 (18.2)	13 (33.3)	7 (14.9)	131 (15.8)
Enterobacter species	48 (12)	27 (11)	9 (9.1)	3 (7.7)	2 (4.3)	89 (10.7)
Klebsiella species	60 (15)	27 (11)	16 (16.2)	4 (10.3)	10 (21.3)	117 (14.1)
Other	169 (42)	114 (48)	44 (44.4)	12 (30.8)	20 (42.6)	359 (43.3)
Total VAP isolates	405	240	99	39	47	830

TABLE 30-2 **Pathogen Distribution for Ventilator-Associated Pneumonia by Birth Weight**

The predominant pathogens associated with VAP among neonatal intensive care unit patients from the Centers for Disease Control and Prevention National Healthcare Safety Network surveillance system from 2006 through 2008 are shown. *VAP*, ventilator-associated pneumonia.
Data from Hocevar et al. Device-associated infections among neonatal intensive care unit patients. Infection Control and Hospital Epidemiology, 33(12), December 2012, pp 1200-1206.

Cernada et al. used a nonbronchoscopic BAL technique to identify 18 episodes of VAP in 16 neonates.[29] There were no complications with the invasive, blind BAL technique; however, four patients considered too unstable were excluded from the analysis. The presence of purulent tracheal aspirates may not be a reliable marker of VAP. Cordero et al.[45] demonstrated that the majority (71%) of infants with purulent "tracheal aspirates" were asymptomatic. Furthermore, radiologically documented VAP occurred in 7% of very low birth-weight infants who never had a purulent tracheal aspirate and in 5% who did. Purulence on a tracheal smear was directly related to the duration of endotracheal intubation. In a 2015 study by Seligman et al., the absence of gram-positive cocci on samples obtained from an endotracheal aspirate was of value in excluding *Staphylococcus* as a potential pathogen.[46] However, the Canadian Critical Care Trials group found no benefit to Gram stain of endotracheal aspirates and BAL specimens, with only a limited role in guiding therapy.[47] Similarly, a meta-analysis published in 2012[48] noted a limited agreement between Gram stain and culture (mostly BAL specimens) and concluded that the Gram stain should not be used to narrow antiinfective therapy until culture results become available. In the only study of preterm infants with VAP[49] the authors concluded that a Gram stain from a tracheal aspirate was useful in predicting classes of culturable microorganisms and for guiding appropriate initial antibiotic therapy. The use of biochemical markers (e.g., C-reactive protein and procalcitonin) has been investigated in adults,[50] but has not been of much value. Traditional markers (neutrophil indices and acute-phase reactants) are of value in infants who are bacteremic, but that represents a minority of the infants with VAP.

PREVENTION

Prevention of VAP in adult populations has been primarily achieved by the use of "bundles" of multiple concurrent preventive interventions for all patients, often aided by tools such as checklists. In some cases there is only theoretical evidence or biologic plausibility for one or more of the elements of the bundle being effective, but application of these bundles is widely used and is considered to be highly successful.[21] Prevention strategies for VAP in adult populations generally include four core interventions: elevation of the head of the bed, assessment of readiness to extubate, peptic ulcer disease (PUD) prophylaxis, and deep venous thrombosis (DVT) prophylaxis.[51] Additional strategies recommended by the CDC include staff education, surveillance, and feedback of VAP rates to clinicians; implementing a comprehensive oral-hygiene program; ensuring proper sterilization of reusable respiratory care equipment; using sterile water in humidification systems; periodic drainage of condensate from breathing circuits; hand hygiene before and after contact with a patient who has an endotracheal tube, as well as before and after contact with respiratory equipment; vaccination against pneumococcal and influenza disease; and prevention of aspiration by avoiding intubation using noninvasive ventilation.[51] Many of the individual interventions as well as the bundles themselves have been extrapolated from the adult population and are less well studied in the pediatric population, especially neonates.[52]

Head-of-the-bed elevation has been effective in reducing VAP in adult populations, presumably by reducing reflux and aspiration. The logic of head-of-the-bed elevation is sound and it is found in almost every VAP reduction bundle, but the physical characteristics of neonates and their support equipment may make its implementation challenging. Another positioning strategy has been proposed, based on an animal model, in which intubated neonates are positioned in the lateral, rather than supine, position. One group of authors hypothesized that such positioning would make use of gravity to help to avoid tracheal contamination from oral secretions. In a prospective randomized trial in Egypt, Aly et al. demonstrated a 50% lower incidence of positive tracheal cultures in the lateral position group.[53] Whether the optimal position of the intubated neonate is with the head of the bed up, lateral, or otherwise needs further research.

Assessment of readiness to extubate is standard in most VAP reduction bundles. Some variation on this practice is reasonable for the neonatal population. In almost all cases, practitioners would agree that extubation is a critical goal, and obviously VAP will not occur in the absence of mechanical ventilation. Noninvasive respiratory support such as NCPAP is becoming more common; the evidence for its safety and efficacy even in the tiniest infants is mounting; and its use should reduce VAP rates.[14]

DVT prophylaxis is not used in neonates, although it is included in most adult VAP reduction bundles.

PUD prophylaxis is another standard intervention in adult VAP reduction bundles. Applying PUD prophylaxis is considered an appropriate intervention in the adult ICU setting because of the higher incidence of stress ulceration in critical illness. In addition, increasing the pH of gastric contents may protect against a greater pulmonary inflammatory response to aspiration of gastrointestinal contents, because the effects of aspirating acidic contents may be worse than those with a higher pH. H_2-receptor blockade is often used in neonates who are not yet being enterally fed (for gastric protection) and also in those infants who are thought to have significant gastrointestinal reflux. However, H_2 blockade in neonates is not without risks. Normally acidic stomach contents are thought to decrease colonization with bacteria; reversing this innate defense has potential to cause harm. There have been several studies in adult populations examining the use of sucralfate, which provides gastric protection, but does not change pH. Very little evidence exists on the question of PUD prophylaxis reducing VAP in pediatric populations and none for neonatal populations. Data from the pediatric population show no change in VAP rates between pediatric ICU (PICU) patients treated with an H_2-receptor antagonist, sucralfate, or placebo.[54] Additionally, H_2 blockade has been shown to be associated with increased rates of both gram-negative bacteremia and candidemia in the neonatal population.[55,56] At this time, there can be no recommendation for routine use of PUD prophylaxis for the purpose of VAP reduction in the neonatal population.

Selective decontamination of the digestive tract (SDD) involves the enteral administration of nonabsorbable antimicrobials for the purpose of decreasing gastrointestinal colonization and, therefore, potentially decreasing respiratory infections because aspirated gastric contents would be less likely to carry contagion. SDD has also been proposed as a preventive strategy for many infections: sepsis, surgical site infections, and others. Although data in adult ICU populations are generally supportive of the role of SDD in VAP reduction, pediatric data are less robust. A prospective randomized trial of colistin, tobramycin, and nystatin administered orally in a PICU population demonstrated a lower rate of pneumonia (VAP was not separated from other types of pneumonia) in the treatment group.[57] A smaller trial of severely burned PICU patients showed no efficacy for a polymyxin E, tobramycin, and amphotericin B regimen.[58] The only study of neonatal patients was a prospective nonrandomized trial of polymyxin E, tobramycin, and nystatin; the treatment group had a statistically significant decrease in infections caused by organisms of intestinal origin; this decrease encompassed respiratory tract infections, sepsis, wound infections, and others. VAP was not reported separately so the results are not clearly indicative of success in its reduction.[59] SDD may have potential in reducing many infections, but carries risk of increased antibiotic resistance; additionally, the long-term effects of manipulation of the neonatal microbiome have not been evaluated rigorously enough to consider its use in neonates outside of a clinical trial.

The CDC recommends a comprehensive oral hygiene care (OHC) program to prevent VAP in adult patients. A Cochrane meta-analysis of OHC, including chlorhexidine gluconate (CHG), has shown significant reductions in VAP rates in adult patients.[60] There are no data in neonates on the benefits of using oral CHG to decrease the risk of VAP. Furthermore, the pathogenesis of VAP may be very different in edentulous neonates and adults who may have gingivitis or other dental disease predisposing them to abnormal oral colonization. In addition, CHG is not licensed for use in children less than 2 months of age. However, human milk is known to facilitate mucosal lining function and immune response in both term and preterm infants; oropharyngeal administration of human milk has been used safely as part of a bundle strategy to reduce VAP in infants less than 1500 g.[61] In a small randomized controlled trial, Lee et al.[62] noted a decrease in the incidence of clinical sepsis (but not VAP) with oropharyngeal administration of colostrum to infants born at <28 weeks' gestation without adverse events. A pilot trial of oral care using a commercial gel containing certain constituents of breast milk, such as lysozyme and lactoferrin, in infants of less than 28 weeks' gestation showed no adverse effects but was not effective in reducing VAP, although the trial was not designed or powered for such outcomes.[63] The appropriate OHC regimen for the purpose of VAP reduction in the neonatal population requires further study.

There is unequivocal evidence that hand hygiene is the most important infection control intervention in all health care settings, but also one of the most difficult infection reduction strategies to maintain. The majority of VAP is polymicrobial and caused by *S. aureus* and a variety of gram-negative organisms. All of these pathogens are carried on the hands of health care workers and are found in the infants' gastrointestinal tracts. Those sites are likely to be the reservoir for gram-negative organisms, especially antibiotic-resistant ones, which are spread between patients, first causing colonization and then disease.[64,65] Respiratory care equipment may be colonized with these organisms as well.[66] Hand hygiene (with an alcohol-based hand sanitizer unless hands are visibly soiled) before and after contact with every patient is clearly a practice that should reduce VAP.[12] Given that the organisms that contaminate respiratory equipment are found in the sputum and oropharynx of patients, hand hygiene before and after contact with respiratory equipment and thorough and regular cleaning of the environment and equipment should be part of comprehensive care plans to reduce VAP. Of note, CDC guidelines do not recommend changing the breathing circuit unless it is visibly soiled or mechanically malfunctioning.

Closed endotracheal suctioning systems, which allow multiple episodes of suctioning without disconnection of the patient from mechanical ventilation, may reduce environmental contamination that occurs with frequent disconnection and manipulation of the ventilatory apparatus. Conversely, such systems may increase the likelihood of reintroduction of contaminated secretions on the multiuse suction catheter into the lower respiratory tract. These systems are increasingly implemented in the NICU, as they may help prevent physiologic derangements that occur when an infant is disconnected from the ventilator and allow for frequent suctioning during high-frequency oscillatory ventilation.[67] Despite their widespread use, the impact of closed suctioning systems on VAP in the neonate has not been adequately studied.[68]

Improvements to the equipment used to mechanically ventilate adult patients have the potential to reduce VAP. One prospective randomized trial in adult patients demonstrated an approximately 35% risk reduction when a silver-coated endotracheal tube was used compared with a conventional one.[69] The authors hypothesized that the silver coating would reduce biofilm formation and bacterial colonization, thus reducing VAP. Similar changes have been made to central venous catheters to reduce catheter-related bloodstream infections, with generally positive results. However, further study of this and other technologies in pediatric and neonatal populations is needed.

Although many health care institutions have developed VAP prevention bundles, in which several of the above interventions are simultaneously and reliably used for all mechanically ventilated patients, no single set of VAP prevention interventions has been adequately studied in the neonatal (or pediatric) population. Given the scant literature regarding all of these measures, a neonatal VAP prevention bundle should contain interventions with biologic plausibility and low likelihood of causing harm. Attempting to elevate the head of the bed (reasonable in infants who tolerate that position), consistent hand hygiene practices, avoiding contamination of suction equipment (such as catheters), avoiding accidental disconnections of the ventilator circuit, and daily assessment of the need for continued mechanical ventilation with extubation as soon as possible comprise a reasonable neonatal VAP bundle. Further studies of H_2 blockade, sucralfate, SDD, and oral care are all warranted in the neonatal population.

TREATMENT

As with many of the diagnostic and preventative strategies discussed above, there are no clear consensus guidelines or studies as to the optimum treatment for neonatal VAP. Treatment recommendations can be extrapolated from adult guidelines and supported by standard epidemiologic principles. In general, treatment of suspected VAP should start with initial broad empirical therapy. The American Thoracic Society and Infectious Disease Society of America have clear treatment guidelines for VAP in adults.[39] These include early empiric broad-spectrum antibiotics (ideally from a class different from that of the antibiotics that the patient has recently received), a careful account of such factors as local epidemiology and the patient's own risk for antibiotic-resistant organisms

(AROs), such as methicillin-resistant *S. aureus* (MRSA) and multidrug-resistant (MDR) gram-negative organisms, and narrowing coverage based on culture results and clinical improvement. Early initiation of appropriate therapy for VAP (and most health care–associated infections) is logical and has been shown to improve outcomes. However, the desire to provide early broad coverage carries the risk of overuse and inappropriate use of antibiotics leading to increased resistance, toxicity, and cost. One study in a combined neonatal and pediatric ICU setting demonstrated that antibiotics for suspected VAP accounted for up to one-third of inappropriate use in this setting.[70]

When selecting empiric therapy, the likely flora and resistance patterns must be known; local epidemiologic data and known risk factors can inform this selection. Risk factors for infection with AROs vary among adults, children, and neonates but have common themes: prolonged hospitalizations, prolonged mechanical ventilation, prior exposure to broad-spectrum antibiotics, more severe and multisystem illness, and immunosuppressive disease.[21,71,72] In adult patients, empiric monotherapy is recommended for those with uncomplicated VAP who are unlikely to be infected with MDR pathogens. In contrast, combination therapy is recommended for more complicated disease or in those likely to be infected with MDR pathogens.

Guidelines for adult VAP treatment suggest that initial empiric therapy should be tailored or discontinued based on culture results and clinical status. The technical difficulties of obtaining lower respiratory tract cultures and the general difficulty in diagnosing VAP (especially as the diagnosis may be made without definitive microbiologic criteria) make this desired deescalation in neonates difficult. The majority of neonates with VAP have multiple risk factors for ARO infection; however, there is no validated clinical scoring system for VAP severity and improvement. Therefore, despite concerns about antimicrobial resistance, most neonates with VAP will receive a full course (7 to 10 days) of empiric broad-spectrum treatment.

As shown in Table 30-2, the majority of neonatal VAP episodes involve *Pseudomonas* or *S. aureus*. Empiric therapy needs to address this epidemiology. In general, an antipseudomonal β-lactam/β-lactamase combination such as piperacillin/tazobactam provides excellent therapy for most gram-negative organisms and many gram-positives and also provides excellent anaerobic coverage. In NICUs where colonization with extended-spectrum β-lactamase-producing organisms is common, a carbapenem such as meropenem would be a more appropriate choice. There is a small amount of evidence that therapy with the fourth-generation cephalosporin cefepime provides adequate coverage.[73] It is controversial whether an additional gram-negative agent such as an aminoglycoside is necessary; this therapy is recommended primarily when there is concern for a carbapenemase-producing gram-negative organism, as these bacteria may retain susceptibility to aminoglycosides. One way to make this decision is to assess the likelihood of concomitant bacteremia or more severe systemic disease (need for blood pressure support, increased transfusion requirements, elevated inflammatory markers, extremes of white blood cell count). Although deescalating therapy in a neonate with VAP can be difficult, the removal of an aminoglycoside when blood cultures are shown to be negative is preferable.

The need for dedicated gram-positive coverage for organisms resistant to the above agents is dependent on local epidemiology. If a given NICU has significant numbers of infants colonized or infected with MRSA, then such therapy is indicated. This treatment has traditionally been given as vancomycin, but there is mounting evidence that linezolid may result in better outcomes for MRSA pneumonia, possibly because of superior lung penetration of linezolid noted in pharmacokinetic studies.[74] It may be possible to discontinue this arm of treatment if no resistant gram-positive organisms are detected, depending on the quality and type of respiratory specimen obtained.

Aerosolized antibiotics are a theoretically attractive therapeutic modality. The only Food and Drug Administration–approved aerosolized antibiotic is tobramycin for cystic fibrosis patients; however, there are case reports of systemic absorption with possible toxicity in preterm infants receiving this therapy.[75] Aerosolized colistin is also now being examined as an option for infants with VAP due to highly resistant gram-negative organisms who are at risk for systemic toxicity with other agents.[76] Further study and product development are needed in this area.

Several novel approaches to neonatal pneumonia have been studied including the administration of exogenous surfactant. One study used surfactant and a specific ventilatory strategy to reduce atelectasis and subsequent bacterial growth and translocation in an animal model of group B *Streptococcus* (GBS) pneumonia.[77] In another animal model of GBS pneumonia, exogenous surfactant administration with specific inhaled immunoglobulin was used.[78] Both of these studies showed promising results and deserve further inquiry.

CONCLUSION

VAP contributes to the substantial burden of hospital-acquired infections in the neonatal intensive care population. Diagnostic accuracy in neonates (and children) is challenging given that obtaining lower respiratory tract specimens is problematic with currently available equipment. In addition, radiographic studies may be difficult to interpret.

Prevention strategies are less well defined than in adults. A VAP prevention bundle for neonates based on available data, biologic plausibility, and consideration of risk/benefit should include elevating the head of the bed for infants who tolerate that position, consistent oral hygiene, excellent hand hygiene, and daily assessment of the need for continued mechanical ventilation. Further studies of other prevention strategies are clearly warranted.

Treatment with broad-spectrum antimicrobials of a class different from what the patient has recently been exposed to for a defined amount of time is a reasonable practice. Changing to more narrowly directed therapy is hampered by the inability to reliably obtain high-quality lower tract cultures. The choice of drugs and the need for MRSA coverage should be informed by local epidemiology.

REFERENCES

A complete reference list is available at https://expertconsult.inkling.com/.

31

Pharmacologic Therapies I: Surfactant Therapy

Gautham K. Suresh, MD, DM, MS, FAAP, Roger F. Soll, MD, and George T. Mandy, MD

The development of exogenous surfactant therapy in the early 1990s was a historic advance in neonatology that led to significant reductions in neonatal mortality.[1-3] Exogenous surfactant therapy is now routinely used in the management of respiratory distress syndrome (RDS) in preterm infants and increasingly in other neonatal respiratory disorders such as meconium aspiration syndrome (MAS). This chapter provides an evidence-based overview of the use of exogenous surfactant therapy in neonatal respiratory disorders.

HISTORY

The development of effective surfactant preparations was the culmination of a series of investigations by pioneers of surfactant research, who described the existence and composition of surfactant, the role of surfactant in lowering surface tension, and the role of surfactant in maintaining alveolar stability.[4,5] A landmark in our understanding of RDS was the demonstration of surfactant deficiency in the lungs of infants dying of extreme prematurity or hyaline membrane disease.[6] Although the introduction of surface-active substances into the lung was suggested as early as 1947,[7] the initial attempts to provide exogenous surfactant therapy for immature lungs were unsuccessful.[8,9] These were followed several years later by successful attempts in animals[10] and then in human neonates.[11] After these initial efforts, numerous animal experiments and human clinical trials were conducted to study the efficacy of surfactant therapy, the relative efficacies of different surfactant preparations, the optimal timing of administration, the optimal dosage, and other aspects of exogenous surfactant therapy. The history and evolution of surfactant therapy have been reviewed in detail by several authors.[12-17]

SURFACTANT FUNCTION, COMPOSITION, AND METABOLISM

The function, composition, secretion, and metabolism of mammalian surfactant have been reviewed by several authors[18-20] and are summarized below.

Function

Pulmonary alveoli, where gas exchange occurs, are bubble-shaped and have a high degree of curvature. The surface tension of the moist inner surface is due to the attraction between the molecules in the alveolar fluid and tends to make the alveoli contract. Unchecked, this tendency would result in lung collapse. Surfactant greatly reduces the surface tension on the inner surface of the alveoli, thus preventing the alveoli from collapsing during expiration.

Composition

An accurate determination of the composition of pulmonary surfactant is difficult. To obtain surfactant for analysis, one must either wash out lungs (with the possible limitation of leaving important components behind) or extract surfactant from minced lungs (with the possible problem of adding cellular contaminants). Mammalian surfactant obtained by lung lavage consists of 80% phospholipids, 8% neutral lipids, and 12% protein. The predominant class of phospholipid (nearly 60%) is dipalmitoyl phosphatidylcholine (DPPC), with lesser amounts of unsaturated phosphatidylcholine compounds (25%), phosphatidylglycerol (15%), and phosphatidylinositol. Of all the constituents of surfactant, DPPC alone has the appropriate properties to reduce alveolar surface tension. However, DPPC alone is a poor surfactant because it adsorbs very slowly to air–liquid interfaces. Surfactant proteins or other lipids facilitate its adsorption.

Approximately half the protein in surfactant consists of contaminating protein from the plasma or lung tissue.[20] The remaining proteins include four unique surfactant-associated apoproteins: SP-A, SP-B, SP-C, and SP-D. SP-A and SP-D are hydrophilic proteins and belong to a subgroup of mammalian lectins called *collectins*. They may play important roles in the defense against inhaled pathogens, and SP-A may have a regulatory function in the formation of the monolayer that lowers the surface tension.[18] SP-B and SP-C are hydrophobic proteins and are required to enhance spreading of phospholipid in the airspaces. SP-B promotes phospholipid adsorption and induces the insertion of phospholipids into the monolayer, thus enhancing the formation of a stable surface film.[18] SP-C enhances phospholipid adsorption, stimulates the insertion of phospholipids out of the subphase into the air–liquid interface, and may increase the resistance of surfactant to inhibition by serum proteins or by edema fluid.[18,19]

Secretion and Metabolism

Surfactant is produced in the type II cells of the alveoli (Fig. 31-1). It is assembled and stored in the lamellar bodies, which consist of concentric or parallel lamellae, predominantly composed of phospholipid bilayers. Lamellar bodies are extruded into the fluid layer lining the alveoli by exocytosis and form structures known as *tubular myelin*. Tubular myelin consists of long stacked tubes composed mainly of phospholipid bilayers, the corners of which appear fused, resulting in a lattice-like

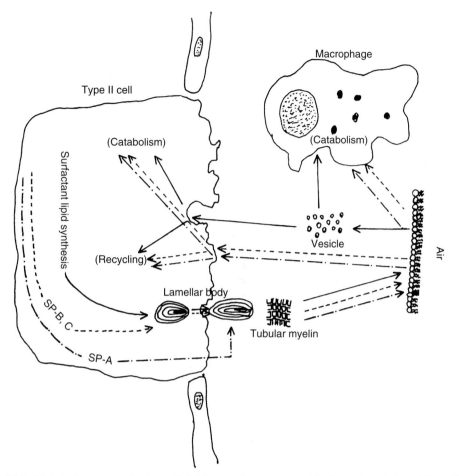

FIG 31-1 Metabolism of surfactant. *Solid line,* surfactant + liquid; *dashed and dotted line,* SP-A; *dashed line,* SP-B, SP-C. (From Jobe AH, Ikegami M. *Clin Perinatol.* 28:655, 2001.)

appearance on cross section. Tubular myelin is thought to be the major source of the monolayer surface film lining the air–liquid interface in the alveoli, in which the hydrophobic fatty acyl groups of the phospholipids extend into the air, whereas the hydrophilic polar head groups bind water.[21] This surfactant monolayer lowers the surface tension at the air–liquid interface by replacing water at the surface.[21] The phospholipid from the monolayer eventually reenters the type II cells through endocytosis and forms multivesicular bodies. These multivesicular bodies are either "recycled" by rapid incorporation into the lamellar bodies or degraded in lysosomes. Of note, all critical components of surfactant (DPPC, phosphatidylglycerol, SP-A, SP-B, and SP-C) are recycled.[20]

TYPES OF SURFACTANT

Three types of exogenous surfactant are available: (1) surfactant derived from animal sources, (2) synthetic surfactant without protein components, and (3) synthetic surfactant with protein components.

Animal-Derived Surfactants

Current commercially made animal-derived surfactants are obtained from either bovine or porcine lungs. Beractant (Survanta) and surfactant TA (Surfacten) are lipid extracts of bovine lung mince with added DPPC, tripalmitoylglycerol, and palmitic acid. Calf lung surfactant extract (calfactant, Infasurf), SF-RI 1 (Alveofact), and bovine lipid extract surfactant (BLES) are bovine lung washes subjected to chloroform–methanol extraction. Poractant (Curosurf) is a porcine lung mince that has been subjected to chloroform–methanol extraction and further purified by liquid–gel chromatography. It consists of approximately 99% polar lipids (mainly phospholipids) and 1% hydrophobic, low-molecular-weight proteins (SP-B and SP-C).[22] All the animal-derived surfactants contain SP-B and SP-C, but the lung mince extracts (Survanta and Curosurf) contain less than 10% of the SP-B that is found in the lung-wash extracts (Infasurf, Alveofact, and BLES).[23] The purification procedure including extraction with organic solvents removes the hydrophilic proteins SP-A and SP-D, leaving a material containing only lipids and small amounts of hydrophobic proteins. Poractant, which is further purified by liquid–gel chromatography, contains only polar lipids and about 1% hydrophobic proteins (SP-B and SP-C in an approximate molar ratio of 1:2).[24] None of the commercial preparations contain SP-A.[23] A surfactant obtained from human amniotic fluid was originally tested in clinical trials[25,26] but is not used as of this writing.

Synthetic Surfactants without Protein Components

The original exogenous products tested in the 1960s were synthetic surfactants composed solely of DPPC, which by itself cannot perform all the functions required of pulmonary surfactant.

Current synthetic surfactants without protein are mixtures of a variety of surface-active phospholipids (principally DPPC) and spreading agents to facilitate surface adsorption. These products include Exosurf and ALEC (artificial lung-expanding compound). Colfosceril palmitate, hexadecanol, tyloxapol (Exosurf) consists of 85% DPPC, 9% hexadecanol, and 6% tyloxapol (a spreading agent). ALEC (pumactant), which is no longer manufactured,[27] was a 7:3 mixture of DPPC and phosphatidylglycerol. These synthetic surfactants lack many of the components of animal-derived surfactant, particularly the hydrophobic surfactant proteins B and C.

Protein-Containing Synthetic Surfactants

The protein-containing synthetic surfactants contain synthetic phospholipids and proteins produced through peptide synthesis and recombinant technology that function similar to the hydrophobic proteins (SP-B and SP-C) of native human surfactant. Research is in progress to develop component protein analogues of the hydrophilic proteins SP-A and SP-D as well.

Of the surfactants containing SP-B analogues, the best studied is lucinactant (Surfaxin), which contains a mimic of SP-B called *sinapultide* or *KL4 peptide*. KL4 is a 21-residue peptide consisting of repeated units of four hydrophobic leucine (L) residues, bound by basic polar lysine (K) residues arranged in the following order: KLLLLKLLLLKLLLLKLLLLK. This structure mimics the repeating pattern of hydrophobic and hydrophilic residues in the C-terminal part of SP-B and stabilizes the phospholipid layer by interactions with the lipid heads and the acyl chains.[28] In lucinactant, sinapultide is combined with DPPC, palmitoyl-oleoyl-phosphatidylglycerol, and palmitic acid.[28,29] Other synthetic surfactants containing SP-B and SP-C analogues have also been tested in animal studies.[30-32]

Of the surfactants containing SP-C analogues, recombinant SP-C (rSP-C) surfactant or lusupultide (Venticute) has been studied in vitro and in animals and has shown efficacy. It contains rSP-C combined with DPPC, palmitoyloleoylphosphatidylglycerol, palmitic acid, and calcium chloride.[33,34] rSP-C is similar to the 34-amino-acid human SP-C sequence, except that it contains cysteine (in place of phenylalanine) in positions 4 and 5 and contains isoleucine (instead of methionine) in position 32.

ACUTE PULMONARY AND CARDIAC EFFECTS OF SURFACTANT THERAPY

Immediate Pulmonary Effects of Surfactant Therapy

In animal models of RDS, administration of exogenous surfactant results in improved lung function (Fig. 31-2)[35] and improved alveolar expansion (Fig. 31-3).[36] Several studies in human neonates have shown that the administration of exogenous surfactant therapy leads to rapid improvement in oxygenation and a decrease in the degree of support provided by mechanical ventilation (Fig. 31-4).[37] These rapid changes are accompanied by an increase in the functional residual capacity and are followed by a slower and variable increase in lung compliance.[38-40] A decrease in pulmonary ventilation–perfusion mismatch has also been reported.[41-43]

Immediate Effects on Pulmonary Circulation

The effect of surfactant treatment on the pulmonary circulation is unclear. In three studies pulmonary blood flow was unchanged with surfactant therapy.[44-46] In contrast, others have

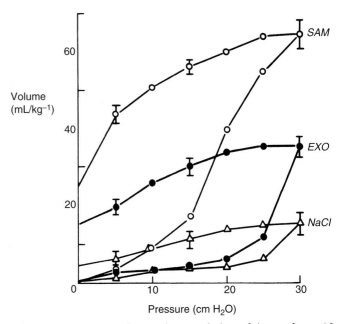

FIG 31-2 Pressure–volume characteristics of lungs from 10 matched prematurely delivered rabbits after treatment with saline (*NaCl*), Exosurf (*EXO*), or surface-active material obtained by lavaging lungs of young adult rabbits with saline (*SAM*), plus ventilation for 30 minutes. Measurements were made 10 minutes after the animals died and their lungs were allowed to degas spontaneously. (From Tooley WH, Clements JA, Muramatsu K, et al. *Am Rev Respir Dis.* 136:651, 1987.)

reported a decrease in pulmonary artery pressure or an increase in pulmonary artery flow with surfactant therapy,[47-50] as well as an increase in the ductal flow velocity from the systemic to the pulmonary circuit.[49] It is uncertain whether these changes in pulmonary circulation are related to ventilation practices, blood gas status, or the surfactant treatment itself.[51]

Radiographic Changes

In addition to these physiologic changes, treatment with exogenous surfactant also results in radiologic improvement, with chest radiographs after treatment often (but not always) showing a decrease in the signs of RDS. This clearing of the lungs can be uniform, patchy, or asymmetric, sometimes with disproportionate improvement of radiologic changes in the right lung.[52-56]

CLINICAL TRIALS OF SURFACTANT THERAPY

Surfactant therapy is one of the best-studied interventions in neonatology and has been subjected to numerous randomized controlled trials comparing various treatment strategies. The findings from these trials, many of which are included in multiple systematic reviews in the Cochrane Database of Systematic Reviews, are summarized in the following sections. The results of meta-analyses are presented as the "typical" or "pooled" estimates of relative risk (RR) and absolute risk difference (ARD), with 95% confidence intervals (CI).

Surfactant Therapy Compared to Placebo or No Therapy

Many of the early trials in the late 1980s and early 1990s studied the effects of surfactant therapy compared to placebo or no

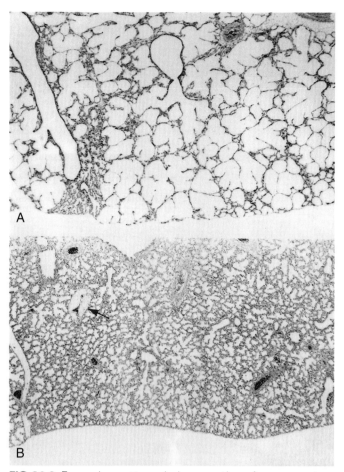

FIG 31-3 Expansion patterns in lung sections from premature rabbits. **A,** Well-expanded area in surfactant-treated fetus. The rounded appearance of the aerated alveoli contrasts with the pattern in **B** and with the wedge of unexpanded parenchyma (lower left). **B,** "Unexpanded" lung in control fetus that did not receive surfactant. The configuration of the alveoli reflects the fluid-filled state. Note abundant interstitial fluid around a pulmonary vein (*arrow*) (hematoxylin and eosin, original magnification ×27). (From Robertson B, Enhorning G. *Lab Invest.* 31:54, 1974.)

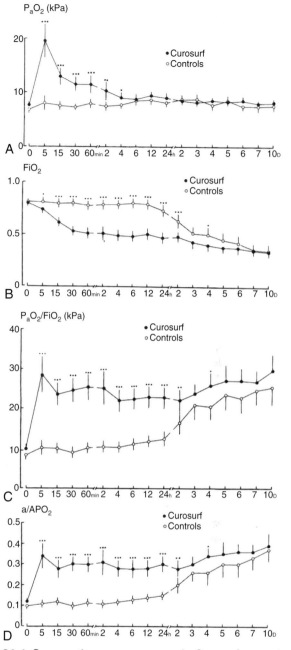

FIG 31-4 Oxygenation measurements in Curosurf-treated and control infants at various intervals after randomization. Results are mean values and 95% confidence intervals. If confidence intervals are overlapping, bars are shown on only one side of the data point. Note that the time scale is not linear. Conversion factor: 1 kPa = 7.52 mm Hg. $*p < 0.05$; $**p < 0.01$; $***p < 0.001$. **A,** Partial pressure of oxygen; **B,** Fraction of inspired oxygen; **C,** Ratio of partial pressure of oxygen to fraction of inspired oxygen; **D,** Arterio-alveolar oxygen ratio. (From Collaborative European Multicenter Study Group. *Pediatrics.* 82:683, 1988.)

therapy. Some of these trials studied the effects of prophylactic administration of surfactant to preterm infants at risk for developing RDS (prophylactic or prevention trials). Others studied the effects of treatment with surfactant in preterm infants with clinical and/or radiologic features of RDS (rescue or treatment trials). Some of these studies used animal-derived surfactant and others used synthetic surfactant. Systematic reviews of these trials[57-60] show that, compared to placebo or no therapy, surfactant treatment or prophylaxis (with either animal-derived or synthetic surfactant) decreases the risk of pneumothorax and of mortality. Estimates from the meta-analyses indicate that there is a 30% to 65% relative reduction in the risk of pneumothorax and up to a 40% relative reduction in the risk of mortality. There were no consistent effects on other clinical outcomes such as chronic lung disease, patent ductus arteriosus, and intraventricular hemorrhage.

Further evidence of the benefits of surfactant therapy is derived from studies demonstrating decreased mortality and morbidity in very low birth-weight infants after the introduction of surfactant therapy into practice.[1,3,61,62]

Prophylactic Surfactant Administration Compared to Postbirth Stabilization on Continuous Positive Airway Pressure and Selective Surfactant Administration

The rationale for prophylactic administration of surfactant is provided by the observation that in animal studies a more uniform and homogeneous distribution of surfactant is achieved when it is administered into a fluid-filled lung[63,64] and by the belief that administration of surfactant into a previously unventilated or minimally ventilated lung will diminish acute lung injury. Even brief (15 to 30 minutes) periods of mechanical ventilation prior to surfactant administration have been shown, in animal models, to cause acute lung injury resulting in alveolar-capillary damage, leakage of proteinaceous fluid into the alveolar space, and release of inflammatory mediators,[65-67] and to decrease the subsequent response to surfactant replacement.[68,69] Surfactant-deficient animals who receive assisted ventilation develop necrosis and desquamation of the bronchiolar epithelium as early as 5 minutes after onset of ventilation.[70] Prophylactic surfactant has been administered after intubating the infant immediately after birth ("before the first breath"). However, administration after initial resuscitation and confirmation of endotracheal tube position was found in a randomized trial to be equivalent or superior to immediate administration.[71]

A systematic review[72] included 11 randomized controlled trials that compared prophylactic surfactant administration to selective surfactant treatment, i.e., treatment of established RDS. All these trials used animal-derived surfactant. The selective treatment group had two categories of infants—those who were routinely stabilized on nasal CPAP immediately after birth and received surfactant if CPAP "failed" (more recent, larger studies with a high rate of maternal antenatal steroid administration) and those who were not stabilized on CPAP and received surfactant treatment at anywhere from 1.5 to 7.4 hours of age (older studies with a low rate of maternal steroid administration). Meta-analysis of studies without routine application of CPAP in controls demonstrated benefits with the use of prophylactic surfactant—a decrease in the risk of air leak and neonatal mortality. However, the analyses of studies that allowed for routine stabilization on CPAP demonstrated a decrease in the risk of chronic lung disease or death in infants stabilized on CPAP. When all studies were evaluated together, no benefits of prophylactic surfactant could be demonstrated. Furthermore, infants receiving prophylactic surfactant had a higher incidence of bronchopulmonary dysplasia (BPD) or death than did infants stabilized on CPAP (RR 1.12; 95% CI 1.02–1.24). Therefore in extremely preterm infants, the early use of CPAP with subsequent selective surfactant administration is the preferred management immediately after birth.[73] Infants managed with CPAP should be monitored closely after birth, and those who show evidence of progressive respiratory failure from RDS should be intubated and given surfactant treatment early without delay. Administration of surfactant should preferably be followed by rapid extubation, and prolonged ventilation should be avoided.

In preterm infants who do not receive prophylaxis, early surfactant treatment of those with signs and symptoms of RDS is preferred. Six randomized controlled trials, including the largest randomized trial conducted in neonatology (the OSIRIS trial), have evaluated early versus delayed selective surfactant administration. The results of these trials are summarized in a systematic review.[74] Of note, this is a comparison of what to do once an infant is intubated and not a decision about when to intubate for surfactant treatment. In these trials, early administration of surfactant consisted of administration of the first dose within the first 30 minutes to 2 hours of life. Two of the trials utilized synthetic surfactant (Exosurf Neonatal) and four utilized animal-derived surfactant preparations. The meta-analyses demonstrate significant benefits to early treatment of intubated infants with RDS:

reductions in the risk of neonatal mortality (typical RR 0.84, 95% CI 0.74 to 0.95; typical risk difference [RD] −0.04, 95% CI −0.06 to −0.01)à, chronic lung disease (typical RR 0.69, 95% CI 0.55-0.86; typical RD −0.04, 95% CI −0.06 to −0.01), and chronic lung disease or death at 36 weeks (typical RR 0.83, 95% CI 0.75-0.91; typical RD −0.06, 95% CI −0.09 to −0.03). Intubated infants randomized to early selective surfactant administration also demonstrated a decreased risk of acute lung injury including a decreased risk of pneumothorax (typical RR 0.69, 95% CI 0.59-0.82; typical RD −0.05, 95% CI −0.08 to −0.03), pulmonary interstitial emphysema (typical RR 0.60, 95% CI 0.41-0.89; typical RD −0.06, 95% CI −0.10 to −0.02), and overall air-leak syndromes (typical RR 0.61, 95% CI 0.48-0.78; typical RD −0.18, 95% CI −0.26 to −0.09). A trend toward risk reduction for BPD or death at 28 days was also evident (typical RR 0.94, 95% CI 0.88-1.00; typical RD −0.04, 95% CI −0.07 to −0.00). No differences in other complications of RDS or prematurity were noted. Therefore preterm infants who do not receive prophylactic surfactant and exhibit the signs and symptoms of RDS should receive the first dose of surfactant as early as possible. Outborn infants are at highest risk of delayed administration. Tertiary referral units accepting outborn infants should attempt to develop systems to ensure that surfactant is administered as early as possible to these infants, either by the transporting team or, if appropriate, by the referring hospital. In inborn infants, delays in administration of surfactant occur if other admission procedures such as line placement, radiographs, and nursing procedures are allowed to take precedence over surfactant dosing soon after birth. Surfactant administration should be given priority over other admission procedures.

Early Surfactant Administration Followed Immediately by Extubation to Nasal Continuous Positive Airway Pressure

When surfactant therapy was first used, infants were maintained on mechanical ventilation after surfactant administration, ventilator support was gradually weaned as the pulmonary status improved, and the infant was extubated from low ventilator settings. This approach has been compared to a strategy of surfactant administration followed immediately (within 1 hour) by extubation to nasal CPAP (NCPAP) to prevent ventilator-induced lung injury (VILI) that can result from even brief periods of mechanical ventilation.[75,76] This approach has been called the INSURE technique (*in*tubate, *sur*factant, *e*xtubate to CPAP). Six randomized trials, all of which were trials of rescue surfactant administration, have compared the INSURE approach in spontaneously breathing infants with signs of RDS to later, selective administration of surfactant in infants with respiratory insufficiency related to RDS, followed by continued mechanical ventilation and extubation from low respiratory support. These trials are summarized in a systematic review.[77] Most of these studies included infants with a gestation of 35 weeks or less and a birth weight of 2500 g or less. The meta-analysis in this review showed that compared to the traditional management strategy of gradual weaning, the INSURE approach reduced the need for mechanical ventilation (typical RR 0.67, 95% CI 0.57-0.79), air-leak syndromes (typical RR 0.52, 95% CI 0.28-0.96), and BPD (oxygen at 28 days, typical RR 0.51, 95% CI 0.26-0.99). A lower threshold for treatment at study entry (FiO_2 less than 0.45) resulted in a lower incidence of air leak (typical RR 0.46, 95% CI 0.23-0.93) and BPD (typical RR 0.43, 95% CI 0.20-0.92). A higher treatment threshold (FiO_2 greater than 0.45) at study entry was associated with a higher incidence of patent ductus arteriosus requiring treatment (typical RR 2.15, 95% CI 1.09-4.13). Since this systematic review two large randomized controlled trials were published. In a randomized trial by the Colombian Neonatal Research Network,[78] 279 infants of 27 to 31 weeks' gestation with RDS who were randomly assigned within the first hour of life to intubation, very early surfactant, extubation, and NCPAP required less ventilation and had a lower incidence of mortality and air leaks (pneumothorax and pulmonary interstitial emphysema) than infants assigned to nasal continuous airway pressure alone. In a large trial utilizing the INSURE technique the Vermont Oxford Network[79] randomized 648 infants to prophylactic surfactant followed by a period of mechanical ventilation (PS), prophylactic surfactant with rapid extubation to bubble NCPAP (ISX), or initial management with bubble NCPAP and selective surfactant treatment (NCPAP). Compared with the PS group, the RR of BPD or death was 0.78 (95% CI 0.59-1.03) for the ISX group and 0.83 (95% CI 0.64-1.09) for the NCPAP group. There were no statistically significant differences in mortality or other complications of prematurity. In the NCPAP group, 48% were managed without intubation and ventilation, and 54% without surfactant treatment. These data suggest that spontaneously breathing preterm infants who show early signs of RDS should be given surfactant at a low threshold, after which they can be quickly extubated and placed on NCPAP to reduce VILI.

Targeted Surfactant Therapy

Several studies have addressed the use of rapid bedside tests such as the click test, lamellar body count, or stable microbubble test on a tracheal aspirate or a gastric aspirate specimen.[80-83] Such tests can potentially supplement the use of clinical criteria in selecting preterm infants whose likelihood of RDS is high enough to merit surfactant therapy and perhaps avoid needless intubations and, in those already intubated, needless surfactant therapy. However, it is unclear whether the logistic challenges of performing these tests are worth the additional refinements in decision making.

Single versus Multiple Surfactant Doses

Many of the initial trials of surfactant therapy tested a single dose of surfactant. However, surfactant may become rapidly metabolized, and functional inactivation of surfactant can result from the action of soluble proteins and other factors in the small airways and alveoli.[20] The ability to administer repeat or subsequent doses of surfactant is thought to be useful in overcoming such inactivation. The results of two randomized controlled trials that compared multiple dosing regimens to single-dose regimens of animal-derived surfactant extract for treatment of established RDS have been evaluated in a systematic review.[84] In one study,[85] after the initial dose of BLES, infants assigned to the multiple-dose group could receive up to three additional doses of surfactant during the first 72 hours of life if they had a respiratory deterioration, provided they had shown a positive response to the first dose and a pneumothorax had been eliminated as the cause of the respiratory deterioration. In the other study,[86] infants in the multiple-dose group received additional doses of poractant at 12 and 24 hours after the initial dose if they still needed supplemental oxygen and mechanical ventilation. Approximately 70% of the infants randomized to the multiple-dose regimen received multiple doses. The meta-analysis supports a decreased risk of pneumothorax associated with multiple-dose surfactant therapy (typical

RR 0.51, 95% CI 0.30-0.88; typical ARD 0.09, 95% CI 0.15-0.02). There was also a trend toward decreased mortality (typical RR 0.63, 95% CI 0.39-1.02; typical ARD 0.07, 95% CI 0.14-0.00). No differences were detected in other clinical outcomes. No complications associated with multiple-dose treatment were reported in these trials. In a third study, in which synthetic surfactant was used in a prophylactic manner, the use of two doses of surfactant in addition to the prophylactic dose led to a decrease in mortality, respiratory support, necrotizing enterocolitis, and other outcomes compared to a single prophylactic dose.[87] In the OSIRIS trial, which used synthetic surfactant, a two-dose treatment schedule was found to be equivalent to a treatment schedule permitting up to four doses of surfactant.[88]

Criteria for Repeat Doses of Surfactant

The use of a higher threshold for re-treatment with surfactant appears to be as effective as a low threshold and can result in significant savings in costs of the drug. The criteria for administration of repeat doses of surfactant have been investigated in two studies, both of which used animal-derived surfactant. In one study[89] the re-treatment criteria compared were an increase in the fraction of inspired oxygen by 0.1 over the lowest baseline value (standard re-treatment) versus a sustained increase of just 0.01 (liberal re-treatment). There were no differences in complications of prematurity or duration of respiratory support. However, short-term benefits in oxygen requirement and degree of ventilator support were noted in the liberal re-treatment group.

In another study,[90] re-treatment at a low threshold (FiO$_2$ greater than 30%, still requiring endotracheal intubation) was compared to re-treatment at a high threshold (FiO$_2$ greater than 40%, mean airway pressure greater than 7 cm H$_2$O). Again, there were minor short-term benefits to using a low threshold with no differences in major clinical outcomes. However, in a subgroup of infants with RDS complicated by perinatal compromise or infection, infants in the high-threshold group had a trend toward higher mortality than the low-threshold group. Based on current evidence, it appears appropriate to use persistent or worsening signs of RDS as criteria for re-treatment with surfactant. A low threshold for repeat dosing should be used for infants with RDS who have perinatal depression or infection.

METHODS OF ADMINISTRATION OF SURFACTANT

A theoretical model for the transport of exogenous surfactant through the airways has been proposed,[91] consisting of four distinct mechanisms: (1) the instilled bolus may create a liquid plug that occludes the large airways but is forced peripherally during mechanical ventilation; (2) the bolus creates a deposited film on the airway walls, either from the liquid plug transport or from direct coating, that drains under the influence of gravity through the first few airway generations; (3) in smaller airways, surfactant species form a surface layer that spreads because of surface-tension gradients, that is, Marangoni flows; and (4) the surfactant finally reaches the alveolar compartment where it is cleared according to first-order kinetics.

Administration through Catheter, Side Port, or Suction Valve

According to the manufacturers' recommendations, beractant and poractant should be administered through a catheter inserted into the endotracheal tube; colfosceril should be administered through a side-port adapter attached to the endotracheal tube, and calf lung surfactant extract can be administered either through a catheter or through a side-port adapter. Other methods of administration of surfactant have been tested in randomized trials. In one randomized trial, the administration of beractant through a catheter inserted through a neonatal suction valve without detachment of the neonate from the ventilator was compared to the administration of the dose (with detachment from the ventilator) in two aliquots through a catheter and to the standard technique of administration of the dose in four aliquots through a catheter.[92] Administration through the suction valve led to less dosing-related oxygen desaturation but more reflux of beractant than the two-aliquot catheter technique. In another study,[93] the administration of poractant as a bolus was compared in a randomized trial to administration via a catheter introduced through a side hole in the tracheal tube adaptor without changing the infant's position or interrupting ventilation. The numbers of episodes of hypoxia and/or bradycardia, as well as other outcomes, were similar in both groups. A slight and transient increase in $PaCO_2$ was observed in the side-hole group.

Administration through Dual-Lumen Endotracheal Tube

The administration of poractant through a dual-lumen endotracheal tube without a change in position or interruption of mechanical ventilation was compared to bolus instillation in a randomized trial.[94] The dual-lumen group had fewer episodes of dosing-related hypoxia, a smaller decrease in heart rate and oxygen saturation, and a shorter total time in increased supplemental oxygen than the bolus group. The dual-lumen method has also been compared to the side-port method of administration of colfosceril in a randomized trial.[95] No difference was found between the two methods in dosing-related hypoxemia.

Administration through a Laryngeal Mask Airway

Surfactant administration through a laryngeal mask airway (LMA) is noninvasive, avoids endotracheal intubation, and potentially avoids the complications associated with intubation. It has been reported in a series of eight preterm infants (mean birth weight 1700 g) with RDS managed with NCPAP.[96] The mean arterial-to-alveolar oxygen tension ratio improved significantly after the treatment, and no complications were reported. Moreover, although the smallest infant in this study was 880 g, the use of the currently available LMA is recommended only for babies above 1500 g. A randomized controlled trial of 26 infants resulted in reduction of FiO_2 in the first 12 hours after surfactant administration, but later no significant difference was found in subsequent need for mechanical ventilation or BPD. However, this study reported several adverse events with the use of LMA.[97] Another randomized trial of 61 patients found that surfactant administration through an LMA reduced the proportion of preterm infants with moderate RDS who required mechanical ventilation compared with standard endotracheal administration following intubation with premedication. The efficacy of surfactant in decreasing RDS severity was similar with both methods.[98] Another randomized trial of 70 infants utilized i-gel for surfactant administration.[99] I-gel is a laryngeal device modeled on the LMA. The study resulted in significantly higher a-APO$_2$ after treatment with i-gel compared to INSURE in

controls. Thus, although there is accumulating evidence for the administration of surfactant through an LMA or similar device, further research is required to establish the efficacy and risk-versus-benefit ratio of these methods.

Nasopharyngeal Administration of Surfactant

Another noninvasive method of surfactant administration is instillation of surfactant into the nasopharynx during or immediately after delivery and before the first breath. Such instillation is thought to cause the surfactant to be aspirated into the fluid-filled airway as an air–fluid interface is established. A case series[100] of 23 preterm infants of 27 to 30 weeks' gestation receiving such intrapartum nasopharyngeal instillation of surfactant followed by placement on CPAP immediately after birth (mask CPAP initially followed by NCPAP) demonstrated the feasibility of such administration. However, more evidence is required to prove the efficacy of this approach before it can be used or recommended.

Thin Catheter Endotracheal Administration (Less-Invasive Surfactant Administration)

Instead of an endotracheal tube, this method utilizes a thin catheter that is inserted into the trachea while the patient is spontaneously breathing on a CPAP tube and surfactant is administered through this thin tube, after which the tube is removed. Two systematic reviews summarized the results of individual studies. There was no significant difference regarding mortality or BPD but there was a potential reduction in the need for mechanical ventilation within 72 hours.[101,102] The Nonintubated Surfactant Application (NINSAPP) multicenter randomized trial[103] found that the intervention did not increase survival without BPD. However, it was associated with increased survival without major complications, specifically a significant reduction of pneumothorax and intraventricular hemorrhage, less need for intubation, and fewer days on mechanical ventilation. Less-invasive surfactant administration is a promising mode of administration of surfactant for the treatment of extremely preterm infants, and the research in this area is active. As of this writing a large randomized multicenter trial (OPTIMIST-A) is being conducted to compare catheter administration of surfactant to sham administration. The trial is expected to conclude in late 2017.

Other Methods

In one randomized clinical trial,[104] the slow infusion of colfosceril using a microinfusion syringe pump over 10 to 20 minutes was compared to manual instillation over 2 minutes. Pump administration resulted in fewer infants with loss of chest wall movement during dosing as well as a smaller increase in peak inspiratory pressure than with hand administration. However, in animals, slow infusion of surfactant into the endotracheal tube results in nonhomogeneous distribution of surfactant in the lung.[105,106] Therefore, currently, bolus administration of surfactant is preferred. Other methods of administration, such as nebulization or aerosolization[107-110] and in utero administration to the human fetus,[111,112] have also been reported. These methods require further clinical testing and may require specialized nebulization equipment. The use of vibrating membrane nebulizers, coupled with appropriate positioning of the interface device, may result in efficient delivery of aerosolized surfactant,[113] but this method also requires further testing and validation.

Chest Position during Administration of Surfactant

In a study in rabbits, pulmonary distribution of intratracheally instilled surfactant was largely determined by gravity, and changing the chest position after instillation did not result in any redistribution of the surfactant. Therefore, for neonates receiving surfactant, keeping the chest in the horizontal position may result in the most even distribution of the surfactant in the two lungs.[114]

Summary of Administration Methods

In summary, based on available evidence, surfactant should be administered in the standard method of aliquots instilled into an endotracheal tube. There is evidence to suggest that the administration of surfactant using a dual-lumen endotracheal tube or through a catheter passed through a suction valve is effective and may cause less dosing-related adverse events than standard methods. The side-port method of administration and the catheter method of administration through the endotracheal tube appear to be equivalent. Less-invasive surfactant administration is a promising method to improve the outcome of extremely preterm infants. More studies are required before firm conclusions can be drawn about the optimal method of administration of surfactant and whether the optimal method is different for different types of surfactant.

CHOICE OF SURFACTANT PRODUCT

Comparison of Animal-Derived Surfactant Extract versus Protein-Free Synthetic Surfactant for the Prevention and Treatment of Respiratory Distress Syndrome

Although both synthetic and animal-derived surfactants are effective, their compositions differ. Animal-derived surfactant extracts contain surfactant-specific proteins that aid in surfactant adsorption and resist surfactant inactivation. Fifteen randomized trials have compared the effects of animal-derived and protein-free synthetic surfactants in the treatment or prevention of RDS. More than 5000 infants were studied in these trials. A systematic review of these trials is available.[115]

Compared to synthetic surfactant without protein, treatment with animal-derived surfactant extracts resulted in a significant reduction in the risk of pneumothorax (typical RR 0.65, 95% CI 0.55-0.77; typical ARD −0.04, 95% CI −0.06 to −0.02) and the risk of mortality (typical RR 0.89, 95% CI 0.79-0.99; typical ARD −0.02, 95% CI −0.04 to 0.00). Animal-derived surfactant extract is associated with an increase in the risk of necrotizing enterocolitis (typical RR 1.38, 95% CI 1.08-1.76; typical ARD 0.02, 95% CI 0.01-0.04) and borderline significant increase in the risk of intraventricular hemorrhage (typical RR 1.07, 95% CI 0.99-1.15; typical ARD 0.02, 95% CI 0.00-0.05), but no increase in grade 3 or 4 intraventricular hemorrhage (typical RR 1.08, 95% CI 0.91-1.27; typical ARD 0.01, 95% CI −0.01 to 0.03). The meta-analysis also supports a marginal decrease in the risk of BPD or mortality associated with the use of animal-derived surfactant preparations (typical RR 0.95, 95% CI 0.91-1.00; typical ARD −0.03, 95% CI −0.06 to 0.00).

In addition to these benefits, animal-derived surfactants have a more rapid onset of action, allowing ventilator settings and inspired oxygen concentrations to be lowered more quickly than with synthetic surfactant.[116-120] A comparison of physical properties and the results of animal studies also suggest that animal-derived surfactants have advantages over protein-free synthetic surfactants.[121] These properties are attributed to the presence of the surfactant proteins SP-B and SP-C in certain animal-derived surfactants.[122]

The use of animal-derived surfactant preparations should be favored in most clinical situations, because their use results in greater clinical benefits than synthetic surfactants.

Comparison of Protein-Containing Synthetic Surfactant versus Animal-Derived Surfactant Extract for the Prevention and Treatment of Respiratory Distress Syndrome

Clinical trials have compared the effects of synthetic surfactants containing peptides to animal-derived surfactant preparations. These synthetic surfactants do not have the theoretical concerns associated with animal-derived surfactants, namely, transmission of microorganisms, exposure to animal proteins and inflammatory mediators, susceptibility to inactivation, and inconsistent content.[123] Lucinactant, the synthetic surfactant containing an analogue of SP-B, sinapultide, has been compared with beractant in the safety and effectiveness of lucinactant versus Exosurf in a clinical trial of RDS in premature infants (SELECT), a multicenter, masked randomized trial of surfactant prophylaxis in infants of 24 to 32 weeks' gestation.[124] Lucinactant was also compared with poractant in Surfaxin therapy against RDS, in a multicenter randomized trial (STAR) of surfactant prophylaxis in infants of 24 to 28 weeks' gestation that was structured as a noninferiority trial.[125] A meta-analysis of these two studies[126] found no significant differences in outcomes between lucinactant and the compared animal-derived surfactant in mortality at 36 weeks' postmenstrual age (typical RR 0.81, 95% CI 0.64-1.03), chronic lung disease at 36 weeks' postmenstrual age (typical RR 0.99, 95% CI 0.84-1.18), the composite outcome of mortality or chronic lung disease at 36 weeks' postmenstrual age (typical RR 0.96, 95% CI 0.82-1.12), or other respiratory outcomes. A decreased risk of necrotizing enterocolitis, a secondary outcome, was noted in infants receiving lucinactant (typical RR 0.60, 95% CI 0.42-0.86; typical RD −0.06, 95% CI −0.10 to −0.01).

However, both trials of lucinactant described above had multiple methodologic problems[127] that undermined their validity, and as of this writing there is no clear evidence of the equivalence or superiority of lucinactant over any animal-derived surfactant product.[128] In March 2012, the Food and Drug Administration approved lucinactant for use in the United States. Further research is required to elucidate the role of newer surfactants in the prevention or treatment of RDS.

Comparison of Protein-Containing Synthetic Surfactant versus Protein-Free Synthetic Surfactant for the Prevention and Treatment of Respiratory Distress Syndrome

In the SELECT trial,[124] the randomized trial of lucinactant, in which lucinactant was compared with beractant, lucinactant was also compared to colfosceril. Infants who received protein-containing synthetic surfactant compared to protein-free synthetic surfactant did not demonstrate significantly different risks of mortality at 36 weeks' postmenstrual age (PMA) (RR 0.89, 95% CI 0.71-1.11), chronic lung disease at 36 weeks' PMA (RR 0.89, 95% CI 0.78-1.03), or the combined outcome of mortality or chronic lung disease at 36 weeks' PMA (RR 0.88, 95% CI 0.77-1.01). Regarding the secondary outcome of RDS at 24 hours of age, a decrease in the incidence was demonstrated in the group that received lucinactant (RR 0.83, 95% CI 0.72-0.95).[129]

Comparison of Different Types of Bovine Surfactants

Two prevention studies and seven treatment studies compared bovine lung lavage surfactant extract to modified bovine minced lung surfactant extract. The meta-analysis[130] of the prevention trials, representing high-quality evidence, found no significant difference in death or chronic lung disease (typical RR 1.02, 95% CI 0.89-1.17; typical RD 0.01, 95% CI −0.05 to 0.06). Analysis of the treatment trials also found no significant differences between these two types of bovine surfactants in death or chronic lung disease (typical RR 0.95, 95% CI 0.86-1.06; typical RD −0.02, 95% CI −0.06 to 0.02, high-quality evidence).

Comparison of Porcine and Bovine Surfactants

Nine treatment studies compared modified bovine minced lung surfactant extract with porcine minced lung surfactant extract. A meta-analysis of these studies[130] found a significant increase in mortality prior to hospital discharge (typical RR 1.44, 95% CI 1.04-2.00; typical RD 0.05, 95% CI 0.01-0.10) in patients treated with modified bovine surfactant extract compared with porcine minced lung surfactant extract. Other outcome parameters like death or oxygen requirement at 36 weeks' PMA (typical RR 1.30, 95% CI 1.04-1.64; typical RD 0.11, 95% CI 0.02-0.20), receiving more than one dose of surfactant (typical RR 1.57, 95% CI 1.29-1.92; typical RD 0.14, 95% CI 0.08-0.20), and patent ductus arteriosus requiring treatment (typical RR 1.86, 95% CI 1.28-2.70; typical RD 0.28, 95% CI 0.13-0.43) also favored treatment with porcine minced lung surfactant. The dose of beractant was uniformly 100 mg/kg across all five studies. When only studies that used a 100 mg/kg dose of poractant were considered, the reduction in mortality prior to discharge and risk of death or oxygen requirement at 36 weeks' PMA were not statistically significant. It is uncertain that the statistical difference between the two types of surfactants was related to the source of extraction (porcine vs bovine) or to the higher initial dose of porcine surfactant.

ADVERSE EFFECTS OF SURFACTANT THERAPY

Transient hypoxia and bradycardia can occur as a result of acute airway obstruction immediately after surfactant instillation.[92,131] Other acute adverse effects of surfactant administration include reflux of surfactant into the pharynx from the endotracheal tube, increase in transcutaneous carbon dioxide tension, tachycardia, gagging, and mucous plugging of the endotracheal tube. These complications of surfactant administration generally respond to a slower rate of surfactant administration or to an increase in the airway pressure or FiO_2 during administration. Rapid improvement in oxygenation after surfactant administration necessitates close monitoring and appropriate reduction of ventilatory parameters.

Several authors have reported a transient decrease in blood pressure,[132-134] a transient decrease in cerebral blood flow velocity,[135-137] a transient decrease in cerebral oxyhemoglobin concentration,[137] and a transient decrease in cerebral activity on amplitude-integrated electroencephalography[132] immediately after surfactant administration. The electroencephalogram (EEG) depression observed after surfactant instillation is not caused by cerebral ischemia,[138] and the EEG suppression

is not directly related to alterations in blood gases or systemic circulation.[139] The clinical significance of these findings is uncertain. One study[140] reported an increase in the incidence of intraventricular hemorrhage, and a case report documents a temporal association between the development of intraventricular hemorrhage and the administration of surfactant TA to improve respiratory failure caused by pulmonary hemorrhage.[141] However, the meta-analyses of multiple trials do not show an increase in the risk of intraventricular hemorrhage with surfactant therapy compared to placebo.[57-60]

There is a well-described increase in the risk of pulmonary hemorrhage with surfactant therapy.[142,143] Although trials in which animal-derived surfactants were used reported a higher incidence (5% to 6%) of pulmonary hemorrhage than trials of synthetic surfactant (1% to 3%), direct comparison of the two types of surfactants demonstrates no difference in the risk of pulmonary hemorrhage. The overall incidence of pulmonary hemorrhage was low, and the absolute magnitude of the increased risk is small.[142] However, moderate and severe pulmonary hemorrhage is associated with an increased risk of death and short-term morbidity. It is not associated with increased long-term morbidity.[144] The occurrence of pulmonary hemorrhage may be related to the presence of a hemodynamically significant patent ductus arteriosus.[145,146] Seppanen studied the association of neonatal complications with the Doppler-derived aortopulmonary pressure gradient (APPG) across the ductus arteriosus, which reflects pulmonary artery pressure during the first day of life. Infants in whom the APPG decreased after birth had a lower frequency of patent ductus arteriosus and pulmonary hemorrhage[147] than those whose APPG remained low. Another mechanism for pulmonary hemorrhage may be a direct cytotoxicity, which has been demonstrated in in vitro studies and appears to be different for different surfactants and different dosages.[148]

When surfactant initially became available for clinical testing, there was concern that the introduction of foreign proteins from animal-based lung surfactants into the lungs of preterm infants could lead to immunologic responses. Two studies did not find antibodies specific to surfactant protein in the sera of preterm infants treated with bovine surfactant.[149,150] In other studies, immune complexes or antibodies to the protein in exogenous porcine, bovine, or human surfactant have been identified in the sera of neonates with RDS. However, similar immune complexes or antibodies were also noted in control infants who did not receive surfactant. Positive enzyme-linked immunosorbent assay values with regard to SP-A, and IgM against SP-A and SP-B and C, were more frequently found in the control group than in the surfactant-treated group in sera from neonates at 1 week of age.[147,151,152] This occurrence was less frequent in surfactant-treated neonates, suggesting that surfactant treatment reduces leakage of these proteins in the circulation.[151]

With animal-derived surfactants, there is a theoretical risk of the transmission of infectious agents, including bovine spongiform encephalitis, with surfactants derived from bovine sources and other viral infections in swine. Organic solvent processing of phospholipids, terminal sterilization techniques, and screening of animal sources have been used to minimize this risk.

ECONOMIC ASPECTS OF SURFACTANT THERAPY

With the introduction of surfactant therapy, there was concern that the increased number of survivors and a possible increase in the length of hospital stay would lead to an increase in the overall cost of neonatal care.[153] These increased costs can be offset to a variable extent by the fact that surfactant therapy can lead to lower hospital charges,[154] reduce the costs or charges per survivor of neonatal intensive care,[3,155,156] and reduce the charges for infants who ultimately die.[3] In an economic analysis for a hypothetic cohort of infants weighing 700 to 1350 g and treated with synthetic surfactant, based on the results of a randomized controlled trial,[157] the total hospital charges through 1 year adjusted age were similar to those for a comparable cohort of infants receiving air placebo, despite the fact that more babies in the synthetic surfactant cohort survived and thus required prolonged hospital care during their first year of life. The incremental cost per survivor estimated in this study was $1585 (in 1995 dollars).

In 1990, the cost per quality-adjusted life year (QALY) with surfactant therapy was estimated in one study to be $1500[158] and in another study to be £710.[159] From a societal perspective, the cost-effectiveness of surfactant therapy is more favorable than that of health care interventions such as renal transplantation, coronary bypass surgery, and dialysis.[159] In a geographically defined, population-based study from Australia, cost-effectiveness and cost-utility ratios in pre-surfactant and post-surfactant periods were compared for 500- to 999-g birth-weight infants. When costs incurred during the primary hospitalization were considered, both of these ratios were lower (i.e., economically better) in the post-surfactant era than in the pre-surfactant era (pre-surfactant vs post-surfactant, $7040 vs $4040 per life year gained; $6700 vs $5360 per QALY). Both ratios fell with increasing birth weight. With costs for long-term care of severely disabled children added, both cost ratios were higher in the post-surfactant era.

FACTORS AFFECTING THE RESPONSE TO SURFACTANT THERAPY

Several factors have been reported by various authors to be associated with a poor response to surfactant therapy, either in terms of immediate pulmonary response or in terms of later morbidity and mortality. These factors include high total fluid and colloid intake in the first days of life;[160] a low mean airway pressure relative to the FiO_2;[160] the presence of an additional pulmonary disorder such as infection;[161] perinatal asphyxia, infection, or other complications of prematurity;[162] and high fraction of inspired oxygen requirement at entry (had a negative impact on a-APO_2 6 and 24 hours after treatment), lower birth weight, male sex, outborn status, perinatal asphyxia, and high airway pressure requirement at entry.[163] Low birth weight, low Apgar scores, and initial disease severity were associated with an increased mortality.[164]

A high pulmonary resistance prior to therapy was associated with a poor response to therapy at 24 and 48 hours.[165] In addition, the immediate response to surfactant therapy itself has been reported to be a significant prognostic indicator for mortality and morbidity.[166] In animal studies poor response to surfactant has been associated with delayed administration[64] and the leakage of proteinaceous fluid into the alveolar spaces. Within some multicenter trials, significant differences in outcomes of surfactant-treated infants have been noted between participating hospitals,[163,164] suggesting that variations in patient care practices have an important influence on the outcomes of surfactant-treated infants.

As noted earlier, observational studies have demonstrated a decrease in mortality and morbidity for such infants after the introduction of surfactant therapy. However, racial differences in this decline in mortality have been reported. In one study, the overall neonatal mortality for black very low birth-weight (VLBW) infants did not change after the introduction of surfactant therapy,[62] and in another study, declines in neonatal mortality risks caused by RDS and all respiratory causes were greater for non-Hispanic white VLBW infants than for black VLBW infants.[167] Although such racial differences have been noted at a population level, the role of racial factors in the response pattern of individual infants with RDS to exogenous surfactant therapy is unknown.

LONG-TERM OUTCOMES AFTER SURFACTANT THERAPY

Long-term outcomes after surfactant therapy have been well studied for synthetic surfactant. Follow-up studies of long-term outcomes after animal-derived surfactant therapy have consisted of small numbers of patients, with a variable proportion of survivors being tested. For both synthetic and animal-derived surfactant, the long-term outcomes reported consist of outcomes predominantly in the first 3 years of life, with very few reports of outcomes at school age or higher. Given these limitations, the evidence suggests that not only do more infants survive from surfactant therapy, but also they are at no selective disadvantage for neurodevelopmental sequelae due to the surfactant therapy. Most comparisons of long-term outcomes have been between infants treated with surfactant and placebo. There are few or no comparisons of long-term outcomes between infants treated with different types of surfactant or different regimens of the same surfactant. The following sections mainly address comparisons between infants treated with surfactant and placebo.

Neurodevelopmental Outcomes

No significant differences have been reported in the long-term neurodevelopmental outcomes of infants treated with surfactant compared to those treated with placebo, either with synthetic surfactant[87,168,169] or with animal-derived surfactant.[170-174]

Long-Term Respiratory Outcomes

Compared to infants treated with placebo, infants treated with surfactant in the neonatal period have been reported either to have improved[175-177] or to have equivalent[178-180] results on pulmonary function testing. Some studies have reported a lower frequency of subsequent clinical respiratory disorders in surfactant-treated infants compared to placebo,[181,182] whereas others have reported no difference[147,168,170,175] or a trend toward an increase in allergic manifestations.[174]

Physical Growth

No significant differences have been reported in weight or height outcomes between surfactant-treated and placebo-treated infants on follow-up.[147,169,174-176,182]

Outcomes of Prophylactic versus Rescue Treatment Strategies

Two studies compared the long-term outcomes of infants treated with prophylactic surfactant to those treated with a "rescue" strategy. In one, there were no differences at school age in neurodevelopmental outcome or in the results of pulmonary function testing between the two groups, although infants who had received prophylactic surfactant showed fewer clinical pulmonary problems than those who received rescue treatment.[183] In another study in which there was significant loss of infants to follow-up (and therefore a high likelihood of attrition bias), the mean scores on the Bayley scales of infant development at 12 months' adjusted age were higher in the rescue group than in the prophylactic group.[181]

EXOGENOUS SURFACTANT THERAPY FOR CONDITIONS OTHER THAN RESPIRATORY DISTRESS SYNDROME

Exogenous surfactant therapy has been attempted in a variety of neonatal respiratory disorders other than RDS, with variable quality of evidence and variable efficacy.[184]

Meconium Aspiration Syndrome

In vitro studies[185,186] and animal studies[187,188] have demonstrated that meconium inhibits surfactant function and is likely to be partially responsible for alveolar collapse in MAS. Components of meconium that may contribute to altered surfactant function include cholesterol, free fatty acids, bile salts, bilirubin, and proteolytic enzymes.[185-187]

In uncontrolled studies of human infants with MAS, improved oxygenation has been reported with exogenous surfactant therapy.[189-191] A randomized trial in infants of greater than 34 weeks' gestation with severe respiratory failure on extracorporeal membrane oxygenation (ECMO) (including infants with MAS) showed that infants treated with beractant had improved lung function, a shorter duration of ECMO, and fewer complications after ECMO.[192]

Four randomized trials[193-196] have studied the effects of animal-derived surfactant in term infants with MAS and are included in a systematic review. In these trials, surfactant therapy was administered as a continuous infusion over 20 minutes[194] or as a bolus. A systematic review and meta-analysis of these four trials[197] showed a decreased need for ECMO with surfactant therapy (typical RR 0.64, 95% CI 0.46-0.91; typical ARD −0.17; 95% CI −0.30 to −0.04). One trial reported a reduction in the length of hospital stay (mean difference = 8 days; 95% CI, −14 to −3 days). There were no statistically significant effects on mortality (typical RR 0.98, 95% CI 0.41-2.39; typical RD 0.00, 95% CI −0.05 to 0.05) or other outcomes (duration of assisted ventilation, duration of supplemental oxygen, pneumothorax, pulmonary interstitial emphysema, air leaks, chronic lung disease, need for oxygen at discharge, or intraventricular hemorrhage).

In summary, infants with severe MAS are likely to benefit from treatment with animal-derived surfactants. Multiple doses are usually required in such infants. Only animal-derived surfactants have been tested in human clinical trials in this setting, and the efficacy of synthetic surfactants is unknown. Each dose should be administered cautiously, with close cardiac, respiratory, and oxygen saturation monitoring, because surfactant can aggravate preexisting airway obstruction from meconium, and transient oxygen desaturation and endotracheal tube obstruction have been reported with bolus administration in nearly one-third of infants.[193]

Investigators have also attempted to treat MAS by lavaging the airways with diluted surfactant solutions to wash out residual meconium.[198] This approach to surfactant treatment requires further study before it can be recommended.

Acute Respiratory Distress Syndrome

Surfactant dysfunction is well described in acute lung injury.[199] Therefore, surfactant replacement has been proposed as a treatment for patients with acute lung injury and acute RDS (ARDS), which, although more common in adults and older children, can occur in term neonates.[200,201] Exogenous surfactant therapy has been attempted in ARDS in adults, but the results of clinical trials have not been promising.[202] There are no randomized trials of exogenous surfactant therapy specifically for ARDS in neonates, but in older children with acute respiratory failure, surfactant use decreased mortality and duration of ventilation.[203,204] Extrapolating from these pediatric studies, and based on the pathophysiologic, clinical, and radiologic similarities between RDS and ARDS, term infants with clinical and radiologic features of ARDS (severe respiratory failure with pulmonary opacification and air bronchograms on chest radiographs) are often treated with exogenous surfactant.[205]

Other Conditions

There are reports (anecdotal or case series) of the use of exogenous surfactant therapy in human infants for the management of pulmonary hemorrhage[206,207] and neonatal pneumonia.[189,208-210] However, the efficacy of surfactant in these conditions is uncertain, and its routine use in these conditions cannot be recommended. Surfactant therapy for infants with congenital diaphragmatic hernia has also been attempted[211-217] but actually resulted in worse outcomes, and therefore is not recommended.

CONCLUSION

Exogenous surfactant therapy has been a significant advance in the management of preterm infants with RDS and has become established as a standard part of the management of such infants. Both animal-derived and synthetic surfactants lead to clinical improvement and decreased mortality, with animal-derived surfactants having advantages over synthetic surfactants. The use of prophylactic surfactant, administered after initial stabilization at birth, to infants at risk for RDS has benefits over rescue surfactant given to treat infants with established RDS. In infants who do not receive prophylaxis, earlier treatment (before 2 hours) has benefits over later treatment. The use of multiple doses of surfactant as needed is superior to the use of a single dose, and the use of a higher threshold for re-treatment appears to be as effective as a low threshold. Adverse effects of surfactant therapy are infrequent and usually not serious; long-term follow-up of infants treated with surfactant in the neonatal period is reassuring. New protein-containing synthetic surfactants are becoming available and show promise. Further research is required on the optimal use of surfactant in conjunction with other respiratory interventions.

REFERENCES

A complete reference list is available at https://expertconsult.inkling.com/.

32

Pharmacologic Therapies II: Inhaled Nitric Oxide

John P. Kinsella, MD

Endogenous nitric oxide (NO) is important for the regulation of vascular tone. The enzyme NO synthase generates NO from L-arginine. NO then activates guanyl cyclase and increases the production of cyclic guanosine monophosphate (cGMP). This in turn activates a cascade of GMP-dependent protein kinases resulting in an efflux of calcium from cells and in the relaxation of the vascular smooth muscle. Inhaled nitric oxide (iNO) reaches the alveolar space and diffuses into vascular smooth muscle of the adjacent pulmonary arteries, where it causes vasodilation. When iNO enters the vascular lumen it is rapidly bound to hemoglobin, restricting its effect to the pulmonary circulation. iNO is distributed to the ventilated segments of the lungs and causes increased perfusion in those areas, leading to an improved ventilation/perfusion ratio and improved oxygenation.

iNO therapy causes potent, selective, sustained pulmonary vasodilation and improves oxygenation in term newborns with severe hypoxemic respiratory failure and persistent pulmonary hypertension.[1-6] Multicenter randomized clinical studies have demonstrated that iNO therapy reduces the need for extracorporeal membrane oxygenation (ECMO) treatment in term neonates with hypoxemic respiratory failure.[7,8]

The role of iNO therapy has been extensively studied, leading to regulatory approval in 1999 by the U.S. Food and Drug Administration of the treatment of near-term and term newborns with hypoxemic respiratory failure and evidence of persistent pulmonary hypertension of the newborn (PPHN). In this chapter, we review an approach to the initial evaluation of the hypoxemic newborn for treatment with iNO, summarize the clinical experience with iNO in near-term and term newborns, and propose guidelines for the use of iNO in this population. We also review controversies and current evidence for the use of iNO in the premature newborn, although its use remains investigational in this population.[9,10]

BACKGROUND

The physiologic rationale for iNO therapy in the treatment of neonatal hypoxemic respiratory failure is based upon its ability to achieve potent and sustained pulmonary vasodilation without decreasing systemic vascular tone (Fig. 32-1).[11] PPHN[12] is a syndrome associated with diverse neonatal cardiac and pulmonary disorders that are characterized by high pulmonary vascular resistance (PVR) causing extrapulmonary right-to-left shunting of blood across the ductus arteriosus and/or foramen ovale (see Chapter 33) (Fig. 32-2).[13,14] Extrapulmonary shunting due to high PVR in severe PPHN can cause critical hypoxemia that is poorly responsive to inspired oxygen or pharmacologic vasodilation. Vasodilator drugs administered intravenously in the past to lower PVR, such as tolazoline and sodium nitroprusside, were often unsuccessful because of systemic hypotension and an inability to achieve or sustain pulmonary vasodilation.[15,16] Thus the ability of iNO therapy to selectively lower PVR and decrease extrapulmonary venoarterial admixture without affecting blood pressure accounts for the acute improvement in oxygenation observed in newborns with PPHN.[17]

As described in children[18] and adults with severe respiratory failure,[19] oxygenation can improve during iNO therapy in some newborns who do not have extrapulmonary right-to-left shunting. Hypoxemia in these cases is primarily due to intrapulmonary shunting caused by continued perfusion of lung units that lack ventilation (e.g., atelectasis), with variable contributions from ventilation–perfusion inequality. Distinct from its ability to decrease extrapulmonary right-to-left shunting by reducing PVR, low-dose iNO therapy can improve oxygenation by redirecting blood from poorly aerated or diseased lung regions to better aerated distal air spaces ("microselective effect").[20]

In addition to its effects on vascular tone and reactivity, other physiologic targets for iNO therapy in hypoxemic respiratory failure may include direct effects of NO on lung inflammation, vascular permeability, and thrombosis in situ. Although some laboratory studies have suggested that NO can potentiate lung injury by promoting oxidative or nitrosative stress,[21] inactivating surfactant, and stimulating inflammation,[22] other studies have demonstrated striking antioxidant and antiinflammatory effects in models of lung injury.[23-25] Thus clinical benefits of low-dose iNO therapy may include reduced lung inflammation and edema, as well as potential protective effects on surfactant function,[26] but these effects remain clinically unproven (Box 32-1).

Finally, the diagnostic value of iNO therapy is important because failure to respond to iNO raises important questions about the specific mechanism of hypoxemia. Poor responses to iNO should lead to further diagnostic evaluation for "unsuspected" anatomic cardiovascular or pulmonary disease.

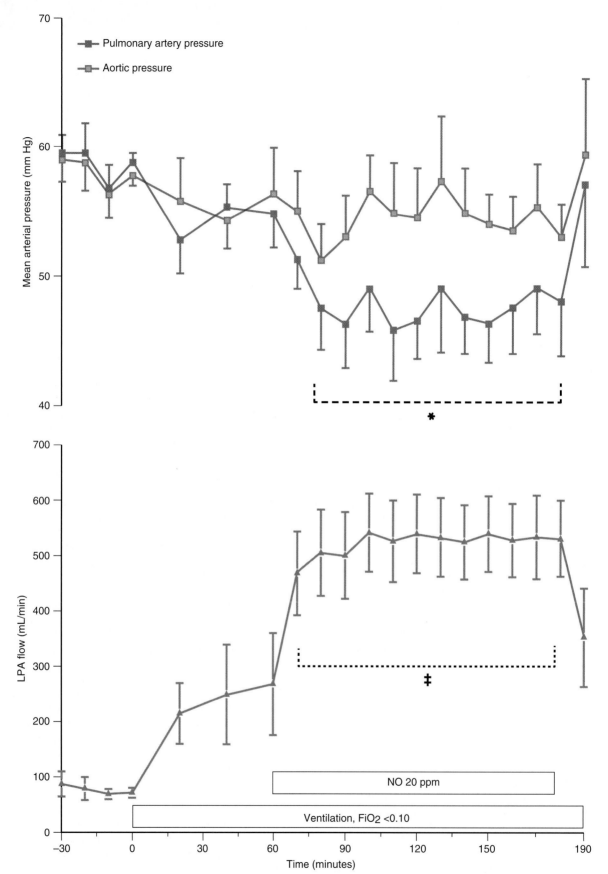

FIG 32-1 Inhaled nitric oxide (*NO*) causes selective and sustained pulmonary vasodilation. *LPA,* left pulmonary artery. (From Kinsella JP, Abman SH. *J Pediatr.* 136:717-726, 2000.)

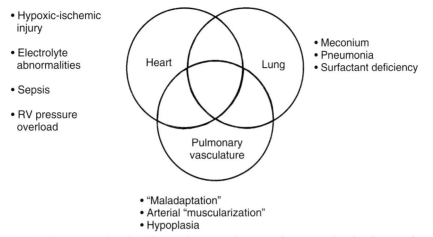

FIG 32-2 Disorders associated with persistent pulmonary hypertension in the newborn. *RV,* right ventricular.

BOX 32-1 Potential Beneficial Effects of Low-Dose Inhaled Nitric Oxide in Hypoxemic Respiratory Failure

1. Pulmonary vasodilation→decreased extrapulmonary right-to-left shunting
2. Enhanced matching of alveolar ventilation with perfusion
3. ↓ Inflammation (↓ lung neutrophil accumulation)
4. ↓ Vascular leak and lung edema
5. Preservation of surfactant function
6. ↓ Oxidant injury (inhibition of lipid oxidation)
7. Preservation of vascular endothelial growth factor expression
8. Altered proinflammatory gene expression

PHYSIOLOGY OF NITRIC OXIDE IN THE PULMONARY CIRCULATION

The fetal circulation is characterized by high PVR. Pulmonary blood flow accounts for less than 10% of combined ventricular output in the late-gestation ovine fetus.[27] Mechanisms responsible for maintaining high fetal PVR and causing sustained pulmonary vasodilation at birth are incompletely understood; however, studies in fetal and transitional pulmonary vasoregulation have led to increased understanding of the normal physiologic control of PVR. Fetal and neonatal pulmonary vascular tone is modulated through a balance between vasoconstrictor and vasodilator stimuli, including mechanical factors (e.g., lung volume) and endogenous mediators.

The pharmacologic activity of nitrovasodilators derives from the release of NO, which was recognized as a potent vascular smooth muscle relaxant as early as 1979.[28] In 1987 investigators from two separate laboratories reported that the endothelium-derived relaxing factor was NO or an NO-containing substance.[29,30] NO modulates basal pulmonary vascular tone in the late-gestation fetus; pharmacologic NO blockade inhibits endothelium-dependent pulmonary vasodilation and attenuates the rise in pulmonary blood flow at delivery, implicating endogenous NO formation in postnatal adaptation after birth.[31] Increased fetal oxygen tension augments endogenous NO release,[32,33] and the increases in pulmonary blood flow in response to rhythmic distension of the lung and high inspired oxygen concentrations are mediated in part by endogenous NO release.[34] However, in these studies the pulmonary circulation was structurally normal. Studies using a model of PPHN in which marked structural pulmonary vascular changes are induced by prolonged fetal ductus arteriosus compression demonstrated that the structurally abnormal pulmonary circulation also was functionally abnormal.[35,36] Despite the progressive loss of endothelium-dependent (acetylcholine) vasodilation with prolonged ductus compression in this model, the response to endothelium-independent (atrial natriuretic peptide, NO) vasodilation was intact.

Exogenous (inhaled) NO causes potent, sustained, selective pulmonary vasodilation in the late-gestation ovine fetus.[11] Based on the chronic ambient levels considered to be safe for adults by regulatory agencies in the United States,[37] studies were performed in near-term lambs using iNO at doses of 5, 10, and 20 ppm. iNO caused a dose-dependent increase in pulmonary blood flow in mechanically ventilated newborn lambs.[11] iNO at 20 ppm did not decrease coronary arterial or cerebral blood flow in this model.

Roberts et al.[38] studied the effects of iNO on pulmonary hemodynamics in mechanically ventilated newborn lambs. iNO reversed hypoxic pulmonary vasoconstriction, and maximum vasodilation occurred at doses greater than 80 ppm. They also found that the vasodilation caused by iNO during hypoxia was not attenuated by respiratory acidosis in this model. Berger et al.[39] investigated the effects of iNO on pulmonary vasodilation during group B streptococcal sepsis in piglets. iNO at 150 ppm for 30 minutes caused marked pulmonary vasodilation but was associated with physiologically significant increases in methemoglobin concentrations. Corroborating studies in other animal models support the observations that iNO is a selective pulmonary vasodilator at low doses (less than 20 ppm).[40-42]

INITIAL EVALUATION OF THE TERM NEWBORN FOR INHALED NITRIC OXIDE THERAPY

Although extensive reference material is available to the clinician when a specific diagnosis has been determined for the hypoxemic term newborn, an approach to the initial evaluation of the cyanotic newborn has received less attention. In this section, we propose an approach to the evaluation of the hypoxemic newborn that may be useful in clarifying the etiology of hypoxemia and in assessing the need for iNO treatment (Fig. 32-3).

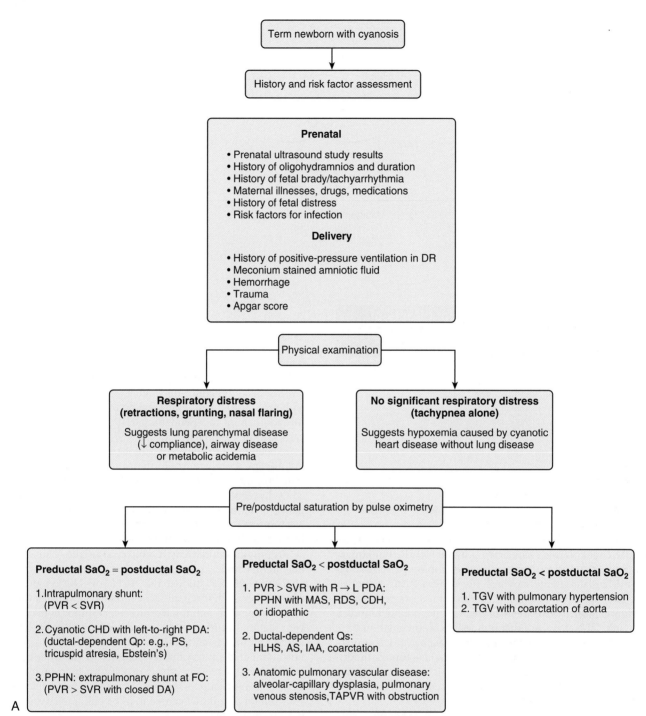

FIG 32-3 An approach to evaluation for inhaled nitric oxide therapy in the cyanotic newborn. *ABG,* arterial blood gas; *AS,* aortic stenosis; *CBC,* complete blood count; *CDH,* congenital diaphragmatic hernia; *CHD,* congenital heart disease; *DA,* ductus arteriosus; *DR,* delivery room; *FO,* foramen ovale; *HLHS,* hypoplastic left-heart syndrome; *IAA,* interrupted aortic arch; *LV,* left ventricular; *MAS,* meconium aspiration syndrome; *PDA,* patent ductus arteriosus; *PPHN,* persistent pulmonary hypertension of the newborn; *PS,* pulmonary stenosis; *PVR,* pulmonary vascular resistance; *R→L,* right-to-left; *RDS,* respiratory distress syndrome; *RV,* right ventricular; *SVR,* systemic vascular resistance; *TAPVR,* total anomalous pulmonary venous return; *TGV,* transposition of the great vessels; *4ext. BP,* four extremity blood pressure.

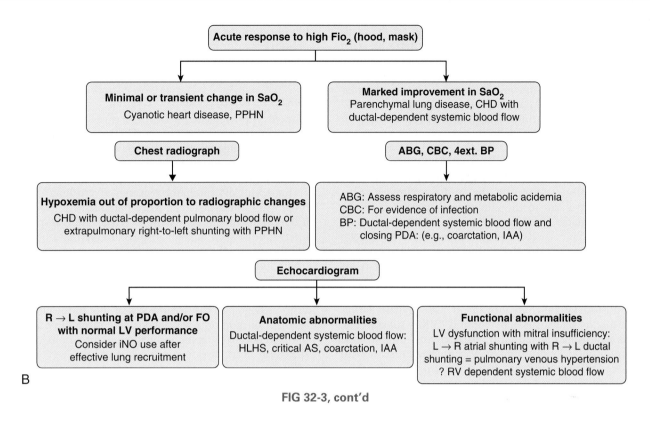

FIG 32-3, cont'd

History

Evaluation of the newborn with cyanosis begins with an approach designed to assess the primary cause of hypoxemia. Marked hypoxemia in the newborn can be caused by parenchymal lung disease with mismatch or intrapulmonary shunting, pulmonary vascular disease causing extrapulmonary right-to-left shunting (PPHN), or anatomic right-to-left shunting associated with congenital heart disease. Evaluation should begin with the history and assessment of risk factors for hypoxemic respiratory failure. Relevant history may include the results of prenatal ultrasound studies. Lesions such as congenital diaphragmatic hernia (CDH) and congenital cystic adenomatoid malformation are diagnosed prenatally with increasing frequency. Although many anatomic congenital heart diseases can be diagnosed prenatally, vascular abnormalities (e.g., coarctation of the aorta, total anomalous pulmonary venous return) are more difficult to diagnose with prenatal ultrasound. A history of a structurally normal heart by fetal ultrasonography should be confirmed by echocardiography in the newborn with cyanosis (see Chapter 33).

Other historical information that may be important in the evaluation of the cyanotic newborn includes a history of severe and prolonged oligohydramnios causing pulmonary hypoplasia. Absent or a marked decrease in fetal movement over several days and a nonreactive fetal heart rate from time of admission may be indicators of chronic fetal hypoxia and acidosis. Prolonged fetal bradyarrhythmia and/or tachyarrhythmia and marked anemia (caused by hemolysis, twin–twin transfusion, or chronic hemorrhage) may cause congestive heart failure, pulmonary edema, and respiratory distress. Maternal illness (e.g., diabetes mellitus), medication use (e.g., aspirin or medications containing nonsteroidal antiinflammatory drugs causing premature constriction of the ductus arteriosus, association of Ebstein malformation with maternal lithium use), and drug use may contribute to acute cardiopulmonary distress in the newborn. Risk factors for infection that cause sepsis/pneumonia should be considered, including premature or prolonged rupture of membranes, fetal tachycardia, maternal leukocytosis, uterine tenderness, and other signs of intra-amniotic infection.

Events at delivery may provide clues to the etiology of hypoxemic respiratory failure in the newborn. For example, if positive-pressure ventilation is required in the delivery room, the risk of pneumothorax increases. A history of meconium-stained amniotic fluid, particularly if meconium is present below the cords, is the *sine qua non* of meconium aspiration syndrome. Birth trauma (e.g., clavicular fracture, phrenic nerve injury) or acute fetomaternal or fetoplacental hemorrhage may cause respiratory distress in the newborn.

Physical Examination

The initial physical examination provides important clues to the etiology of cyanosis. Marked respiratory distress in the newborn (retractions, grunting, nasal flaring) suggests the presence of pulmonary parenchymal disease with decreased lung compliance. However, it is important to recognize that upper airway obstruction (e.g., Pierre Robin sequence or choanal atresia) and metabolic acidemia also can cause severe respiratory distress. In contrast, the newborn with cyanosis alone or cyanosis plus tachypnea ("nondistressed tachypnea") typically has cyanotic congenital heart disease, most commonly transposition of the great vessels (TGV) or idiopathic PPHN.

The presence of a heart murmur in the first hours of life is an important sign in the newborn with cyanosis or respiratory distress. In that setting, it is unusual for the common left-to-right shunt lesions (patent ductus arteriosus, atrial septal defect, ventricular septal defect) to produce an audible murmur because PVR remains high and little turbulence is created across the defect. A murmur that sounds like a ventricular septal defect in the first hours of life is most commonly caused by tricuspid regurgitation (associated with PPHN or asphyxiated myocardium).

Interpretation of Pulse Oximetry Measurements

The interpretation of preductal (right hand) and postductal (lower extremity) saturation by pulse oximetry provides important clues to the etiology of hypoxemia in the newborn. Right-to-left shunting across the ductus arteriosus (but not the patent foramen ovale) causes postductal desaturation (i.e., greater than 5% difference). However, it is important to recognize that variability in oximetry readings may be related to differences in available devices and affected by local perfusion. If the measurements of preductal and postductal SaO_2 are equivalent, this suggests either that the ductus arteriosus is patent and PVR is subsystemic (i.e., the hypoxemia is caused by parenchymal lung disease with intrapulmonary shunting or cyanotic heart disease with ductal-dependent pulmonary blood flow) or that the ductus arteriosus is closed (precluding any interpretation of pulmonary artery pressure without echocardiography). It is uncommon for the ductus arteriosus to close in the first hours of life in the presence of systemic or suprasystemic pulmonary artery pressures.

The most common cause of preductal–postductal gradients in oxygenation is suprasystemic PVR in PPHN. However, ductal-dependent systemic blood flow lesions (hypoplastic left-heart syndrome, critical aortic stenosis, interrupted aortic arch, coarctation) may also present with postductal desaturation. Moreover, anatomic pulmonary vascular disease (alveolar–capillary dysplasia, pulmonary venous stenosis, anomalous venous return with obstruction) can cause suprasystemic PVR with right-to-left shunting across the ductus arteriosus and postductal desaturation.

Finally, the unusual occurrence of markedly lower preductal SaO_2 compared to postductal measurements suggests one of two diagnoses: TGV with pulmonary hypertension or TGV with coarctation of the aorta.

Laboratory and Radiologic Evaluation

One of the most important tests to perform in the evaluation of the newborn with cyanosis is the chest radiograph (CXR). The CXR can demonstrate the classic findings of respiratory distress syndrome (air bronchograms, diffuse granularity, underinflation), diffuse parenchymal lung disease in pneumonia, meconium aspiration syndrome, and CDH. Perhaps the most important question to ask when viewing the CXR is whether the severity of hypoxemia is out of proportion to the radiographic changes (Table 32-1). In other words, marked hypoxemia despite supplemental oxygen in the absence of severe pulmonary parenchymal disease radiographically suggests the presence of an extrapulmonary right-to-left shunt (idiopathic PPHN or cyanotic heart disease). The diagnosis of PPHN without CXR evidence of pulmonary parenchymal disease is sometimes called *black lung PPHN*.

Other essential measurements include an arterial blood gas to determine the blood gas tensions and pH, a complete blood count to evaluate for signs of infection, and blood pressure measurements in the right arm and a lower extremity to determine aortic obstruction (interrupted aortic arch, coarctation).

Response to Supplemental Oxygen

Marked improvement in SaO_2 (increase to 100%) with supplemental oxygen (100% oxygen by hood, mask, or endotracheal tube) suggests the presence of intrapulmonary shunt or mismatch resulting from lung disease or reactive PPHN. The response to mask continuous positive airway pressure is also a useful discriminator between severe lung disease and other causes of hypoxemia. Most patients with PPHN have at least a transient improvement in oxygenation in response to interventions such as high inspired oxygen and/or mechanical ventilation. If the preductal SaO_2 never reaches 100%, the likelihood of cyanotic heart disease is high.

Echocardiography

Echocardiography has become a vital tool in the clinical management of newborns with hypoxemic respiratory failure. The initial echocardiographic evaluation is important to rule out structural heart disease causing hypoxemia (e.g., coarctation of the aorta, total anomalous pulmonary venous return). Moreover, it is critically important to diagnose congenital heart lesions for which iNO treatment would be contraindicated. In addition to the lesions mentioned earlier, congenital heart diseases that can present with hypoxemia unresponsive to high inspired oxygen concentrations (i.e., dependent on right-to-left shunting across the ductus arteriosus) include critical aortic stenosis, interrupted aortic arch, and hypoplastic left-heart syndrome. Decreasing PVR with iNO in these conditions could lead to systemic hypoperfusion, worsening the clinical course and delaying definitive diagnosis.

Echocardiographic evaluation is an essential component in the initial evaluation and ongoing management of

TABLE 32-1 **Mechanisms of Hypoxemia in the Term Newborn with Respiratory Failure**

Mechanism	Associated Conditions	Response to 100% Oxygen
Ventilation–perfusion disturbances (high ratios indicate increased dead space; low ratios indicate alveolar underventilation)	Meconium aspiration, retained lung fluid, pulmonary interstitial emphysema, effects of positioning on gas exchange (i.e., decreased ventilation in dependent lung)	PaO_2 ⇈
Intrapulmonary right-to-left shunt (= 0, blood that passes through nonventilated segments of lung)	Atelectasis, alveolar filling (meconium, blood), bronchial collateral circulation	Little change in PaO_2
Extrapulmonary right-to-left shunt	PPHN (right-to-left shunting at FO and DA), cyanotic heart disease	Little change in PaO_2

DA, ductus arteriosus; *FO,* foramen ovale; *PPHN,* persistent pulmonary hypertension of the newborn.

the hypoxemic newborn. Not all hypoxemic term newborns have echocardiographic signs of PPHN. As noted earlier, hypoxemia can be caused by intrapulmonary right-to-left shunting or disturbances associated with severe lung disease. In unusual circumstances, right-to-left shunting can occur across pulmonary-to-systemic collaterals. However, extrapulmonary right-to-left shunting at the foramen ovale and/or ductus arteriosus (PPHN) also complicates hypoxemic respiratory failure and must be assessed to determine initial treatments and evaluate the response to those therapies.

PPHN is defined by the echocardiographic determination of extrapulmonary venoarterial admixture (right-to-left shunting at the foramen ovale and/or ductus arteriosus), not simply evidence of increased PVR (i.e., elevated PVR without extrapulmonary shunting does not directly cause hypoxemia). Echocardiographic signs suggestive of pulmonary hypertension (e.g., increased right ventricular systolic time intervals, septal flattening) are less helpful (Table 32-2).

Doppler measurements of atrial and ductal level shunts provide essential information when managing a newborn with hypoxemic respiratory failure. For example, left-to-right shunting at the foramen ovale and ductus arteriosus with marked hypoxemia suggests predominant intrapulmonary shunting, and interventions should be directed at optimizing lung inflation.

Finally, the measurements made with echocardiography can be used to predict or interpret the response or lack of response to various treatments. For example, in the presence of severe left ventricular dysfunction with pulmonary hypertension, pulmonary vasodilation alone may be ineffective in improving oxygenation. The echocardiographic findings in this setting include right-to-left ductal shunting (caused by suprasystemic PVR) and mitral insufficiency with left-to-right atrial shunting. In this setting, efforts to reduce PVR should be accompanied by targeted therapies to increase cardiac performance and decrease left ventricular afterload.

This constellation of findings suggests that left ventricular dysfunction may contribute to pulmonary venous hypertension, such as occurs in congestive heart failure. In this setting, pulmonary vasodilation alone (without improving cardiac performance) will not cause sustained improvement in oxygenation.

Careful echocardiographic assessment will provide invaluable information about the underlying pathophysiology and help guide the course of treatment.

The initial echocardiographic evaluation determines both structural and functional (i.e., extrapulmonary right-to-left shunting in PPHN, left ventricular performance) causes of hypoxemia. Serial echocardiography is important to determine the response to interventions (e.g., pulmonary vasodilators) and to reevaluate cases in which specific interventions have not resulted in improvement or have resulted in progressive clinical deterioration. For example, in a patient with extrapulmonary right-to-left shunting and severe lung disease, pulmonary vasodilation might reverse the right-to-left venous admixture with little improvement in systemic oxygenation. These observations unmask the critically important contribution of intrapulmonary shunting to hypoxemia (see also the discussion in Chapter 26).

WHOM TO TREAT

Guidelines for the use of iNO therapy are given in Box 32-2.

Diseases

Because of its selective pulmonary vasodilator effects, iNO therapy is an important adjunct to available treatments for term newborns with hypoxemic respiratory failure. However, hypoxemic respiratory failure in the term newborn represents a heterogeneous group of disorders, and disease-specific responses have clearly been described.[3]

Several pathophysiologic disturbances contribute to hypoxemia in the newborn infant, including cardiac dysfunction, airway and pulmonary parenchymal abnormalities, and pulmonary vascular disorders. In some newborns with hypoxemic respiratory failure a single mechanism predominates (e.g., extrapulmonary right-to-left shunting in idiopathic PPHN), but more commonly several of these mechanisms contribute to hypoxemia. For example, in a newborn with meconium aspiration syndrome, meconium may obstruct some airways, decreasing ratios and increasing intrapulmonary shunting. Other lung segments may be overventilated relative to perfusion and increase physiologic dead space. Moreover, the same patient may have severe pulmonary hypertension with extrapulmonary right-to-left shunting at the ductus arteriosus and foramen

TABLE 32-2 Echocardiographic Findings in Persistent Pulmonary Hypertension of the Newborn

Measurement	Findings in PPHN
Estimate of PA pressure using Doppler estimate of tricuspid regurgitation jet: $4(V^2)$ + CVP, where V is the peak velocity of tricuspid regurgitation jet (in m/s) and CVP is the central venous pressure	Elevated PA pressure reliably estimated (mm Hg); compare with simultaneous systemic pressure
Direction of PDA shunt (by pulsed and color Doppler)	Right-to-left or bidirectional PDA shunting
Direction of atrial shunt (by pulsed and color Doppler)	Right-to-left or bidirectional shunting through PFO

PA, pulmonary artery; *PDA*, patent ductus arteriosus; *PFO*, patent foramen ovale; *PPHN*, persistent pulmonary hypertension of the newborn.

BOX 32-2 Guidelines for Use of Inhaled Nitric Oxide Therapy

Patient profile: Near-term/term newborn of 34 weeks' or greater gestation in the first week of life with echocardiographic evidence of extrapulmonary right-to-left shunting and OI greater than 25 after effective lung recruitment.
Starting dose: 20 ppm
Monitoring for methemoglobinemia: Monitor percentage methemoglobin by co-oximetry within 4 hours of starting iNO and at 24-hour intervals.
Duration of treatment: Typically less than 5 days.
Discontinuation: FiO_2 less than 0.60 with increase in FiO_2 of less than 0.15 after discontinuation.
ECMO availability: If used in a non-ECMO center, arrangements should be in place to continue iNO during transport.

ECMO, extracorporeal membrane oxygenation; *iNO*, inhaled nitric oxide; *OI*, oxygenation index.

ovale. Not only does the overlap of these mechanisms complicate clinical management, but time-dependent changes in the relative contribution of each mechanism to hypoxemia require continued vigilance as the disease progresses. Therefore, understanding the relative contribution of these different causes of hypoxemia becomes critically important as the inventory of therapeutic options expands.

Considering the important role of parenchymal lung disease in many cases of PPHN, pharmacologic pulmonary vasodilation alone would not be expected to cause sustained clinical improvement. The effects of iNO may be suboptimal when lung volume is decreased in association with pulmonary parenchymal disease.[43] Atelectasis and airspace disease (e.g., pneumonia, pulmonary edema) will decrease effective delivery of iNO to its site of action in terminal lung units, and PVR increases at lung volumes above and below functional residual capacity. In PPHN associated with heterogeneous ("patchy") parenchymal lung disease, iNO may be effective in optimizing matching by preferentially causing vasodilation within lung units that are well ventilated. The effects of iNO on matching appear to be optimal at low doses (less than 20 ppm).[18,19] However, in cases complicated by homogeneous (diffuse) parenchymal lung disease and underinflation, pulmonary hypertension may be exacerbated because of the adverse mechanical effects of underinflation on PVR. In this setting, effective treatment of the underlying lung disease is essential (and sometimes sufficient) to resolve the accompanying pulmonary hypertension (Fig. 32-4).

Clinical Criteria
Gestational and Postnatal Age
Available evidence from clinical trials supports the use of iNO in late preterm (greater than 34 weeks' gestation) and term newborns.[7,8] The use of iNO in infants of less than 34 weeks' gestation remains investigational. Clinical trials of iNO in the newborn have incorporated ECMO treatment as

an endpoint. Most patients were enrolled in the first few days of life. Although one of the pivotal studies used to support the new drug application for iNO therapy included as an entry criterion a postnatal age of up to 14 days, the average age at enrollment in that study was 1.7 days.[7] Currently, clinical trials support the use of iNO before treatment with ECMO, usually within the first week of life. However, clinical experience suggests that iNO may be of benefit as an adjuvant treatment after ECMO therapy in patients with sustained pulmonary hypertension (e.g., CDH). Thus postnatal age alone should not define the duration of therapy in cases in which prolonged treatment could be beneficial.

Severity of Illness
Studies support the use of iNO in infants who have hypoxemic respiratory failure with evidence of PPHN and require mechanical ventilation and high inspired oxygen concentrations. The most common criterion used has been the oxygenation index (OI). Although clinical trials commonly allowed for enrollment of patients with OI levels greater than 25, the mean OI at study entry in multicenter trials was approximately 40.[3,7] It is unclear whether infants with less severe hypoxemia would benefit from iNO therapy. Davidson et al.[6] reported a controlled clinical trial in which the average OI at study entry was 49. Unlike other trials, however, iNO treatment in this study did not reduce ECMO use. In addition, although entry criteria for this trial included echocardiographic evidence of pulmonary hypertension, only 9% of the patients had clinical evidence of right-to-left ductal shunting. Because of the mechanism of action of iNO as a selective pulmonary vasodilator, it is likely that acute improvement in oxygenation caused by decreased PVR and reduced extrapulmonary right-to-left shunting would be most predictive of clinical improvement.[7] Konduri et al. tested the hypothesis that treatment of newborns with less severe hypoxemic respiratory failure (OI 15 to 25) with iNO would improve outcomes.[44] However, they found no

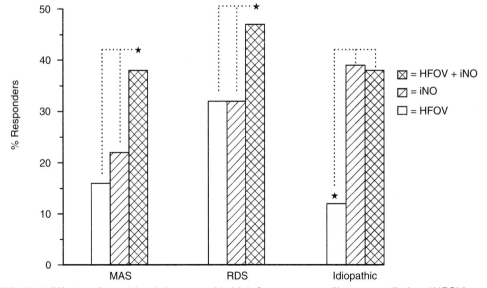

FIG 32-4 Effects of combined therapy with high-frequency oscillatory ventilation (*HFOV*) and inhaled nitric oxide (*iNO*) in term newborns with persistent pulmonary hypertension of the newborn (PPHN). HFOV augments the response to iNO in newborns with PPHN and parenchymal lung disease. *MAS*, meconium aspiration syndrome; *RDS*, respiratory distress syndrome.

differences in the need for ECMO or mortality with early vs late initiation of iNO therapy. More recent multicenter studies suggest that indications for treatment with iNO may include an OI greater than 25 with echocardiographic evidence of extrapulmonary right-to-left shunting.

Treatment Strategies

Delivery of Nitric Oxide during Mechanical Ventilation

Early studies of NO treatment in newborns used simple two-stage regulators with low-flow meters that were manually adjusted to deliver finely regulated flow rates of NO gas into the circuit of continuous-flow neonatal ventilators. Monitoring of NO/NO_2 was performed using chemiluminescence analyzers.[2] This configuration was inexpensive and reliable but lacked an alarm system to detect high/low delivered gas errors. As of this writing, gas for NO therapy in the United States is provided by a single manufacturer (Ikaria, Madison, Wisconsin, USA) and is linked to a single delivery system.

The INOvent delivery system uses an inline sensor to detect flow rates of gas through the ventilator circuit and a mass-flow controller for delivery of NO gas to yield the desired NO concentration. This device allows for stable NO delivery in ventilator systems that do not use continuous flow throughout the inspiratory/expiratory cycle. The range of NO delivery is 0 to 80 ppm, and the system includes NO/NO_2 alarms that use electrochemical sensors. This device also has a manual NO delivery unit for use during bag ventilation.

Dose

The first studies of iNO treatment in term newborns reported initial doses that ranged from 80[1] to 6 to 20 ppm.[2] The rationale for doses used in these clinical trials was based on concentrations that previously had been found to be effective in animal experiments by the same investigators.[11,38] Roberts et al.[1] reported that brief (30 minutes) inhalation of NO at 80 ppm improved oxygenation in patients with PPHN, but this response was sustained in only one patient after NO was discontinued. In the second report, rapid improvement in oxygenation in neonates with severe PPHN also was demonstrated, but this was achieved at lower doses (20 ppm) for 4 hours.[2] This study also reported that decreasing the iNO dose to 6 ppm for the duration of treatment provided sustained improvement in oxygenation. The relative effectiveness of low-dose iNO in improving oxygenation in patients with severe PPHN was corroborated in a study by Finer et al.[45] Acute improvement in oxygenation during treatment was not different with doses of iNO ranging from 5 to 80 ppm.

These laboratory and clinical studies established the boundaries of iNO dosing protocols for subsequent randomized clinical trials in newborns.[3-5] Increasing the dose to 40 ppm does not generally improve oxygenation in patients who do not respond to the lower dose of 20 ppm.[3] The initial dose in the Neonatal Inhaled Nitric Oxide Study (NINOS) trial was 20 ppm, but the dose was increased to 80 ppm if the improvement in PaO_2 was less than 20 torr.[7] In this study, only 3 (6%) of 53 infants who had little response to 20 ppm had an increase in PaO_2 greater than 20 torr when treated with 80 ppm iNO. Whether a progressive increase in PaO_2 would have occurred with continued exposure to 20 ppm could not be determined with this study design. Roberts et al.[4] initiated treatment with 80 ppm NO and subsequently weaned the iNO concentration if oxygenation improved; thus the effects of lower initial iNO

doses could not be evaluated and the effects on ECMO use were not evaluated.

The effects of sustained exposure to different doses of iNO in separate treatment groups of newborns were evaluated by Davidson et al.[6] These investigators reported the results of a randomized, controlled, dose–response trial in term newborns with hypoxemic respiratory failure. In this study, patients were randomized to treatment with 0 (placebo), 5, 20, or 80 ppm NO. Each iNO dose improved oxygenation compared to placebo, but there was no difference in responses among groups. However, at 80 ppm, methemoglobinemia (blood levels greater than 7%) occurred in 13 (35%) of 37 patients and high inspired NO_2 concentrations (greater than 3 ppm) were reported in 7 (19%) of 37 patients. Thus iNO at a dose of 80 ppm was not more effective in improving oxygenation than 5 or 20 ppm and was associated with adverse effects.

The available evidence supports the use of doses of iNO beginning at 20 ppm in term newborns with PPHN, because this strategy decreased ECMO use without an increased incidence of adverse effects. Although brief exposures to higher doses (40 to 80 ppm) appear to be safe, sustained treatment with 80 ppm NO increases the risk of methemoglobinemia.

Duration of Treatment

In multicenter clinical trials of iNO therapy, the typical duration of iNO treatment has been less than 5 days, which parallels the clinical resolution of PPHN. However, individual exceptions occur, particularly in cases of pulmonary hypoplasia.[46] If iNO is required for more than 5 days, investigations into other causes of pulmonary hypertension should be considered (e.g., alveolar capillary dysplasia), particularly if discontinuation of iNO results in suprasystemic elevations of pulmonary artery pressure noted by echocardiography. In our practice, we discontinue iNO if FiO_2 is less than 0.60 and PaO_2 is greater than 60 without evidence of rebound pulmonary hypertension or an increase in FiO_2 greater than 15% after iNO withdrawal.

In the pre-iNO era, concerns were raised about delaying ECMO therapy if conventional treatment was prolonged. However, these retrospective data do not account for recent changes in management strategies, which include newer ventilator devices and exogenous surfactant therapy. Moreover, decreased ECMO use with iNO treatment in more recent multicenter controlled trials has not been associated with an increased incidence of chronic lung disease.[7] In the most recent trial as of this writing, iNO treatment was associated with improved pulmonary outcomes.[8] No controlled data are available to determine the maximal safe duration of iNO therapy.

Weaning

After improvement in oxygenation occurs with the onset of iNO therapy, strategies for weaning from the iNO dose become important. Numerous approaches have been used, and few differences have been noted until final discontinuation of iNO treatment. In one study, iNO was reduced from 20 to 6 ppm after 4 hours of treatment without acute changes in oxygenation. In another trial, iNO was reduced in a stepwise fashion to as low as 1 ppm without changes in oxygenation.[47] Weaning from iNO has different physiologic consequences compared to discontinuation of iNO therapy (see discussion below).

Discontinuation of Inhaled Nitric Oxide Therapy

Early clinical studies reported rapid and sometimes dramatic decreases in oxygenation and increases in PVR after abrupt withdrawal of iNO during prolonged therapy.[15] These responses often are mild and transient, and many patients with decreased oxygenation after iNO withdrawal will respond to brief elevations of FiO_2 and careful observation. In patients with a persistent need for treatment with higher inspired oxygen concentrations or increased pulmonary hypertension after iNO withdrawal, restarting iNO treatment will generally cause rapid clinical improvement. Clinical experience with postoperative cardiac patients suggests that children with higher pulmonary artery pressure at the time of iNO withdrawal may be at greatest risk for adverse hemodynamic effects. In general, this so-called "rebound" response appears to decrease over time after more prolonged therapy. However, iNO withdrawal can be associated with life-threatening elevations of PVR, profound desaturation, and systemic hypotension due to decreased cardiac output.

Mechanisms that contribute to these "rebound" effects are uncertain but include several factors. First, exogenous NO may downregulate endogenous NO production, which contributes directly to the severity of vasospasm after iNO withdrawal. For example, exposure of normal adult rats to iNO (40 ppm) for 2 days potentiated the pressor response to angiotensin II and hypoxia and selectively impaired endothelium-dependent vasodilation.[48] This response also occurred at low doses of iNO (1 ppm) and reversed after discontinuation of iNO for 8 hours. Because lung endothelial NO synthase (NOS) protein content was unchanged, these authors speculated that iNO decreased NOS activity by an alternate mechanism. Second, decreased vascular sensitivity to NO due to alterations in other components of the NO–cGMP pathway, such as decreased soluble guanylate cyclase or enhanced phosphodiesterase (PDE5) activities, may contribute to vasospasm after NO withdrawal. For example, in a prospective study of postoperative cardiac patients with marked hemodynamic changes after iNO withdrawal, dipyridamole (a cGMP-specific PDE type V inhibitor) inhibited the adverse effects of acute iNO withdrawal.[49] These findings led to the speculation that dipyridamole may sustain smooth muscle cGMP content and that persistent PDE5 activity may contribute to rebound pulmonary hypertension after iNO withdrawal.

Alternatively, the rise in PVR and drop in oxygenation after iNO withdrawal may simply represent the presence of more severe underlying pulmonary vascular disease with loss of the treatment effect of iNO. Increasing pulmonary blood flow into a hypertensive vascular bed with decreased NOS activity may augment myogenic responses or stimulate vasoconstrictor products (such as endothelin) that increase vascular tone.[50] The sudden increase in pulmonary artery pressure after rapid withdrawal of vasodilator therapy is not unique to iNO; it has been observed in other clinical settings, such as prostacyclin withdrawal in adults with primary pulmonary hypertension and in postoperative cardiac patients.

Monitoring

Early experience suggested that careful monitoring of NO and NO_2 levels should be done with chemiluminescence devices. It now has become clear that NO_2 levels remain low at delivered iNO doses within the recommended ranges and that electrochemical devices are reliable. The currently available systems use electrochemical cells and appear to be reliable when they are used appropriately. However, the response time of electrochemical sensors is relatively slow, and these devices are not accurate when measurement of acute changes in NO concentrations is desired.

Methemoglobinemia occurs after exposure to high concentrations of iNO (80 ppm).[6] (Because there is no proven advantage to iNO at this high dose, this concentration is not recommended.) This complication has not been reported at lower doses of iNO (less than 20 ppm). Because methemoglobin reductase deficiency may occur unpredictably, it is reasonable to measure methemoglobin levels by co-oximetry within 4 hours of starting iNO therapy and subsequently at 24-hour intervals.

Ventilator Management

Along with iNO treatment, other therapeutic strategies have emerged for the management of the term infant with hypoxemic respiratory failure. Considering the important role of parenchymal lung disease in specific disorders included in the syndrome of PPHN, pharmacologic pulmonary vasodilation alone should not be expected to cause sustained clinical improvement in many cases.[14] Moreover, patients who do not respond to iNO can show marked improvement in oxygenation with adequate lung inflation alone.[23] High success rates in early studies were achieved by withholding iNO treatment until aggressive attempts were made to optimize ventilation and lung inflation with mechanical ventilation. These early studies demonstrated that the effects of iNO may be suboptimal when lung volume is decreased in association with pulmonary parenchymal disease, for several reasons. First, atelectasis and airspace disease (pneumonia, pulmonary edema) may decrease the effective delivery of iNO to its site of action in terminal lung units. Second, in cases complicated by severe lung disease and underinflation, pulmonary hypertension may be exacerbated because of the adverse mechanical effects of underinflation on PVR. Third, attention must be given to minimize overinflation to avoid inadvertent positive end-expiratory pressure and gas trapping that may elevate PVR from vascular compression. This commonly complicates the management of infants with asymmetric lung disease or airways obstruction as observed in meconium aspiration syndrome.

In newborns with severe lung disease, high-frequency oscillatory ventilation (HFOV) frequently is used to optimize lung inflation and minimize lung injury (see Chapter 22).[51] In clinical pilot studies using iNO, we found that the combination of HFOV and iNO resulted in the greatest improvement in oxygenation in some newborns who had severe PPHN complicated by diffuse parenchymal lung disease and underinflation (e.g., respiratory distress syndrome, pneumonia).[52,53] A randomized multicenter trial demonstrated that treatment with HFOV + iNO often was successful in patients who failed to respond to HFOV alone or iNO with conventional mechanical ventilation in severe PPHN, and differences in responses were related to the specific disease associated with the complex disorders of PPHN[3] (see Fig. 32-4). For patients with PPHN complicated by severe lung disease, response rates for HFOV + iNO were better than with HFOV alone or iNO with conventional ventilation. In contrast, for patients without significant parenchymal lung disease, both iNO and HFOV + iNO were more effective than HFOV alone. This response to combined treatment with HFOV + iNO probably reflects both improvement in intrapulmonary shunting in patients with severe lung disease and PPHN (using a strategy designed to recruit and sustain lung volume rather than to hyperventilate) and augmented NO delivery to its site of action. Although iNO may be an effective treatment for PPHN, it should be considered as only part of an overall clinical strategy that cautiously manages parenchymal lung disease, cardiac performance, and systemic hemodynamics.

ROLE OF INHALED NITRIC OXIDE IN NEWBORNS WITH CONGENITAL DIAPHRAGMATIC HERNIA

CDH is a complex syndrome that causes severe hypoxemic respiratory failure and is associated with a high mortality rate.[54] In the most severely affected subset of newborns, CDH is characterized by pulmonary hypoplasia, pulmonary hypertension with structural and functional pulmonary vascular abnormalities, and disturbances in cardiac performance.

iNO was considered a promising therapy for the treatment of acute pulmonary hypertension in CDH, and the first report of the use of iNO in newborns with CDH suggested that early, acute improvement in oxygenation was possible when adequate lung inflation was first achieved.[55] However, the largest randomized, controlled trial of early iNO treatment in patients with CDH found no difference in the combined endpoint of death and/or ECMO use between iNO-treated and control infants.[56] Moreover, in this trial, ECMO use was higher in the iNO-treated group. In retrospect, this observation was perhaps predictable, because an often unrecognized physiologic perturbation caused by CDH is severe left ventricular (LV) systolic and diastolic dysfunction early in the course of treatment. In this setting, pulmonary vasodilation with iNO might not be beneficial. Indeed, decreasing PVR and increasing preload to a left ventricle that is incapable of responding with increased stroke volume could be detrimental by worsening pulmonary venous hypertension. Moreover, some patients with CDH and severe LV dysfunction actually benefit from pulmonary hypertension by allowing the right ventricle to serve as a systemic pump through the contribution of right-to-left ductal shunting (in the most extreme cases, similar to hypoplastic left-heart syndrome). Thus patients with severe CDH are poor responders as a group. Available evidence suggests that iNO therapy in patients with CDH should not be routinely used; rather, its use should be limited to patients with suprasystemic PVR after establishing optimal lung inflation and demonstrating adequate LV performance (i.e., without ductal-dependent systemic blood flow).

However, there is clearly a role for iNO therapy in the treatment of late pulmonary hypertension (PH) in patients with CDH. Often clinically evident protracted or late PH leads to prolonged mechanical ventilation, a second course of ECMO, or death.[57-61] Late PH in newborns with CDH is clinically evident when PVR becomes suprasystemic with right-to-left venoarterial admixture of blood across the foramen ovale and/or the ductus arteriosus causing hypoxemia. However, suprasystemic levels of PVR may be masked during treatment with ECMO or iNO, and subsystemic levels of PVR can be determined only by direct pulmonary artery measurements or echocardiography. Moreover, some newborns with CDH may have persistent pulmonary vascular abnormalities despite marked improvements in respiratory function, necessitating pulmonary vasodilator therapy to reduce PVR even when mechanical ventilation is no longer required. Thus targeting late PH may be an effective approach to reducing mortality in a subset of newborns with CDH.[62]

THE PREMATURE NEWBORN

Early reports of iNO therapy in a premature newborn with PH demonstrated marked improvement in oxygenation caused by effective treatment of severe PH and resolution of extrapulmonary right-to-left shunting;[63] improvement was also noted in other preterm infants with severe respiratory failure.[64,65] Subsequently, several randomized, controlled trials (RCTs) have confirmed the acute improvement in oxygenation caused by iNO treatment. However, in contrast to the direct pulmonary vasodilator effects of iNO, the focus of the most recently published studies was on the potential beneficial effects of prolonged iNO administration on lung parenchymal and vascular development.[66]

In preterm infants, iNO can be used for acute treatment of severe PPHN (as in term infants), management of chronic PH in evolving or established BPD, and for prevention of BPD). Several case series have reported improved oxygenation and less PH by echocardiographic parameters in preterm infants with severe acute hypoxemic respiratory failure and PPHN physiology. Often, the preterm infants who were treated had clinical courses complicated by suspected lung hypoplasia due to preterm and prolonged rupture of membranes causing oligohydramnios. In other studies, iNO therapy acutely lowered pulmonary artery pressure and improved gas exchange in preterm infants with established BPD. However, these studies remain observational only and as of this writing we lack RCT data to substantiate the use of iNO in these settings. In contrast, several multicenter RCTs have been performed to explore the potential role for iNO therapy in the prevention of BPD with early use. We briefly summarize and discuss these studies below.

In a small, unmasked, randomized trial of iNO (20 ppm) and dexamethasone treatment, Subhedar et al.[67] reported no differences in survival, chronic lung disease, or intracranial hemorrhage (ICH) between iNO-treated infants and controls. In a randomized, masked, multicenter clinical trial of low-dose iNO therapy (5 ppm) in severely ill premature newborns with respiratory distress syndrome who had marked hypoxemia despite surfactant therapy (a/A O_2 ratio less than 0.10), iNO acutely improved PaO_2, but did not reduce the incidence of mortality or BPD.[68] Notably, there was no increase in the incidence or severity of ICH in this trial, and the incidence of the most severe ICH (grade 4) was 19% for the iNO group and 29% for the control group. The Franco-Belgium study group reported the results of an acute iNO response study (2-hour oxygenation endpoint); however, the brief duration of therapy and a high rate of crossover before the 2-hour trial endpoint compromised the interpretation of late outcome measures.[69] Hascoet et al.[70] reported the results of an unmasked, randomized trial of iNO in 145 premature newborns with hypoxemic respiratory failure. They found no difference between the iNO and the control group in the primary outcome measure (intact survival at 28 days) and no differences in adverse events. As noted by Finer[71] in an accompanying editorial, interpretation of the findings is limited by a relatively high rate of "open-label" iNO use and the lack of important outcomes such as death before discharge and BPD incidence at 36 weeks.[72] However, these investigators also studied the effect of low-dose iNO on serum markers of oxidative stress and found that iNO treatment apparently reduced signs of oxidative stress in these patients. Field et al.[73] described the findings of the U.K. INNOVO trial. In this unblinded study, 108 premature infants with severe hypoxemic respiratory failure were randomized to receive or not receive iNO. There was no difference between the iNO and the control group in the main outcome measure (death or severe disability at 1 year corrected age) and no difference in adverse events. Limitations of the study included an 8% crossover to iNO treatment and treatment with other pulmonary vasodilators in 30% of the control group. Moreover, Field[74] described a lack of equipoise among investigators demonstrated by the observation that 75 infants eligible for enrollment were treated with iNO outside of the trial, leaving only infants with very severe lung disease enrolled in the study.

The largest trials of iNO therapy in premature newborns reported as of this writing include the single-center study of Schreiber et al.[75] and the multicenter trials of Van Meurs et al.,[76] Ballard et al.,[77] and Kinsella et al.[78] and the Ikaria-sponsored EUNO study.[79] All of these studies were randomized, controlled, and masked, but have key differences in patient population, disease severity, dose and duration of therapy, and other factors.

Schreiber et al.[75] randomized 207 infants to treatment with iNO or placebo. The main finding of the trial was a reduction in the incidence of BPD and death by 24% in the iNO group. These benefits appeared to accrue predominantly from the subset of newborns with relatively mild respiratory failure (OI less than 6.94). However, in addition to apparent pulmonary benefit caused by low-dose iNO, these authors also reported a 47% decrease in the incidence of severe ICH and periventricular leukomalacia (PVL). Moreover, in a subsequent report, the same group showed that the early decrease in ICH/PVL associated with iNO treatment manifested in improved neurodevelopmental outcome on follow-up examinations of this population.[80] In this follow-up study, 138 children (82% of survivors of the RCT) were evaluated for neurodevelopmental outcome at 2 years of age. In the group treated with iNO in the newborn period, 24% had abnormal outcomes (defined as cerebral palsy, blindness, hearing loss, or one score of less than 70 on the Bayley Scales of Infant Development II), in contrast to 46% in the control group.

Van Meurs et al.[76] enrolled 420 newborns (401 to 1500 g birth weight) in a multicenter RCT. Although the focus of this study was on premature newborns and the major outcome measure was BPD, the design of the trial was similar to the previous NINOS trial in which term newborns were enrolled and acute changes in oxygenation determined continued treatment with study gas. That is, an acute dose–response study was performed and only patients who showed significant improvement in PaO_2 were continued on study gas. In striking contrast to other studies, the average duration of iNO treatment was only 76 hours. Overall, they found no difference in the incidence of death/BPD between the iNO and the control group. However, in post hoc analyses, infants with birth weight greater than 1000 g showed a reduction in death/BPD after treatment with iNO (50% iNO vs 69% control). But a worrisome outcome was suggested in a post hoc analysis of newborns weighing less than 1000 g. This analysis showed an increased risk of ICH/PVL (43% iNO vs 33% control). However, as noted in an editorial by Martin and Walsh,[81] baseline ultrasound examinations were not performed, and it cannot be determined whether these very severely ill infants had ICH

before iNO was initiated. Indeed, the severity of illness of the infants in this trial of Van Meurs et al.[76] was also markedly different from that of the study of Schreiber et al.[75] In the Van Meurs trial, the mean OI at enrollment for the iNO group was 23, compared to the median OI of 7.3 in the Schreiber study. This suggests that the degree of illness based upon the severity of respiratory failure may be related to iNO safety and efficacy in this population; however, an increased risk of ICH/PVL was not observed in a previous trial of iNO in premature newborns with severe hypoxemic respiratory failure (OI = 30).[82] Other differences between these two trials may offer insights into the disparate outcomes, including the duration of iNO treatment (3 days vs 7 days), birth weight (839 g vs 992 g), and gestational age (26 weeks vs 27.4 weeks). Thus Van Meurs et al.[76] enrolled smaller, more immature infants with severe respiratory failure who were treated relatively briefly with iNO, making direct comparisons between these two trials problematic.

Ballard et al.[77] randomized 582 premature newborns with birth weights of 500 to 1250 g who required ventilatory support between 7 and 21 days of age. Infants were treated with study gas for a minimum of 24 days and had an estimated OI of 7. They found that the incidence of survival without BPD was increased in the iNO treatment group (43.9%) compared to controls (36.8%) ($p = 0.042$). A major finding of this trial was that the benefit of BPD reduction derived almost entirely from the subset of patients enrolled between 7 and 14 days, suggesting that early treatment is important to prevent BPD. There were no differences between the iNO and the control group in adverse events, including medical or surgical treatment of patent ductus arteriosus (PDA). A trial sponsored by Ikaria, Inc., and designed to test the efficacy of iNO in a population similar to that of Ballard et al. has been completed and preliminary results presented.[83] Yoder et al. randomized 451 mechanically ventilated premature newborns with birth weight less than 1250 g at 7 to 21 days after birth to treatment with iNO or placebo gas. They found no differences in survival without BPD, severity of BPD, or adverse events between the two groups.

Kinsella et al. randomized 793 premature newborns with birth weights of 500 to 1250 g and requiring mechanical ventilation in the first 48 hours of life to treatment with 5 ppm iNO or placebo gas and treated for 21 days or until extubated.[78] Overall, there was no difference in the incidence of death or BPD between groups; however, iNO therapy reduced the incidence of BPD for infants with birth weight greater than 1000 g by 50% ($p = 0.001$). Low-dose iNO therapy reduced the incidence of PVL ($p = 0.048$), as well as the combined endpoints of ICH, PVL, and ventriculomegaly for the entire study population ($p = 0.032$). iNO therapy did not increase the incidence of adverse events, including mortality, ICH, PVL, pulmonary hemorrhage, and PDA treatment, in any subgroup. In this trial there was no relationship between OI and brain injury risk, in contrast to the findings of Van Meurs et al.[76] Mechanisms through which iNO therapy might provide neuroprotection in the premature newborn are uncertain and warrant further study. Based on laboratory studies, several possibilities exist that include modulation of circulating cells (including neutrophils, monocytes, and platelets) that may occur during NO exposure as they transit the pulmonary circulation. Alternatively, iNO-induced downregulation of lung-derived cytokines may also reduce distant organ injury.[82,84,85] Another possible mechanism may relate to distal delivery of NO or NO-related metabolites through the systemic circulation through red blood cell- or protein-mediated pathways.[86,87] Although the findings of this clinical trial are intriguing, using a similar study design, the EUNO study group did not confirm these findings.[79]

The effects of iNO in the premature newborn may depend on the timing, dose, and duration of therapy and the nature of the underlying disease. The available evidence from clinical trials suggests that low-dose iNO may be safe and effective in reducing the risk of death/BPD for a subset of premature newborns, in particular infants with birth weights greater than 1000 g. A neuroprotective effect of iNO has been demonstrated in large RCTs, but the relationship of disease severity and ICH/PVL risk is uncertain. Treatment of premature newborns with respiratory failure between 7 and 14 days after birth appears to be safe and effective in reducing the incidence of BPD; however, these results were not confirmed in a second trial. Early concerns about the potential adverse effects of iNO on surfactant function and PDA risk have been effectively eliminated with the cumulative results of clinical trials; however, routine use of iNO in premature newborns cannot be recommended. A consensus conference that was sponsored by the NICHD suggested that there are insufficient data to support the use of iNO therapy for the prevention of BPD; however, the proceedings of this meeting further state that future studies are needed to determine its role in preterm infants with severe PPHN and respiratory failure or for the use of iNO in subgroups that appeared responsive in the course of other large trials.[10]

SUMMARY

iNO improves oxygenation and decreases ECMO use in term newborns with PPHN. From the available information, a reasonable recommendation for starting dose of iNO in the term infant is 20 ppm, with reductions in dose over time. Toxicity is apparent at a dose of 80 ppm, which causes increases in methemoglobinemia and inspired NO_2. High doses (greater than 20 ppm) of iNO may prolong bleeding time, but clinically significant increases in bleeding complications have not been reported in term newborns. The use of iNO in non-ECMO centers must be done cautiously, with arrangements in place for transport to an ECMO center without interruption of iNO delivery in patients with suboptimal acute responses. Finally, there is conflicting evidence for the potential role of iNO in premature newborns for the prevention of BPD. Low-dose iNO causes acute improvement in oxygenation in preterm infants with severe respiratory failure and PPHN and may prove to be useful as a lung-specific antiinflammatory therapy; however, clinical application as of this writing should be limited to controlled trials that target outcomes of both safety and efficacy.

REFERENCES

A complete reference list is available at https://expertconsult.inkling.com/.

33

Pharmacologic Therapies III: Cardiovascular Therapy and Persistent Pulmonary Hypertension of the Newborn

Keith J. Barrington, MB,ChB, and Eugene M. Dempsey, MBBCH BAO, FRCPI, MD, MSc

INTRODUCTION

Hemodynamic problems are frequent in infants undergoing neonatal intensive care. The evaluation and treatment of such problems must take into account the developmental physiology of the neonatal cardiovascular system, cardiac structure, microstructure, and function, which in neonates differ in many important and fundamental ways from those of mature humans. For example, the myocardium of the newborn has a greater concentration of noncontractile elements, such as mitochondria, and an irregular orientation of the myofibrils.[1] The neonatal myocardium utilizes glucose and lactate[2] rather than the preferential metabolism of fatty acids of the mature myocardium. Calcium-induced calcium release, which marks the function of the sarcoplasmic reticulum, is absent in immature myofibrils.[1]

As a result of its structural and metabolic immaturity, the neonatal heart is functionally limited; basal contractility is already close to maximal levels, and therefore there is little "contractile reserve," and the neonatal myocardium is largely incapable of responding to further demands on its function.[3] One important implication of this is the afterload sensitivity of the circulation. An increase in afterload commonly leads to a reduction in cardiac output.[4] Many inotropic/vasopressor agents directly increase afterload and may therefore result in a decrease, rather than an increase, in systemic perfusion. Responses to all cardiovascular medications are affected by the metabolic immaturity, functional immaturity, and pharmacokinetic differences. Some drugs that are positive inotropes in the mature myocardium have negative inotropic effects on the immature one. Milrinone and other phosphodiesterase-3 inhibitors act by blocking the third fraction of phosphodiesterase; however, phosphodiesterases 3 and 4 are unbalanced in immature myocardium,[5] and therefore blocking phosphodiesterase-3 may have relatively unpredictable effects in a neonate.[6] Extrapolation from studies in older subjects is of little or no value, only studies investigating specifically neonatal populations are relevant.[7]

Similarly, immature responses are also seen in the neonatal vasculature. We have little information about the development of the adrenergic vascular receptors, which are responsible for the responses to catecholamines. Vasoconstrictors, like dopamine, have been shown to increase systemic vascular resistance in the preterm newborn[8]; however, the stage of maturation at which such responses appear and the gestational age at which vasodilator responses may appear in response to other agents are unknown.

Another important factor that limits extrapolation of data from older patients is the presence of shunts. Both ductal and intracardiac shunts are frequent; there is therefore no single value for "cardiac output" in the sick neonate; left ventricular output, right ventricular output, systemic perfusion, and pulmonary blood flow are all potentially different numbers. In addition, interventions that differentially affect systemic and pulmonary vascular resistance may significantly affect systemic perfusion. Total systemic perfusion is equal to systemic venous return, that is, the sum of superior and inferior vena caval flow; pulmonary blood flow is equal to the sum of all of the pulmonary venous return to the left atrium. So in the absence of an intracardiac shunt, we have what seems initially to be paradoxical; systemic perfusion is equal to right ventricular output, whereas pulmonary blood flow is equal to left ventricular output; when there are significant shunts across the foramen ovale these statements have to be modified. Finally, left ventricular output is equivalent to systemic perfusion only when the ductus arteriosus has closed.[9]

NORMAL TRANSITION

Pulmonary vascular resistance (PVR) is very high before birth, and less than 15% of the combined ventricular output perfuses the lungs during most of gestation; in human fetuses this proportion may increase prior to delivery at term. Right ventricular output mostly crosses the ductus arteriosus (from right to left) and perfuses the lower body and the low-resistance placental circulation. Right ventricular afterload is therefore low in utero; afterload increases at birth with clamping of the cord and then falls again as the PVR decreases with respiration.

Physiologic investigations have shown that clamping of the umbilical cord prior to initiation of breathing in a neonatal lamb model, when the PVR is still high, causes a reduction in left ventricular preload, in addition to the increase in right ventricular afterload. Delaying clamping until after breathing has commenced may avoid these changes, thus avoiding cardiovascular compromise around the time of birth. Further work confirming clinical benefits of delayed clamping in the very preterm infant is required.[10]

HEMODYNAMIC PROBLEMS IN THE NEONATE

Persistent Pulmonary Hypertension of the Newborn

When PVR is persistently increased, or when it increases after an initial fall, there may be clinical consequences, known as persistent pulmonary hypertension of the newborn (PPHN). The most common underlying pulmonary disorders causing PPHN are meconium aspiration, septicemia, pneumonia, and pulmonary hypoplasia. In addition it can be seen occasionally in neonates with clear chest X-rays, as so-called primary or idiopathic PPHN.

Clinical Evaluation

The clinical presentation is hypoxic respiratory failure with the clinical signs of one of the underlying pulmonary conditions detailed above. In some patients this may be accompanied, if the ductus arteriosus is open, by a gradient in the saturations from pre- to postductal sites, indicating bidirectional or right-to-left ductal shunting, usually in the most severely affected patients.

On echocardiography many infants will be shown to have intracardiac shunting across a patent foramen ovale or they may have hypoxia from intrapulmonary shunting, that is, ventilation–perfusion mismatch.[10] Intra-atrial shunting will occur when right atrial pressure is above left atrial pressure; right atrial pressures increase when right ventricular failure occurs, usually as a result of high right ventricular afterload. Studies have shown that right ventricular function is an important predictor of good outcome in infants with this condition.[10]

Intervention

Initial interventions should be supportive, including oxygen, fluid administration, warmth, minimal handling, and assisted ventilation. Infants who are agitated may benefit from sedation.

Oxygen should be given to achieve normal saturations, but hyperoxia should be avoided. Oxygen is toxic when given in higher concentrations, may increase pulmonary vascular reactivity,[11] and may even decrease the response of the pulmonary circulation to nitric oxide.[12] It does not appear that increasing FiO_2 beyond that required to achieve normal saturations has any effect on decreasing PVR. As for sedation, it is not clear which sedative agent is preferable. A hemodynamic study of infants with pulmonary artery catheters undergoing surgery showed that fentanyl reduces pulmonary vascular responses to endotracheal suctioning,[13] which suggests that fentanyl may reduce pulmonary vasoreactivity and have a benefit in some infants with PPHN.

Hyperventilation should be avoided as it risks increasing pulmonary damage and causes cerebral vasoconstriction. Persistent respiratory alkalosis seems to cause progressive systemic hypotension, at least in some animal models.[14] It also may cause potential adverse long-term neurodevelopmental effects and hearing loss. Bicarbonate should be avoided, as its use has been associated with an increase in mortality and an increased need for extracorporeal membrane oxygenation (ECMO).[15] Optimizing lung inflation and ventilation to achieve a "normal" pH is reasonable, but going beyond this to alkalinize the patient, even if this might lead to a short-term improvement in Po_2, is not supported by any evidence.

Specific Therapy

The only specific evidence-based therapy for PPHN is inhaled nitric oxide.[16] Nitric oxide can be commenced at between 2 and 20 ppm[17]; there is little evidence that increasing beyond the initial concentration improves any clinical responses. More than 50% of children with PPHN will have a definite increase in the oxygen saturation after starting nitric oxide. Nitric oxide decreases the number of infants who will deteriorate to the point of needing ECMO; the number needed to treat to prevent one case of ECMO, among term newborns and late preterms with hypoxic respiratory failure who have reached an oxygenation index of 25, is 5.[16]

Cardiovascular Support

Cardiovascular support including the use of inotropes may be required for infants with PPHN, but there is little evidence to support a choice of one agent over another. The most appropriate agent would have no pulmonary vasoconstrictor effects, or be a pulmonary vasodilator, one that would increase contractility and cardiac output without increasing vascular resistance. No agent is known to have all these effects.

In animal models dopamine increases both systemic vascular resistance (SVR) and PVR equally, unless enormous doses are used,[18] suggesting that it may not be the best choice. In some animal models epinephrine has a greater systemic than pulmonary pressor effect. Norepinephrine also may be reasonable choice; a small observational study in full-term infants showed a good response to norepinephrine.[19] Other agents such as milrinone[20] and levosimendan[21] have been suggested, and some animal models do show possible pulmonary vasodilatation with milrinone,[22] but there is limited clinical research data to support their use. Evidence for the use of milrinone in PPHN is limited to case series demonstrating an improvement in oxygenation when used in infants failing to respond to inhaled nitric oxide. Milrinone is thus a potential candidate in this setting that deserves further investigation. If investigation of the hemodynamic responses in the sick newborn with PPHN confirms the potential inotropic, lusitropic, and pulmonary vasodilator responses, this should then be followed by investigation of the clinical outcomes.

Research Needs

Comparative studies of various agents among those who require hemodynamic support are needed. It will be important to determine which agents increase systemic pressures more than pulmonary pressures, which increase systemic perfusion, and most importantly if any choice of agent affects clinical outcomes.

Septic Shock

The hemodynamic features of septic shock in the newborn have not been well described. Adults with gram-negative septic shock often present with so-called warm shock; this is a combination of excessive vasodilatation with incomplete cardiac response; cardiac output may be increased or within the normal range, and the patient often presents with hypotension; many of the changes are due to the endotoxins (in particular lipopolysaccharides) produced by the responsible organisms. Newborn infants with their different cardiovascular physiology and different bacteriology may present with a more variable profile. Newborn animals (such as piglets) with group B streptococcus more commonly have cold shock, with marked reductions in cardiac function (as a result of exotoxins produced by the organisms), and blood pressure is maintained initially with profound vasoconstriction, hypotension being a preterminal event.[23] Some infants with *Escherichia coli* or other gram-negative sepsis seem to present with typical warm shock, but there are very few descriptions of the hemodynamics of sepsis in the literature. One study described hemodynamic features in several septic infants,[24] but only a minority had signs of circulatory compromise or shock, as evidenced by the fact that several received neither fluid boluses nor inotropes. The organisms involved were variable; the infants tended to have low SVR and relatively high left- and right ventricular outputs. A more recent study of infants with septic shock suggested that the infants had mostly warm shock, but this study had a number of limitations.[25]

Clinical Evaluation

If the above considerations are appropriate, we can divide the clinical presentations into warm and cold shock: Infants with sepsis and cold shock are vasoconstricted with prolonged capillary filling, adequate blood pressure, and oliguria. They are often lethargic and may have biochemical signs of poor oxygen delivery. Infants with warm shock on the other hand have bounding pulses, hypotension, and normal capillary filling, but may also be oliguric with lactic acidosis.

Evaluation of the circulatory status with echocardiography may well be important in such patients and may aid in targeted management strategies. Echocardiographic evaluation should include an analysis of cardiac filling, contractility, and systemic blood flow. Although such an evaluation may aid in providing more rational treatment, there is no clear evidence that it improves outcomes, and it is uncertain how echocardiographic findings should guide the selection of specific interventions.

A reasonable therapeutic approach is to use physiology-based medicine. This implies examining the abnormalities found on clinical evaluation combined with echocardiography. Therefore an infant with echocardiographic signs of reduced cardiac filling should receive a fluid bolus; an infant with reduced perfusion but adequate blood pressure may benefit from dobutamine or very low-dose epinephrine (which increases systemic perfusion with little effect on blood pressure). Infants with shock and hypotension may receive a moderate dose of epinephrine, which appears to increase both blood pressure and systemic perfusion. Norepinephrine has been little studied in the newborn, but one published study[26] and our own experience[27] suggest that it may have a very favorable hemodynamic profile.

The pharmacokinetics of the drugs is extremely variable; in addition, the concentration, affinity, and activity of the adrenoceptors are extremely variable. There is no consistent relationship between plasma catecholamine concentration and target-organ effect. Thus, in general, for individual catecholamine infusions, the hemodynamic response to therapy is not related to plasma concentrations in a simple linear fashion. The response to a particular plasma catecholamine concentration varies with the functional state and density of adrenergic receptors and the capacity of the target organs to respond. This means that dose responses are unpredictable and doses should be individualized.

Norepinephrine is now the first-line inotropic agent advocated in adult sepsis. However, a systematic review of data from adults with septic shock showed no difference in survival or other important outcomes from trials comparing inotropic agents, despite differences in short-term hemodynamic responses. There are no such trials of norepinephrine in the newborn.

Even in the absence of signs of inadequate preload, septic patients are often considered to have "functional hypovolemia." They therefore receive fluid boluses, often multiple. However, a trial in older infants showed an increase in mortality in the group of children with early septic shock who were randomized to a fluid bolus, compared to controls who were not,[28] calling into question this common practice. If we decide to give a fluid bolus, what fluid should we use? Acute responses to crystalloids and to colloids are different; the increase in systemic perfusion with colloids appears to be greater and more prolonged compared to saline. There is, however, no evidence that clinical outcomes are different,[29] and several trials are currently under way to try to answer this question. The choice of fluid in the newborn is uncertain.

Research Needs

Further studies are clearly needed. Interventions for septic shock will probably need to be individualized according to the hemodynamic profile of the patient. Mortality from septic shock in the newborn is very high,[30] so research in this area is clearly warranted. These studies should determine whether gram-negative and gram-positive shock have similar or differing profiles in the newborn. The role of bedside targeted neonatal echocardiography in the setting of neonatal sepsis needs to be investigated. The place of fluid-bolus therapy in the newborn needs to be evaluated, and the hemodynamic effects and clinical responses to various agents need to be evaluated. Finally the role and place of steroids, which are often given in treatment of septic shock, should be determined.

Hypoxic–Ischemic Encephalopathy

Infants with hypoxic–ischemic encephalopathy (HIE) may have a number of serious cardiovascular challenges, with myocardial insufficiency, leading to cardiogenic shock, as well as bradycardia, hypotension, and pulmonary hypertension. Infants with HIE often receive therapy with hypothermia, which leads to a further reduction in heart rate and blood pressure, and may be associated with a worsening of pulmonary hypertension. Infants undergoing hypothermia therefore are more likely to receive inotrope/vasopressor therapy, but it is not clear what the effects of hypothermia are on the pharmacokinetics and pharmacodynamics of the commonly used agents. Thresholds for (and goals of) intervention during hypothermia treatment are also not certain. Cardiovascular instability potentially leading to impairment of brain blood flow may contribute to adverse outcome, including mortality and adverse neurodevelopmental outcome. Therefore treatment aimed at preventing hypotension, poor myocardial contractility, and reduced cardiac output may have long-term benefits.

Cardiogenic Shock

Cardiogenic shock is encountered most commonly after perinatal asphyxia. Other causes include following cardiac surgery or infants with hypoplastic left heart syndrome who may have profound shock, usually following closure of the ductus arteriosus. Aberrant coronary artery origins, although rare, should be considered in the absence of other clear etiology. Other causes such as cardiomyopathy and myocarditis are also possible but uncommon.

Usually such infants have poor perfusion and are often tachycardic (not always in the asphyxiated infant); increasing serum lactate, often leading to a frank acidosis, and oligoanuria may occur. This is one situation in which echocardiography is essential. As well as an analysis of cardiac function, the cardiac structure, including a verification of normal coronary artery distribution, should be examined.

As mentioned, even the healthy neonatal myocardium is intolerant of increases in afterload. When the primary problem is cardiac dysfunction it is essential to avoid increasing afterload. Agents that support cardiac function and decrease afterload, such as dobutamine and low-dose epinephrine, are reasonable first choices. Newer agents such as levosimendan, and perhaps milrinone, at least in the full-term infant, warrant further investigation. Excessive fluid administration should be avoided; even single fluid boluses should be carefully considered and given only if there is a good reason to suppose that there is hypovolemia.

Hypotension in the Extremely Low Gestational Age Newborn

In the first few days of life, preterm infants of less than 28 weeks' gestation are often treated with fluid boluses and inotropes after a diagnosis of hypotension. One large prospective cohort study[31] showed that, among infants born at 23 weeks' gestation, 93% received a fluid bolus and over half were treated with an inotrope (usually dopamine). Even at 27 weeks 73% received a fluid bolus and 25% were treated with dopamine.[31] There was huge variation between the 14 hospital centers, but the variation was not related to differences in patient characteristics, rather to variations in practice patterns.[31] The most consistent finding of this study is that in the majority of circumstances intervention commenced on the first day of life (90%, 89%, 91%, and 89% of infants born at 23 to 24, 25, 26, and 27 weeks of gestation). This is a time period in which notable cardiorespiratory changes occur. Long-term outcome data from the same cohort show no evidence of benefit from more aggressive treatment of hypotension.[32,33]

Many of these extremely immature babies are being treated with fluid boluses and inotropic agents despite there being no clinical or other objective evidence that they are underperfused. A number of studies have shown a poor correlation between indicators of systemic blood flow or oxygen delivery and mean arterial blood pressure in the preterm infant.[34] Most hypotensive preterm infants have flows in the superior vena cava and/or right ventricular output that are within the normal range.[35] The converse of this is that infants with low systemic flow may well have normal blood pressure, and thus patients who may benefit most from appropriate intervention are often underrecognized.

The combination of low numeric blood pressure with adequate systemic flow means that the SVR is low. On the first day of life this low SVR is unlikely to be due to an open ductus arteriosus, PVR is high, and shunting across the ductus is relatively limited for the most part. A low SVR with adequate oxygen delivery appears therefore to be part of the normal postnatal adaptation of the (very abnormal) extremely low gestational age newborn. Low numeric blood pressure without signs of poor perfusion may well not require any treatment; a small retrospective cohort study showed that good results can be seen with a permissive approach, avoiding active intervention for well-perfused infants who have low blood pressure.[36] Treating normal transition may not be the best course of action.

Intervention algorithms and surveys of practice are characterized by a very similar approach, volume administration followed by dopamine. However, we need evidence whether treating low blood pressure as such in the preterm infant is beneficial and safe. Prospective randomized trials of intervention based on currently commonly used thresholds for intervention are warranted; some of these are under way as of this writing. The European Commission has funded two of these studies in an attempt to determine the efficacy of dopamine and dobutamine in the extremely preterm infant. The HIP trial is enrolling as of this writing to determine whether a standard approach to management of hypotension with volume and dopamine, versus a more observational approach, will result in an improved outcome.[37] The Neocirc group will determine if dobutamine therapy results in an improvement in outcome in preterm infants with low flow. The TOHOP study is currently enrolling patients with low blood pressure and is attempting to evaluate the role of near-infrared spectroscopy as an adjunct in the management of low blood pressure. It is hoped that these studies will provide the clinician with evidence to direct therapy in preterm infants in the first few days of life.

CONCLUSION

Hemodynamic problems are frequent in the neonate who requires respiratory support. Unfortunately, evidence-based recommendations for therapy are limited. Although the patients involved are often unstable, research networks must be created to perform the trials that will form the basis of future evidence-based practice.

REFERENCES

A complete reference list is available at https://expertconsult.inkling.com/.

34

Pharmacologic Therapies IV: Other Medications

Jegen Kandasamy, MBBS, MD and Waldemar A. Carlo, MD

INTRODUCTION

Pharmacologic agents are often used during mechanical ventilation of newborn infants to achieve various therapeutic goals including sedation and analgesia, neuromuscular paralysis, maintenance of fluid balance, and treatment of ventilator-associated inflammatory injury. Dosing, frequency, duration of use, and adverse effect profiles have not been studied well for most drugs used in neonates. Neonatal pharmacokinetics and pharmacodynamics exhibit considerable interindividual variability among neonates, and also differ considerably from those of adults, so extrapolation of animal and adult studies to this age group is often fraught with errors.[1] Because of the limited data from studies, many of these drugs are used off-label as they have not undergone the rigorous testing in this age group required by the U.S. Food and Drug Administration (FDA).[2] This chapter deals with several pharmacologic adjuncts to neonatal mechanical ventilation that are not covered in more detail elsewhere in the book.

STEROIDS

Maternal antenatal steroid administration for pregnancies at risk for preterm delivery to improve fetal lung maturity has become a well-established practice and has led to interest in using steroids postnatally for mechanically ventilated preterm infants at risk for bronchopulmonary dysplasia (BPD). Prolonged mechanical ventilation and its associated complications of volutrauma and biotrauma are some of the most important etiologic factors in the initiation and augmentation of the inflammatory processes that contribute to BPD.[3] As potent anti-inflammatory agents, corticosteroids can potentially play a role in reducing its incidence and severity; indirect evidence for such a role is seen in infants with adrenal insufficiency, who have been shown to be at higher risk for developing BPD.[4] Steroids act through several mechanisms to reduce inflammation. They increase the synthesis of annexin-1, a protein that inhibits phospholipase A2-induced release of arachidonic acid, the source of eicosanoid inflammatory mediators such as prostaglandins and leukotrienes.[5] Steroids also inhibit other enzymes such as cyclooxygenases 1 and 2, which are also involved in eicosanoid synthesis[6] and the influx of innate immune cells such as eosinophils into the pulmonary epithelium, thereby reducing inflammation and the concentration of inflammatory cytokines such as interleukin-1 in bronchoalveolar lavage.[7] Steroids accelerate lung maturation by promoting alveolar wall thinning and microvascular maturation and promote surfactant production, especially when given during the first week after birth.[8,9]

They decrease elastase activity and collagen formation in the developing lung and increase antioxidant status and activity.[10,11] Postnatal steroid regimens have been categorized as early (less than 8 days, postnatal age) or late (greater than or equal to 8 days of life) depending on the timing of their initiation.

Early Postnatal (<8 Days) Steroid Therapy for Prevention of Bronchopulmonary Dysplasia

Though adopted enthusiastically by many clinicians in the late 1980s, early steroid therapy has become more controversial today, with the results of several studies raising concern for neurodevelopmental sequelae. The vast majority of these studies evaluated dexamethasone, which is a more potent steroid compared to hydrocortisone. In a large trial, 384 infants of less than 30 weeks' gestation were randomized to receive an early short course (two doses beginning at 12 hours of age) of dexamethasone or placebo.[12] This trial showed that a short course of early dexamethasone reduced later prolonged dexamethasone treatment and ventilator and/or oxygen use but did not reduce death or BPD at 36 weeks of gestation. The largest trial that evaluated early dexamethasone was conducted in 2001 by the Vermont Oxford Network. In this multicenter trial, 542 extremely low birth-weight (ELBW) infants on mechanical ventilation soon after birth were randomized to receive either dexamethasone or placebo for 12 days with the first dose administered at 12 hours of age.[13] The trial had to be stopped early before the completion of the predetermined sample size because of an increased incidence of complications including gastrointestinal perforation, hyperglycemia, poor weight gain, and hypertension in the early dexamethasone group. Furthermore, this trial also showed that early dexamethasone therapy increased periventricular leukomalacia and did not decrease the risk for BPD or death. Studies of early hydrocortisone therapy to prevent BPD were also carried out around this time. A multicenter trial randomized 360 mechanically ventilated ELBW infants at 12 to 48 hours of life to receive either hydrocortisone or placebo for 15 days.[14] This trial, which was also stopped early as the authors discovered increased incidence of gastrointestinal perforation in the hydrocortisone group, found that survival without BPD and mortality were similar between the two groups.

A recent Cochrane Collaboration systematic review that identified 29 such trials of the early use of postnatal steroids for preterm infants at risk for developing BPD concluded that early (<8 days) steroid treatment (either hydrocortisone or dexamethasone) decreases BPD at 36 weeks' postmenstrual age and facilitates extubation but also increases the risk for complications including intestinal perforation, hypertension, gastrointestinal bleeding, hyperglycemia, cardiomyopathy, and growth failure.[15] More important, the meta-analysis also found that long-term follow-up studies of infants from the early steroid trials showed an increased risk for abnormal neurologic examination and cerebral palsy. Based on these findings the authors concluded that routine use of early steroids cannot be recommended for preterm infants at this time. However, because only a small number of trials reported follow-up data the authors of the meta-analysis also felt there was a compelling need for more extensive follow-up data regarding long-term neurodevelopmental outcomes from these studies.

Late (≥8 Days) Postnatal Steroid Therapy for Prevention or Therapy of Bronchopulmonary Dysplasia in Preterm Infants

The Cochrane Collaboration systematic review[16] that included 21 trials with a total of 1424 infants who were randomized to receive steroids or placebo when older than a week concluded that steroid regimens initiated on or after 8 days of life reduced neonatal mortality rate at 28 days' and at 36 weeks' postmenstrual age (PMA) and decreased BPD at 36 weeks' PMA in addition to facilitating earlier extubation. Although there was a trend toward an increase in cerebral palsy rates, there was also an opposing and larger trend for decreased mortality in the steroid group at the latest follow-up. The review concluded that corticosteroid therapy should be restricted to infants who are unable to be weaned off mechanical ventilation and that such exposure be limited to minimal dosing and duration of treatment. The Canadian Pediatric Society has also taken a similar stand on the use of postnatal corticosteroids, by recommending against the use of routine dexamethasone or hydrocortisone therapy for ventilated infants.[17] These authors suggest short-term low-dose dexamethasone therapy as an alternative for infants with BPD who are on maximal ventilator and oxygen therapy, and further, that such therapy be initiated only after providing parents of such infants with information about the known short-term and long-term risks of such therapy. As of this writing, a large multicenter trial of a 10-day course of hydrocortisone for infants who are less than 30 weeks' gestational age (GA) and unable to wean off mechanical ventilation at 14 to 28 days' postnatal age is being conducted by the Neonatal Research Network. The primary outcome of this trial is survival without BPD as well as survival without neurodevelopmental impairment at 22 to 26 months' corrected age.

In addition to management of BPD, steroids have also been used in attempts to facilitate and improve success rates of extubation for mechanically ventilated preterm infants. Studies have used up to three doses of 0.25 to 0.5 mg/kg dexamethasone given intravenously for this purpose. Infants included in these studies weighed at least 1 kg, had a mean GA greater than 30 weeks, and had been intubated for at least 7 days.[18-20] A Cochrane Collaboration systematic review that analyzed these studies concluded that because dexamethasone use for facilitating extubation has not been adequately evaluated in ELBW infants and is associated with adverse effects such as hyperglycemia, its use can be approved only for infants at high risk for airway edema and obstruction such as those with repeated or prolonged intubations.[21]

As an alternative to systemic steroid therapy, inhaled corticosteroids (ICS) offer the advantage of minimal or limited adverse systemic effects. A survey found that ICS therapy has been utilized for infants with BPD in 25% of U.S. children's hospitals.[22] However, variable and inefficient drug delivery and deposition in the lower airways of premature infants, secondary to factors such as small endotracheal tube diameters, short inspiratory times, and device limitations (type and placement of nebulizer used, particle size, aerosol flow, and other factors) have been serious limitations to the use of ICS for preterm infants.[23] Although previously available data (Table 34-1) suggested that the use of ICS does not prevent BPD, either compared to placebo or with systemic steroid use, a large multinational clinical trial in which infants were randomized to receive either inhaled budesonide or placebo has found that ICS therapy does reduce BPD incidence in ELBW infants. However, this study also found an increased rate of mortality, albeit statistically nonsignificant, in the inhaled steroid group compared to the placebo group.[24,242] Further follow-up of the neurodevelopmental outcomes of infants enrolled in this study is being conducted as of this writing. More evidence regarding the effectiveness and safety of such early and prolonged use of ICS is required before their routine use can be recommended for the ELBW infant population.

SEDATION AND ANALGESIA

About 20% of all infants and 50% of all ELBW infants admitted to tertiary neonatal intensive care units (NICUs) receive endotracheal intubation and/or mechanical ventilation.[25-27] Sedation and analgesia may be important for the management of pain in neonates receiving respiratory support. In a 1997 survey neonatologists and nurses rated their assessment of pain for intubation and endotracheal suctioning in neonates at 2 on a scale of 4 (not painful to very painful).[28] Consequences of episodic pain related to procedures like intubation include physiologic responses such as hypoxemia; pulmonary and systemic hypertension; release of stress hormones like cortisol, catecholamines, and glucagon; and increased markers of oxidative stress such as malondialdehyde.[29-35] In addition, agitation during endotracheal intubation can cause increased intracranial pressures that can lead to intraventricular hemorrhage; trauma to gingival, orolabial, and glottic structures; and increased number of attempts required for any provider irrespective of their level of training and experience.[34,36-41]

Despite the potential for adverse effects of pain during respiratory support, the management of procedural pain and sedation during endotracheal intubation remains an area of controversy and debate. For example, in a survey, only 44% of U.S. neonatal units reported routine use of premedication for elective intubations.[42] First, pain assessment in the neonate is imperfect, and there is a poor correlation between individual tools that are used to attempt to objectively estimate pain.[43,44] Facial expressions of pain, high activity levels, poor response to routine care, and poor ventilator synchrony were associated with inadequate analgesia in one study of preterm ventilated infants.[45] Second, there are limited safety data regarding most drugs used for sedation and analgesia, especially regarding long-term neurodevelopmental outcomes when such medications are used for extremely premature infants.[46,47] An American Academy of Pediatrics guidance statement published in 2010 recommends routine administration of premedication, including sedatives and analgesics, for infants that undergo nonemergent intubations but also recognizes these and other knowledge gaps and stresses the importance of continued research before

TABLE 34-1 Published Randomized, Placebo-Controlled Trials of Inhaled Steroids

Reference	Sample Size	Dosage	Recruitment Criteria	Delivery Method	Placebo	Positive Results in Steroid-Treated Infants
Laforce et al.	13	Beclomethasone 3 × 50 mg for 28 days	>14 days, CXR BPD, VLBW	Nebulization through ventilator circuit or face mask	No blinded placebo	CRS; R(aw); no difference in infection
Geip et al.	19	Beclomethasone 1000 mg daily for 7 days or until extubated	>14 days, VLBW CXR BPD	MDI + spacer	Double blind	Extubation
Arnon et al.	20	Budesonide 600 mg twice daily for 7 days	14 days, BW <2000 g, IPPV	MDI + spacer	Double blind	Significant PIP; no difference in serum cortisol levels
Ng et al.	25	Fluticasone propionate 1000 mg per day for 14 days	First 24 hr, <32 weeks' GA, VLBW	MDI + spacer	Double blind	Basal and poststimulation plasma ACTH and serum plasma cortisol concentrations significantly suppressed
Fok	53	Fluticasone 500 mg bid for 14 days	<24 h, VLBW MDI + spacer IPPV		Double blind	17/27 vs 8/26 extubated at 14 days; CRS
Cole et al.	253	Beclomethasone 40 mg/kg/ day, decreasing to 5 mg/kg over 4 weeks	3-14 days, <33 weeks' GA, ≤1250 g, IPPV	MDI + spacer neonatal anesthesia bag + ET tube (even when extubated)	Double blind	Rescue dexamethasone, RR 0.6 (0.4-1.0); IPPV at 28 days, RR 0.8 (0.6-1.0) at 28 days
Jangaard et al.[241]	60	Beclomethasone (250 μg/ puff), 1-2 puffs every 6-8 hr depending on birth weight	28 days	Inline in respiratory limb of ventilator circuit with Medilife spacer via aerochamber with mask	Double blind	Similar incidence of growth failure, IVH, infection as well as long-term outcomes including NDI compared to placebo
Bassler et al.	863	Budesonide (200 μg/puff), 2 puffs every 12 hr for first 14 days, followed by 1 puff every 12 hr from day 15 until enrolled infant no longer required PPV or reached 32 weeks' PMA	<12 hr, ELBW requiring PPV	MDI + spacer, inserted into ventilator circuit or face mask	Double blind	Reduced BPD incidence in the inhaled steroid group, RR 0.74 (0.6-0.91), p < 0.05, accompanied by increased mortality, RR 1.24 (0.91-1.69), p > 0.1

ACTH, adrenocorticotropic hormone; *bid*, twice a day; *BW*, birth weight; *CRS*, compliance; *CXR BPD*, chest radiograph appearance consistent with bronchopulmonary dysplasia; *ELBS*, extremely low birth weight; *ET*, endotracheal; *GA*, gestational age; *IPPV*, ventilator dependent (intermittent positive-pressure ventilation); *IVH*, intraventricular hemorrhage; *MDI*, metered-dose inhaler; *NDI*, neurodevelopmental impairment; *PIP*, peak inspiratory pressure; *PMA*, postmenstrual age; *PPV*, positive-pressure ventilation; *R(aw)*, airway resistance; *RR*, relative risk, *VLBW*, very low birth weight.
(Data from Greenough A. *Neonat Respir Dis.* 2000;10:1-7.)

such practice can become routine in all facilities that take care of such critically ill neonates.[48]

Invasive mechanical ventilation in infants appears to be associated with chronic pain and/or stress, as supported by the increased serum levels of β-endorphins.[32] Stress can lead to long-term consequences such as impaired motor and cognitive development at 8 and 18 months of corrected GA, lower IQ at 7 years, as well as internalizing behaviors at 18 months of age and decreased pain thresholds in adult life.[49-52] These outcomes are thought to be secondary to frontoparietal cortical thinning, reduced development of white matter and subcortical gray matter, and increased activation of the somatosensory cortex associated with repeated or prolonged exposure to painful stimuli, especially in the early neonatal period.[53,54] On the other hand, prolonged or repeated analgesic exposure can lead to excessive and prolonged need for ventilation, hypotension, and enhanced neuronal cell death.[55-59] Current evidence indicates that the use of sedatives and analgesic agents for premature neonates should be a carefully considered decision that takes into account the safety and effectiveness of such agents. Nonpharmacologic interventions such as administration of oral sucrose, swaddling, containment, kangaroo care, facilitated tucking, and reduction of environmental stressors such as light and noise along with intermittent music therapy are variously effective for reducing stress associated with acutely painful procedures such as endotracheal suctioning and can be attempted as adjuncts or as first-line measures prior to the use of pharmacologic agents.[60-64] However, there are limited data regarding the utility of these nonpharmacologic interventions for infants on mechanical ventilation. Typical dosages for sedatives and analgesics used in neonates are listed in Table 34-2. Individual drugs are discussed below.

Opioids

From the time it was first isolated from *Papaver somniferum* in 1803, the alkaloid opioid morphine and its related drugs have been the standard against which all other agents with analgesic effects have been measured. The analgesic effect of opioids is due to their activation of the endorphin μ, κ, and/or δ receptors in the central nervous system, which initiates signal transduction and activation of inhibitory G proteins and reduction of cyclic adenosine monophosphate (cAMP) levels, leading to reduced neuronal excitability and decreased neurotransmitter release.[65] Spinal and supraspinal activation of these pathways

TABLE 34-2 Sedation and Analgesia for Neonates

Agent	Bolus Dose	Dose Frequency	Infusion Dose
Sedation			
Lorazepam	0.05-0.1 mg/kg	4-12 hr	Not recommended
Midazolam	0.05-0.15 mg/kg	2-4 hr	10-60 mg/kg/hr
Analgesia			
Morphine	0.05-0.2 mg/kg	2-4 hr	10-15 μg/kg/hr
Fentanyl	1-4 mg/kg*	2-4 hr	1-2 mg/kg/hr

*Slowly, over approximately 5 minutes.

inhibits ascending nociceptive pathways, reduces pain thresholds, and alters the individual's perception of pain.[65,66]

Morphine

Morphine is one of the first-line agents for analgesia in adults and is also one of the most frequently used agents for this purpose in neonates. Morphine is a strong agonist of the μ opioid receptor (MOR) through which it mediates effects such as analgesia and respiratory depression.[65] Tolerance of and dependence on morphine are also mediated through this receptor.[67] Morphine acts as a weak agonist of the κ and the δ opioid receptors, unlike naturally occurring endorphins, which mediate most of their effects through these receptors rather than the MOR. The major effects of morphine are on the central nervous system (CNS) and organs containing smooth muscle such as the gastrointestinal and urinary tracts.[65,66,68]

While morphine can be administered through oral, subcutaneous, and rectal routes, intravenous administration is the most common route of use for premature infants. Morphine has a quick onset of action and peaks at about 1 hour after injection.[66] Its duration of action in neonates may be 2 to 4 hours.[69] After an initial loading infusion of 100 mcg/kg over the first hour, standard doses used for continuous infusion range between 5 and 15 mcg/kg/h. Analgesia, the primary therapeutic indication for morphine, is achieved with morphine plasma concentrations of 15 to 20 ng/mL; some studies, however, suggest that the effective plasma morphine concentration to produce analgesia may be variable in preterm neonates.[70] However, respiratory depression is often noted at levels not much more than this range in young infants ages 2 to 570 days.[69,71,72] Respiratory depression, which is due to effects on respiratory centers in the brain stem, may be marked but is not usually of clinical significance in ventilated infants unless weaning from the ventilator is anticipated. Sedation, another therapeutic effect of morphine, occurs at much higher plasma levels (125 ng/mL), so morphine does not provide sedation at doses that are used to provide analgesia.[73]

Rapid morphine bolus infusions can induce histamine release from mast cells, a common effect seen with other opioids as well, leading to vasodilation, hypotension, and bradycardia.[66] Morphine infusions can be used safely for most preterm infants, but caution is required for infants of 23 to 26 weeks' gestation, especially those with preexisting hypotension (Hall et al.).[56,74] There are both interindividual and intraindividual variations in the effects of morphine. The metabolism of morphine matures with increasing GA; therefore, morphine infusion should be carefully titrated to the effect in preterm infants.[70,75] Other effects of morphine include bronchoconstriction, decreased

gastric motility, and increased anal sphincter tone and urinary tract smooth muscle tone. With prolonged morphine administration, some degree of tolerance develops, necessitating an increase in dosage.[67,76] Following extended use, a weaning regimen that reduces the dose by 10% to 20% per day is recommended to prevent withdrawal symptoms. Morphine effects can be reversed by a naloxone dose of 0.1 mg/kg.[65] Hepatic UDP-glucuronosyl transferase 2B7 converts morphine into morphine 6-glucuronide (responsible for both the analgesic and the respiratory depressant effects of morphine) and morphine 3-glucuronide (M3G), which acts as an antagonist to morphine and contributes to morphine tolerance.[71,77] Both metabolites are eliminated through urinary and biliary excretion. Data suggest that preterm neonates metabolize morphine to form the M3G derivative predominantly, because of which accelerated development of tachyphylaxis to continuous morphine infusion may be noted.[78] Morphine clearance reaches adult rates only at 6 to 12 months corrected postconceptual age.[79] Morphine is not highly protein-bound even in adults, so its metabolism is relatively unaffected by plasma protein levels, but whether this is also true in preterm infants, who often have decreased albumin levels, remains unclear.[80,81]

The effectiveness and safety of morphine as a continuous infusion in ventilated infants remain to be established. The Neurologic Outcomes and Preemptive Analgesia in Neonates (NEOPAIN) trial was a large multicenter study that randomized 212 infants undergoing mechanical ventilation to receive placebo or morphine infusions (ranging from 10 to 30 mcg/kg/h), along with open-label intermittent morphine used for additional analgesia based on physician discretion. Reduction of pain score and smaller increases in heart rate and respiratory rate were noted in the morphine group. However, these infants took longer to tolerate full enteral feeds, had significant hypotension more often, and required mechanical ventilation for longer duration than infants in the placebo group. Mortality rates, the primary outcome of the NEOPAIN study, and morbidities related to prematurity such as intraventricular hemorrhage (IVH) and periventricular leukomalacia (PVL) were similar between the two groups.[55] Neurologic outcomes also did not differ between the infants given morphine (up to 10 mcg/kg/h) or placebo in another study of 150 ventilated term and preterm infants.[82] A systematic meta-analysis of 13 studies (1505 infants) found that the reduction in pain scores achieved with continuous morphine infusion was clinically insignificant. This analysis also found that very preterm infants who received morphine took longer to achieve full enteral feeds and had more hypotensive episodes that required treatment. Other outcomes such as mortality, duration of mechanical ventilation, BPD, IVH, and PVL did not differ between infants who received morphine and those who received placebo. Overall, the systematic review concluded that there was insufficient evidence to recommend routine use of continuous morphine infusions for infants undergoing mechanical ventilation.[83]

Preclinical animal studies have provided evidence that morphine can alter hippocampal development in the developing brain.[84] Data regarding the impact of routine morphine use for preterm infants with regard to their long-term neurodevelopmental outcomes have shown that while overall intelligence may not be affected, effects on other neurodevelopmental outcomes may be of concern. A follow-up study of 19 infants who were part of the NEOPAIN trial showed that while there were no differences in IQ or school performance between the groups, head circumference was lower for infants who received morphine compared to those who received placebo. Infants from the morphine group also required longer time to complete tasks compared to those from the placebo group.[85] A 5-year follow-up of mechanically ventilated preterm infants who were randomized to receive continuous morphine infusion or placebo also found that overall IQ scores, executive function, visual–motor integration, and intelligence did not differ between the morphine and the control groups, but the visual analysis subtest component score was noted to be lower for infants from the morphine group.[82,86] Other studies have also highlighted subtle adverse effects on long-term motor development and neurobehavior when morphine was routinely used for analgesia for preterm infants.[52,87]

Thus, based on the currently available data, morphine administration, especially as a continuous infusion, should not be considered routine for mechanically ventilated infants. Instead, opioids such as morphine should be used judiciously, either as intermittent doses or as continuous infusions, appropriately titrated for each infant to measurements of pain based on well-validated scales.

Fentanyl

Fentanyl is a synthetic opioid with higher lipophilicity compared to morphine. This higher lipid solubility allows fentanyl to cross the blood–cerebrospinal fluid barrier more rapidly and produce analgesic effects more quickly than morphine. In addition, the analgesic effects of fentanyl are 80 to 100 times more potent than the morphine effects. Fentanyl is oxidized by hepatic microsomal cytochrome P450 into norfentanyl, an inactive metabolite that is then renally excreted.[65,66] Fentanyl clearance matures quickly after birth, reaching 70% of adult levels by 2 weeks' postnatal age in term infants.[88,89] Clearance of fentanyl can be reduced secondary to decreased hepatic blood flow.[90] Owing to faster redistribution and an elimination half-life of 4 hours, fentanyl also has a shorter duration of action (30 to 40 min) than morphine, making it ideal for scenarios like intubation that require rapid induction and recovery from sedation and analgesia.[91,92] Fentanyl also has reduced propensity to cause histamine release from mast cells, as well as decreased activity on the vasomotor center. These advantages of fentanyl make it theoretically less likely to cause significant hypotension compared to morphine.[93,94] In addition, when used prior to endotracheal suctioning fentanyl blunts increases in pulmonary arterial pressure, as shown in a study of infants recovering from cardiac surgery, who are often prone to such crises.[95] In contrast to morphine, studies of fentanyl pharmacodynamics also show that its therapeutic effects may be more predictable using serum levels.[89] Because of these advantages, fentanyl has emerged as the most commonly used synthetic opioid for procedural analgesia in neonates.[48]

Continuous fentanyl infusion is also often used to achieve more prolonged analgesia for mechanically ventilated infants. Currently available data suggest that fentanyl offers analgesia equivalent to that produced by morphine, as shown in a trial of 163 mechanically ventilated newborn infants between 29 and 37 weeks' gestation at birth randomized to receive continuous infusions of either fentanyl or morphine in the first 2 days of life. Adverse effects such as decreased gastrointestinal motility were also less commonly observed in the fentanyl group.[96] However, similar needs for vasopressors to treat hypotension were observed in both groups. Another important, though rare, disadvantage that appears to be more common with fentanyl

use than with morphine is chest wall rigidity, especially when it is administered as a rapid bolus infusion.[97] In addition, when used as a continuous infusion the serum half-life of fentanyl is prolonged in preterm infants.[98] This may be secondary to the high lipid solubility of fentanyl that allows it to accumulate in adipose and other lipid-rich tissue. When discontinued after prolonged use, redistribution of fentanyl from such stores can prolong respiratory depression and delay the recovery from sedation.[91] Severe gastrointestinal adverse effects can also be seen with fentanyl, showing that the choice of fentanyl over morphine for analgesia may not be as advantageous as is sometimes believed.[99]

Prolonged opioid use can lead to the development of tolerance, tachyphylaxis, and withdrawal symptoms when such use is discontinued. In one study of infants on extracorporeal membrane oxygenation, fentanyl infusion was associated with more rapid development of tolerance and requirement for higher doses over time, along with increased incidence and severity of withdrawal effects, leading to significantly longer hospital stay compared to continuous morphine infusion.[76] Fentanyl use is also associated with more severe tachyphylaxis compared to morphine.[100] In another study, a fentanyl total dose greater than 415 mcg/kg predicted withdrawal with 70% sensitivity and 78% specificity, whereas a fentanyl infusion duration greater than 8 days predicted withdrawal with 90% sensitivity and 67% specificity.[101] Both fentanyl and morphine require weaning from the total daily dose by 10% to 20% per day to prevent such withdrawal.

As an analgesic agent, fentanyl is associated with disadvantages as shown in several trials that compared it to placebo. Fentanyl was noted to be associated with a need for higher, rather than lower, ventilator support in a randomized trial of 20 infants with respiratory distress syndrome, possibly secondary to decreased chest wall compliance due to fentanyl-induced chest wall rigidity.[102] In a multicenter trial of 131 mechanically ventilated infants between 22 and 32 weeks' GA at birth randomized to receive either fentanyl or placebo, short-term pain scores were lower for infants who received fentanyl, but there were no long-term differences in either the pain scores or the need for open-label fentanyl use, which was also similar between the two groups. Fentanyl use also prolonged the duration of mechanical ventilation and the time to first meconium passage in this study.[103] Data available from a randomized placebo-controlled trial of 27 preterm ventilated infants regarding the impact of fentanyl infusion on mortality or the incidence of short-term adverse neurologic effects such as IVH indicate it has no advantages over placebo; as of this writing there are no data regarding its effects on long-term neurodevelopmental outcomes.[104]

Dexmedetomidine

As an analgesic agent with additional anxiolytic and sedative properties and the additional advantage of very minimal potential to cause respiratory depression, dexmedetomidine has been extensively used in adults, often beyond the 24 hours of use that it has been approved for by the FDA.[105] Dexmedetomidine is an imidazole derivative and the active isomer of medetomidine. It is a selective central α_2-adrenergic receptor agonist. α_2-Adrenergic receptors are found in a number of supraspinal and spinal neuronal sites in the central and peripheral nervous systems where they modulate both presynaptic and postsynaptic sympathetic output. One of the areas of the CNS with a high density of this receptor is the locus coeruleus, the primary site of norepinephrine synthesis in the brain, with functions that include maintenance of sleep–wake cycle, attention, memory, and arousal. Blocking sympathetic outflow from the locus coeruleus is the primary mechanism behind the sedative and analgesic effects of dexmedetomidine. This area is also the origin of several descending spinal nociceptive pathways that converge on the substantia gelatinosa in the dorsal horn of the spinal cord. At this level, dexmedetomidine stimulates α_2 receptors to inhibit release of substance P, a nociceptive mediator.[106] While other drugs that act on α_2-adrenergic receptors such as clonidine exist, dexmedetomidine is unique in its high specificity for the α_{2A} subtype of this receptor which is primarily responsible for its very effective sedative and analgesic effects.[107,108]

Dexmedetomidine is increasingly being used in the pediatric population, especially in the postoperative cardiac intensive care environment.[109] In the first-ever study of its use in preterm infants a study with historic controls (for whom fentanyl had been used as analgesic) assessed the use of dexmedetomidine in 24 preterm infants with a mean GA of 25 weeks.[110] This study showed that dexmedetomidine use was associated with less need for adjunctive sedation, shorter duration of mechanical ventilation, and lower incidence of culture-positive sepsis episodes compared to fentanyl use. The lower incidence of sepsis noted with dexmedetomidine is believed to be secondary to its promotion of macrophage activity and reduction of inflammatory mediators such as tumor necrosis factor-α and interleukin-6 that has been noted in animal studies.[111,112] This anti-inflammatory effect of dexmedetomidine, if confirmed in large randomized trials, may be a significant advantage for mechanically ventilated preterm infants who are very often prone to developing BPD. Another difference was the lack of signs of withdrawal for infants in the dexmedetomidine group, whereas infants in the fentanyl group often required slower weaning.

Other potential advantages of dexmedetomidine use in preterm mechanically ventilated infants may include its minimal potential to cause respiratory depression and gastrointestinal dysmotility.[113] Adverse effects associated with dexmedetomidine also are a result of its α_2-adrenergic agonist activity. Like clonidine, which has similar receptor activity albeit with lesser specificity, dexmedetomidine can cause hypotension, bradycardia, decreased secretion, bowel motility, and excessive diuresis.[114] In the study of dexmedetomidine use in preterm infants, the incidence of significant hypotension or bradycardia was similar between the dexmedetomidine group and the control group (fentanyl), indicating that dexmedetomidine may not be inferior to other currently used sedatives and analgesics with respect to this adverse effect. While no differences were noted between the two groups with respect to short-term neurologic outcomes such as IVH, large randomized trials that include long-term neurodevelopmental outcomes of its use need to be conducted before dexmedetomidine can be recommended for use in premature infants without reservation.[110]

Benzodiazepines

As sedative–hypnotics, the benzodiazepines cause CNS depression to reduce anxiety, produce drowsiness, and maintain a state of reduced awareness. Benzodiazepines are widely used for such purposes in the NICU. However, benzodiazepines do not possess analgesic effects. By increasing the affinity of γ-amino butyric acid (GABA) binding to the GABA-A receptors, benzodiazepines increase neuronal inhibition at various levels of the nervous system including the cerebral cortex, hypothalamus, hippocampus, and substantia nigra. Side effects of benzodiazepine use include respiratory depression and, especially in infants with hypovolemia or impaired cardiac function, hypotension.[115] The most commonly used benzodiazepines in the NICU are discussed here.

Midazolam

Because of its pH-dependent water and lipid solubility, midazolam combines decreased incidence of thrombophlebitis or discomfort during intravenous administration with rapid onset of action (less than 3 minutes) and time to peak sedative effects (less than 20 minutes) compared to other benzodiazepines, making it a preferred drug for use in emergent situations in which rapid onset and termination of sedative effects may be required.[116,117] It is also frequently used as a continuous infusion for sedation of mechanically ventilated neonates. Midazolam is converted by hepatic cytochrome P450 3A4 hydroxylation to form active and inactive metabolites. Owing to relatively lower levels of this enzyme at birth, midazolam has a longer elimination half-life (6.3 hours) and lower clearance rate (1.8 mL/kg/min) in healthy neonates.[118,119] In a study of 187 neonates between 26 and 42 weeks' GA who underwent mechanical ventilation, the midazolam elimination half-life was 1.6-fold greater than normal.[120] Preterm infants have a longer elimination half-life compared to term infants, indicating that midazolam clearance increases with postnatal age and is decreased by critical illness as well as mechanical ventilation.[121] Oral midazolam use in neonates is rare and associated with reduced clearance; bioavailability via the oral route was estimated to be around 50% in one study.[122] Midazolam is highly protein bound; low serum albumin concentrations may lead to increased fractions of unbound midazolam available to enter the CNS and potentiate its therapeutic as well as adverse effects.[123]

The adverse effects of midazolam in neonates include respiratory depression, hypotension, hypotonia, hypertonia, dyskinetic movements, myoclonus, and paradoxic agitation.[124] The decreased number of GABA-A receptors seen in the neonate is believed to be the cause of the hyperexcitability instead of sedation that is often seen with midazolam use. Young age, female gender, and reduced serum albumin levels have been reported to be risk factors for the development of such adverse short-term neurologic effects.[125] Withdrawal associated with discontinuation of midazolam use has been noted in rodent studies and may be the cause of the neurologic adverse effects seen in older infants, children, and adults.[126] Finally, the usual parenteral preparation contains 1% benzyl alcohol as a preservative; this may need to be taken into consideration when dosing this drug. Use of the more concentrated 5 mg/mL preparation will reduce exposure to benzyl alcohol per milligram of midazolam used. Newer preparations of midazolam are preservative-free.[116]

A randomized trial of the use of continuous midazolam infusion as sedation for mechanical ventilation in 46 preterm infants found that while midazolam was an effective sedative compared to placebo, it did not reduce duration of ventilation, supplemental oxygen use, or incidence of severe lung disease or mortality compared to placebo. In addition, midazolam use prolonged NICU stay and tended to increase the incidence of hypotension and bradycardia in preterm infants when its use was continued beyond 48 hours.[127] Another multicenter study of sedation in the NICU randomized 67 mechanically ventilated infants between 24 and 32 weeks' GA to receive morphine, midazolam, or dextrose placebo infusions for up to 14 days (the Neonatal Outcome and Prolonged Analgesia in Neonates trial). In addition to finding results similar to those of the previous study, this trial also found that midazolam use led to increased incidence of neurologic adverse effects such as IVH and PVL compared to morphine or placebo use.[57] A meta-analysis of such studies by Ng et al.[128] concluded that in light of the currently available evidence, the increased risks of adverse neurologic effects seen with midazolam use outweigh any benefits and therefore preclude its recommendation for use as a continuous infusion for sedation in the preterm infant.

Lorazepam

Lorazepam is a longer acting, highly lipophilic benzodiazepine compared to midazolam with a serum half-life of 24 to 56 hours and a duration of action of 8 to 12 hours in critically ill neonates.[129] Lorazepam is metabolized by hepatic glucuronidation into inactive metabolites, which are then eliminated through biliary excretion.[115] Apnea, somnolence, and stereotypic movements are complications associated with lorazepam use in neonates.[130,131] In adults and older children, prolonged administration or continuous infusion of lorazepam causes metabolic acidosis secondary to accumulation of toxic alcohols such as propylene glycol, an agent that is used to increase the solubility of lorazepam in currently available lorazepam formulations.[132] Therefore, lorazepam cannot be recommended for administration as a continuous infusion in neonates. As lorazepam is a longer acting agent, prolonged sedation can be achieved with intermittent dosing to achieve sedation in mechanically ventilated infants. However, like other benzodiazepines, routine use of lorazepam for sedation in preterm infants has not been adequately characterized with respect to its long-term neurodevelopmental effects and cannot be recommended at this time.

Diazepam

Diazepam has anxiolytic, hypnotic, anticonvulsant, muscle relaxant, and amnesic effects that are characteristic of benzodiazepines and, like other benzodiazepines, has no analgesic properties. Diazepam is absorbed rapidly after oral administration but irregularly after intramuscular administration. The elimination half-life approximates 75 hours in preterm infants and 30 hours in term infants.[133] Diazepam is metabolized in the liver and, along with its metabolites, is slowly excreted in the urine. Simple correlations do not exist between plasma level and clinical response. Diazepam can cause respiratory depression, which may actually help infants to "settle" on the ventilator. Diazepam can be useful as a long-acting sedative when given in doses ranging from 0.10 to 0.25 mg/kg every 6 hours.

Other Sedative Agents

Propofol is an intravenous alkylphenol sedative–hypnotic without analgesic effects. It is a rapid-acting agent with short half-life and low propensity to cause respiratory depression.[134] A study of 63 neonates that compared a combination of succinylcholine, atropine, and morphine to the use of only propofol for sedation prior to intubation found that propofol use led to shorter time required for successful intubation and less associated oral/nasal trauma as well as shorter recovery times. Infants in the propofol group also experienced less hypoxemic events during the endotracheal intubation attempts.[135] Despite these advantages, the use of propofol in neonates as an induction agent for endotracheal intubation has been associated with a high incidence of hypotension.[248] In addition, continuous infusion of propofol has been associated with fatal complications secondary to metabolic acidosis, bradycardia, rhabdomyolysis, and renal failure (the propofol infusion syndrome) when used in children and adults.[136] Thus, continuous infusion of propofol for sedation is strongly discouraged.

Chloral hydrate, a commonly used sedative agent, has the major advantages of excellent oral bioavailability and minimal respiratory depression.[59,137] While it is well suited to procedural sedation, particularly for radiologic procedures, electroencephalography, and echocardiography, with prolonged use accumulation of trichloroethanol leads to life-threatening arrhythmias, hypotension, and paradoxic CNS stimulation.[138] This disadvantage of chloral hydrate, along with its tendency to displace various drugs and bilirubin from their protein-bound sites, as well as its propensity to cause direct hyperbilirubinemia,[139] preclude its use for sedation in neonates.

MUSCLE RELAXANTS

Neuromuscular blockade is sometimes required for the care of critically ill infants, especially during procedures that often require their immobilization. Such blockade can be achieved either through excessive depolarization at the neuromuscular junction (depolarizing agents) or through a blockade of transmission at the neuromuscular junction achieved by acetylcholine antagonists (nondepolarizing agents). The use of muscle relaxants is not routinely indicated during mechanical ventilation of neonates, but muscle relaxants are sometimes used as part of premedication regimens and in certain patient populations such as infants with persistent pulmonary hypertension of the newborn (PPHN).[140] Although paralysis may improve oxygenation and ventilation of severely hypoxemic term infants with PPHN, it may have adverse effects on preterm infants with respiratory distress syndrome.[141] The use of synchronized ventilation using ventilator rates above the spontaneous rate of the patient frequently will accomplish the goals of paralysis (see Chapter 18).[142] Muscle relaxants may be useful in selected preterm infants whose own respiratory efforts interfere with ventilation and may reduce the incidence of pneumothorax in these infants.[143]

Perlman et al. demonstrated that the elimination of fluctuating cerebral blood flow velocity by muscle paralysis reduced the incidence of IVH in selected preterm infants with respiratory distress syndrome (RDS), but this has not been tested in a large trial and is not practiced commonly. As muscle paralysis may reduce oxygen consumption, paralysis may be advantageous to infants with compromised oxygenation.[144,145] Prolonged paralysis of greater than 2 weeks' duration has been associated with disuse atrophy and subsequent skeletal muscle growth failure. Importantly, in terms of pulmonary mechanics, Bhutani et al.[146] have shown a decrease in dynamic lung compliance and an increase in total pulmonary resistance only after more than 48 hours of continuous paralysis with pancuronium. Both parameters improved by 41% to 43% at 6 to 18 hours after discontinuation of paralysis.

Spontaneous respiratory efforts appear to contribute little to minute ventilation in the severely ill preterm infant with very low lung compliance.[145] These infants are at risk of decreased functional residual capacity after paralysis, possibly through loss of upper airway braking mechanisms.[141] In infants with

TABLE 34-3 Neuromuscular Blocking Agents for Neonates

Agent	Initial Dose (mg/kg)	Dose Frequency	Infusion Dose (mg/kg/hr)
Pancuronium	0.04-0.15	1-4 hr	Not recommended
Vecuronium	0.03-0.15	1-2 hr	0.05-0.10
Rocuronium	0.3-0.6	0.5-1 hr	0.4-0.6

lung compliance that is less compromised and in larger infants, spontaneous respiratory efforts contribute markedly to total ventilation. Thus, ventilator adjustments (usually increases in rate) are necessary to prevent significant hypoventilation when paralysis is instituted. Monitoring gas exchange is recommended. Although loss of intercostal muscle tone may lead to an increase in intrathoracic pressure, this does not appear to cause an increase in respiratory resistance.[147]

The primary hazard during paralysis appears to be accidental inconspicuous extubation. The paralyzed neonate is entirely dependent on mechanical ventilation, and careful observation is required. Also, paralysis obscures a variety of clinical signs whose expression depends on muscle tone and movement, such as seizures. Finally, paralysis does not alter the sensation of pain; thus, analgesics should be administered under circumstances in which their use would be indicated in a nonparalyzed infant.

In practice, the decision to administer a muscle relaxant is most often based on clinical observation of an infant in combination with arterial blood gas measurements. Muscle relaxants are used frequently to facilitate hyperventilation therapy (see Chapter 18 and the section entitled Persistent Pulmonary Hypertension of the Newborn in Chapter 23). Analysis of ventilator or esophageal pressure waveforms is a more objective method of assessing whether an infant is in phase with the ventilator and whether mean intrathoracic pressure is increased.[143] However, there is no reliable way of predicting which infants in this circumstance will benefit from paralysis. Thus, muscle relaxants should be administered as a therapeutic trial and their use continued if blood gas values improve during the trial, if nursing care is greatly simplified, or if there is obvious improvement in patient synchrony with the ventilator and comfort. If the complications of prolonged paralysis are to be prevented, periodic assessment of the infant in the nonparalyzed state is essential. The short-acting depolarizing muscle relaxant succinylcholine is infrequently used in the care of neonates, except when paralysis for intubation is necessary; therefore, only the commonly used nondepolarizing agents are discussed in this section. Recommended dosages are listed in Table 34-3.

Pancuronium

Pancuronium bromide, a long-acting, competitive neuromuscular blocking agent, is the muscle relaxant most frequently used in neonates. Gallamine and D-tubocurarine are seldom used because of significant cardiovascular effects, sympathetic ganglionic blockade, and, in the case of the former, obligatory renal excretion. All of these agents block transmission at the neuromuscular junction by competing with acetylcholine for receptor sites on the postjunctional membrane.[148] Pancuronium has vagolytic effects, and an increase in heart rate is commonly observed during its use. Administered intravenously, pancuronium produces maximum paralysis within 2 to 4 minutes. The duration of apnea after a single dose is variable and prolonged

in neonates and can last from one to several hours. Incremental doses increase the duration of respiratory paralysis. In addition, the duration of paralysis is prolonged by acidosis, hypokalemia, use of aminoglycoside antibiotics, and decreased renal function. Alkalosis can be expected to antagonize blockade. Although renal excretion is the major route of elimination of pancuronium, hepatobiliary excretion and metabolism may account for the elimination of a significant portion of an administered dose.

The recommended dosage of pancuronium in neonates varies from 0.06 to 0.10 mg/kg.[148] Although it is customary to administer repeat doses that are of the same magnitude as the initial dose, subsequent doses of half the initial dose may be effective in prolonging paralysis when muscular activity or spontaneous respiration returns. Continuous infusion of pancuronium in neonates is associated with the potential for accumulation because of these patients' slow rate of excretion; thus this method of administration is best avoided unless electrophysiologic monitoring is available.

The long-term benefits of respiratory paralysis need to be balanced with potential complications. Prolonged use of pancuronium bromide has been implicated in sensorineural hearing loss in childhood survivors of congenital diaphragmatic hernia.[149,150] In a cohort study of head trauma patients in a pediatric intensive care unit setting, patients treated with and without pancuronium were compared.[151] In the 15 patients with isolated intracranial pathology who received continuous paralysis, compliance progressively dropped by 50% over 4 days. Compliance normalized after discontinuation of paralysis. Compliance did not change in the patients who were ventilated but not paralyzed. The paralyzed patients required mechanical ventilation longer than the nonparalyzed patients, and 26% of these patients developed nosocomial pneumonia, a complication that was not seen in the nonparalyzed patients. Prolonged use of pancuronium has also been associated with weight gain and third-space accumulation from lack of movement and urinary retention.

Despite the reported complications, pancuronium is still frequently used in the NICU population.[152] A systematic review[153] summarized the literature by stating that in ventilated preterm infants with evidence of asynchronous respiratory efforts, neuromuscular paralysis with pancuronium seems to be associated with less IVH and possibly less pulmonary air leak. The authors went on to stress that long-term pulmonary and neurologic effects are uncertain.

The effects of pancuronium can be rapidly reversed with the use of the anticholinesterase agent neostigmine at 0.08 mg/kg intravenously, preceded by the administration of glycopyrrolate at 2.5 to 5 mcg/kg, which blocks the muscarinic side effects. Although rapid reversal is seldom needed for medical reasons in neonates receiving assisted ventilation, reversal may occasionally be useful diagnostically in infants considered to have suffered a CNS insult during paralysis.

Vecuronium

Vecuronium is a short-acting nondepolarizing muscle relaxant that is structurally related to pancuronium, with time to onset of action of 1.5 to 2.0 minutes after intravenous bolus infusion, with a duration of effect that lasts only 30 to 40 minutes.[148] It has few cardiovascular side effects and is cleared rapidly by biliary excretion. Thus, it is safer than pancuronium in the presence of renal failure. Interference with excretion or potentiation of effect has been suggested when vecuronium is used in combination with metronidazole, aminoglycosides, and hydantoins.

However, no problems have been observed in infants receiving these agents and vecuronium in its usual dosage.[148] Acidosis can be expected to enhance the neuromuscular blockade provided by vecuronium and alkalosis to antagonize it.

Vecuronium usually is given by continuous intravenous infusion at a rate of 0.1 mg/kg/hr after an initial paralyzing bolus dose of 0.1 mg/kg. Intermittent bolus dosing would need to be so frequent (i.e., every 30 to 60 minutes) that this type of regimen usually is impractical. Continuous infusion is preferred for certain postoperative cardiac patients whose respiratory or other muscular movement may jeopardize the success of the repair. The effects of vecuronium can be reversed by neostigmine administration, as described earlier for pancuronium.

Rocuronium

Rocuronium is a rapid-acting but less potent desacetoxy analogue of vecuronium. Like other steroidal drugs it is mostly (70% to 90%) metabolized in the liver and excreted through the biliary tract, which accounts for its shorter duration of action, reported to be 20 to 35 minutes, compared to agents that are mostly excreted through the renal system.[243] A trial of 44 intubations in preterm infants who were randomized to receive either atropine or fentanyl alone or rocuronium added to these agents found that infants in the latter group were more likely to be successfully intubated on the first attempt. Onset of paralysis was 22 to 106 seconds after administration of a 0.5-mg/kg dose of rocuronium. Complete paralysis was noted to last for 3 to 29 minutes after administration of the above dose. Adverse effects noted in this study included transient tachycardia (7%) and bronchospasm in one infant.[244] Recommended dosages for rocuronium can be found in Table 34-3.

Cisatracurium

Atracurium is an isoquinoline nondepolarizing neuromuscular blocker that is metabolized mostly by Hofmann elimination, a nonenzymatic spontaneous degradation process that occurs at physiologic pH and temperature. Cisatracurium is an enantiomer of atracurium that is four times more potent, slower in its onset of action, but similar to atracurium in its duration of action. Like atracurium it undergoes Hofmann elimination but is not hydrolyzed by plasma cholinesterase. Unlike atracurium, cisatracurium does not provoke histamine release, thereby minimizing adverse effects such as hypotension and bradycardia. Its metabolism also produces less laudanosine, a CNS stimulant that can provoke seizures.[243] A study of continuous cisatracurium infusion for neuromuscular blockade compared to vecuronium in 19 infants recovering from cardiac surgery found that infants in the cisatracurium group recovered their neuromuscular function faster compared to infants in the vecuronium group. This study used doses of cisatracurium ranging between 0.75 and 4.5 mcg/kg/min. In these dosage ranges, cisatracurium had an elimination half-life between 15 and 468 minutes for the nine infants in this study.[245] Routine use of cisatracurium in newborn infants, especially for ELBW premature infants, requires more evidence regarding its pharmacokinetic and pharmacodynamic profiles in this patient group.

BRONCHODILATORS AND MUCOLYTIC AGENTS

Bronchospasm was long believed to play a minimal if any role in contributing to airway resistance in the newborn, especially in preterm infants. Anatomic studies that demonstrated lack

TABLE 34-4		Aerosolized Medications for Neonates		
Agent	Dose	Dose Frequency	Comments	
Salbutamol	0.20 mg/kg	Every 3-6 hr	With 0.5% solution, dilute 0.04 mL/kg in 1.5 mL NS 18-mg/puff, 1 or 2 puffs/dose with metered-dose inhaler*	
Ipratropium bromide	0.025 mg/kg	Every 8 hr		
N-acetylcysteine	10-20 mg	Every 6-8 hr	Add bronchodilator if bronchospasm occurs; restricted use advised in view of undesirable effects	
Cromoglycic acid (cromolyn sodium)	10 mg	Every 6 hr	Dilute 1 mL of 10-mg/mL solution up to 1.5 mL NS	

*Only available metered-dose inhaler in the United States.
NS, normal saline.

of smooth muscle in the distal airways of premature infants strengthened this opinion.[154] However, studies that confirmed the presence of airway smooth muscle even in the lungs of 23-week gestation infants have disproved such misconceptions. The airways of 25-week-old infants have smooth muscle relative to airway circumference that is similar to that of term infants, indicating that bronchospasm is possible in preterm infants within the first few days after birth.[155] It is now known that mechanically ventilated infants with BPD have airway smooth muscle hypertrophy that often plays a significant role in increasing airway resistance.[156] In addition to contributing to resistance to airflow, the tracheobronchial tree of preterm infants compared to term infants and adults also possesses a relatively higher number of goblet cells that express mucus and fewer ciliated airway cells to assist in the mobilization of airway secretions and mucus.[157] In addition to effecting bronchodilation, some agents such as aminophylline improve diaphragmatic and inspiratory muscle contractility, which may result in both improved ventilation and a greater likelihood of successful and earlier extubation, the goals for which the clinician should be striving.[158] Thus, bronchodilators to decrease airway resistance and mucolytic agents that promote mucin breakdown are often used as aids to mechanical ventilation of the neonate. Typical dosages for commonly used aerosolized medications are listed in Table 34-4.

Albuterol (Salbutamol)

Albuterol is a selective β_2-adrenergic agonist. By enhancing cAMP production, which then decreases intracellular calcium in smooth muscle cells, albuterol causes bronchodilation. While other formulations exist, albuterol is primarily used as an aerosol, further enhancing its selectivity.[159,160] At high doses, inhaled albuterol loses such bronchial β_2 selectivity and leads to adverse effects such as vasodilation, hypotension, reflex tachycardia, hyperglycemia, and hypokalemia, secondary to its effects on other β_2-adrenergic receptor systems.[161]

Infants with established or developing BPD often have increased airflow resistance, decreased forced expiratory flow, and increased functional reserve capacity compared to normal cohorts.[162,163] Albuterol improves static lung compliance in very low birth-weight infants as early as the second postnatal week.[164] Thirty-five percent of infants with BPD, especially those with clinically noted symptoms such as wheezing, exhibited responsiveness to albuterol inhalation.[163]

Most of the above-mentioned studies, however, did not assess longer-term clinical outcomes of albuterol therapy for premature infants with BPD. In the only study as of this writing that assessed longer term outcomes in 173 infants of less than 28 weeks' GA, albuterol treatment started on day 11 and continued for 28 days did not reduce supplemental oxygen or mechanical ventilation, mortality, or the severity of BPD.[165] An important caveat to note is that all of these studies predate the use of surfactant and antenatal steroids and may not be applicable to infants with "new BPD." Controversy also exists regarding long-term β-agonist stimulation of nonpulmonary tissues, possible adverse effects of long-term bronchodilation on healing lung tissue, and theoretical concerns over the development of tolerance.[166] A 2012 Cochrane collaboration systematic review also concluded that because of the paucity of clinical trials that have examined the effectiveness of albuterol in improving clinical outcomes for infants with BPD, its use should be limited to clinical trial settings only.[167]

Cromoglycic Acid

Cromoglycic acid (cromolyn sodium) is an anti-inflammatory agent that prevents mast cell activation and degranulation by inhibiting chloride transport and protein kinase C. Cromoglycic acid can also inhibit neutrophil chemotaxis and free radical-induced neutrophil NADPH oxidase.[168] As cromoglycic acid is a highly ionized water-soluble compound, it does not cross cell membranes and can be effectively administered only by inhalation.[169] Interest in using cromolyn as a therapy for mechanically ventilated infants was created by a small cohort study that found that cromolyn sodium therapy administered to infants with BPD was associated with decreased need for invasive ventilation and an increase in dynamic lung compliance.[170] The anti-inflammatory effects of cromolyn sodium that were postulated in this study led to two small trials that attempted to use cromolyn early in life for preterm infants to mitigate their risk for lung inflammation. In the first of these small studies, a trial of 38 infants with mean GA of 26 weeks who required mechanical ventilation at birth, nebulized cromolyn sodium given every 6 hours for the duration that the infants remained intubated did not reduce risk for BPD or mortality compared to placebo.[171] Another small trial of 26 infants randomized to receive either cromolyn or placebo for 28 days after birth also showed no difference in BPD or death.[172] Neither study found beneficial effects for the anti-inflammatory effects of cromolyn for outcomes such as IVH, sepsis, necrotizing enterocolitis, or patent ductus arteriosus (PDA). A Cochrane review that included both of these studies found no evidence to recommend routine use of cromolyn sodium for prevention of BPD in preterm infants.[173] As there is some evidence for a decrease in inflammatory markers associated with BPD when sodium cromolyn is used in conjunction with surfactant, diuretics, and steroids, cromolyn sodium may be an important adjunct therapy when used with other agents such as steroids and warrants further clinical trials.[174]

Ipratropium Bromide

Atropine, a potent inhibitor of acetylcholine at postganglionic muscarinic receptors, is known to produce bronchodilation and reduce the production of airway mucin. Ipratropium bromide is a quaternary ammonium derivative of atropine that when administered by inhalation into the airways is poorly absorbed

into the circulation and can be used as a selective bronchodilator.[161] Because functional muscarinic airway receptors have been demonstrated in the airways of premature infants, ipratropium bromide has been used as a bronchodilator for infants with BPD.[175] A study that used inhaled ipratropium bromide for infants with BPD found that muscarinic receptors contributed to the increased bronchomotor tone seen in these infants and that a combination of ipratropium and albuterol produced effective and long-lasting bronchodilation.[176] However, similar to inhaled β agonists, there is no evidence as of this writing for long-term benefits of ipratropium bromide use for the natural course of BPD in preterm infants.

Racemic Epinephrine

The subglottis is the narrowest portion of the airway in neonates. The presence of a foreign body, as occurs with prolonged intubation, produces edema in the subglottic region, which can produce further narrowing of the airway when the neonate is extubated. Racemic epinephrine stimulates both α- and β-adrenergic receptors. It acts on vascular smooth muscle to produce vasoconstriction, which markedly decreases blood flow at the capillary level. This shrinks upper respiratory mucosa and reduces edema. Racemic epinephrine is a useful agent in patients with established postextubation stridor; however, its efficacy for prevention of postextubation stridor has not been proven.[177] Racemic epinephrine may also be considered as an adjunct to therapy for pulmonary hemorrhage.[178] When using racemic epinephrine, one should be aware of the side effects, which include tachycardia, arrhythmias, hypertension, peripheral vasoconstriction, hyperglycemia, hyperkalemia, metabolic acidosis, and leukocytosis.[177]

N-Acetylcysteine

N-Acetylcysteine (NAC) is a well-known thiol compound that possesses a free sulfhydryl group through which it reduces disulfide bonds present in mucoproteins, thereby reducing the elasticity and viscosity of mucus.[179] NAC also interacts directly with oxidants such as hydrogen peroxide and the hydroxyl radical through its role as a modulator of cellular redox status.[180] This role may also contribute to the efficacy of NAC in improving lung function in adults with chronic obstructive pulmonary disease.[181] However, experience with the use of NAC in neonates is fairly limited. A small study of NAC found that hourly doses of up to 0.2 mL of endotracheally administered NAC did not alter postmortem histology of trachea or bronchi in preterm infants.[182] Another study evaluated the effects of intratracheal NAC administration on lung function in mechanically ventilated infants with a mean GA of 27 weeks and mean postnatal age of 22 weeks. This study found that NAC administration was associated with an increase in airway resistance by the third day of treatment. The authors concluded that NAC administration was not associated with any improvement in lung function for infants with BPD and also that its administration may indeed be associated with adverse effects such as increased airway resistance and cyanotic spells.[183] Thus the use of NAC in preterm infants should be undertaken cautiously, and when used, NAC should be administered along with bronchodilators to offset these reported adverse effects.

While NAC held promise as an effective anti-inflammatory agent secondary to its antioxidant properties, this too has not been borne out in studies. A study of 33 preterm infants between 24 and 28 weeks of gestation randomized them to receive either

NAC or placebo during the first week of life. Measurements of lung function conducted when these infants were close to discharge from the NICU did not show any differences between the groups. The authors concluded that prophylactic NAC treatment for preterm infants at risk for BPD does not improve their lung function at term.[184]

Combination Therapies

In addition to the use of bronchodilators and ICS in isolation, their use in combination, using delivery devices like metered-dose inhalers (MDIs) and jet nebulizers, as therapy for BPD has also been evaluated. In a study of 173 infants of less than 31 weeks' GA randomized to receive albuterol, beclomethasone, their combination, or placebo delivered through an MDI or a jet nebulizer, no differences in the duration of oxygen therapy or ventilator support, or the incidence and severity of BPD, were noted among the various groups.[165] In addition the combined use of such medication may not provide any additional effects than when administered individually, as was shown by a small study of 15 infants in which combined administration of β agonists and anticholinergics failed to demonstrate any synergy between these two agents in improving airway function.[246]

In summary, as concluded by a review that reported on 22 trials involving the use of inhaled β agonists, anticholinergics, and corticosteroids for infants with BPD, no clear long-term benefits have been demonstrated as of this writing.[247] Newer modalities of drug-delivery devices and combinations of such medications need to be evaluated, and as suggested by the authors of the review, stratification of infants who respond to such medications could help identify specific infant subgroups that could benefit from such therapy.

DIURETICS

Neonates have increased alveolar and interstitial fluid in the lungs. "Classic" BPD has also been associated with the exudative–inflammatory process in its earliest stages. Such excessive pulmonary interstitial fluid reduces lung compliance, increases airway resistance, and is followed by subacute and chronic fibroproliferative changes that further exacerbate its pathogenesis.[185] Factors responsible for this excessive pulmonary fluid accumulation include increased pulmonary epithelial, capillary permeability, and overcirculation secondary to a persistent PDA.[186,187] Diuretics decrease work of breathing and aid mechanical ventilation by decreasing pulmonary interstitial fluid and improving lung compliance.[188,189] In a 2013 survey, wide between-hospital variations for overall diuretic usage as well as specific agents used for infants under 29 weeks' GA were reported.[190] Although several classes of diuretics exist, the most commonly used agents in premature infants include the loop diuretic furosemide and the thiazides.

Furosemide

Furosemide is a sulfonamide derivative and is the most commonly used diuretic in the neonate. By blocking the NaCl reabsorption by the Na/K/2Cl symporter in the thick ascending loop of Henle (TAL), furosemide and other similar "loop" diuretics can produce highly efficacious diuresis. In addition, furosemide induces increased prostaglandin E2 (PGE2) synthesis by renal cyclo-oxygenase 2.[191] PGE2 is also a direct inhibitor of salt transport across the TAL and also acts as a vasodilator to increase renal blood flow and glomerular filtration, thereby enhancing

the diuretic actions of furosemide.[192] Through such diuresis, furosemide decreases intravascular volume, increases systemic venous capacitance, and decreases lung lymph flow to decrease pulmonary interstitial fluid accumulation.[193] In addition to its diuretic effect furosemide-induced PGE2 synthesis also causes pulmonary vasodilation and decreases pulmonary interstitial fluid accumulation.[194] Additionally, furosemide decreases inflammatory mediators such as leukotrienes and histamine in lung tissue.[195] Furosemide can be administered through enteral, intravenous, or intramuscular routes; oral bioavailability has been reported to be about 84% in term newborn infants.[196] The usual dosage is 1 to 2 mg/kg intravenously, but it may also be given intramuscularly or orally. A study of 10 preterm infants whose mean GA at birth was 27 weeks showed that plasma $T_{1/2}$ was greater than 24 hours in infants under 32 weeks and declined to approximately 4 hours by term corrected age, implying that furosemide clearance increases with maturity.[197]

Major adverse effects include hypokalemia, hypocalcemia, hypercalciuria, nephrocalcinosis (risk is especially higher with exposure to more than 10 mg/kg cumulative dose of furosemide in preterm infants), hypomagnesemia, hypochloremic alkalosis, and hyponatremia.[198] Coadministration of a thiazide diuretic along with furosemide can decrease the incidence of nephrocalcinosis.[199] Ototoxicity has been reported with furosemide exposure especially in preterm infants for whom a 12-hour interval dosing of furosemide often produced furosemide accumulation to potentially ototoxic levels (greater than 25 mcg/mL).[196] Though such hearing loss is often transient and reversible, additive damage secondary to concomitant use of other ototoxic agents such as gentamicin should be taken into consideration during furosemide pharmacotherapy.[200] In addition, infants with BPD are often fluid restricted in an attempt to reduce pulmonary edema, and brisk diuresis with furosemide administration has the potential to cause hypotension in these infants. Elevated PGE2 levels secondary to furosemide use can also decrease closure of the ductus arteriosus and increase risk for hemodynamically significant PDA.[201,202] In addition, chronic use of loop diuretics may have the paradoxic effect of raising P_{CO_2} because they work by retaining bicarbonate at the expense of the excretion of chloride.

Furosemide-induced diuresis for preterm infants with RDS who required mechanical ventilation has been shown to improve lung compliance, improve functional residual capacity, and reduce peak inspiratory pressure required for ventilation.[203] Daily furosemide use for 3 days at 1 mg/kg/day improved diuresis and facilitated quicker extubation in a trial of 57 low birth-weight infants who required mechanical ventilation for RDS.[204] In another randomized trial of 99 infants of less than 30 weeks, furosemide use led to decreased duration of mechanical ventilation and increased survival compared to thiazide-use or no-diuretic-use groups.[205] However, these investigators found in a subsequent study that routine use of prophylactic furosemide for infants with RDS did not improve pulmonary outcomes and, furthermore, led to volume depletion and increased requirement for vasopressors.[206] The most recent Cochrane review of diuretic use for preterm infants with RDS concluded that the risk of clinically significant hypotension and PDA associated with furosemide use outweighed the benefits of improved short-term pulmonary outcomes and recommends against the routine use of furosemide for infants with RDS.[207]

Similar to its effects on pulmonary function in younger infants with RDS, furosemide may also improve pulmonary compliance, airway conductance, and resistance in older infants with established BPD. A small randomized study in which pulmonary function of 17 infants with BPD was measured before and after administration of daily doses of 1 mg/kg of furosemide or placebo for 7 days found decreased ventilator requirements, increased pulmonary compliance, and improved alveolar ventilation for infants in the furosemide group but not for those in the placebo group.[208] However, a Cochrane review of loop diuretic use for infants with BPD concluded that all six studies eligible to be included in the review focused only on pathophysiologic parameters and not long-term clinical outcomes. Despite finding that long-term administration of furosemide did improve oxygenation and lung compliance, the authors do not recommend routine use of long-term furosemide to prevent or treat BPD.[209]

Furosemide has also been administered as an aerosol to preterm infants with BPD. When administered directly to the lung as an aerosol furosemide has been shown to decrease bronchospasm by decreasing smooth muscle contractility through several possible mechanisms that include modification of mast cell and sensory epithelial activation in the airways, decreased release of inflammatory mediators such as leukotrienes and histamine, increased vascular endothelial release of prostaglandins, and inhibition of cholinergic bronchoconstriction.[195,210-212] This mode of delivery offers the advantage of possibly decreasing systemic side effects while maintaining desired pulmonary effects. However, in view of the lack of data from randomized trials on the effects of aerosolized loop diuretics on important clinical outcomes, routine or sustained use of this mode of delivery cannot be justified based on the current evidence.[213]

Bumetanide

Bumetanide is also a loop diuretic, about 40 times more potent than furosemide. Owing to its high lipid solubility, bumetanide is able to diffuse passively to its site of action, unlike furosemide, which requires active tubular secretion. Bumetanide is highly effective in producing rapid diuresis and relieving pulmonary edema. Bumetanide also causes less renal potassium loss and is less ototoxic compared to furosemide. In a study of bumetanide metabolism in 14 neonates between 26 and 40 weeks' GA, its half-life was noted to be about 1.74 to 7 hours and the volume of distribution was 0.22 L/kg (range 0.11 to 0.32 L/kg).[214] The authors suggest that bumetanide dosing may need to be higher and the dosing interval prolonged for neonates compared to adults. At plasma concentrations above those achieved during routine therapeutic use, the binding of bumetanide to neonatal plasma proteins is approximately 97%. Hence, saturation of albumin-binding sites is unlikely at therapeutic doses.[215] Nonrenal clearance is responsible for 58% to 97% of bumetanide metabolism. In a random crossover trial of 17 premature infants, bumetanide was found to produce lower sodium loss per urine volume, but higher urinary calcium loss, compared to furosemide.[216] There are currently no randomized trials that have compared bumetanide to furosemide use with respect to their safety profiles or their efficacy in preventing or reducing the severity of BPD in ventilated preterm neonates.

Thiazides and Potassium-Sparing Diuretics

Derived from sulfonamides, the thiazides are less potent diuretics compared to furosemide. They act at the distal tubule to inhibit reabsorption of NaCl through the apical luminal transporter. Because 90% of sodium reabsorption occurs proximal to their site of action in the distal nephron, thiazides are only

moderately effective diuretics compared to the more potent loop diuretics. Spironolactone, a potassium-sparing diuretic, competes with aldosterone in the distal convoluted tubule. Because of the nature of aldosterone's mode of action, which is dependent on protein synthesis, the onset of action of spironolactone is delayed. In addition to increasing renal sodium excretion, thiazides can also cause hypokalemia, hypomagnesemia, and hypophosphatemia by increasing urinary loss of these electrolytes. However, in contrast to the loop diuretics, thiazides and spironolactone do not cause increased urinary calcium loss. Serum electrolyte monitoring should be considered when long-term use of thiazide diuretics is required. The usual dosages of chlorothiazide and spironolactone are 10 to 20 and 1 to 2 mg/kg, respectively.

Thiazide diuretic use for infants with BPD has become widespread. In one survey of diuretic use in children's hospitals in the United States, chlorothiazide was found to be the diuretic with the longest median duration of use, approximately 21 days.[190] A study that assessed the effect of combined chlorothiazide and spironolactone in 10 nonventilated infants with BPD found that the use of these diuretics was associated with decreased airway resistance and improved lung compliance compared to placebo.[217] Several other small studies have also concluded that thiazide diuretics improve lung function. A Cochrane collaboration systematic review included six such studies to assess the impact of distal renal tubular diuretic use in improving outcomes for infants with BPD. As most of these studies focused on pathophysiologic parameters and did not sufficiently assess clinical outcomes or potential complications related to diuretic therapy, the reviewers concluded that there is no strong evidence for benefit from the routine use of thiazide diuretic therapy in preterm infants with BPD.[218]

RESPIRATORY STIMULANTS

Whereas apnea of prematurity continues to remain the primary indication for the use of respiratory stimulants such as caffeine in the NICU, these agents have shown benefits for other outcomes such as duration of mechanical ventilation, need for PDA ligation, and incidence of BPD at 36 weeks.[219] This has expanded their indications for use to include assistance with weaning mechanical ventilation and facilitating earlier extubation in neonatal units around the United States.[220] Methylxanthines, including caffeine and theophylline, are the most commonly used respiratory stimulants for treatment of apnea. By inhibiting phosphodiesterase (PDE) enzyme isoforms (especially PDE4) and through cell surface adenosine receptor antagonism, methylxanthines stimulate the medullary respiratory center and therefore increase minute ventilation. They also cause bronchodilation and enhanced diaphragmatic contractility. Research also suggests that methylxanthines enhance histone deacetylation, an epigenetic process that decreases genetic transcription.[161] Because some of the anti-inflammatory effects of corticosteroids are mediated by histone deacetylation of several inflammatory genes, methylxanthines could enhance the effects of corticosteroids when these two therapies are used together, as is often the case in premature infants with BPD.[221,222] The pharmacology of theophylline and caffeine, the major methylxanthines in therapeutic use, and doxapram, which is a nonmethylxanthine respiratory stimulant, are discussed in detail below, and the usual dosages for methylxanthines are listed in Table 34-5.

		TABLE 34-5 Methylxanthines for Neonatal Apnea		
Drug	Loading Dose (IV, mg/kg)	Maintenance Dosage (IV)*	Plasma Concentration (mg/L)	Toxicity
Theophylline	5.5-6.0	1 mg/kg every 8 hr or 2 mg/kg every 12 hr	7-20[†] (~10 ideal)	Cardiovascular: tachycardia CNS stimulation: seizures, jitteriness Gastrointestinal: vomiting, distention
Caffeine	10	2.5-5 mg/kg every 24 hr	7-20[†]	Unlikely with plasma levels <50 mg/L
Caffeine citrate	20	5-10 mg/kg every 24 hr		As for caffeine

*Oral dosage = intravenous (IV) dosage × 1.25.
[†]Monitor levels and screen for signs of toxicity.

Theophylline

Theophylline is a methylated xanthine alkaloid (1,3-dimethyl-xanthine) that is found naturally in tea. Its half-life is approximately 30 hours in the neonate, compared to 7 hours in adults.[223] Theophylline has more potent inotropic, vasodilator, bronchodilator, and diuretic actions compared to caffeine because of its more efficacious PDE inhibition and adenosine antagonism. Theophylline may cause less respiratory center stimulation than caffeine but enhances diaphragmatic contractility to a greater extent by facilitating increased neuromuscular transmission with increased tidal volumes.[158] It is also an inhibitor of lymphocyte function as well as mast cell histamine release; by these mechanisms it can reduce airway inflammation.[224] In the adult, theophylline is eliminated by hepatic biotransformation and urinary excretion. In the newborn, however, the hepatic biotransformation with *N*-demethylation is absent; instead, the occurrence of *N*-7-methylation produces caffeine.[225] The therapeutic plasma concentration is about 7 to 20 mg/L. In one study, levels greater than 6.6 mg/L controlled apneic spells, whereas cardiovascular toxicity with tachycardia was noted only at levels greater than 13.0 mg/L.[226] Some newborns manifested toxicity at levels of 9.0 mg/L of transplacentally acquired theophylline. Because of the problems at these lower levels and because of the potential additive effects of the caffeine produced from theophylline, 10 mg/L may be a desirable level. Signs of toxicity may include irritability, diaphoresis, diarrhea, seizures, gastroesophageal reflux, and tachycardia.[227] The usual intravenous loading dose of theophylline is 4.0 to 6.0 mg/kg, with a maintenance dose of 1 mg/kg every 8 hours or 2 mg/kg every 12 hours. Its low cost makes its use especially advantageous in low-resource settings.

Caffeine

The addition of another methyl group to theophylline produces caffeine (1,3,7-trimethylxanthine), an agent with a plasma half-life of approximately 100 hours, because of which it can be administered once daily compared to theophylline, which needs to be administered two or three times daily.[224] Preterm infants have limited capacity to metabolize caffeine through the hepatic cytochrome P450 pathway; therefore most of the drug is excreted unchanged in the urine. Caffeine has similar efficacy compared to theophylline for most therapeutic effects, but may have less propensity for adverse effects such as tachycardia. Plasma levels of 5 to 20 mg/L are considered therapeutic, and studies suggest that higher levels (up to 50 mg/L) may not be associated with adverse effects.[225] Toxic manifestations of caffeine include excessive jitteriness and rarely seizures. The usual loading dose of caffeine is 10 mg/kg, with a daily maintenance dose of 2.5 to 5 mg/kg. The usual form of caffeine, the citrate in a 20-mg/mL solution, is equivalent to a 10-mg/mL solution of the base and may be administered intravenously or orally.[225]

A 2010 meta-analysis that reviewed five trials comparing theophylline and caffeine for apnea of prematurity found reduced risk of tachycardia and feeding intolerance for caffeine (relative risk 0.17 (CI: 0.04 to 0.72)).[228] Because of these advantages, caffeine has become the most commonly used methylxanthine in the NICU.[152] In a study of 234 infants randomized to receive low-dose (2.5 mg/kg/day) versus high-dose (10 mg/kg/day) caffeine, significantly lower risk for extubation failure and disability at 12 months as well as documented apneic events was noted for infants who received the higher dose. However, risk for BPD remained similar between the two groups.[229] The largest study of the effects of caffeine use in preterm neonates was the Caffeine for Apnea of Prematurity (CAP) trial, which enrolled 2006 infants to receive either caffeine or placebo when caffeine was indicated.[230] This study found that caffeine use led to reduced requirements for various forms of respiratory support, including intubation, positive-pressure support, and need for supplemental oxygen. Decreased duration of mechanical ventilation was another significant advantage noted with early initiation of caffeine therapy (up to 3 days of life), a benefit that was lost when caffeine was started beyond this age. In addition, caffeine use also reduced the incidence of BPD as well as the need for surgical ligation of PDA compared to placebo in infants with indications to give caffeine. One of the initial follow-up studies of the CAP trial showed that caffeine offered a significant benefit in reducing risk for death or disability at 18 months' corrected GA as well as reducing the risk for cerebral palsy compared to placebo.[231] Infants receiving respiratory support appeared to derive more neurodevelopmental benefits from caffeine than infants not receiving support.[232] However, a follow-up study of these infants at 5 years of age somewhat dampened the initial enthusiasm by showing no significant differences in neurodevelopmental indices between the two groups of infants at this age.[233]

Doxapram

Doxapram is a pyrrolidinone derivative with CNS-stimulant (analeptic) effects. Its mechanism of action, though still unclear, is believed to involve stimulation of both central and peripheral chemoreceptors, which then leads to stimulation of ventral brainstem nuclei and subsequent increased depth and rate of respiration.[234] In a study of 83 full-term infants, doxapram given at doses of 2 to 3 mg/kg immediately after birth hastened the recovery from respiratory depression secondary to maternal narcotic or anesthetic exposure.[235] Another study of 31 infants with apnea of prematurity with a mean GA of 30 weeks that randomized them to receive placebo, theophylline, or doxapram showed fewer treatment failures with theophylline or doxapram compared to placebo.[236] A smaller study of 15 infants showed that although both doxapram and aminophylline were equally efficacious for treatment of apnea of prematurity, of 10 infants who failed treatment with aminophylline, eight responded to the addition of doxapram with complete cessation of apnea.[237] There are, however, no large trials of doxapram vs aminophylline or caffeine use for premature infants with apnea. A Cochrane Collaboration systematic review concluded that there are insufficient data to recommend doxapram for use as treatment to reduce apneic episodes in premature infants.[238]

Doxapram has been used primarily as a second-line agent in addition to methylxanthines for refractory apnea of prematurity. It is most often administered as a continuous intravenous infusion, though an intermittent intravenous bolus regimen has been proposed. Loading doses of 2.5 to 3 mg/kg are used, followed by maintenance infusion of 0.5 to 2.5 mg/kg/hr. Because many doxapram preparations contain benzyl alcohol or butorphanol, the use of doxapram should be exercised with caution. Ideal plasma therapeutic levels have been suggested to be between 2 and 5 mg/L with adverse effects seen beyond this level. Potential side effects include hypertension, gastrointestinal disturbances that can lead to emesis and feeding intolerance, hypokalemia, jitteriness, hyperglycemia, and glycosuria.[239,240]

SUMMARY

The goal of mechanical ventilation for neonates, especially ELBW infants, should be to provide the least support required for adequate support of their cardiorespiratory status. Such a strategy will reduce the lung injury that accrues from volutrauma and barotrauma associated with mechanical ventilation. Pharmacologic adjuncts that are used to support mechanical ventilation such as sedative and analgesic agents should be used sparingly and with judiciousness to prevent prolonged mechanical ventilation. With the exception of caffeine and, to a limited extent, late administration of corticosteroids and thiazide diuretics, none of the other drug classes has proven effective in reducing ventilator-associated lung injury or BPD to date. More important, several of these agents have not yet been adequately evaluated for their efficacy as aids to mechanical ventilation and in reducing the severity or incidence of BPD in large randomized trials. Well-designed trials for these drugs that are adequately powered to test for differences in long-term outcomes such as BPD or neurodevelopmental impairment are required to make further recommendations regarding these medications. Until then all of the drugs discussed should be dispensed by personnel who are competent in their administration, know their effects, and are aware of the attention required for patient monitoring. Techniques for the monitoring of many serum drug levels now are available in many centers. The information that such monitoring provides may allow the clinician to use these agents with greater accuracy and safety.

REFERENCES

A complete reference list is available at https://expertconsult.inkling.com.

35

Management of the Infant with Bronchopulmonary Dysplasia

Huayan Zhang, MD, and William W. Fox, MD

INTRODUCTION

Infant chronic lung disease, or bronchopulmonary dysplasia (BPD), is a debilitating lung disease that occurs in premature infants. Since the nineteen seventies, advances in neonatal intensive care have led to the survival of smaller and extremely immature infants at a critical stage of lung development. As the survival of very preterm infants improved, the rate of BPD has increased. Survivors with BPD have serious consequences ranging from chronic cardiopulmonary impairment to growth failure, developmental delay, and impaired social functioning of the patient and family. Lengthy hospitalizations, persistent respiratory illness, pulmonary hypertension, delayed growth and development, and poor long-term neurodevelopmental outcomes are common in this population.[1-3] Currently there is no definitive treatment or prevention for BPD. Many clinical practices currently used in the care of these infants are inadequately studied to ensure safety or efficacy, with potentially serious consequences. The lack of an evidence base has led to large practice variations between neonatal intensive care units and within individual centers. Therefore management of infants with BPD, especially the ones with severe disease, can be extremely challenging to clinicians. This chapter will focus on the respiratory management of patients with established BPD.

EPIDEMIOLOGY, PATHOPHYSIOLOGY AND DIAGNOSIS OF BRONCHOPULMONARY DYSPLASIA

Despite the efforts to reduce premature birth, there are still over 75,000 infants born at less than 32 weeks' postmenstrual age (PMA) each year in the United States. Over 50,000 are very low birth-weight (VLBW) infants, born with birth weight <1500 g.[4] BPD is the most prevalent sequela of preterm birth, affecting 10,000-15,000 infants annually in the United States.[5] The Israeli, Canadian, and Japanese Neonatal Networks reported rates of BPD in VLBW infants of 13.7%, 12.3%, and 14.6%, respectively.[6,7]

Traditionally, the diagnosis of BPD has been based on the presence of chronic respiratory insufficiency with persistent oxygen requirement and abnormal chest radiograph at 1 month of age or at 36 weeks' PMA. Over the years, many diagnostic criteria for BPD have been developed. Currently the most widely adopted criterion is the severity-based National Institutes of Health (NIH) consensus definition.[8] In this definition, the diagnosis of BPD is first based on treatment with >21% oxygen for at least 28 accumulative days after birth, and then the severity of BPD is based on oxygen level and respiratory support level at 36 weeks' PMA. However, there is significant center-to-center variability in oxygen use due to the ongoing controversy of appropriate oxygen saturation limits for preterm infants. To decrease this variability, Walsh et al. have proposed a "physiologic" definition of BPD that utilizes an oxygen reduction test to determine oxygen dependency at 36 weeks' PMA in infants receiving ≤30% supplemental oxygen.[9] Depending on the diagnostic criteria used, the rate of BPD in extremely preterm infants of 22 to 28 weeks' gestation in the National Institute of Child Health and Human Development (NICHD) Neonatal Research Network centers varies from 68% by NIH consensus definition, to 42% defined as supplemental oxygen use at 36 weeks' PMA, to 40% by the physiologic definition.[5]

The etiology of BPD is multifactorial, and many potential risk factors for BPD have been identified. Some commonly discussed risk factors for BPD are listed in Table 35-1.[10,11] The most important risk factor for developing BPD is extreme prematurity. The incidence of BPD in VLBW infants ranges between 15% and 65%, and this incidence increases as the gestational age (GA) decreases.[5,12] In a large cohort study of over 15,000 infants born between 22 and 29 weeks' GA with birth weight of 401 to 1500 g, Lapcharoensap et al.[11] reported an overall rate of BPD among survivors to 36 weeks' PMA of 33.1%. However, rates of BPD were as high as 80.7% for infants born at <750 g and 93.8% for those with GA of <24 weeks.

Northway et al. first described BPD in a group of preterm infants who died after receiving mechanical ventilation and oxygen therapy for respiratory distress syndrome (RDS) in 1967. This was later named as the "classic" or the "old BPD," as it occurred mainly in relatively large premature newborns (born at 30-34 weeks' GA) and with pathological features characterized by extensive heterogeneous lung injury with alternating areas of atelectasis, cystic changes and fibrosis, pulmonary artery muscularization, and severe large airway injury.[13] Over the past 40 years, there have been significant advancements in the care of premature infants, including the routine use of surfactant replacement and antenatal steroids as well as the introduction of gentler ventilation modalities. As a result, smaller and more immature infants born at late canalicular or early saccular stages of lung development are surviving. These infants are born several weeks before alveolarization begins, and their lungs are therefore extremely prone to injury. However, with the advances in clinical care, many of these premature infants have a much milder clinical course, and the concept of "new BPD" was proposed in the 1990s.[14,15] The effects of various injuries on the developing lung give rise to a pathologic picture characterized by impaired alveolar and pulmonary vascular development but less heterogeneous lung injury. These

injurious stimuli include inflammation, oxidative stress, ventilator-induced lung injury, infection, drugs, and other factors such as maternal smoking.[16] In recent years, BPD has become a much less common event in infants born at over 30 weeks' GA and much of the discussion has focused on the new BPD. However, with the prolonged survival of the smallest and sickest premature infants, we have seen a slow increase in the number of infants with extremely severe BPD. At autopsy, the lung histology of those infants who die with the extremely severe lung disease displays a mixed feature of severely delayed lung development and significant lung injury, features seen in both the old and the new BPD (Fig. 35-1).

CLINICAL PRESENTATION OF ESTABLISHED BRONCHOPULMONARY DYSPLASIA

With the widespread use of antenatal steroids and postnatal surfactant, many small premature infants exhibit a milder course of BPD. These infants often start out with only minimal or mild RDS requiring a low level of respiratory support and then display deterioration in lung function with increased respiratory support and/or oxygen requirements within a few days or weeks after birth. The typical radiographic changes in these patients are usually mild diffuse haziness that persists over time and the pathologic findings are those of typical "new" BPD. With proper nutritional and respiratory support, prevention and control of infection, and other management, such as control of pulmonary overflow through persistent patent ductus arteriosus (PDA), most of these infants will demonstrate slow but steady improvement in their lung function and radiographic changes. After a variable period of time, they can be weaned off respiratory and oxygen support.

Despite the therapeutic improvements, however, we still see infants with severe BPD (sBPD). Using data from the NICHD Neonatal Research Network Generic Database, Natarajan et al. found that 537 of 1159, or 46.3%, infants with birth weights of 401 to 1000 g (born between January 1, 2006, and June 30,

TABLE 35-1	**Risk Factors for Bronchopulmonary Dysplasia**
Prenatal risk factors	Intrauterine growth restriction
	Lack of antenatal corticosteroids
	Maternal chorioamnionitis, smoking, or preeclampsia
	Genetic predisposition
Risk factors at birth	Low gestational age
	Low birth weight
	Male gender
	Lower level of neonatal intensive care at birth hospital
	Lower Apgar scores
	Perinatal asphyxia
Postnatal risk factors	Mechanical ventilation
	Supplemental oxygen
	Patent ductus arteriosus
	Sepsis and systemic inflammatory response
	Gastroesophageal reflux

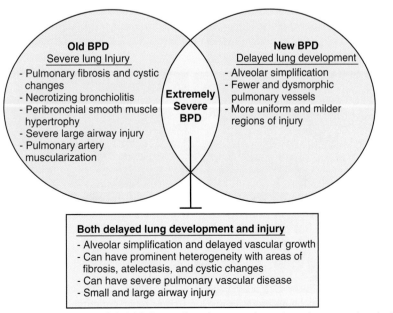

FIG 35-1 Pathologic features of "old," "new," and severe bronchopulmonary dysplasia (BPD). Severe BPD demonstrates mixed pathologic features from both "old" and "new" BPD, with arrest in lung development as well as significant lung injury.

2007) still required mechanical ventilation or continuous positive airway pressure (CPAP) or supplemental oxygen with an effective FiO_2 >30% at 36 weeks' PMA.[17] Many of these infants require high levels of respiratory support and high concentrations of inspired oxygen from the first week of life. Their initial postnatal courses are frequently complicated by severe RDS, pneumothorax, pulmonary interstitial emphysema, and pulmonary hemorrhage. Some infants may have a milder initial course but have significant deterioration after infections or due to pulmonary edema secondary to PDA. As described earlier in this chapter, the pathologic feature of their lung disease is a combination of delayed lung development and severe injury.

Since the establishment of the Newborn and Infant Chronic Lung Disease Program at the Children's Hospital of Philadelphia in September 2010, we have treated over 200 premature infants with sBPD. The majority of these patients are older former premature infants with extremely severe lung disease that results in high rates of mortality and long-term ventilation needs. However, although all patients have the same diagnosis

of sBPD, they can have very different clinical presentations. This is probably due to different lung developmental stages at which the injuries occurred and the interaction between injuries and host response. We have observed three major phenotypical variants—namely, (1) severe lung parenchyma disease, (2) pulmonary vascular disease, mainly manifests as pulmonary hypertension (PH), and (3) severe airway disease, as the leading features of sBPD (Fig. 35-2). In addition, each of these phenotypes has various subtypes, and an individual patient may have overlapping clinical features from different phenotypes.

Severe Lung Parenchyma Disease as the Leading Feature of Severe Bronchopulmonary Dysplasia

The underlying pathologic changes in these patients may range from homogeneous alveolar simplification (Fig. 35-3, *A*) to heterogeneous micro-/macrocystic changes with areas of fibrosis and/or atelectasis. The radiographic appearance therefore varies from generalized parenchymal opacification to a bubble-like pattern to mixed areas of hyperinflation, cystic changes, and opacifications (Fig. 35-3, *B*).

Pulmonary Hypertension as the Leading Feature of Severe Bronchopulmonary Dysplasia

PH often complicates the course of BPD and contributes to late morbidity and mortality during infancy.[18] Some patients with relatively mild lung disease develop PH, and other infants with severe lung disease may or may not have PH. Nonetheless, this group of patients presents with significant or worsening PH as their key clinical feature in addition to various degrees of lung parenchyma disease. The pulmonary vasculature of these patients is not only underdeveloped and hyperactive but is also undergoing remodeling. Clinically, these infants often present with chronic respiratory insufficiency with oxygen dependency, intermittent cyanotic or life-threatening episodes ("BPD spells") when agitated, and poor growth. These symptoms are typically not seen until 3 to 4 months after birth, when the patient starts to "outgrow" his or her own pulmonary vascular supply. At this time, significant pulmonary vascular "pruning" can be seen in these patients. As the long-term morbidity and mortality of patients with PH are extremely high, it is very important to identify these infants early so that we can deliver

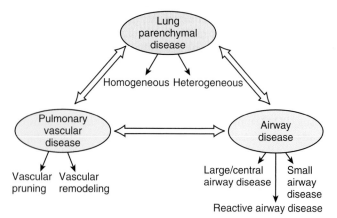

FIG 35-2 Three main phenotypical presentations as the leading clinical feature of severe bronchopulmonary dysplasia. (1) Severe lung parenchymal disease, (2) pulmonary vascular disease, (3) airway disease. Each phenotype has various subtypes, and an individual patient may have overlapping clinical features from different phenotypes.

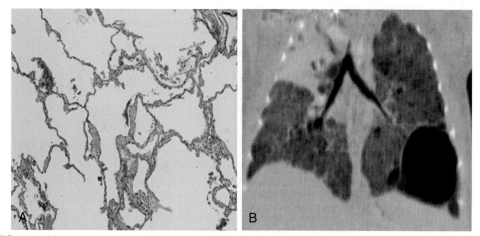

FIG 35-3 Homogeneous or heterogeneous lung disease in patients with severe lung parenchymal disease. **A,** Lung biopsy sample demonstrating homogeneous alveoli simplification at 50 weeks' PMA. **B,** Chest computed tomography scan of an infant with heterogeneous lung disease demonstrating areas of opacification and cystic changes.

adequate respiratory and other support and provide appropriate follow-up for this population.

Airway Disease as the Leading Feature of Severe Bronchopulmonary Dysplasia

These patients have striking airway abnormalities in addition to varying degrees of lung disease. The central and upper airways abnormalities—for example, glottic/subglottic stenosis and tracheal stenosis—are well-known complications from tracheal intubation and prolonged mechanical ventilation. However, the importance of tracheobronchomalacia and acquired tracheomegaly is less recognized. BPD spells in many patients are caused by airway collapse instead of PH crisis, and therefore the treatment strategy is vastly different from that for someone with PH. Patients with BPD often have asthma-like symptoms, many due to increased small airway reactivity. However, chronic wheezing in some of these patients may be associated with airway obstruction due to malacia and therefore may be unresponsive to bronchodilator therapy.

PHYSIOLOGIC BASIS FOR RESPIRTORY SUPPORT IN INFANTS WITH ESTABLISHED BRONCHOPULMONARY DYSPLASIA

Ventilatory Control in Infants with Bronchopulmonary Dysplasia

Carotid body function plays an important role in the normal ventilatory response to hypoxia or hyperoxia. The perinatal environment has been shown to affect the development of normal carotid body morphometry and function. Supplemental oxygen at birth profoundly blunts future carotid body development. In rodent BPD models, perinatal hyperoxia causes impaired oxygen sensitivity, carotid body hypoplasia, and decreased total afferent neuron number.[19] Infants with BPD have been shown to have decreased response to both hypoxia-induced increase in ventilation[20] and hyperoxia ventilation depression compared to premature infants who did not need mechanical ventilation or supplemental oxygen.[21] In infants with BPD, ventilation control dysfunction, in combination with decreased efficiency in gas exchange, muscle immaturity, and increased work of breathing, may contribute to both difficulties with oral feeding[22] and disordered breathing during sleep, with more central and obstructive apneas[23] in these infants. Because these infants have been exposed to prolonged hypercarbia, the control of P_{CO_2} is reset, and they can appear comfortable at higher than normal P_{CO_2} levels.

Pulmonary Mechanics in Infants with Bronchopulmonary Dysplasia

Many methods have been used to evaluate pulmonary mechanics in infants with established BPD. For example, resistance and compliance can be measured using an esophageal pressure catheter or the single-breath occlusion method, plethysmography or nitrogen washout and gas dilution methods can be used to measure functional residual capacity (FRC), and the rapid thoracic compression method has been used in the measurement of forced flows. Each of these methods has its own advantages and limitations,[24] and accurate measurements in the unstable infants can be difficult to achieve. In general, infants with established BPD have been found to have decreased compliance, increased resistance with decreased conductance, reduced FRC, and reduced forced flows. These abnormalities may improve over time in the first 3 years of life, but many persist until adolescence and even young adulthood.[14,25,26] Many modern ventilators have resistance, compliance, and pressure–volume (P-V) loops displayed. Although the resistance and compliance values may not be absolute, they can be used to trend the patient. Monitoring the changes in resistance and compliance while adjusting ventilator settings at the bedside can be a valuable tool.

In many patients with severe BPD, there are heterogeneous cystic changes with areas of atelectasis in the lung. Ventilation in these patients is not uniform throughout the lung fields, and the time constant is different in different parts of the lung. The respiratory system mechanics in these patients are therefore better explained by a two-compartment (fast and slow) model, rather than a linear one-compartment model.[27] With similar compliance, the slow compartment has a much higher resistance and therefore results in significantly longer time constants compared to the fast compartment. The utility of the two-compartment model in severe BPD has been explained in detail by Castile and Nelin.[28] In addition, current data suggest that infants with established BPD mainly have obstructive rather than restrictive disease and small airways are the primary contributor to the obstruction.[29] Follow-up studies have demonstrated that this obstructive airway disease with air trapping persists over time despite continued increase in the total lung capacity over the first 2 years of life.[30] These changes in lung mechanics need to be taken into consideration when deciding the best respiratory support strategies in the patients with severe BPD.

RESPIRATORY MANAGEMENT IN INFANTS WITH ESTABLISHED BRONCHOPULMONARY DYSPLASIA

Over the years, multiple strategies have been tried to prevent BPD with variable success. The major changes in the respiratory support strategies include an attempt to redefine the goals for "adequate gas exchange," allowing for permissive hypercarbia[31,32] and permissive hypoxemia,[33] and the widespread use of noninvasive ventilation.[34,35] These strategies are aimed at minimizing exposure to mechanical ventilation whenever possible. However, in the population with established sBPD, the focus of respiratory support is no longer on the prevention of BPD, as in the newly born premature infants, but rather on how to provide adequate support and minimize V/Q mismatch to promote lung growth while preventing further lung injury.

Noninvasive ventilation

In recent years, noninvasive respiratory support modalities, including nasal intermittent positive-pressure ventilation (NIPPV), nasal CPAP (NCPAP), or high-flow nasal cannula (HFNC), have been used as first-line respiratory therapies in premature infants after birth and following mechanical ventilation. Current pooled data from multiple randomized trials have shown a significant benefit for the combined outcome of death and BPD at 36 weeks' corrected gestation in premature infants treated with NCPAP, with a number needed to treat of 25.[36] Other studies have demonstrated that noninvasive support modalities such as NIPPV or HFNC may have similar effects compared to NCPAP.[37,38] With these data, there was widespread use of noninvasive respiratory strategies as a way to avoid or limit duration of intubated respiratory support, and this has also been quickly extended beyond the immediate neonatal period.

Despite a lack of convincing data demonstrating the efficacy of noninvasive respiratory support modalities in infants with established BPD, many neonatologists will extubate or be reluctant to reintubate infants with chronic respiratory insufficiency and keep them on high levels of noninvasive support. In infants with typical "new" BPD who have mild respiratory insufficiency, noninvasive support may be able to adequately support these infants, and over time they can gradually wean off support. Unfortunately, in infants with sBPD, prolonged periods of undersupport may bring severe consequences, including poor growth (both somatic and alveolar/pulmonary vascular growth) and persistent V/Q mismatch contributing to lung injury and the development of PH. Figure 35-4 shows the computed tomography (CT) scan of a 6-month infant born at 26 weeks' GA. She received about 6 weeks of mechanical ventilation followed by 4 months of noninvasive support. Despite chronic respiratory failure with Pco_2 in the 80- to 100-mm Hg range, she was maintained on noninvasive support with chronic diuretics and systemic steroids. Physicians were reluctant to change her from 7-L/min HFNC to intubated mechanical ventilation when she was unable to maintain oxygen saturation above 70%, with Pco_2 over 110 mm Hg, persistent tachycardia over 200, evidence of PH, and severe growth failure at 52 weeks' PMA. Many neonatologists think that weaning the patient to lower respiratory support modalities—namely, CPAP or HFNC—is being successful. However, this may not be true in this group of patients. Although this may be an extremely severe case, it reflects the current trend of relying on noninvasive support and a fear of intubation and mechanical ventilation. Indeed, we have been seeing more patients with sBPD transferred to our center on very high levels of noninvasive support, such as NCPAP >10 cm H_2O or HFNC >5 L/min or high settings of NIPPV. In a retrospective cohort study of infants who were referred to our center with severe BPD between 2010 and 2013,[39] we found 45% (32 of 71 patients) were on noninvasive respiratory support when they were transferred to our center at 40 to 45 weeks' PMA. In these patients, 28% either died (9%) or required tracheostomy placement for long-term respiratory support (19%). Fifty-three percent of patients discharged without tracheostomy were discharged on supplemental oxygen. These data highlight the fact that prolonged noninvasive support may not necessarily translate into better pulmonary outcome in infants with severe BPD.

The mechanism of action for noninvasive support may be related to its ability to provide continuous positive pressure and to flush the dead space of the nasopharyngeal cavity, hence improving alveolar ventilation. The goal of noninvasive support in infants with established BPD needs to be providing adequate support to minimize V/Q mismatch and promote growth rather than the sole purpose of avoiding intubation. Therefore some authors have advocated using more objective tools such as esophageal and gastric pressure monitoring to help titrate CPAP pressure.[40] Although there is no consensus on the best methods of titrating the noninvasive support levels, the cardiorespiratory status, overall health, and tolerance to activities, as well as growth, need to be closely monitored and taken into consideration during the duration of noninvasive support. In patients who are not adequately supported by noninvasive support methods, mechanical ventilation (MV), via either endotracheal tube or tracheostomy, needs to be considered.

Mechanical Ventilation

Despite the advancements in respiratory care, a subset of infants with sBPD continues to require prolonged MV. Severe ventilator-dependent BPD is uncommon in most delivery centers but is not rare in many major referral centers. The BPD Collaborative Group reported data from eight U.S. academic centers and showed that 28% of infants with sBPD were on invasive MV at a mean PMA of 47 weeks (range 36 to 86 weeks).[41] Currently there is a dearth of evidence from clinical trials to guide the optimal ventilator management in patients with established BPD. Similar to noninvasive support, the goal of MV should be improving V/Q matching and promoting optimal growth. MV strategies therefore need to be selected based on the lung physiology and pathologic changes of each patient. Identifying phenotypical presentation of sBPD and determining the underlying lung pathology may therefore be the first important step in determining the appropriate management strategy in each patient.

Conventional Mechanical Ventilation

Intermittent mandatory ventilation with time-cycled, pressure-limited ventilation has been the main mode of conventional MV for many years. Advances in ventilation techniques in recent years include volume-targeted ventilation, patient-triggered ventilation including synchronized intermittent mandatory ventilation (SIMV), assist/control ventilation, pressure support ventilation (PSV), and flow-cycled ventilation (mainly used in PSV). In addition, real-time graphic monitoring is now available in the newer ventilators, enabling clinicians to visualize respiratory mechanics on a breath-to-breath basis. Unfortunately, most of the ventilation data for preterm infants, especially high-quality randomized trials, is concentrated in the early postnatal period with RDS, and there is no clear evidence for an optimal ventilator strategy in infants with established BPD. Because of the lack of evidence in this population, our group evolved the following care strategies after caring for several

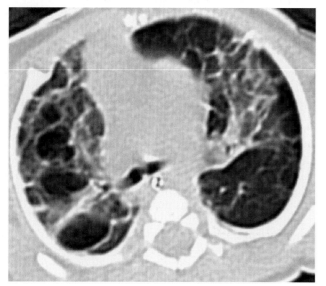

FIG 35-4 Chest computed tomography scan of an infant after 4 months of noninvasive ventilation. Born at 26 weeks' GA, the infant received mechanical ventilation for 6 weeks after birth followed by prolonged noninvasive ventilation. She was maintained on 7 L/min high-flow nasal cannula at 52 weeks' PMA despite chronic respiratory failure, progressively worsening PH, and severe growth failure.

hundred infants with sBPD since 2010. Summarized below are three guiding principles to use when trying to provide optimum ventilator support for these patients:

1. The main goal of MV in this population is to provide sufficient support that the patient needs, rather than weaning.
2. Make sure the alveoli are well recruited—that is, use an open lung strategy.
3. Ensure adequate expiration to minimize air trapping.

Here we use the SIMV + PSV mode as an example to discuss the methods we can use to follow the above guiding principles. Main parameters to adjust in this mode include tidal volume (V_T) or peak inflating pressure (PIP) to achieve the targeted V_T, mandatory ventilator rate, inspiration time (i-time), positive end-expiratory pressure (PEEP), and pressure support (PS). The targets and strategies used to set the ventilator parameters are summarized in Table 35-2. Other ventilator modes may also be used successfully in infants with sBPD; however, the same guiding principles and targets should be followed.

When adjusting the ventilator parameters to achieve these targets, it is important to remember there is interplay of the targets. Therefore adjusting one or two parameters may produce a profound impact in one area but may not result in overall improvement. In the following paragraphs, we will discuss each key parameter in more detail.

Setting the target tidal volume. Because volutrauma has been associated with the development of lung injury, volume-targeted ventilation has been advocated in neonatal MV in recent years.[42,43] In the early postnatal days, reported benefits of volume-targeted ventilation included tighter V_T and carbon dioxide control, fewer pneumothoraces, fewer days of ventilation, reduction in severe intraventricular hemorrhage, and, most important, decreased death or BPD.[44,45] As patients with sBPD often have marked variability in compliance and resistance over time, they may benefit from volume-targeted

or patient-initiated pressure-regulated and volume-controlled ventilation to ensure delivery of adequate V_T with the least pressure. Unfortunately, currently there is no specific evidence to guide the use of volume-targeted ventilation in patients with sBPD. In our experience, these patients may need much higher V_Ts (8 to 12 mL/kg) compared to younger preterm infants. High enough V_T, in conjunction with adequate support during spontaneous breath, can ensure adequate minute ventilation and improve a patient's comfort, which in turn will contribute to improvement in the increased work of breathing and tachypnea often seen in this population.

Owing to issues of high airway resistance and distended trachea with prolonged intubation, many infants with sBPD have significant leak around the endotracheal tube (ETT), often over 50%, and the amount of leak varies from inflation to inflation. This poses challenges to effective volume ventilation. In the presence of ETT leak, the gas leaving the lung most closely represents the V_T that entered the lung. Targeting the expired V_T may be the best way to control the delivered V_T in these patients. Luckily many newer ventilators now have the flow sensor at the "Y" connector and are able to measure and display the V_T in and out of the baby. This improvement enables the ventilator to provide better leak compensation, and clinicians are able to achieve tighter control of the expired V_T. However, in cases of severe leak and when the newer ventilators are not available, volume ventilation may not be feasible. In these cases, patients may need high PIP settings in the 30- to 40-cm H_2O range, given their stiff lungs with poor lung compliance.

Finding appropriate rate and inspiration time. The majority of patients with sBPD have heterogeneous lung disease (see Fig. 35-3, *B*), with both collapsed and overinflated areas in their lungs, causing significant maldistribution of ventilation. As discussed earlier, the lung mechanics in these patients are better explained by a two-compartment model with different time constants in different parts of the lung. To ensure adequate gas exchange and emptying of the slower compartment, which contributes to the majority of the exhaled V_T, we elect to use a low rate and long inspiratory time strategy. This strategy has been used successfully in several centers that treat infants with sBPD.[28] Patients with sBPD often breathe fast with a short i-time. Setting a long i-time during mandatory ventilator breaths therefore is needed to ensure air entry into the slow compartments. However, these slow compartments also need long expiration time for alveolar pressure to equilibrate with upper airway pressure. Therefore, a slow rate allowing enough time during expiration for the slow compartments to empty is critical in minimizing gas trapping. To ensure an overall slow respiratory rate and a good composite inspiratory-to-expiratory (I:E) ratio, we advocate using a slow ventilator rate (10 to 20) with adequate V_T and PS. Adding adequate PS to the spontaneous breath will help prevent underventilation of the fast compartment. The combined effort of improving ventilation in both the slow and the fast compartments often results in improved minute ventilation and patient comfort, which in turn helps to slow down the breathing rate and further minimize air trapping.

The slow-rate, long i-time ventilation plus adequate PS strategy may be an effective way of ventilating the majority of infants with sBPD. In a patient with uniform lung disease, however (see Fig. 35-3, *A*), who has a homogeneous hazy chest radiographic appearance and underlying pathologic feature of generalized alveolar simplification, respiratory insufficiency is probably due

Target	Strategies
TABLE 35-2 **Targets and Strategies for Setting Ventilator Support under Synchronized Intermittent Mandatory Ventilation Plus Pressure Support Ventilation Mode**	
Establish optimum lung volume	• May need higher tidal volume of 8-12 mL/kg • Provide adequate PEEP (may need PEEP >10-15 cm H_2O) • Adequate PS to support spontaneous breath (may be as high as the PIP needed on the mandatory vent breath)
Promote even distribution of ventilation	• Long i-time and e-time to adequately ventilate the slow compartments (i-time may be >0.5-0.8 s) • Low vent rate (10-20/min) to ensure long enough e-time • Adequate PS to help maintain minute ventilation and achieve overall low respiratory rate
Maintain open airway	• Inspiration phase: Enough pressure from both vent breath PIP and PS • Exhalation phase: Adequate PEEP

e-time, Expiration time; *i-time*, inspiration time; *PEEP*, positive end-expiratory pressure; *PIP*, peak inflating pressure; *PS*, pressure support.

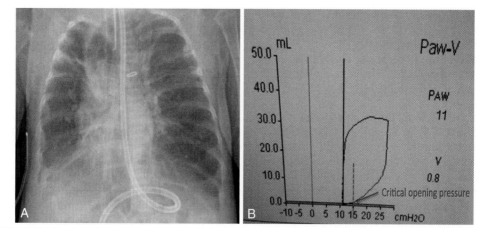

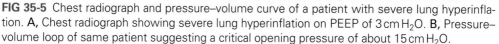

FIG 35-5 Chest radiograph and pressure–volume curve of a patient with severe lung hyperinflation. **A,** Chest radiograph showing severe lung hyperinflation on PEEP of 3 cm H_2O. **B,** Pressure–volume loop of same patient suggesting a critical opening pressure of about 15 cm H_2O.

to decreased alveoli surface area rather than having a maldistribution of ventilation. The lung compliance would be fairly consistent throughout the lung fields, and the time constant is usually relatively short. These patients may do better with faster rate and shorter i-time.

Setting optimum PEEP. Setting an appropriate PEEP is an important component of ventilator management. An appropriate level of PEEP can increase FRC, promote alveoli recruitment, reduce work of breathing, and improve V/Q matching.[46,47] Animal studies have suggested that very low PEEP will lead to impaired gas exchange and increased risk of lung injury,[48,49] whereas open lung ventilation improves gas exchange and attenuates secondary lung injury.[50] Major concerns about high PEEP level mainly come from the worry that high PEEP may decrease tidal and minute ventilation; impair expiration, causing gas trapping; and impair venous return, resulting in decreased cardiac output.[51,52] Randomized clinical trials comparing different PEEP levels have been performed in both adults and neonates with acute RDS but not in infants with BPD.[53,54]

Paradoxically, increased PEEP may be indicated when overexpansion of the lungs is observed. This is contrary to common practice but is based on sound pathophysiologic principles. As described earlier, infants with established BPD have been found to have decreased lung compliance, increased resistance, reduced FRC, and obstructive lung disease. In addition, many patients with sBPD have issues with tracheobronchomalacia, resulting in dynamic airway collapse. These airway and pulmonary mechanical characteristics put them at increased risk of developing inadvertent or intrinsic PEEP ($PEEP_i$). When the set ventilator PEEP is less than $PEEP_i$, the nonparalyzed infant must first overcome the imposed elastic load of the $PEEP_i$ before any inspiratory flow can be generated. This means that the infant often cannot generate enough inspiratory flow to trigger the ventilator in the normal respiratory cycle, resulting in ineffective inspiratory efforts, loss of patient–ventilator synchrony, air hunger, and excessive respiratory work.[55,56] This may also be the source of some BPD spells (desaturation episodes), as the infant's ineffective efforts cause greater air hunger and hypoxemia. The poorly supported floppy airways of infants with sBPD are susceptible to collapse in the later phase of exhalation as lung volume decreases, especially when the infant is agitated.

It is imperative that an individual level of PEEP be established for each patient and changes made as the disease changes. We have learned that this individualized PEEP level can be found based on possible underlying pathology and ventilator P–V curves[57] of each patient. Finding this optimum PEEP may help break the cycle of alveolar collapse and airway instability. Figure 35-5 shows the admission chest radiograph of an infant with sBPD who was transferred to our center for management of ventilator failure. She had persistent hyperinflation of her lungs despite decreasing PEEP to 3 cm H_2O and required 100% oxygen for several weeks prior to her transfer. Based on P–V curve changes with different levels of PEEP, we determined that this patient required a PEEP of 14 to 15 cm H_2O (see Fig. 35-5, right). A bedside bronchoscopy demonstrated that her bilateral bronchus completely collapsed when PEEP was decreased to less than 8 cm H_2O. Her oxygenation improved dramatically, and the lung hyperinflation gradually decreased with the higher PEEP. We have attempted using a PEEP grid to identify optimum PEEP in each patient. Figure 35-6 demonstrates the identification of peak and plateau pressure, peak flow, and volume under a PEEP of 12 cm H_2O during a PEEP grid testing. Compliance and resistance under different levels of PEEP (5-18 cm H_2O) were calculated based on the identified values. Airway malacia can be documented using full-inflation and end-exhalation controlled-ventilation chest CT or bedside flexible bronchoscopy.[58-60] In addition, PEEP level can be titrated at the bedside with the use of bronchoscopy by applying a stepwise increase/decrease in PEEP to the airways and directly visualizing and determining the effect of increased PEEP on airway collapse. The challenge in using these methods is that the patient needs to be quiet and often sedated to obtain an accurate value. PEEP requirements in these patients are also dynamic and may vary from day to day, during agitation, or when the disease process changes. The optimal PEEP is determined by the interplay between the severity of airway collapse or tracheobronchomalacia and the severity of parenchymal lung disease.

A high rate, short inspiratory time, and low V_T approach is often employed early in the course in preterm infants. Transition from this mode to a mode that addresses the complex interaction between small and large airway disease as well as the heterogeneity of lung parenchymal disease may be indicated with the development of established BPD. Optimally utilizing a

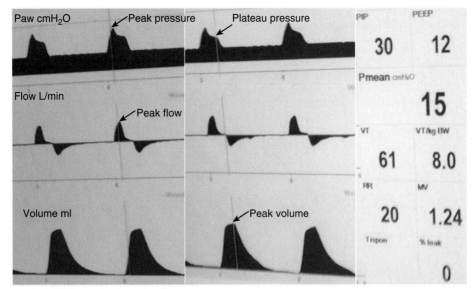

FIG 35-6 Identifying optimum PEEP with PEEP grid. PEEP grid was done on a Dräger V500 ventilator under pediatric volume mode and with fixed flow rate. Peak and plateau pressure and peak volume were measured under different PEEP levels. Compliance and resistance were calculated and optimum PEEP was selected based on the PEEP level that produces the best compliance and lowest resistance.

low rate, high inspiratory time with larger V$_T$, and adequate PS to offset the effects of a lower rate will compensate for increased dead space with acquired airway obstruction and allow for more even gas distribution throughout the lung. This often results in significant improvements in gas exchange and clinical stability.

High-frequency ventilation. High-frequency ventilation (HFV) delivers very small V$_T$s with rapid rates. This may avoid large volume changes associated with conventional ventilation and therefore decrease the incidence and severity of lung injury. The main forms of HFV include high-frequency oscillatory ventilation (HFOV) and high-frequency jet ventilation (HFJV).

HFOV delivers extremely small V$_T$s at rates of 6 to 15 Hz. There have been a number of clinical trials comparing HFOV with conventional MV in preterm infants with RDS with differing results.[61-64] Although some studies suggest early HFOV use in the course of RDS may reduce the incidence of BPD,[61,64] as of this writing there are no data supporting the use of HFOV in infants with established BPD. In BPD infants with heterogeneous lung disease who have poorly supported, floppy airways, there is a concern that active exhalation and relatively high I:E ratio (1:2) of HFOV may cause further air trapping and exacerbate respiratory failure in these infants. In contrast, the much lower achievable I:E ratio on HFJV (1:7 to 1:11) may minimize gas trapping and improve gas exchange in such patients. In one retrospective study, Friedlich et al.[65] found that HFJV improves hypoxemic respiratory failure unresponsive to HFOV in preterm infants requiring MV for at least 4 weeks. In a small prospective pilot trial, Plavka et al.[66] demonstrated that HFJV improved gas exchange and facilitated weaning from MV in preterm infants with evolving BPD. In recent years, lower jet rate in the range of 260 to 320 has been suggested for infants with established BPD with a goal of lengthening expiration time. However, the efficacy of this strategy is unclear.

The mechanism of gas transport during HFV may facilitate diffusion and gas exchange in compartments with different time constants and therefore may be beneficial in infants with established BPD. However, the specific mode of HFV, the optimal timing and settings of HFV, as well as the impact on long-term outcomes in this population need further investigation.

ADJUNCT THERAPIES FOR THE RESPIRATORY SUPPORT OF INFANTS WITH ESTABLISHED BRONCHOPULMONARY DYSPLASIA

Heliox

In cases of airway obstruction, heliox, the helium–oxygen gas mixture, with its reduced density, may improve gas flow in the airways and increase oxygen and carbon dioxide diffusion in the alveoli by reducing turbulence. Given this property, it has been hypothesized that heliox may be particularly beneficial in BPD infants with heterogeneous lung inflation. Beneficial effects including decreased pulmonary resistance, reduced work of breathing, and improvements in V$_T$ and oxygenation have been reported in BPD infants both on noninvasive respiratory support[67] and on MV.[68] However, although heliox was well tolerated in these small studies (12 to 15 patients), poor tolerance with changes in behavior, a decrease in skin temperature, and hypoxia have been observed in some other studies.[69,70] Szczapa et al.[68] have suggested heliox should be used in BPD patients during exacerbations to minimize further injury to the lung associated with MV and stopped when lung function improves. However, conclusions cannot be drawn regarding the efficacy, safety, dose, timing, and duration of heliox use based on current available data.

Pharmacotherapy

Medical therapies such as corticosteroids, bronchodilators, and diuretics are frequently used in conjunction with respiratory support modalities in infants with BPD. These commonly used drug therapies are summarized in Table 35-3. Unfortunately, randomized controlled trials in this population are rare, and

TABLE 35-3	Frequently Used Medications in Infants with Severe Bronchopulmonary Dysplasia	
Class of Therapy	**Potential Benefits**	**Concerns**
Methylxanthines • Caffeine • Theophylline	Central respiratory stimulants, decrease diaphragmatic fatigability, weak bronchodilators and diuretics	Decrease incidence of BPD[128] but no data for established BPD
Diuretics • Furosemide • Spironolactone • Thiazides	Improve lung mechanics and oxygenation, may decrease extubation failure[129]	• Electrolyte and acid–base imbalance, osteopenia and/or nephrocalcinosis, endocrine and metabolic effects of spironolactone • Few RCTs with small number of patients • No evidence to support benefit in nonintubated patients[129]
Systemic steroids	• Antiinflammatories • Facilitate weaning down or off mechanical ventilation	• Variable dosing, duration, and timing • Concerns about adverse neurodevelopmental outcomes[130] • Benefit likely to outweigh risk when risk of BPD is high[131]
Inhaled steroids	• Decrease pulmonary inflammation • Trend toward reduced use of systemic steroids[132]	• Low number of patients in RCTs • Unclear efficacy • Paucity of data on adverse effects
β agonists	• Increase bronchodilation and decrease airway resistance • Improve dynamic compliance	Limited RCT data on efficacy or adverse effects[133]
Anticholinergics	• Often used with β agonists • Increase bronchodilation, decrease respiratory resistance, and increase compliance[134,135]	Limited data on efficacy or adverse effects

BPD, Bronchopulmonary dysplasia; *RCT*, randomized controlled trial.

definitive evidence of efficacy and/or safety for many of these drugs is lacking. Data on other potentially beneficial medications such as superoxide dismutase, leukotriene receptor antagonist, citrulline, and inositol are also very limited. This lack of evidence probably contributed to the observed significant variation in medication use in infants with sBPD.[41,71] When deciding on the choice of medication and the dose and duration of therapy, clinicians need to carefully weigh the potential benefit against possible adverse effects of the medications. Well-designed clinical studies examining efficacy, safety, and long-term effects of these medications are urgently needed.

Management of Pulmonary Hypertension

PH contributes to morbidity and mortality in infants with BPD.[72,73] Reported incidence ranges from 16% from a prospective study screening all extremely preterm infants[73] to 25% in a retrospective study of infants with BPD.[74] However, the optimum timing and methods to diagnose and monitor the progression of PH in these patients remain unclear at this time. Echocardiography is currently the most commonly used method. Although noninvasive and widely available, echocardiography can be especially challenging in infants with BPD owing to the presence of lung hyperinflation, expansion of the thoracic cage, and heart rotation. In a retrospective study of infants with chronic lung disease, Mourani et al. found that echocardiography was able to detect a measurable tricuspid regurgitant jet velocity (TRJV) in only 61% of the patients. More important, compared to subsequent cardiac catheterization, echocardiography was able to determine the severity of PH correctly in only 47% of the studies even in the presence of measurable TRJV. In addition, it failed to diagnose PH in 11% and inaccurately diagnosed PH in 11% of patients.[75] Given the limitations in echocardiography, some groups have adopted the use of brain-type natriuretic peptide (BNP) as an adjunct method for the screening and follow-up of BPD-associated PH, as BNP and N-terminal pro-BNP have been shown to correlate with mean pulmonary artery pressure, pulmonary vascular resistance, and

right atrial pressure in both adult and pediatric populations.[76,77] However, elevated BNP in BPD can be related to PH, left-ventricular dysfunction, or chronic pulmonary disease itself. It is therefore unclear whether BNP levels can be used to directly diagnose PH or assess the severity of PH. Higher BNP levels have been found both at 36 weeks' PMA and at the time of discharge in preterm infants with BPD compared to those without BPD and also correlate with severity of BPD.[78] In a retrospective cohort study, a BNP value of 220 pg/mL has been found to have 90% sensitivity and 65% specificity in predicting mortality in infants with BPD-associated PH.[79] BNP level therefore can be a useful biomarker for disease severity and prognosis. Currently most clinicians use serial BNP levels in combination with other clinical and echocardiographic data to monitor trends in disease progression.

As of this writing, treatment of PH in these infants mainly focuses on pharmacologic treatment with vasodilators such as inhaled nitric oxide and sildenafil.[80] However, PH that complicates BPD is often multifactorial. Therefore, pursuing vasodilation without understanding the underlying pathophysiology frequently will not achieve anticipated results and may even be detrimental. Figure 35-7 shows a chest radiograph of an infant with severe PH. He had severe work of breathing with frequent desaturation episodes, poor growth, and signs of heart failure on noninvasive respiratory support using NIPPV. His PH and right-heart failure improved dramatically after intubation. Further examination by bronchoscopy found that the patient had severe tracheobronchomalacia with frequent airway collapse despite being on high settings of noninvasive support. Key treatment in this patient was therefore adequate PEEP support rather than PH medications.

Both frequent hypoxemia events and exposure to increased oxygen concentration can induce pulmonary vascular constriction and remodeling. However, vasodilators can only dilate existing vessels in the lung, and vasodilation in poorly ventilated areas may worsen V/Q mismatch and exacerbate hypoxemia in these patients. Therefore, one of the most important

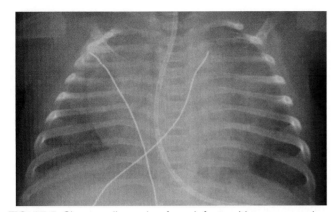

FIG 35-7 Chest radiograph of an infant with severe pulmonary hypertension. He was found to have severe tracheobronchomalacia. A high level of nasal intermittent positive-pressure ventilation (PIP of 28 and PEEP of 14) was unable to maintain an open airway in this patient. His pulmonary hypertension quickly improved after intubation, and he was eventually discharged home on room air with PEEP/pressure support via tracheostomy.

aspects of PH management in BPD infants is adequate respiratory support and oxygen therapy. Well-supported infants will have better lung growth, improved gas exchange, less agitation, and intermittent hypoxia, which will facilitate lung vascular growth and decrease pulmonary vasoconstriction. Rushing to wean a patient off of supplemental oxygen may have detrimental effects, as previous studies have shown that the pulmonary vascular resistance in BPD is responsive to hypoxia and oxygen.[81,82] Some centers therefore advocate maintaining oxygen saturation in the range of 91% to 95%. However, the optimum oxygen saturation target in this population is currently unknown.

Management of Patent Ductus Arteriosus

Persistent PDA is very common in premature infants. Although the open ductus protects the developing pulmonary circulation from overflow in the fetus, PDA after birth has multiple effects on the developing lung that contribute to the development or worsening of BPD. These include (1) higher driving pressures and excessive blood flow from PDA that negatively affect the development of the pulmonary vasculature and induce endothelial injury[83-85]; (2) increased level of inflammatory cytokines such as tumor necrosis factor-α, platelet-activating factor, and activated neutrophils[86-88]; (3) increased vascular resistance and decreased dynamic lung compliance, which may result in higher levels and longer duration of ventilatory support[89,90]; and (4) inhibition of alveolarization in preterm baboons[91,92]. Consistent with the experimental evidence, several studies found an increased risk of BPD in infants with symptomatic PDA.[93] However, to date, there are scarce data from prospective clinical trials to confirm this association. In contrast, clinical trials have failed to demonstrate a meaningful long-term benefit of PDA closure,[94-96] and several studies have suggested that early surgical PDA ligation is an independent risk factor for the development of BPD.[97,98] With the ongoing controversy regarding the efficacy and safety of PDA treatment, we have seen a shift in clinical practice from early aggressive therapy to selective treatment of hemodynamically significant PDA (HSDA).[99] Unfortunately, as of this writing, there are no high-quality data to guide the diagnosis, timing, and methods of treatment of this

HSDA. In patients with established sBPD, closure of the ductus may result in significant clinical improvement, and delayed treatment may result in progressively worsened pulmonary mechanics as well as contribute to the development of severe PH. However, when severe PH is already developed, with significant right-to-left shunting and right-ventricular (RV) dysfunction, closing the ductus may severely increase RV pressure by eliminating the "pop-off" mechanism through the ductus. Thus, clinicians need to carefully evaluate the risks and benefits of ductus closure in these infants. In older infants with sBPD, our center has tried using cardiac catheterization to first evaluate pulmonary hemodynamics and then, in selected patients, close the ductus in the cardiac catheterization laboratory with a coil or plug. These patients in general have favorable clinical responses to the ductus closure and fast recovery from the procedure. However, this method is not feasible in smaller centers, and the role of cardiac catheterization in the management of PH complicating BPD needs to be further studied.

Nutritional Support

Infants with sBPD face nutritional challenges due to increased energy expenditure from increased respiratory demands and generalized growth suppression from chronic stress, inflammation, and medication use.[100,101] Data from the Children's Hospital Neonatal Consortium Database reported that more than half of infants with sBPD had postnatal growth failure at 36 weeks' PMA, and rates continued to increase in those hospitalized beyond 36 weeks' PMA.[101] Associated with poor overall nutritional status, infants with sBPD have also been reported to have high incidence of metabolic bone disease.[102] Undernutrition has several important impacts on the outcome of infants with BPD: (1) it affects both somatic and lung growth, possibly by limiting vital pulmonary cell signaling in cell multiplication, differentiation, growth, and extracellular matrix protein deposition[103-106]; (2) it affects lung function through the breakdown of connective tissue fibers, leading to emphysema and inadequate ossification of the bony skeleton and fractures causing decreased stability of the thoracic cage[107,108]; (3) it decreases antioxidant enzymes and increases susceptibility to hyperoxic injury[109,110]; (4) it affects alveolar fluid balance by contributing to pulmonary edema[111,112]; (5) it increases susceptibility to infection and predisposes to pulmonary infection[113]; and (6) poor linear growth is associated with reduced lean body mass accretion and poor brain growth and development.[114] In light of this information, the delivery of adequate and titrated nutrients according to the individual patient's needs to achieve a "progrowth" state with balanced weight and linear growth should be the focus of nutritional management in infants with BPD. To achieve this "progrowth" state, rather than focusing solely on increased calories, attention should be given to ways of providing balanced nutrition, decreasing energy expenditure, and facilitating physical activities, such as providing adequate respiratory support, avoiding deficiency of vitamins/minerals, and decreasing stress of the intensive care unit environment.

Minimizing Pulmonary Microaspiration

Pulmonary aspiration may exacerbate lung disease in infants with BPD.[115] Gastroesophageal reflux (GER) is commonly seen in preterm infants, especially infants with BPD. Increased work of breathing and frequent transient increases in intra-abdominal pressure due to coughing, agitation, and airflow obstruction in infants with BPD can lead to a decrease in lower esophageal sphincter (LES) tone and LES relaxation, which probably contribute to the increased risk of GER.[116] Studies have reported increased frequencies of GER events (especially acid reflux-related events), longer acid clearance time, and higher symptom sensitivity index scores in infants with BPD compared to infants without BPD. In addition, Jadcherla et al. also reported that acid reflux events in the pharynx were associated with increased symptom occurrence and delayed symptom clearance.[117-119] Improvement in respiratory status has been reported in infants with BPD after medical or surgical antireflux therapy.[102,117,118,120] However, there are increasing concerns about the safety and efficacy of antireflux drugs among preterm infants, and there are currently no reliable diagnostic or clinical criteria to guide antireflux surgery. In our center, we would consider a trial of postpyloric feeds in infants with sBPD. Some infants demonstrated significant clinical improvement with decreased respiratory distress, fewer agitation and hypoxia events, and decreased oxygen requirement. Many patients were able to transition back to gastric feeds after their respiratory status improved, and the ones who failed tolerating gastric feeds were considered for antireflux surgery. The majority of our patients needing surgery underwent laparoscopic fundoplication with gastric tube placement, and our data indicated that the procedure could be safely performed in infants with sBPD.[102] Considering the current deficiency in reliable diagnostic tools and the risk of treatment, coordinated multicenter studies in the optimum management of GER in infants with sBPD are needed.

As previously discussed, chemoreceptor hypersensitivity may contribute to feeding difficulties in infants with BPD. In addition, infants with sBPD have decreased opportunity to develop oral motor and swallowing skills and have lower tolerance for breathing pause during sucking and swallowing. All these put them at higher risk for aspiration during oral feeding. Therefore, safety of oral feeding needs to be established and frequently reevaluated when trying to promote oral feedings in these patients. This can be achieved through a multidisciplinary coordinated approach.[121]

Role of Tracheostomy in Infants Requiring Long-Term Support

BPD is an independent risk factor for neurodevelopmental impairment in VLBW infants.[122] Furthermore, a protracted course of MV is associated with increased mortality and neurodevelopmental disability in this population.[123] Although tracheostomy is commonly viewed as a negative event, it may be unavoidable in infants with sBPD. In fact, sBPD requiring long-term MV has been reported as the most common reason for tracheostomy in preterm infants.[124] We have observed, in our center, that tracheostomy placement in infants with sBPD may be associated with better proportional growth and increased participation in age-appropriate developmental activities. This is consistent with data from DeMauro et al., who found a possible association between earlier (<120 days) tracheostomy and better neurodevelopmental outcomes in infants in whom tracheostomy was unavoidable.[125] Tracheostomy does not treat lung disease; however, it provides a stable airway that allows the clinicians to transition their treatment focus from weaning off ventilator support to providing adequate support and developmental enrichment. In our experience, and also reported by Mandy et al., tracheostomy placement is safe even in infants needing high ventilator support. Mandy et al. have suggested that chronically ventilated infants should be evaluated for tracheostomy placement at around or shortly after 40 weeks' corrected gestation.[126] When clinicians and parents try to decide whether to place a tracheostomy, the beneficial effects, especially the benefits on growth and development, need to be taken into consideration and balanced against the risks and caregiver burden of tracheostomy.

PULMONRY OUTCOMES IN INFANTS WITH BRONCHOPULMONARY DYSPLASIA

Reports suggest that infants with BPD continue to have significant pulmonary sequelae during childhood and adolescence. These include persistence of respiratory symptoms with increased rehospitalization for respiratory illness, decreased pulmonary function, persistent small and large airway dysfunction, and decreased respiratory reserve. However, the frequency of respiratory symptoms and rehospitalization decreases over the first few years, and pulmonary mechanics normalizes and lung volume improves over time.[127] These data suggest that with proper management, infants with BPD may have a reasonable long-term outcome; however, continued surveillance of young adults with BPD is critical. The reader is referred to Chapter 43 for a more complete discussion of pulmonary outcomes of ventilated neonates.

CONCLUSIONS

In infants with established BPD, treatment should be focused on promoting growth while minimizing further lung injuries. To achieve this goal, it is important to understand the underlying pathophysiology and clinical presentation of each patient and provide adequate respiratory and multisystem support accordingly. An interdisciplinary approach that provides comprehensive support from multiple disciplines is extremely beneficial for these patients. High-quality multicenter research data are urgently needed to guide the optimum care strategies in this patient population. In addition, long-term airway, pulmonary, and neurodevelopmental follow-up is critical in ensuring optimum long-term outcomes and also providing further information on this special patient population.

REFERENCES

A complete reference list is available at https://expertconsult.inkling.com/

36

Medical and Surgical Interventions for Respiratory Distress and Airway Management

Jonathan F. Bean, MD, Robert M. Arensman, BS, MD, Nishant Srinivasan, MD, Akhil Maheshwari, MD, and Namasivayam Ambalavanan, MBBS, MD

INTRODUCTION

The advent of the specialty of neonatology has promoted the care and survival of ever-increasing numbers of extremely small newborns. These patients have a whole host of complex anatomic problems. Consequently, neonatologists and pediatric surgeons face vast challenges in the management of problems with the airway and lungs. In this chapter, we look first at medical management of the neonatal airway and then progress to the supporting role of pediatric surgeons and otolaryngologists in the diagnosis and management of complex airway problems.

MEDICAL MANAGEMENT OF THE NEONATAL AIRWAY

Maintenance of the airway in sick neonates is critical for ensuring their survival. A compromised airway such as a partial obstruction could potentially lead to gas trapping and ventilatory problems.[1] This in turn can lead to hypoxia, hypercarbia, and serious hemodynamic disturbances. Successful airway management in neonates involves accurate and continuous assessment of the patient by a team of skilled care providers. Adequate preparation prior to performing airway securing procedures is vital to avoid complications associated with artificial airway maintenance. Adequate preparation includes checking all required equipment for availability and full functionality, utilization of resources available in the neonatal intensive care unit (NICU) such as nurses and respiratory therapists, and last, but not least, due diligence on the part of the neonatologist to anticipate and prepare for complications (see Chapter 27, Pulmonary Care).

Typically, the neonatal airway is managed by a team of physicians, respiratory therapists, and nurses in the NICU. The NICU has developed into a unit that provides care not only for premature infants but also for infants with surgical or cardiac problems. Airway needs and indications for interventions may be completely different in such situations and may require the intervention of airway experts such as otolaryngologists and pediatric surgeons. In this section we will discuss the challenges involved in management of the neonatal airway and the medical interventions performed for airway maintenance prior to seeking surgical support.

ANATOMIC DISADVANTAGES OF THE NEONATAL AIRWAY

The neonatal airway is distinctly different from the adult airway. The anatomic disadvantages begin with the shape of the head in neonates, who have a larger occiput. The large occiput in a supine posture naturally places the infant's neck in a flexed position that may cause kinking of the airway and potentially lead to obstruction. This may also obscure visualization of the larynx during intubation, which may require a shoulder roll to reduce neck flexion. A "sniffing posture" with slight extension of the neck when the infant is supine is often required to align the airway axis to achieve unobstructed air entry.

Neonates are obligate nasal breathers, which makes their nasopharynx a vital conduit for ventilation. Secretions and mucosal edema causing impediment to airflow at the level of the nasopharynx can significantly compromise the neonate's airway. Therefore care providers managing the airway of neonates should not only be proactive about clearing secretions but also use extreme caution during airway toileting procedures to avoid iatrogenic nasal mucosal edema.

Hypopharyngeal structures such as the vallecula, the epiglottis, and the laryngeal structures such as arytenoids that commonly serve as landmarks during laryngoscopy and intubation also differ in neonates. The epiglottis is omega-shaped and is generally longer, larger, and less flexible in infants, making this structure more susceptible to injury during intubation and suctioning. Abnormalities of the epiglottis or swelling associated with certain conditions in newborns, such as trauma, and in infants and older children, such as epiglottitis, may make endotracheal intubation extremely challenging. The soft tissue structures of the hypopharynx and larynx follow the physical principles of Bernoulli and the Venturi effect and collapse easily. Bernoulli's principle states that, when these structures are subjected to fast airflow, a low pressure is exerted on the walls of the tube. The Venturi effect is seen during inspiration when these low-pressure walls collapse. Conditions such as laryngomalacia may exaggerate these effects and compromise the airway further.

The lower airway in the premature infant is significantly smaller compared to that of older children and adults. In 1982 Wailoo and Emery described the normal development of the trachea from 28 weeks to 14 years of age based on quantitative assessment of the trachea obtained postmortem.[2] It was observed that the trachea is funnel-shaped, with the upper end wider than the lower end in the neonatal period. It becomes cylindrical with increasing age. This discrepancy was found to be inversely proportional to the gestational age of the infant.[2] The narrowest part of the infant's trachea is considered to be at the level of the cricoid cartilage, whereas in an adult it is at the level of the epiglottis.[2] The unique funnel-shaped trachea with a natural subglottic narrowing places neonates at a certain disadvantage and at higher risk for further airway compromise, especially with development of mucosal edema following prolonged intubations. The cricoid cartilage is composed of two parts: a posterior plate-like portion that forms the posterior wall of the larynx and an inferior ring. In neonates, the plate is inclined posteriorly, with the narrowest part of the funneled trachea at the level of the cricoid ring.

As the infant grows the cricoid plate becomes vertical, the ring enlarges, and the point of narrowing at the funnel spout disappears. In addition to the anatomic orientation of the trachea, the susceptibility of the subglottic area to mucosal edema is related to the difference in cellular lining. The lining above the cords is resilient squamous epithelium, whereas below the cords it is ciliated columnar epithelium that is loosely attached to the submucosal tissue and can be easily infiltrated by fluid to form edema. This alters the internal diameter of the already narrow subglottic trachea. As explained by Poiseuille's law, the resistance to airflow is inversely proportional to the fourth power of the radius of the airway during laminar airflow and to the fifth power during turbulent flow. When the internal diameter of the neonatal airway is decreased to 50% in conditions such as mucosal edema, the resistance to airflow is increased 16-fold.[3] This highlights the importance of timely assessments of airway status and suitable interventions to prevent obstruction to airflow.

Infants with airway narrowing or obstruction may require immediate airway assistance. Interventions are aimed at splinting the airway open for unobstructed airflow. Use of nasal continuous positive airway pressure (CPAP) has gained popularity among neonatologists because of its noninvasiveness and ability to splint the airway effectively, especially in premature infants.[4] However, tracheal intubation with an endotracheal tube (ETT) is sometimes essential to quickly resuscitate an infant.

MEDICAL MANAGEMENT OF NEONATES WITH COMMON RESPIRATORY DISORDERS REQUIRING SURGICAL INTERVENTION

With increasing emphasis on prenatal care and availability of fetal ultrasonography, a large number of congenital respiratory disorders are being detected during fetal life. Availability of early diagnosis provides ample opportunity to plan the early neonatal and preoperative management to reduce the risk of surgical complications and improve postoperative outcomes. Planning often involves availability of medical personnel, which includes neonatologists, respiratory therapists, skilled nurses, pediatric surgeons, otolaryngologists, and bronchoscopists; availability of all required equipment and infrastructure, which includes operating rooms, bronchoscope, and tertiary-level NICU; and ability to perform extracorporeal membrane oxygenation (ECMO) or rapidly transfer the baby to a center with such capabilities. However, a lack of prenatal diagnosis may result in quick decompensation of the neonate, which in turn might create challenges in the surgical management and long-term outcomes of the infant. Most of these neonatal conditions may require specific corrective or palliative interventions. However, the overall management of the infant prior to surgery often follows common principles.

Congenital Airway Disorders

Congenital respiratory or airway disorders such as laryngomalacia, macroglossia, retrognathia or micrognathia, neck masses, hydrops fetalis with neck swelling, congenital diaphragmatic hernia, cystic adenomatoid malformation, congenital lobar emphysema, and similar anomalies can lead to rapid respiratory failure and hemodynamic instability in infants. Stabilization of the infant in the delivery room and a well-planned and well-executed initial management in the NICU may minimize further complications. The airway should be assessed immediately upon delivery for patency. Secretions should be cleared using bulb suction or other suction devices if needed. Studies by Velaphi et al. have shown that wiping could be as effective as suctioning in certain cases.[5] In many circumstances, infants with congenital respiratory disorders will require assisted forms of ventilation, and each infant should be individually assessed and managed. In less severe cases, noninvasive ventilation such as nasal CPAP or nasal intermittent mandatory ventilation may be adequate to achieve target oxygenation and ventilation parameters. However, in more severe cases, tracheal intubation through oral or sometimes even nasal routes may be necessary. Difficult intubations may require the use of fiber-optic laryngoscopes.

Persistent hypoxemia or hypercarbia as a result of inadequate ventilation can result in failure of the infant to transition from the fetal to the neonatal circulation, resulting in persistent pulmonary hypertension of the newborn (PPHN). It is important to closely monitor blood gases and chest X-ray to optimize ventilation. Certain airway disorders lead to persistent hypoxia that in turn can activate various pathways in the lung that result in airway and pulmonary vascular remodeling. These infants may require alternate modes of tissue oxygenation such as ECMO. Ideally, infants should be adequately ventilated and oxygenated (although with caution in premature infants to minimize risks of oxygen toxicity) to avoid complications such as persistent hypoxia, acidosis, or PPHN. At the same time, extreme caution should be taken to avoid volutrauma, oxytrauma, and barotrauma, which are commonly associated with assisted invasive ventilation. This can be achieved by adopting gentle ventilation strategies and permissive hypercarbia.

Once the infant is stabilized, a formal consultation with the surgical specialty should be arranged and appropriate imaging studies ordered to confirm the diagnosis. Frequently, chest X-ray is the initial study of choice to assess lung expansion and extent of abnormality. Other studies that are commonly used are chest ultrasonography, computed tomography (CT), or magnetic resonance imaging (MRI). Infants should always be accompanied to these studies by a provider capable of intubation and resuscitation. Sedation for long procedures is commonly done by the neonatologist or anesthesiologist. In recent times, infant immobilizing devices have been used as a safer alternative to sedation for imaging procedures.[6]

Nutrition plays a major role in preparing these infants for surgery. Although the caloric requirement is better met with enteral feeding, in some infants with respiratory disorders requiring ventilatory support, enteral feeding may not be feasible. Parenteral forms of nutrition are preferred in such infants and instituted early, typically within 24 hours of birth, to provide necessary proteins and lipids that could contribute to growth and body building. Lower total body fat mass and acute and chronic malnourishment are associated with worse clinical outcomes in children undergoing major surgeries.

Acquired Airway Disorders

Acquired airway disorders commonly seen in neonates are often secondary to traumatic laryngoscopic procedures, prolonged intubation, and chronic irritation from a hard nasal cannula. The most vulnerable site for problems in the neonatal airway appears to be the subglottic portion of the trachea at the level of the cricoid ring because of the above-mentioned anatomy and physiologic mechanisms. These complications can be avoided by using gentle techniques during naso-oropharyngeal suctioning and endotracheal intubation. Longer length of intubation time and multiple reintubations frequently result in subglottic stenosis, which makes it more challenging to extubate. Infants who require prolonged ventilation should be intubated only with uncuffed ETTs. This could potentially minimize an inflammatory response in the surrounding walls of the subglottic trachea. However, with prolonged duration of intubation these changes might become inevitable. These neonates should be evaluated at regular intervals for signs of obstruction or airway edema. Currently used ventilators provide information on expiratory flow leak and tidal volume. Infants with significant airway edema tend to have low airflow leak estimations. In some cases altered breath sounds such as stridor, crowing, or dysphonic or raspy cry in association with respiratory distress, which are signs of airway edema, are identified only post extubation. The goal, however, should be to identify infants at risk for development of airway edema prior to extubation. Cautiously planned and timely efforts to extubate infants to a noninvasive form of ventilation are needed. The provision of positive end-expiratory pressure in some form (CPAP, high-flow nasal cannula, noninvasive ventilation) is often helpful in avoiding extubation failure. Use of a short course of dexamethasone in high-risk cases is frequently recommended prior to extubation to reduce airway edema and risk of reintubation.[7] Also racemic epinephrine may be used with caution to decrease the vascular congestion in the trachea and improve stridor post extubation.[8] Reflux precautions in these infants can also be helpful in preventing caustic damage to the airway by stomach acid. However, use of antireflux medications generally should be avoided and reserved for infants with unique anatomic problems such as tracheoesophageal fistula. Unfortunately, some infants are exceedingly dependent on artificial airways and may eventually require surgical interventions such as a tracheostomy as a long-term solution.

SURGICAL MANAGEMENT OF THE NEONATAL AIRWAY

Respiratory distress in the neonate has a variety of causes (Box 36-1), and pediatric surgeons and otolaryngologists are increasingly becoming involved in the care of these patients. The ability to intubate, mechanically ventilate, and thereby prolong the lives of children with neonatal asphyxia, congenital anomalies, or other causes of respiratory distress redefines the role of the surgeon as part of the neonatal management team.

The role of the surgeon is twofold: (1) as a diagnostician and therapist for those infants who manifest respiratory distress from an anatomic problem or who present with congenital airway obstruction (i.e., congenital stridor [Box 36-2]) and (2) as a consultant for neonates undergoing medical treatment requiring long-term intubation of their airways.

THE PEDIATRIC SURGEON/OTOLARYNGOLOGIST AS DIAGNOSTICIAN AND THERAPIST

The role of the pediatric surgeon/otolaryngologist is often defined by the anatomic abnormalities present in any given infant. For purposes of organization, material presented here is divided into developmental abnormalities of (1) the airway, (2) the lung, (3) the diaphragm, and (4) the skeleton.

Developmental Abnormalities of the Airway
Tracheal Obstruction

Nasopharyngeal Obstruction. The presence of stridor signals a need for urgent diagnosis and possible intervention due to the narrow size of the infant airway and the ease at which it can reach critical narrowing. The severity of neonatal stridor can vary. Some cases may be managed medically, whereas other cases may represent impending total obstruction; therefore, the approach to diagnosis is deliberate (Fig. 36-1).

BOX 36-1 Indications for Neonatal Bronchoscopy

- Prolonged intubation (6 to 8 weeks)
- Repetitive failure of extubations
- Inability to aerate all lobes of the lung (persistent atelectasis)
- Clinical need for cultures or bronchial washings
- Suspicion of necrotizing tracheobronchitis
- Evaluation of stridor

BOX 36-2 Differential Diagnosis of Neonatal Stridor (Anatomic Approach)

Nasopharynx
Choanal atresia

Tongue
Idiopathic
Beckwith-Wiedemann syndrome
Metabolic disorders
    Hypothyroidism/lingual thyroid
    Glycogen storage disease
Down syndrome

Oropharynx (Micrognathia and Glossoptosis)
Pierre Robin sequence
Treacher Collins syndrome
Hallermann-Streiff syndrome
Möbius syndrome
Freeman-Sheldon syndrome
Nager syndrome

Larynx
Laryngeal atresia
Laryngeal web
Vocal cord paralysis
Laryngomalacia
Subglottic stenosis
    Congenital/traumatic
Laryngocele
Laryngeal cleft
Subglottic hemangioma

Trachea
Intrinsic compression
    Tracheomalacia
    Tracheal stenosis
    Necrotizing tracheobronchitis
Extrinsic compression
    Cystic hygroma
    Vascular rings

A differential diagnosis for neonatal upper airway obstruction can be formulated by approaching the subject anatomically, beginning in the nasopharynx and oropharynx and progressing down through the respiratory tract.

Choanal Atresia. Choanal atresia, a rare anomaly, with a reported incidence of 1 in 8000 births, involves occlusion of the posterior nares by a membranous (10%) or bony (90%) septum (Fig. 36-2). Unilateral lesions typically can be asymptomatic, but bilateral lesions may cause total airway obstruction because

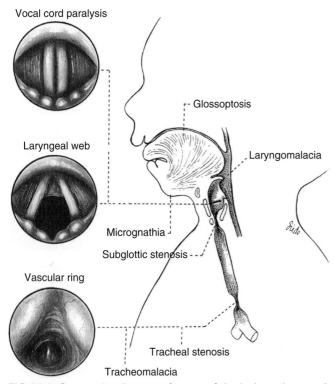

FIG 36-1 Composite diagram of some of the lesions that result in neonatal stridor (proceeding downward through the respiratory passages).

neonates are preferential nasal breathers. Symptoms are most evident when a baby is at rest, because when agitated and crying, the infant breathes via the oropharynx. Associated anomalies include esophageal atresia, congenital cardiac lesions, colobomata, and Treacher Collins syndrome, among a large number of rarer associations.[9-14] Diagnosis can be made by the inability to pass a catheter through the nostrils into the oropharynx. Management ranges from simple placement of an oropharyngeal airway to operative opening of the occlusion with placement of stents. Rarely, tracheostomy may be needed if definitive surgical correction cannot be performed in the neonatal period.[15]

Oropharyngeal Obstruction

Macroglossia. The tongue is often a site of obstruction. Stridor in a neonate can occur if the tongue is disproportionately larger than the infant's oropharynx. Physical examination confirms the diagnosis. Insertion of an oral airway is usually successful in treating this type of airway obstruction. Several well-known syndromes include macroglossia as a component.

Beckwith-Wiedemann Syndrome. Severe hypoglycemia, in many cases secondary to hyperinsulinemia, initially brought these examples of infantile gigantism to medical attention. Macroglossia secondary to muscular hypertrophy, visceromegaly, microcephaly, and a series of umbilical abnormalities ranging from congenital umbilical hernia to omphalocele also compose this syndrome. Affected infants may also demonstrate a facial nevus flammeus, renal medullary dysplasia, and a characteristic pit on the tragus of the ear. These babies are typically large for gestational age. The congenital stridor resulting from the enlarged tongue usually resolves rapidly with the insertion of an oropharyngeal airway. Little further diagnostic workup of the airway is necessary if the child is identified as having this syndrome.[16-20]

Metabolic Disorders. Several neonatal metabolic disorders cause macroglossia and result in congenital stridor, the best known of which are hypothyroidism and glycogen storage disease. The large tongue, high nature of the airway obstruction, and findings consistent with the underlying condition should suggest the diagnosis and appropriate workup early in the

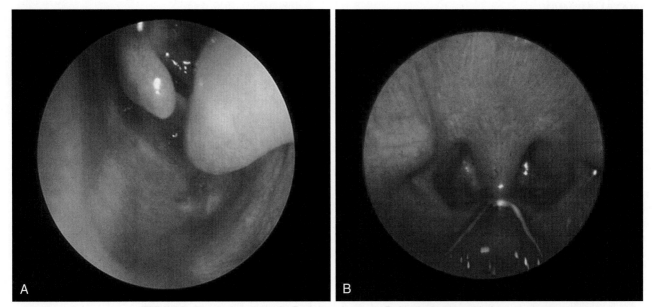

FIG 36-2 Choanal atresia. **A,** Endoscopic view. **B,** Nasopharyngeal view.

course of the disease. The stridor in these babies is generally mild, usually successfully treated with an oropharyngeal airway, and disappears shortly after birth as the underlying condition is successfully treated. Diagnostic evaluation in these patients should be directed at the underlying metabolic disorder; little additional diagnostic work is needed for the tracheobronchial tree.

Down Syndrome (Trisomy 21). Children affected by Down syndrome are easily identified by their constellation of abnormalities. Their relative macroglossia may result in a mild congenital stridor. Because of the reported association between Down syndrome and congenital subglottic stenosis, endoscopy may be necessary to establish the cause of the stridor.[21]

Lingual Thyroid. Lingual thyroid can be a rare cause of oropharyngeal obstruction.[22–24] Stertor in the presence of hypothyroidism, detected by persistent elevation of thyroid-stimulating hormone on routine neonatal screening, raises the suspicion of lingual thyroid, although other lesions are more commonly responsible. This condition occurs in just over 1 in 10,000 births.

Laryngoscopy is used to confirm a mass at the base of the tongue. Further characterization by CT scan and thyroid scintigraphy should be performed. Of note, the thyroid may continue to hypertrophy during early infancy and childhood. Respiratory complications associated with hypothyroidism, such as respiratory depression, may not occur until later.

Severe Bronchopulmonary Dysplasia. Although not generally reported and not often appreciated, macroglossia can develop in infants with severe bronchopulmonary dysplasia and worsen the chronic pulmonary compromise. The obstruction caused by this condition is the result of chronic hypoxia (similar to clubbing of the fingernails) and often heralds a poor outcome. The condition often contributes to compensated respiratory acidosis and is best treated by tracheostomy as opposed to surgical reduction of the tongue.

Craniofacial Dysmorphology Syndromes. The craniofacial dysmorphology syndromes range from unusual to extremely rare. All result in an obstruction located in the oropharynx. This is secondary to micrognathia with glossoptosis.[25] Stridor varies from mild to severe, and it is important to identify the underlying problem, which is often genetic. More complete descriptions of these conditions can be found in texts on congenital malformations.

Pierre Robin Syndrome. Pierre Robin syndrome[26-31] represents the most common craniofacial dysmorphology with micrognathia and glossoptosis. In addition to the aforementioned characteristics, approximately half of these babies also have cleft palates/cleft lip anomalies, perhaps attributable to protrusion of the tongue between the posterior palatine plates during embryologic development. This protrusion results in failure of normal midline fusion. Furthermore, the tongue often prolapses posteriorly, resulting in partial obstruction of the upper airway. During inspiration, negative pressure in the pharynx retrodisplaces the already enlarged tongue and this increases the degree of pharyngeal obstruction. Stridor consequently results in children with Pierre Robin syndrome, and they have particular difficulty with inspiration. The airway obstruction is usually resolved with insertion of an oropharyngeal airway, and these patients tend to breathe more comfortably in a prone position. Feeding may create further problems for these babies and necessitate special nipples or gavage nutrition.

Tracheostomies are rarely necessary in these cases and are to be avoided if at all possible because of the risks of airway occlusion and death. Surgical procedures such as glossopexy or creation of a lingual flap have been described as alternatives but are also seldom needed except in the most severe cases. The first few months of life are critical in determining the severity of a particular infant's anomaly and its importance in the overall prognosis.

Treacher Collins Syndrome. Treacher Collins syndrome,[32] also known as *mandibulofacial dysostosis*, is a variable and diffuse group of craniofacial anomalies. This syndrome is characterized by downward-sloping palpebral fissures, colobomata of the lower lids, sunken cheek bones, and blind fistulae on an angle between the mouth and the ears (Fig. 36-3). Pinnae may be deformed, deafness is common, and micrognathia is part of the syndrome (usually less severe than that seen in Pierre Robin syndrome). The presumed genetic defect is autosomal dominant, with mutation in the *TCOF1* gene at chromosome 5q32-q33.1.

The hypopharynx is the location of the obstruction in these children (as in children with Pierre Robin syndrome), owing to the disproportionate relationship between the small jaw and the large tongue. These cases of stridor can most often be managed medically, often with simple insertion of an oropharyngeal airway, and tracheostomy is seldom necessary. Rarely, bronchoscopy may be indicated if associated tracheobronchial tree anomalies are a concern, but these are quite unusual.

Hallermann-Streiff Syndrome. The Hallermann-Streiff syndrome[33,34] is a rare syndrome that consists of microphthalmia, cataracts, blue sclerae, and nystagmus. Associated anomalies include a pinched nose, micrognathia, and hypertrichosis of the scalp, eyebrows, and eyelashes (Fig. 36-4). Transmission is presumed to be autosomal dominant, although most cases are thought to represent de novo mutations. Congenital stridor in these infants arises from micrognathia with relative glossoptosis, and treatment is similar to that outlined for Pierre Robin or Treacher Collins syndrome.

Möbius Syndrome. Infants with the Möbius syndrome[35,36] have a characteristic absence or maldevelopment of various cranial nerve nuclei. Cranial nerve VII (facial nerve) is the most commonly involved, but other cranial nerves such as cranial nerves V, VI, and VIII may also be affected. Common findings include facial paralysis, ptosis, ophthalmoplegia, clubbed feet, and syndactyly. It is presumed that this condition is inherited in an autosomal dominant manner.

Paralysis of the facial nerve is the cause of upper airway obstruction as well as difficulties with mastication and deglutition. Both inspiratory and expiratory components of stridor result from the relatively fixed nature of the obstruction. Tracheostomy may be required in severe cases. Many children, however, can be successfully treated by parental instruction in very careful feeding techniques.

Freeman-Sheldon Syndrome. Infants with Freeman-Sheldon syndrome[37,38] are often called "whistling-faced" children. They have hypoplastic alae nasi, clubbed feet, and masklike whistling facies. Their eyes are deep set with blepharophimosis, ptosis, and strabismus. Transmission is autosomal dominant with some variations that transmit as autosomal recessive. Chromosomal abnormalities have been reported at both 11p15.5 and 17p13.1. These children are classified as having a type of distal arthrogryposis.

Stridor in these children is the result of air passage through a narrow channel. Although the sound may be alarming, it usually does not require intervention.

Nager Syndrome. Nager syndrome[39–44] is a rare acrofacial dysostosis that presents with upper limb malformation, mandibular and malar hypoplasia, downward-slanting palpebral fissures, absent eyelashes in the medial third of the lower lids, dysplastic ears with conductive deafness, and variable degrees of palatal clefting. This syndrome is associated with chromosome 9 defects. Airway obstruction in these patients is related to posterior tongue displacement due to hypoplasia of the mandible. Acute management often requires early tracheostomy, and subsequent mandibular distraction is eventually needed to correct the defect.

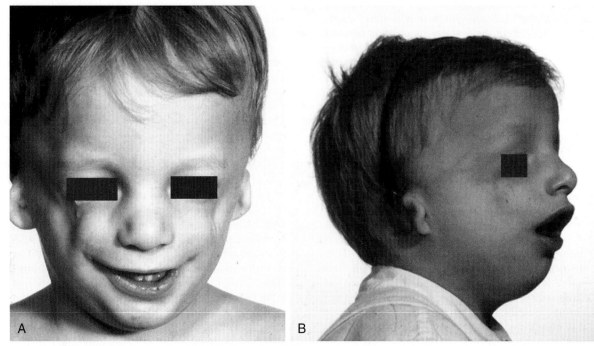

FIG 36-3 Example of a child with Treacher Collins syndrome demonstrating sunken cheek bones, downward sloping palpebral fissures, and micrognathia.

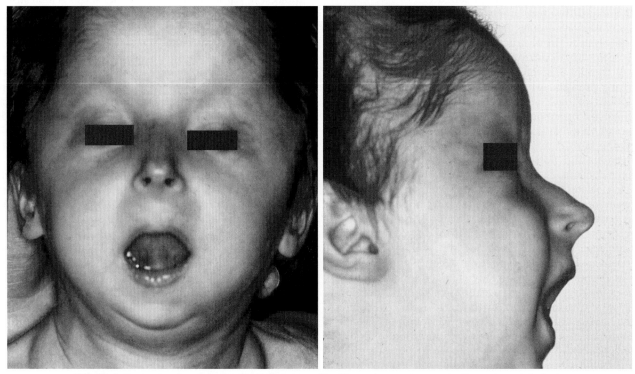

FIG 36-4 Example of an infant with Hallermann-Streiff syndrome demonstrating microphthalmia, pinched nose, micrognathia, and hypertrichosis of the scalp.

Laryngeal Anomalies. An infant's larynx is the next site of possible obstruction, and laryngeal anomalies account for the majority of cases of stridor in newborns.

Laryngeal Atresia. The most extreme form of obstruction at this level, laryngeal atresia, results in a desperate emergency during the first few moments of life. This lesion was originally described in 1826, but only 51 cases were reported in the subsequent 160 years. Very few of these patients survive because surgical intervention to secure a definitive airway must occur within 2 to 5 minutes of clamping of the umbilical cord.[45]

The most dramatic physical finding is that the child is aphonic, with absence of any cry or gasp at birth. If the lesion is immediately recognized on direct laryngoscopy, an emergency cricothyroidotomy should be performed. Diagnosis of laryngeal atresia has now been reported prenatally,[46] and in the future, clinicians may be able to prepare for emergent airway management at birth or schedule the child for an ex utero intrapartum treatment procedure followed by emergent airway opening.

Laryngeal Web. Laryngeal webs account for approximately 5% of laryngeal anomalies (Fig. 36-5). These lesions arise about the 10th week of intrauterine life and probably represent an arrest of the development of the larynx in the area near the vocal cords. Seventy-five percent of these lesions occur at the level of the cords; the rest are subglottic or supraglottic in about equal numbers. The web generally occurs anteriorly, and the lesions are often asymptomatic if they extend less than halfway back along the cords. Because the glottic area is triangular, these anteriorly placed webs reduce the glottic area by only 15% to 20% and are usually not sufficient to cause stridor.[47]

If the web extends posteriorly, the symptoms may be marked. The stridor is primarily inspiratory but often has an expiratory component. The affected infant's cry is hoarse and weak; the child is rarely aphonic and often is dyspneic at rest.

Laryngoscopy and bronchoscopy should be performed as soon as possible. If a thin, transparent web is encountered at the level of the cords, it may be easily swept away with the bronchoscope, completely correcting the problem. Completion of the bronchoscopy should be performed to rule out associated anomalies beneath the area of the web.

If the web is thick and fibrous, no attempt should be made to force the bronchoscope through the area. This kind of web is often encountered in the subglottic region. Tracheostomy is the treatment of choice if the child is dyspneic and unable to tolerate the web. If aeration of the child is satisfactory despite the stridor, as evidenced by arterial blood gas determinations, simple observation may be sufficient management until the baby is able to undergo surgical repair. This is usually deferred until the child is 18 to 24 months of age. The best results to date have been achieved in those children who undergo a meticulous removal of the thick fibrotic web.[48] Depending on the thickness of the web, laser therapy is an alternative and may yield superior results in the future.

Congenital Vocal Cord Paralysis. Congenital vocal cord paralysis is the second most common cause of congenital stridor. In the past, birth trauma was frequently implicated in the etiology of the paralysis but now appears to be a declining cause. Intracranial lesions and the possibility of congenital cardiac lesions, especially one impinging on the recurrent laryngeal nerve, must be considered.[49]

Fortunately, paralysis is unilateral in 70% to 80% of cases. Some studies report that both sides are equally involved,[50] but left-sided paralysis is typically associated with underlying congenital cardiac anomalies. These infants have a hoarse and weak cry, and if the paralysis is bilateral, these children may be truly aphonic. The inspiratory stridor is obviously worse in bilateral paralysis. Marked suprasternal and intercostal retractions may be present in these children.

Diagnosis is rapidly made by laryngoscopy, and treatment depends on the severity of the problem. In a unilateral paralysis with minimal or no dyspnea, simple observation is appropriate. Bilateral paralysis, generally associated with severe symptoms, necessitates tracheostomy. Once the airway is adequately secured, the cause of the paralysis can be explored. If the causal lesion can be identified and corrected, the stridor may improve. If no lesion can be found or if it cannot be safely corrected, later fixation of the arytenoids with the vocal cord in abduction may result in satisfactory control of the stridor and decannulation.

Laryngomalacia. Laryngomalacia is the most common cause of congenital stridor, accounting for 60% to 75% of cases of stridor in newborns. It also accounts for three-fourths of the congenital laryngeal abnormalities. The pathophysiology of this condition involves an immature, floppy larynx that collapses during each inspiration (Fig. 36-6), producing an inspiratory stridor of varying severity that is often much worse when the baby is agitated or screaming. Some infants improve at night, but others experience a worsening of their respiratory sounds.

Laryngomalacia occurs with a 2:1 male-to-female predominance and is usually present at birth. Despite most cases being present at birth, for up to a quarter of patients, the first symptoms appear during the first or second week of life. Many cases are reported to have micrognathia, and some may be confused with Pierre Robin syndrome.

Diagnosis is made easily by laryngoscopy, which shows a soft, enfolded epiglottis. The larynx is often difficult to expose and is found high under the tongue. Bronchoscopy should accompany laryngoscopy to rule out associated anomalies or extensive malacia, such as tracheomalacia and/or bronchomalacia.

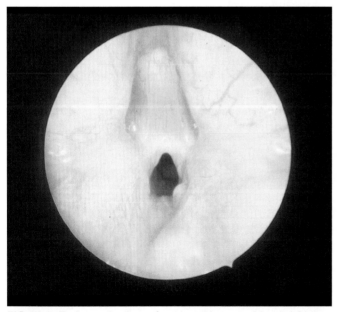

FIG 36-5 Endoscopic view of neonatal larynx with partial laryngeal atresia and a laryngeal web partially obstructing the laryngeal orifice.

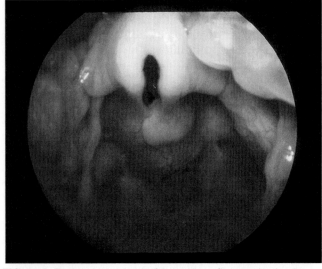

FIG 36-6 Endoscopic view of immature floppy glottis characteristic of laryngomalacia. Dynamic examination demonstrates downward placement of glottis into larynx with inspiration.

Maturation of the epiglottis by the age of 18 to 24 months usually results in resolution of the stridor. Accordingly, tracheostomy is not typically necessary in the final treatment of this disorder.

Congenital Subglottic Stenosis. The overall incidence of congenital subglottic stenosis is unknown because many such cases remain undiagnosed. It has been estimated that 39% of all subglottic stenoses are congenital (the remaining group being acquired).[51] The stenotic area is typically found 2 to 3 mm below the vocal cords and may reduce the subglottic area to 3 to 3.5 mm. The proposed cause of the congenital group is arrested development of the conus elasticus or the cricoid.[52]

The stridor, if present at all, is usually biphasic and sometimes arises during the first or second month of life. Respiratory distress after an upper respiratory tract infection is typically the presenting symptom. These patients are generally unable to clear the resultant increased secretions found in association with infection. Affected children are often treated for recurrent pneumonias or prolonged tracheobronchitis. Many cases are not discovered until a severe episode of croup or epiglottitis results in emergency intubation or tracheostomy.[21]

Mild lesions should be observed, and antibiotic therapy should be added during periods of upper respiratory tract infection. Tracheostomy is necessary in more than half the cases of children with severe stenosis and marked symptoms.[53] Once the tracheostomy is in place, dilation during monthly serial laryngoscopy under general anesthesia often results in improvement. The dilation must be gentle to prevent further damage or fibrosis of the subglottic region. For more severe degrees of stenosis, open surgical intervention may be necessary. The outcome in this congenital group of subglottic stenosis is quite good, with 82% of patients in one large series successfully decannulated after one procedure.[51]

Acquired Subglottic Stenosis. Acquired subglottic stenosis is most often caused by prolonged endotracheal intubation. Because of the increased survival of neonates with respiratory difficulties requiring intubation (especially extremely low birthweight infants), this lesion is increasing in frequency as a cause of stridor. A protracted form of acquired subglottic stenosis was found to occur in 8.3% of neonates surviving a period of endotracheal intubation in one study.[54] In its mildest form, the stenosis consists of laryngeal edema and has been reported in 30% of infants immediately after intubation. Stridor in these patients is inspiratory and presents with the first breaths after tube removal. This usually resolves within 72 hours. During this 3-day period, head elevation, humidified air, racemic epinephrine, nasal CPAP or noninvasive nasal ventilation, and occasionally systemic steroids are used to treat the mild form of this disorder.

In its most severe form, acquired stenosis is a dense scar of well-organized fibrous tissue. This lesion may require tracheostomy before the actual stenosis can safely be manipulated. Initial treatment includes graded, gentle dilation with or without intralesional steroids. As many as half of the stenotic scars will improve and often stabilize after four to six treatments. Failure to achieve significant improvement by then indicates the need for more aggressive treatment such as cryosurgery, laser ablation, cricoid split procedure, or resection and reconstruction with stents. There have been reasonable results with the cricoid split procedure and intubation during healing rather than recourse to tracheostomy, and this alternative should always be considered.

Laryngeal Cleft. Although laryngeal clefts were once considered extremely rare lesions, they have frequently been reported since 1990.[55] This is probably a result of enhanced endoscopy techniques and improved ability to make the diagnosis in the antemortem period. The lesion forms owing to a failure of dorsal fusion during the chondrification of the cricoid cartilage.[56] A midline cleft thus remains posteriorly and extends down between the arytenoids into the upper portion of the esophagus and trachea. Affected children are often very stridorous at birth, and many have died in the past because of inadequate resuscitation. In addition to their respiratory difficulties, aspiration and pneumonitis occur if these patients are fed without regard for their clefts. Consequently, they require recognition, intubation, and stabilization. A feeding gastrostomy and possible fundoplication are often necessary until definitive repair can be performed. Once extubation is accomplished, close observation is necessary to ensure that upper airway secretions do not continuously pass into the lungs. If this proves to be a severe and ongoing problem that precipitates recurrent pneumonia and respiratory distress, it may be necessary to place a tracheostomy until surgical closure of the cleft can be achieved.

Subglottic Hemangioma. Hemangiomas are another cause of congenital subglottic obstruction. The onset of symptoms is variable, as symptomatology is related to the growth and development of these lesions. The lesions are at first quite small and may have a period of rather rapid growth, followed by a long plateau and slow involution. Time to presentation for patients with subglottic hemangiomas depends upon the age at which the hemangioma develops. If the hemangioma develops early in fetal life, then the patient will become symptomatic earlier in life. On the other hand, if the subglottic hemangioma develops after birth, there may be several months' lag in the time to presentation of symptoms. Hemangiomas on other areas of the body suggest the possibility of subglottic hemangioma; definitive diagnosis is made by laryngoscopic and bronchoscopic examination.[57]

A bronchoscopic finding of a red or purple mass just beneath the cords is generally considered diagnostic. Most pediatric

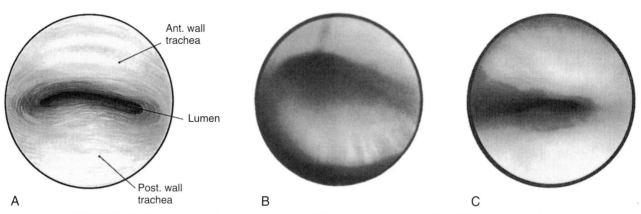

FIG 36-7 Tracheomalacia showing collapse of the trachea on expiration. The lumen is almost obliterated as the anterior (Ant.) wall approaches the posterior (Post.) wall. **A,** Artist's drawing. **B** and **C,** Photographs.

surgeons believe that biopsy is contraindicated when such findings are seen, because hemorrhage necessitating emergent surgery is a distinct possibility after biopsy. Once the diagnosis is established, appropriate therapy is chosen according to the severity of symptoms. If the child is stable and has normal blood gas values at rest, observation is sufficient. If the obstruction is significant enough to result in dyspnea, severe stridor, and possibly abnormal blood gas values, tracheostomy below the lesion should be considered. One must also be aware of the possibility of platelet trapping (Kasabach-Merritt syndrome) before surgical intervention.

It is questionable whether radiation should be used in the treatment of these children today because of the risk of thyroid malignancy. Prednisone, 2 to 4 mg/kg per day, and β-blockers, such as propranolol, are quite beneficial if the hemangioma is growing quickly and causing thrombocytopenia. The side effects of interferon-α are so substantial as to preclude use in most cases as of this writing. Dramatic regression of the hemangioma and prompt correction of the thrombocytopenia with the use of these agents have been reported, although both have also been associated with significant side effects.[58]

Tracheal Anomalies

Intrinsic Tracheal Compression

Tracheomalacia. Tracheomalacia results from a failure of the cartilaginous rings to fully support the round shape of the normal trachea. The cartilages are hypoplastic and allow the trachea to collapse, especially during expiration (Fig. 36-7). This condition is commonly seen in babies and children undergoing bronchoscopic evaluation but is only incidentally responsible for stridor in a moderate number of them. Because obstruction of the airway tends to occur as the trachea collapses with expiration, stridor occurs at that time. The condition is diffuse and usually occurs throughout the length of the trachea.

Diagnosis is most simply achieved by bronchoscopy. After the scope is passed through the vocal cords, the trachea assumes a transverse or ovoid appearance, which is accentuated as expiration takes place. It is frequently difficult to see the carina as the scope advances through the trachea because of the collapse of the anterior wall. Despite some rather marked findings in some children, this lesion rarely necessitates any treatment, and it can be expected to resolve spontaneously with growth and maturation.

Tracheal Stenosis. Tracheal stenosis can involve either a short stenotic segment in an otherwise normal trachea or the entire trachea with a cylindrical tapering from the subglottic region (Fig. 36-8).[59] Either form may demonstrate a fixed

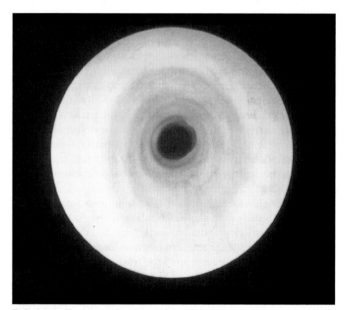

FIG 36-8 Endoscopic view of tracheal stenosis as a result of complete tracheal rings tapering to a narrow lumen.

obstruction resulting in inspiratory and expiratory stridor. Tracheal cartilages are often absent when this occurs, and instability of the tracheal lumen is not uncommon.

Depending on the severity of the stenosis and its length, affected children may have severe respiratory distress with cyanosis. Respiratory sounds may be weak, and the danger of sudden and acute obstruction is quite possible. Bronchoscopy is the best study to confirm the diagnosis.

Necrotizing Tracheobronchitis. The necrotizing tracheobronchitis lesion is mainly of historical interest after having been reported in two relatively large series from two different institutions, and numerous case reports and a small series have followed.[60,61] It is a necrotizing process that results in sloughing of the tracheal mucosa. Although the cause is unknown, it seems to be associated with hypoperfusion (such as a difficult birth requiring extensive resuscitation) and the use of high-frequency ventilators. With improvement of ventilator humidification, very few cases have been reported recently.

Clinical presentation primarily involves deterioration of respiratory status. Affected babies generally manifest sudden carbon dioxide retention that fails to respond to changes in ventilator settings, change of ETT, or intratracheal suctioning. Mortality is high unless suspicion of the lesion leads to bronchoscopy and mechanical clearing of the airway.[62] Moreover, even if a child is able to recover from an acute episode, recurrent necrotizing tracheobronchitis or chronic strictures may result.[63]

Extrinsic Tracheal Compression

Cystic Hygroma. Cystic hygromas have been reported to reach sufficient size and extension to result in compression of the trachea, thus resulting in stridor.[64] When these lesions are severe enough to result in stridor, they almost always produce respiratory distress and require surgical intervention. The goal of the initial treatment is to relieve the compression, which may be achieved by simple aspiration of fluid from the cyst. This can be followed by bronchoscopy to rule out the possibility of associated laryngotracheal anomaly and by surgical extirpation of the cyst.[57] Cystic hygromas are benign lesions, and as such, critical structures must be preserved during resection whenever possible.

Vascular Rings. Vascular rings arise from anomalous formation of the great vessels that cross over or encircle the trachea and the esophagus. The variety of anomalies is quite extensive, but the few categories that commonly occur and lead to problems can be classified under four to six headings. Those structures usually responsible for congenital stridor are the double aortic arch, the right aortic arch with left ductus arteriosus or ligamentum arteriosum, and the anomalous innominate artery. More rarely, an anomalous right subclavian artery (Fig. 36-9), an anomalous left pulmonary artery sling, or an anomalous left common carotid artery may give rise to symptoms. For technical accuracy, only a few of these conditions should be considered true vascular rings that are complete encirclement of the trachea and esophagus by vascular structures. Specifically, these lesions include the double aortic arch and the right aortic arch with left ductus. The others are more correctly referred to as *slings* because they pass around the trachea or esophagus and compress one or the other, but do not completely encircle them. Stridor in affected neonates is present at birth or by 1 to 2 months of age. With the fixed nature of the obstruction, stridor is both inspiratory and expiratory. Afflicted infants have a brassy, barking cough. If the compression of the vascular anomaly affects the esophagus, as it does in a few cases, the neonate may have associated problems with deglutition, such as regurgitation, vomiting, and aspiration.

Evaluation of these infants begins with a barium swallow, which usually shows a single or double oblique indentation on the esophagus.[65] Subsequent bronchoscopy often reveals the pulsatile compressing mass passing over the anterior portion of the trachea on either the right or the left side.[66] Depending on the location of the indentation, a presumptive diagnosis can be made. Also, one can occasionally compress the pulsatile area to check for disappearance of pulses to suggest which of the vascular anomalies is present. In most of these cases, CT or MRI with contrast materials gives wonderfully accurate pictures of the exact anatomy.

Treatment of these lesions[67] is essentially surgical division of the ring when one is present. In cases of double aortic arch or right arch with left ductus arteriosus, division of the ring at its narrowest portion or ductal ligation and division usually result in considerable improvement. In the case of sling lesions, the offending vessel may be divided (as in treatment of the anomalous right subclavian artery) with or without reanastomosis. If transection alone does not relieve the obstruction, dissection of the trachea and esophagus with vessel suspension to the anterior chest wall has been performed with considerable improvement of symptoms.

All of these operations may be performed through a standard left thoracotomy, and results have been quite acceptable in several large review series.[68-70] The anomalous left pulmonary artery sling is fortunately one of the rarest of the vascular slings and continues to be the most difficult to handle surgically, with consequently a greater surgical morbidity/mortality rate.[71,72]

Families must be warned that a residual tracheal deformity and tracheomalacia will persist after surgery and that stridor may not abate for 6 to 24 months.

Developmental Abnormalities of the Lung
Pulmonary and Lobar Agenesis

In intrauterine life, an entire lung or a portion of a lung may fail to develop. The etiology is not definitively known, but sufficient cases have been reported in neonates to document that little effect is seen with lobar agenesis. However, a right or left pulmonary agenesis generally creates respiratory distress and has a significant mortality. Interestingly, mortality seems to be greatest when the lung missing is the right lung. Numerous associated anomalies have been reported in all the organ systems.

Generally, a neonate born with this problem requires immediate intubation. Chest radiograph shows an opaque hemithorax with narrowed rib spaces and variable mediastinal shift. If the chest radiograph has been sufficiently penetrating, it may be possible to see the absence of a carina or a blind-ended bronchial stump. Endoscopy confirms the agenesis.

After intubation and stabilization, attempts are made to wean the neonate from ventilatory support. In the event of success and survival, the neonate is at risk for recurrent pulmonary infection.

Pulmonary Hypoplasia

Pulmonary hypoplasia is discussed elsewhere in this text in terms of ventilatory management (Chapters 14 and 32). However, there are several lesions that are well known to produce pulmonary hypoplasia from lung compression. The most recognized is the diaphragmatic hernia, but large intrauterine tumors such as tonsillar or head/neck teratomas can produce the same result. In

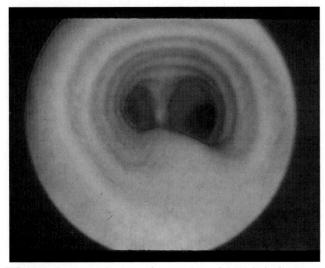

FIG 36-9 Endoscopic view of anomalous right subclavian artery with impingement on the tracheal membrane.

cases such as diaphragmatic hernia, surgical intervention may be necessary, but the airway is usually not involved.

Congenital Lobar Emphysema

Congenital lobar emphysema,[73,74] frequently referred to as CLE, is extremely rare, usually present at birth or apparent within the first 6 months, and is of unknown etiology. The mechanism of development is a ball–valve obstruction leading to overinflation of a lung lobe. This obstruction is attributed to deficient cartilage formation in the bronchi accompanied by bronchomalacia. However, fully half of the lungs removed as therapy fail to show any significant anatomic abnormality other than hyperinflation. Most series report a male preponderance of 2:1.

The pattern of involvement is surprisingly consistent, involving the upper lobes, first the left upper lobe (40% to 45% of cases), then the right middle lobe (30% to 35% of cases), and finally the right upper lobe (20% to 25% of cases). Rarely, two lobes are affected at the same time, and a few reports of metachronous involvement of two lobes have been described.

Respiratory distress, possibly with cyanosis, is the presenting symptom. Intubation may stabilize the situation, especially if the intubation is bronchial in the unaffected lung. In fact, bronchial intubation may result in resolution of hyperinflation that fails to return when the endobronchial tube is removed. Mild cases may be observed, but severe distress requires thoracotomy and lobectomy. Chest X-ray alone is often sufficient for the diagnosis, based on hyperinflation, widened rib space, mediastinal shift, and collapse of the other lung. CT and V̇/Q̇ scanning have been advocated to confirm the diagnosis and add anatomic information, but in most cases these modalities are not necessary.

Congenital Cystic Adenomatoid Malformation

Congenital cystic adenomatoid malformation (CCAM) is, again, a rare pulmonary malformation that affects all lobes, affects both sexes, and produces nonfunctional pulmonary tissue that has cysts, increased amounts of cellular elements, and abnormalities of cartilage, elastin, and other tissues.[75-77] The cystic component may be microcystic or macrocystic. The respiratory compromise is caused by space occupation with nonfunctioning pulmonary tissue that produces respiratory distress and a predilection for infection (Fig. 36-10).

All lobes may be involved with this process; there is no sex preponderance. Maternal polyhydramnios is common, and one in four neonates affected will die from nonimmune hydrops. The clinical presentation of these patients is quite variable. Some neonates have no symptoms at birth; others are severely compromised. Many of these infants are now diagnosed with prenatal ultrasound, so planning can be done to support the newborn at birth in case respiratory compromise is severe.

Space occupation and mediastinal shift may compromise a neonate at birth. Resection and removal may be completely curative therapy, but many of these infants have mild or severe pulmonary hypoplasia and pulmonary hypertension. Surgery will not solve these problems, so recourse to extracorporeal life support (ECMO), long-term ventilation, and all the various modalities of ventilation and pharmacologic therapies may be necessary. Despite this gamut of therapies, some children have inadequate lung volume for survival (particularly those with severe mediastinal shift and marked polyhydramnios in utero).

Sequestration

Sequestrations[78-81] are masses of pulmonary tissue that do not attach to the bronchopulmonary tree. In other words, they are sequestered segments of mesoderm that should have contributed to the alveolar mass of the lung on the side where they are found. The exact etiology is unknown, but this lesion seems to affect males three or four to one over females, involves the lower lobes more frequently than the upper, has a systemic arterial blood supply, and often has an anomalous venous drainage system.

Symptoms occur when these sequestrations become infected or attain a size that results in significant space occupation (often because they have become a huge intrathoracic abscess). Antibiotic therapy and fluid resuscitation may be the initial treatment, but surgical resection is eventually necessary.

Sequestrations are often divided into two groups depending on the proximity of the sequestered mass to the actual lung. Those immediately adjacent or within a lobe are called *intralobar* (Fig. 36-11). Those more remote and often with a complete pleura covering are called *extralobar*. The latter group is often seen with other anomalies; about half of the extralobar type occur around the opening of a diaphragmatic hernia.

These lesions have a systemic arterial blood supply, generally arising as a direct branch from the aorta. Often, this systemic arterial supply originates from the thoracic aorta and traverses the diaphragm. This is also frequently seen with CCAM, and the similarity of some of these characteristics has led to the

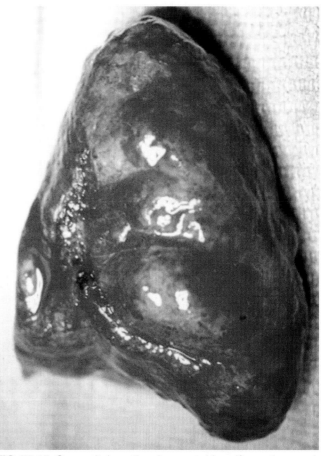

FIG 36-10 Congenital cystic adenomatoid malformation—red, beefy lobe from lung with increased terminal alveolar tissue.

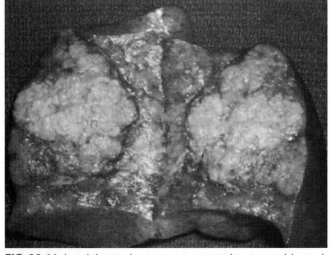

FIG 36-11 Intralobar pulmonary sequestration treated by pulmonary lobectomy.

suggestion that these lesions may represent a spectrum of developmental pulmonopathy.

Pulmonary Cystic Lesions

Pulmonary cystic lesions[82-84] may be developmental or acquired. Within the first group are the bronchogenic cysts and the duplication cysts. In all these lesions, sequestration or maldevelopment of some portion of the tracheobronchial tree or foregut results in the development of a cystic lesion that may grow over time, especially if there is a secretory lining. Within the group of acquired lesions are the cysts that result from barotrauma secondary to prolonged intubation, ventilation, suctioning, and recurrent infection. These often appear later in the neonatal course, having not been evident on X-ray at birth.

Size can vary from small to enormous, and these can essentially replace an entire lung. Symptoms result from space occupation or infection. Often infection creates the increase in size (abscess) that finally leads to the diagnosis of the lesion. Plain radiography is generally sufficient to make this diagnosis, but barium swallow, CT, and MRI may all occasionally be needed.

Generally, surgical resection is the best solution because it eliminates the chance of infection and prevents any further enlargement and anatomic displacement. If the baby is ventilator dependent on high settings, a ventilation strategy such as low-volume high-frequency ventilation may be necessary to prevent a recurrence in other areas of the lung postoperatively.

Developmental Abnormalities of the Diaphragm

Only three conditions need be considered here: diaphragmatic hernia, diaphragmatic paralysis, and diaphragmatic eventration. Concerning diaphragmatic hernias, only the congenital diaphragmatic hernia of Bochdalek is of concern clinically because the other hernias are rare, and seldom do any of them create major respiratory problems in the neonatal period.

Diaphragmatic Hernia of Bochdalek

The posterolateral diaphragmatic hernia, most common on the left as described by Bochdalek, occurs in approximately 1 in 5000 live births.[85-88] The etiology is unclear but we now have a rat model in which the diaphragmatic defect and the pulmonary hypoplasia can be induced by maternal ingestion of the teratogen Nitrofan

(2,4-dichlorophenyl-p-nitrophenyl ether; generic name nitrofurantoin). The diaphragmatic hernia is complicated by serious pulmonary hypoplasia that exists not only on the side of the diaphragmatic defect but is also often found in the contralateral lung.

Many neonates afflicted with this problem have associated anomalies and die in utero. Those who survive to term are generally fairly large and surprisingly free of other problems. Males comprise about two-thirds of the reported cases.

Many of these cases are now diagnosed prenatally, and sufficient data are now available to prognosticate on ultimate outcome in a general fashion. Neonates who have a small chest consistent with pulmonary hypoplasia; large amounts of abdominal viscera within the chest, particularly the left lobe of the liver; and marked mediastinal shift can be expected to have severe problems at the time of birth and often are nonsurvivors. In marked contrast are the babies born without symptoms or babies who are not diagnosed until 1 to 2 months of age. Virtually all of these children are survivors.

Presentation is generally some degree of respiratory distress that requires intubation at birth or shortly thereafter. Those who are tolerating the lesions without problems or who have minimal symptoms are brought to elective repair when other anomalies have been excluded and pulmonary hypertension has had a chance to abate. For those who require immediate intubation, a large number of therapeutic ventilation programs with the addition of nitric oxide have proven quite successful.

Those who fail these modalities can be taken to ECMO with ultimate repair on the pump or after successful decannulation (see Chapter 40), although the latter approach may have advantages of diminished hemorrhage after completion of anticoagulation. Use of all the modalities has produced survival rates that are near 80% today compared to historical reports of 40% survival.

Diaphragmatic Paralysis/Eventration

Diaphragmatic paralysis and eventration can be lumped together because it is virtually impossible to distinguish them from each other. They look alike and act in a similar fashion. If a neonate has had a traumatic birth and has other neurologic deficits or if the baby has undergone intrathoracic surgery, it is reasonable to assume that the child has paralysis. If those conditions are not met, it is just as likely to be one lesion as the other.

In both conditions, one or both diaphragms assume a high position on chest X-ray and may compromise function of the lung. Fluoroscopy for paradoxical motion suggests paralysis, but a thin, attenuated muscle may give very similar results. In addition to the space problems, the paradoxical motion creates increased work of breathing, tires the baby, and makes effective spontaneous ventilation difficult.

If either of these conditions is present but asymptomatic, the situation can be observed. Obviously, if the baby needs ventilation, some future action may be needed. The literature is replete with recommendations, none based on any good objective data, that suggest diaphragmatic plication be done in 3 to 6 weeks if the neonate cannot be weaned from ventilation. These recommendations do not seem unreasonable because intubation and ventilation are not without their own risks and complications. The folding and suturing of the diaphragm creates a stable platform against which the other diaphragm can effectively achieve normal or near-normal breathing.

Developmental Abnormalities of the Skeleton

There are a host of skeletal anomalies that result in thoracic asphyxiation at the time of birth or shortly thereafter. These are beyond the scope of this chapter, but the reader should be aware that there are some surgical expansion procedures offered in a limited number of institutions in the United States that can increase thoracic volume and hold some small promise for some of these children.

THE PEDIATRIC SURGEON/OTOLARYNGOLOGIST AS CONSULTANT

Neonatal Bronchoscopy

The increased frequency of long-term neonatal intubation and the survival of children with severe respiratory difficulties have been associated with increased airway complications. The pediatric surgeon has an important role in the evaluation of congenital stridor, persistent atelectasis, and ETT position or patency and as an aid in difficult intubations.[89]

Anatomic Considerations

A neonate's air passages are obviously smaller than those of an adult or a larger child, and this increases their vulnerability to obstruction.[90] Care must be observed during bronchoscopy because the mucosa of these patients is softer, looser, and more fragile. The location of the epiglottis and larynx of the neonate's airway is more cephalad and anterior than an adult's. Of note, the cricoid cartilage is the narrowest point in an infant's upper airway. This feature not only makes the use of a cuffed ETT usually unnecessary in this population but also increases the risk of the complication of subglottic stenosis from pressure during prolonged intubation. Furthermore, at an infant's carina, the main stem bronchi angulate almost symmetrically, unlike the anatomy in older children and adults.

Pathophysiology

Edema is the minimum adverse effect of endotracheal intubation. If intubation continues for longer than a few hours, acute inflammation becomes superimposed on edema. This proceeds over days and weeks to mucosal ulceration, submucosal inflammation, chondritis, cartilage fragmentation, and tracheomalacia. The body's reparative response to these changes is fibrosis and scarring, which, if severe, results in laryngotracheal stenosis.

To minimize this cycle of destruction when intubation is mandatory, an ETT of appropriate size should be used. Furthermore, the ETT should be fixed in position to minimize lateral or horizontal motion. Finally, all attempts should be made to shorten the time necessary for intubation. Some clinicians advocate nasotracheal intubation and fixation for prolonged intubation, but this technique has the same serious adverse sequelae associated with orotracheal intubation and has the added risk of nasopharyngeal trauma and potential for sinusitis.

Evaluation of Intubation

Because the majority of patients admitted to most NICUs for intubation and ventilatory support are treated medically, the role of the surgeon is primarily one of consultation. Improved techniques for orotracheal and nasotracheal intubation and the use of noninvasive ventilation and nasal CPAP have shortened the time of intubation in most units. The development of better neonatal ventilators makes it quite possible to maintain most infants safely on respiratory support for 6 to 8 weeks with minimal concern for permanent pressure damage to the airway. After 6 to 8 weeks of endotracheal intubation, one should consider bronchoscopic evaluation to determine whether damage

has occurred and whether continued intubation is appropriate management (see Tracheostomy). For a list of other indications for diagnostic bronchoscopy, see Box 36-1.

Endoscopes

Excellent rigid and flexible endoscopes are now available for examination of the neonatal airway. In addition, ultrathin flexible bronchoscopes are available that allow examination of the tracheobronchial tree through ETTs. The scopes are available in diameters from 1.3 to 2.7 mm.[91,92] They allow bronchoscopic examination without major disruption to positive-pressure ventilation when a Y-adaptor (Vigo, France) is used between the ETT and the ventilator. These scopes are easy to maneuver, and serious complications such as perforation are unlikely. As such, these procedures are as safe to perform in the NICU as in the operative theater. Unfortunately, the majority of these scopes do not provide capabilities for significant lavage or suction, and their resolution is somewhat limited. Furthermore, scopes of sizes smaller than 2.7 mm do not have flexible tips.

One role for flexible bronchoscopy is aiding in difficult intubations of a neonate. With the new ultrathin flexible endoscopes, it is possible to place an ETT under direct vision by passing the tube over the bronchoscope. This can be particularly useful in neonates with congenital airway obstruction or craniofacial anomalies. The flexible endoscopes can also rapidly provide information about ETT position and patency. For major diagnostic and all therapeutic procedures, however, rigid bronchoscopy performed by an experienced bronchoscopist provides the maximum yield. Performed with appropriate anesthesia, lighting, and suction, rigid bronchoscopy is associated with minimal morbidity and mortality.

Rigid scopes, such as those provided by Storz equipped with Hopkins telescopes, are available for neonates in sizes from 2.5 to 4.0 mm. These provide superb illumination and magnification for inspection as well as an adequate lumen through which to insert tubes or instruments. A technique for using the Hopkins telescope without the sheath but instead inserting it directly through an ETT via a Y-adapter has also been described and allows continuation of endotracheal intubation and positive-pressure ventilation throughout the procedure.[93]

Both flexible and rigid scopes can easily be used in the NICU when the condition of a baby precludes moving him or her to the operating room; consequently, it is rare for an infant to be denied an endoscopic examination when diagnostic or therapeutic benefits are likely.

If an ETT has been in place for several weeks, mucosal edema, petechiae, and erythema are inevitable. The finding of worse sequelae of intubation indicates that these patients should undergo tracheostomy. Mucosal erosion, granulation and early fibrosis, and ultimately stricture are ominous signs and will probably progress if irritation from the ETT continues.

Tracheostomy

Although physicians at some centers would continue endotracheal intubation if no damage is encountered on evaluation of the airway, many clinicians would proceed with neonatal tracheostomy after prolonged periods of continuous intubation (generally 6 to 8 weeks). Such a procedure helps respiratory function by decreasing the work of breathing and reducing dead space and makes oral motor activity possible for the baby. Tracheostomy should also be seriously considered for infants who manifest central nervous system failure, severe bronchopulmonary dysplasia, or complex cardiovascular disease or in whom an ETT is inadequate for maintaining pulmonary toilet.

The specific technique of neonatal tracheostomy varies little from a well-performed tracheostomy at any age. Except in dire emergency, when a needle cricothyroidotomy is the preferred approach, neonatal tracheostomy should be performed under operating room conditions, and the infant should be intubated before the surgical procedure begins.

Procedure

After the landmarks of the anterior triangle of the neck are well established, a transverse or midline skin incision can be made (Fig. 36-12). The choice of skin incision used appears to make little difference in the overall outcome and should reflect the preference and experience of the operating surgeon. Once the skin and subcutaneous tissues have been opened, midline dissection is mandatory to prevent damage to vascular or neural structures. Division of the thyroid isthmus may occasionally be necessary and can easily be performed with electrocautery (Fig. 36-13). Either a simple transverse[94] or a T-type tracheal incision is performed in neonatal cases (Fig. 36-14). Stay sutures, often called *trapdoor* sutures, are placed through the cartilages of the tracheostomy site at the time the initial incision into the trachea

is made. If reintubation in the early postoperative period is necessary, these sutures aid the replacement, decrease the trauma of replacement, and may prevent placement into subcutaneous tissues. At no time should cartilaginous rings or portions of them be removed, because this almost inevitably results in stricture formation if decannulation is successful in the future.[95–99]

Because a neonatal tracheostomy is performed over an ETT if possible, the ETT is removed under direct vision as the tracheostomy tube is inserted (Fig. 36-15). This ensures control of the neonatal airway throughout the entire procedure. Finally, fixation of the tube is critical, because dislodgment in the postoperative period can be fatal if experienced personnel are unable to reinsert the tube immediately. Consequently, the tube must be tied securely by those familiar with this technique; alternatively,

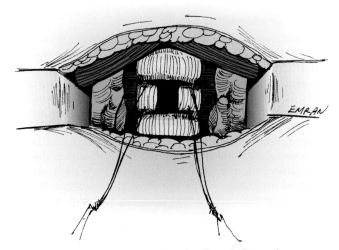

FIG 36-14 The tracheal opening is dilated. Retention sutures are sewn through the cartilages to aid postoperative reinsertion if necessary. No tracheal cartilage is removed at any time.

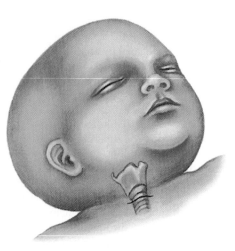

FIG 36-12 Transverse skin incision over tracheal rings (1 to 3).

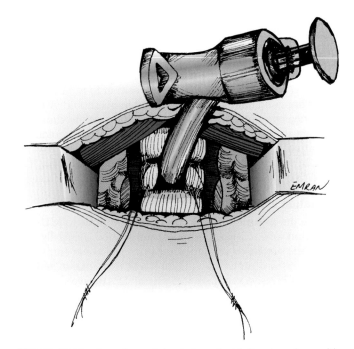

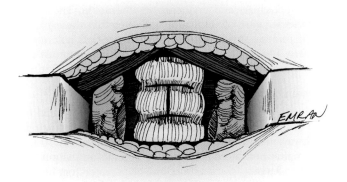

FIG 36-13 Platysma and strap muscles retracted laterally to allow midline dissection to the trachea. The thyroid isthmus is retracted or cut as necessary.

FIG 36-15 Tracheostomy tube is inserted following slow withdrawal of the endotracheal tube under direct vision.

the tube may be sutured directly to the lateral aspects of the neck (Fig. 36-16).

Despite all efforts to prevent tracheostomy dislodgment, these events still occur. If the tracheostomy becomes dislodged in the perioperative period prior to maturation of the tracheostomy tract, replacement of the tracheostomy tube can be quite difficult despite the presence of stay sutures. Recannulation of the trachea through the neck wound can be attempted and if successful resolves the problem. It should be noted, though, that if recannulation through the neck wound is unsuccessful, then definitive airway control should be obtained through orotracheal intubation. In the meantime until definitive airway control is obtained, patients can be bag–valve ventilated as a sufficient temporizing measure with simple digital occlusion of the neck wound/tracheotomy to prevent loss of the tidal volumes through the neck wound.

Anterior Cricoid Split Procedure

The improved survival of premature infants who require prolonged intubation has increased the incidence of complications associated with long-term intubation. As an alternative method of management, instead of tracheostomy in neonates with early stages of subglottic stenosis, Cotton and Seid[100] have recommended an anterior cricoid split procedure performed over an ETT. This procedure involves a transverse skin incision and a longitudinal incision through the cricoid cartilage and upper two tracheal rings as well as through the underlying mucosa (Fig. 36-17). The soft tissues of the neck are then reapproximated over the defect via a single-layer (skin) closure. After this procedure, the patient remains intubated for several weeks, during which time the mucosa heals by fibrosis, and tracheal stability is reestablished (Fig. 36-18). Finally, extubation is attempted when the trachea is healed.

Experience with this technique has shown it to be a reasonable alternative to tracheostomy in the treatment of subglottic stenosis. Its use results in about a 75% rate of successful extubation. Unfortunately, reintubation and positive-pressure ventilation put the patient at risk of potential aerocele or fistulas if he or she subsequently undergoes respiratory failure once again.[101,102] Therefore, these patients should be carefully selected for the anterior cricoid split procedure. Tracheostomy should remain the gold standard of treatment for the majority of neonates with complications associated with prolonged endotracheal intubation.

Tracheostomy Tubes

The choice of an appropriate tracheostomy tube is as important as the correct technique of tracheostomy placement. The soft, pliable, polyvinyl chloride tubes manufactured under the Shiley and Portex trade names are best suited to the neonatal

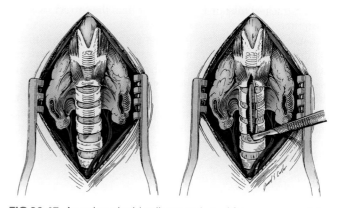

FIG 36-17 Anterior cricoid split procedure. After exposure of the anterior surface of the cricoid cartilage and upper two tracheal rings, a vertical incision is made through the cricoid and tracheal rings. Exposure of the endotracheal tube along the length of the split indicates completion of the procedure. (From Drake AF, Babyak JW, Niparko JK, et al. The anterior cricoid split: clinical experience with extended indications. *Arch Otolaryngol Head Neck Surg.* 1988;114:1405. [Copyright 1988, American Medical Association.])

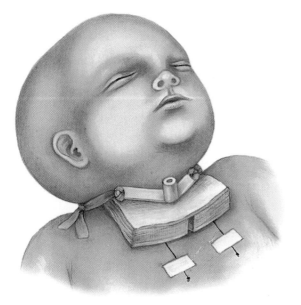

FIG 36-16 Completed tracheostomy with dressing and tapes in place.

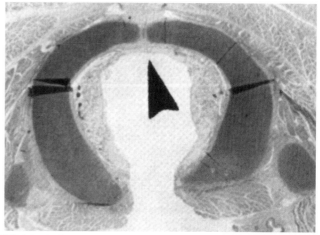

FIG 36-18 Cross-sectional specimen obtained at autopsy from a patient who had previously undergone an anterior cricoid split. The *arrow* indicates the site of the cricoid split (the posterior opening was created by the pathologist during autopsy). (From Cotton RT, Seid AB. Management of the extubation problem in the premature child: anterior cricoid split as an alternative to tracheostomy. *Ann Otol Rhinol Laryngol.* 1980;89:510.)

airway. The Aberdeen tube, a silicone elastomer tube, is also an excellent alternative but is available in fewer sizes. These tubes remain pliable at physiologic body temperature and conform well to individual anatomy. Additionally, the balloons associated with cuffed tracheostomy tubes are designed to exert less pressure on the tracheal walls. These factors reduce trauma and the risk of subsequent stricture formation in cases of prolonged mechanical ventilation. Additionally, the softer tubes are more comfortable for a patient and reduce the chances of cervical skin irritation or abrasions from sharp metal edges. Rigid metal tracheostomy tubes are contraindicated in this population.

If a patient undergoing tracheostomy has an ETT in place, the size of the ETT can be used to guide the selection of a tracheostomy tube of appropriate size. A reasonably reliable rule is that the tracheostomy tube can be 0.5 mm larger than the correct orotracheal tube or 1.0 mm larger than the correct nasotracheal tube.

Choosing a tube of proper length is usually more difficult than finding the proper diameter. At birth, tracheal length for the normal term birth-weight infants is a maximum of 5 to 6 cm. Even a very short tracheostomy tube may lie dangerously close to the carina and risk right or left main stem bronchus intubation with subsequent exclusion of the other bronchus and lung. Alternatively, if the tube is too short and lies high in the neck, the chance of dislodgment is increased. Generally pediatric tubes are 3 to 6 mm longer than neonatal tubes of the same diameter and can be used if the neonatal tube of the appropriate width is too short. Today, all the manufacturers will provide custom-constructed tubes, usually with only a 2- to 3-day delay in delivery. Consequently, it is possible to request the appropriately sized tube.

Once a tracheostomy is in place with adequate tract formation, daily changing of the dressing and weekly changing of the tube seem adequate when coupled with fastidious tracheostomy care provided by the nursing staff. Generally, it is best to have the surgeon or his or her service make the first tracheostomy tube change. Once it has been established that the tract is well healed and tubes can be removed and replaced without major problems, the nurse and family members may assume this task. An alternative tube should always be available at the bedside. This is cleansed with soap and water, stored in a clean container, and used in the event that sudden replacement is necessary. Suctioning is performed as necessary to keep the airway clear of secretions to maintain adequate pulmonary hygiene and decrease the risk of pulmonary infectious complications, and details of suctioning are similar to those for ETTs (see Chapter 12).

REFERENCES

A complete reference list is available at https://expertconsult.inkling.com/.

37

Intraoperative Management of the Neonate

Christopher E. Colby, MD, and Malinda N. Harris, MD

The neonatal patient requiring surgery presents a unique challenge in the delivery of safe and effective airway management, ventilation, sedation, and anesthesia. The physiology of the neonate is unique and cannot simply be extrapolated from experiences with the older pediatric surgical patient. This chapter will begin with a review of fetal lung development, transitional physiology, and congenital anomalies as they pertain to the development of operative ventilation strategies. The remainder of the chapter will explore the procedural components that may improve patient safety and outcomes such as a risk and facilities assessment to determine if the patient is best served by undergoing the operation in the intensive care unit or the standard operating theater.

When considering operative intervention for the neonate, a multidisciplinary preoperative review of clinical status, with consideration given to anatomic complexities, current modality and degree of respiratory support, medications, and recent laboratory and radiographic data, should be performed. In preparation for the operation, a thoughtful approach to premedication for intubation and selection of the appropriate endotracheal tube is recommended. The use of a standardized checklist in the perioperative period may facilitate enhancing the situational awareness of the patient's condition during these important transitions of care (Table 37-1). During the operation, ventilation of the patient may be performed successfully using vigilant monitoring of the vital signs and blood gas parameters.

"Children are not simply small adults" is a tenet within pediatrics. An accurate reinterpretation of this maxim could be "Neonates are not simply small children." The acutely ill newborn population is often cohorted in the neonatal intensive care unit (NICU) until the first discharge from the hospital. Despite the commonality of location, the physiology and developmental status of the pulmonary system for patients within the NICU are heterogeneous. A fetus delivered at a gestational age considered at the margin of viability will have lungs with marked developmental immaturities. The pulmonary system of this patient may be in the canalicular stage of development, reliant on newly formed acini as the basic structure for gas exchange with a paucity of both alveolar development and surfactant production by type II pneumocytes. Unique physiology is also encountered in the NICU. The transition from fetal to extrauterine circulation may occur without interruption after birth or may present ongoing management challenges for the patient who requires surgery during the first several days of life. Concerns for pulmonary hypertension may persist for some neonates as a sequela of ventilator dependence, birth depression, prematurity, or congenital anomalies. Finally, congenital anomalies requiring surgical intervention necessitate a disease- and patient-specific management plan to account for challenges that may be encountered during the operation.

TRANSITIONAL PHYSIOLOGY AND PULMONARY HYPERTENSION

During pregnancy the fetus is dependent on gas exchange, which occurs at the level of the placenta. For centuries, the uterus had been referred to as the *uterine lung*.[1] This description is appropriate, as development of the fetus requires oxygen delivery and elimination of carbon dioxide through the placenta. Both maternal and fetal blood flow to the placenta increases throughout gestation. Oxygenated blood is supplied to the fetus through the umbilical vein and returns to the placenta through the umbilical arteries. This unique circulation results in an oxygen saturation of approximately 60% in the term fetus prior to delivery.[2]

Once the baby is delivered and the umbilical cord is clamped, the newborn is dependent on ventilation occurring at the level of the alveolar capillary interface. With spontaneous breathing, the lungs become inflated and stretch receptors are activated, which promote pulmonary vasodilation. Inspired oxygen and the newborn's production of endogenous nitric oxide result in a decrease in pulmonary vascular resistance. Shunts at the level of the foramen ovale and ductus arteriosus, which had previously been very important in fetal development, close. The transition from fetal to extrauterine circulation is clinically apparent within the first 10 minutes of life. The immediate newborn oxygen saturation level will reflect the native fetal oxygen saturation of approximately 60%, but by 10 minutes of life the preductal oxygen saturation should increase to greater than 90%.

This transition to extrauterine circulation can be delayed in some newborns. The diagnosis of persistent pulmonary hypertension (historically referred to as persistent fetal circulation) should be suspected if the baby does not have primary lung disease (e.g., surfactant deficiency, aspiration syndrome) and is requiring additional oxygen to maintain ideal oxygen saturations and if there is a significant difference in oximetry measured in the preductal (right hand) and postductal location (left hand or either foot). The differential diagnosis for persistent pulmonary hypertension of the newborn (PPHN) is found in Table 37-2 (and further discussed in Chapters 14 and 32). Pulmonary vascular resistance will often decrease throughout the first several days of life. This can be assessed through serial echocardiography, the difference in pre- and postductal saturation levels, and a bedside evaluation of the fraction of inspired oxygen required to maintain ideal preductal saturations.

TABLE 37-1   Perioperative Checklist to Facilitate Transitions of Care

Presurgical	Postsurgical
Gestational age	Estimated blood loss
Pertinent medical history	Modifications to preoperative mode of ventilation
Current mode of ventilation	Description of intraoperative patient stability
Review of recent labs and radiographs	Medications administered during operation
Medication list and dosing	Intraoperative blood gas review
Airway status including type and depth of artificial airway	Challenges or complications that occurred intraoperatively
Confirm consent has been obtained	Operation performed
	Status of parental postoperative update

TABLE 37-2   Differential Diagnosis of Pulmonary Hypertension

Persistent fetal circulation (idiopathic)	Respiratory distress syndrome
	Hypothermia
Meconium aspiration	Chronic lung disease
Blood aspiration	Maternal medications
Pulmonary hypoplasia	• Nonsteroidal antiinflammatories
Congenital diaphragmatic hernia	• Selective serotonin reuptake inhibitors
Pneumonia/sepsis	

This is clinically relevant for the anesthetist when surgery is considered in the first postnatal days for a baby diagnosed with primary pulmonary disease with or without PPHN. If the baby is improving from the perspective of pulmonary hypertension, waiting to perform a nonemergent procedure may allow a greater margin for safety and effective ventilation during the case. Preoperative identification of a patient with a history of PPHN or lung disease who may develop PPHN intraoperatively allows the anesthetist to predict risk for rebound pulmonary hypertension and be prepared to recognize and initiate appropriate therapies.

The diagnosis of pulmonary hypertension may also become clinically relevant in the former premature infant with bronchopulmonary dysplasia (BPD). Premature infants with BPD are at risk for concomitant pulmonary hypertension, though it remains unclear which of the two is the principal diagnosis.[3-5] In most cases, infants with BPD and associated pulmonary hypertension will continue to require oxygen and sometimes diuretic supplementation for several months after birth. In severe cases, medications such as sildenafil may also be prescribed. These infants may present to the anesthetist just prior to discharge from the initial hospitalization for procedures including gastrostomy tube placement, inguinal herniorrhaphy, and intervention for progressive retinopathy of prematurity.

There are special considerations for the surgical patient with pulmonary hypertension. Ventilation strategies that were being utilized in the NICU prior to the operation may continue to be effective during the operation. These strategies typically include avoidance of hypoxemia and acidosis. Hypoxemia and acidosis increase pulmonary vascular resistance, placing strain on the right ventricle and worsening pulmonary hypertension. Pharmacologic and nonpharmacologic interventions to decrease pain and agitation are indicated. Inhaled nitric oxide, a selective pulmonary vasodilator, may be a component of the ventilation strategy utilized in the NICU and should be continued throughout the operation. Alternatively, it may be considered as an intraoperative rescue strategy through the mechanical ventilation circuit. Additional therapies considered in the treatment of pulmonary hypertension include milrinone or vasopressin as adjunctive intravenous infusions that may provide additional pulmonary vasodilatory effects. Milrinone may also affect systemic vascular resistance, necessitating vigilant blood pressure monitoring.

Key Points

- Common causes of pulmonary hypertension in the infant are delayed transition to extrauterine life, prematurity, and primary pulmonary disease.
- Suspect pulmonary hypertension if there is a significant difference in pre- and postductal oxygen saturation and an increased oxygen requirement.
- Intraoperative treatment strategies for patients with PPHN include avoidance of hypoxemia and acidosis, adequate sedation, and utilization of inhaled nitric oxide.

PULMONARY DEVELOPMENT AND LUNG INJURY

The diversity of size of patients within the NICU is remarkable. There may be a tenfold difference in weight of the smallest to largest patient. Beyond the marked variation in the birth weight of this population, the individual patients are at different stages of the lung development continuum. The smallest and often most premature babies are dependent on primordial gas exchange units within the lungs, whereas the largest patients may have progressed toward a fully developed alveolar capillary interface. Additionally, a patient who began life as a fragile extremely low birth-weight newborn may have developed BPD while hospitalized. Despite the appearance of a now robust infant approaching or past the estimated due date, the pulmonary system of the former premature patient may be markedly abnormal. Recognition of normal lung development stages and potential abnormal pathophysiology will allow the anesthetist to develop a ventilation strategy appropriate for the individual patient.

The respiratory system of many premature babies in the NICU may be at the canalicular stage, which typically occurs between 16 and 25 weeks of gestation. Characteristics of this stage of lung development include the formation of the earliest gas exchange units and early evidence of surfactant production by the type II pneumocytes. The lungs begin to develop both respiratory and nonrespiratory bronchioli. During this developmental stage, an extensive capillary network becomes progressively approximated to the epithelium of the developing airspaces.

Beyond 25 weeks the lung enters into the terminal sac stage of development. The appearance of mature alveoli may be seen as early as 28 weeks' gestation. Lung volume and surface area increase throughout this stage to allow for sufficient gas exchange.

Premature infants are at risk for the development of BPD, a disease in which there is arrest of lung maturation[6] (see Chapter 35). A multitude of factors may contribute to this pathology including the administration of exogenous corticosteroids, exposure to prolonged mechanical ventilation, and inadequate postnatal nutrition. Following the initial injury, further exposure to excessive oxygen delivered to the developing airway, mechanical ventilation, and barotrauma may activate release of cytokines, thus contributing to continued airway inflammation. BPD is characterized by reduced lung compliance and increased airway resistance. Radiographically, a heterogeneous appearance to the lung, with areas of atelectasis and hyperinflation, may be observed.

The patient may have a chronic supplemental oxygen requirement to achieve target oxygen saturations. Often the blood gas of infants with BPD will demonstrate a markedly compensated respiratory acidosis, with serum bicarbonate levels significantly above expected values. Blood gases in the operating room probably will continue to reflect a long-standing compensated hypercarbic baseline. Operative strategies to support adequate gas exchange while minimizing risks to the developing lung, such as utilizing lower tidal volumes and proper oxygen saturation limits, being used in the NICU may remain a viable option during the procedure.

Key Points

- Postnatally, premature infants continue to develop sufficient gas exchange by maturation of the alveolar capillary interface.
- Premature infants are at risk for BPD and require lung-protective ventilatory strategies such as lower tidal volumes and oxygen saturation limits to prevent exposure to barotraumas and excess oxygen exposure.
- Infants with BPD have reduced lung compliance and increased airway resistance; they may require supplemental oxygen and unique ventilator strategies intraoperatively.

Intraoperative homeostasis for a chronic BPD patient may be to replicate the compensated respiratory acidosis from the preoperative state rather than the achievement of "normal" blood gases.

ANATOMIC CONSIDERATIONS

A variety of congenital anomalies requiring operative intervention shortly after birth are commonly encountered in the NICU. In the case of a thoracic anomaly, the lungs may be smaller than those of an equivalently aged healthy infant. Alternately, infants born with abdominal wall defects may have healthy lungs equivalent to those of healthy newborns, but the operation to repair the defect may cause a temporary reduction in total lung capacity and loss of functional residual capacity due to displacement of the diaphragm cephalad after restoration of the contents to an intra-abdominal position (Fig. 37-1).

Intrathoracic Masses

Infants with a prenatally diagnosed intrathoracic mass, such as a congenital diaphragmatic hernia (CDH) or a congenital pulmonary adenomatous malformation, are at high risk for pulmonary hypoplasia owing to abnormal fetal lung development. Pulmonary hypoplasia is most typically encountered in the lung ipsilateral to the mass, but in severe cases, both lungs may be significantly hypoplastic. In addition to pulmonary hypoplasia, a patient with CDH may have marked developmental abnormalities of the smooth muscle of the pulmonary vasculature leading to a severe form of PPHN. When viewed microscopically, the lungs of infants with CDH have fewer alveoli, increased interstitial tissue, thickened alveolar walls,[7] and pulmonary arteries

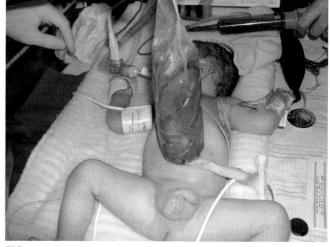

FIG 37-1 Newborn with gastroschisis. Compare the amount of intestine in the silo to the small abdominal cavity.

with increased medial and adventitial tissue present.[8] These findings and altered autonomic regulation are likely to unite to create higher pulmonary pressures, which are often "fixed," or not responsive to typical pulmonary vasodilators like inhaled nitric oxide.[9,10] In fact, the largest study as of this writing investigating the role of inhaled nitric oxide in patients with CDH demonstrated immediate short-term improvements in oxygenation in some treated infants but no reduction in the need for ECMO or death.[11]

Following delivery, infants with CDH are often ventilated over several days with a lung-protective strategy, minimizing exposure to barotrauma,[12] until pulmonary vascular resistance has decreased prior to operative interventions.[13-15] High-frequency ventilation with a high-frequency oscillator or jet ventilation may be considered. It is appropriate during the surgical repair of CDH to continue a lung-protective strategy while being mindful of recurrence of pulmonary hypertension. Although the entirety of the pulmonary hypertension in these patients may not be responsive to acute modulation, avoidance of hypoxemia and acidosis is recommended while monitoring for acute pulmonary vasculature hyperreactivity. Pulmonary hypertension in the setting of operative stress or alterations in pH and carbon dioxide levels may be recognized by continuous intraoperative monitoring of pre- and postductal saturations as well as continuous transcutaneous P_{CO_2} levels. An increasing difference between pre- and postductal saturations during the case suggests a right-to-left shunting of deoxygenated blood through the patent ductus arteriosus. At the time of hernia reduction, it is also important to maintain awareness of thoracic anatomy and recognize that as the tracheobronchial tree shifts toward midline, tube displacement could potentially occur, resulting in the tip of the endotracheal tube becoming located within the right main stem bronchus. This scenario should be considered if the patient develops worsening respiratory stability after the bowel has been reduced and the hernia repaired. Following the reduction of intestine and repair of the hernia, a "potential" space within the thoracic cavity remains on the affected side. In concept, this can be considered a pneumothorax ex vacuo, and this space will fill with fluid postoperatively. The decision to leave a chest tube in place at the end of the operation is dependent more on the surgeon's preference than evidence. Increasingly, pediatric surgeons are no longer leaving chest tubes in place following these types of repairs, which may prevent potential exposure of the hypoplastic lung to excess distention by allowing some fluid to accumulate in the intrapleural space.[16]

Abdominal Wall Defects

Infants with omphalocele and gastroschisis often have normal fetal lung development. Infants with giant omphaloceles are at risk for pulmonary hypoplasia,[17] most likely due to abnormal thoracic cage development related to liver displacement.[18,19] However, most often infants with abdominal wall defects are born at term, require no significant respiratory intervention at the time of birth, and remain without respiratory support until the time of surgery.

Some lesions, depending on the amount of displaced bowel content, can be replaced intra-abdominally in the first few hours of life. However, larger lesions may require a staged approach. Over the first days to week of life, attempts are made to reduce the bowel slowly into the relatively hypoplastic abdominal cavity through a silastic silo created soon after birth.[20] When the surgeon determines that bowel reduction from the silastic silo into the peritoneum is adequate, complete operative reduction and abdominal wall closure occur. Once the abdominal contents are reduced, intraperitoneal pressure increases, resulting in a reduction of total lung capacity and functional residual capacity (FRC). With a reduction in FRC, lung compliance decreases and the infant may require increased peak inspiratory pressures to maintain adequate minute ventilation. Positive end-expiratory pressure (PEEP) may need to be increased once the bowel has been reduced to preserve FRC. Maintaining appropriate minute ventilation may also be addressed by increasing the mandatory rate or through high-frequency ventilation. Postoperatively the use of pulmonary function studies may help guide ventilator management.

Key Points

- Intraoperative ventilation strategies for the patient with congenital anomalies should include consideration of how the anatomy may influence respiratory mechanics.
- Infants with thoracic anomalies are at high risk for pulmonary hypoplasia and require a lung-protective ventilatory strategy that minimizes barotrauma.
- Infants with abdominal wall defects can develop reduced total lung capacity following surgery and may require a ventilatory strategy that focuses on maintaining minute ventilation. This can be accomplished by an increased ventilation rate and lung recruitment through increased PEEP.
- An operative ventilatory strategy should include close monitoring for pulmonary vascular hyperreactivity for infants with pulmonary hypoplasia who are at high risk for pulmonary hypertension.

LOCATION OF OPERATION

Performing neonatal surgery in the intensive care unit is well described.[21-23] One of the primary incentives for operating at the patient's bedside is the inherent risk associated with transporting the unstable neonatal patient between the intensive care unit and the operating room. In addition to central line placement, the two most common neonatal surgeries that occur at the patient bedside are ligation of the patent ductus arteriosus

and laparotomy or peritoneal drain placement for necrotizing enterocolitis.[24,25] Other surgeries frequently performed at the bedside include reservoir placement for posthemorrhagic hydrocephalus and surgeries associated with extracorporeal membrane oxygenation including cannulation and decannulation. Though it may seem desirable to bring the surgeon to the baby's bedside, there is concern for and increased risk for infection and, of most concern, inadequate lighting in the operative field. At centers with experience bringing the operating team and requisite equipment to the intensive care unit, these interventions have been performed safely and with outcomes at least equivalent to, if not better than, transporting the patient to the operating room. The provider who will direct the ventilation during the operation will need to become familiar with mechanical ventilators that may not be commonly used in the operating room. This can be achieved by performing a presurgical briefing between the anesthesia team that will be managing the case and the neonatology team that has been providing care for the patient preoperatively. The mode of ventilation and recent blood gases should be discussed collaboratively to determine if change is necessary and anticipated prior to surgery. Once the operation has finished, a similar postsurgical debriefing should occur between teams to ensure a safe transition of care.

Premedication for Intubation

Neonatal tracheal intubation and mechanical ventilation support will probably be necessary for the operative procedure. Recent position statements recognize that intubation may need to proceed without premedication during an emergent resuscitation or in certain neonates with airway anomalies.[26,27] However, most presurgical neonatal intubations present an opportunity to provide premedication prior to insertion of the endotracheal tube. This painful procedure is known to induce apnea, hypoxemia, and bradycardia while causing increases in systemic and intracranial pressure.[28,29] Along with the technical skill required to successfully intubate, an evidence-based approach to selection of analgesia, sedation, vagolytics, and muscle relaxants is essential to optimize the quality of this procedure.

Providing adequate analgesia for this invasive procedure is indicated to provide patient comfort, avoid hypertension, and optimize intubation conditions. The ideal analgesic would be fast acting, with a short half-life and minimal side effects.

The opioids most commonly considered for neonatal premedication include natural (morphine) as well as synthetic (fentanyl and remifentanil) opioids. Administration of intravenous morphine results in peak analgesia in 15 minutes.[30] The clearance of morphine is gestational age dependent, with a longer half-life observed in premature infants compared to term.[31] Fentanyl has a rapid onset of action within 2 to 3 minutes and a short duration of action of 60 minutes.[32] Clearance of fentanyl is also positively correlated with gestational age and birth weight.[33] Remifentanil has an immediate onset of action, has a half-life of less than 5 minutes, and has been used in the term and preterm populations.[34-36] Benzodiazepines and barbiturates have been investigated as classes of medications that may be used for premedication because of their sedative effects. Midazolam is the most widely used benzodiazepine for premedication for endotracheal intubation. Pharmacokinetics varies among individual neonates, and clearance appears to be positively correlated with gestational age.[37] Propofol is an amnestic sedative that appears to have several mechanisms of action including activation of γ-aminobutyric acid receptors, inhibition of *N*-methyl-D-aspartate receptors, modulation of calcium influx through slow calcium ion channel activity, and sodium channel blockade.[38,39] Early reports of the use of propofol as an induction agent for endotracheal intubation in preterm infants with gestational ages of 25 to 30 weeks suggested a reassuring safety profile.[40] However, more recent data suggest that propofol use for this indication in this population should be approached with caution owing to its significant cardiovascular side effects.[41,42]

Vagolytic agents have been investigated as medications to be used for premedication because of the ability to reduce vagal-induced bradycardia and to decrease oral secretions. Both atropine and glycopyrrolate have been shown to be effective in preventing vagal bradycardia during endotracheal intubation in neonates.[43-45]

Muscle relaxation is another component of optimizing intubation conditions. The intended effect is primarily to decrease patient movement, allowing the provider to have a more controlled field for visualization. The secondary effect of neuromuscular blockade is a decrease in intracranial pressure.[44,46] These medications act at the end plate of the neuromuscular junction to block transmission between motor nerve endings, causing paralysis of the skeletal muscles to facilitate endotracheal intubation. Neuromuscular blockers can be classified as nondepolarizing (atracurium, mivacurium, vecuronium, rocuronium, and pancuronium) and depolarizing (succinylcholine). Succinylcholine should be approached with caution in patients with hyperkalemia or a family history of malignant hyperthermia.

It is recommended to use premedication for nonurgent neonatal intubations, including analgesic agents or an anesthetic dose of hypnotic drugs. Vagolytic agents and rapid-onset muscle relaxants should be considered. Use of sedatives alone such as benzodiazepines without analgesics should be avoided, and muscle relaxants should be given only after an analgesic agent has been used (Table 37-3).

Selection and Placement of the Endotracheal Tube

The anatomy and dimensions of the neonatal airway differ from those of the adult. Historically, the neonatal airway has been described as being conical in the anterior-posterior (AP) dimension, with the cricoid ring being the narrowest portion of the airway and circular in the transverse dimension. More recent studies utilizing advanced airway imaging such as magnetic resonance and computed tomography in sedated as well as spontaneously breathing subjects have found that the airway of a neonate is in fact elliptical in the transverse dimension, with the larynx most closely resembling a cylinder in the AP dimension. The smallest part of the airway is at the level of the vocal cords and subvocal cords.[47,48] These differences raise legitimate questions regarding our choices of endotracheal tubes that are used during an operation. An appropriately sized uncuffed endotracheal tube will have a leak as the circular tube is inserted into an elliptical airway. It is likely, given the anatomy of the airway, that a tube with no leak may be placing excess pressure on the lateral walls of the airway.

This problem is not fully solved with the use of a cuffed tube, as a cuffed tube may still not prevent an air leak from occurring, though the pressure exerted on the lateral walls may be lessened. Advantages to using a cuffed endotracheal tube include more consistent sealing of the airway, thus providing (1) accuracy in quantitative measurements of ventilation, (2) prevention of aspiration of gastric contents into the lungs, and (3) accurate

end-tidal carbon dioxide monitoring.[48] However, hesitation occurs frequently on the part of the neonatal provider in utilizing a cuffed endotracheal tube owing to concerns including excess cuff pressure placed on the developing airway, as well as the size of the tube, as a smaller tube may inhibit suctioning and increase airway resistance. Studies of cuffed versus uncuffed endotracheal tubes have not demonstrated postextubation stridor in subjects with a cuffed endotracheal tube.[49,50] The elliptical anatomy suggests that pressure exerted on the airway is likely to be higher in those who are intubated with an uncuffed endotracheal tube.

A cuffed endotracheal tube may be considered in larger newborns, as there would probably be little impact on ventilation and oxygenation from airway resistance related to tube size in a baby of term or near-term size. However, in growth-restricted infants or infants born prematurely, a cuffed tube may be too large for the airway. In the case of premature infants, an uncuffed tube may be utilized while recognizing that ventilation and oxygenation may be a challenge and quantitative end-tidal carbon dioxide monitoring will not be accurate if there is a substantial air leak. This strategy may require transcutaneous or blood gas measurement of carbon dioxide.

Identification of the correct depth of insertion of the endotracheal tube can also be a challenge. The "7-8-9 rule" is widely utilized within neonatology and endorsed by the American Academy of Pediatrics and the Neonatal Resuscitation Program. This rule entails adding the infant's weight in kilograms to 6, resulting in the appropriate depth in centimeters from the tip of the tube to the vermilion border of the lips. This has been found to be particularly inaccurate in infants weighing <750 g, though the accuracy improves as birth weight increases.[51] The risks of inappropriate tube depth include accidental extubation if too shallow, as well as barotrauma, pneumothorax, and poor ventilation if too deep. Methods of assessing adequate depth, such as auscultating bilateral breath sounds, have been found to be inaccurate in 30% of subjects, the majority of which were infants and children.[52] Alternative approaches have been suggested, and one that has been successful has been utilizing the distance between the base of the nasal septum and the tip of the tragus to estimate tube depth. In this method the appropriate depth of the tube when secured at the lip is equivalent to the nasal–tragus length + 1.[53-55] When utilized in the study setting, this method was >90% accurate. We recommend that consideration be given to utilizing nasal–tragus length as a method of estimating tube depth, particularly in those infants of <750 g in which the "7-8-9 rule" may not be as accurate (Fig. 37-2). Some institutions intubate surgical babies in the NICU and confirm placement with a chest X-ray prior to transport to the operating room. This strategy may improve safety and efficiency once the final confirmation of the surgical case has occurred.

Key Points

- Consideration should be given to performing selective operative procedures in the NICU on critically ill infants.
- Elective intubation of the neonate should include premedication with an appropriately dosed analgesic and/or hypnotic agent. Consideration should be given to the use of vagolytic agents and muscle relaxants.
- Use of a cuffed endotracheal tube in term and term-sized infants may improve oxygenation and ventilation strategies operatively and potentially reduce adverse events related to intubation. Use of a cuffed endotracheal tube is not indicated in premature infants.

TABLE 37-3   Medications for Elective Intubation

Drug	Dose (IV)	Onset of Action	Common Adverse Effects
Analgesic			
Fentanyl	1-4 μg/kg	Almost immediate	Apnea, hypotension, CNS depression, chest wall rigidity—give slowly
Remifentanil	1-3 μg/kg	Almost immediate	Apnea, hypotension, CNS depression, chest wall rigidity
Morphine	0.05-0.1 mg/kg	5-15 min	Apnea, hypotension, CNS depression
Hypnotic/Sedative			
Midazolam	0.05-0.1 mg/kg	5-10 min	Apnea, hypotension, CNS depression
Propofol	2.5 mg/kg	30 s to 10 min	Histamine release Apnea Bronchospasm Bradycardia
Muscle Relaxant			
Pancuronium	0.05-0.1 mg/kg	1-3 min	Hypertension Tachycardia Bronchospasm Salivation
Vecuronium	0.1 mg/kg	2-3 min	Hypertension/ hypotension Tachycardia Bronchospasm Arrhythmias
Rocuronium	0.6-1.2 mg/kg	1-2 min	Hypertension/ hypotension Tachycardia Bronchospasm Arrhythmias
Vagolytic			
Atropine	0.02 mg/kg	1-2 min	Dry hot skin Tachycardia
Glycopyrrolate	4-10 μg/kg	1-10 min	Dry hot skin Tachycardia

CNS, Central nervous system.

OPERATIVE MANAGEMENT

The ventilator aspects of operative management of a neonate can be subdivided into three distinct domains. The first is selection of appropriate mode of ventilation. The second is that of vital sign monitoring, including respiratory rate, heart rate, blood pressure, and oxygen saturation as well as periodic measurements of serum pH and carbon dioxide levels. Finally, consideration must be given to ongoing operative ventilation management and troubleshooting.

Ventilator Mode

An almost infinite number of ventilator modes are available for use in neonates through adults. This is another opportunity to resist the temptation to simply apply adult principles to newborns. Effective intraoperative ventilator management is optimal when the neonatal patient is recognized as requiring specific

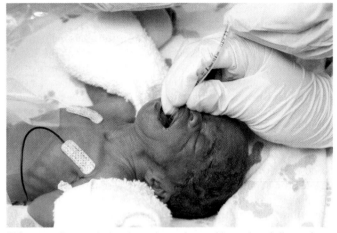

FIG 37-2 Recently intubated newborn. Note the delicate handling of the patient and the endotracheal tube. While waiting for the endotracheal tube to be secured, the proceduralist holds the endotracheal tube against the patient's hard palate. This will reduce the likelihood of tube displacement.

strategies to safely support the patient through the operation but also reduces the risk of ventilator- or oxygen-associated lung injury. Historically, pressure-targeted ventilation was used in NICUs as it was the only type of ventilation available. As ventilators evolved, volume-targeted, pressure-controlled ventilation was demonstrated to decrease morbidities such as pneumothorax and intracranial hemorrhage among premature neonates.[56,57] This technology has become widely utilized within the NICU.

For most commercially available patient ventilators, the lowest set tidal volume is 2.5 to 3 mL. If these target tidal volumes are used for our smallest patients (e.g., <500 g), the patient may be exposed to barotrauma as the milliliters per kilogram per breath may exceed our typical target of 4 to 6 mL/kg. The performance characteristics of many ventilators may make volume-targeted, pressure-controlled ventilation a challenge in patients who weigh <500 g. Additionally, these ventilators may be found only in the NICU and not be available in the operating room. This reason alone may lead to performing a procedure in the NICU rather than the operating theater or bringing the mechanical ventilator from the NICU to the operating room with the patient who requires surgery.

If volume-targeted, pressure-controlled ventilation cannot be utilized, pressure-controlled ventilation may be used while monitoring "in-line" exhaled tidal volumes and adjusting both the PEEP and the peak inspiratory pressure to deliver 4- to 6-mL/kg tidal volumes where appropriate. Hyperventilation from excess minute ventilation may result in hypocarbia, a risk factor for white matter injury and neurodevelopmental impairment, especially in very low birth-weight (VLBW) infants.[58,59] Providing manual ventilation ("hand bagging") of the neonate should be avoided owing to the great variability in rate, peak inspiratory pressure, PEEP, and tidal volumes delivered.

There has been increasing suggestion that neonates may not need to be intubated and mechanically ventilated for all procedures. A prime example of this is the performance of laser surgery for retinopathy of prematurity while maintaining neonates on continuous positive airway pressure only or with the use of a laryngeal mask airway. While there is appeal in the less invasive nature of this approach to decrease ventilator-induced lung injury, there is insufficient evidence to recommend this strategy routinely. However, in time, noninvasive ventilatory support during less complex operative procedures may become more common.

Vital Signs

The set mandatory rate of mechanical breaths for a sedated and paralyzed neonate may range anywhere from 35 to 75 inflations per minute, depending on severity of lung disease, degree of pulmonary insufficiency, and gestational age. The preoperative briefing and evaluation will probably yield important information on the patient's recent respiratory support requirements.

The patient's heart rate and blood pressure parameters will require frequent monitoring throughout the case. While both may vary because of the ongoing operation, changes in oxygenation and ventilation status may affect each other as well. Blood pressures may trend downward if the ventilator mean airway pressures remain too high, thus limiting venous return to the heart. The heart rate may become quite elevated if the patient is uncomfortable because of inadequate sedation or inadequate ventilation.

Of particular importance in the premature neonate is recognition of hyperoxia and the adverse effects of prolonged exposure to hyperoxia. Neonatologists have long recognized that newborn infants exposed to excess oxygen are at higher risk for retinopathy of prematurity (the leading cause of blindness in the premature population) and chronic lung disease. Prolonged exposure of the developing neonatal lungs, brain, and eyes to oxygen free radicals may result in damage to the developing vasculature and tissue of the respective organ systems. The field of neonatology has focused on identifying the optimal amount of oxygen to provide adequate oxygen delivery in premature neonates while recognizing a higher risk of morbidity related to excess oxygen exposure. Evidence suggesting that consistent exposure to higher oxygen saturations led to an increased risk of retinopathy of prematurity[60] resulted in the adoption of lower oxygen saturation limits (i.e., 85% to 92%) in many NICUs. However, a meta-analysis of three international trials (SUPPORT, BOOST II, and COT) concluded that, while targeting a lower oxygen saturation limit did reduce the risk of retinopathy of prematurity, it increased the risk of necrotizing enterocolitis and death. The authors concluded that a target oxygen saturation of 90% to 95% should be utilized.[61] This sentiment has been supported by expert opinion.[62,63] It would stand to reason that these saturation targets would be equally appropriate during operative interventions in an effort to avoid prolonged periods of hyperoxia while delivering adequate oxygen content to the developing tissues. Because of this, it is of utmost importance that an oxygen blender is available in the operating room as well as in transport to and from that location. The preoperative briefing should include the oxygen saturation range goal utilized in the NICU, and that goal range should be maintained throughout the procedure, promoting consistency in care between the NICU and the operating room. Exposure to hyperoxia during surgery may have little recognized morbidity in older patients, but in neonates it may contribute to an already higher risk of long-term morbidity.

In an attempt to mitigate morbidities such as BPD, permissive hypercarbia increases the efficiency of CO_2 removal,[64] improves ventilation–perfusion matching in the lung,[65] and potentially increases respiratory drive, resulting in less apnea,[66] of which premature infants already have a higher risk. Previous studies in neonates have indicated that this strategy may reduce the risk of death or BPD and reduce mechanical ventilation days overall.[67-70] This strategy tolerates higher serum carbon dioxide values and lower serum pH values to reduce exposure of the neonatal lung to barotrauma as a result of aggressive mechanical ventilation.[64] The details of ranges tolerated may be unit-specific but may incorporate tolerating arterial CO_2 levels of up to 65 mm Hg and serum pH of 7.25 to 7.35 (see Chapter 19).

End-tidal CO_2 measurements may be inaccurate in premature infants, particularly those with an uncuffed endotracheal tube. The anesthetist may wish to trial the use of an end-tidal CO_2 detector or transcutaneous CO_2 detector, but correlation should be made with serum values, particularly when the CO_2 value shown appears out of target range or appears to be varying considerably throughout the procedure. Hypocarbia (CO_2 values <35 mm Hg) during the operation should also be avoided as prolonged exposure to hypocarbia can result in cerebral vasoconstriction and has been shown to have an impact on the risk of neurodevelopmental impairments such as cerebral palsy, especially in VLBW infants.[58,59]

Intraoperative Fluid Management and Electrolyte Management

Appropriate intravenous fluid administration among ill neonates, particularly those who are premature, is a key management tactic that influences all other areas of management. Exposing critically ill neonates to excess fluid can result in volume overload, which causes significant capillary leak, particularly in the lungs, and in worsening of respiratory distress. Providing too little intravenous fluid can result in tachycardia, poor urine output, acute kidney injury, acidosis, and hypotension. Several factors are taken into consideration when selecting the typical daily intravenous fluid prescription for each neonate. These factors include gestational age, postnatal day, current weight, postnatal growth, urine output, vital sign parameters, ventilatory requirements, and oxygen requirements. In an otherwise well infant undergoing a routine procedure (i.e., herniorrhaphy, etc.) during which fluid resuscitation is not expected, it could be considered prudent of the anesthetist to leave the neonate on the intravenous fluids prescribed by the neonatologist, as that volume is probably adequate for needs. If the infant does require a fluid bolus—for example, because of hypotension as a result of anesthesia induction—a small (10 mL/kg) bolus of normal saline or lactated Ringer's solution could be given. This can be repeated if no improvement is seen. Care should also be taken not to expose the neonate to excess intravenous fluid when unneeded. Placing a peripheral intravenous tube (IV) and running TKO ("to keep open") fluids at 2 mL/hr may be common in older children, but that rate of fluid can add up to a great deal of fluids in proportion to a neonate's body size. Depending on institutional practice, peripheral IVs may be heparin-locked when not in use or run at a lower rate (i.e., 1 mL/hr).

In a more critically ill neonate, undergoing a procedure such as an abdominal laparotomy or cardiac surgery, during which consistent fluid resuscitation is expected, it may be indicated to continue the intravenous fluids with which the patient arrives at the operating room. However, through the course of the operation, events may arise that may require discontinuation of fluids owing to their content (i.e., potassium-containing maintenance intravenous fluids or total parenteral nutrition). In this event, it is imperative that the anesthesia team recognize that any new fluids

TABLE 37-4   Electrolyte Imbalances

	Risk Factor(s)	Intervention
Glucose		
Hypoglycemia	Infant of a diabetic mother Small for gestational age Sepsis Insufficient glucose infusion rate in maintenance fluids	200 mg/kg (2 mL/kg D10W) infusion and increase basal glucose infusion rate
Hyperglycemia	Surgical stress Corticosteroid therapy	Examine current glucose infusion rate to determine if it could be decreased. If glucose infusion rate is ≤4 mg/kg/min, consider insulin infusion
Calcium		
Hypocalcemia	Prematurity Small or large for gestational age DiGeorge syndrome	Calcium chloride (10-20 mg/kg) or calcium gluconate (100-200 mg/kg) Note: Should be given through central venous access*
Sodium		
Hyponatremia	Excess free water administration	Examine current fluid infusion rate. Determine if maintenance fluid rate could be **decreased**
Hypernatremia	Dehydration	Examine current fluid infusion rate. Determine if maintenance fluid rate could be **increased**
Potassium		
Hypokalemia	Furosemide	Consider potassium chloride infusion (1 mEq/kg)
Hyperkalemia	Prematurity	Examine intravenous fluid composition and remove potassium. Consider calcium (above), sodium bicarbonate (1 mEq/kg), and insulin infusion if hyperkalemia persists

*D10W, 10% Dextrose Water.

utilized must contain an adequate amount of dextrose to maintain euglycemia. If dextrose concentration is changed during the procedure, the anesthetist should regularly check blood glucose values so that unrecognized hypoglycemia does not occur.

There are several electrolyte abnormalities that may be observed in neonates in the intensive care and operating room setting. The provider may correctly anticipate these findings based on risk factor assessment and respond appropriately (Table 37-4).

Key Points
- Volume-targeted, pressure-controlled ventilation is preferable when the weight of the patient allows for accurate volume delivery.
- Operative ventilatory strategy for premature neonates should include strict avoidance of hyperoxia and hypocarbia and may incorporate permissive hypercarbia.
- End-tidal carbon dioxide measurements should be correlated with serum values in neonates with uncuffed endotracheal tubes.

TABLE 37-5   Hypothermia

Causes	Treatment Considerations
Cold exposure	Maintain operating room temperature between 27°C and 29°C Warm blankets Radiant heaters Warming mattresses Frequent intraoperative core temperature monitoring (bladder, esophageal, rectal)
Skin preparation with cold solutions	Consider warming antiseptic solutions before application
Infusion of cold intravenous solutions	Warm intravenous fluids
Irrigation of wounds with cold solution	Warm irrigation fluids before instillation
Dry gases through mechanical ventilation circuit	Heated and humidified gases

- Intraoperative ventilation of the neonate is best provided by a mechanical ventilator for consistent and accurate volume delivery.
- Intravenous fluids should be provided cautiously and with recognition of the risk of fluid overload in neonates.

TROUBLESHOOTING

Sudden, unexplained decompensation of the neonatal patient during surgery should lead the anesthetist to the DOPE mnemonic. Tube *displacement* is the most likely complication in this situation. Given the small length of airway available in the neonate, it would take a minimal change in depth to cause either a main stem intubation or extubation. In a surgery such as CDH repair, in which tracheal position may change throughout the procedure, this potential complication may arise. Tube depth should be evaluated as well as capnography and potentially direct visualization via laryngoscopy. Tube *obstruction* is a potential problem given the small size of endotracheal tube often used in neonates, particularly those preterm. The tube should be suctioned carefully to evaluate for excessive secretions or plugging. An acute *pneumothorax* is less likely but certainly a potential problem if the patient has had a main stem intubation or has been requiring higher peak inspiratory pressures during the procedure (an indication intraoperatively that the tube may have been at the carina). Finally, faulty *equipment* should be evaluated by removing the infant from the ventilator and hand bagging. Again, care should be taken not to expose the infant to excess pressure or volume during manual ventilation.

ADDITIONAL OPERATIVE CONSIDERATIONS

Temperature Regulation

Neonates are prone to heat loss because of their large body surface area-to-mass ratio and limited subcutaneous fat. They lose heat by radiation, conduction, convection, and evaporation. Hypothermia leads to increased oxygen and glucose consumption, inadequate oxygen delivery, hypoventilation, apnea, acidosis, and, if untreated, cardiovascular collapse. Sources of cold stress and management considerations are noted in Table 37-5.

TABLE 37-6 Intravenous Anesthetic Drugs for the Neonate: Dosages

Anesthetic Agents	Premedication (mg/kg)	Induction (mg/kg)	Maintenance (µg/kg)	Intubation (mg/kg)	Reversal (mg/kg)
Anticholinergics					
Atropine	0.01-0.02				
Glycopyrrolate	0.005-0.01				
Hypnotics					
Propofol		2.5-3.0			
Thiopental		4-6			
Ketamine		0.5-2.0			
Midazolam		0.02-0.05			
Opioids					
Fentanyl		0.005-0.010	1-2 µg/kg/h		
Morphine		0.05-0.1	10-50 µg/kg/h		
Sufentanil		0.0001-0.0002	0.05-0.1 µg/kg/h		
Remifentanil		0.0001	1.5-3 µg/kg/min		
Muscle Relaxants					
Succinylcholine				1-2	
Pancuronium				0.05-0.1	
Vecuronium				0.1-0.15	
Rocuronium				0.8-1.2	
Anticholinesterases					
Neostigmine					0.05-0.08
Pyridostigmine					0.02-0.03
Narcotic Antagonist					
Naloxone					0.005-0.01

Neonate Pain Perception

Although an extensive presentation of intraoperative anesthetic management is beyond the scope of this textbook, commonly used medications are listed in Table 37-6. Providers should be mindful that any neonate who will undergo surgical intervention is capable of feeling pain irrespective of gestational age. Poor pain control may lead to an increase in morbidity and mortality as well as potentially life-altering longitudinal complications for the newborn including intraventricular hemorrhage and subsequent sequelae. Operative management may be complicated by inadequate pain control including acute onset of pulmonary hypertension, systemic hypertension, and exaggerated stress responses. Validated and standardized pain assessment tools are widely available, and each institution should select one instrument to facilitate appropriate evaluation and management of intraoperative and postoperative pain.

CONCLUSION

Delivering safe and effective mechanical ventilation for neonates requiring surgery is an important aspect of operative care. While it is important to understand the unique physiology, stages of lung development, and anatomic considerations for neonatal patients, utilization of neonatal-specific devices and application of lung-protective strategies intraoperatively will help providers achieve optimal outcomes.

REFERENCES

A complete reference list is available at https://expertconsult.inkling.com/.

38

Neonatal Respiratory Care in Resource-Limited Countries

Amuchou S. Soraisham, MBBS, MD, DM, MS, FRCPC, FAAP, and Nalini Singhal, MBBS, MD, FRCPC

The first chapter in this book describes the historical origins of neonatal ventilation in the Western world. Despite rapid growth in the developed countries, neonatal intensive care units (NICUs) and high-technology care such as neonatal respiratory support have evolved more slowly in resource-limited countries since 1975. Multiple factors such as poor economy, lack of skilled personnel, lack of equipment, and failure to develop structured programs have been responsible for the delayed progress. Furthermore, countries with high neonatal and infant mortality rates have rightfully focused more on prevention of common public health issues and simple programs for resuscitation and essential care of the newborn rather than on establishing expensive NICUs with ventilator care facilities. However, in recent years, globalization has increased access to new medical knowledge and technology for many developing countries.[1] The twenty-first century will see rapid progression of respiratory support programs in neonatal units around the world, although progress will be uneven. The Every Newborn Action Plan calls for an end to preventable newborn deaths.[2] To accomplish this goal, some babies will need the assistance of more advanced respiratory care, including continuous positive airway pressure (CPAP) and neonatal-specific ventilators.

In this chapter we review the current status of NICUs in resource-limited countries, barriers to development of respiratory care programs, and possible strategies to overcome these barriers to develop functional respiratory care programs appropriate to the region.

SCOPE OF THE NEED

High neonatal mortality rates (NMRs) and infant mortality rates (IMR) constitute major health problems in low- and middle-income countries. According to the World Bank classification system, a country with a gross national per capita income of less than US $12,746 in 2013 is considered a low- and middle-income or developing country.[3] Globally, nearly 3 million babies die in the neonatal period (during the first 28 days of life), and 2.6 million babies are stillborn each year.[4] Most newborn deaths occur in low- and middle-income countries. Three causes accounted for more than 80% of neonatal mortality in 2012: complications of prematurity, intrapartum-related neonatal deaths (including birth asphyxia), and neonatal infections. Complications of

prematurity are the second leading cause of all deaths under 5 years of age. Newborn resuscitation programs such as Helping Babies Breathe[5] have demonstrated a reduction in neonatal mortality.[6] Resuscitation training in resource-limited facilities can reduce intrapartum-related neonatal death by 30% and early neonatal death by 38%.[7] However, after newborn resuscitation, some newborns may require CPAP or assisted ventilation. An estimated 21% of babies presenting with illness in the first 6 days of life have respiratory symptoms that may require respiratory support.[8] In low- and middle-income countries, there is a need for neonatal care programs equipped with proper respiratory equipment and trained personnel. Facilities need tools such as oxygen, resuscitation bags and masks, and possibly CPAP to provide basic respiratory support. The higher level care hospitals should have the capabilities of CPAP and mechanical ventilation. To provide CPAP and assisted ventilation, the health facilities must be staffed by well-trained medical and nursing personnel.

The information about level II and III units in resource-limited countries is scanty. As expected, these countries have the highest NMRs and IMRs and therefore have the greatest needs. For example, India, with an NMR of 29 in 1000[9] and 25 million births per year would require hundreds of level III and perhaps thousands of level II NICUs. It is estimated that in India, with approximately 1.2 billion people, one level III NICU with 30 beds is required for every 1 million population[10] with additional level II health facilities. Ideally, to be effective there should be a cooperative regional perinatal program that is responsible for the coordination of clinical activities, education, resource use, quality improvement, and development of evidence-based clinical pathways for best practices.

A parallel improvement in hospital-based prenatal and neonatal care is required for further reduction in the NMR. Because respiratory compromise is common in all three important causes of neonatal mortality (prematurity, birth asphyxia, and neonatal infections), effective programs for managing respiratory distress could have a major impact on NMRs.[11]

LIMITING FACTORS

Major barriers to developing regional respiratory care programs in resource-limited countries include limited infrastructure and availability of equipment, properly trained staff, and quality improvement programs and the absence of coordinated systems. Health facilities in many resource-limited countries do not meet the basic needs of newborn care such as provision of warmth, a clean environment, and breast milk. Yet ironically, some of these countries are

Acknowledgment: We would like to acknowledge Dr. Dharmapuri Vidyasagar for his contributions in the earlier edition of this chapter.

beginning to open level III units in their district hospitals.[12] Some district-level hospitals are equipped with oxygen and suction; however, resuscitation bags and radiant warmers are often not present, and oxygen hoods are infrequently available.[12] Even when resuscitation bags are available, there is often no system in place to clean and store them in an appropriate place. The primary health centers, each of which serves a population of 10,000 to 15,000 and provides basic maternity services, have practically no equipment. There is an urgent need to improve these deficiencies. Respiratory support is either limited to a very few hospitals or is available only in the private sector and hence not accessible to most babies.

There are several barriers to developing respiratory care services at all levels in resource-limited countries.[13] Some of these barriers are described below.

Respiratory Care Program Barrier

There is a lack of structured respiratory care programs with quality improvement initiatives. There are essentially few or no policies or guidelines either for clinical care or for maintenance of equipment. Even if equipment is said to be available, it may not be functioning or may be locked away and unavailable.

Infrastructure

Appropriate physical infrastructure is lacking. The hospitals do not have properly designed intensive care units for adults, much less for newborns. Even in district and teaching hospitals, the space for the management of high-risk infants is arbitrarily allocated and may lack the basic requirements of running water, a consistent supply of electricity, and a controlled environment. There are problems maintaining a consistent supply of oxygen and/or compressed air. Many units depend on cylinders for air and oxygen. Maintenance of equipment is irregular at the best hospitals and nonexistent in most units.

Skilled Health Care Personnel

There is a shortage of skilled medical and nursing staff in resource-limited countries. These limitations put constraints on patient care. Even if nurses are trained, they are variably assigned to different units so that there is a constant turnover of staff. Physicians have to assume many responsibilities for which they are ill equipped, such as manipulations of the ventilator. In the absence of trained neonatologists, care is performed by general pediatricians who usually are not familiar with ventilator management. A few are able to manage mild cases of respiratory distress with oxygen. For the most part, physicians are not trained to provide CPAP, endotracheal tube placement, or ventilation. Most NICUs are managed by general pediatricians who have a special interest or have had some previous experience in assisted ventilation. Nurses and pediatricians in most resource-limited countries do not have degrees of training and proficiency in managing neonatal respiratory support similar to those of workers in developed countries.

Developing countries also face shortages of doctors and nursing staff because of widespread emigration of skilled health care personnel to the developed world, known euphemistically as the "Brain Drain."[14] Innovative programs are needed to retain skilled workers in resource-limited countries.

Support Equipment

Ancillary services such as blood gas machines, portable radiology machines, microchemistry laboratories, oxygen saturation monitors, and heart rate monitors are not available in most of the NICUs.

CURRENT STATUS

During the last quarter of the twentieth century, many resource-limited countries successfully developed a few model NICUs with outcomes comparable to those of the developed world. These unique programs were developed mainly through the efforts of committed individuals and concerted efforts of professional organizations. NICU development was complemented by the phenomenon of "globalization and diffusion of technology" during the past three decades.[1] It is recognized that widespread implementation of low-cost, robust respiratory technologies (e.g., oxygen concentrators, oxygen saturation monitoring, bubble CPAP) could save the lives of many newborns admitted to facilities in resource-limited nations.[11] The evolution of neonatal intensive care and specifically ventilatory care is described below for a few select regions of the world.

China

The neonatal intensive care program in China was established by the Ministry of Health and the United Nations Children's Fund in the early 1980s.[15] Since then the infant mortality and morbidity rates in China have declined steadily. However, the incidence of low-birth-weight (LBW) infants is reported to have increased from 4% to 6% in the 1990s to 10.2% in 2002.[15] LBW infants constitute most of the NICU admissions at all medical centers. Continuing advances in neonatal intensive care, especially the introduction of mechanical ventilation and surfactant administration, have increased the survival of preterm infants in China.

The Neonatal Resuscitation Program was introduced into China in the 1990s, decreasing delivery room deaths and the incidence of Apgar ≤7 at 1 minute.[16] Babies requiring further care are usually transferred to level III hospitals to receive additional treatment.

The levels of care in the NICUs differ across the country. Nasal CPAP is most often used earlier in babies with respiratory distress syndrome (RDS) or spontaneously breathing premature infants when oxygen requirements are less than 50%. CPAP is also used for weaning infants from ventilators and in preterm babies with recurrent apnea. Limited data are available regarding the best ways to use CPAP in the country. It is now common practice to intubate and ventilate as an elective procedure in the early stage of most forms of severe neonatal respiratory disease. Synchronized intermittent mandatory ventilation is one of the most widely used modalities of respiratory support. Li and Wei[15] showed that the use of pulmonary mechanics measurement was helpful in guiding the use of ventilator adjustment and decreased ventilator-associated lung injury in neonatal RDS. High-frequency oscillatory ventilation (HFOV) and high-frequency jet ventilation are used in only a few units when infants with respiratory failure do not respond to conventional ventilation. A study from China showed that, compared with conventional mechanical ventilation, HFOV was associated with lower mortality (2.3% vs 7.3%), bronchopulmonary dysplasia (BPD) (7.5% vs 16.9%), and BPD or death (9.6% vs 29.3%) in preterm infants of <32 weeks.[17]

In a survey of 23 NICUs done in 2004-2005, with a total of 13,070 admissions, 1722 (13%) babies were treated with mechanical ventilation for respiratory failure, with the predominant diagnoses of RDS, pneumonia/sepsis, and meconium aspiration syndrome (MAS).[18] The mortality rate of ventilated infants was 32%. The mean length of hospital stay for all infants treated with ventilation was 19.2 ± 14.6 days. The median length of stay for survivors was 70 days. Mean hospital cost per survivor was $14,966 \pm 13,465$ yuans (equivalent to approximately US$2138). An updated survey in 2010 revealed that the incidence of neonatal respiratory failure in NICUs had increased from 13% to 19.7%, and the overall mortality had decreased from 32% to 24.7%; the overall mortality for MAS fell from 39.3% to 29.7%; and the overall mortality for pneumonia/sepsis decreased from 33.8% to 28.6%.[19]

With increasing use of ventilatory support in premature infants and increasing survival, the incidence of chronic lung disease (CLD) in China is increasing.[15] In view of increasing CLD and concerns of pulmonary oxygen toxicity, the government of China has developed guidelines for oxygen therapy in the neonatal period. These guidelines call for strict indications for the use of oxygen and using the lowest supplemental FiO_2 to maintain oxygenation saturation between 90% and 95% with pulse oximetry.

India

The development of neonatal intensive care in India has been slow because of constraints[20] such as availability of required technology and skilled personnel. Economic constraints prevent the development of expensive high-technology NICUs in the country. Faced with high NMR and IMR, policy makers thought it prudent to invest in improving overall health rather than in high-technology medicine. The concept of providing good level II care to premature and LBW infants was well in place as early as the 1950s. Respiratory support was limited to providing oxygen in addition to providing thermal care and intravenous (IV) fluids. It was not until the mid-1970s and early 1980s that NICUs in India began to provide ventilator support.

A major impetus to the nationwide growth of neonatal intensive care and therefore neonatal ventilation in India came from the professional organization, National Neonatology Forum (NNF), which was established in 1980.[21] The NNF focused on developing policy guidelines and standardization of care (bedside monitoring, equipment use, evidence-based guidelines, and assisted ventilation), designation of levels of care, and an accreditation process for neonatal and perinatal care in the country. The organization also placed a great emphasis on the education and training of pediatricians and nurses. Surveys by the NNF demonstrated a gradual improvement in the availability of equipment and staffs.[20,22,23]

Since 1995, several neonatal units providing complete care with ventilatory capabilities have evolved, primarily in private settings. The results in these units managed by highly qualified staffs are comparable to those of Western units for almost all birth-weight groups (Table 38-1). In a survey of 70 neonatal units in India, there was significant progress in infrastructure and availability of equipment and trained workers, supporting staff, and services.[24] The units had mechanical ventilators but very few had blood gas machines, in-house X-ray facilities, invasive blood pressure monitoring, and ophthalmology support. High-frequency ventilation to provide respiratory support is limited to a few centers.

The progress in neonatal ventilation can be indirectly assessed by the number of ventilators purchased in the country. The data provided by Marketstrat, Inc.,[25] a company that analyzes such global information, shows that the number of ventilator purchases in India has been increasing at a steady rate of 3% to 4% per year. This is somewhat higher than the rate of ventilator growth projected in China (2%-3%/year). Based on the large numbers of births and high rates of birth asphyxia, LBW, and prematurely born infants (estimated 7% of births or 1.75 million per year), there is a greater need for further development of NICUs across the country. With nearly 548 special care newborn units in district hospitals, 1810 newborn stabilization units at subdistrict hospitals, and 0.9 million Accredited Social Health Activist workers in the community, the country is gearing up to face the enormous task of providing health care to 26 million neonates born each year.[26] Low-cost and innovative methods to provide respiratory support (such as bubble CPAP) short of mechanical ventilation at subdistrict and district hospitals are also being initiated.[27]

Some privately run NICUs in India meet all of the international standards in space, equipment, and skilled medical and nursing staff. A few hospitals in developing countries have been accredited by The Joint Commission.[28] The high cost of care in these hospitals precludes access by the majority of the country's population.

Other Countries

Bhutta et al.[29] reported an encouraging experience in Pakistan. The provision of ventilatory support to infants with RDS in Pakistan resulted in increased survival specifically in infants weighing more than 1000 g. The authors concluded that respiratory care can be developed in selected hospitals to successfully manage neonates with RDS. With the establishment of NICUs,

TABLE 38-1	Neonatal Survival Rates by Birth-Weight Category in 1995, 2010, and 2014 at All India Institute of Medical Sciences, New Delhi		
Birth Weight (g)	1995 $n=1672$ (%)	2010 $n=2191$ (%)	2014 $n=2631$ (%)
<750	0	38.5	43.5
750-999	73.3	69.0	80.6
1000-1249	77.8	78.9	84.4
1250-1499	95.5	97.8	90.9
1500-1749	85.3	93.9	97.0
1750-1999	96.2	94.6	95.7
2000-2499	98.4	97.8	98.6
2500-2999	99.3	99.9	99.4
3000-3999	100.0	99.1	99.5
4000 or more	100.0	100.0	100.0

Ho and Chang[30] from Malaysia reported that the survival of all very low birth-weight (VLBW) infants in one NICU improved from 69% in 1993 to 81% in 2003. Among ventilated VLBW babies, survival improved from 53% to 93%. Interestingly, there was no significant improvement in mortality of nonventilated babies, suggesting that neonatal ventilation significantly contributed to increased survival among VLBW infants in this unit.

Latin America has high NMRs and IMRs with significant disparities among the countries. In some Latin American countries (e.g., Cuba, Chile, Costa Rica, Jamaica), the NMR ranges from 3 to 11 in 1000 births, whereas other countries (Mexico) report IMRs as high as 25 in 1000 births. Similar to other resource-limited countries in the world, the major cause of neonatal mortality is respiratory diseases. Most newborns who die do so within days of birth, mostly from inadequate resuscitation at birth and lack of respiratory support after admission to the ward. The majority of these deaths could be prevented with development of facilities that provide adequate resuscitation and respiratory support. In 1980, Ventura-Junca et al. showed the effectiveness of NICU care in reducing neonatal mortality in Chile.[31] However, such facilities are available mainly in private hospitals. In a multicenter study from South American NICUs, infants randomized to bubble CPAP had significant reduction in need for mechanical ventilation and surfactant therapy compared to hood oxygen alone.[32]

Malawi has the highest rate of preterm births in the world: 18.1% of all newborns in Malawi are born prematurely[33] with a not surprisingly high NMR. The current standard of care in Malawi for babies with any type of respiratory difficulty is nasal oxygen therapy. However, the use of bubble CPAP to treat babies with RDS resulted in 27% absolute improvement in survival to discharge.[34] Only 24% of neonates with RDS treated with nasal oxygen survived to discharge compared to 65% receiving bubble CPAP. Introduction of CPAP in Fiji was associated with a 50% reduction in the need for mechanical ventilation, thereby demonstrating that CPAP for resource-limited settings may be a viable and relatively inexpensive option to decrease neonatal mortality.[35] Moreover, the staff nurses were able to safely apply bubble CPAP after 1 to 2 months of training.[36]

On the basis of reported national NMR, Paul and Singh proposed a stepwise approach to neonatal health care strategies in developing countries.[37] For countries with neonatal mortality of more than 25 per 1000 live births, the focus should be on community-based care. Once the mortality is less than 25 per 1000 live births, perinatal care should be provided by a network of facilities close to the community managed by midwives, nurses, and physicians. At this stage widespread implementation of low-cost, robust respiratory technologies (e.g., oxygen concentrators, oxygen saturation monitoring, and bubble CPAP) could save the lives of many newborn infants admitted to the facilities.[11] The projected needs for respiratory support to save lives in resource-limited countries are presented in Figure 38-1.

ESTABLISHING RESPIRATORY CARE PROGRAMS

There is a great interest among pediatricians and neonatologists in resource-limited countries to establish respiratory care programs for critically ill newborns and save many more babies. However, establishing a respiratory care unit requires a major commitment of funds, resources, personnel, and time that would have to be diverted away from other health care needs. A one-time capital investment for the purchase of equipment

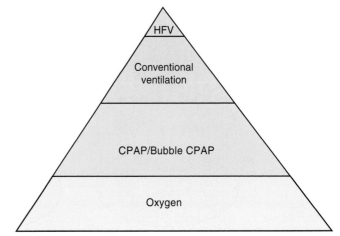

FIG 38-1 Projected need for respiratory support to save lives in resource-limited countries. *CPAP*, Continuous positive airway pressure; *HFV*, high-frequency ventilation.

would seem reasonable. However, it should be understood that establishing a respiratory care program requires more than equipment, including development of clinical care pathways, maintenance of the equipment, ability to obtain replacement parts, ongoing professional development programs for all levels of providers, full-fledged ancillary support systems (e.g., laboratory, radiology), and a regional system of referral that promotes centralized ventilator care. To be cost-effective, regional centers that serve large populations should develop assisted ventilation support systems. A regionalized perinatal center requires a well-developed and efficient transport system for in utero transport as well as newborn emergency transport.

However, the introduction of CPAP/bubble CPAP may be appropriate for level II units in these settings. Fernandez and Mondkar[10] suggest establishing one tertiary care NICU providing assisted ventilation per 1 million population in resource-limited countries. To establish a strong respiratory care program, the following components are necessary (Fig. 38-2):

(a) Leadership and partnership
(b) Implementation
(c) Education
(d) Evaluation and monitoring

Leadership and Partnership

In the past the leadership has consisted of a small group of technical experts or champions. There is a need for engagement of active stakeholders at all levels of government. They can advocate and set a course of action that is supported at national and local levels. In addition, families are an important partner who can assist with taking care of their baby, recognizing that respiratory care saves lives, and publicly advocating for the provision of these services. Governments respond to increases in demand, and it will be easier to develop regionalized services with families as partners.

Implementation

Implementation of respiratory services needs adequate infrastructure, resources (equipment and human), clinical care monitoring systems, and ongoing quality improvement programs. Policies have to be developed based on local evidence. Proper infrastructure should be made available depending on

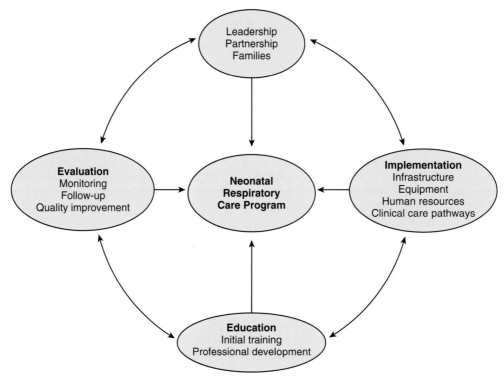

FIG 38-2 Basic components of a neonatal respiratory care program.

the size of the unit. In addition, medications such as antibiotics and surfactant should be readily available.

Infrastructure

It is the ultimate goal of pediatricians and neonatologists around the world to be able to establish an NICU providing ventilator care. To be successful and cost-effective, the planners must consider certain criteria before attempting to establish a neonatal respiratory care program. Box 38-1 lists some basic requirements for establishing a respiratory care program in any hospital. It describes the operational needs, costs, and criteria for choosing a ventilator. In addition to the provision of basic needs such as space and an uninterrupted supply of power, water, and gases, the availability of appropriate equipment and skilled staff is critical to the successful operation of any respiratory care program.

Resources

Critical to the success of improving neonatal respiratory care in resource-limited countries is training of bedside health care personnel in the early recognition of and ability to manage respiratory distress. Because most of the facilities have minimal or no equipment, health care personnel must be trained in clinical skills that help identify infants at risk who require immediate respiratory support, including appropriate resuscitation and stabilization until the infant can be transferred to a higher level of care. Transport facilities for sick neonates requiring a higher level of care must be developed. Worldwide there is an acute shortage of trained health care personnel particularly in resource-limited countries.[13] Establishment of neonatal respiratory care programs requires innovative methods to overcome this problem. Sen et al.[27] described how a rural district hospital under government auspices was transformed into a functioning regional center for neonatal intensive care, including respiratory care, by improving physical facilities and training of locally

| BOX 38-1 | Guidelines for Setting up a Respiratory Care Program |

A. Operational Considerations
- Availability of adequate space
- Uninterrupted availability of power and running water
- Continuous availability of a pediatrician trained in ventilator care
- Availability of sufficient nursing staff trained in ventilator care in the ratio of one nurse to two or three patients
- Availability of maintenance staff trained in ventilator repair
- Continuing education of staff
- Acquisition, review, and analysis of data for quality improvement

B. Typical Cost in U.S. Dollars of a Ventilator in a Resource-Limited Country
- Cost of ventilator: $30,000
- Cost of disposables per year: $250
- Cost of service contract: $200
- First-year cost: $30,450
- Recurrent yearly cost: $450

C. Choosing a Ventilator
- Simplicity of operation
- Cost considerations
- Ease of maintenance, availability of replacement parts
- Brand name
- Lower overall cost of ownership and life-cycle cost

(Data from Marketstrat, Inc. These cost estimates do not include costs of oxygen supply or delivery systems such as continuous positive airway pressure devices or high-flow devices; 2005.)

available health care workers to care for infants admitted to the NICU. Over a 2-year period they were able to demonstrate a significant decrease in neonatal mortality in a cost-effective manner. Many of the traditional roles of medical providers were modified in what has become known as "the Purolia Model." This experience may serve as a model for others contemplating the creation or improvement of intensive care programs.

Equipment for Respiratory Care Programs

The basic principles of management of an at-risk infant include provision of warmth and nutritional support. Basic respiratory care services include availability of oxygen, compressed air, blenders, suction devices, bags and masks, oxygen hoods, nasal cannulae, nasal prongs, face masks, CPAP devices, ventilators, pulse oximeters, cardiorespiratory monitoring devices, disposable gas and suction circuits, other noninvasive monitoring devices, and possibly oxygen analyzers. Lack of essential equipment may allow for the delivery of oxygen without appropriate monitoring and result in significant complications (e.g., retinopathy of prematurity) or death. With globalization and increasing diffusion of technology since 1995, some resource-poor countries have obtained incubators, electronic monitoring systems, pulse oximetry, IV fluids, CPAP devices, and neonatal ventilators.[1] But they experience difficulty in obtaining consumable commodities such as oxygen and have difficulty in maintaining equipment in working order, both of which are vital to the management of infants in respiratory distress. The lack of readily available oxygen has been reported as a major cause of death in Africa and other developing areas.[38]

In developed countries, oxygen is stored at -183°C (-297.4°F) and is supplied via wall outlets. This requires highly sophisticated cryotechnology. In resource-limited countries, oxygen is supplied in pressurized tanks. This is an expensive method and lacks the reliability of a constant supply in remote health facilities with poor transport systems. Appropriate methods for administering oxygen are often also lacking. Oxygen is administered in the nursery by different techniques—commonly by an oxygen hood. The oxygen hood cannot ensure the delivery of an intended concentration of oxygen, especially when there is no oxygen analyzer. It is difficult to achieve oxygen concentrations greater than 40% unless the hood has minimal leakage. There is also a great wastage of oxygen, which adds to the cost. Delivery of oxygen by nasal cannulae minimizes loss of oxygen and ensures direct delivery even at low flow rates. In the absence of nasal cannulae, oxygen can be delivered by face mask. Commercially available face masks, infrequently used in NICUs in the developed world, come in different sizes for term and premature infants.

Physicians and health care workers can use commercially available equipment (nasal cannulae, oxygen hoods, and CPAP devices) where feasible and affordable or develop innovative methods using basic principles of physics and physiology combined with ingenuity. Nasal prongs are simple to use and ensure effective oxygen delivery. Judicious application of CPAP in infants in respiratory distress has been shown to be very effective in managing infants with RDS in resource-poor countries. Sahni and Wung[39] have demonstrated that CPAP devices are important tools in the management of RDS in this environment. The techniques of oxygen delivery and application of CPAP are well described elsewhere in this book.

Bubble CPAP for resource-limited areas of the world is a good low-cost alternative for providing respiratory support. A study in Iran demonstrated better survival with bubble CPAP (100%) compared to ventilator-derived CPAP (71%).[40] Similarly, bubble CPAP had a higher success rate than ventilator-derived CPAP in a study from India.[41] In Malawi there was a 27% absolute improvement in survival using bubble CPAP.[35] Introduction of CPAP in a level II unit significantly reduced the need for transfer of infants to tertiary care units in India.[42] In a systematic review, bubble CPAP was reported to be safe

and reduced the need for mechanical ventilation in neonates with respiratory distress in tertiary referral hospitals in low- and middle-income countries.[43] Moreover, bubble CPAP has been effectively applied by nurses and other health care workers to improve neonatal survival and quality of neonatal care in these settings.[32,36] Hence in resource-limited countries, starting bubble CPAP services in special care newborn units with good level II care may be a better option than mechanical ventilation and parallels recent thinking in developed regions of the world, where mechanical ventilators are freely available, but attempts are being made to reduce ventilator-induced lung injury by using CPAP. There are a number of commercially marketed CPAP devices manufactured in the United States and the United Kingdom that are available to resource-limited countries. However, the cost of commercially available CPAP devices and circuits could be as high as seven times that of indigenously made CPAP devices. The costs of home-made bubble CPAP devices range from as little as US$10 for simple devices to US$6000 for commercial units. Bubble CPAP is cheaper, less invasive, and more accessible and requires less technical skill for application than currently available commercial ventilators.[43]

Ventilators

The purchase of ventilators is a major investment for hospitals in resource-limited countries. The initial cost is a major determining factor in establishing a ventilator care program. The typical costs of ventilator and supplies are shown in Box 38-1 based on the data provided by Marketstrat, Inc.[25] Often physicians and hospital administrators are pressured into buying expensive equipment based on brand name recognition. Health professionals and administrators must consider some basic guidelines, shown in Box 38-1, in selecting a particular brand of ventilator. In addition to a well-recognized brand name, simplicity of operation and ease of maintenance and availability of spare parts should be the important considerations in selecting a specific ventilator. Because of limited funding, ventilators that can serve various age groups may be more economical. The ventilator should have an overall low life-cycle cost. In addition to the purchase of the ventilator, the purchase of disposables and service contracts is to be taken into consideration to maintain a functioning program. Most programs fail to maintain service contracts because of yearly budget constraints, a major barrier faced in all low- and middle-income countries. Once purchased, the unit should designate a professional (doctor/nurse) in the unit with the responsibility of maintenance and ordering disposable supplies. Regular maintenance checkups of the ventilators are essential.

Clinical Care Pathways

Pathways for clinical management, including management of babies on CPAP or assisted ventilation, skin-to-skin care, monitoring for ventilator-associated infections, nosocomial infections, blood gases, and nutritional support, are essential parts of establishing respiratory care programs. Standardizing care and developing clinical care pathways can be helpful in day-to-day management. An increase in the use of evidence-based practices has been associated with an increase in survival.[30] As the babies will need continuous support and the most senior person is not at the bedside at all times, having clinical care pathways that are evidence based helps the bedside provider manage the patient. Nurses in India report having to manage problems with very little support at night.[44]

Some institutes in India have developed protocols for management of sick neonates in the NICU.[45]

Clinical Monitoring

Monitoring of critically ill infants in resource-poor countries is based mainly on clinical observation because very few electronic monitors are available. Several investigators have adopted different methods to train health care personnel in assessing clinical hypoxemia. Bang et al.[46] have shown that lay village workers can be trained to recognize infants in respiratory distress in the community. However, no such studies have been done in the immediate neonatal period.

Downes et al.[47] published a clinical scoring system, the "RDS score," which correlated with blood gas measurements. The original Downes score consisted of hourly assessment of five clinical signs: respiratory rate, grunting, color, retractions, and breath sounds on auscultation. Later this evaluation was modified by including gestational age and oxygen requirement in the Acute Care of At-Risk Newborns Respiratory Score[48] (Table 38-2). The score is simple and can be learned by almost any health professional; it requires no electronic or biochemical monitoring and provides a guideline of changing clinical status to initiate interventions when required. Based on total score, respiratory distress can be divided into mild, moderate, and severe if the score is <5, 5 to 8, or >8, respectively. Babies with a respiratory score of <5 in the first 4 hours need close observation and possible oxygen supplementation. Babies with moderate respiratory distress (i.e., score of 5 to 8) may need some degree of respiratory support such as CPAP and sometimes mechanical ventilation to prevent progression into severe respiratory distress and respiratory failure. Babies with severe respiratory distress (score >8) require immediate intubation and assisted ventilation. A modified Downes score has been adopted in several resource-poor countries including Indonesia and the Russian Federation States.[49] The respiratory score is used to clinically evaluate hypoxemia in neonates with respiratory distress in resource-poor countries where pulse oximetry and blood gas analysis is not available.

Education

To sustain respiratory care services, there should be a program for training all health care providers. Nurses require orientation for care of the newborn[44] and then require ongoing support from the medical staff to care for these fragile babies. The training should be done during the initial orientation to the unit. Ongoing educational programs and professional development training programs should be available to enhance the skill and knowledge of health care workers concurrent with the implementation of evidence-based practices. Clinical care teams at health facilities need to be trained in monitoring and improving quality of care by conducting PDSA (plan–do–study–act) cycles for performance improvement.

Evaluation

Those units undertaking neonatal respiratory care should also develop database systems for frequent auditing, maintaining quality control, and addressing ongoing quality improvement of services provided. Ongoing evaluation should consist of data collection, monitoring systems for implementing change, and follow-up.

One of the complications of enhanced respiratory care programs is the emergence of retinopathy of prematurity (ROP) as a major cause of blindness in children in the low- and middle-income countries of Latin American and Asia, where advanced intensive care services have improved the survival of high-risk neonates.[50-53] About 65% of those visually impaired from ROP were born in resource-limited countries.[54] Approximately 6% of all ROP visually impaired infants were born at >32 weeks. It appears that the overzealous administration of oxygen without appropriate monitoring in addition to the survival of more VLBW infants is responsible for this phenomenon. Therefore improved oxygen delivery and monitoring, along with locally adapted screening/treatment programs, are necessary when considering management of respiratory care services.

Health-care-associated infection and ventilator-associated pneumonia (VAP) are common and serious problems among mechanically ventilated neonates. The incidence of VAP is reported to be 17.3% to 57.1% in resource-limited countries.[55-58] Factors such as prolonged NICU stay, reintubation, parenteral nutrition, and blood transfusion are additional risk factors for VAP.[59] There is a need for quality improvement initiatives to monitor and decrease important morbidities such as health-care-associated infections, VAP, ROP, and CLD.

PROJECTED GROWTH IN NEONATAL VENTILATION—A GLOBAL PERSPECTIVE

Despite all of the aforementioned difficulties, there is steady growth of the neonatal ventilator market worldwide. Research data from Marketstrat, Inc.,[25] reveal an increasing awareness and interest in the purchase and use of ventilator support for adults and newborns around the world. Their global market survey shows that although the developed countries have the greatest proportion of the ventilator market share, there has been a rapid and progressive increase in ventilator purchases in low- and middle-income countries, especially China, Latin

TABLE 38-2	Acute Care of At-Risk Newborns Respiratory Distress Score System		
Score	0	1	2
Respiratory rate	40-60/min	60-80/min	>80/min
Oxygen requirement*	None	≤50%	>50%
Retractions	None	Mild to moderate	Severe
Grunting	None	With stimulation	Continuous at rest
Breath sounds on auscultation	Easily heard throughout	Decreased	Barely heard
Prematurity	>34 weeks	30-34 weeks	<30 weeks

*A baby receiving oxygen prior to setup of oxygen analyzer should be assigned a score of 1.
(Adapted from Downes JJ, Vidyasagar D, Boggs TR Jr, Morrow GM 3rd. Respiratory distress syndrome of newborn infants. I. New clinical scoring system (RDS score) with acid–base and blood gas correlations. *Clin Pediatr.* 1970;9(6):325-331.)

America, and India. The total world market sales for mechanical ventilators (adults and neonates) and associated disposable and maintenance services have increased significantly since 1995. The neonatal ventilator market is also expected to grow steadily. The United States is the largest market, whereas India is the fastest growing, followed by Latin America.

Globally, neonatal ventilators account for about 10% to 11% of all ventilators sold. Sales of high-frequency ventilator units are expected to grow at a rate of 1.3% per year. The Americas have the largest market share, followed by Europe, and then the Asian Pacific countries.

Even though neonatal ventilator purchases are increasing in resource-limited countries, these acquisitions are far fewer than these countries need. With the current projected rate of purchase, India will have one ventilator per 80,000 live-born babies; China will have one ventilator per 30,000 live births, compared to one ventilator per 500 births in the United States. Considering higher neonatal morbidity from LBW and birth asphyxia rates in India and China, the requirements for ventilators are many times higher than the above estimates. The current estimated rate of purchases of 100 ventilators per year in each country is grossly insufficient to meet current and future needs.

OUTCOMES OF NEONATAL VENTILATION

The outcomes of neonates treated with ventilation in resource-limited countries have been published in recent years. Investigators of the National Neonatal–Perinatal Database[60] from India reported that 45% of outborn babies admitted to the NICU required oxygen therapy, and 16% required assisted ventilation. Of the 3831 newborns admitted to NICUs, 87% were delivered at small private hospitals and 68% of admissions were male. Half of the admissions were LBW, 32% were preterm, and 7.5% left against medical advice. Common causes of death included sepsis (36%), prematurity (26%), and perinatal asphyxia (10%). The survival rate of ventilated infants in India ranges from 46% to 58%.[61-64] As expected increasing gestational age and birth weight were significantly associated with improved survival rates.

A study from China reported 18-month outcomes of 288 preterm infants mechanically ventilated for RDS. The incidence of cerebral palsy (CP) among study subjects was 17%, 5%, and 2% in infants less than 28, 28 to 30, and 30 to 32 weeks, respectively.[65] The incidence of Mental Developmental Index (MDI) score <70 was 49%, 24%, and 13% in infants less than 28, 28 to 30, and 30 to 32 weeks, respectively. Infants ventilated by conventional mode had significantly higher incidences of CP and cognitive delay (MDI <70) compared to those ventilated on HFOV. Longer duration of mechanical ventilation and blood transfusions was associated with an increased risk of having an MDI of <70 or CP.

In a study from Pakistan, of the 200 babies admitted to NICUs with RDS, 79% required assisted ventilation, with an overall mortality of 39%.[30] The mortality rate for infants weighing less than 1000 g was 70% but only 30% for infants weighing greater than 1000 g.

A report from Ghana showed that establishment of a ventilator support program in the NICU at a teaching hospital led to a dramatic decrease in mortality of infants admitted to the unit.[66] The significant finding of this report was that the major single intervention in an already existing NICU was the addition of ventilators and improved physical facilities. This was a one-time capital budget commitment. No new nurses were added; however, the existing staff was given on-site additional training in ventilator care. These observations suggest that it is possible to develop NICUs with ventilatory support even in developing countries with minimum investments.

Initiating ventilatory support is associated with emergence of new morbidities, specifically CLD and ROP. Wei in China noted that improved survival of infants weighing less than 1500 g was associated with an increase in CLD.[15] Similarly, there are reports of increasing occurrence of ROP in survivors after ventilation in resource-poor countries.[50-53,67] However, the programs in these resource-poor countries lack the required pediatric ophthalmologic services for screening or ROP surgery. Considering these limitations, one should take a cautious approach in developing ventilator care programs in resource-limited countries.

ETHICAL DILEMMAS

The introduction of neonatal and critical care services poses several economic and ethical dilemmas. In a national study in India, 7.5% of NICU infants were discharged against physician advice.[60] These discharges were most likely due to economic, social, and family reasons. Moazam and Lakhani[68] discussed the dilemmas of providing neonatal intensive care in a resource-limited country. Their concerns were related to the high cost of NICU care. Narang et al.[69] reported that the average total cost of care for a baby less than 1000 g in India was Rs 168,000 (US$3800), Rs 88,300 (US$2000) for babies 1000 to 1250 g, and Rs 41,700 (US$950) for those between 1250 and 1500 g. In addition, there is considerable disease burden secondary to associated morbidities of CLD, ROP, and neurodevelopmental disabilities in resource-limited countries. The ethical question is, "Is it justifiable to invest a country's meager health care resources to benefit a few sick infants?" With increasing awareness of available technologies to save critically ill infants, parents have higher expectations. But daily expenses incurred for the care given in the NICU challenge the parental support. The mounting daily hospital costs may exceed the capabilities of the family. Therefore every attempt should be made to honor distributive justice.

Physicians and health care administrators in these regions should define priorities and decide the level of care based on the resources available. All babies must be given the basic care available in the country. Decisions to offer ventilator care should be based not only on immediate clinical needs but also on the implications of long-term needs of health care and the availability of support systems in the community once the infant recovers from the acute illness.[70] Singh,[70] in an article on ethical and social issues in the care of the newborn in resource-limited countries, offers some suggestions regarding the ethical issues faced by pediatric and neonatal practitioners in these countries (Box 38-2). Clearly, each society must develop guidelines based on its local values, cultural variations, and resources.

CONCLUSIONS

It is clear that resource-limited countries have the highest neonatal and infant mortality from respiratory problems and that there is a great unmet need for respiratory care and ventilatory support. Yet these are the same countries that lack the most essential minimum equipment such as bags and masks

BOX 38-2   Ethical Questions to Consider in Resource-Limited Countries

- Should the best interest of the baby or the global interest of the family determine the care given?
- Should each country decide a cutoff weight (or gestational age) below which no NICU care is given?
- Should NICU ventilator care be denied to those who cannot afford to pay?
- Can therapy be stopped when a family cannot afford to pay for further care?
- Should expensive NICU care be given to extremely or very low birth-weight infants of parents who do not have basic amenities at home and where social support from the government is not available?

for resuscitation, continuous supplies of oxygen, and oxygen delivery devices. It is suggested that the World Health Organization (WHO) designate this life-saving equipment as part of essential equipment, similar to the WHO Essential Drug List.[71] Such policies would make a major impact on neonatal survival internationally. Health care workers at primary health care centers and hospitals should be trained in providing basic respiratory care, including clinical assessment using the RDS score, basic principles of care including clearing the airway, bag and mask ventilation, and proper oxygen therapy. The staff at level II units must be routinely trained in providing oxygen therapy and applying CPAP. Staff in level III units should be capable of providing ventilatory support using mechanical ventilation.

Countries with high birth rates and high NMRs require the establishment of regional NICUs with ventilatory support. These centers of excellence must provide nationwide training of health care personnel in basic resuscitation, stabilization with nasal CPAP, and triage and transport to hospitals that can provide higher levels of respiratory care. The market research data also show that developing countries are rapidly acquiring neonatal ventilators; however, there is a lack of concurrent development of respiratory care programs. China has developed a model in which health policies are implemented in a top-down fashion by the government. The NNF of India provides a model in which a professional physician organization has started a major initiative to improve newborn care in the country. Other countries have developed individual NICUs. A combination of varying models may work well for other resource-limited countries.

Because of the large global need, it is important that professionals, organizations, institutions, and government agencies in developed countries extend their services and participate in global programs to accelerate the transfer of knowledge and skills of respiratory care to resource-limited countries. These goals can be achieved through bilateral exchange of medical faculty and nurses between institutions in resource-limited and developed countries. In our own experience, these approaches have made an enormous impact in several countries.

REFERENCES

A complete reference list is available at https://expertconsult .inkling.com/.

39

Transport of the Ventilated Infant

Robert M. Insoft, MD

IMPORTANT ROLE OF THE TRANSPORT TEAM

The widespread development of both regional perinatal centers and interhospital transport services for critically ill newborns and infants has been an important factor in decreasing perinatal morbidity and mortality. Starting in the 1970s, the growing recognition that regionalization of care improved patient outcomes resulted in the formation of regionalized centers for perinatal and neonatal care. With this development of regionalized care, the need for skilled transport teams was realized. Today, as advanced technologies have become more available and portable, the transport team has become an extension of the intensive care unit, and transport teams now initiate the comprehensive specialized care in the referral hospital that will be continued in the tertiary care center. Transport teams bring the intensive care environment to the infant, even starting care in the referring hospital's delivery room, stabilizing the infant to ensure a safe and effective transfer.

As advanced technologies have been approved and adopted, sophisticated treatments such as high-frequency ventilation (HFV) and inhaled nitric oxide (iNO) are now frequently initiated in many level III units. When these therapies fail to stabilize the infant in intensive care units that do not offer extracorporeal membrane oxygenation (ECMO), transport to a quaternary neonatal care unit is often necessary. Transfer of these highly complex neonates requires a sophisticated and skilled transport team and may be aided by real-time audio and video cell phone capabilities and wireless electronic medical records.

The modern transport team has adapted to meet the needs of these complex infants. Teams now have the ability to provide intensive therapies such as surfactant therapy, HFV, iNO, passive or active therapeutic hypothermia, and even mobile ECMO in some cases. Team members competent in the critical care of an ill newborn must be able to provide a rapid response to the referral hospitals who request their services. They must provide appropriate stabilization for transport in an expedient and safe manner. Importantly, as the skills and technologies of transport teams continue to change and develop, it is becoming evident that comprehensive care and therapies initiated during transport can improve patient outcomes.

REGIONALIZED CARE

In the early 1970s, clinicians recognized that neonates treated at tertiary centers had improved outcomes, and the push for regionalized care began. Usher[1] demonstrated a 50% reduction in mortality for critically ill newborns who received care at tertiary centers. Other studies confirmed these results and also showed improved mortality rates for infants transported to regional care centers.[2-3]

Although the previous studies supported the early transfer of high-risk mothers and fetuses to tertiary centers, the birth of high-risk infants in nontertiary centers has continued to occur, and data suggest that 14% to 30% of very low birth-weight (VLBW) infants are delivered in nontertiary hospitals.[4-6] Studies of such infants further support the fact that outborn infants experience significantly higher morbidity and mortality compared to infants delivered at tertiary perinatal centers. Chien et al.[7] found that outborn infants were at higher risk of death, severe intraventricular hemorrhage (IVH), patent ductus arteriosus, respiratory distress syndrome (RDS), and nosocomial infections, even after adjusting for perinatal risks and illness severity.

Lui et al.[8] performed an interesting study comparing inborn and outborn infants born between 23 weeks and 28 weeks 6 days of gestation before and after the development of regionalized care. They compared outcomes for infants born from 1992 to 1995 to those born from 1997 to 2002. They showed that optimization of in utero transfers resulted in 25% fewer nontertiary hospital births and that with provision of perinatal consults, increased provision of antenatal steroids, and centralization of the neonatal retrieval system, outborn mortality rates decreased significantly from 39.4% to 25.1%. Rates of severe IVH and necrotizing enterocolitis (NEC) also decreased in outborn infants between the two periods after interventions were started. Importantly, however, morbidity for outborn infants continued to be significantly higher than that for inborn infants, especially with regard to severe (grade 3 or 4) IVH (19.4% outborn vs 10% inborn, $p = 0.002$) and radiologically or surgically proven NEC (7.2% outborn vs 1.7% inborn, $p < 0.001$). These data demonstrate that implementation of a coordinated system to provide perinatal consults and appropriate neonatal transport improves outcomes, but outborn infants continue to face higher morbidity despite these interventions. Thus in utero transfer of high-risk pregnancies to a tertiary center remains the best option. When maternal transfer cannot be accomplished because of rapid labor progression, pending delivery, or fetal or maternal compromise, the specialized services offered by the neonatal transport team play an important role in optimizing outborn infant care. Many teams will even now offer to attend unexpected high-risk deliveries in community settings if a maternal transport is prohibited.

Acknowledgment: We would like to acknowledge Dr. Kristen Melton and Dr. Gary Pettett for their contributions in the earlier edition of this chapter.

TRANSPORT TEAM COMPOSITION

Multiple approaches have been used when determining the makeup of the ideal transport team. Each institution must determine the most appropriate model for their facility based on the volume, types of transport (ground vs rotor wing vs fixed wing), travel times, skills required for efficient and safe transfers, availability of team members, and overall costs. The American Academy of Pediatrics (AAP) has recommended that transport teams consist of at least two providers, with one member being a nurse who has 5 years or more of nursing experience.[9] Team members can include emergency or intensive care nurses, nurse practitioners (NPs), pediatric respiratory therapists (RTs), paramedics, and physicians, including attending staff, fellows, or residents in training. Most commonly teams are made up of RT/nurse pairs or nurse/nurse pairs with paramedic support. Given the significant number of neonatal transports requiring respiratory interventions, many teams find the skills of an RT helpful and often necessary. However, all transport team members should be cross-trained and capable of supporting all transport procedures and interventions.

Karlsen et al.[10] have studied transport volume and various team models and their effects on patient care outcomes. Karlsen's survey found wide variation in many aspects of team organization, including team configuration, staff orientation, and use of protocols as well as quality improvement methodologies. Consistent with previous work, Karlsen found no difference in patient care outcomes when comparing variations in team members, including RN/RT, NP/RT, and MD/RN/RT. The presence of a physician did not alter patient outcomes in this study.

Multiple other studies have supported the idea that nonphysician teams are capable of providing care that is effective, and potentially timelier, than teams accompanied by a physician. Beyer et al.[11] demonstrated that nonphysician teams were able to provide care and transport intubated neonates without problems. In their cohort, 20% of infants were intubated by a transport nurse or RT at the referring facility. They concluded that there was a low incidence of complications in intubated neonates when transported by personnel trained in intubation and neonatal resuscitation. Leslie and Stephenson[12] found that transports directed by advanced neonatal NPs were as effective as those directed by physicians, and King et al.[13] found that there was no change in mortality or complications when teams were converted from nurse/physician teams to nurse/nurse teams but that response time did improve. Voluntary reporting by pediatric and neonatal transport teams to the AAP Section of Transport Medicine team database indicates that almost half of the teams providing information (37 of 82 teams) do not include physicians on transport.[14] Thus with a well-trained, experienced transport team, availability of a medical control physician by telephone may be all that is required.

Regardless of the model chosen, however, team members should be specialists in neonatal and pediatric care because specialized teams have been shown to make a significant difference in outcome. Early studies demonstrated that dedicated neonatal transport teams reduced both morbidity and mortality in VLBW infants who required transfer to a tertiary center[15,16] and that outborn infants who were not transferred by a specialized transport team experienced a 60% greater mortality rate.[17]

More recent studies confirm that the incidence of transport-related morbidity increases when personnel without specific pediatric training transport critically ill children. A study by Edge et al.[18] demonstrated that adverse events during interhospital transport, such as accidental extubation or intravenous (IV) access problems, were significantly higher in transports performed by a nonspecialized team (20%) compared to transports performed by a specialized pediatric team (2%). Similarly, Macnab[19] demonstrated a higher rate of secondary complications in infants transported by nonspecialized transport teams compared to pediatric transport teams.

High-volume transport programs have the advantage of being able to develop full-time transport teams dedicated solely to neonatal transport, in which experience is greater and skills are more easily maintained. Smaller services that use team members on a more infrequent basis must invest significantly in continuing education to maintain their knowledge base and technical skills to provide specialized services. Data from the ongoing AAP voluntary registration of transport teams suggest that the majority of teams provide combined pediatric and neonatal transport services.[14] Although this is often necessary and allows the maintenance of a dedicated team, team members should track the number of neonatal transports they perform to be sure they are maintaining adequate exposure to the unique circumstances involved in neonatal resuscitation and transport. A lack of exposure should be offset by continuing education including in-unit training and simulation.

Transport teams are frequently called to attend and participate in the deliveries of high-risk preterm infants that occur outside of the tertiary center. Although all delivery hospitals should have at least one attendant certified in neonatal resuscitation available at all times, transport personnel may be asked to support referral staff or, in some cases, may be the primary resuscitator at a preterm delivery. Although this is often a stressful situation, data demonstrate that the presence of a dedicated neonatal retrieval team can improve delivery room resuscitation of these outborn premature infants.[6] In this study, neonates who were resuscitated by a specialized transport team were intubated more promptly with fewer attempts, had fewer accidental extubations, and were more likely to receive surfactant therapy in a timely manner.

Neonates cared for only by the referring hospital team had higher rates of hypothermia, lack of vascular access, and more extensive resuscitation. Despite having the same average gestational age, infants resuscitated by the referral team received longer chest compressions (6 min vs 0.5 min), longer bag–mask ventilation (13.5 min vs 7 min), and longer continuous positive airway pressure (CPAP) (14 min vs 2 min), all of which may reflect a delay in intubation by the referral team. These differences are not surprising, because referral hospitals that appropriately transfer high-risk mothers and fetuses lack a critical mass of preterm births and experience in resuscitation of extremely low birth-weight (ELBW) and VLBW preterm infants.

Dedicated teams with specialized training and increased experience are able to provide better specialized care and resuscitation. Given the evidence that the first few minutes of resuscitation and early oxygen exposure can influence long-term outcome, the need to optimize resuscitation is evident.[20-22] These studies reinforce the fact that transport teams should be made up of clinicians with specific training in comprehensive neonatal care and resuscitation and also suggest that the use of the transport team as a neonatal resuscitation team for outborn infants may be optimal.

TRANSPORT EDUCATION

The need for extensive education of team members who transport neonates is obvious, because team members are expected to recognize and treat a wide array of disorders. They must be able to resuscitate and stabilize neonates in critical condition and ensure their safe transport, often under conditions that may be suboptimal. Although no standard curriculum exists, guidelines for team education have been published by the AAP Section on Transport Medicine.[23] Education of transport team members includes a requirement for resuscitation training through the Neonatal Resuscitation Program (AAP and American Heart Association provider course) or a similar program, as well as continuing education in neonatal pathology and disease. Continuing medical education (CME) and transport review conferences ensure that team members maintain their skills in neonatal stabilization and expose them to new topics in neonatal care. CME opportunities should include skills lab, with stations focusing on skilled intubation, effective bag–mask ventilation, handling of the difficult airway, chest tube placement, and vascular access, including IV line placement, umbilical line placement, and intraosseous line placement. In addition, simulation-based exercises should be employed when possible.

Unique to transport team education are the requirements for basic knowledge about flight physiology and its contribution to disease states, the physical and mental stresses of transport, and the need for a significant focus on safety that includes both team and patient safety. Given the many unique challenges encountered during transport (excessive noise, vibration and rotation forces, low-level lighting, variable ambient temperatures/humidity, and the need for specific safety measures), team members should receive extensive supervised orientation and then must participate in transports with sufficient regularity to maintain their skills in all transport settings. Team members may also benefit from training on ethical and legal issues such as the withdrawal of support, because they may be involved in situations in which support is stopped after resuscitation or in which infants are deemed appropriate for withdrawal of care at the referring facility, in which the family can participate, rather than for transport to a distant facility. Training should also be given regarding the social aspects of transport to help team members work more compassionately with families and help raise team awareness of the many emotional issues that are faced by parents and family members during the crisis precipitated by a neonatal transport.

TRANSPORT PHYSIOLOGY

The effects of altitude and the stresses of flight can have a significant impact on the neonate during fixed-wing or helicopter transport, especially in the already compromised infant. The transport environment itself, including ground transport, introduces unique stressors such as noise, vibration, and temperature variation. Transport team members must understand altitude physiology and the physiologic stresses of neonatal transport to anticipate and properly treat problems that may occur during transport. Each of these factors can affect team members as well. The most significant concerns include the following:

1. Hypoxia
2. Air expansion
3. Noise and vibration
4. Thermoregulation

Hypoxia

As an aircraft ascends, the partial pressure of gas decreases. As the altitude above sea level increases, the barometric pressure falls, and the partial pressure of ambient oxygen and thus the alveolar oxygen partial pressure decrease. During this time, infants may develop hypoxia. This is demonstrated using the simplified alveolar gas equation, $P_{AO_2} = (P_B - 47) \times FiO_2 - PaCO_2/0.8$, where P_{AO_2} is the partial pressure of alveolar oxygen, P_B is the barometric pressure, 47 is the partial pressure of water vapor, FiO_2 is the inspired oxygen concentration, $PaCO_2$ is the partial pressure of arterial CO_2, and 0.8 is the respiratory quotient. If an infant receiving 50% inspired oxygen with a $PaCO_2$ of 50 is transported from sea level (barometric pressure = 760) in a nonpressurized plane that must achieve 8000 feet for the transfer (barometric pressure = 570), then the alveolar oxygen partial pressure will drop from 294 at sea level to 199 at altitude, if you assume no change in minute ventilation, FiO_2, or $PaCO_2$. In reality, the partial pressure of arterial CO_2 will decrease at altitude as well, making the alveolar oxygen partial pressure slightly greater than that calculated by the following equation:

$$P_{AO_2} \text{ (sea level)} = (760 - 47) \times 0.5 - 50/0.8 = 294$$

$$P_{AO_2} \text{ (8000 ft)} = (570 - 47) \times 0.5 - 50/0.8 = 199$$

Preterm infants, infants with respiratory diseases, and infants with high oxygen demands (sepsis, shock) are at particular risk of developing hypoxia. Careful monitoring of oxygen saturation helps with identification of infants experiencing hypoxia, who usually respond to increased FiO_2 levels or increased positive end-expiratory pressure (PEEP). For infants already receiving oxygen prior to transport, the need for increased oxygen during flight should be anticipated. The anticipated adjustment in oxygen administration can be calculated using the following equation:

$$\text{Adjusted } FiO_2 = (FiO_2 \times P_{B1})/P_{B2}$$

where FiO_2 represents the current FiO_2 being administered, P_{B1} is the current barometric pressure, and P_{B2} is the barometric pressure at the highest anticipated altitude during transport.

Air Expansion

As an aircraft ascends and barometric pressure falls, the volume of gas within a closed space expands. Gas in an enclosed space at sea level (i.e., a pneumothorax) will expand by a factor of 1.5 at 10,000 feet. This is most significant for the infant with a pneumothorax or a pneumopericardium, although it may influence the status of the infant with a pneumoperitoneum or pneumatosis as well. Ideally, air leaks are treated prior to flight because of the concern of further expansion at higher altitudes.

Noise and Vibration

Noise and vibration are significant problems encountered during both air and ground transports. Studies have shown that neonates are exposed to very high levels of sound during transport and that mean sound levels for all modes of transport exceed the recommended levels for neonatal intensive care.[24,25] Similarly, neonates experience high vibration accelerations within the transport incubator.[25] Configuration of the transport unit should be optimized to reduce vibration, and ear protection should be considered for neonates during transport, particularly during air transport, in which sound exposure is greatest.

Thermoregulation

Ambient temperatures change significantly with altitude variation and with seasonal variation during ground transport. Proper thermoregulation has been shown to be critical for the intact survival of VLBW infants,[26,27] whereas hyperthermia can be detrimental to infants with perinatal acidosis and hypoxic–ischemic encephalopathy.[28,29] Temperature variation will also increase metabolic and oxygen demands, which can cause further compromise in the hypoxic or septic patient. Transport members must be thoughtful about optimizing the thermal factors they can control. Conductive heat loss can be minimized by preheating the transport incubator and blankets and using a chemical heating mattress. Evaporative heat losses are minimized by keeping the skin surface dry, using a polyethylene bag for ELBW/VLBW infants, and heating and humidifying inspired gases. Additional efforts to control cabin temperature may be required during specific seasons.

STABILIZATION

The goal of the transport team is to initiate definitive care for the ill neonate and to bring the resources of the tertiary center to the infant. Ideally neonates should be transported when they are stable, so that transport can occur in a safe and controlled manner. This means that the ill neonate should be stabilized as much as possible in the referring hospital environment, which offers the advantages of space; easy access to the infant; better lighting and visibility; access to personnel, equipment, and support (laboratory and radiology); thermal stability for the infant; and ease of communication with the tertiary center neonatologist. Stabilization involves identifying and treating factors that could lead to deterioration of the infant's condition. Procedures or interventions that are needed, such as intubation, chest tube placement, or vascular access, should be anticipated as much as possible and performed prior to transport. Given the limitations of the transport space, and the complexity added to the transport environment by vibration and noise, only rarely should a major intervention such as intubation need to be performed during the course of transport itself. Despite the inherent desire to expedite the transport process, time spent stabilizing an infant at the referring facility is an important investment to ensure a safe and effective transport. There are rare situations (e.g., transposition of the great vessels with intact ventricular septum) in which definitive treatment can be offered only at the tertiary institution and the benefit of rapid transport outweighs the risk of transporting an unstable infant.

CLINICAL ISSUES

The members of a specialized transport team must recognize and treat a wide array of neonatal disorders. Although each transport is different, there is a standard set of broad issues that must be addressed in every neonatal transport. These include the following:
1. Respiratory support and airway issues
2. Cardiovascular support
3. Vascular access
4. Glucose stability
5. Thermal regulation
6. Infection risks and treatment

The most common problem encountered by neonatal transport personnel is respiratory distress. Multiple studies[30] have found that over 85% of neonates that are transported received some form of assisted ventilation, and transport teams performed intubation as well as initiating ventilation in a vast majority of transported infants. Newborns most commonly present with respiratory diseases, so it is not surprising that airway interventions (intubation, mechanical ventilation including CPAP) are the most common interventions performed by the transport team.[30,31] Transport personnel must be skilled in establishing and maintaining an airway in a neonate. Airway skills should include not only intubation but also appropriate bag–valve mask ventilation, use of nasal and oral airways, placement of CPAP prongs, use of a laryngeal mask airway (LMA), and options for handling a difficult airway. Skills in basic chest X-ray interpretation are needed for diagnosis and optimal management of respiratory diseases.

Transport personnel must also understand the concepts of mechanical ventilation. They should be able to recognize and treat complications encountered with the use of positive pressure and an endotracheal tube, because endotracheal tube or ventilator problems occur in almost 10% of transports.[32] Priority must be given to properly securing the endotracheal tube to avoid accidental extubation in transit. Team members should be able to recognize and treat pulmonary air leaks of various forms and need to have experience in needle thoracentesis or chest tube placement. Optimization of ventilation and oxygenation prior to and during transport are important for maintaining stabilization and for achieving the goal of providing comprehensive care. There is room for improvement in transport ventilator management; studies have shown that 15% to 25% of transported infants have suboptimal pH or Pco_2 levels at tertiary center arrival.[33,34]

From a cardiovascular standpoint, transport personnel must be able to recognize and appropriately stabilize infants with congenital heart disease. Differentiating severe pulmonary disease from cyanotic congenital heart disease can be difficult, but proper recognition and initiation of prostaglandin can significantly influence outcome. Team members must be well versed in the use of prostaglandin and its complications. Teams in communication with medical control must make a decision about intubation of infants on prostaglandin E_1 (PGE_1) based on the stability of the infant, the dose of medication being used, and the length and mode of transport. Limited evidence exists regarding the need for intubation of infants on PGE_1 prior to transport. Apnea has been reported to occur in 12% to 30% of infants treated with PGE_1, but the incidence can be as high as 42% in infants weighing less than 2 kg.[35,36] Browning-Carmo et al.[37] evaluated 93 of 300 infants with congenital heart disease undergoing transport who did not have mechanical ventilation initiated at the beginning of the PGE_1 infusion. Of these infants, 17% went on to require intubation for apnea within 1 hour of PGE_1 initiation, and 2.6% of the remaining infants developed apnea during transport. Overall, 25% of infants were able to be successfully transported without intubation, but these infants were receiving very low doses of PGE_1, less than 0.015 µg/kg/min. Although each situation must be individually assessed, in general, term infants who are receiving standard PGE_1 doses may be transported short distances safely without intubation. Transport teams also have the ability to supply nitrogen or CO_2 to unstable infants with hypoplastic left heart physiology during transport, but extensive education is needed before this approach is implemented.

The ability to establish vascular access is a critical skill for transport team members to possess. Team personnel must be able to place an umbilical venous line emergently during resuscitation for the purpose of administering epinephrine and volume, as well as nonemergently for administration of IV fluids, medications, or blood products. Some centers expect that transport personnel will be able to place umbilical arterial lines as well; however, the time necessary for umbilical arterial line placement should be weighed against earlier transport to the tertiary center where the procedure can be done under more ideal circumstances. Unless central blood pressure and/or arterial blood gas monitoring is needed on transport, this procedure is typically deferred to the tertiary center. Team members also should have the training and skills required for intraosseous line placement for emergent situations.

Maintenance of normal glucose levels and maintenance of thermal stability have both been shown to be critical for neonatal morbidity and mortality prevention.[26,28,38] Transport team members must recognize the importance of glucose stability and thermal stability in neonates and should have protocols that address these two key issues for every transport. Although glucose and temperature alterations are problems that are usually easily treated or controlled, they are also easily overlooked. Several studies evaluating optimization during transport have shown that approximately 10% of neonates have hypothermia, and 10% of neonates have hypoglycemia on arrival following transport.[32,34]

Ongoing quality improvement is an essential piece to transport management. Lee et al.[33] first validated a physiology-based scoring system for assessment of neonatal transport. The Transport Risk Index of Physiologic Stability (TRIPS) allows for prediction of 7-day mortality following transport, neonatal intensive care unit (NICU) mortality, and severe intraventricular hemorrhage. Recently, Schwartz et al.[39] demonstrated widespread agreement on the basic key quality metrics to ensure the success of a high-reliability program. His studies showed that transport metrics can be grouped into the following five basic categories: (1) effectiveness (intubation success rates), (2) safety metrics (medication administration errors), (3) efficiency (standardized patient handoff), (4) family/patient centeredness (family members on transport), and (5) timeliness (mobilization times). In addition, these investigators demonstrated that patient acuity scoring is relatively new to this field and has shown mixed benefits in clinical practice compared to the NICU or pediatric intensive care unit.

Finally, the suspicion of or true incidence of infection in newborn infants is high, and transport teams must consider these risks in order to perform appropriate evaluations and testing and initiate antibacterial or antiviral therapy in a timely manner.

EQUIPMENT

The equipment carried by the transport team must be lightweight, durable, compact, and easily secured, but most of all it must be complete to meet the safety needs of transport. The assumption should be made that the referring hospital will not have equipment needed to stabilize the neonate prior to transport. Medications and basic support supplies for interhospital transport are listed in Boxes 39-1 and 39-2. A variety of durable equipment bags exist for organizing consumable supplies and medications. Supply bags should be checked and replenished after every transport.

Transport systems have now been specifically designed to incorporate all of the critical life support systems and technology in a single mobile unit, including the transport incubator,

ventilator, monitoring systems, suction apparatus, and infusion pumps. Medical gas tanks are usually stowed on the bottom of the transport sled to provide compact storage but easy accessibility. Equipment used during transport can be run via an AC/DC power source or via internal battery if necessary. Transport ventilators may be powered pneumatically or by AC/DC power with battery backup. These complete systems have been designed to promote ease of movement, security within the transport vehicle to minimize the effects of vibration and motion, clear visualization of both monitors and the baby, and easy access to the infant.

Monitoring during transport of the ventilated infant has become significantly easier with the development of the pulse oximeter. Current models available provide adequate readouts despite the vibration contributed by the transport environment. Monitoring with pulse oximetry and electrocardiograph leads is standard during all transports. Target ranges for oxygen saturation should be adhered to during transport, especially for the ELBW infant. Several teams have also used noninvasive end-tidal CO_2 detectors or transcutaneous CO_2 monitors for evaluation during transport and found them to be effective, although some have noted problems with specific monitors being cumbersome and difficult to secure during transport.[40-42] Tingay et al.,[43] however, found that end-tidal CO_2 monitoring underestimated arterial CO_2 levels and did not trend reliably over time. Transport teams must still evaluate these adjuncts individually to determine their benefit, because no single standard has been adopted. Colorimetric CO_2 monitors that are placed briefly on the end of the endotracheal tube have been more universally adopted and have proven useful for confirming initial endotracheal intubation and continued intubation after movement from the isolette to the warmer and back during transport.[42] Quality of care and efficiency during transport have been greatly improved by the use of point-of-care devices, a handheld device that allows point-of-care analysis of blood gases, hematocrit, glucose, electrolytes, and ionized calcium on a small amount of blood (0.3 mL). Compact and easy to use, this instrument is easily carried in the equipment pack and provides rapid analysis at outlying hospitals, where blood

---

BOX 39-1   Suggested Medications for Interhospital Transport

Adenosine 6 mg/2 mL	Gentamicin 10 mg/mL
Albumin 5%	Heparinized saline
Alprostadil (PGE$_1$) 500 μg/mL	Lacri-Lube
Ampicillin 100 mg/mL	Lidocaine 1% 10 mg/mL
Atropine 0.1 mg/mL	Lorazepam (Ativan) 2 mg/mL
Calcium chloride 10% 100 mg/mL	Magnesium sulfate 1 g/2 mL
Calcium gluconate 10% 100 mg/mL	Midazolam (Versed) 1 mg/mL
Cefotaxime 100 mg/mL	Morphine 2 mg/mL
Clindamycin 150 mg/mL	Naloxone (Narcan) 1 mg/mL
D10W 250 mL	Nipride 50 mg/2 mL
Digoxin 100 μg/mL	Normal saline
Dobutamine 250 mg/20 mL	Phenobarbital 65 mg/mL
Dopamine 400 mg/5 mL	Rocuronium 10 mg/mL
Epinephrine 1:1000	Sodium bicarbonate 4.2%
Epinephrine 1:10,000	Sodium chloride, 3 mEq/mL
Fentanyl 0.05 mg/mL	Sterile water
Flumazenil 0.5 mg/5 mL	Surfactant
Fosphenytoin 100 mg/2 mL	Vecuronium 1 mg/mL
Furosemide (Lasix) 10 mg/mL	

gas measurements may be difficult to obtain in a timely manner. Macnab et al.[44] demonstrated that there is significant cost efficacy with the use of this technology and that use of point-of-care testing can reduce stabilization times and improve quality of care.

One piece of equipment not carried by all transport teams is the LMA. The laryngeal mask is a supraglottic airway device that fits over the laryngeal inlet to provide a means for positive-pressure ventilation. The deflated mask is inserted into the mouth of the infant using two fingers and is guided blindly along the hard palate without laryngoscopy or instrumentation.

Once resistance is met, the mask is seated by inflating the rim with 2 to 4 mL of air, occluding the esophagus while covering the laryngeal opening. The most frequently reported use of laryngeal masks in neonates is for airway rescue when face-mask ventilation and endotracheal intubation have failed. Multiple single-case reports or small retrospective series have described successful use of a laryngeal mask as a lifesaving maneuver during management of a difficult airway. In a meta-analysis, Mora and Weiner[45] concluded that a fairly strong recommendation could be made to attempt laryngeal mask ventilation during resuscitation when other methods fail, based on the fact that placement of the laryngeal mask is fairly noninvasive, is easily done by most providers, has a relatively low incidence of reported complications, and may be lifesaving.

There are several case reports on the use of the LMA during transport. These case reports have documented the use of the LMA to resuscitate, and in some cases transport, infants with congenital anomalies and difficult airways, including descriptions of its successful use for choanal atresia,[46] severe micrognathia,[46] and laryngotracheoesophageal clefts.[47] The International Guidelines for Neonatal Resuscitation state that the LMA may be an effective alternative for establishing an airway if bag–mask ventilation is ineffective or attempts at intubation have failed, but routine use of the LMA is not currently recommended.[48] Given the unpredictable nature of difficult airway presentations and the challenge of providing optimal resuscitation under sometimes suboptimal conditions, transport teams may consider including an LMA in their equipment box and providing training to personnel in the use of the LMA. The smallest size LMA (size 1) is appropriate for most term and larger preterm neonates but is too large for infants weighing less than 1500 g.

Transport Ventilators

The Bio-Med MVP-10 ventilator has been the prototypic ventilator used for transport for some time. It is still the "workhorse" ventilator used by many transport teams and is configured into many modular transport incubators (Bio-Med Devices, Inc., Guilford, Conn., USA). The MVP-10 is a pneumatically powered ventilator that provides time-cycled pressure-limited ventilation. It is capable of meeting standard ventilation needs and provides intermittent mandatory ventilation (IMV), PEEP, and CPAP. A number of other ventilators are now available for use on transport.

Previously, transport ventilators lacked the versatility and mobility found in ventilators used in the intensive care nursery. Today, however, most ventilator modes can be replicated in transport, and ventilators providing pressure or volume ventilation with control, assist/control, synchronized IMV, PEEP, CPAP, and pressure support modes are all available. Patient-triggered systems that respond to pressure or flow are also available. Ventilators may be pneumatically powered or have AC/DC operation with internal battery backup.

During transport, it is essential to be able to deliver oxygen concentrations between 21% and 100%, to limit oxygen exposure for preterm infants and infants with congenital heart disease, yet provide high oxygen concentrations for infants with pulmonary hypertension and hypoxic respiratory failure. Air–oxygen blenders are available and should be used to adjust oxygen delivery. Medical gases for the ventilator are provided by cylinders mounted on the transport system frame during transfer or by larger cylinders that are part of the ambulance

BOX 39-2 Suggested Supplies for Interhospital Transport

Intravenous Supplies	Airway Supplies
Alcohol and Betadine swabs	Resuscitation masks (various sizes)
Chlorhexidine preparation	Anesthesia bag
Gauze (2 × 2 and 4 × 4)	Endotracheal tubes (2.5, 3.0, 3.5, and 4.0)
Cotton balls	Stylet
Band-Aids	Skin protector (DuoDERM)
Label tape	Adhesive and adhesive remover
Clear tape (½ inch, 1 inch)	Adhesive tape
Self-adherent wrap (1 inch)	CO$_2$ detector
Tegaderm, small and large	Suction catheters (6, 8, and 10 Fr)
Needles (23 gauge, 19 gauge)	Laryngoscope and blades (00, 0, and 1)
Intraosseous needles (18 gauge)	Spare laryngoscope bulb and batteries
Intravenous catheters (14, 16, 18, and 24 gauge)	Magill forceps
Butterfly needles (19, 23, and 25 gauge)	Nasal continuous positive airway pressure prongs (10.5, 12, and 15 Fr)
Syringes (blood gas, 1, 3, 5, 10, and 30 mL)	Endotracheal tube bridge
Arm board	Laryngeal mask airway (1 and 1.5)
Intravenous extension tubing	Nasal trumpet
Y-adapter and T-connector	Oral airway (50 mm)
Intravenous pump tubing	Thoracostomy tubes (8, 10, and 12 Fr)
Three-way stopcock	Thoracostomy tray
Heparin lock	Heimlich valve
Catheter adapters (18, 20, and 21)	5-to-1 (Christmas tree) adapter
Umbilical line supplies	Vaseline gauze
Catheters (3.5 and 5 Fr with double lumen 5 Fr)	Nasal cannula
Umbilical tape	Normal saline bullets
Umbilical line tray	Bulb syringe
Suture	Meconium aspirator
Umbilical line bridges	Gastrointestinal supplies
Phlebotomy supplies	Replogle catheters (6, 8, 10, and 12 Fr)
Lancets	Feeding tubes (5, 6.5, and 8 Fr)
Capillary tubes	Sterile specimen (bowel) bag
Heparin tubes	Other
Tourniquet	Soft restraints
Blood culture bottles	Stockinette cap
Chemstrips	Safety pins
Chemical warmers, small	Rubber bands
Monitoring supplies	Scissors
Electrocardiography leads	Hemostats
Oximeter probe	Penlight
Blood pressure cuffs (1, 2, 3, and 4)	Flashlight
Thermometer	Sterile gloves

or aircraft configuration during transport itself. Table 39-1 lists the characteristics and expected life of various gas cylinders at differing flow rates. Team members should be familiar with cylinder capacity and the number of hours of flow provided, particularly for long transports or for infants requiring high concentrations and high flows of inspired oxygen.

High-Frequency Ventilation

HFV has been shown to be useful for the treatment of many respiratory disorders, including RDS, air leaks, meconium aspiration syndrome, and persistent pulmonary hypertension.[49-51] Many intensive care nurseries use HFV for infants who have failed conventional management, whereas others use it as their primary ventilator strategy for preterm infants at risk for chronic lung injury (see Chapter 22). Delivery of iNO has been shown to be more effective with high-frequency oscillatory ventilation (HFOV) for infants with hypoxic respiratory failure,[52] and it is this scenario that can pose difficulties for transport, when an unstable infant must be converted from HFV to conventional ventilation for transfer. Risks associated with such a conversion include loss of lung recruitment, atelectasis, and subsequent hypoxic respiratory failure. To maintain stability for infants already being treated with HFV at the outlying institution, as well as to extend a standard tertiary resource out to the transport environment, high-frequency ventilators providing high-frequency jet ventilation (HFJV) or high-frequency flow interruption are now available for use on transport.

Although high-frequency ventilators are now available, few studies have been performed to evaluate the risks and benefits of transport HFV. In a retrospective study, Mainali et al.[53] compared the use of HFJV, with or without iNO, to that of conventional ventilation. Twelve infants were transported on HFJV alone, 17 on HFJV with iNO, and 9 on conventional ventilation with iNO. The infants transported on HFJV, regardless of the use of nitric oxide, demonstrated significant improvement in ventilation during transport after conversion to HFJV without an escalation in support. This included infants converted from conventional ventilation and HFOV. Infants on HFJV also demonstrated a trend toward improved oxygenation and oxygen index, but this did not reach statistical significance. It is important to note, however, that there was an increased incidence of pneumothorax both pre- and posttransport in the infants who received HFV compared to those receiving conventional ventilation (7/29 HFJV vs 1/9 conventional pretransport and 3/29 HFJV vs 0/9 conventional posttransport), although the presence of a pneumothorax pretransport may have biased decision making toward the use of HFJV. The authors concluded that HFJV with or without iNO is safe and efficacious during transport and may even be preferred to conventional ventilation.

Honey et al.[54] reported their experience transporting 134 infants using HFV with flow interruption. Sixty percent of the infants were less than 37 weeks', and 16% were less than 28 weeks' gestational age. Infants were successfully transported on HFV 96% of the time. Reassuringly, there were no pneumothoraces in any of the transported infants. For the small number of infants who had pre- and posttransport blood gases available ($n = 24$), pH improved significantly after the initiation of HFV,

TABLE 39-1 Characteristics of Portable Gas Cylinders

SPECIFICATIONS OF OXYGEN CYLINDERS

Cylinder Type	CAPACITY (cu/ft)	(gal)	(L)	Height (in)	Diameter (in)	Weight of Full Tank (lb)
E	22	165	620	20	4¼	15
M	122	900	3450	46	7⅛	86
H	244	1800	6900	55	9	130

VOLUME AND FLOW DURATION OF OXYGEN IN THREE CYLINDER SIZES

Cylinder Type	FULL E	M	H	¾ E	M	H	½ E	M	H	¼ E	M	H
Contents (cu/ft)	22	107	244	16.5	80.2	193	11	53.5	122	5.5	26.8	6
Liters	622	3028	6900	466.5	2271	5175	311	1514	3450	155.5	757	172
Pressure (psi)		2000			1500			1000			500	

APPROXIMATE NUMBER OF HOURS OF FLOW IN THREE CYLINDER SIZES

Cylinder Type	FULL E	M	H	¾ E	M	H	½ E	M	H	¼ E	M	H
Flow Rate (L/min)												
2	5.1	25	56	3.8	18.5	42	2.5	12.5	28	1.3	6	14
4	2.5	12.6	28	1.8	10.4	21	1.2	6.3	14	0.6	3.1	7
6	1.7	8.4	18.5	1.3	6.3	13.7	0.9	4.2	9.2	0.4	2.1	4.5
8	1.2	6.3	14	0.9	4.6	10.5	0.6	3.1	7	0.3	1.5	3.5
10	1	5	11	0.7	3.7	8.2	0.5	2.5	5.5	0.2	1.2	2.7
12	0.8	4.2	9.2	0.6	3	6.7	0.4	2.1	4.5	0.2	1	2.2
15	0.6	3.4	7.2	0.4	2.5	5.5	0.3	1.7	3.5	0.1	0.8	1.7

whereas oxygenation and ventilation remained stable. Insights that were provided by the study include the fact that extensive training and education are needed for implementation of HFV on transport and that there is a steep learning curve with its use. Differences in ventilator readouts and the need for fine-tuning of ventilator settings further complicate training, even for those with prior experience using HFV. Finally, point-of-care testing for blood gas analysis and complete cardiorespiratory, O_2 saturation, and CO_2 monitoring are necessary for optimal management of an infant on transport HFV. Our own institutional experience mirrors these insights. We have found frequent blood gas analysis to be essential, with overventilation being a common problem encountered during the use of HFV (Children's Mercy Hospital Transport, Kansas City, Mo.).

Continuous Positive Airway Pressure

The increasing use of CPAP for the respiratory support of newborn infants has necessitated that transport teams become more familiar and facile with its use. Despite a large body of evidence supporting the use of CPAP in the delivery room and intensive care unit, few data exist regarding its use during transport. The few studies that have been done suggest that CPAP can be delivered safely and effectively in appropriately selected infants during transport. Simpson et al.[55] reported their experience with seven preterm neonates and reported no complications during transport. Bomont et al.[56] reviewed their experience with 100 infants transferred on CPAP. Infants required minimal intervention during transport and were safely transported on CPAP with adequate blood gases on arrival. Five of 100 infants required stimulation or prong repositioning for apnea, bradycardia, and desaturation, but no major intervention was needed.

Several limitations of the transport environment make the use of CPAP more difficult, however. Visual and auditory assessment is limited in the transport environment, and it can be difficult to achieve proper infant positioning in the transport isolette for adequate CPAP delivery. The use of more extensive transcutaneous or end-tidal CO_2 monitoring may facilitate the evaluation of the infant on transport CPAP. Owing to these limitations, however, careful consideration must be given to the safety and stability of an infant being transported on CPAP, and factors such as the length of transport, mode of transport, and gestational and chronologic age of the infant may all influence decision making regarding the appropriateness of CPAP in transport. Given the increasing use of CPAP in the delivery room for preterm infants, further study of the safety and efficacy of CPAP on transport should be undertaken.

Surfactant Administration

The administration of surfactant to infants with surfactant deficiency has had a significant impact on the morbidity and mortality of infants with RDS.[57,58] Experience with surfactant replacement in the transport environment has not been widely reported but has been adopted as part of the standard care offered by most transport teams. Costakos et al.[59] found that surfactant could be administered safely prior to the interhospital transport of preterm infants but was unable to identify significant benefits in terms of ventilator days, time to discharge, or incidence of bronchopulmonary dysplasia for infants who received surfactant prior to transport.[59] Endotracheal administration of surfactant is associated with the risk of respiratory compromise (desaturation, hypoxemia, bradycardia)[60] and

should be performed by personnel with adequate experience in administration. Moreover, the change in lung compliance that usually follows surfactant administration should be carefully monitored by the transport team; however, it may be difficult to discern in a transport vehicle.

Inhaled Nitric Oxide

iNO has been shown to improve oxygenation and reduce the need for ECMO in near-term and term infants with persistent pulmonary hypertension of the newborn (PPHN) and hypoxemic respiratory failure.[52,61,62] Since the U.S. Food and Drug Administration (FDA) approved use of iNO for respiratory failure, iNO has become available at most level III NICUs. Although this benefits most infants, 30% to 40% of infants fail to show a sustained response to iNO and may require transport to an ECMO center.[63] Further, rapid withdrawal of iNO can precipitate rebound hypoxemia, thereby further compromising an already unstable infant.[64] The need to continue iNO initiated at the outlying institution has prompted most transport teams to become capable of delivering iNO during transfer.

Several studies have evaluated the use of iNO during transport.[63,65-67] Kinsella et al.[65] and Goldman et al.[66] first demonstrated that critically ill infants with hypoxemic respiratory failure could be safely transported on iNO and that ambient levels of the gas were maintained well below levels of risk in a closed transport vehicle. Since that time, all studies have demonstrated safe transfer of infants on iNO. Kinsella et al.[65] was able to show that iNO acutely improved oxygenation in hypoxemic infants and that the effect was sustained during transport. iNO was also used to support the conversion from HFOV to conventional ventilation, because it minimized the pulmonary vasoreactivity associated with the change and decreased the lability associated with PPHN. These results were confirmed by Westrope et al.,[67] who retrospectively reviewed their experience in transporting 55 patients on iNO to a tertiary center for ECMO consideration. They found that oxygenation improved after the initiation of iNO, as demonstrated by significant improvement in both PaO_2 and oxygen saturations, and that iNO delivered in transport maintained the stability of patients previously on iNO.

Therapies should be initiated on transport with the goal of providing appropriate stabilization for safe transport but ultimately with the goal of improving patient outcome. With this in mind, Lowe et al.[68] evaluated whether iNO initiated during transport showed benefit compared to iNO initiated at arrival at the receiving facility. Although they found no difference in mortality rates or the need for ECMO for infants who received iNO prior to transfer, they did find a significantly shorter hospital stay for survivors who had iNO initiated in the field, suggesting that iNO initiated in transport may be cost saving.

For teams that decide to offer iNO, two FDA-approved delivery systems are commercially available—the AeroNOx device (Pulmonox Group of Companies, Edmonton, Alberta, Canada) and the inhaled nitric oxide delivery system (Mallinckrodt, St. Louis, MO). Safety during transport is of the utmost importance, and teams must be careful when transporting with a hazardous gas. Kinsella et al.[63] has shown that in a worst-case scenario, in which a full D cylinder of nitric oxide is completely released, maximum concentrations of nitric oxide would be 25.3, 34, and 94 ppm in a fixed-wing jet, ambulance, and helicopter, respectively. Maximum allowable transient exposures are 25 to 100 ppm, and in a helicopter, completely released levels approach Occupational Safety and Health and National

Institute for Occupational Safety and Health levels that pose an immediate danger to life or health.[69] Transport teams should develop a system in which the choice to carry nitric oxide can be made during the preparation for the transport run, to avoid carrying a hazardous gas unnecessarily for all neonatal transports.

Extracorporeal Membrane Oxygenation

Uncommonly, a neonate may require transport while receiving ECMO. This occurs most often when an infant is unable to be weaned off ECMO but requires specialized services at another institution. It also may occur when an infant is too unstable to survive transport, necessitating cannulation at the referring facility prior to transport. Currently 12 centers in the United States offer transport ECMO. Wilford Hall Medical Center provides global transport ECMO and have reported their 22-year experience with 68 children transported on ECMO by ground or fixed-wing aircraft.[70] All children survived transport. Survival to discharge was 65% for transported ECMO infants, which was equivalent to a survival rate of 70% for in-house patients receiving ECMO. Given the increasing use of extracorporeal cardiopulmonary resuscitation,[71,72] the need for transport ECMO may increase in the future but will probably continue to be a specialized service offered by only a few institutions with specialized training.

Hypothermia for Hypoxic Ischemic Encephalopathy

Therapeutic hypothermia (either by whole body or selective head cooling methods) is now the standard of care for selected newborn infants with moderate to severe hypoxic–ischemic encephalopathy (HIE). Multiple studies have shown that efficacy of treatment is enhanced by meeting early inclusion criteria and starting cooling before 6 hours of life. Therefore, starting cooling prior to and on transport is a natural extension, because in many cases, the appropriate window to commence treatment may already pass before a neonate is transported and admitted to a tertiary center. There are limited data suggesting how to perform cooling during transport, either passively or by certain manufactured or home-built cooling methods. Programs should work in close connection with their neurologists and intensivists to arrive at an agreed-on method, and appropriate training should be documented for all team personnel.[73] Through outreach education, referring centers should be aware of uniform inclusion criteria and delivery methods. The largest study published in 2013 by the California Perinatal Quality Care Collaborative confirmed earlier observations that there is variability in delivery methods; most patients do not achieve target temperature by the time of arrival at the accepting cooling center. Manufactured cooling devices and not passive cooling methods are the recommended mode on transport. Outcome studies now show that infants with moderate HIE may benefit more than those with severe HIE.[31,73]

FUTURE DIRECTIONS

The neonatal transport team plays a critical role in providing optimal care to the ill outborn neonate. The role of the transport team has expanded as technology has advanced and has made it possible to deliver sophisticated therapies to infants out in the field. The integration of wireless Web-based cellular technology and telemedicine allows tertiary centers to observe and interact with the transport team in real time. We have now begun to consider that earlier initiation of specific therapies, beginning in transport, may influence long-term outcomes. Although it is more difficult to conduct studies in the transport arena, prospective studies are possible and are now being done. The transport environment will continue to change as new technology and therapies develop. The expanding use of clinical simulators should be useful for transport team education and should be used to promote technical and clinical skill maintenance for team members. The emerging use of telemedicine, and its use on transport, may significantly change interactions with outlying practitioners and team communication with medical control. As changes come, the neonatal transport team will continue to play a vital role in stabilizing and transferring infants who require specialized care.

REFERENCES

A complete reference list is available at https://expertconsult.inkling.com/.

40

Extracorporeal Membrane Oxygenation

Robert M. Arensman, BS, MD, Billie Lou Short, MD, and Daniel Stephens, MD

Advances in the field of assisted ventilation include computer-assisted ventilators with an ever-increasing number of modalities, bedside pulmonary function measurements, and graphics and drugs to modulate the pulmonary vascular bed and alveoli and manage the complications of ventilation. Despite the use of these advances, some neonates fail to improve and die of respiratory failure unless alternative treatment is available. Persistent pulmonary hypertension of the newborn (PPHN) and congenital diaphragmatic hernia (CDH) may not respond to assisted ventilation and require alternative therapy.

In addition to nonsurvival, many children who receive aggressive ventilatory support continue to experience unacceptably high rates of ventilator-induced pulmonary complications: barotrauma including pulmonary air leak, bronchopulmonary dysplasia, and chronic lung disease. These subsequent complications of ventilation impose increased rates of morbidity and mortality even after the newborn period. For all these reasons, judicious use of cardiopulmonary bypass techniques for temporary respiratory support of selected term and near-term newborns is needed and useful (Figs. 40-1 and 40-2).

This technique is most frequently referred to as *extracorporeal membrane oxygenation* (ECMO), a name that unfortunately puts an undue emphasis on the role of oxygen support. Equally important may be the role of carbon dioxide extraction, cessation of toxic ventilatory settings, and cardiovascular support. Consequently, these processes of support may be referred to instead as *extracorporeal life support* (ECLS). ECLS expands the definition of extracorporeal support to include many newer cardiac support systems such as ventricular assist devices and pumpless extracorporeal support with membrane lungs only. In reality, both terms are frequently used when discussing neonatal support systems.

HISTORY OF CARDIOPULMONARY BYPASS

Artificial maintenance of circulation was pioneered by John and Mary Gibbon beginning in 1934[1]; it was first reported in 1937 but not used in a widespread fashion by cardiac surgeons until the 1950s. It was soon discovered that if used for more than 1 to 2 hours, the device itself was lethal because of protein denaturation,[2] which was thought to be caused by the gas exchange device. This finding led to the use of the biologic lung as the oxygenator for extracorporeal circulation, as described by Lillehei and colleagues.[3] Because the major problem with artificial circulation was the oxygenator, many new devices were developed, including the membrane oxygenator[4] and the bubble oxygenator,[5] which became the standard for cardiac surgery.

During attempts to use these oxygenators for prolonged bypass, it was noted that the oxygenator, which directly exposes blood to oxygen (O_2), damages cells and proteins. Manifesting as coagulopathy and anemia, this effect is apparent within a few hours of initiating bypass. The large reservoir used for oxygenation also complicated management of volume and necessitated complete suppression of coagulation in the low-flow component.

Development of Membrane Oxygenators

Streamlined units that had no reservoir and incorporated a membrane oxygenator instead of a bubble oxygenator eliminated the direct blood–gas interface (Fig. 40-3). The first membranes were made of polyethylene and Teflon but required large surface areas for adequate oxygenation.[6] In 1957, Kammermeyer[7] first reported the excellent gas transfer properties of a polymer of dimethylsiloxane, commonly known as silicone (Fig. 40-4). This led to the development of many oxygenators and to the first trials in infants.[8]

Once these membrane lungs and the circuits that bring blood to and take blood from them become coated with a protein monolayer, the blood is no longer in direct contact with a thrombogenic foreign surface. This allows for prolonged gas exchange with minimal cellular trauma, as well as elimination of the reservoir and the use of high-dose anticoagulation. For most patients, bleeding events are reduced and manageable.

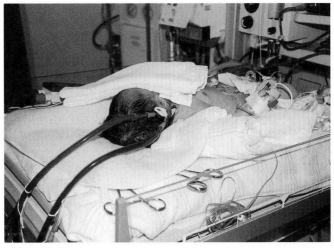

FIG 40-1 Photograph of a neonate on extracorporeal membrane oxygenation.

Development of a Pump

In the development of neonatal ECMO, most devices were readily adapted from devices already in use by the cardiac surgery teams. Consequently, multiactivated Sigma motor pumps were used initially. Soon thereafter, roller pumps gained popularity because of their reliability and ease of use. With these devices, blood-conducting tubing is compressed, and the fluid is forced forward. To prevent increased hemolysis of red blood cells, partially occluding systems are used. More recently, the centrifugal pump has gained popularity. This type of pump has the advantages of low hemolysis, usability over a wide range of flows, and little risk for air pumping (air embolus); thus it has become the most common form of pump currently utilized in most ECMO centers.

The great disadvantage of all of the pumps in use as of this writing is the lack of pulsatile blood flow to the patient. This variation from the normal cardiac flow has physiologic effects on the end organs. Consequently, the use of venovenous bypass whenever possible with preservation of endogenous pulsatile flow may confer advantage to the sick neonate (see further discussion of venovenous cannulation later in this chapter).

Vascular Access

The last major problem to be overcome in the quest to perform successful bypass in the neonate was vascular access. Early investigators used umbilical vessels, which did not provide adequate flow for substantial respiratory and cardiac support. Later, investigators cannulated the internal jugular vein and the common carotid artery. These sites allow sufficient flow to permit near-total cardiopulmonary bypass if needed. The successful solution of these multiple problems enabled Bartlett and his colleagues[9] to complete the first successful application of ECMO for respiratory failure in a neonate in 1975.

PHYSIOLOGY OF EXTRACORPOREAL CIRCULATION

Membrane Lung

The membrane lungs in use as of this writing are the diffusion, hollow-fiber membrane oxygenators. Unlike other hollow-fiber oxygenators, the fibers are made of poly-4-methyl-1-pentene and are nonporous. These membranes are therefore a "true" membrane lung, as was the older version of the silicone membrane (no longer manufactured), and will not develop a plasma leak like the microporous hollow fiber oxygenators. Oxygen and carbon dioxide (CO_2) diffuse across the membrane at the molecular level (Fig. 40-5, shown for a silicone membrane; hollow-fiber membrane is essentially the same process). The gradient for O_2 diffusion across the membrane is the difference between the O_2 content in the ventilating gas and that in the venous blood of the patient.

Oxygen and Carbon Dioxide Transfer

The red blood cells closest to the membrane fibers become saturated with oxygen first, and the local partial pressure of

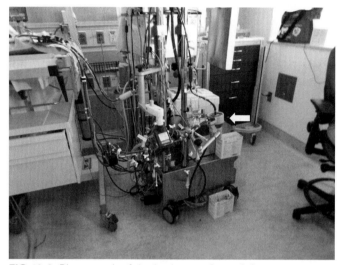

FIG 40-2 Photograph of the bed space for an infant on extracorporeal membrane oxygenation (ECMO) showing a centrifugal ECMO pump in the foreground.

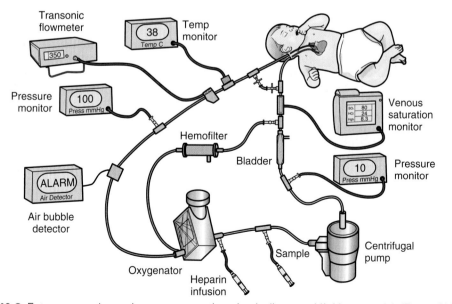

FIG 40-3 Extracorporeal membrane oxygenation circuit diagram. *VA,* Venoarterial. (From *CNMC ECMO Training Manual.* Ann Arbor, Michigan; 1980-2014; 2014.)

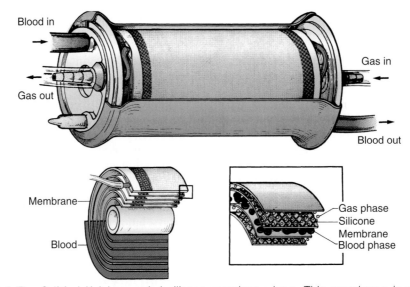

FIG 40-4 The SciMed Kolobow spiral silicone membrane lung. This membrane is no longer manufactured.

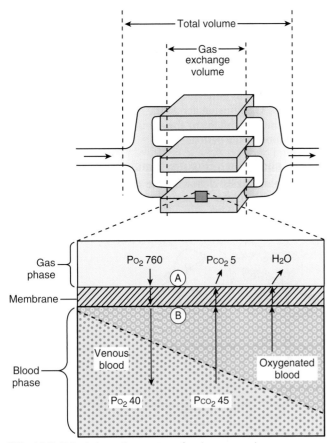

FIG 40-5 Principles of gas transfer in a membrane oxygenator. This expanded view shows interactions across the gas-exchange membrane. Venous blood enters from the left and becomes arterialized as O_2 diffuses through the membrane and blood film and as CO_2 diffuses from the blood film into the gas phase. (From Bartlett RH, Gassaniga AB. Extracorporeal circulation for cardiopulmonary failure. *Curr Prob Surg.* 1978;15:9.)

O_2 (Po_2) increases. Dissolved O_2 then diffuses deeper into the blood film, saturating more red blood cells. The bundled fibers provide adequate surface area for gas exchange. For complete saturation of the blood film to occur, it must remain in contact with the membrane long enough for O_2 to diffuse to the center of the film. For any given membrane lung, the amount of venous blood that can be completely saturated is a function of the O_2 content of the venous blood returning to the membrane and the amount of time spent in the membrane. As the flow increases, blood spends less time in the membrane. Oxygen transfer increases in proportion to the flow rate until a limitation to O_2 transfer is imposed by the thickness of the blood film. When venous blood entering the membrane is 75% saturated, the flow rate at which blood leaving the membrane is 95% saturated is termed the *rated flow* of that device, a number that allows for standardization of various membrane lungs (Fig. 40-6).[10] If it is assumed that the membrane is large enough, the amount of O_2 that can be delivered is dependent on the blood flow available, not on the capacity of the membrane to transfer O_2.

Carbon dioxide is much more diffusible through plasma than O_2, and CO_2 transfer is limited by its diffusion rate across the membrane. The newer hollow-fiber membranes have such excellent gas transfer at low gas flow rates, 0.25 to 0.5 L/min, that it is unusual to require addition of CO_2 gas to the membrane gas mixture going across the membrane, as was usual with the older silicone membrane lung. Because CO_2 transfer is independent of blood flow but dependent on the surface area of the membrane, an increasing partial CO_2 pressure (Pco_2) can be a sensitive indicator of loss of surface area and oxygenator function, which generally indicates clot formation or water in the gas phase.

Blood flow to the membrane is limited by the total circulating blood volume and the diameter of the venous catheter. The system must allow at least 120 mL/kg/min of flow to achieve support of cardiorespiratory function. The ECMO circuit is designed to permit this blood flow volume, with the membrane lung having a greater rated flow.

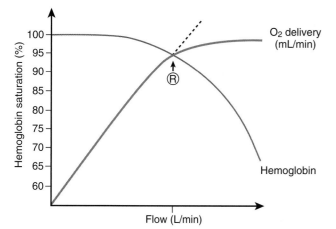

FIG 40-6 Rated flow. As flow through the membrane increases, actual O_2 transfer increases proportionally until the residence time of the venous return prevents complete hemoglobin saturation. At this point, the absolute O_2 transfer becomes fixed, but as the flow continues to increase, a smaller percentage of the venous return to the membrane becomes saturated. ® represents the rated flow, which is the flow at which the blood leaving the membrane is 95% saturated. (Adapted from Galletti PM, Richardson PD, Snider MT. A standardised method for defining the overall gas transfer performance of artificial lungs. *Trans Am Soc Artif Intern Organs.* 1972;18:359.)

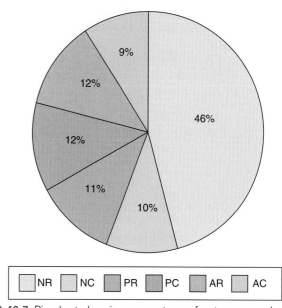

FIG 40-7 Pie chart showing percentage of extracorporeal membrane oxygenation patients by category. *NR,* neonatal respiratory; *NC,* neonatal cardiac; *PR,* pediatric respiratory; *PC,* pediatric cardiac; *AR,* adult respiratory; *AC,* adult cardiac. (Data from the ECMO Registry of the Extracorporeal Life Support Organization. Ann Arbor, Michigan; 1980-2014. Data from 2014 are incomplete.)

PATIENT SELECTION

There are two critical questions in the application of ECMO: (1) Which patients can be helped, or alternatively, who is likely to die without this therapy? (2) When should this therapy be instituted? Because this is an invasive procedure, great effort to determine appropriate entry criteria for it should be undertaken before its institution.

Disease States

The major criterion for ECMO selection is that the disease process must be reversible, usually within 2 to 4 weeks. ECLS beyond this time is difficult but has been successfully done for up to 2 months. Disease processes that lend themselves to ECMO therapy include meconium aspiration syndrome, pneumonia, neonatal sepsis, primary and secondary PPHN,[10-12] CDH, perinatal asphyxia, respiratory distress syndrome, barotrauma with air-leak syndrome, and perioperative support of newborns with congenital cardiac lesions. ECMO has expanded from the newborn population to older children and adults (Fig. 40-7).

In general, congenital cardiac defects can be identified and corrected without the need for ECMO. One cardiac condition that causes PPHN and may mimic some of the other conditions listed above is total anomalous pulmonary venous return. Unless there is an associated intracardiac defect, the heart itself may appear normal on a two-dimensional echocardiogram. The common pulmonary venous channel and absence of pulmonary veins entering the left atrium can only sometimes be demonstrated with noninvasive techniques. If the anomalous pulmonary venous drainage is obstructed, most commonly in the infradiaphragmatic variety, then pulmonary hypertension results.[13]

ECMO may be useful for perioperative stabilization of very seriously ill infants with this condition and allows for completion of the workup and preparation for surgery in a more hemodynamically stable patient. ECMO can also be used as a ventricular assist device in the management of infants with perioperative ventricular failure, often allowing babies who would otherwise be unable to come off operative bypass to survive.

Selection Criteria

In theory, selection criteria for ECMO would allow providers to predict which patients will not tolerate traditional therapy before they develop life-threatening complications or irreversible lung injury. These patients would escape to ECMO at the point when the risks of conventional therapy outweighed the risks of ECMO. In practice, however, it has been difficult to determine this set point. Box 40-1 describes criteria used for scoring systems at a number of centers. While variation exists, these systems at the least provide guidance for when a discussion of ECMO use should occur.[14]

Alveolar–Arterial Oxygen Gradient

One of the original, and therefore the oldest, predictors of mortality in the neonate with respiratory failure is the alveolar–arterial O_2 gradient:

$$A\text{-}a_{DO_2} = P_{AO_2} - P_{aO_2} \tag{1}$$

where P_{AO_2} is the alveolar O_2 tension and P_{aO_2} is the arterial O_2 tension.

The P_{aO_2} is measured directly from a postductal arterial blood sample, and the P_{AO_2} can be calculated from the alveolar air equation:

$$P_{AO_2} = P_{IO_2} - P_{ACO_2}/R + P_{aCO_2} \times F_{IO_2}\,(1-R)/R \tag{2}$$

where P_{IO_2} is the partial pressure of inspired O_2 and is calculated by the following equation:

$$P_{IO_2} = F_{IO_2} \times (P_{ATM} - P_{H_2O}) \tag{3}$$

BOX 40-1 Extracorporeal Membrane Oxygenation Selection Criteria

Indications

- $A–aD_{O_2}$ greater than 610×8 hours or greater than 605×4 hours, if PIP is greater than $38\,cm\,H_2O$
- Oxygen index greater than 40
- Acute deterioration with PaO_2 less than 40×2 hours and/or pH less than 7.15×2 hours
- Unresponsive to treatment: PaO_2 less than 55 and pH less than 7.4×3 hours
- Barotrauma (any four concurrently)
  Pulmonary interstitial emphysema
  Pneumothorax or pneumomediastinum
  Pneumoperitoneum
  Pneumopericardium
  Subcutaneous emphysema
  Persistent air leak for more than 24 hours
  MAP greater than $15\,cm\,H_2O$ and subcutaneous emphysema
- Postoperative cardiac dysfunction
- Bridge to cardiac transplantation

Relative Contraindications

- Prolonged severe hypoxia
- Prolonged mechanical ventilation for longer than 7 days

- Structural cardiac disease
- History or evidence of ischemic neurologic damage
- Lack of parental consent

Absolute Contraindications

- Lack of parental consent
- Inadequate conventional therapy
- Weight less than 2000 g
- Gestational age less than 35 weeks
- Contraindications to anticoagulation
  Severe pulmonary hemorrhage
  IVH grade II or greater
  Gastrointestinal hemorrhage
  Head trauma
- Prolonged mechanical ventilation longer than 7 to 14 days
- History of severe asphyxia or severe global cerebral ischemia
- Lethal genetic condition or unrelated fatal diagnosis (trisomy 13, trisomy 18, untreatable malignancy)
- Untreatable nonpulmonary disease, significant untreatable congenital cardiac malformation or disease

ECMO, Extracorporeal membrane oxygenation; *IVH*, intraventricular hemorrhage; *MAP*, mean airway pressure; *PIP*, peak inspiratory pressure.

---

where P_{ATM} is the atmospheric pressure, P_{H_2O} is the partial pressure of water vapor, P_{ACO_2} is the alveolar CO_2 tension, and R is the respiratory exchange ratio.

If it is assumed that the FiO_2 is 1.0 during maximum ventilation therapy, that the P_{ACO_2} is equal to the $PaCO_2$, and that R is 1.0, substitution of Eqns. (2) and (3) into Eqn. (1) yields a simplified equation for calculation of the gradient[15]:

$$P_{AO_2} - PaO_2 = (P_{ATM} - P_{H_2O}) - (PaO_2 + PaCO_2) \quad (4)$$

Krummel et al.[16] and Ormazabal et al.[17] showed that a gradient greater than 620 mm Hg for 12 consecutive hours predicted a 100% mortality rate, even in the presence of maximum conventional therapy, including alkalinization and tolazoline (Priscoline®; no longer available). However, by the time one-third of patients met this criterion, they were so moribund that ECMO salvage was no longer possible. A gradient of greater than 600 mm Hg for 12 consecutive hours predicted a mortality rate of 94%. Beck et al.,[18] in a retrospective study of 30 infants with PPHN, found that a gradient of 610 mm Hg for 8 consecutive hours predicted a mortality rate of 79% (see Box 40-1). Others have studied babies within their own institutions and found this criterion has a different value, but there is little doubt that high figures over prolonged times indicate high probability of a poor outcome.

Oxygenation Index

The ventilatory management improvements in the 1980s made the alveolar–arterial O_2 gradient somewhat less sensitive as a predictor of outcome. Dworetz et al.[19] showed that the previous gradient criterion predicted only 10% mortality for their cohort of patients. Thus other investigators attempted to develop new indices, none perfect, but with somewhat greater precision. Today, probably the most used index in most ECMO centers is the oxygenation index (OI). This criterion assesses a neonate's oxygenation status but also accounts for the amount of ventilator support needed to achieve it by measuring the mean airway pressure (MAP) on conventional ventilation.

The OI is calculated by dividing the product of the FiO_2 (times 100) and the MAP by the postductal PaO_2:

$$OI = FiO_2 \times MAP \times 100/PaO_2 \quad (5)$$

If it is assumed that the FiO_2 is 1.0, as it is in most patients who are candidates for ECMO, the equation can be simplified to read as follows:

$$OI = \frac{MAP \times 100}{PaO_2} \quad (6)$$

Ortega and colleagues[20] found that an OI greater than 40 for 2 hours in patients who were candidates for ECMO predicted an 82% mortality rate even though the alveolar–arterial O_2 gradient in the same population was not an accurate measure. This had been correlated by Ortiz and colleagues,[21] who found an 80% to 90% mortality rate for patients with an OI of 40 or more for greater than 2 hours. It should be stressed that reliance on these or any historical criteria has pitfalls, and each ECMO center should constantly reassess the criteria they are employing for entry into ECMO therapy.

Acute Deterioration

A term or near-term neonate who was previously doing well may have a sudden and drastic deterioration. Such an infant may not survive the necessary 3 to 12 hours needed to calculate the alveolar–arterial O_2 gradient or OI. Therefore, many ECMO centers have adopted criteria to alleviate this problem. The most common criteria considered are a pH less than 7.15 and a PaO_2 less than 40 mm Hg. If an infant has one or both of these measures for 2 consecutive hours, he or she is considered a candidate for ECMO.[22] In addition, if the baby is in severe distress or cardiac arrest, clinical judgment supervenes, and a decision must be made as to whether ECMO may be used to attempt life salvage.

Barotrauma

In addition to the criteria that are used to evaluate an infant's oxygenation, criteria have been designed to take into account the effect that mechanical ventilation has on a baby's lungs, in particular, if evidence of barotrauma is identified. Barotrauma is pulmonary injury caused by the high pressure or volume created by the ventilator. Indicators of barotrauma are as follows:

1. Pulmonary interstitial emphysema or pseudocyst
2. Pneumothorax or pneumomediastinum
3. Pneumoperitoneum
4. Pneumopericardium
5. Subcutaneous emphysema
6. Persistent air leak for 24 hours
7. MAP of 15 cm H_2O or greater

If a neonate meets four or more of these criteria, significant barotrauma is present. The barotrauma not only increases the mortality rate but also significantly increases the morbidity. If pulmonary damage and chronic lung disease are to be prevented, a neonate demonstrating these problems should be seriously considered for ECMO therapy.

Contraindications

The contraindications to ECMO are those clinical situations that preclude either a quality outcome or a successful ECMO run (see Box 40-1). Weight less than 2000 g is associated with an increased risk of intraventricular hemorrhage. Infants with this characteristic are generally premature and have an immature germinal matrix that is susceptible to vascular rupture.[23] In their initial pilot study, Bartlett and Andrews[24] treated 15 infants weighing less than 2000 g and had only 3 (20%) survivors. Patients with an estimated gestational age of less than 35 weeks have been found to have an almost 100% incidence of intracranial hemorrhage (ICH).[25] Evaluations in two later periods have shown survival in this population between 40% and 70% and an ICH rate between 40% and 50%.[26,27] Most centers still consider these high-risk patients and continue to use a cutoff of 2000 g and/or 34 weeks' gestation.

Generally, neonates with chromosomal abnormalities or syndromes known to be associated with profound retardation or a fatal outcome in infancy should be excluded from ECMO therapy. In addition, children with already existing, severe ICH should be excluded, although many centers will accept children with a grade I or II hemorrhage. These neonates, if very closely monitored (low activated clotting times and high platelet counts), may undergo ECMO without extension of the bleed. It is difficult to determine if a patient has hypoplastic lungs to the degree that ECMO will not change their outcome. Some centers have used the inability to reduce $PaCO_2$ to <70 to 80 pre-ECMO as a measure of hypoplastic lungs. Many still place these patients on ECMO but counsel the parents on the high risk of irreversibility of the lung disease. To date there are no specific criteria for the use of $PaCO_2$, just institutional experience.

Evaluation before Extracorporeal Membrane Oxygenation

When an infant is considered for ECMO, special attention must be directed toward the cardiovascular and neurologic systems. A thorough physical examination is mandatory to exclude congenital defects. Although any abnormality in laboratory analyses rarely precludes ECMO, baseline values, such as initial platelet count and coagulation studies, are important for management.

A cardiovascular evaluation is performed to rule out congenital heart disease (CHD). Two-dimensional echocardiography is performed to demonstrate signs of pulmonary hypertension: elevated right-sided heart pressure, septal bulging, tricuspid valve regurgitation, and right-to-left shunting at the ductal or foramen ovale sites. The degree of ventricular dysfunction and the presence of any structural abnormalities are noted. Poor ventricular function secondary to hypoxia coexisting with pulmonary hypertension is frequently seen and is not a contraindication to ECMO. In babies with this problem, ECMO increases the myocardial oxygen supply and decreases the ventricular workload by decreasing preload, which usually improves the hypokinesia. If CHD is strongly suspected, the patient should be placed on ECMO in most circumstances with plans for a reevaluation on ECMO for CHD including a potential cardiac catheterization. Most patients are too ill to tolerate a cardiac catheterization prior to being placed on ECMO. If a congenital cardiac lesion is found, then discussion should be undertaken with the cardiac surgery team to determine the timing of the operation and the value of ECMO in the perioperative period.

The degree of ischemic neurologic damage before ECMO can be very difficult to determine. When Apgar scores are evaluated, three important points must be considered. First, Apgar scores often do not correlate with intrauterine asphyxia.[28] Second, neonatal asphyxia is not the only cause of depressed Apgar scores.[29] Third, because an infant can have good Apgar scores and then experience a prolonged period of asphyxia, Apgar scores cannot predict neurologic outcome and are of limited value in the determination of candidates for ECMO.[30]

Seizure activity and focal neurologic deficits can be difficult to assess because most infants who are candidates for ECMO are paralyzed, sedated, or both, for the purpose of better ventilator management. Cranial ultrasound is done to rule out ICH but may not detect ischemic lesions. If an ICH is found, reconsideration of the procedure should occur because there may be rapid extension of the hemorrhage from systemic anticoagulation. Von Allmen and colleagues[31] showed that grade I ICH is not associated with a significant risk for major intracranial complications after ECMO but that severe edema and periventricular leukomalacia are associated with a 63% incidence of major intracranial complications. Grade II hemorrhage requires close anticoagulation management and close observation using head ultrasound studies daily. Any bleed greater than grade II should not be considered for ECMO secondary to risk for rapid increase in the hemorrhage and associated major morbidity and/or mortality.

In the paralyzed term infant, the most reliable readily obtainable bedside indicator of hypoxic–ischemic encephalopathy is the electroencephalogram (EEG). The presence of low-voltage, burst-suppression or isoelectric patterns on the EEG indicates a poor neurologic outcome[32] and is therefore a relative contraindication to ECMO. Seizure activity on the EEG is not an absolute contraindication to ECMO if none of the already mentioned underlying ominous patterns is present. Consultation with a pediatric neurologist is helpful in questionable cases.

TECHNIQUE FOR BEGINNING ECMO

Before Cannulation

When an infant appears to be a candidate for ECMO, the perfusion team and operating crew are notified and put on standby while the workup is completed. Blood samples are sent to the blood bank for preparation of the blood components necessary for the priming solution.

When a child meets criteria for ECMO, parental consent is obtained. Special attention is devoted to ensuring that the parents are well informed about the possible complications and various outcomes, including neurologic deficits, chronic lung disease, and death. Next, the preparation of the patient for bypass and the final priming of the ECMO circuit are carried out simultaneously. The circuits are preassembled and sterilized. The components consist of polyvinyl chloride tubing and incorporate a polypentane hollow-fiber membrane, a small venous bladder or compliance chamber, multiple ports for sampling and infusions, heat exchanger, and computer-aided perfusion system (several models are available). The tubing runs through a 5-inch roller pump or a centrifugal pump (personal choice of the perfusion team, ECMO team, ECMO director), which is servo regulated by the venous return in the bladder reservoir. If the bladder collapses because of inadequate venous return, the pump is automatically retarded or shut off; this prevents the system from creating a negative pressure and sucking in air if a roller pump is being used.

Today very sophisticated systems are commercially available to monitor pressure throughout the system, such as the transmembrane pressure, Δ pressure, inlet and outlet pressure, bladder volumes, and so on. These systems can adjust the flow very minutely to match the volumes available for perfusion.

The ECMO circuit is primed with packed cells, fresh-frozen plasma, and platelets. The pH and electrolytes in the priming solutions are corrected as time allows so that an adverse reaction in the neonate can be prevented, because priming volumes may be two to three times the neonatal blood volume.

Venoarterial versus Venovenous Cannulation

ECMO can be done via a double cannula venoarterial (VA) (Fig. 40-8) or a single cannula (double lumen) venovenous (VV) (Fig. 40-9) approach. A combination of techniques may also be used. VA bypass is used when cardiac function is a concern because single-catheter VV bypass requires good cardiac function.

In VA bypass, venous outflow is established from the right atrium via the internal jugular vein with a 10- to 16-French cannula. Blood is returned to the aortic arch through an 8- to 12-French cannula within the right common carotid artery. This method allows support of cardiac function and oxygenation; therefore, in the very sick neonate with an asphyxiated myocardium or in a baby requiring maximum pressor support, this is generally the procedure of choice.

VV ECMO functions to oxygenate the blood but relies on the neonate's cardiac output. VV ECMO also does not decompress the pulmonary circulation to the same extent as does VA ECMO. Infants undergoing VV ECMO can be more difficult to manage and may have to be converted to VA ECMO if cardiac failure ensues. Thus this modality is often best used in those infants who come early to ECMO, are in the more stable category, and require help primarily with gas exchange.

Venous outflow is still via the internal jugular vein with a 12- to 16-French cannula, and venous return is via the second lumen of the double-lumen cannula. Alternatively, one can, in extraordinary cases, return the blood via a femoral vein. There is now sufficient experience with both techniques to prove them both efficacious. Clearly, VV is less invasive than VA, so that approach should be the determinant choice, unless there is a clear advantage or need to have VA bypass.

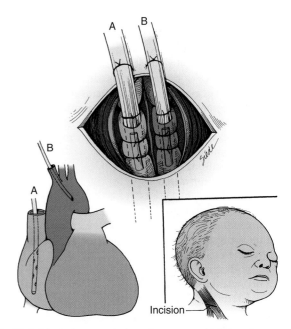

FIG 40-8 Vessel cannulation for venoarterial extracorporeal membrane oxygenation. Both the internal jugular vein (**A**) and the carotid artery (**B**) are ligated. The cannulae are then secured in the vessels with two ligatures over a small piece of vessel loop. When these ligatures are removed, they are cut over the vessel loop without risking damage to the vessels or the cannulae. Both cannulae are also secured to the skin of the neck.

Operative Procedure

The operative procedure is usually performed in the intensive care nursery with operating room personnel in attendance. Surgeons generally have magnifying loupes, headlights, and electrocautery on hand as necessary. The patient is positioned under a radiant warmer during the procedure to prevent hypothermia. If not done previously, the infant is paralyzed to prevent spontaneous respiration and air embolism during venous catheter insertion. In addition, local anesthesia or morphine is given.

Incision is made over the right sternocleidomastoid muscle and the carotid sheath is exposed. The vessels are isolated from surrounding tissues, taking care to preserve the vagus nerve that also runs within the carotid sheath. The neonate is given an intravenous bolus of heparin at a dose of 100 to 200 units/kg.

For VA bypass, the common carotid artery is ligated distally and controlled proximally with a clamp and suture ties. Through a transverse arteriotomy, the arterial cannula is passed a premeasured distance into the common carotid artery almost or just to the aortic arch. The cannula is tied securely in position. The venous cannula is then passed in a similar fashion into the right atrium through the internal jugular vein. During venous cannulation, care is taken to prevent air embolization from occurring.

For VV bypass, the procedure is much the same. The carotid artery is visualized but left in place; only the jugular vein is opened. Care is used to place the double-lumen venous cannula so that the blood-return orifices are directed toward the tricuspid valve. Cannulae are secured to vessels, skin, and scalp and to the patient bed, because dislodgment often will prove fatal to the child (Table 40-1).

A chest radiogram is needed to confirm correct placement. If further information is needed, an echocardiogram is very useful,

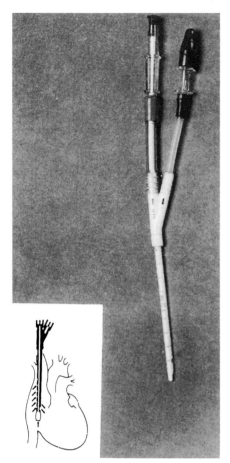

FIG 40-9 Double-lumen venovenous catheter for single-site access. The indwelling obturator is seen in the venous drainage lumen. The two lumens, separated by an eccentrically located septum, allow both venous blood drainage and reinfusion of warmed oxygenated blood. The catheter is inserted through a venotomy in the internal jugular vein such that the tip of the catheter, and thus the reinfusion port, is located in the right atrium (*inset*). (From Anderson HL, Snedecor SM, Otsu T, et al. Multicenter comparison of conventional venoarterial access versus venovenous double-lumen catheter access in newborn infants undergoing extracorporeal membrane oxygenation. *J Pediatr Surg.* 1993;28:530.)

especially to ensure that a cannula or the cannula flow is not across or directed at the aortic valve. The arrow notes the tip of the venous catheter, which has a small metal dot at the end (Fig. 40-10).

DAILY MANAGEMENT

Once bypass is established, ventilator settings are reduced to allow lung rest. Typically, the FiO_2 is reduced to 0.21 to 0.40; the respiratory rate is set to 10 to 20 breaths per minute with a peak inspiratory pressure of 15 to 20 cm H_2O and a positive end-expiratory pressure (PEEP) of 5 to 6 cm H_2O. Ventilator settings generally remain low throughout an ECMO run because gas manipulation now occurs via the ECMO circuit.

Typically, during the first 1 to 2 days on ECMO therapy, the infant's pulmonary status worsens, and almost no gas exchange occurs within the lungs. Keszler et al.,[33] in a multicenter randomized study, evaluated the effect of increased PEEP on lung function during ECMO. They found that patients treated with higher levels of PEEP had a significantly shorter course of

TABLE 40-1   Comparison of Venovenous and Venoarterial Extracorporeal Membrane Oxygenation

VV ECMO	VA ECMO
Advantages	
• Requires venous access only	• Good oxygenation and CO_2 removal
• Pulsatile flow to organs preserved via native cardiac function in series with ECMO circuit	• ECMO circuit both in parallel and in series with native cardiopulmonary circuit. The fraction of blood flowing in parallel is dependent upon the ECMO pump velocity.
• Good CO_2 removal	• Can provide partial cardiac bypass and cardiac rest
• Easy to wean off ECMO support	• Rapid wean off ventilator, inotropes, and pressors
Disadvantages	
• Dependence on native cardiac function for cardiac output	• Nonpulsatile pump flow
• Flow through circuit may be limited by smaller cannula compared to single-lumen VA venous cannula	• Cannulation of right carotid artery support
	• Somewhat more difficult to wean off ECMO
• Decreased oxygen delivery to periphery compared to VA ECMO	
• Decreased flow if mediastinum is displaced	

ECMO, Extracorporeal membrane oxygenation; *VA,* venoarterial; *VV,* venovenous.

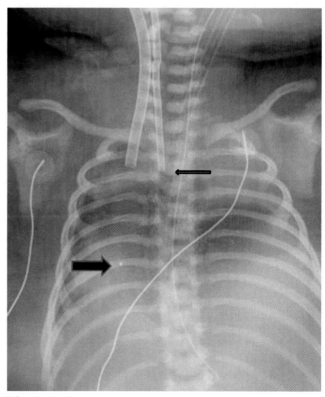

FIG 40-10 Chest radiograph of venoarterial extracorporeal membrane oxygenation patient showing the venous cannula tip (*large arrow*) in the right atrium, with the tip at the right atrium–inferior vena cava junction, and the arterial cannula (*small arrow*) in the aortic arch.

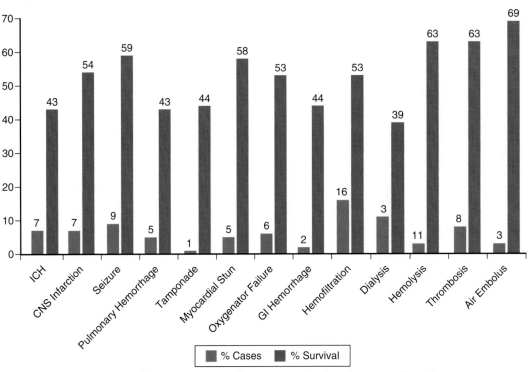

FIG 40-11 Incidences of the most commonly seen complications in neonatal respiratory extracorporeal membrane oxygenation. *ICH,* Intracranial hemorrhage; *CNS,* central nervous system; *GI,* gastrointestinal. (Data from the ECMO Registry of the Extracorporeal Life Support Organization. Ann Arbor, Michigan; 1980-2014. Data from 2014 are incomplete.)

ECMO therapy and demonstrated measurably better lung compliance in the first 72 hours of bypass. In addition, the high-PEEP group had overall fewer complications than the low-PEEP group. Consequently, some centers manipulate this parameter to try to improve lung function more quickly.

Activated clotting times are measured hourly at the bedside and are maintained at approximately two times normal values (160 to 200 seconds) by variations in the rate of a continuous heparin infusion. The usual heparin dose is 25 to 50 units/kg/hr. Good correlation has been found between the activated clotting time and the blood heparin levels in patients undergoing ECMO.[34] The hematocrit is maintained at between 35% and 45% with transfusions of saline-washed packed red blood cells. Platelet counts are maintained at greater than 75,000/mm³ with infusion of platelet concentrates as needed. This level may be increased to more than 100,000 to 125,000/mm³ in patients with bleeding problems or in those for whom surgical intervention is planned. Fibrinogen levels are maintained with infusion of cryoprecipitate as needed, and other clotting factors are given with fresh-frozen plasma if active bleeding is excessive.

Complete nutritional support is established with standard hyperalimentation techniques that provide trace elements, multivitamins, and lipids in addition to protein and carbohydrate. When the volume administration is determined, insensible water losses across the membrane must be taken into consideration. These losses can be up to 5 to 7 mL H₂O/m²/4.0-mL thickness per hour at 37° C. Excessive free water loss can occur if this is not remembered and added to the calculation as necessary. Electrolyte values are determined daily, and adjustments are made according to laboratory results.

During bypass, prophylactic antibiotics are given by many ECMO centers. Some provide antibiotics throughout an ECMO run; others provide coverage only for the first few days. Cultures of blood, sputum, urine, and tube insertion sites are frequently required, and antibiotics are determined by culture results. All other medications are given as needed. Sedation is almost routinely and universally given.

Echocardiography is extremely useful during ECMO therapy. This modality is an excellent tool for determining correct placement of cannulae. Serial evaluation of pulmonary vascular resistance, the direction and location of shunts, ventricular function, and atrial size contribute greatly to clinical management. For example, resolution of pulmonary artery hypertension, with reversal of shunt flow, indicates success and the ability to wean from ECMO. One group of patients in whom this principle may not be applicable is the CDH patients, who routinely come off ECMO with high pulmonary artery pressures that resolve with time.[35]

Similarly, serial cranial ultrasound examinations are used to screen for ICH during ECMO. These exams are done fairly routinely for the first 5 to 7 days. Some centers will then discontinue them on the basis of studies that suggest that most intracranial bleeds will occur within that time frame if they are going to occur. Other centers continue twice-weekly screening throughout the ECMO run. Of course, a study should be performed whenever clinical evidence suggests a sudden change that might indicate a fresh bleed (seizure, bulging fontanelle, sudden unexplained fall in hematocrit). A severe bleed is an indication for the cessation of ECMO. Small bleeds or initiation of therapy with a grade I–II bleed requires close control of anticoagulation and maintenance of a higher platelet count throughout the ECMO period. Figure 40-11 shows that many of the complications seen on ECMO are related to either bleeding or clotting complications.

Respiratory support continues during ECMO as stated earlier. Chest X-rays are generally a daily event to monitor progress and catheter and endotracheal tube placement. Even with initiation of ECMO, barotrauma events may occur and will need therapeutic intervention if they do occur. Pneumothorax can occur on ECMO. Decisions on treatment include monitoring with no chest tube placement or evacuation with a chest tube. Most nonsymptomatic pneumothoraces can be monitored and will resolve on ECMO without placement of a chest tube. If surgical intervention is required while a baby is on ECMO, meticulous hemostatic techniques with special emphasis on maintenance of adequate platelet levels and very close attention to the anticoagulation status of the child are required.

WEANING

Total flow through the bypass circuit controls the patient's mixed PaO_2 by varying the relative contributions from the pump and the infant's heart and lungs. Arterial O_2 content, as measured in the distal aorta (from umbilical artery catheters), represents a mixture of pump blood and the blood that traverses the pulmonary circuit. Because the pump blood is greater than 99% saturated, any increase in distal aorta PaO_2 represents an increase in the contribution of the patient's cardiovascular system (provided the pump flow remains constant). Early in the course of ECMO, when the infant's lungs provide little or no function, the circuit flow is maintained at 100 to 120 mL/kg/min, which is adequate to achieve near-total gas exchange via the oxygenator. As the infant's lungs improve, the additional oxygenation taking place via the lungs increases the systemic PaO_2, which allows the flow through the extracorporeal circuit to be reduced. This process continues stepwise, gradually decreasing the extracorporeal support, until the child can maintain adequate blood gas levels with a total bypass flow of 50 to 80 mL/min. In some centers, this flow rate, called *idling*, is maintained for 4 to 6 hours. If stable blood gases are seen during this time, the baby can be decannulated. Other centers like to test the patient off ECMO with the catheters left in place. At this point, the baby is excluded from the circuit by clamping the cannulae but not removing them. If the vital signs are stable and the arterial blood gas values remain acceptable for some time at low ventilator settings, the patient is ready for decannulation. At decannulation, the vessels are ligated or repaired. The wound is then closed. During the exclusion from the pump, if the infant's condition deteriorates, then bypass is reestablished, the infant is stabilized, and the weaning process is begun again.

The infant's volume status is monitored by evaluation of several parameters, including blood pressure, heart rate, capillary refill, skin turgor and color, urine output, and venous blood gas levels. Venous pH and O_2 content are sensitive indicators of adequate perfusion (aerobic cellular respiration), and changes in these parameters may be seen before any changes in arterial blood gas values. Blood volume can be increased or decreased simply with the infusion or withdrawal of blood from the ECMO circuit. In general, an increase in total body water (specifically, an increase in extracellular fluid) occurs; this increase is manifested by an increase in weight and often visible edema.[36] When natural diuresis occurs, pulmonary status generally improves, and weaning can begin.

Carotid Artery Repair

For many years, the carotid artery has been ligated at the time of decannulation. This practice is still probably the norm at most

TABLE 40-2 Rationale for Carotid Artery Repair versus Ligation

Carotid Ligation	Carotid Artery Repair
Benefits	
• Faster decannulation procedure	• Restore normal flow to vessel
• No worry about future stenosis, aneurysm, or leak	• No need to rely on collateral perfusion from circle of Willis or vertebrobasilar system
• No vascular repair in contaminated wound	
• No risk of air or thrombus embolism during repair	
• No evidence that repair has clear benefit	
• No need for follow-up vascular studies	
• As child grows, remaining vasculature will compensate and deliver needed flow	
Risks	
• Permanently remove right carotid artery from circulation	• Blowout at repair site from ischemic vessel at arteriotomy or rupture of repair from tension after segmental resection
• Risk of relative ischemia of right cerebral hemisphere	• Future stenosis or aneurysm, with alteration of flow or showers of emboli
	• Need for serial follow-up vascular studies to evaluate flow and rule out stenosis

centers. Although studies have shown retrograde flow from the external carotid artery on the right side to the internal carotid artery after ligation,[37] there is still an inherent fear that ligation of one of the major blood vessels to the brain may create long-term problems in these neonates. Therefore, attempts have been undertaken to reconstruct the carotid artery after ECMO decannulation. For carotid artery repair, the cannula is removed, and the proximal vessel is controlled with a vascular clamp. The distal ligature on the artery is then removed; the distal aspect of the artery is also controlled with a vascular clamp. Backbleeding is allowed, both to prevent emboli from reaching the brain and to assess adequacy of distal blood flow. The artery is then repaired with a variety of techniques. Adolph and colleagues[38] use a longitudinal arteriotomy at the time of cannulation and then close the site transversely to prevent stricture formation. Moulton and colleagues[39] found that on histologic section, the vessel wall had undergone greater than 50% transmural necrosis, and they advocate resection of the involved segment (between the distal and the proximal ligatures) with primary anastomosis. Both techniques have met with good results on preliminary evaluation. Other methods have suggested simple closure of a transverse arteriotomy with Gore-Tex® patching of the artery (Table 40-2).

OUTCOME

To date, the Extracorporeal Life Support Organization Registry has recorded 27,728 neonates with respiratory failure having been treated with ECMO; 84% were successfully decannulated and 74% survived to discharge.[40] The cumulative survival statistics are highest for meconium aspiration syndrome at 94%

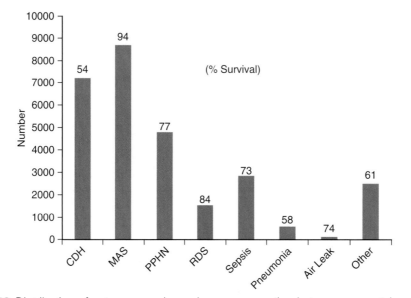

FIG 40-12 Distribution of extracorporeal membrane oxygenation between neonatal respiratory diagnoses and survival rates to hospital discharge with each diagnosis. *CDH*, Congenital diaphragmatic hernia; *MAS*, meconium aspiration syndrome; *PPHN*, persistent pulmonary hypertension of the newborn; *RDS*, respiratory distress syndrome. (Data from the ECMO Registry of the Extracorporeal Life Support Organization. Ann Arbor, Michigan; 1980-2014. Data from 2014 are incomplete.)

and lowest for CDH at 51% (Fig. 40-12). Changes in intensive care and the introduction of new therapies such as surfactant, selective antibiotic prophylaxis for mothers and babies, high-frequency ventilation, and inhaled nitric oxide have reduced the numbers of infants who require ECMO annually. As of this writing approximately 800 infants per year are placed on ECMO for respiratory failure. Newer therapies and the greater use of a gentle ventilation approach have reduced the number of CDH infants requiring ECMO.[41]

Medical and neurodevelopmental outcomes of the ECMO patient are encouraging considering the severity of illness in the newborn period. Analysis of outcome studies performed in PPHN survivors treated with conventional medical therapy, inhaled nitric oxide, and ECMO yield grossly equivalent morbidities and longer term outcomes.[42] This suggests that neurodevelopmental outcome is more related to the underlying illness than to the therapeutic interventions used.

Chronic lung disease (defined as oxygen use at 28 days) is seen in 15% of ECMO survivors, but long-term oxygen use is uncommon except in infants with CDH. Hospitalization for respiratory problems in the first year of life is needed in approximately 25% of survivors.[43] Normal somatic growth is seen in ECMO-treated children except those with CDH.

Progressive high-frequency sensorineural hearing loss is seen in 3% to 21% of ECMO-treated infants.[44] An important aspect of this morbidity is the delayed onset, making diagnosis problematic. The position statement by the Joint Committee on Infant Hearing in 2000 added PPHN and ECMO as risk indicators for hearing loss and stated that babies with these risk factors should receive audiologic evaluation every 6 months until 3 years of age.[45]

Numerous investigators have studied the neurodevelopmental outcomes of ECMO patients and consistently report Bayley scores in the normal range in the first 2 years of life.[46-49] Fewer studies of ECMO survivors at older ages have been performed.

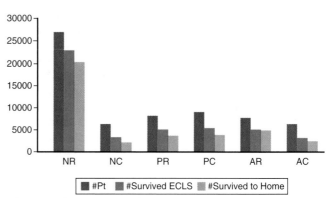

FIG 40-13 Distribution of extracorporeal membrane oxygenation between patient categories and survival rates to decannulation and discharge within each category. *ECLS*, Extracorporeal life support. (Data from the ECMO Registry of the Extracorporeal Life Support Organization. Ann Arbor, Michigan; 1980-2014. Data from 2014 are incomplete.)

By 5 years of age, mean IQ scores remain in the normal range but are lower than normal controls (96 vs 115, $p < 0.001$).[49] Glass et al.[49] reported that approximately 15% of ECMO survivors at age 5 years had a major handicap, most commonly mental retardation, whereas less than 5% had severe or profound impairment. Nevertheless, 50% of ECMO survivors have an increased risk of learning and behavioral problems compared to normal controls. As a result of these deficits, ECMO survivors are vulnerable to academic and psychosocial difficulties. All ECMO patients and the near-miss ECMO population should be followed closely into school age so that interventions can be started early if needed. But, in general, the ECMO population is doing quite well and if patients are selected appropriately, the risk of short-term and long-term morbidities and mortality should not deter the initiation of this procedure (Figs. 40-13 and 40-14).

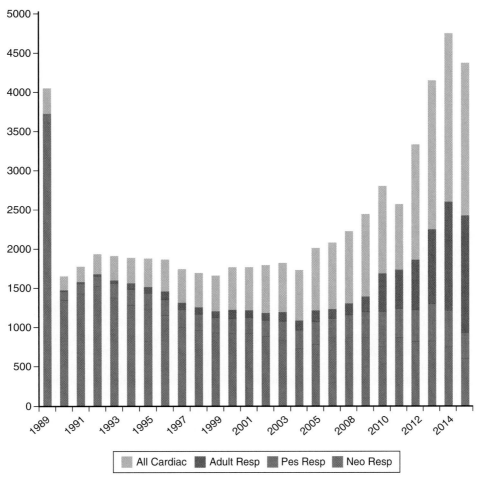

FIG 40-14 Number of extracorporeal membrane oxygenation (ECMO) runs each year by patient category. There is a steady decline over the past several years in neonatal respiratory ECMO cases. (Data from the ECMO Registry of the Extracorporeal Life Support Organization. Ann Arbor, Michigan; 1980-2014. Data from 2014 are incomplete.)

REFERENCES

A complete reference list is available at https://expertconsult.inkling.com/.

41

Discharge and Transition to Home Care

Lawrence Rhein, MD

The discharge readiness of infants is usually determined by the demonstration of achieving several minimum functional competencies. These competencies include (1) thermoregulation; (2) control of breathing without apnea, bradycardia, or desaturation; (3) respiratory stability with adequate oxygen saturation and ventilation; and (4) sustained weight gain.[1,2] With improvements in neonatal intensive care leading to increased survival of very preterm and very ill infants, a growing number of infants may not achieve these minimum competencies, especially those involving adequate respiratory function, in a reasonable time frame without requiring especially prolonged hospitalization or without use of technology.[3-8]

Prolonged use of technology to support respiration results in difficult choices about disposition. Simply extending hospitalization allows continuity of care. However, prolonging inpatient hospitalization has several significant disadvantages. These include:

1. Increasing the period of separation of infants from their families. Several studies have shown that decreased visitation by parents during the neonatal intensive care unit (NICU) hospitalization results in decreased bonding.[9-14]
2. Increasing the risks of hospital-acquired morbidities, such as hospital-acquired infections.[15]
3. Decreased availability of required developmental therapies. Most infants who require technology to support breathing are in acute-care facilities. Such facilities tend to dedicate fewer resources to rehabilitation services (occupational therapy, physical therapy, etc.) that growing infants often require to optimize neurodevelopment.

Depending on the capabilities of home caretakers and the resources in the community, pediatric home ventilation may be a feasible option in certain situations because of improvements in ventilator technology and increased prevalence of outpatient follow-up support.[16-18] However, to minimize risks, careful planning is required.

The goal of this chapter is to review the factors to consider when deciding to discharge a technology-dependent infant to home, as well as providing guidelines to accomplish a safe transition.

FACTORS TO CONSIDER WHEN DETERMINING READINESS FOR DISCHARGE

Determining the appropriate timing to safely discharge a technology-dependent infant from the hospital after a stay in the NICU can be complicated. This decision is made primarily on the basis of the infant's medical status but requires consideration of several additional factors (Table 41-1). These factors include:

1. Medical stability of the child. Infants need to be clinically stable for a minimum of 2 to 4 weeks. Clinically stable means no major diagnostic or therapeutic changes in the management, with stable ventilator settings and oxygen requirement. There is no absolute maximum level of support that precludes discharge,[19] but typically the oxygen requirement includes $FiO_2 \leq 40\%$ and peak inflation pressure (PIP) $<30\,cm\,H_2O$ for pressure-limited ventilation. Infants with higher pressure limits (close to but $<30\,cm\,H_2O$) should meet all other safety criteria (i.e., no requirement to increase settings within 2 weeks, dedicated caregiver, etc.) as described in this section. For all parameters (PIP, oxygen concentration, etc.) there needs to be an ability to increase levels at home without automatically requiring a visit to the emergency department. In addition, the infant needs to be able to tolerate a nutritional regimen that allows adequate growth.
2. Availability of care providers. The level of care/support required at home varies with each child. Usually, at least one parent must be dedicated to the care of the child. Families of technology-dependent children qualify for home nursing support, but the number of hours filled often falls short of those eligible or those deemed necessary. Especially in households with other siblings, the increased care needs of the technology-dependent child often require a caregiver without other distracting responsibilities.
3. Seasonal factors. While technology-dependent infants can be discharged in any season, the risk of rehospitalization due to viral infection is increased in the fall and winter months. If available, transition to a rehabilitation facility during the peak viral season may be desirable not only to minimize infectious risk but also to allow additional training and potential improvement in medical stability.

Most important, the decision to initiate transfer of a ventilated patient to home (instead of extension of hospitalization in an acute-care facility or transfer to a rehabilitation facility) requires confirmation that the patient's needs can be balanced with resources at home. The needs to be considered include physician availability and care (including pulmonary subspecialist care) and appropriate equipment and personnel (nursing care, respiratory care, personal care attendants, and family members). The remainder of this chapter describes guidelines to facilitate a successful transition to home and also provides guidance regarding the discharge of infants on home oxygen therapy.

TABLE 41-1	Discharge Criteria
Medical Stability	
Treatment plan for all medical conditions is in place, will not require frequent changes, and can be implemented at home	
Adequate nutritional plan in place	
Respiratory Stability	
Safe and secure airway: Tracheostomy with sufficiently mature stoma to allow tube changes or stabilized on regimen of non-invasive ventilation (NIV) with minimal risk for aspiration	
Able to clear secretions, spontaneously or with assistance	
Oxygenation stable, including during suctioning and repositioning	
Stable $FiO_2 \leq 0.4$ with positive end-expiratory pressure $\leq 8\,cm\,H_2O$	
Stable ventilator settings with peak inflation pressure $\leq 30\,cm$	
Stability criteria met for 2-4 weeks	
Home Stability	
Stable home and family setting	
Willing and able caregivers identified and trained prior to discharge	
Adequate financial resources and mechanisms for reimbursement identified prior to discharge	

DISCHARGE TEAM

Discharge of the ventilator-dependent child requires a multidisciplinary approach.[20-23] The team needs to include hospital and community-based personnel, including those who will continue to monitor the patient in the outpatient setting. Although there is no standard method for coordinating the discharge, we recommend a collaborative team approach that includes the following components:

Family caregivers: Clearly, the most important decision makers in the process of discharging ventilated patients are the family members themselves, who need to be involved in all aspects and fully able to medically care for the patient.

Medical discharge coordinator: Hospital discharge planners have specific expertise with reimbursement-related issues, specifically the financial issues including coverage of durable medical equipment (DME) by health care benefits and coverage of nursing personnel. Discharge planners assist families in the identification of all health care benefits covered by third party insurers, entitlements, and assistance from federal, state, or local agencies.

Bedside clinical nursing staff: Prior to discharge, the bedside nursing team needs to identify all potential physician subspecialist caregivers (potentially pulmonology, otolaryngologist, and certainly the primary care pediatrician) to confirm that all discharge criteria for each specialty have been met and to arrange appropriate follow-up visit schedules. In addition, bedside nursing is often responsible for the direct teaching of basic nursing care skills to the home caregivers.

Respiratory care clinicians: Whereas the bedside nursing staff is responsible for teaching nursing care, the respiratory care therapist provides the specific teaching regarding the operation and use of the ventilator.

DME provider: DME providers are responsible for providing the ventilators and associated supplies to patients on long-term ventilation.

Primary outpatient physician: For most patients, even those with complex medical needs, the primary leader of the outpatient team is the primary care pediatrician. For ventilator-dependent patients, a specialist (pulmonologist or home ventilator team clinician) should be included as a primary consultant for families.

PREDISCHARGE NEEDS ASSESSMENT

Prior to discharge to home, all infants require an assessment to ensure that they are in fact ready for discharge. The components of a comprehensive assessment include the home environment, the availability of necessary equipment, and the availability of personnel resources to allow safe care. The level of support required at home will vary with each child and family. Factors to consider include level of medical care required, including (1) time dependent on ventilator, (2) the amount of "reserve" in the event of ventilator failure or disconnection or airway obstruction, (3) other care needs related to feeding issues, and (4) other demands on the family's time, particularly the presence of other children and work commitments. Although children can be discharged to home at any time of the year, sometimes discharges in the peak of viral season, when infectious risks are highest, may be deferred. Finally, the availability of nonfamily assistance (home nursing) has to be a primary consideration.

HOME ENVIRONMENT

The home environment needs to include sufficient space for all of the medical equipment and supplies, including the ventilator. The home environment needs to have appropriate power supplies for all the equipment, and accessibility to emergency medical services needs to be ensured through the presence of a working telephone. Power companies should be notified of the electrical requirements and location of persons who require mechanical ventilation.

EQUIPMENT AND SUPPLIES

All children should be trialed on the equipment designated for home use while still in the hospital. Of note, most ventilators are not approved for use in infants below a minimum weight (5 kg), so discharge may need to be deferred until the infant has achieved this minimal weight to utilize an approved ventilator.

In addition to the ventilator, an itemized equipment list should be prepared and checked by the team (Table 41-2). A monthly estimate of disposable supplies and consumables also needs to be provided.

A second ventilator is required for any child who is unable to cope for 6 hours off the ventilator. In the event of power failure, it is critical to have an alternative power source available, in the form of either batteries or a generator.

PERSONNEL RESOURCES

DME providers should have personnel trained to manage ventilator-assisted patients in the home.

In combination with the hospital-based respiratory therapist and bedside nursing staff, DME providers assist in training the family regarding the use and maintenance of the ventilator, as well as in some of the care techniques, such as suctioning and tracheostomy care. The DME provider should have backup equipment ready at all times to handle emergencies. The DME provider should also have an emergency response time clearly defined.

TABLE 41-2   Equipment and Supplies to Be Considered for Ventilator-Assisted Patients

Mechanical ventilator (also need backup)
Exhalation valve
Tracheostomy tube adapter/connector
Humidifier and heater
Humidifier bracket
Heat and moisture exchanger
Manual resuscitator
Oxygen supply system (stationary and portable)
Oxygen bleed-in adapter to ventilator
Noninvasive patient interfaces
Face mask
Nasal mask or nasal pillows
Suction machine (stationary and portable)
Suction catheters
Connecting tubing
Suction collection container
Gloves
Other secretion clearance aids such as cough in-exsufflator
Spare tracheostomy tube (including next smaller size)
10-mL syringe used only to inflate or deflate cuff (for cuffed tracheostomy tubes)
Velcro tracheostomy tube strap
Tracheostomy tape
Sterile saline solution
Antibiotic ointment
Cotton-tipped applicators
Compressor for aerosolized medications

HOME NURSING

The agency selected to provide home health care should have adequate staff available and have a nurse case manager to follow the patient and the nursing care and staffing provided. Families may also contract with private-duty nursing, but this also requires coordination with the discharge planners.

EMERGENCY PLANNING

Parents or caregivers need to be instructed on common potential scenarios that require urgent intervention. They should be able to recognize early signs and symptoms of illness and know how to respond. Local rescue and ambulance service should be informed that a technology-dependent child is in their region, so they can be prepared to provide emergency treatment or transport. In many cases, the closest hospital to a patient's home may not have pediatric expertise. Still, the local hospital must be notified of potential emergency needs, because in many cases, transport to the local hospital is necessary, with subsequent transport to a more specialized pediatric facility via a trained pediatric transport team.

The discharging facility should provide parents with a printed summary of medical issues, ventilator settings, and medications to provide to emergency responders.[24] If limits to resuscitation have been discussed, these also should be documented to avoid unwanted interventions.

POSTDISCHARGE FOLLOW-UP

A primary responsible caregiver needs to be clearly identified to assist in the ongoing management of the technology-dependent child. This may be the child's primary care pediatrician, a pulmonary specialist, or another pediatric specialist. The parents/guardians must be able to identify the individual whom they can contact to seek advice, both during normal working hours and after hours, and should be able to identify indications for seeking help (Table 41-3). Ongoing follow-up to monitor growth,[25] stability of respiratory status, and neurodevelopment is critical.

In summary, transition of the ventilator-dependent infant from hospital to home requires advance planning, teaching resources, and a collaborative team willing to partner with families. This chapter highlights some of the considerations required to ensure optimal outcomes and help infants to thrive in their home environment.

TABLE 41-3   Indications for Seeking Additional Assistance

Persistent symptoms of respiratory distress (tachypnea, grunting/flaring/retractions)
Oxygen desaturation
Ventilator alarms (low-minute ventilation, apnea, etc.)
Fever
Lethargy
Feeding intolerance
Pallor/cyanosis
Tachycardia or bradycardia

TRACHEOSTOMY CARE

Most infants who require ventilator support at home have tracheostomies, although noninvasive ventilation (BiPAP) may be effective in rare select cases (infants who do not require ventilation support when awake).

Optimal care of a tracheostomy requires effective suctioning technique at appropriate frequency, as well as appropriate tracheostomy changes.

CHANGING TRACHEOSTOMY TUBES

The frequency of tracheostomy changes is determined by physician preference and availability of tubes. Increased frequency of changes may decrease infectious risk, but it may also cause increased granuloma formation.

Ideally, elective tracheostomy changes should occur prior to feeding to minimize the possibility of emesis. An emergency tracheostomy change may need to occur if:
- The tracheostomy tube is blocked,
- The tracheostomy tube slips out of the trachea,
- A suction catheter is unable to pass through the tracheostomy tube,
- The tracheostomy tube/cuff is not able to stay inflated,
- There are symptoms of respiratory distress, including pallor or cyanosis, retractions, nasal flaring, or ineffective chest wall rise.

Prior to changing the tracheostomy tube, caregivers must prepare the following supplies:
- Oximeter
- Self-inflating bag with pop-off/mask
- Oxygen
- Suction with appropriate catheter
- Two tracheostomy tubes: one that is the current size and one that is a size smaller

- Tracheostomy tie
- Stoma dressing
- Syringe
- Water-soluble lubricant
- Scissors
- Clean moistened gauze

To change the tracheostomy tube, caregivers should carry out the following steps:

1. Suction if secretions are present.
2. Check new tube with cuff inflation (if applicable).
3. Remeasure the suction depth with a sterile catheter, adding 1 cm to the measured length.
4. Prepare the tracheostomy tie and stoma dressing.
5. Put the tie onto the new tracheostomy tube.
6. Apply water-soluble lubricant to the end of the tube and obturator.
7. Position the child with stoma exposed by putting a rolled towel under the child's shoulders to access the site.
8. Unfasten the tracheostomy tie while holding the tube in place.
9. Deflate the cuff (if applicable).
10. Remove the tracheostomy tube.
11. Wipe the stoma with moistened gauze.
12. Check the stoma site for any areas that may look not normal.
13. Place the new tube with obturator in the stoma following the curve of the airway.
14. Immediately remove the obturator while holding the tracheostomy tube in place.
15. Place the child back on support, such as ventilator, oxygen, etc.
16. Inflate the cuff (if applicable).

Optimal outpatient management includes follow-up with a multidisciplinary team, including pulmonary specialists, respiratory therapists, and otorhinolaryngology surgeons.

OUTPATIENT MANAGEMENT OF SUPPLEMENTAL OXYGEN THERAPY

A subset of infants with bronchopulmonary dysplasia (BPD) meet all other discharge criteria but remain hypoxic, requiring supplemental oxygen to maintain adequate saturations. For many such infants, the decision to use home oxygen therapy (HOT) is an acceptable and desirable option. HOT has been shown to decrease health care costs[26-31] and to improve patient satisfaction compared to prolonged hospitalization.[28,32]

In the next section, we review the indications for HOT and strategies for safe discontinuation of HOT.

INDICATIONS FOR HOME OXYGEN THERAPY

Hypoxemia

The most common indication for HOT is persistent hypoxemia due to diffusion abnormality or parenchymal lung disease. It is important to note that not all causes of hypoxemia are treated with oxygen therapy. Specifically, infants with hypoventilation as a primary cause for their hypoxemia may be harmed by supplemental oxygen because of impairment of the respiratory drive to breathe, which may worsen hypoxemia.

No randomized controlled trials have been performed to determine what pulse oximeter saturation (SpO_2) criteria should be used for the initiation and management of HOT for BPD. As a result, there is little consensus regarding specific indications for its use.[33-36]

Most reviews suggest that HOT should be considered in infants whose room air SpO_2 is <92% to 95%, with target saturations >94%.[34-37] When considering these targets, it may be reasonable to consider adjusting the target based on whether the infant still has either pulmonary hypertension or retinopathy of prematurity. Target saturations in infants with pulmonary hypertension should be slightly higher in those infants with BPD complicated by pulmonary hypertension. In contrast, the use of oxygen may need to be more restrictive, with lower tolerable target SpO_2 in infants whose eyes are not yet mature.

Growth Failure

Several studies have shown that HOT improves weight gain.

Groothuis and Rosenberg found that when parents prematurely discontinued supplemental oxygen against medical advice, mean daily weight gain fell significantly and improved once HOT was resumed. Other studies have replicated this finding.[38-40]

Intermittent Hypoxia and Pulmonary Hypertension

Oxygen supplementation has been shown to decrease episodes of intermittent desaturation,[41] which are known to be extremely common even in otherwise "healthy" preterm infants.[42]

Oxygen is also a potent pulmonary vasodilator. Several studies have shown that supplemental oxygen can decrease pulmonary artery pressure in infants with severe BPD.[43,44]

OXYGEN DELIVERY SYSTEMS FOR HOME OXYGEN THERAPY

There are three basic home oxygen delivery systems: (1) oxygen concentrators, (2) liquid oxygen units, and (3) high-pressure cylinders.

OXYGEN CONCENTRATOR

A concentrator is a device that separates oxygen from room air. It is small, reliable, and relatively inexpensive. Maximum flow rate is normally 5 to 6 L/min. Concentrators have a unique advantage in that they are the only approved device for air travel for commercial flights.

LIQUID OXYGEN

Liquid oxygen is the most highly efficient means of transporting oxygen. One liter of liquid oxygen equals 860 gaseous liters. Liquid oxygen is approximately −297°F and when kept under pressure of 18 to 22 psi will remain in a liquid state. Conventional liquid oxygen vessels require no power source to operate, making it an appropriate choice for patients in areas with frequent power outages. Conventional liquid oxygen systems are quiet and have no major moving parts. Unfortunately, liquid oxygen is significantly more expensive than other oxygen delivery options.

HIGH-PRESSURE SYSTEMS

Cylinders of varying sizes are available. Such systems take up significantly more space, and larger cylinders can be very heavy. Smaller cylinders allow more portability but drain more quickly and so require more frequent replacement.

Strategies for Discontinuation of Home Oxygen Therapy

Blending oxygen with room air allows delivery of a wider range of oxygen concentrations but requires blending of varying ratios of 100% oxygen with 21% oxygen. This is impractical in the home setting, so only 100% oxygen is delivered in the outpatient setting. Therefore, the primary variable that influences "effective" oxygen delivery, or the concentration of oxygen seen by the lungs, is the flow rate. Few studies have been performed to determine the appropriate flow rate from which oxygen can be safely discontinued. In a small prospective study, Simoes et al. demonstrated that infants on 20 cc/kg or less of oxygen were more successful at weaning to room air.[45] Other studies have suggested that an FiO_2 of 24% oxygen is the appropriate amount of oxygen from which oxygen weaning can safely be started. Finer et al. evaluated the effective oxygen concentration in infants of different sizes, with variable oxygen delivery flow rates.[46] For infants of minimum size for outpatient care (2 kg), a flow rate of 125 cc/min achieves an effective oxygen delivery of less than 24%, so this flow rate is an appropriate rate from which to begin a discontinuation plan.[47]

For infants who are discharged home on supplemental oxygen at flow rates greater than 125 cc/min, we evaluate saturations in the clinic for 20-minute intervals, and if saturations can be maintained above 93% for 20 minutes, we decrease oxygen flow rates by 50%, as usually the regulators allow changes in only such increments (1 L/min, 500, 250, and 125 cc/min). Once infants can maintain stats at 125 cc/min, we trial a sprint off oxygen for 20 minutes.

Simoes et al. suggested that a 40-minute room air trial predicted successful discontinuation off oxygen.[45] In our clinic, we initiate sprints off oxygen in increments of 1 to 2 hours and allow extension of sprints every 3 to 4 days. During the sprints to room air, infants should stay on an oximeter to confirm their ability to maintain saturations above 93%. Assuming uninterrupted successful biweekly extensions of the sprints, infants should be able to remain off oxygen for 12 hours during the day within 3 weeks of starting the sprints. Once this is achieved, we perform a recorded oximetry study off oxygen to confirm that the infants can maintain acceptable saturations >93% off oxygen for a minimum of 8 hours. This is consistent with many other institutions in the United States.[48] If infants can maintain saturations >93% for >95% of the recorded time, then the oxygen is discontinued. However, if growth is not maintained, then nocturnal oxygen use may be extended. It is important to note that not only oxygen saturation but also adequate somatic growth and normalization of pulmonary pressures are important outcomes to consider prior to discontinuing supplemental oxygen therapy.

Newer technology now allows for more convenient long-term recording of patient oxygen saturations. Studies are under way to determine if such data may improve outpatient weaning protocols.

In summary, for many infants with BPD, safe outpatient use of supplemental oxygen can allow infants to continue to progress in the home environment rather than in the NICU. Further research is needed to determine optimal weaning strategies, but recent published case series can provide guidance until more definitive studies are completed.

REFERENCES

A complete reference list is available at https://expertconsult.inkling.com.

42

Neurologic Effects of Respiratory Support

Matthew A. Rainaldi, MD, and Jeffrey M. Perlman, MBChB

The use of respiratory support in the neonatal intensive care unit (NICU) to treat a variety of newborn respiratory conditions (e.g., respiratory distress syndrome and chronic lung disease) is quite common. Both the respiratory pathologies and the interventions used to treat these conditions have been linked to brain injury in preterm and term neonates. This chapter reviews (1) the basic physiology of cerebral blood flow in the neonate; (2) the common causes of neonatal brain injury, including their pathophysiology; (3) how carbon dioxide and oxygen influence brain injury; (4) how mechanical aspects distinct to the mode of ventilation affect brain injury; and (5) how medications used in respiratory management can modulate brain injury. The focus will be on preterm infants, as this is the population at the highest risk for permanent brain injury.

CEREBRAL BLOOD FLOW IN THE NEONATE

Cerebral blood flow (CBF) is tightly linked to cerebral metabolic demands in the normal brain.[1-3] In the newborn infant, CBF is low, which corresponds to low neuronal activity in this patient population.[4] Various methods of evaluation, including positron emission tomography, xenon clearance technique, ultrasound flowmetry, magnetic resonance imaging, and near-infrared spectroscopy (NIRS), indicate a wide range of CBF values of between 10 and 20 mL/100 g/min.[5-7] These values are approximately one-third of the value for a healthy adult brain.[1,8] A low CBF value in this patient population does not imply poor outcome, as the lower threshold required to maintain neuronal viability remains unknown.[9] Interestingly, on the first day of life, CBF in preterm infants can be lower than the minimal CBF necessary to preserve viability and metabolism in the adult brain.[10]

CBF is a function of cerebral perfusion pressure (CPP) and cerebrovascular resistance (CVR) as follows: CBF = CPP/CVR.[2,3] Total and regional CBF, coupled with cerebral oxygen consumption, increases with postconceptual and postnatal age corresponding to increases in cerebral metabolic rates and energy demands.[2,11] This increase is most prominent in the first day of life and probably represents a normal adaptive response of the cerebral circulation to postnatal life.[7,9] Regional differences in CBF also reflect varying metabolic demands. For instance, blood flow to parasagittal and periventricular white matter is lower relative to that of other regions such as the cerebellum and basal ganglia.[2]

Cerebral Autoregulation and Pressure-Passive Circulation

Cerebral autoregulation is the normal intrinsic ability of the cerebral blood vessels to maintain relatively constant CBF over a range of mean arterial blood pressures (MABPs) (Fig. 42-1). As CPP decreases, CVR also decreases by way of alterations in the diameter of the precapillary arterioles, thus maintaining CBF.[4] This adaptive ability has a limited capacity and will result in a decrease of CBF when the blood pressure falls below a certain threshold and, conversely, will increase when blood pressure reaches an upper threshold.[12] This is referred to as a loss of autoregulation, or a pressure-passive state.[12]

Cerebral autoregulation appears to be intact in fetal and neonatal animal models.[2,13] It also appears to be intact in the stable human preterm infant. In a study of extremely preterm infants with median gestational age of 24 weeks, CBF was found to be low (range of 4.4 to 11 mL/100 g/min), with no relationship of CBF to systemic blood pressure, suggesting intact autoregulation.[9] In another study of preterm infants with a mean gestational age of 26 weeks, normotensive infants (MABP 37 ± 2 mm Hg) were shown to have intact autoregulation, although there was a loss of autoregulation in those who became hypotensive (MABP 25 ± 1 mm Hg). This study also identified an MABP threshold of ~30 mm Hg, below which the CBF became pressure passive.[14] However, a definition of this lower threshold remains elusive. Victor et al. analyzed electroencephalography (EEG) patterns in 35 preterm infants (median gestational age 27 weeks) daily until day 4 of life.[15] Notably, four infants had abnormal EEGs, and the MABPs in these infants were significantly lower than those with normal EEGs (22 vs 33 mm Hg, $p < 0.001$). This suggests that the lower limit of MABP for autoregulation was in the range of 22 to 33 mm Hg in this cohort. Another study showed no difference in CBF between a group of preterm infants with MABP of less than 30 mm Hg and another group with MABP greater than 30 mm Hg.[16]

In summary, although cerebral autoregulation has been documented in the premature infant, it appears to function within a limited blood pressure range and is impaired or absent in the sick hypotensive preterm infant.[17-19] This vulnerable state places the developing brain at extraordinary risk for injury during times of hypotension and/or elevated blood pressures. As such, CBF is one of the most important factors contributing to the major forms of preterm brain injury, as will be detailed subsequently.

BRAIN INJURY IN THE PRETERM INFANT

The most common forms of brain injury in the underdeveloped premature brain are periventricular–intraventricular hemorrhage (IVH, including periventricular hemorrhagic infarction [PVI]) and periventricular leukomalacia (PVL). These lesions are more likely to occur in the smallest, most immature infants with respiratory distress syndrome requiring mechanical

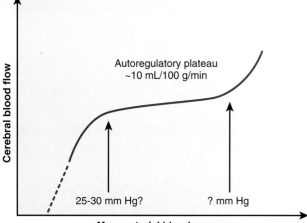

FIG 42-1 Schematic depiction of the relationship between cerebral blood flow and mean arterial blood pressure. Note the autoregulatory plateau. The precise range of blood pressures in which this occurs for preterm neonates is unknown.

ventilation. The majority of permanent long-term neurologic sequelae in preterm infants are a result of these two forms of brain injury.[20,21]

Periventricular–Intraventricular Hemorrhage

The overall incidence of IVH has declined over the past few decades, although severe hemorrhage continues to be a significant morbidity in the increasing population of very low birth-weight (VLBW) survivors.[21,22] The incidence and severity of IVH are inversely proportional to gestational age. About 25% of infants between 501 and 750 g and 14% between 751 and 1000 g still develop the most severe forms of hemorrhage, with the incidence remaining essentially unchanged since the mid-1990s.[21]

The primary lesion in IVH is bleeding from the periventricular subependymal germinal matrix. This matrix is a transitional region of neuronal and glial precursor cells that migrate to other regions of the cerebrum. Notably, it is highly cellular, richly vascularized, and gelatinous in texture.[2] It is located between the caudate nucleus and the thalamus at the level of, or slightly posterior to, the foramen of Monro.[22] It begins to involute after 34 weeks, and by term gestation, it is essentially absent. Destruction of the germinal matrix may result in impairment of myelination, brain growth, and cortical development.[2]

Reviewing the vascular supply of the germinal matrix is crucial to understanding its propensity to bleed. The immature capillary network of the germinal matrix is primarily supplied by a branch of the anterior cerebral artery (Heubner's artery), striate branches of the middle cerebral artery, and the anterior choroidal artery. Venous drainage incorporates a system of medullary, choroidal, and thalamostriate veins that link to form the terminal vein. Where the terminal vein and the internal cerebral vein join, the venous flow makes a striking U-turn before continuing on to join the vein of Galen. The venous anatomy suggests that elevated venous pressure secondary to obstruction of the venous drainage may lead to venous distention and rupture (Fig. 42-2).[2] Moreover, hypotension leading to decreased CBF probably also plays a role in the genesis of IVH in some infants. This presumably occurs via a mechanism of ischemia–reperfusion with rupture of blood vessels upon

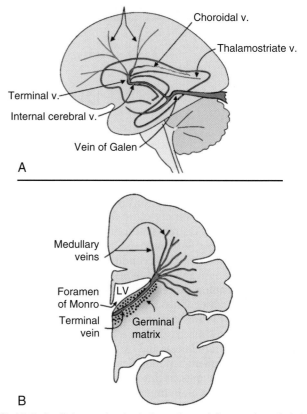

FIG 42-2 **A,** Schematic depiction of medullary veins draining into the terminal vein (v.), sagittal view. Note the U-turn the terminal vein takes before draining into the internal cerebral vein, a potential site for increasing venous pressure. **B,** Coronal view representing the medullary veins draining into the terminal vein and traveling directly through the germinal matrix. *LV,* lateral ventricle. (Adapted from Volpe JJ. *Neurology of the Newborn.* 5th ed. Philadelphia: Saunders/Elsevier; 2008 [xiv, 1094 p.].)

reperfusion. Precise description of the vasculature of the germinal matrix has been elusive because the small capillaries, venules, and arterioles that populate the matrix are hard to distinguish from one another histologically due to their relatively simple endothelial wall structure.

The physiologic factors contributing to increased risk of IVH are complex and incorporate a combination of vascular, intravascular, and extravascular influences (Box 42-1).[22] Intravascular factors, especially those that involve perturbations in CBF and volume, play a critical role in the development of hemorrhage. A pressure-passive circulation in the sick preterm brain leads to direct changes in CBF with changes in systemic blood pressure. Acute changes in blood pressure and cerebral perfusion are likely to lead to disruption of the vulnerable blood vessels in the germinal matrix. Fluctuating CBF velocity in the VLBW infant also predisposes the infant to hemorrhage.[23,24] Physiologic increases in cerebral venous pressure exacerbate the already compromised venous drainage of the terminal vein. These physiologic disturbances may be from a variety of factors, such as the labor and delivery process and intrathoracic pressure changes induced by the ventilator or air leaks. Intrathoracic pressure is directly transmitted to cerebral vessels, and these fluctuations are applied to vessels probably already maximally dilated with little autoregulation. Another intravascular component that has been implicated in playing a role in IVH is inflammation, which has been correlated with increased risk of IVH.[25,26] Although precise mechanisms are unclear, increased interleukin (IL)-1β, IL-6, and IL-8; mononuclear cells; and other inflammatory markers have been increased in the fetal and neonatal period in infants with IVH.[27-31] Similarly, both clinical and histologic chorioamnionitis have been associated with hemorrhage.[30,32] Conversely, antenatal steroids decrease the risk. The protective effect of steroids may in part be related to enhanced support for the blood vessels within the germinal matrix.[22] The general vascular support of the germinal matrix capillaries is poor, with increased fibrinolytic activity and decreased glial stabilization. Finally, the germinal matrix capillaries themselves are quite tenuous, as they are in a constant state of involution and remodeling. Their vascular lining is deficient, and they reside in an end-arterial zone between the striate and the thalamic arterial distribution.[2]

In most cases the diagnosis of IVH is made with screening ultrasound. The most vulnerable period is the first few postnatal days, with greater than 50% occurring in the first 24 hours and 90% in the first 72 hours of life.[26] Risk factors associated with the development of IVH include low birth weight and gestational age, maternal smoking, breech presentation, premature rupture of membranes, postnatal resuscitation and intubation,

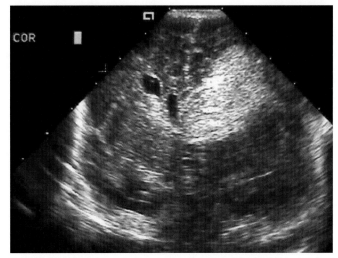

FIG 42-3 Coronal head ultrasound—intraventricular hemorrhage/periventricular infarction. Note the increased echodense area in the left frontal white matter approximating the distribution of the medullary veins.

early-onset sepsis, respiratory distress syndrome (RDS), pulmonary air leaks, metabolic acidosis, and rapid bicarbonate infusions.[33] Extremes of arterial $PaCO_2$ in the first 4 days of life are also associated with severe IVH (see below).[34]

Periventricular Hemorrhagic Infarction (Grade 4 Intraventricular Hemorrhage)

One of the complications of IVH is PVI, also termed *grade 4 IVH.* PVI is a hemorrhagic venous infarction that is associated with severe and usually asymmetric bleeding. It occurs in about 15% of infants with IVH, particularly the smallest, most immature ones. On brain imaging, there is often a large, fan-shaped region of hemorrhagic necrosis in the periventricular white matter, invariably on the side with the larger amount of intraventricular blood (Fig. 42-3). A variety of studies have shown that this lesion is not merely an extension of IVH. Instead, the likely mechanism is the obstruction of the medullary and terminal veins by the intraventricular and germinal matrix blood clot, leading to venous congestion in the periventricular white matter with subsequent hemorrhage and ischemia. PVI is associated with a high rate of mortality (40% to 60%), with survivors being at very high risk of cerebral palsy (CP) (66% in one study) and other neurologic abnormalities.[35,36]

Periventricular Leukomalacia and Diffuse White Matter Injury

Focal and diffuse white matter injury (WMI) may occur adjacent to the lateral ventricles with or without associated hemorrhage—a condition referred to as *PVL* (Fig. 42-4). The sonographic findings include cyst formation, ventriculomegaly, and diffuse WMI. This last form often manifests with ventriculomegaly in the absence of cyst formation and occurs most commonly in premature infants who require prolonged ventilator support.[37] The pathogenesis of WMI is complex and involves vascular factors, as well as the intrinsic vulnerability of oligodendrocytes to noxious substances. The vascular factors include the following: (1) The white matter resides in a border zone region, which increases the likelihood of injury during periods of systemic hypotension (Fig. 42-5). (2) The risk for injury to

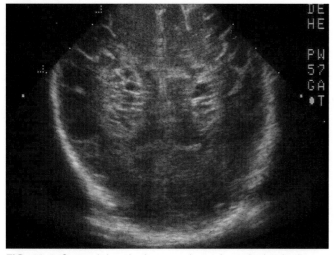

FIG 42-4 Coronal head ultrasound—periventricular leukomalacia. Note the bilateral cystic areas within the periventricular white matter.

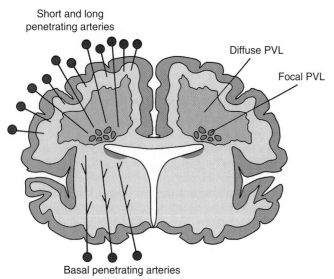

FIG 42-5 Schematic depiction of focal and diffuse periventricular leukomalacia (*PVL*). Note the penetrating arteries and the distribution of the leukomalacia in the vascular border zones. (Adapted from Volpe JJ. *Neurology of the Newborn.* 5th ed. Philadelphia: Saunders/Elsevier; 2008 [xiv, 1094 p.].)

these regions is increased in the face of a pressure-passive circulation as discussed above. (3) There is a limited vasodilatory response to $PaCO_2$ of those vessels supplying the white matter.

The intrinsic vulnerability of the early differentiating oligodendrocyte has been established in studies that show that these cells are sensitive to injury secondary to the release of numerous factors, including free radicals, excitotoxins (glutamate), and cytokines, as well as a lack of growth factors.[20] The importance of intrinsic vulnerability is suggested from a report of 14 of 632 infants (2.3%) weighing less than 1750 g at birth who developed bilateral cystic PVL.[38] Overt hypotension occurred in only four of the babies with PVL, mostly in the immediate postnatal period. In the other 10 cases, PVL was seen in infants with mild to moderate lung disease without hypotension and was detected only on routine ultrasound screening. Two conditions

were found to be significantly associated with development of PVL in this cohort—chorioamnionitis and prolonged rupture of membranes. Other conditions that have been associated with the development of PVL include hypocarbia, meningitis, and recurrent severe apnea and bradycardia.[2] Surviving preterm infants with PVL are at risk for CP (primarily spastic diplegia) and other motor deficits. Cognitive problems are also common, along with more subtle behavioral and attention disturbances.[2]

INFLUENCE OF OXYGEN CONCENTRATION AND CARBON DIOXIDE ON CEREBRAL BLOOD FLOW

As discussed above, abnormal CBF is one of the most important pathophysiologic factors in preterm brain injury. The cerebral circulation of the healthy newborn infant, and even in the very preterm infant, responds to physiologic stimuli in much the same way as in the adult. Cerebral blood vessels are sensitive to changes in $PaCO_2$, arterial oxygen concentration (Cao_2), and pH.[1] In pathologic situations, a pressure-passive state occurs and cerebral blood vessels may not react to chemical or metabolic stimuli. These infants are at increased risk for developing hemorrhagic and/or ischemic cerebral injury.

Oxygen and Hemoglobin

CBF increases when arterial oxygen tension decreases markedly in the human infant and in neonatal animal models.[1,3,20] CBF is regulated by Cao_2, which in turn is determined by hemoglobin concentration, oxygen affinity to hemoglobin, and PaO_2.[1,13] In preterm infants studied in the first 3 days of life, it has been shown that CBF increases by approximately 12% for every 1-mM decrease in hemoglobin concentration.[39] There is also a direct relationship of CBF with the relative proportion of fetal hemoglobin, probably due to the stronger affinity of fetal hemoglobin for oxygen.

Cerebrovascular dilation occurs within 30 to 60 seconds in response to hypoxia.[1] At lower blood pressures, the vasodilator response to hypoxia may be impaired. Conversely, hyperoxia induces a fall in CBF in preterm infants through cerebral vasoconstriction.[1] Median reduction was found to be 0.06 cm/s for every 1-kPa increase in oxygen tension. When 80% oxygen was given during resuscitation at birth, preterm infants were subsequently shown to have a 25% reduction in CBF velocity versus those infants given room air.[40]

Carbon Dioxide

The fetal and neonatal brain remains sensitive to changes in $PaCO_2$; hypocarbia decreases CBF through vasoconstriction of cerebral arteries and hypercarbia has a relaxant effect.[1,3,41,42] The primary mediator linking arterial CO_2 tension and cerebral vasoreactivity may be pH. In one study performed on isolated dog cerebral arteries, hypercarbia-induced cerebral arterial relaxation was shown to be mediated mainly with a fall of extracellular pH.[43] Because CO_2 crosses the blood–brain barrier readily, abrupt changes in CO_2 tension may also cause a rapid change in vascular reactivity within 1 to 2 minutes. This acute effect is then actively regulated by perivascular pH causing the vessel diameter to normalize gradually during the next 24 hours.[1]

In the healthy adult, CBF changes by a mean of approximately 30% for every 1-kPa change in $PaCO_2$. Similarly, in spontaneously breathing preterm infants studied at 2 to 3 hours after birth, CBF–carbon dioxide reactivity was shown to be approximately 30% per 1-kPa change in $PaCO_2$. In mechanically ventilated preterm infants, this reactivity was much less, that is, ~11% per 1-kPa change in $PaCO_2$ when studied shortly after birth, although it increased to near-adult levels by the second day of life. In the infants in whom severe intracranial hemorrhage subsequently developed, there was a loss of CBF reactivity to changes in $PaCO_2$, implying an impairment of CBF regulation before hemorrhage.[39]

LINKING CHANGES IN CARBON DIOXIDE AND OXYGEN CONCENTRATION TO HEMORRHAGIC–ISCHEMIC INJURY

Hypocarbia and White Matter Injury

Hypocarbia is a common occurrence in the ventilated preterm infant. It may be seen as a result of improved lung compliance and/or function or with aggressive ventilator support (either unintentional or intentional). Several studies have reported the association of hypocarbia with PVL, neurodevelopmental problems, and CP.[42,44,45] In one study, time-averaged $PaCO_2$ on the third day of life was lower in preterm infants who developed PVL than in those who did not develop PVL.[46] Others have supported a similar dose-dependent effect of hypocarbia, with longer and more frequent episodes of hypocarbia associated with more severe brain injury.[45,47] In full-term infants, hypocarbia following perinatal hypoxia–ischemia is associated with adverse outcomes, as evidenced by a retrospective study of nearly 250 newborns.[48] This was also noted in the National Institute of Child Health and Human Development Neonatal Research Network's trial of whole-body hypothermia.[49] When early blood gases were examined (from birth through 12 hours of hypothermia), infants with death or disability had significantly lower minimum Pco_2 concentrations (median 22 vs 26 mm Hg, $p = 0.15$), and this was a predictor of outcome.[50] This relationship also held true in those infants exposed to a higher cumulative duration of hypocarbia, as they also had worse outcomes. Despite these correlations, it remains unclear whether hypocarbia leads to brain injury or is merely an early marker of increased risk.

Hypercarbia and Intraventricular Hemorrhage

Permissive hypercarbia has been advocated as a ventilatory strategy to minimize barotrauma and volutrauma to the lungs of preterm infants and thus prevent evolution to chronic lung disease.[51] Although there may be beneficial effects in terms of lung injury, the risks of elevated $PaCO_2$ to the brain must not be ignored. As reviewed earlier, hypercarbia is associated with both an increase in CBF and an impairment of cerebral autoregulation in ventilated VLBW infants.[51] In a study undertaken in the first week of life in VLBW infants of gestational age 26.9 ± 2.3 weeks, increasing $PaCO_2$ resulted in increasing impairment of cerebral autoregulation.[52] Hypercarbia, defined by the maximum $PaCO_2$ recorded during the first 3 days of life, was also associated with severe IVH in a retrospective cohort study of 574 VLBW infants.[53] As maximum $PaCO_2$ increased from 40 to 100 mm Hg, the probability of severe IVH increased from 8% to 21%. A retrospective review of 849 infants weighing less than 1250 g suggested that extremes in $PaCO_2$, both hypocarbia and hypercarbia, as well as fluctuations in $PaCO_2$ during the first 4 days of life, increased the risk of severe IVH.[34] In this analysis, infants who developed severe IVH had higher maximum $PaCO_2$ (median: 72 vs 59 mm Hg, $p < 0.001$), lower minimal $PaCO_2$ (median: 32 vs 39 mm Hg, $p < 0.001$), and a greater range between maximum and minimum $PaCO_2$ values (median: 39 vs 21 mm Hg, $p < 0.001$). This was reinforced in a reanalysis of data from the SUPPORT trial.[54,55] In over 1300 infants from 24 to 27 6/7 weeks, severe IVH was increased in those with $PaCO_2$ levels in the highest quartile. These infants were also at increased risk of neurodevelopmental impairment. Similarly, infants with a large range between maximum and minimum $PaCO_2$ (i.e., fluctuators) had increased incidences of neurodevelopmental impairment as well as bronchopulmonary dysplasia (BPD). Comparable results linking increased $PaCO_2$ fluctuations with IVH were shown in a retrospective analysis by Altaany et al.[56] Taken together, these studies indicate that extremes in $PaCO_2$ should be avoided during the period in which infants are at high risk of IVH.

Oxygen and Brain Injury

Fraction of inspired oxygen (FiO_2) is a parameter that must be chosen by the provider when respiratory support is initiated—this may range from room air to 100% O_2. Clinicians often use oxygen saturation (SpO_2) and PaO_2 to subsequently guide their administration, varying their targets based on factors such as gestational age, risk of retinopathy of prematurity, and heart and lung disease. Although the optimal saturation range of preterm infants is unclear, it is known that the extremes of both hypoxia and hyperoxia can have adverse effects on the developing brain.[57,58] The SUPPORT trial randomized infants to SpO_2 targets of either 85% to 89% or 91% to 95% to address this question.[55] Although there were no differences in IVH or PVL, the lower oxygen-saturation group had an increased incidence of death (19.9% vs 16.2%; $p = 0.04$), and the higher oxygen-saturation group had an increased incidence of severe retinopathy (17.9% vs 8.6%; $p < 0.001$).

The effect of hyperoxia on the preterm infant has received considerable attention. As reviewed earlier, Cao_2 is a primary regulator of CBF. The preterm infant often has labile oxygen saturations and therefore CBF, which increases the risk of IVH. At a biochemical level, hyperoxia has also been shown to have deleterious effects on the preterm brain through mechanisms of inflammation, apoptosis, and oxidative stress.[57] Excess oxygen can lead to the generation of reactive oxygen species. These free radicals can be harmful to preterm infants because of their already low antioxidant defense compared to term infants. Of particular importance, premyelinating, or immature, oligodendrocytes are vulnerable to oxidative injury, which may be a potent contributor to PVL in a preterm infant receiving excessive oxygen therapy.[59,60]

In addition to SpO_2 and PaO_2, the measurement of regional tissue hemoglobin oxygen saturation ($rSto_2$) has been gaining popularity. Using NIRS, $rSto_2$ can be measured noninvasively in various circulatory regions (e.g., cerebral, splanchnic, etc.). A trial of 166 preterm infants of less than 28 weeks' gestation randomized subjects to visible or blinded cerebral NIRS monitoring for the first 3 days of life.[61] The visible NIRS subjects were managed with the goal of maintaining $rSto_2$ between 55% and 85% by targeting respiratory and circulatory parameters. While the treatment group did maintain $rSto_2$ in the target range better than the control group, no significant differences in clinical outcomes were found.

In summary, both low and high blood oxygen concentrations have harmful effects on the brain. Pulse oximetry and

PaO_2 are the mainstays of adjusting oxygen therapy, but new technologies, such as NIRS, may have a prominent role in the future.

MODE OF VENTILATION AND BRAIN INJURY

Mechanical factors related to the delivery of inhaled gas have also been implicated in causing brain injury. Driving gas via positive pressure into the lungs is fundamentally different from inhalation via negative pressure. Such pressure changes in the thorax can disrupt hemodynamics, increase venous pressure, and therefore alter CBF. This section focuses on the most common methods of respiratory support and how they relate to brain injury.

Continuous Positive Airway Pressure

Continuous positive airway pressure (CPAP) is a commonly used noninvasive mode of respiratory support that can improve ventilation by maintaining functional residual capacity. In a model of chronic lung disease in which preterm baboons were mechanically ventilated, Loeliger et al. weaned one group to CPAP at 24 hours of life and another at 5 days of life.[62] Both groups showed diffuse brain injury, but the early CPAP group had less severe injury. This link between longer duration of mechanical ventilation and worse neurologic outcome has also been shown in human studies.[63,64] Mechanical ventilation compared to CPAP has been associated with lower developmental scores, more disruptions in CBF, increased IVH, and a higher incidence of death.[63,64] However, infants receiving mechanical ventilation are likely to be sicker, and as a consequence it is difficult to implicate ventilator support versus the underlying disease.

Conventional Mechanical Ventilation

Mechanical ventilation can affect CBF by impeding venous return or through changes in the acid–base balance (see above). Elevated mean airway pressure can increase central venous pressure, thereby decreasing superior vena cava return and increasing the risk for IVH. This will in turn decrease cardiac output, increasing the risk of cerebral hypoperfusion.[65,66] This puts the vulnerable areas of the premature brain, such as the periventricular white matter, at risk for injury.

Exposure to fluctuations of CBF with prolonged mechanical ventilation presumably results in repeated insults throughout the course of intensive care. Walsh et al. demonstrated that extremely low birth-weight infants who are ventilated longer, probably representing the sickest of the cohort, have increased incidence of CP.[67] All surviving infants who were ventilated for 120 or more days had neurologic impairment.

High-Frequency Oscillatory Ventilation

Physiologically, continuous sustained lung inflation as seen with high-frequency oscillatory ventilation (HFOV) can lead to a higher mean airway pressure. This is associated with an increased risk of venous distention, particularly to the medullary veins in the periventricular white matter (see above). However, when the lungs are poorly inflated, complications may result secondary to poor ventilation and low oxygenation. Thus, there is likely to be an optimal mean airway pressure to be achieved for each infant receiving high-frequency ventilation. How to define this value for the individual infant remains unclear.

In a meta-analysis of 17 studies involving a total of 3652 preterm infants, HFOV compared with conventional ventilation did not affect neonatal mortality, IVH, or PVL.[68] Although HFOV has been associated with short-term neurologic morbidity in some studies, this has not been a consistent finding.[69] As of this writing, the cumulative data indicate that longer term neurologic morbidities are not increased with the use of HFOV.[70]

MEDICATIONS USED TO TREAT RESPIRATORY CONDITIONS

Surfactant

In the presurfactant era, VLBW infants, especially those that developed pneumothorax, had increased risk of IVH. Because surfactant reduced the severity of RDS and the rate of pneumothorax, it was postulated that it would also lead to a decrease in the rates of IVH. However, this has not been borne out in the many surfactant trials. A 2012 Cochrane review evaluated IVH as a secondary outcome when comparing prophylactic surfactant to CPAP with selective use of surfactant.[71] There was a trend toward decreased risk of IVH in those infants who received prophylactic surfactant (RR 0.91, 95% CI 0.82 to 1.0). Despite the many trials of surfactant and regardless of the type of intervention—prophylactic versus rescue—or the type of surfactant used—synthetic versus natural—no consistent effect on IVH has been observed.[72] This lack of effect has been attributed to the impact of surfactant administration on fluctuations in CBF in sick preterm infants who have pressure-passive circulations and the rapid changes in $PaCO_2$ and PaO_2 that may subsequently lead to brain injury.[73] There are multiple studies on the effects of surfactant administration on CBF. The results have been equivocal, with both human and animal data demonstrating conflicting results.

Methylxanthines

Methylxanthines have been used in neonatology as a respiratory stimulant since the 1970s, with caffeine being one of most frequently prescribed medications in neonatal intensive care.[74] Caffeine has been found to decrease the frequency of apnea of prematurity as well as decrease the need for mechanical ventilation. The mechanism of action remains unclear, but it is likely related to an increase in chemoreceptor responsiveness, enhanced respiratory musculature performance, and generalized central nervous system excitation.[75] The most likely pathway is as an antagonist of adenosine receptors at the cell membrane. There were concerns regarding the central nervous system effects of caffeine because adenosine is protective of the brain during experimental hypoxia and ischemia.[76]

The Caffeine for Apnea of Prematurity Trial Group reported on the short- and long-term effects of caffeine (Table 42-1). In this randomized, placebo-controlled trial of VLBW infants initially followed postnatally up to 18 to 21 months, it was found that there was a decreased rate of death or survival with a neurodevelopmental disability in the caffeine-treated group (40% vs 46%, OR 0.77; 95% CI 0.64 to 0.93, $p = 0.008$). The study also demonstrated less CP (4.4% vs 7.3%, OR 0.58; 95% CI 0.39 to 0.87, $p = 0.0009$), fewer cognitively affected infants (33.8% vs 38.3%, OR 0.81; 95% CI 0.66 to 0.99, $p = 0.04$), and even decreased incidence of severe retinopathy of prematurity in the treatment group (5.1% vs 7.9%, OR 0.61; 95% CI 0.42

TABLE 42-1	Long-Term Effects of Caffeine Therapy			
	Outcome	Caffeine (*n*=833)	Placebo (*n*=807)	*p* value
18 months	Death or disability	307 (38.1%)	352 (45.1%)	0.006
	Cerebral palsy	33 (4.3%)	57 (7.7%)	0.006
	Severe cognitive delay*	88 (11.9%)	116 (16.2%)	0.02
5 years	Death or disability	176 (21.1%)	200 (24.8%)	0.09
	Motor impairment[†]	13 (1.6%)	21 (2.7%)	0.2
	Severe cognitive impairment[‡]	38 (4.9%)	38 (5.1%)	0.89

Data from Schmidt B, et al. Survival without disability to age 5 years after neonatal caffeine therapy for apnea of prematurity. *JAMA.* 2012;307(3):275-282.
*Mental developmental index <70.
[†]Gross motor function classification scale level >2.
[‡]Full scale IQ <70.

to 0.89, $p = 0.01$). Subsequently, the results of a 5-year follow-up of nearly 85% of these infants were not as notable.[77] At that time, 21% of caffeine-treated infants suffered death or disability versus 25% in the placebo group (OR 0.82; 95% CI 0.65 to 1.0, $p = 0.09$). In a secondary analysis of these infants, gross motor function was improved in the caffeine-treated infants (OR 0.64; 95% CI 0.47 to 0.88, $p = 0.006$). Also, a subset of caffeine-treated infants showed lower rates of developmental coordination disorder (11.3% vs 15.2%, OR 0.71; 95% CI 0.52 to 0.97, $p = 0.03$), which has been associated with CP.[78] Overall, the striking differences in neurologic outcomes at 18 months did not persist at 5 years. Two recent studies showed that early caffeine (i.e., within the first 2-3 days of life) was associated with a combined reduction in death and BPD, but one reported a higher incidence of death in the early treatment group.[79,80]

The clinical indication for caffeine varies among providers and NICUs but is often guided by gestational age and apneic symptoms. The traditional practice is to prescribe caffeine for infants approaching extubation and/or those infants at high risk of apnea of prematurity. Some providers have expanded their use of caffeine beyond this as a potential neuroprotective agent—for example, prescribing early caffeine (at initiation of ventilator support or at less than 3 days of age) to a preterm infant who remains intubated and is not having apnea.[80] As described above, evidence supporting long-term benefits of caffeine is conflicting, so the risks and benefits must be considered. At the current time, caffeine has an excellent safety profile, and thus the risks are likely to be low in most cases.[76,81]

Inhaled Nitric Oxide

Inhaled nitric oxide (iNO) is commonly used to treat hypoxemic respiratory failure in term neonates. Its use has expanded to preterm neonates, primarily as an adjunct therapy to improve pulmonary blood flow and therefore oxygenation. There has been emerging evidence regarding potential neuroprotective effects of iNO, as it has been shown to influence both CBF and the inflammatory cascade.[82]

In an initial clinical evaluation, 207 premature infants were randomized to receive either iNO or placebo.[83] Treatment with iNO significantly reduced the risk of death or chronic lung disease (49% vs 64%, RR 0.76; 95% CI 0.60 to 0.97; $p = 0.03$). In this study, the risk of severe IVH or PVL was significantly lower with iNO than with placebo (12% vs 24%; RR 0.53; 95% CI 0.28 to 0.98; $p = 0.04$). While this seemed promising for a neuroprotective role, subsequent studies were conflicting.[67,84,85] Some even demonstrated a worsening of neurologic injury with iNO, such as a multicenter study by Van Meurs et al., which reported that severe IVH and death were higher with iNO than with placebo in a 1000 g or less subgroup.[84] Unfortunately, comparisons across these studies are difficult, given differences in study populations and treatment paradigms.

Similarly, no definitive conclusion regarding the effects of iNO on long-term neurodevelopmental outcomes can be drawn. In a 2005 study, a total of 138 children (82% of survivors) were assessed at 2 years of age.[86] Treatment with iNO was associated with a lower risk of abnormal neurodevelopmental outcome (disability or delay) compared with placebo (24% vs 46%, RR 0.53; 95% CI 0.33 to 0.87, $p = 0.01$). A 1-year follow-up of infants randomized to iNO or placebo showed greater survival free of neurodevelopmental impairment in a subset weighing 750 to 999 g (67.9% vs 55.6%, $p = 0.04$).[85] But this did not hold true for smaller infants, who had more oxygen dependence as well as a significant increase in cost of care. Finally, a 2-year follow-up of the NO CLD Trial (in which iNO was associated with increased survival without BPD) did not show a difference in neurodevelopmental outcomes.[87]

Postnatal Steroids

The use of postnatal systemic glucocorticoids, particularly high-dose dexamethasone, to prevent or treat chronic lung disease in the preterm infant has been shown to be associated with increased risk of CP and neurodevelopmental impairment.[88] Other strategies, such as lower dose dexamethasone for BPD, hydrocortisone for BPD, or short-course steroids for airway edema, may have fewer adverse effects, but current data are insufficient to provide recommendations.[88] The American Academy of Pediatrics' 2010 policy statement cited insufficient evidence to make recommendations regarding other steroid protocols.[89] Our practice is to reserve the use of systemic glucocorticoids to facilitate extubation of select infants who remain intubated beyond 3 to 4 weeks of life—that is, those at highest risk of developing BPD. This individualized decision should be made in conjunction with the family and involve a thorough analysis of the potential risks and benefits.

SUMMARY

The developing brain of the fetus and newborn is extremely vulnerable to injury in the form of IVH and/or PVL. There is an intimate relationship between neonatal respiratory disease and risk of brain injury in the premature infant. This relationship is a result of both the disease process and the interventions we use to treat respiratory conditions. There are a plethora of variables related to respiratory support that, either in combination or in isolation, may increase the risk for brain injury (physiologic variables such as acid–base disturbances, carbon dioxide, oxygen, positive-pressure mechanical ventilation, commonly used respiratory medications, air leaks, etc.). In the management of a sick newborn with respiratory distress, the risk/benefit ratio of any intervention that is being pursued for its pulmonary effect must be weighed against its potential central nervous system effects. Hemorrhagic–ischemic injury should be considered in each case to minimize such injury and thus improve long-term neurodevelopmental outcome.

REFERENCES

A complete reference list is available at https://expertconsult.inkling.com/.

43

Pulmonary and Neurodevelopmental Outcomes Following Ventilation

Andrea N. Trembath, MD, MPH, Allison H. Payne, MD, MSCR, and Michele C. Walsh, MD, MSEpi

INTRODUCTION

The outcomes of neonates after assisted ventilation are highly variable. Even among infants who require minimal respiratory support, predicting long-term lung and developmental outcomes is complex. Whether the result is respiratory distress syndrome (RDS), genetic predisposition, or postnatal management, prematurity remains the strongest predictor of chronic lung disease and developmental delays. In this chapter we will discuss the key drivers for long-term pulmonary morbidity among premature infants, subsequent pulmonary disease, and the associated neurodevelopmental outcomes.

BRONCHOPULMONARY DYSPLASIA

Prematurity, as defined by birth prior to 37 weeks' gestation, is an important risk factor for the development of lung disease. Despite significant advances in the respiratory care of neonates, bronchopulmonary dysplasia (BPD) remains the most common serious pulmonary morbidity in premature infants. Attempts at eliminating BPD have been largely unsuccessful, and the incidence of BPD is widely variable among sites, even after adjusting for potential risk factors. Among Vermont Oxford Network (VON) sites the rates of BPD range from 12% to over 40% among infants born at less than 32 weeks' gestation. Data from a 2010 VON report suggest that the incidence of BPD appears to have plateaued and the absolute number of premature infants with BPD may be increasing. A potential cause for the increase may be the improvement in the survival of extremely preterm and extremely low birth-weight (ELBW) infants, leading to an increase in the numbers of preterm infants who survive to be classified as having BPD.[1,2]

The contemporary definitions, predictors, and outcomes of BPD have changed.[1,3] BPD, as recognized and described by William Northway, a pediatric radiologist, was based largely on radiographic evidence of lung disease in infants who survived RDS. Chest radiography demonstrated areas of diffuse heterogeneity and coarse opacities in the most severe of cases. Northway recognized that the key component was a history of mechanical ventilation, a technology not available only several years prior to Northway's observations. The infants were moderately to late premature infants, and the management of these infants included exposure to prolonged mechanical ventilation, high airway pressures, and oxygen. Histologically, characteristic areas of hyperinflation alternating with areas of focal collapse were found. Hyperplasia of the bronchial epithelium was present and extensive fibrosis was also noted.[4]

The current landscape in which BPD occurs is distinct from that of Northway. "Classic" or "old" BPD has now been replaced by a "new" form of the disease. "New" BPD is found primarily among extremely low gestational age neonates, defined as <28 weeks' gestational age, and ELBW (i.e., <1000 g birth weight) infants with a history of RDS. These infants are almost uniformly exposed to antenatal steroids and frequently treated with exogenous surfactant therapy. Even the most premature infants may receive only limited exposure to conventional mechanical ventilation but may be exposed to other noninvasive respiratory support such as intermittent positive pressure ventilation, continuous positive airway pressure, or high-flow nasal cannula. The trend in respiratory management has resulted in fewer days on positive pressure ventilation, less time on endotracheal intubation, and less exposure to supplemental oxygen. Chest radiography of new BPD is characterized by diffuse hazy opacities and minimal hyperinflation. In addition, the histology of new BPD shows a reduction in alveoli and capillaries, but minimal fibrosis.[5,6]

Definitions of Bronchopulmonary Dysplasia

The definition and classification of BPD have evolved as the disease itself has changed. The hallmark feature of BPD that remains constant is the receipt of oxygen therapy or positive pressure for a period of time or on a specific day of life. There are three commonly used definitions: (1) receipt of oxygen at 28 days, (2) need for supplemental oxygen at 36 weeks' postmenstrual age, and (3) the physiologic definition. The first two definitions, though simple, are limited by the various developmental considerations of infants born at different gestational ages (i.e., 23 weeks vs 28 weeks), site variation in defining need for supplemental oxygen (i.e., oxygen targets), or the use of therapies targeted at reducing oxygen requirements (i.e., diuretics, steroids, high-flow nasal cannulae).

In 2000 a workshop to clarify the definition of BPD was held by the National Institute of Child Health and Human Development (NICHD). At that time the NICHD recognized the importance of distinguishing BPD from the large heterogeneous group of chronic lung disease.[7] This workshop proposed a severity-based definition classifying BPD into mild, moderate, or severe based on either postnatal age or postmenstrual age (PMA) (Table 43-1). Mild BPD was defined as a need for supplemental oxygen (O_2) for ≥28 days but not at 36 weeks' PMA or discharge, moderate BPD as O_2 for ≥28 days plus treatment with <30% O_2 at 36 weeks' PMA, and severe BPD as O_2 for ≥28 days plus ≥30% O_2 and/or positive pressure at 36 weeks' PMA.

The severity-based definition of BPD was validated by Ehrenkranz et al.[8] by comparing it to the other commonly used definitions such as supplemental oxygen at 28 days and at 36 weeks' PMA. Overall, the NICHD consensus severity-based scale identified infants most at risk for poor pulmonary outcomes as well as neurodevelopment impairment better than the common definitions[8] (Table 43-2).

The physiologic definition of BPD, as developed by Walsh, defines BPD at 36 weeks' adjusted age. Unit-specific rates of BPD among premature infants weighing 501 to 1249 g were compared using the traditional oxygen at 36 weeks' PMA definition (15-66%) and compared to rates of BPD using the physiologic definition (9-57%). The physiologic definition reduces the between-center variability in the diagnosis of BPD and reduces the diagnosis as much as 10% at individual centers. The physiologic definition has also been validated and shown to be independently predictive of cognitive impairment in infants with BPD.[9] The physiologic definition is used in many clinical trials throughout the United States.

Some clinicians have questioned whether all the definitions are needed. There is merit to the severity classification introduced with the National Institutes of Health (NIH) consensus definition, rather than a binary outcome of yes or no. There is also merit to the more objective criteria introduced by the physiologic definition with the room air challenge. The two definitions are easily combined to merge the best of both (Table 43-3).

PULMONARY OUTCOMES

It is time for careful consideration of the validity, relevance, and limitations of commonly targeted short-term and long-term outcomes in neonatal clinical trials. The ideal primary outcomes are those that are objective rather than subjective, occur with sufficient frequency to offer practical enrollment targets, and are important to the child's long-term quality of life. RDS mortality, for example, no longer serves as a relevant primary outcome. Death from RDS in the first week or two of life is an infrequent occurrence in contemporary neonatal intensive care units (NICUs). Death before discharge, while clearly objective and relevant, is influenced by comorbidities and ethical considerations and would be an applicable endpoint only for infants with birth weights less than 800 g, as death occurs infrequently in larger preterm infants and is more often attributable to nonrespiratory causes.

TABLE 43-1 NIH Consensus Definition of Bronchopulmonary Dysplasia

	Respiratory Support at 28 Days of Age	Respiratory Support at 36 Weeks' PMA
No BPD	Room air	Room air
Mild BPD	Respiratory support	Room air
Moderate BPD	Respiratory support	Respiratory support (FiO_2 <30%)
Severe BPD	Respiratory support	Respiratory support (≥30%)

Modified from Jobe AH, Bancalari E. Bronchopulmonary dysplasia. *Am J Respir Crit Care Med.* 2001;163:1723-1729.
BPD, Bronchopulmonary dysplasia; PMA, postmenstrual age.

TABLE 43-2 Respiratory Outcomes of Infants at 18 to 22 Months' Corrected Age as Classified by the NIH Consensus Definition of Bronchopulmonary Dysplasia*

BPD Definition	NICU Infants, n (%; n=4866)	Follow-up Infants, n (%; n=3848)	Pulmonary Medications (% of Follow-up[†])	Rehospitalized Pulmonary Cause (% of Follow-up[†])	RSV Prophylaxis (% of Follow-up[†])
Consensus					
None	1124 (23.1)	876 (22.8)	27.2	23.9	12.5
Mild	1473 (30.3)	1186 (30.8)	29.7	26.7	16.6
Moderate	1471 (30.2)	1143 (29.7)	40.8	33.5	19.2
Severe	798 (16.4)	643 (16.7)	46.6[‡]	39.4[‡]	28.4[‡]

Modified from Ehrenkranz RA, Walsh MC, Vohr BR, et al. Validation of the National Institutes of Health Consensus definition of bronchopulmonary dysplasia. *Pediatrics.* 2005;116:1353-1360.
BPD, Bronchopulmonary dysplasia; CXR, chest x-ray; NICU, neonatal intensive care unit; RSV, respiratory syncytial virus.
*Missing data: 28 days–CXR, 17 infants (13 for follow-up cohort); 36 weeks–CXR, 12 infants (8 for follow-up cohort); pulmonary medications, 17; rehospitalizations for pulmonary causes, 35; RSV prophylaxis, 17.
[†]Cohort of infants who were seen at 18 to 22 months' corrected age.
[‡]$p < 0.0001$, §$p < 0.001$ versus no BPD for the 28 days, 28 days–CXR, 36 weeks, and 36 weeks–CXR definitions, Mantel-Haenszel Π^2 for linear association across the categories of the consensus definition (none to severe), Mantel-Haenszel Π^2.

TABLE 43-3 An Approach to Combining the NIH Consensus Definition with the Physiologic Definition

Respiratory Support at 28 Days of Age	Respiratory Support at 36 Weeks' PMA	BPD Definition	
Room air	Room air	No BPD	
Any respiratory support	Room air	Mild BPD	
Any respiratory support	Respiratory support with FiO_2 <0.30	Room air challenge needed	Challenge passed, mild BPD
			Challenge failed, moderate BPD
Any respiratory support	Respiratory support with FiO_2 ≥0.30	Severe BPD	

BPD, Bronchopulmonary dysplasia; PMA, postmenstrual age.

Composite outcomes are frequently used in contemporary neonatal clinical trials. The value of such combined outcomes as death or BPD (or its counterpart, survival without BPD) becomes clear when considering an intervention that may increase the percentage of survivors without BPD by increasing the mortality among the sickest or most vulnerable infants. Such composite outcomes also adjust for differences among centers in their willingness to withdraw support from infants with a poor neurodevelopmental prognosis.

Although BPD, as diagnosed near term gestation, cannot be considered a long-term outcome, the incidence of BPD remains a very relevant endpoint for clinical trials of respiratory management in preterm infants. BPD is an important cause of morbidity and mortality, has been associated with prolonged and recurrent hospitalizations, and is linked to higher rates of other serious complications of prematurity.[10] Its incidence is high, with 7000 to 10,000 new cases each year in the United States alone, and has not been reduced by numerous interventions, including surfactant replacement therapy. The prevalence of BPD has actually increased since 2005 as more ELBW infants survive to discharge.[11] Long-term follow-up suggests that, compared with gestational age-matched infants without BPD, infants with BPD have lifelong alterations in lung function[12,13] and an increased incidence of cerebral palsy and neurodevelopmental delays.[14,15]

Pulmonary Function Testing and Imaging

In the future it would be desirable to directly assess an infant's functional respiratory status with bedside pulmonary function tests during the acute hospitalization. Such tests are currently feasible in intubated neonates and in older, nonintubated infants as young as 4 months of age and have revolutionized the care of neonates with cystic fibrosis.[16] Unfortunately, the currently available tests for nonintubated older infants require sedation and are appropriate only for those over 4 months of age. It would be highly desirable to develop such techniques to study nonintubated convalescent premature infants.

The primary pulmonary function abnormality in survivors of preterm lung disease is reduced forced flows and forced expiratory volume in the presence of normal forced vital capacity, which did not normalize later in infancy in infants either with or without BPD.[17,18] Many investigators have documented limitations in airflow that may, in part, be reversible with bronchodilators.[18-21] In the original descriptions by Northway, persistent abnormalities were detected into adulthood.[22]

In the modern era, however, most studies suggest that, with growth, pulmonary function can improve or even normalize. Narayanan and colleagues used the magnetic resonance imaging to demonstrate that former infants with BPD who were evaluated at 10 to 14 years of age had alveolar dimensions similar to those of term controls and of preterm infants without BPD.[23] This suggests an ability to normalize alveolarization with continued development.

Sophisticated imaging techniques to study pulmonary structure have improved the care of neonates with cystic fibrosis.[24] The use of advanced imaging systems, such as high-resolution computerized tomography (CT) and dynamic imaging magnetic resonance, has allowed detailed imaging of the airways, has improved understanding of the pathophysiologic derangements in cystic fibrosis, and is beginning to be applied to BPD. Sarria and colleagues used thin-slice high-resolution CT scan to evaluate the airways and lung parenchyma in 38 survivors

of preterm birth (25-29 weeks) compared to full-term infants who had sedated CT scans for nonpulmonary reasons.[25] They found structural differences in both airways and parenchyma. Airway changes were the most marked, while reductions in lung volume were shown only among those with moderate or severe BPD. Increased heterogeneity within the parenchyma was seen in all survivors of BPD. Remarkably, they also found a negative impact of exposure to maternal smoking, with smaller airways in both BPD and control infants and toddlers. Additional information on the long-term impact of these airway and parenchymal changes is emerging. Wong and colleagues studied 21 adult nonsmoking survivors of BPD with CT scan. All of those studied had parenchymal abnormalities, with some showing severe emphysematous changes (Figs. 43-1 and 43-2). These changes were correlated with reductions in pulmonary function tests.[26] Taken together, these findings provide cause for concern about the future pulmonary function of survivors.

Respiratory Illnesses/Wheezing or Asthma

The disruption in the pulmonary function and respiratory outcomes of premature infants persists long after discharge from the NICU. Overall, preterm infants are at increased risk of wheezing-related illnesses as children and young adults, thought in part to be due to an imbalance in the relationship between airway reactivity (smooth muscle structure and function) and airway compliance (connective tissues and parenchyma).[27] In the first year of life, preterm infants, compared to term infants, have higher rates of wheezing (44% vs 21%), are more likely to be rehospitalized for respiratory symptoms (25% vs 1.5%), and are more likely to receive an inhalation medication (13%).[28,29] At early school age these differences result in decreased peak expiratory flow and high rates of asthma diagnosis (36%) among former premature infants even without the diagnosis of BPD at hospital discharge. The prevalence of medication use for respiratory illnesses, wheezing events, and rehospitalizations was noted to decrease, however, from 30 months to 6 years.[30] Among ELBW children with a diagnosis of BPD at discharge, evaluation at 8

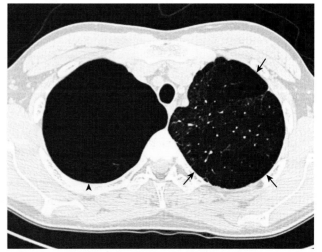

FIG 43-1 Computed tomography scan of the chest of a 20-year-old nonsmoking male born at 28 weeks' gestation, showing severe emphysema and large bulla (*arrows*). (From Wong M, Lees AN, Louw J, et al. Emphysema in young adult survivors of moderate-to-severe bronchopulmonary dysplasia. *Eur Respir J.* 2008;32:321-328.)

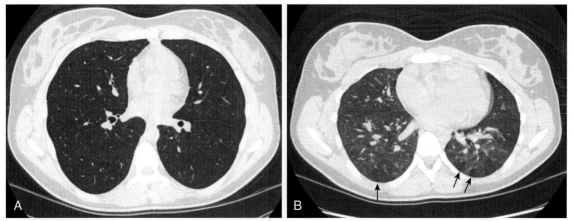

FIG 43-2 Computed tomography scans (**A**, inspiratory; **B**, expiratory) of the chest of a 19-year-old nonsmoking female born at 25 weeks' gestation, showing minimal emphysema and moderate multilobar air trapping (*arrows*). (From Wong M, Lees AN, Louw J, et al. Emphysema in young adult survivors of moderate-to-severe bronchopulmonary dysplasia. *Eur Respir J.* 2008;32:321-328.)

and 14 years revealed rates of asthma medication use unchanged (23%), though overall rates of asthma medication use increased among matched controls. This suggests a stability in wheezing prevalence among ELBW children as they age.[31]

HEALTH CARE UTILIZATION

Premature infants with BPD have a longer initial hospitalization than their peers without BPD,[32] and BPD remains a substantial lifelong burden. The costs of the disorder are both social and economic and are measured in impaired childhood health and quality of life, family stress and economic hardship, and increased health care costs.[33-35] Lodha and colleagues documented in a cohort of preterm infants of <1250 g that at 4, 8, and 18 months of follow-up, the use of respiratory medications and supplemental oxygen was significantly higher in infants who had BPD compared to those with no BPD.[36] More physician visits and higher use of respiratory medications and supplemental oxygen continued through the third year of life.

These findings must be taken in the context that even low-risk preterm infants without BPD have worse respiratory outcomes compared to a full-term cohort.[37]

NEURODEVELOPMENTAL OUTCOMES AND BRONCHOPULMONARY DYSPLASIA

Infants with BPD have more neurodevelopmental sequelae in the forms of cognitive, language, motor, hearing, and vision deficits and cerebral palsy than matched gestational-age controls without BPD, even after controlling for confounding variables. Gregoire et al.[38] showed that at 18 months, the use of the 36 weeks' qualifier in determining severity of BPD was a better predictor of neurodevelopmental outcome than the older 28 days' definition, with a significant decrease in developmental quotient for those infants with severe BPD, although the scores were still within normal range. Lodha and colleagues found that at 3 years of age, children with BPD with or without need for chronic supplemental oxygen had higher odds of neurodevelopmental disability compared to those without BPD (odds ratio 1.9; 95% confidence interval

1.1 to 3.5).[39] These changes persist to 8 years of age, with 54% requiring special education classes compared with 37% of very low birth-weight survivors without BPD.[40] Early and middle school age studies suggest BPD is associated with higher rates of subtle neurologic deficits and behavioral difficulties, as well as deficits in perceptual motor integration, motor coordination, and processing speeds.[41-43] In one of the first assessments of executive functioning in adult survivors of BPD, Gough and coworkers showed deficits in problem solving, awareness of behavior, and organization.[44] It is not clear whether BPD per se is responsible for these deficits or rather the prolonged illness and hospitalization, negative impact of medications such as corticosteroids and sedatives, and poor nutrition are the primary culprits.

Because inflammation had been shown to be a prominent component in BPD, there was great enthusiasm in the 1990s for the use of corticosteroids, especially dexamethasone, on the basis of several small case series. By 2001 numerous authors raised concern over neurotoxicity. Barrington completed a meta-analysis of available studies and concluded that the relative risk for developing cerebral palsy was 1.92 in those exposed to dexamethasone compared to controls.[45] By 2002 both the American Academy of Pediatrics and the Canadian Paediatric Society advised against the routine use of systemic dexamethasone.[46] Postnatal dexamethasone exposure has been associated with smaller total brain tissue volumes, which persist into adolescence.[47]

A 2014 Cochrane review of late (>7 days) postnatal corticosteroids for chronic lung disease in preterm infants compiling data from 21 randomized trials showed that composite outcomes of death or cerebral palsy and of death or major neurosensory disability were not significantly different between steroid and control groups.[48] These results may suggest a role for postnatal corticosteroids in preterm neonates over 1 week of age. However, the meta-analysis includes studies of significant heterogeneity, use of antenatal corticosteroids, and varying dosing regimens of corticosteroids. Neonatologists continue to struggle to balance the risks of continued mechanical ventilation against the potential harm of corticosteroid exposure. A randomized trial of hydrocortisone is in progress as of this writing and may provide an answer.

OUTCOMES AFTER NEONATAL HYPOXIC RESPIRATORY FAILURE

Inhaled Nitric Oxide

The best studied pulmonary vasodilator used in hypoxic respiratory failure in term and near-term infants is inhaled nitric oxide (iNO) (see Chapter 32). Fourteen randomized trials have been published with remarkably consistent findings.[49,50] The largest of these is the NINOS Trial conducted by the NICHD Neonatal Research Network in which 235 infants were randomized to iNO versus standard ventilator management.[51] The primary outcome was death or extracorporeal membrane oxygenation (ECMO). There was no difference in the occurrence of death, but there was a 40% reduction in the use of ECMO in those infants treated with iNO. Follow-up at 2 years of age showed similar neurodevelopmental outcomes in the two groups.[52] In a meta-analysis of the results from all 14 randomized trials, 50% of all infants treated responded to iNO, with an average increase in PaO$_2$ of 53 mm Hg.[53]

Lipkin and coworkers followed 133 full-term infants treated with iNO for respiratory failure to 1 year of age. There were no significant differences between the placebo and the iNO groups in any pulmonary or neurodevelopmental outcome. Rehospitalization occurred in 22% of the cohort. Forty-six percent of the cohort showed either neurodevelopmental or audiologic outcomes. Major neurologic abnormalities occurred in 13%, cognitive delays in 30%, and hearing loss in 19% of infants.[54]

iNO has also been used in preterm infants. When used early in the course with severely ill preterm infants, there was an increased rate of intraventricular hemorrhage. Attempts to use iNO to prevent the development of BPD have been disappointing. In 2011 the NIH held a consensus conference, which did not endorse the routine use of iNO.[55] However, they acknowledged that there might be individual situations such as pulmonary hypoplasia for which nitric oxide may be beneficial.

Extracorporeal Membrane Oxygenation

Over 27,000 newborns have been treated with ECMO with an overall survival of 74% (see Chapter 40). Infants with meconium aspiration have the highest survival, at over 90%, contrasting with infants with congenital diaphragmatic hernia, whose survival is 51%.[56] Survivors of respiratory failure severe enough to be treated with ECMO are among the most severely ill infants treated by neonatologists. Early reports before the era of nitric oxide comparing those infants treated with ECMO to those who were "near misses" (i.e., not meeting criteria for ECMO cannulation) showed equivalent neurodevelopmental outcomes but worsened pulmonary outcomes in the conventionally treated group.[57,58] The largest randomized trial of ECMO enrolled 100 newborns in the U.K. Collaborative ECMO Trial. At 7 years of age, 90 of 100 survivors were assessed by a team masked to their intervention. Higher rates of respiratory morbidity were found in the conventionally treated group, with 32% having persistent wheezing compared to 11% of the ECMO-treated group.[59]

Within the first few years of life, cognitive scores and motor function for neonatal ECMO survivors overall are similar to those of healthy peers, though a subgroup analysis of ECMO–congenital diaphragmatic hernia survivors suggests these specific infants have motor development indices significantly below age group norms.[60-63] At preschool ages the U.K. ECMO trial showed that 60% of ECMO-exposed children had neuromotor problems at age 4[64]; furthermore, Glass et al.[65] and Dutch studies[66,67] showed gross motor, though not fine motor skills, to be poorer in ECMO-exposed 5-year-olds compared to healthy controls.

Moreover at preschool ages, the U.K. ECMO trial found cognitive scores within normal range in nearly two-thirds of the overall ECMO-exposed group.[64] While Glass et al.[65] also found ECMO-exposed survivors to have cognitive scores in the normal range, the mean scores were significantly lower than those of healthy peers (full-scale IQ 96 compared to 115). However, cognitive scores alone do not give a complete picture, and ECMO survivors may be at risk of academic problems and school failure owing to noncognitive issues. With neuropsychological testing, Glass et al.[65] reported that about 30% of ECMO survivors with normal cognitive scores had problems in at least one domain. In particular, visuospatial ability,[59,66,68] working speed, and working memory[68-70] seem to be problematic. In a Dutch study, 8-year-old ECMO survivors were twice as likely to require either special education or adaptive mainstream education services compared to their peers. Potentially contributing to academic difficulties is an increase in risk of behavioral problems, particularly hyperactivity and attention deficits, in up to 35% of survivors by 5 years of age[59,64,68,71] (Table 43-4).

CONCLUSION

Mechanical ventilation and the development of iNO and ECMO have been major therapeutic advances in neonatal care. Despite impressive improvements in survival, too many of these tiny patients carry both respiratory and neurologic morbidity that persists into school age and adolescence. Ongoing surveillance of these high-risk children is warranted to permit early detection of abnormalities and early intervention to reduce future impairments.

TABLE 43-4 **Overview of Long-Term Outcomes Reported Following Neonatal ECMO Treatment**

	Infancy (<2 yr)	Preschool Age (2-5 yr)	School Age (6-12 yr)	Adolescence (>12 yr)
Medical Outcome				
Lung function	Airflow obstruction,[7,8] normal lung volume,[7,8] and hyperinflation in CDH[9]	–	Airflow obstruction,[10,11,13] air trapping,[10,13] problems mainly in CDH patients[13]	Airflow obstruction and air trapping[10]
Exercise capacity	–	Decreased[14]	Decreased[11,14] to normal	Normal[10]
Growth	Normal[5,7] to slightly decreased weight[8] especially in CDH[9]	Normal[14]	Normal,[12,14] decreased height and weight in CDH[12]	–
SNHL	Prevalence ranging from 3% to 26%, in various studies over time[17-22,33]			
Chronic kidney disease	Abnormal urine protein/creatinine ratio or estimated glomerular filtration rate in 11%[31]			
(Neuro)developmental Outcome				
Motor function	Normal in 84%[32]	Normal in 64-73%[15,36]	Normal in 43%[39] and normal in 71% of CDH patients[36]	–
Cognition	Normal in 92%[32]	Normal average scores[15,33,38,45]	Normal in 68%[39] and normal average scores[43]	–
Neuropsychological tests	–	Decreased scores at verbal, reasoning, and spatial abilities,[22] and neuropsychological deficit at ≤1 domain in 11%[38]	Spatial ability scores below 10th percentile in 26%,[39] visuomotor integration below average in 20%,[43] memory problems in 26-48%,[39] decreased working speed in 70%,[43] and decreased accuracy in 39%[43]	Memory problems in 46-57%[36]
School performance	–	–	Special education 9-20%[39,43]; extra support 20-39%[39,43]	–
Behavior	–	Normal in 48.5-65%,[45,47] more problems compared with controls in social, attention, and hyperactivity domains[38]	Clinical total problems 18%, social problems 5%, and attention problems 6%[43]	Self-reported externalizing problems 6%[36]

From Ijsselstijn H, van Heijst AFJ. Long term outcome of children treated with neonatal extracorporeal membrane oxygenation: Increasing problems with increasing age. *Seminars in Perinatology.* 2014(38):114-121.
CDH, Congenital diaphragmatic hernia; *SNHL,* sensorineural hearing loss.

REFERENCES

A complete reference list is available at https://expertconsult .inkling.com/.

Appendices

Jay P. Goldsmith, MD, FAAP

APPENDIX 1

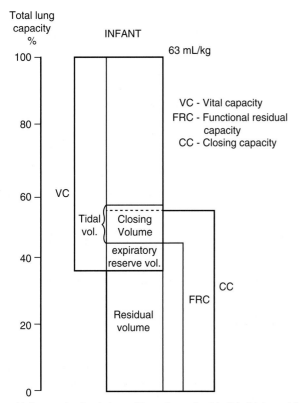

Lung Volumes in the Infant. (Data from Smith CA, Nelson NM. *The Physiology of the Newborn Infant*. 4th ed. Springfield, IL: Charles C Thomas Publisher; 1976.)

APPENDIX 2

Changes in Respiratory System Dimensions with Growth*

	Newborn to 1 month	Infant
Chest Diameter (cm)		
Transverse	10	14
Anteroposterior	7.5	9
Trachea, length (mm)	40/57	42/67
Diameter (mm)	4	5
CSA (mm²)	26	34
Main Stem Bronchi		
Diameter (mm)	4	4
CSA, right/left (mm²)	—	20/13
Bronchioles, diameter (mm)	0.3	0.4
CSA (mm²)	0.07	0.12
Terminal Bronchioles		
Diameter (mm)	0.2	0.3
Internal diameter (mm)	0.1	0.12
CSA	0.03	0.07
Alveoli, diameter (mm)	0.05	0.06-0.07
Surface area (m²)	2.8	6.5
Body length (cm)	50	—
Weight (kg)	3.4	—
Surface area (m²)	0.21	0.3
Lung weight (g)	50	70
Dead space (mL)	7-8	—

(Data from Scarpelli EM, ed. *Pulmonary Physiology of the Fetus, Newborn, and Child.* Philadelphia, Lea & Febiger, 1975.)

* Values are from Engel S (autopsy data) and Fearon S, Whalen JS (living subjects; autopsy/living).

CSA, cross-sectional area.

APPENDIX 3

Effect of Age on Lung Size*

Age	No. of Cases Studied	Alveoli (10⁶)	Respiratory Airways (10⁶)	Air–Tissue Interface (m²)	Body Surface Area (m²)	Generations of Respiratory Airways
Birth	1	24	1.5	2.8	0.21	—
3 months	3	77	2.5	7.2	0.29	21
7 months	1	112	3.7	8.4	0.38	—
13 months	1	129	4.5	12.2	0.45	22
22 months	1	160	7.1	14.2	0.50	—
4 years	1	257	7.9	22.2	0.67	—
8 years	1	280	14.0	32.0	0.92	23
Adult		296	14.0	75.0	1.90	23
Approximate fold increase, birth to adult	—	10	10	21	9	—

(Data from Thibeault DW, Gregory GA, eds. *Neonatal Pulmonary Care*. Menlo Park, Calif., Addison–Wesley Publishing Co., 1979:217-236, and Scarpelli EM, ed. *Pulmonary Physiology of the Fetus, Newborn, and Child*. Philadelphia, Lea & Febiger, 1975.)

* Values are from Dunnill MS.

APPENDIX 4

Normal Lung Function Data for Term Newborns during the Neonatal Period

Measurement	No. of Infants Studied	Mean	Standard Deviation	Range
Tidal volume (mL/kg)	266	4.8	1.0	2.9-7.9
Respiratory rate (bpm)	266	50.9	13.1	25-104
Minute volume (mL/kg/min)	266	232	61.4	0.9-3.7
Dynamic compliance (mL/cm H_2O/kg)	266	1.72	0.5	—
Total pulmonary resistance (cm H_2O)/L/s)	266	42.5	1.6	3.1-171
Work of breathing (G·cm)	266	11.0	7.4	1.1-52.6
Expiratory time (s)	291	0.57	0.17	0.27-1.28
Inspiratory time (s)	291	0.51	0.10	0.28-0.87
Time to maximum expiratory flow/total expiratory time (s)	291	0.51	0.12	0.18-0.83
Static compliance (mL/cm H_2O/kg)	289	1.25	0.41	0.43-2.07
Respiratory system resistance (cm H_2O/L/s)	299	63.4	16.6	34.9-153.3
Time constant of respiratory system (s)	299	0.24	0.10	0.08-1.1
FRCpleth (mL/kg)	271	29.8	6.2	14.5-15.6

FRCpleth, functional residual capacity by body plethysmography. (Data from Milner et al. Effects of smoking in pregnancy on neonatal lung function. *Arch Dis Child.* 1999;80:F8–F14.) The tidal volume and volume were measured using a type 00 Fleisch Pneumotachograph and intrathoracic pressure with a 4-cm esophageal balloon. Babies were supine in quiet sleep. Dead space was eliminated by a bias flow of air.)

APPENDIX 5

Allen's Test

Gently squeeze the hand to partially empty it of blood. Apply pressure to both the ulnar and the radial arteries. Then remove pressure from the hand and the ulnar artery. If the entire hand flushes and fills with blood, the ulnar artery can supply the hand with blood and the radial artery can be safely punctured or cannulated.

APPENDIX 6

Procedure for Obtaining Capillary Blood Gases

Equipment needed:
- 75-μL capillary tube (heparinized)
- Lancet device (3 mm)
- Alcohol sponge
- Metal stirrer and magnet
- Sealing wax

Procedure for obtaining capillary blood gases:
- Wash hands.
- Warm the infant's foot for 3 minutes with water at body temperature or slightly warmer. Use a thermometer. Water temperature should not exceed 39°C (101 to 104°F).
- Cleanse the heel with an alcohol sponge.
- Puncture with a lancet device.
- Wipe away the first drop of blood.
- Collect blood in a sample tube by holding the tube below the level of puncture and allowing blood to flow freely into the tube. Avoid squeezing the heel to fill the tube because this introduces serum and venous blood and renders the sample inaccurate. Avoid introducing air into the tube.
- Hold an alcohol sponge against the puncture site to stop the flow.
- Place a metal stirrer in the tube.
- Slide the magnet along the tube to move the stirrer and mix the blood.
- Seal the ends of the tube.
- Send to the laboratory for analysis.

APPENDIX 7

Normal Umbilical Cord Blood Gas Values

	Venous Blood Normal Range (mean ± 2 SD)	Arterial Blood Normal Range (mean ± 2 SD)
pH	7.25-7.45	7.18-7.38
Pco_2 (mm Hg)	26.8-49.2	32.2-65.8
(kPa)*	*3.57-6.56*	*4.29-8.77*
Po_2 (mm Hg)	17.2-40.8	5.6-30.8
(kPa)*	*2.29-5.44*	*0.75-4.11*
HCO_3^- (mmol/L)	15.8-24.2	17-27
BD† (mmol/L)	0-8	0-8

SD, standard deviation.
*1 kPa = 7.50 mm Hg; 1 mm Hg = 1.33 kPa.
†*BD*, base deficit, estimated from data.
(Data from Yeomans ER, Hauth JC, Gilstrap LC, Strickland DM. Umbilical cord pH, Pco_2, and bicarbonate following uncomplicated term vaginal deliveries. *Am J Obstet Gynecol.* 1985;151:798-800.)

APPENDIX 8

Arterial Blood Gas Values in Normal Full-Term Infants*

		Umbilical Vein (cord)	Umbilical Artery (cord)	5-10 min	20 min	30 min	60 min	5 h	24 h	2 days	3 days	4 days	5 days	6 days	7 days
pH	$\overline{X}$	7.320	7.242	7.207	7.263	7.297	7.332	7.339	7.369	7.365	7.364	7.370	7.371	7.369	7.371
	SD	0.055	0.059	0.051	0.040	0.044	0.031	0.028	0.032	0.028	0.027	0.027	0.031	0.023	0.026
Pco_2 (mm Hg)	$\overline{X}$	37.8	49.1	46.1	40.1	37.7	36.1	35.2	33.4	33.1	33.1	34.3	34.8	34.8	35.9
	SD	5.6	5.8	7.0	6.0	5.7	4.2	3.6	3.1	3.3	3.4	3.8	3.5	3.6	3.1
Po_2 (mm Hg)	$\overline{X}$	27.4	15.9	49.6	50.7	54.1	63.3	73.7	72.7	73.8	75.6	73.3	72.1	69.8	73.1
	SD	5.7	3.8	9.9	11.3	11.5	11.3	12.0	9.5	7.7	11.5	9.3	10.5	9.5	9.7
Standard bicarbonate (mEq/L)	$\overline{X}$	20.0	18.7	16.7	17.5	18.2	19.2	19.4	20.2	19.8	19.7	20.4	20.6	20.6	21.8
	SD	1.4	1.8	1.6	1.3	1.5	1.2	1.2	1.3	1.4	1.4	1.7	1.7	1.9	1.3

(Data from Bancalari E. Pulmonary function testing and other diagnostic laboratory procedures. *J Peds.* 1987;110(3):448-456; Thibeault DW, Gregory GA, eds. *Neonatal Pulmonary Care.* Reading, Mass., Addison–Wesley Publishing Co., 1979:123, Table 7-4.)
*Values from Koch and Wendel. Blood obtained through umbilical artery line. Po_2 and Pco_2 measured with Clark and Severinghaus electrodes.
SD, standard deviation; $\overline{X}$, sample mean.

Arterial Blood Gas Values in Normal Premature Infants*

		3-5 h	6-12 h	13-24 h	25-48 h	3-4 days	5-10 days	11-40 days
pH	$\overline{X}$	7.329	7.425	7.464	7.434	7.425	7.378	7.425
	SD	0.038	0.072	0.064	0.054	0.044	0.043	0.033
Pco_2 (mm Hg)	$\overline{X}$	47.3	28.2	27.2	31.3	31.7	36.4	32.9
	SD	8.5	6.9	8.4	6.7	6.7	4.2	4.0
Po_2 (mm Hg)	$\overline{X}$	59.5	69.7	67.0	72.5	77.8	80.3	77.8
	SD	7.7	11.8	15.2	20.9	16.4	12.0	9.6
Base excess (mEq/L)	$\overline{X}$	-3.7	-4.7	-3.0	-2.3	-2.9	-3.5	-2.1
	SD	1.5	3.1	3.3	3.0	2.3	2.3	2.2

(Data from Bancalari E. Pulmonary function testing and other diagnostic laboratory procedures. In: Thibeault DW, Gregory GA, eds. *Neonatal Pulmonary Care.* Reading, Mass., Addison–Wesley Publishing Co., 1979, 123, Table 7-5.)
*Values from Orzalesi et al. Mean birthweight, 1.76 kg; gestational age, 34.5 wk. Blood obtained from radial, temporal, or umbilical artery. Po_2 measured with Clark electrode, and Pco_2 calculated with use of the Siggaard-Andersen nomogram.
SD, standard deviation; $\overline{X}$, sample mean.

APPENDIX 9

Capillary Blood Gas Reference Values in Healthy Term Neonates

Variable	n	Mean ± SD	2.5 Percentile	97.5 Percentile
pH	119	7.395 ± 0.037	7.312	7.473
Pco₂ (mm Hg)	119	38.7 ± 5.1	28.5	48.7
Po₂ (mm Hg)	119	45.3 ± 7.5	32.8	61.2
Lactate (mmol/L)	114	2.6 ± 0.7	1.4	4.1
Hemoglobin (g/dL)	122	20.4 ± 11.6	14.5	23.9
Glucose (mg/dL)	122	69 ± 14	3.8	96
iCa (mmol/L)	118	1.21 ± 0.07	1.06	1.34

Samples were collected at 48 ± 12 h of life. *SD*, standard deviation; *iCa*, ionized calcium.
(Data from Cousineau J, et al. Neonate capillary blood gas reference values. *Clin Biochem.* 2005;38:906.)

APPENDIX 10

Blood Gas Values in Cord Blood and in Arterial Blood at Various Ages during the Neonatal Period
Oxygen Tension

		UV	UA	5-10 min	20 min	30 min	60 min	5 h	24 h	2 days	3 days	4 days	5 days	6 days	7 days
Po₂ (mm Hg)	$\bar{X}$	15.9	27.4	49.6	50.7	54.1	63.3	73.7	72.7	73.8	75.6	73.3	72.1	69.8	73.1
	SD	3.8	5.7	9.9	11.3	11.5	11.3	12.0	9.5	7.7	11.5	9.3	10.9	9.5	9.7
	Range	7	15	33	31	31	38	55	54	62	56	60	56	55	57
		23	40	75	85	85	83	106	95	91	102	93	102	96	94

SD, standard deviation; *UA*, umbilical artery; *UV*, umbilical vein; $\bar{X}$, sample mean.
(Data from Koch G, Wendel H. Adjustment of arterial blood gases and acid-base balance in the normal newborn infant during the first week of life. *Biol Neonat.* 1968;12:136-161.)

Carbon Dioxide Tension

		UV	UA	5-10 min	20 min	30 min	60 min	5 h	24 h	2 days	3 days	4 days	5 days	6 days	7 days
Pco₂ (mm Hg)	$\bar{X}$	49.1	37.8	46.1	40.1	37.7	36.1	35.2	33.4	33.1	33.1	34.3	34.8	34.8	35.9
	SD	5.8	5.6	7.0	6.0	5.7	4.2	3.6	3.1	3.3	3.4	3.8	3.5	3.6	3.1
	Range	35	26	35	31	28	28	29	27	26	26	27	28	28	30
		60	52	65	58	54	45	45	40	43	40	43	41	42	42

SD, standard deviation; *UA*, umbilical artery; *UV*, umbilical vein; $\bar{X}$, sample mean.
(Data from Koch G, Wendel H. Adjustment of arterial blood gases and acid-base balance in the normal newborn infant during the first week of life. *Biol Neonat.* 1968;12:136-161.)

pH

		UV	UA	5-10 min	20 min	30 min	60 min	5 h	24 h	2 days	3 days	4 days	5 days	6 days	7 days
pH	$\bar{X}$	7.320	7.242	7.207	7.263	7.297	7.332	7.339	7.369	7.365	7.364	7.370	7.371	7.369	7.37
	SD	0.055	0.059	0.051	0.040	0.044	0.031	0.028	0.032	0.028	0.027	0.027	0.031	0.032	0.02
	Range	7.178	7.111	7.091	7.180	7.206	7.261	7.256	7.290	7.314	7.304	7.320	7.296	7.321	7.32
		7.414	7.375	7.302	7.330	7.380	7.394	7.389	7.448	7.438	7.419	7.440	7.430	7.423	7.43

SD, standard deviation; *UA*, umbilical artery; *UV*, umbilical vein; $\bar{X}$, sample mean.
(Data from Koch G, Wendel H. Adjustment of arterial blood gases and acid-base balance in the normal newborn infant during the first week of life. *Biol Neonat.* 1968;12:136-161.)

Base Excess

		UV	UA	5-10 min	20 min	30 min	60 min	5 h	24 h	2 days	3 days	4 days	5 days	6 days	7 days
Base excess	$\bar{X}$	−5.5	−7.2	−9.8	−8.8	−7.8	−6.5	−6.3	−5.2	−5.8	−5.9	−5.0	−4.7	−4.7	−3.2
	SD	1.2	1.7	2.3	1.9	1.7	1.3	1.3	1.1	1.2	1.2	1.1	1.1	1.1	0.6

(Calculated from data in Koch G, Wendel H. Adjustment of arterial blood gases and acid base balance in the normal newborn infant during the first week of life. *Biol Neonate.* 1968;12:136-161. By permission of S. Karger, A.G. Basel.)
SD, standard deviation; *UA*, umbilical artery; *UV*, umbilical vein; $\bar{X}$, sample mean.

APPENDIX 11

Conversion Tables
Torr to Kilopascal

Torr	kPa
20	2.7
25	3.3
30	4.0
35	4.7
40	5.3
45	6.0
50	6.7
55	7.3
60	8.0
65	8.7
70	9.3
75	10.0
80	10.7
85	11.3
90	12.0
95	12.7
100	13.3
105	14.0
110	14.7
115	15.3
120	16.0
125	16.7
130	17.3
135	18.0

Kilopascal to Torr

kPa	Torr
2.5	19
3.0	22.5
3.5	26
4.0	30
4.5	34
5.0	37.5
5.5	41
6.0	45
6.5	49
7.0	52.5
7.5	56
8.0	60
8.5	64
9.0	67.5
9.5	71
10.0	75
10.5	79
11.0	82.5
12.0	90
12.5	94
13.0	97.5
13.5	101
14.0	105

APPENDIX 12

Hemoglobin–Oxygen Dissociation Curves

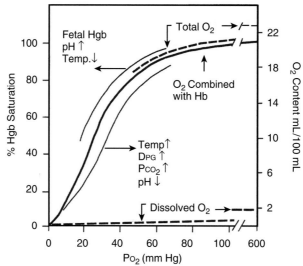

The figure shows the nonlinear or S-shaped oxyhemoglobin curve and the linear or straight-line dissolved oxygen (O_2) relationships between the O_2 saturation (SaO_2) and the O_2 tension (PO_2). Total blood O_2 content is shown with division into a portion combined with hemoglobin and a portion physically dissolved at various levels of PO_2. Also shown are the major factors that change the O_2 affinity for hemoglobin and, thus, shift the oxyhemoglobin dissociation curve either to the left or to the right. *Hgb, Hb,* hemoglobin; *DPG,* diphosphoglyceric acid. (Data from West JB. Respiratory Physiology—the Essentials. 2nd ed. Baltimore, Williams & Wilkins, 1979:71, 73.)

APPENDIX 13

Siggaard–Andersen Alignment Nomogram

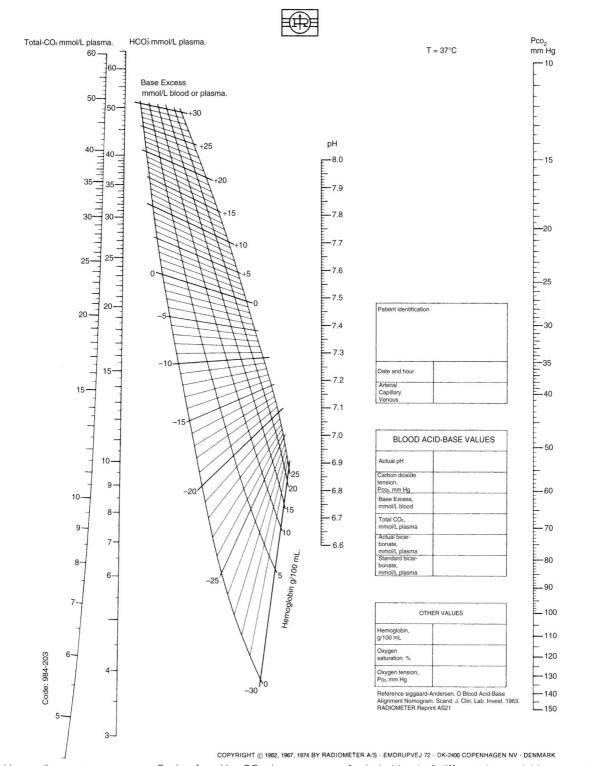

Blood acid-base alignment nomogram: Scales for pH, pCO$_2$, base excess of whole blood of different hemoglobin concentrations, plasma bicarbonate and plasma total CO$_2$.

APPENDIX 14

Systolic, Diastolic, and Mean Blood Pressure by Birth Weight and Gestational Age

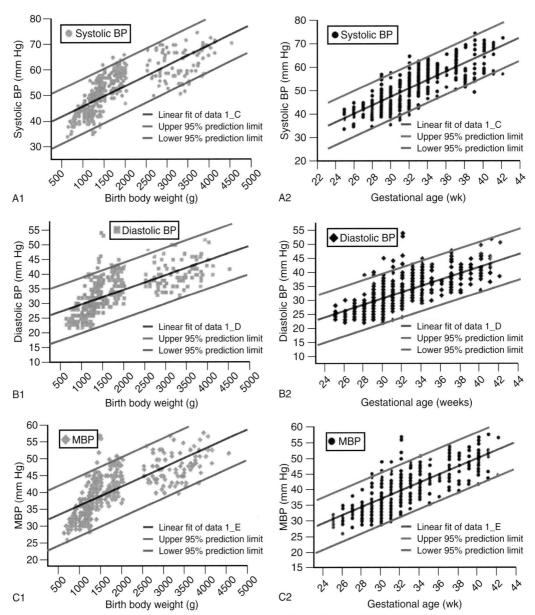

BP, blood pressure; *MBP,* mean blood pressure. (Data from Pejovic B, Peco-Antic A, Marinkoviv-Eri J. Blood pressure in non-critically ill preterm and full-term neonates. *Pediatr Nephrol.* 22:249-257, 2007.)

APPENDIX 15

Systolic and Diastolic Blood Pressure in the First 5 Days of Life

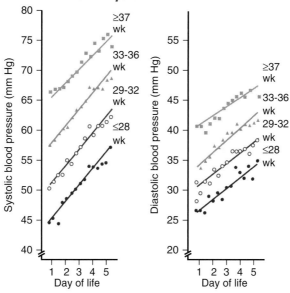

(Zubrow AB, Hulman S, Kushner H, et al. Determinants of blood pressure in infants admitted to neonatal intensive care units: a prospective multicenter study. Philadelphia Neonatal Blood Pressure Study Group. *J Perinatol*. 15:470, 1995.)

APPENDIX 16

Neonatal Resuscitation Record

Patient Name _____ Date _____

Est. Wt. _____ grams   Sex _____   Est. Gest. Age _____

Time of Birth _____ AM/PM

	Min	Heart Rate	Muscle Tone	Reflex Irritability	Color	Resp. Effort	Total
A	1						
P	5						
G	10						
A	15						
R	20						
S	25						

Time Resuscitation Procedures Initiated: _____

Time Resuscitation Procedures Completed: _____

Perinatal History:

Amniotic Fluid: ❑ Clear   ❑ Meconium Stained

PROCEDURES	START	END	BY WHOM	
UVC or UAC				UA/UV size: 3.5 5 8
Intubation				ETT Size: 2.5 3.0 3.5 4.0
Intubation w/Ventilation				
Intubation/Suctioning Only				
Cardiac Compressions				
Positive-Pressure Ventilation				
Free Flow Oxygen @ _____ L/min				
Suction				
O/G Tube In: ❑ Yes ❑ No				

DRUGS	TIME/AMT	TIME/AMT	ROUTE	FLUSH SOLUTIONS
Epinephrine 1:10000 0.1 - 0.3 mL/kg				_____ Normal saline + 1 unit heparin/cc
Volume Expander: 5% Albumin 10 mL/kg Normal saline Ringer's Lactate				_____ 1/2 Normal saline + 1 unit heparin/cc
Sodium Bicarbonate 0.5 mEq/mL 2 mEq/kg (4.2% solution)				_____ Other
Naloxone Hydrochloride 0.4 mg/mL or 0.1 mg/kg 1.0 mg/mL				
Blood Products				
Others				

BASE I.V. SOLUTION	LABS
_____ D_5W	_____ Glucose
_____ $D_{10}W$	

Condition at Completion of Resuscitation: ❑ Good   ❑ Fair   ❑ Guarded   ❑ Expired

Transferred to: ❑ Newborn Nursery   ❑ NICU

Comments: _____
_____
_____

Resuscitation Personnel Signatures:

M.D. _____

NNP _____

R.N. _____

Recording R.N. _____

R.T. _____

APPENDIX 17

Effective FiO₂ Conversion Tables for Infants on Nasal Cannula

1. The tables below are based on those used in the STOP-ROP trials.* The data were derived from Equations (3) and (4) in the paper by Benaron and Benitz, "Maximizing the stability of oxygen delivered by nasal cannula" (*Arch Pediatr Adolesc Med* 148:294-300, 1994).

*The STOP-ROP Multicenter Study Group: Supplemental therapeutic oxygen for prethreshold retinopathy of prematurity (STOP-ROP): a randomized, controlled trial. I: Primary outcomes. *Pediatrics* 105:295-310, 2000.

2. These tables include assumptions made by Benaron and Benitz (that nasal flow is constant over the entire inspiratory cycle and that the upper airway does not act as a reservoir) plus the following assumptions made by the STOP-ROP investigators: inspiration time is 0.3 s, tidal volume is 5 mL/kg, and either inspiration is entirely nasal or cannula flow is sufficiently low such that on each inspiration the infant exhales all output from the cannula.

3. Example: What is the effective FiO₂ in a 2.0-kg infant on 100% cannula at a flow of 0.15 L/min?
Answer: Use 2.0 and 0.15 L/min in Table A-1 to get a factor of 8. Then use Table A-2 and the factor of 8% and 100% oxygen to yield an effective FiO₂ of 27%. Thus the effective oxygen concentration is less than 30% and the infant is eligible for the physiologic evaluation.

TABLE A-1 Factor as a Function of Flow and Weight*,†

Flow (L/min)	Flow (L/min)	WEIGHT (kg)								
		0.7	1.0	1.25	1.5	2	2.5	3	3.5	4
0.01		1	1	1	1	1	0	0	0	0
0.03	¹/₃₂	4	3	2	2	2	1	1	1	1
0.06	¹/₁₆	9	6	5	4	3	2	2	2	2
0.125	¹/₈	18	12	10	8	6	4	4	4	4
0.15		21	15	12	10	8	6	5	4	4
0.25	¹/₄	36	52	20	17	13	10	8	7	6
0.5	¹/₂	71	50	40	33	25	20	17	14	13
0.75	³/₄	100	75	60	50	38	30	25	21	19
1.0	1.0	100	100	80	67	50	40	33	29	25
1.25		100	100	100	83	63	50	42	36	31
1.5		100	100	100	100	75	60	50	43	38
2.0		100	100	100	100	100	80	67	57	50

*Factor = 100 × min (1 U min/kg) (see Table A-2).
†Note: If your patient's exact values are not included in the table, round up or down to find the value closest to that of your patient. If the value is exactly halfway between the two values, round up.

TABLE A-2 Effective FiO$_2$ (× 100) as a Function of Factor and Concentration*

Factor	CONCENTRATION (%)						
	21	22	25	30	40	50	100
0	21	21	21	21	21	21	21
1	21	21	21	21	21	21	22
2	21	21	21	21	21	22	23
3	21	21	21	21	22	22	23
4	21	21	21	21	22	22	24
5	21	21	21	21	22	22	25
6	21	21	21	22	22	23	26
7	21	21	21	22	22	23	27
8	21	21	21	22	23	23	27
9	21	21	21	22	23	24	28
10	21	21	21	22	23	24	29
11	21	21	21	22	23	24	30
12	21	21	21	22	23	24	30
13	21	21	22	22	23	25	31
14	21	21	22	22	24	25	32
15	21	21	22	22	23	25	33
17	21	21	22	23	24	26	34
18	21	21	22	23	24	26	35
19	21	21	22	23	25	27	36
20	21	21	22	23	25	27	37
21	21	21	22	23	25	27	38
22	21	21	22	23	25	27	36
23	21	21	22	23	25	28	39
25	21	21	22	23	25	28	41
27	21	21	22	23	25	29	42
28	21	21	22	24	26	29	43
29	21	21	22	24	27	29	44
30	21	21	22	24	27	30	45
31	21	21	22	24	27	31	47
33	21	21	22	24	27	31	47
36	21	21	22	24	28	31	49
38	21	21	23	24	28	32	51
40	21	21	23	25	29	33	53
42	21	21	23	25	29	33	53
43	21	21	23	25	29	33	55
44	21	21	23	25	29	34	56
50	21	21	23	25	30	35	60
55	21	21	23	26	31	37	64
57	21	22	23	26	32	38	66
60	21	22	23	26	32	38	68
63	21	22	24	27	33	39	71
67	21	22	24	27	34	40	74
71	21	22	24	27	34	42	77
75	21	22	24	28	35	43	80
80	21	22	24	28	36	44	84
83	21	22	24	28	37	45	87
86	21	22	24	29	37	46	89
100	21	22	25	30	40	50	100

*Shaded area signifies FiO$_2$ >3.0 (i.e., concentration >30%).

APPENDIX 18

Neonatal Indications and Doses for Administration of Selected Cardiorespiratory Drugs

Cardiorespiratory Pharmacopeia for the Newborn Period

Dosages and comments about these drugs are based on experience, consensus among neonatologists, and the limited evidence available from studies in neonates. Other styles of treatment are often acceptable and may be superior to those listed.

Administration Routes

ET—endotracheal
IM—intramuscularly
IT—intrathecally or intratracheally
IV—intravenously
PO—by mouth
PR—by rectum
SC—subcutaneously

Drug	Route and Dose	Contraindications and Cautions
Acetazolamide	IV, PO: 5 mg/kg/dose q6-8h; increase as needed to 25 mg/kg/dose (*temporarily effective*), max dose 55 mg/kg/day	Hyperchloremic metabolic acidosis, hypokalemia, drowsiness, paresthesias
Adenosine	Initial: 50 mcg/kg/dose IV as rapidly as possible (1-2 s) followed by saline flush of the line Increase dose by 50 mcg/kg/dose IV and repeat every 1-2 min if there is no response and no AV block	Contraindicated in heart transplant patients; higher dosages needed in patients receiving methylxanthines; antidote for severe bradycardia is aminophylline 5-6 mg/kg over 5 min
Albumin, 5%	IV: 0.5-1 g/kg slowly	Hypervolemia, heart failure; monitor blood pressure
Albuterol	Aerosol: 0.5-1 mg/dose q2-6h PO: 0.1-0.3 mg/kg/dose q6-8h	Tachycardia, arrhythmias, tremor, irritability
Aminophylline	See theophylline	See theophylline
Amiodarone	Loading dose: 5 mg/kg IV over 30-60 min, preferably by central venous catheter Maintenance: Infusion: 7-15 mcg/kg/min; PO: 5-10 mg/kg/dose q12h	Phlebitis, hypotension, bradycardia, liver enzyme elevations, increased and decreased thyroid function, photosensitivity, optic neuritis, pulmonary fibrosis in adults
Amrinone	Initial: 0.75 mg/kg over 2-3 min Maintenance: 3-5 mcg/kg/min	Fluid balance, electrolytes, renal function
Atropine	IV, IM, ET, SC: 0.01-0.03 mg/kg/dose, repeat q10-15 min prn; max total dose of 0.04 mg/kg	Bradycardia
Beractant (Survanta)	IT: *for prophylactic treatment*, give 4 mL/kg as soon as possible; may repeat at 6-h intervals to a maximum of 4 doses in 48 h IT: *for rescue treatment*, give 4 mL/kg as soon as respiratory distress syndrome is diagnosed; may repeat at 6-h intervals to a maximum of 4 doses in 48 h	May give additional doses if infant still has respiratory distress and needs >30% FiO_2 to keep PAo_2 >50 mm Hg Administer each dose as 4 doses of 1 mL/kg each, giving each dose over 2-3 s and turning newborn to a different position after each dose Watch for improved compliance or endotracheal plugging
Bumetanide	IV, PO: 0.005-0.05 mg/kg/dose q6-12h	Loop diuretic that also acts on proximal tubule; 40 times as potent as furosemide; less ototoxicity than furosemide; hypokalemia, hyponatremia, metabolic alkalosis
Caffeine citrate (Cafcit)	PO, IV: loading dose: 20-25 mg/kg; maintenance dose: 5-10 mg/kg/dose q24h	Restlessness, emesis, tachycardia; therapeutic plasma concentration 5-25 mcg/mL
Calcium chloride 10% (27 mg elemental Ca^{2+}/mL)	IV: 0.2 mL (9 mg Ca^{2+})/kg/dose for acute hypocalcemia; repeat q10 min	Bradycardia if injected too quickly; necrosis from extravascular leakage
Calcium gluconate 10% (9.3 mg elemental Ca^{2+}/mL)	IV: 1 mL (9 mg Ca^{2+})/kg/dose for acute hypocalcemia; repeat q10 min PO: 3-9 mg/kg/day in 2-4 divided doses (28-84 mg Ca^{2+}/kg/day) for chronic use	Bradycardia if injected too quickly; necrosis from extravascular leakage
Calfactant (Infasurf)	Initial: IT: 3 mL/kg divided into 2 aliquots repeated up to three times q12h	Do not shake or filter; ventilate for at least 30 s after dose until infant is stable; administer at room temperature

Continued

Drug	Route and Dose	Contraindications and Cautions
Captopril	PO: 0.01-0.05 mg/kg/dose q6-24h; increase dose up to 0.5 mg/kg/dose to control blood pressure	High initial doses may cause hypotension and renal insufficiency
Chlorothiazide	PO: 5-15 mg/kg/dose q12-24h	Hypokalemia; hyponatremia decreases calcium excretion; hyperglycemia
Citric acid/sodium citrate	Dose according to degree of metabolic acidosis; each milliliter is equivalent to 1 mEq HCO$_3$ and contains 1 mEq sodium	Adds sodium and potassium and must be used carefully with renal dysfunction, hyperkalemia, or hypernatremia
Dexamethasone	IM, IV: for bronchopulmonary dysplasia, 0.25 mg/kg/dose q8-12h for 3-7 days; for severe chronic lung, 0.05-0.25 mg/kg/dose q12h IV or PO for 3-7 days	Delayed head growth and developmental delay associated with treatment for as few as 3 days; weigh risk and benefit
Diazepam	PO, IV, IM: as sedative, 0.02-0.3 mg/kg/dose q6-8h; for seizure, 0.1-0.2 mg/kg/dose slow IV push	Diluted injection may precipitate; IM absorption is poor; respiratory depression, hypotension
Digoxin	IV: Acute digitalization *Loading dose* *Prematures* <1.5 kg 10-20 mcg/kg 1.5-2.5 kg 20 mcg/kg *Term newborns* 30 mcg/kg *Infants (1-12 months)* 35 mcg/kg Maintenance dose: ⅛ loading dose q12h Begin 12 h after last digitalization dose	Risk of arrhythmias is increased during digitalization; IV formulation is twice as concentrated as oral; conduction defects, emesis, ventricular arrhythmias
Dobutamine	IV: 2-20 mcg/kg/min by continuous infusion and titrate to desired effect	Tachycardia, hypotension
Dopamine	IV: 2-20 mcg/kg/min by continuous infusion and titrate to desired effect	Extravasation may lead to necrosis (phentolamine is an antidote); high dose may constrict renal arteries, but the dose for this effect is uncertain in neonates
Enalapril (PO), enalaprilat (IV)	IV enalaprilat: for hypertension, 5-10 mcg/kg/dose q8-24h PO enalapril for CHF, 0.1 mg/kg each day to a max of 0.5 mg/kg/day	Reduce dose with renal failure; severe hypotension may occur, especially with volume depletion from diuretic treatment
Epinephrine	Resuscitation: IV: 1:10,000: 0.01-0.03 mg/kg (0.1-0.3 mL/kg) q3-5 min; 0.1 mg/kg via ET if IV not available Hypotension: 0.01-0.1 mcg/kg/min by continuous infusion and titrate to desired effect	Tachycardia, arrhythmia
Fentanyl	IV, IM: 1-2 mcg/kg/dose, q4-6h prn, increase as needed	50-100 times the potency of morphine; muscle rigidity ("stiff man syndrome") may occur with rapid dose infusions; treat with muscle relaxants
Furosemide	IM, IV: 0.5-2 mg/kg/dose q12-24h PO: 1-2 mg/kg/dose q12-24h Bioavailability reduced by cor pulmonale; may require higher dosages	Hypokalemia, hyponatremia, hypochloremia; half-life prolonged in premature newborns
Hydralazine	PO, IM, IV: 0.1-0.5 mg/kg q6h; increase as needed in 0.1-mg/kg increments up to 4 mg/kg/day	Tachycardia, lupus-like reactions
Hydrochlorothiazide	PO: 2.0-4.0 mg/kg/day q12h	Hypercalcemia, hypokalemia, hyperglycemia
Hydrocortisone	Hypotension refractory to pressors, 1 mg/kg/dose IV; acute adrenal insufficiency, 0.25 mg/kg/dose q6h IV; physiologic replacement, 0.3 mg/kg/day IM	Treatment of more than 7-10 days requires gradual dosage reduction to avoid adrenal insufficiency; immunosuppression, hyperglycemia, growth delay, leukocytosis, gastric irritation
Ibuprofen lysine	Initial dose 10 mg/kg; 2nd and 3rd doses 5 mg/kg. Administer IV over 15 min at 24-h intervals	GI perforation; renal impairment. Use cautiously in patients with active bleeding or renal or hepatic dysfunction Avoid in patients with ductal-dependent cardiac malformations
Indomethacin	PO, IV: 0.1-0.2 mg/kg/dose q12-24h for 2-7 days; 0.25 mg/kg/dose, >7 days	Transient renal dysfunction, decreased platelet aggregation; infuse over a minimum of 30-60 min to minimize reduction in CNS and mesenteric perfusion; avoid in patients with ductal-dependent cardiac malformations
Isoproterenol	IV: 0.05-0.5 mcg/kg/min by infusion	Arrhythmias, systemic vasodilation, tachycardia, hypotension, hypoglycemia
Lidocaine	IV: 1 mg/kg infused over 5-10 min; may be repeated q10 min five times, prn; infusion dose 10-50 mcg/kg/min or 1 mg/kg/h	Monitoring of blood levels useful (therapeutic range 1-5 mcg/mL plasma); dilute for ET administration
Lorazepam	IV: 0.05-0.1 mg/kg infused over 2-5 min	Limited data in newborns, preparations may contain benzyl alcohol; dilute
Magnesium sulfate	IM, IV: 25-50 mg/kg q4-6h for 3-4 doses prn; use 50% solution IM, 1% solution IV	Hypotension, CNS depression; monitor serum concentration; calcium gluconate should be available as an antidote

Drug	Route and Dose	Contraindications and Cautions
Methyldopa	IV, PO: 2-3 mg/kg q6-8h; increase as needed at 2-day intervals; maximum dosage 12-15 mg/kg/dose	Sedation, fever, false positive Coombs test, hemolysis; sudden withdrawal of methyldopa may cause rebound hypertension
Methylprednisolone	IV, IM: 0.1-0.4 mg/kg/dose, q6h	Hydrocortisone preferred for physiologic replacement
Metoclopramide	PO, IV: 0.1-0.2 mg/kg/dose q6-8h or prior to each feeding	Dystonic reactions, irritability, diarrhea, decreases glomerular filtration rate in adults Efficacy for GERD shown at >6 months
Midazolam	IV, IM, intranasal: 0.07-0.20 mg/kg/dose q2-4h prn for sedation; infusion dosing: <33 weeks, 30 mcg/kg/h; >33 weeks, 60 mcg/kg/h	Limited experience in newborns; respiratory depression, apnea Rapid infusion doses (<10 min) may cause tonic clonic movements
Morphine sulfate	IV, IM, SC: 0.05-0.1 mg/kg/dose q2-6h prn; 0.1-0.2 mg/kg/dose PO q3-6h	Respiratory depression reversible with naloxone; local urticaria from histamine release
Naloxone	IV, IM, SC: 0.1 mg/kg/dose; may be repeated as necessary; delivery room minimum, 0.5 mg for term newborn	Onset of action may be delayed 15+ min after IM or SC administration; narcotic effects may outlast naloxone antagonism; dilute for ET administration
Neostigmine	IV: Test for myasthenia gravis, 0.02 mg/kg IM: Test for myasthenia gravis, 0.04 mg/kg PO: Treatment for myasthenia gravis, 0.33 mg/kg/day q3-6h	Cholinergic crisis; atropine pretreatment is recommended
Nitroprusside	IV: Begin with dose of 0.25 mcg/kg/min and vary as needed up to 8 mcg/kg/min to control blood pressure	Profound hypotension possible; requires arterial line to monitor blood pressure; thiocyanate toxicity with long-term use or renal insufficiency
Omeprazole	PO: 0.5-1.5 mg/kg/dose each day	Hypergastrinemia; diarrhea; monitor gastric pH
Pancuronium	IV: 0.03-0.1 mg/kg/dose q1-4h prn; titrate to age and effect desired	Ensure adequate oxygenation and ventilation; tachycardia, bradycardia, hypotension, hypertension; potentiated by acidosis, hypothermia, neuromuscular disease, aminoglycoside antibiotics
Phentolamine	SC: Dilute to 0.5 mg/mL, inject 0.2 mL at five sites around α-adrenergic drug infiltration maximum, 2.5 mg total dose	Marked hypotension, tachycardia, arrhythmia Do not treat hypotension with epinephrine, because hypotension may worsen owing to α-adrenergic blockade
Fresh-frozen plasma	IV: 10 mL/kg; repeated prn	Volume overload, viral infection risk
Poractant alfa (Curosurf)	IT: 2.5 mL/kg/dose divided into 2 aliquots, followed by 1.25 mL/kg/dose q12h up to 2 additional doses if needed	Do not filter or shake; suction prior to administration; administer in 2-4 aliquots with positioning of infant to improve distribution within the lungs; ventilate for at least 30 s after dose until infant is stable
Prednisone	PO: 0.5-2 mg/kg/day q6h	Asystole, myocardial depression, anorexia, vomiting, nausea
Procainamide	IV: 1.5-2.5 mg/kg infused over 10-30 min; may be repeated in 30 min if needed; infusion: 20-60 mcg/kg/min PO: 40-60 mg/kg/day q4-6h	Blood level monitoring helpful (therapeutic range: procainamide, 3-10 mcg/mL; N-acetyl procainamide, 10-20 mcg/mL)
Propranolol	IV: 0.01 mg/kg initial dose and 0.01-0.15 mg/kg infused over 10 min; may be repeated in 10 min and then q6-8h to maximum of 0.15 mg/kg/dose PO: 0.05-2 mg/kg q6h	Relatively contraindicated in low-output congestive heart failure and patients with bronchospasm
Prostaglandin E1, alprostadil	IV: 0.03-0.1 mcg/kg/min; often, dose may be reduced by ½ after initial response; intra-arterial infusion offers no advantage	Apnea, seizures, fever, disseminated intravascular coagulation, diarrhea, cutaneous vasodilation, decreased platelet aggregation, cortical bone proliferation during prolonged infusion
Quinidine gluconate	PO, IM: 2-10 mg/kg/dose q2-6h until desired effect or toxicity occurs	Check electrocardiogram before each dose; discontinue if QRS interval increases 50% or more
	IV route not recommended in neonates (dose is specific for the salt form)	Maintain level of 2-6 mcg/mL; nausea, vomiting, diarrhea, fever, atrioventricular block
Sodium bicarbonate (0.5 mEq/mL)	IV: 1-2 mEq/kg/dose infused slowly only if infant ventilated adequately	Intravascular hemolysis may be associated with rapid infusion
Sodium polystyrene sulfonate (Kayexalate)	PO, PR: 1 g/kg; approximately q6h	Usually administered as a solution with 20% sorbitol to prevent intestinal obstruction; 20% sorbitol solution may injure intestinal mucosa of very low birth-weight newborns; may decrease serum calcium or magnesium
Spironolactone	PO: 1-3 mg/kg/day q8-12h	Contraindicated with hyperkalemia; onset of action delayed; drowsiness; nausea; vomiting; diarrhea; androgenic effects in females; gynecomastia in males

Continued

Drug	Route and Dose	Contraindications and Cautions
Theophylline	PO, IV: loading dose 5-6 mg/kg; maintenance dose 1-2.5 mg/kg/dose q6-12h; aminophylline (IV) dose = theophylline (IV) dose × 1.25	Blood level monitoring indicated (therapeutic range: *apnea*, 7-12 mcg/mL; *broncho-spasm*, 10-20 mcg/mL); tachycardia at 15-20 mcg/mL, seizures at >40 g/mL; avoid rectal dosing because of variable absorption, clearance decreased by asphyxia and prematurity; tachycardia
Vecuronium	IV: 0.08-0.1 mg/kg/dose, repeat prn at 0.03-0.15 mg/kg/dose q1-2h; dose to effect	Neuromuscular blockade potentiated by calcium channel blockers such as verapamil and aminoglycoside antibiotics
Verapamil	IV: 0.1-0.2 mg/kg infused over 2 min; if response is inadequate, repeat in 30 min PO: 2-5 mg/kg/day in 3 divided doses	Monitor electrocardiogram during infusion; bradycardia, atrioventricular block, asystole; contraindicated in patients with 2nd- or 3rd-degree atrioventricular block during treatment with β blockers

AV, atrioventricular; *CHF*, congestive heart failure; *CNS*, central nervous system; *GERD*, gastroesophageal reflux disease; *GI*, gastrointestinal; *prn*, pro re nate (as needed).
(Data from Young TE, Mangum B. *Neofax*. ed 27. Montvale N.J., Thomas Reuters, 2014, and McClary J. *Drug Dosing Table. Care of the High Risk Neonate*. 6th ed. Fanaroff AA, Fanaroff JM, eds. 2013.)

APPENDIX 19*

ALVEOLAR–ARTERIAL OXYGEN GRADIENT

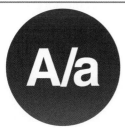

Name of the app: **Alveolar–arterial gradient (A/a)**

How to download the app:

iPhone: Go to the app store, search for Alveolar–arterial gradient and look for the icon, and tap to download.

Android: Go to the play store, search for Alveolar–arterial gradient and look for the icon, and tap to download.

The A/a oxygen gradient is a measure of oxygen transfer across the alveolar capillary membrane ("A" denotes alveolar and "a" denotes arterial oxygenation). It is the difference between the amounts of oxygen in the alveoli and in the arteries.

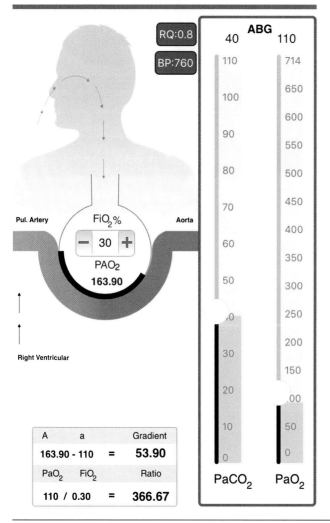

A	a		Gradient
163.90 - 110		=	**53.90**
PaO$_2$	FiO$_2$		Ratio
110 / 0.30		=	**366.67**

Enter

FiO$_2$

PaCO$_2$

PaO$_2$

The app calculates A/a gradient and PaO$_2$/FiO$_2$ ratio

Respiratory Quotient and Barometric Pressure

Respiratory quotient (RQ): RQ can affect A/a gradient and PaO$_2$/FiO$_2$ ratio. The app calculates the correct value for a given RQ.

Barometric pressure (BP): The app can also calculate the correct A/a gradient and PaO$_2$/FiO$_2$ ratio. The app calculates the correct value for a given BP. This is especially useful if the baby has been airlifted.

Information About Alveolar–Arterial Oxygen Gradient and PaO$_2$/FiO$_2$ Ratio

The A/a oxygen gradient is a measure of oxygen transfer across the alveolar capillary membrane ("A" denotes alveolar and "a" denotes arterial oxygenation). It is the difference between the amounts of the oxygen in the alveoli and in the arteries.

PAO$_2$ is the alveolar oxygen tension

PaO$_2$ is the arterial oxygen tension

A/a oxygen gradient = PAO$_2$ − PaO$_2$.

PaO$_2$ is derived from the arterial blood gas (ABG) and PAO$_2$ is calculated as follows:

$$PAo_2 = [FiO_2 \times (P_{atm} - PH_2O)] - (PaCO_2 \div R),$$

where FiO$_2$ is the fraction of inspired oxygen (0.21 at room air), P$_{atm}$ is the atmospheric pressure (760 mm Hg at sea level), PH$_2$O is the partial pressure of water (47 mm Hg), PaCO$_2$ is derived from the ABG, and R is the respiratory quotient (the respiratory quotient is approximately 0.8 at normal physiological state).

The A/a gradient varies with age and can be estimated from the following equation, assuming the patient is breathing room air:

$$A/a \text{ gradient} = 2.5 + 0.21 \times \text{age in years}.$$

The A/a gradient increases with higher FiO$_2$.

The PaO$_2$/FiO$_2$ ratio is a measure of oxygen transfer across the alveolar capillary membrane. The normal PaO$_2$/FiO$_2$ ratio is 300–500 mm Hg, with values less than 300 mm Hg indicating impaired gas exchange and values less than 200 mm Hg indicating severe hypoxemia.

Dr. Satish Deopujari, MD, DNB (Pediatrics)

Founder National Chairperson (Ex) Intensive Care Chapter, Indian Academy of Pediatrics

Professor of Pediatrics (Hon) LMH, Nagpur, India

deopujaris@gmail.com

deopujari@me.com

www.deopujari.com

*Contributed by Satish Deopujari, DCH, MD, MNAMS (Paed), Founder National Chairman, PICC, India; Director, CHILD Hospital and Shree Clinics, Dhantoli, Nagpur, India.

COMPLETE ABG

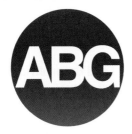

Name of the app: **Complete ABG**

How to download the app:

iPhone: Go to the app store, search for Complete ABG and look for the icon, and tap to download.

Android: Go to the play store, search for Complete ABG and look for the icon, and tap to download.

This dynamic arterial blood gas (ABG) app, assisted by clinical features, is designed to arrive at the complete ABG diagnosis. The app is simple to operate and is also helpful in learning the dynamic physiology of blood gas with all its details. The app is available free on Apple and Android smartphones. The internal consistency of the ABG is also checked by the app by confirming that the measured bicarbonate (shown by the app) corresponds to the depicted bicarbonate value in the ABG report.

At bedside the app also helps in calculations of alveolar/arterial oxygen gradient (A/aDO$_2$) difference and thus helps in evaluation of oxygenation status.

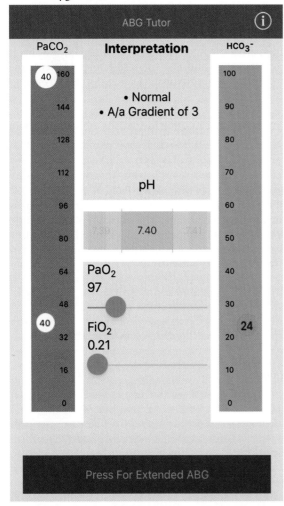

Enter PaCO$_2$ and pH and see the calculated bicarbonate.

Diagnosis is displayed under Interpretation and, depending on the diagnosis, the screen for extended ABG appears.

Enter PaO$_2$ and FiO$_2$ to get the A/a gradient

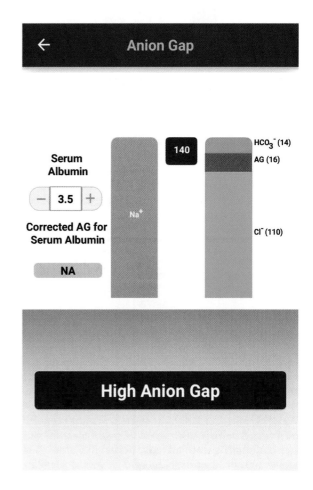

Enter serum sodium, chloride, and albumin to obtain the value of anion gap (AG). Bicarbonate is pulled from the ABG calculations.

With high AG, further evaluation takes the user to Δ/Δ gap and osmolar gap and thus to the complete diagnosis of wide AG acidosis.

With normal AG, the evaluation leads to the diagnosis of renal tubular acidosis (RTA) and the subgroups.

For Metabolic Alkalosis

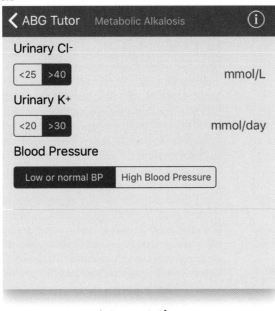

Interpretation

Gitelman Syndrome (low urinary calcium) or
Bartter Syndrome (high urinary calcium)

Press here for algorithm

Enter urinary chloride, potassium, and blood pressure as and when applicable for further workup of metabolic alkalosis.

App Information

Complete ABG: This app helps in the diagnosis of acid–base and oxygenation disorders and makes it easy to understand this complex subject.

It is designed as alphabet H and puts the Henderson–Hasselbalch (HH) equation at center stage.

From the ABG report, enter $PaCO_2$ and pH and see the calculated bicarbonate (do not try to move HCO_3; it is a calculated parameter and varies with $PaCO_2$ and pH). If the displayed bicarbonate does not correspond to that in the ABG report (±3), then the ABG report is not internally consistent.

On the first screen it CLEARLY shows that bicarbonate is a calculated parameter.

Play with the app to understand this relationship between pH, $PaCO_2$, and bicarbonate and by doing this you will actually understand the HH equation.

This app works in three steps:

1. Bedside ABG: This is useful for making decisions at the bedside (point of care). Simple and clear, it tells the user what matters at bedside. It calculates A/aDO_2, on the basis of the entered PaO_2 and FiO_2 values, considering an atmospheric pressure of 760 mm Hg and respiratory quotient of 0.8 (to learn more on A/aDO_2 use the A/a gradient).

2. Extended ABG: Extended interpretation is provided on the basis of AG, Δ/Δ, osmolar gap, urinary AG, and urinary potassium level.

3. Flowchart: This algorithm is available to learn the approach used by this app to arrive at the diagnosis.

This app works on the following equations:

1. HH equation: $\dfrac{[H^+][HCO_3^-]}{PaCO_2} = 24$.

2. $[H_+] = 10^{(9 - pH)}$

3. $AG = (Na^+) - [(Cl^-) + (HCO_3^-)]$

4. Corrected AG for serum albumin $<3.5 = AG + [(3.5 - \text{serum albumin}) \times 2.5]$

5. Delta Delta $= [(AG - 12) - (24 - HCO_3^-)]$

6. Osmolar gap = measured osmolarity − calculated osmolarity

7. Calculated Osmolarity $= \left[(2 \times Sr. Na) + \left(\dfrac{blood\,glucose}{18}\right) + \left(\dfrac{BUN}{2.8}\right)\right]$

8. Urinary AG = Urinary Na^+ + Urinary K^+ − Urinary Cl^-.

Dr. Satish Deopujari, MD, DNB (Pediatrics)
Founder National Chairperson (Ex) Intensive Care Chapter, Indian Academy of Pediatrics
Professor of Pediatrics (Hon) LMH, Nagpur, India
deopujaris@gmail.com
deopujari@me.com
www.deopujari.com
Dr. Lawrence Martin, MD
Professor of Clinical Medicine
Author of the famous and most read book on ABG,
All You Really Need to Know to Interpret Arterial Blood Gases

Case Western Reserve University School of Medicine, Cleveland, OH, USA (retired)

Dr. Vivek K. Shivhare,
MD (Pediatrics)
Fellow Intensivist
Consultant Pediatric Intensivist,
CARE Hospital and Mure Memorial Hospital, Nagpur, India
Dr. Shruti Deopujari, MD
Eastern Virginia Medical School, Norfolk, VA, USA

ETCO₂ TUTOR

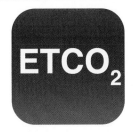

Name of the app: **ETCO₂ Tutor**
How to download the app:
iPhone: Go to app store, search for ETCO₂ Tutor and look for the icon, and tap to download.
Android: Go to play store, search for ETCO₂ Tutor and look for the icon, and tap to download.
ETCO₂ Tutor is a dynamic app and clearly explains the physiological background related to end-tidal CO_2 (ETCO₂) monitoring. Hyper- and hypoventilation affecting the ETCO₂ are clearly shown in the app by altering the respiratory rate. The app shows the various waveforms, in beautiful colors, and the related pathophysiology.

Tap for breathing here and understand the concept of ETCO2

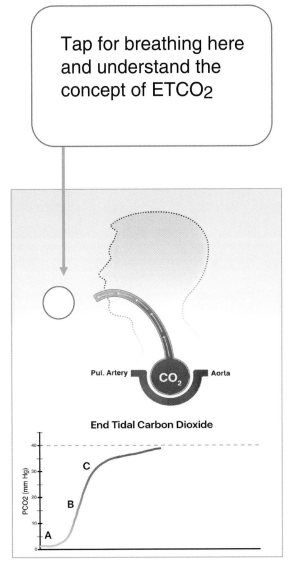

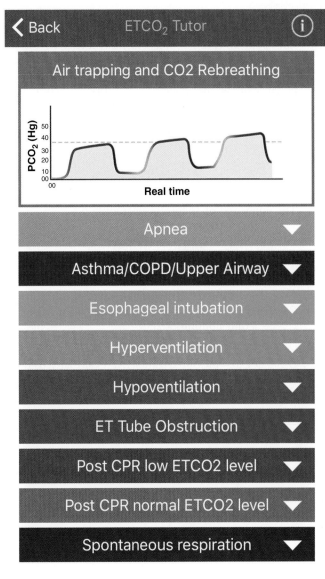

Clicking on the title shows the related graph.
Enter urinary chloride, potassium, and blood pressure as and when applicable for further workup of metabolic alkalosis.

← Press here for algorithm

App Information
Complete ABG: This app helps in the diagnosis of acid–base and oxygenation disorders and makes it easy to understand this complex subject.
It is designed as alphabet H and puts the Henderson–Hasselbalch (HH) equation at center stage.
From the arterial blood gas (ABG) report, enter $PaCO_2$ and pH and see the calculated bicarbonate (do not try to move HCO_3; it is a calculated parameter and varies with $PaCO_2$ and pH). If the displayed bicarbonate does not correspond to that in the ABG report (±3), then the ABG report is not internally consistent.
On the first screen it CLEARLY shows that bicarbonate is a calculated parameter.
Play with the app to understand this relationship between pH, $PaCO_2$, and bicarbonate and by doing this you will actually understand the HH equation.

This app works in three steps

1. Bedside ABG: This is useful for making decisions at the bedside (point of care). Simple and clear, it tells the user what matters at bedside. It calculates A/aDO_2, on the basis of the entered PaO_2 and FiO_2 values, considering an atmospheric pressure of 760 mm Hg and respiratory quotient of 0.8 (to learn more on A/aDO_2 use our app for A/a gradient).

2. Extended ABG: Extended interpretation is provided on the basis of anion gap, Δ/Δ, osmolar gap, urinary anion gap, and urinary potassium level.

3. (📊) Flowchart: This algorithm is available to learn the approach used by this app to arrive at the diagnosis.

This app works on following equations:

1. HH equation: $\dfrac{[H^+][HCO_3^-]}{PaCO_2} = 24$.

2. $[H_+] = 10^{(9-pH)}$

3. $AG = (Na^+) - [(Cl^-) + (HCO_3^-)]$

4. Corrected anion gap for serum albumin $<3.5 = AG + [(3.5 - \text{serum albumin}) \times 2.5]$

5. Delta Delta $= [(AG - 12) - (24 - HCO_3^-)]$

6. Osmolar gap = measured osmolarity − calculated osmolarity

7. Calculated Osmolarity $= \left[(2 \times Sr.\ Na) + \left(\dfrac{\text{bloodglucose}}{18} \right) + \left(\dfrac{BUN}{2.8} \right) \right]$

8. Urinary AG = Urinary Na^+ + Urinary K^+ − Urinary Cl^-.

Dr. Satish Deopujari, MD, DNB (Pediatrics)
Founder National Chairperson (Ex) Intensive Care Chapter, Indian Academy of Pediatrics
Professor of Pediatrics (Hon) LMH, Nagpur, India
deopujaris@gmail.com
deopujari@me.com
www.deopujari.com

Dr. Lawrence Martin, MD
Professor of Clinical Medicine
Case Western Reserve University School of Medicine, Cleveland, OH, USA (retired)

Dr. Vivek K. Shivhare,
MD (Pediatrics)
Fellow Intensivist
Consultant Pediatric Intensivist,
CARE Hospital and Mure Memorial Hospital, Nagpur, India
Dr. Shruti Deopujari, MD
Eastern Virginia Medical School, Norfolk, VA, USA

Note: Page numbers followed by *f* indicate figures, *t* tables, *b* boxes.